Women's Health

Readings on Social, Economic, and Political Issues

Fourth Edition

Edited by

Nancy Worcester and Mariamne H. Whatley

Women's Studies Program
University of Wisconsin—Madison

 **KENDALL/HUNT PUBLISHING COMPANY**
4050 Westmark Drive   Dubuque, Iowa 52002

Book Team

Chairman and Chief Executive Officer   Mark C. Falb
Vice President, Director of National Book Program   Alfred C. Grisanti
Assistant Director of National Book Program   Paul B. Carty
Editorial Developmental Manager   Georgia Botsford
Developmental Editor   Angela Willenbring
Assistant Vice President, Production Services   Christine E. O'Brien
Prepress Project Coordinator   Angela Shaffer
Permissions Specialist   Renae Heacock
Permissions Editor   Corinna Vohl
Design Manager   Deb Howes
Designer   Suzanne Millius
Senior Vice President, College Division   Thomas W. Gantz
Managing Editor, College Field   David Tart
Associate Editor, College Field   Edward Siemek

Contents

Chapter 11 • Childbirth and Lactation 477

Chapter 12 • Aging, Ageism, Mid-life and Older Women's Health Issues 521

Acknowledgments

Each woman who has worked as a part of the Women's Studies 103 teaching team of the University of Wisconsin–Madison has made her own contributions to the course. This book reflects the input of all the women who have worked as Teaching Assistants for WS103 since the course was first taught in 1978.

Book Introduction

Women cannot have control over our own lives until we have control over our bodies; thus, understanding and gaining control over our bodies and our health is essential to taking control of our lives. Consequently, activism around women's health issues has been a central part of the struggles, by women and men, for improving the role of women in society.

The readings in this book are a representation of the exciting range of excellent resources now available on women's health issues. The resource information at the end of the book summarizes many of the sources for the material used in this book and thus serves as a partial list of the periodicals and magazines which regularly feature women's health topics. These articles are examples of the amazing range of women's health writing and organizing being done throughout the world by individuals and groups actively striving for health care systems more appropriate to women's needs.

This collection of readings is designed specifically for use as a part of the women's health course, *Women Studies 103: Women and Their Bodies in Health and Disease,* which is taught to 380–400 students each semester, in the Women's Studies Program at the University of Wisconsin–Madison. (We are delighted to hear that the book is also being used in many other women's health courses throughout the country!) Readings and worksheets are particularly chosen or written to stimulate thought and analysis in preparation for discussion sections. Selections have been made to complement, rather than overlap, material covered in the other books which are required for the course: *Biology of Women* by Ethel Sloane, published by Wiley, *The Black Women's Health Book* edited by Evelyn C. White, published by Seal Press, and *Our Bodies, Ourselves for the New Century* by the Boston Women's Health Book Collective, published by Simon and Schuster.

This is the 4th edition of this book. Reflecting the rapidly changing area of women's health, the tremendous interest shown in women's health in recent years by both health care providers and consumers, and the new national debates, this book contains a very different range of articles than was available for the first three editions. In an effort to provide an historical context to many present debates, we have deliberately added not only new articles but also those with an historical perspective, as well as older articles which we mark as "classics." A goal for this book is to have students learn to value and use women's health "classics" as a part of studying present day issues and developing their own analysis. Often in the field of women's health, earliest articles written on a topic do an excellent job of identifying the crucial issues. Once that basic analysis has been written, other women's health writers are more likely to write an article  which serves to update the information rather than writing an article very similar to the first one. When researching a women's health topic, students are encouraged to read both the "classics" and the most recent information to get the clearest overview of both the fundamental issues and which aspects of the area have and have not changed.

This collection will be regularly updated. We work towards having an anti-racist, cross-cultural perspective on topics, and are eager to find articles which make the connections between social, economic, scientific and political issues and women's mental and physical health. We hope our next book will be even better in looking at health issues related to poverty, ageism, racism, anti-semitism, heterosexism, fatphobia, and what it means to be differently abled. Readers' suggestions or reactions to articles are welcome and valued.

CHAPTER 1

Women and the
Health Care System

The role of women in the health system and the priority given to achieving good mental and physical health for *all* women reflect much about the values of a society. Similarly, the priorities and visions each of us has for how to improve the health care system and women's health reflect much about our personal values and goals in wanting the system to better serve us individually or to work for radical social change. Thus, studying the changing and non-changing roles of women in the health system and grassroots activism and professional organizing to improve women's health becomes an effective lens for viewing societal changes of the last decades.

Since the late 1960's, modern women's health movements have critiqued medical systems, organized for fundamental changes in the system, and worked for the empowerment of women both as consumers and health care providers to be more involved in health care decisions for themselves and the system. Mary Halas's classic 1979 article, "Sexism in Women's Medical Care," sets the scene for the important ongoing discussion of how sexism in medical practice is rooted in the socialization of both women to be passive patients and of doctors (both men and women) to have a lack of respect for women and their right to information about their own bodies. Halas emphasized why it is essential for women to take a more involved role in their own health. The question of how much the sexism of the medical system has changed (or stayed the same) since 1979 will be a theme addressed throughout many specific topics in this book. As reflected in the 1979 Halas article, much of the writing and debates of the 70's and 80's focused largely on why the health system was not adequately serving women and why women's health needed to be taken seriously. Today we can celebrate that women's health movements were extremely successful in many ways. The next two articles, "PRO: Women's Health: Developing a New Interdisciplinary Speciality" and "CON: Women's Health as a Speciality: A Deceptive Solution," demonstrate how the debate increasingly changed from *why* to *how* the health system should take women's health seriously. Both these articles, written by women doctors, center around the specific debate about whether there should be a "women's health speciality" (somewhat more of a "hot" topic in the early 1990's than it is today). These "opposing" articles symbolize that even when providers, consumers, or activists agree that there need to be fundamental changes, we often do not agree on what strategies will be most effective.

The next two articles, "Thinking about Women's Health: The Case for Gender Sensitivity" and "Exploring the Biological Contributions to Human Health: Does Sex Matter?" represent a sophisticated new appreciation for how *both* sex and gender impact on women's, men's, and transgender health. Until recently, the different roles of sex and gender have too often been confused in health research and policies. These two new articles are calling for distinctly different, though potentially complementary, approaches to understanding health issues. Responding to a backlash, which claims that the success of women's health advocacy detracts from men's health, Khoury and Weisman recommend, "that a better framework for addressing both women's health and men's health is one that focuses less on gender equity in access to resources and more on gender-sensitivity—that is, attention to both gender differences and to gender-specific needs in research, practice, and policy." They argue for a gender analysis in understanding patterns of health care utilization and quality. In contrast, the policy paper by the Society for Women's Health Research emphasizes the need for a much more basic understanding of how sex differences operate at the cellular and molecular levels. They say this research will help answer two important questions: "How can information on sex differences be translated into preventative, diagnostic, and therapeutic practice?" and "How can new knowledge about and understandings of biological sex differences and similarities most effectively be used to positively affect patient outcomes and improve health and health care?"

The next three articles in this chapter represent a range of ways that women as consumers and health care practitioners have been working to help women individually and collectively be more informed, active patients and to prepare the health system for consumers who expect a more respectful relationship with their health care providers. The classic, "How to tell Your Doctor a Thing or Two," published by Bread and Roses Women's Health Center (a feminist health center, *by* women, *for* women) is representative of how women's health movements have encouraged women to be a different kind of patient. In this article, Morton Hunt identified changes in medical practices which have caused a deterioration in doctor-patient relationships and proposed a seven-point program for becoming a more active patient. (See "What to Ask Your Gynecologist" on page 599 for a 2000 version of this type of active patient article, specifically focused on asking about sexually transmitted infections.)

From the other end of the speculum, Judy Schmidt's "The Gynecological Exam and the Training of Medical Students" gives an example of a training program which aims to educate physicians to be "patient-orientated." In a more theoretical approach to the same issues, Terri Kapsalis, in "Cadavers, Dolls, and Prostitutes: Medical Pedagogy and the Pelvic Rehearsal," explores how "the types of practice performances adopted reveal and promote specific ideas about female bodies and sexuality held by the medical institution."

The years 1990/1991 are important "turning point" years in the history of women's health movements. Decades of grassroots activism resulted in much visible organizing at the national level. Congressional hearings demonstrated that an embarrassingly small (13%) percentage of the national health research funding was earmarked for women's health and top-level policy makers started seeing the need for increased attention to and funding of women's health issues. The Office of Research on Women's Health was established in 1990 and the US Department of Health and Human Services' Office on Women's Health was established in 1991. Thus, it is fitting here to include the Office of Women's Health's own highlights of the women's health events of the twentieth century. The Ruzek and Becker article, "The Women's Health Movement in the United States: From Grassroots Activism to Professional Agendas," is key to understanding the differences between groups who have worked to improve women's health. Ruzek and Becker contrast the work and philosophies of early grassroots organizations and newer (post-1990) "professionalized" women's health organizations on six important issues. Although these authors present organizational philosophies as "early organizing" versus "today's organizing," this textbook aims to encourage readers to think about how crucial the philosophies of "early organizing" are to today's issues and how we can better incorporate more of those philosophies and activism into present day organizing. An excellent example that grassroots organizations are still alive and well and extremely effective today is the Boston Women's Health Book Collective (BWHBC). Their book, *Our Bodies, Ourselves,* continually updated since 1970, has been described as one of the most influential books ever published. "This book not only had a decisive impact on how generations of American women felt about their bodies, their sexuality and their health, but it was translated and adopted in 20 languages." (Quote from Kathy Davis in an excellent scholarly article on the BWHBC, "Feminist Body/Politics as World Traveller" published by *The European Journal of Women's Studies,* Volume 9 (3), 223–247, 2002.) "Crossing Cultural Borders with 'Our Bodies Ourselves' " summarizes a recent gathering of grassroots feminists from 10 countries as they discussed the development and distribution of culturally appropriate versions of the classic women's health book in very different situations around the world, in many ways reflecting the very different struggles facing women's health organizers around the world.

The next three articles on women doctors provide various perspectives on the question of whether increasing the number of women doctors is important in improving health care for women. Adriane Fugh-Berman's "Tales Out of Medical School" vividly describes some of the traumas facing women trying to become doctors and reminds us that simply getting more women into medicine would do little to make the health system more appropriate for women (or men) until the medical socialization of doctors is changed. We hope many of the problems identified in Fugh-Berman's 1992 article no longer exist, but whether the socialization of health practitioners is suitable for appropriately serving *all* patients remains an important question examined throughout this book. The article "Women in Medicine," written for women physicians, appearing in a medical journal, is particularly useful for identifying issues which may be of concern to some women physicians. Similar to articles which appear in many women's magazines, this article identifies a key issue of how to combine work and family and also issues unique to women physicians, particularly as the field of medicine itself changes. Ironically, one of the changes in medicine which is first identified as distressing and later described as opening up possibilities for women doctors, is the emergence of a new type of patient which this book so proudly identifies as active patients! Considering that the Ruzek and Becker article identifies women physicians as the key players in professionalized women's health organizations, one certainly hopes that women physicians recognize active patients and doctors who work well with active patients as essential to improving health care for women. The "Women in Medicine" article also serves as a reminder of the limitations of looking at gender issues or sexism without looking at interlocking issues. Readers are encouraged to look at the heterosexist and class assumptions of this article and think of how different the article would be if it addressed the issues of balancing work and family for lesbians working in medicine or for lower paid health care workers, including nurses, medical assistants, or dental hygienists.

Dr. Judith Lorber's answers to the question, "What Impacts Have Women Physicians Had on Women's Health?" are both optimistic and realistic in recognizing the obstacles to, and potential for, women to have very positive influences on medicine when and if they are able to move into policy-making positions. (Readers may be interested in other articles in this series on women physicians in the fall 2002, Volume 57, no. 4, edition of *The Journal of the American Medical Women's Association.* The series includes an article, "Differences in Income Between Male and Female Primary Care Physicians," pp. 180–184, showing that women physicians presently earn annual incomes 60–85% lower than men physicians, earn 71–98% as much per hour, but see about 17% more patients per hour.)

Work to improve the health of US women must take place within the context of the most urgent "big picture" issue of work to improve a very sick US medical system/non-system. "Confronting the Myths" shows that the wealthiest country in the world spends twice as much per capita on health care as any other country but leaves out 40+ million people and is ranked as #37 by the World Health Organization. As with other strategies for improving women's health, there need to be debates about the most fundamental changes needed. "Confronting the Myths" provides useful vocabulary and concepts for such discussions. All such debates on improving the US health system (although seldom focusing on women and too often leaving out women's voices) are basically women's health debates because women are overwhelmingly the health care providers and consumers who have the most to gain by meaningful change.

The "Scientific Terms Explained" information is from Adriane Fugh-Berman's excellent *Alternative Medicine: What Works,* a comprehensive easy-to-read review of the scientific literature. This information demystifies many of the terms involved in describing scientific studies and helps the consumer become a better judge of these studies. This chapter ends with essential new consumer literacy information on "Evaluating Online Health Information" from the *Our Bodies, Ourselves* website. This begins to answer to the important question posed to women's health activists by Ruzek and Becker: Who will speak for women in the electronic age?

Sexism in Women's Medical Care

by Mary A. Halas

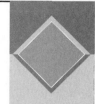

A twenty-seven-year old woman complained that her health had taken a sudden unexplained change for the worse. She had a diffuse sense of not being well, with pains in various parts of her body, weakness, and fatigue. Her gynecologist gave her a physical exam and pronounced her fine. As the symptoms continued, she returned to her physician and also went to several other doctors—meeting reactions of disbelief and even ridicule with increasing frequency. Eventually one specialist recommended she see a counselor, because she obviously had no real physical problems.

That recommendation turned out to be a good one. After a few sessions the counselor concluded that the woman was in good mental health and concentrated on supporting her to continue seeking medical attention to evaluate the sudden change in her physical health.

Finally, months after her symptoms appeared and weeks after her last visit to her gynecologist, the woman had an appointment with a female physician who listened to an exhaustive list of her symptoms and concerns, and gave her an extremely thorough physical examination.

The results: the woman had a large lump in her left breast; after surgery two days later the lump was diagnosed as cancer. No one will ever know whether the lump was already there during her gynecologist's hurried and skeptical exam, but it is certain that the woman might have had a better chance of finding the lump herself if her doctor had ever taught her how to examine her own breasts. According to the woman's oncologist, there is a 70 percent chance that the cancer will recur, because of its type and size at the time of discovery.

Fortunately, the woman's counselor knew that sexism in the medical care system poses particular problems for women. Many physicians see women's physical complaints as trivial, neurotic disorders best treated with placebos or symptomatic therapy. A therapist who had conducted a prolonged analysis of the possible psychological causes of this woman's complaints or had considered the symptoms to be evidence of emotional disturbance would have put her life in even further jeopardy.

The medical needs of women and their problems in getting good health care are key issues. First, many women have psychosomatic illnesses, and counselors get many legitimate referrals from doctors who recognize that there needs to be a psychological as well as medical component to healing women's medical problems. Second, therapists get *too many* referrals from doctors, as the case of the woman with undetected breast cancer illustrates. Serious, treatable problems often progress to irreversible damage or death while a woman is trying to convince her doctor that her problems are not all in her head.

Before the advent of modern medical technology and the professionalization of medicine, women were the primary healers as "witches" and herbalists, and female midwives were the sole practitioners of physical care for women's special concerns—childbirth and gynecology. Now, however, the situation is radically reversed. Although women are the largest single group of health care consumers, 93 percent of all doctors are male, and 97 percent of all gynecologists are male.[1]

Women's experience in obtaining health care is different from men's in that women almost always are putting their bodies in the hands of someone of the opposite sex for medical care. In addition, women make 25 percent more visits to the doctors than men. They also take 50 percent more prescribed drugs than men and are admitted to hospitals more frequently.[2]

Sex-role stereotyping in the socialization of women has skewed the kind of medical care they seek. Women learn to identify themselves in terms of their reproductive potential, and the medical system reinforces this behavior. For example, a majority of women turn to the specialist obstetrician/gynecologist, not as a source of care for specialized problems, but as a first-line source for all medical care—rather than choosing a general practitioner or internist for routine care. A study which Helen Marieskind presented at a 1974 meeting of the American Association of Obstetricians and Gynecologists found that 86 percent of the women in the study saw no doctor other than an obstetrician/gynecologist on a regular, periodic basis.

Socialization of Women as Patients

The socialization of women to be passive recipients of medical care—especially from men—militates against their receiving adequate care. The attitude with which women seek medical care within the male-dominated system is one of subservient dependence on all-knowing authority. This dependence on all-powerful doctors and women's relinquishing of responsibility for their health to male doctors is the result of physician behavior that reduces the patient's sense of autonomy.

For example, a woman having a routine gynecological exam is ushered into the examining room without meeting the physician first in his office and is instructed to take off her clothes. Vulnerable, naked, and draped with a white sheet, she waits an indeterminate period for the doctor to enter. Once he arrives and her feet are in the examining table stirrups, she is literally helpless in his hands and feels this way—naked, supine, being manipulated with fingers and tools in her body by a male hidden behind a sheet. This dependence on male doctors works against women patients' interests. A patient's stereotyped respect for a doctor's wisdom and competence does not make a poor doctor into a good one.

Dependence on doctors also eliminates the woman's own desires and needs from decision-making about her care. Most medical care involves various levels of benefits and risks and choices about them, even when doctors do not allow patients to make those choices. Lack of information about their bodies, plus the dependent, fearful relationship with their physicians, make it difficult for women to find out what is really wrong with them physically and what methods of treatment are possible. In a study on doctor-patient communication, Barbara Korsch and Vida Negrete found that the use of medical jargon which is unintelligible to patients, plus doctors' frequent disregard for patients' concerns and perspectives, were obstacles to effective care.[3]

A logical result of this confusion and failure in doctor-patient communication is that only 42 percent of the women in this study carried out all the medical advice they received; 38 percent complied in part; and 11 percent did not follow instructions at all.

In gynecology and obstetrics the level of communication can be even poorer, because of an attitude generated by the fact that many of the visits are from healthy women. The attitude is that if there is nothing wrong, then there is nothing to tell. In 1970 hearings before the U.S. Senate, a physician who did research on oral contraceptives opposed labeling for these drugs which would inform women of the risks. He said, "A misguided effort to inform such women leads only to anxiety on their part and loss of confidence in the physician. . . . They want him [the doctor] to tell them what to do, not to confuse them by asking them to make decisions beyond their comprehension. . . . The idea of informing such a woman is not possible."[4]

One would hope that this individual doctor's attitude represents an extreme case. However, in general many doctors neglect to give women information they do not ask for, and treat them as if they are not capable of understanding the basis of decisions and treatment. In the view of much of the medical profession, women cannot even be trusted with information about their own conditions or medication.

A graphic illustration of this point is the years-old controversy still raging over the government's proposal to require patient education leaflets on all prescription drugs. In response to tremendous pressure from Congressional advocates and the Food and Drug Administration, the major medical associations reluctantly have endorsed the abstract concept of such leaflets but continue to oppose specific applications.

The specter the medical associations raise in their congressional testimony on patient package inserts for drugs is that if patients are told all that can go wrong with a drug, a disease, or an operation, their hypochondriacal minds will ensure that all these things do go wrong. It is significant that it was a consumer group, the Center for Law and Social Policy, which sparked the government initiative on patient package inserts through a petition—and not the medical profession.

An example in which doctors have not given women information that can have life and death consequences for themselves and their children involves the hormone diethylstilbestrol (DES). During the 1950's many thousands of pregnant women received DES without being informed what the medication was. No one knew until fifteen years later that this drug greatly increased the risk of cancer in their children.

In October 1978, after years of press coverage of DES-caused cancer, the government issued a special letter and bulletin to the country's doctors because of the finding that some doctors were still prescribing DES for pregnant women and many others still were not informing their patients who had taken the drug of possible risks.[5]

Socialization of Doctors

Where do doctors get this lack of respect for a woman's right to information about health care and for her ability to participate intelligently in her medical care? Mary

Howell describes the process of professionalization of doctors in medical school—where they learn attitudes about work and patients—as strongly colored by a demeaning regard for women.[6] Medical schools teach discrimination against women as patients, Howell says, through lack of focus on diseases specific to women, in misogynic comparisons made between male and female patients with similar health problems, and in instructions regarding the appropriate behavior of doctors toward women patients.

In their classes, medical students learn both implicitly and explicitly that women patients have uninteresting illnesses, are unreliable historians of their health, and are beset by such emotionality that their symptoms are unlikely to reflect real disease.

Pauline Bart and Diana Scully reviewed twenty-seven gynecology textbooks published between 1943 and 1972 and found that at least half of the writers stated women are inherently frigid, have less sex drive than men, or are interested in sex only for procreation.[7] Two authors urged physicians to encourage women to simulate orgasm to please their husbands. The core of the female personality as described in these textbooks is narcissistic, masochistic, and passive.

Another much-used vehicle for the socialization of doctors in their attitudes toward women is drug advertisements in medical journals. Many of these ads serve to reinforce the prejudices against women. They teach doctors that women's physical complaints are trivial; their illnesses are irritating to others; and that women are emotional, have psychosomatic illnesses, and are bothersome to doctors.

Many ads for tranquilizers and antidepressants in particular suggest these products as treatment of choice before psychotherapy or social action for life situations and problems beyond the traditional concepts of illness and disease.

In a 1971 review of medical journals, Seidenberg found that misogynic statements in drug advertisements resonate with the bias of the intended observer—the male doctor. He targeted in particular advertisements that recommended doctors use drugs to adjust women to their lot when they are discontented with a humdrum environment. One caption accompanying a portrayal of a woman behind the bars of broom and mop handles read, "you can't set her free, but you can help her feel less anxious."[8]

In 1979 men are beginning to appear more frequently in drug advertisements as patients, but the difference in portrayal of men and women is still striking. Men on antidepressant medications are depicted as, "Alert on the job," and "functioning effectively in daily activities" (Pamelor). Women needing antidepressant medications, however, appear in drug ads as helpless patients under a doctor's care because, "Everything I saw was negative" (Norpramin).

The insidious effects of the sexist bias doctors learn in medical school, the professional literature they read, and the drug advertising they are exposed to are broad-ranging. The bias affects decision-making about individual patients and perpetuates misinformation about women's psychic and physiological processes. Negative consequences of these medical myths about women include the justification of limited opportunities for education, employment, and participation in the political process.

The following three specific issues are examples of sexism in medical care. All pose particular threats to women's well-being and as such are illustrations of medical care delivery to women.

Contraceptive Methods   Every woman has a right to make a free and informed choice about birth control for herself. The information about methods and the freedom of choice are key, because there is no completely satisfactory method of birth control. Each method has a unique range of benefits and risks which will differ for women of various medical histories, personal preferences, income, and health habits.

There are widespread misunderstandings about the risks and failure rates of various methods of contraception.[9] Some of this is caused by unethical advertising by pharmaceutical firms. In addition, the biases of clinics or individual doctors frequently deprive women of complete information on which to base their choices. Planned Parenthood prides itself on giving women unbiased information so they can make choices, but many women have already made up their minds about a method before they come into the clinics. According to the Washington, D.C. Public Interest Research Group, the popularity of the Pill is based on its convenience, and fewer women would expose themselves to its many risks if they took these into account in making their choices. Much of the pro-Pill reasoning is fallacious, especially the comparison of risks of the Pill with risks of pregnancy. Such comparisons assume that women not taking oral contraceptives will become pregnant, whereas they could use other safer contraceptive methods; furthermore, many of the necessary studies on the Pill's long-term safety have not been done, and many complications are never reported, so that valid comparisons between the risks of pregnancy and oral contraceptives cannot be made.

Estrogen Use in Menopause   Uterine cancer used to be rare—about one in 1,000 postmenopausal women who had not had their uteruses surgically removed.

Since 1970, however, the incidence of uterine cancer in women over fifty years of age increased dramatically—by 50 percent for invasive cancer and by 100 percent for localized cancer.[10] It is not a coincidence that in the last ten to fifteen years the use of estrogen has at least tripled, and recent studies have concluded that there is a causal connection, and that the major cause of the increasing rate of uterine cancer in the United States is estrogen therapy. The sharpest rise in uterine cancer rates is among white upper- and middle-class women, who are most likely to take estrogens. Fifty percent of all postmenopausal women have taken estrogens, and approximately half of these women have taken estrogen for more than ten years. The longer the estrogen treatment and the higher the dose, the higher the incidence of uterine cancer. There are strong social pressures causing the high use of estrogen. Unsupported claims that estrogen will retard the aging process, plus the sexism that devalues older women, combine to create strong consumer demand for the drug. This demand reinforces physicians' entrenched prescribing habits, despite new scientific findings.

Six million women are using estrogens, many of them in hopes that the drug will keep them "feminine forever." This attitude, created in large part by irresponsible drug company advertising, is not going to evaporate soon. Also resistant to change are the time-hallowed doctors' attitudes toward menopause as a disease rather than as a normal physiological process.

Psychoactive Drugs   Use of legitimate psychoactive drugs among women is an important issue. An estimated one to two million people in the U.S. from all walks of life and social strata have abuse problems with prescription drugs, according to the National Institute of Drug Abuse's February and April 1978 *Capsules* press releases.

Almost twice as many women as men have had tranquilizers, sedatives, and stimulants prescribed for them. In many cases, there is no medical reason for use of the drugs, but they become a chemical support system to adjust a woman to a frustrating or unfulfilling marriage, divorce, lifestyle, or work situation. Psychoactive drugs become both a substitute and a barrier to use of counseling or other measures to combat or alter the distressing situation or the individual's response to it.

Chemical crutches for women are nothing new. In the 1800's it was common medical custom to prescribe then-legal opium for "female troubles."[11] A wide spread pattern of opium abuse grew among women—outnumbering male opium-eaters three to one in the late nineteenth and early twentieth centuries. In the drug pattern of the 1970's, general practitioners write most of the tranquilizer prescriptions for Valium alone; there were fifty-seven million prescriptions between May 1976 and April 1977.[12]

Doctors get their education about psychoactive drugs primarily from drug companies. A survey of seventy-two medical schools found that only 20 percent had any course in psychopharmacology, and the average time on the subject was seventeen hours in four years.[13] Medical advertising for drugs typically portrays women as frustrated, anxious, neurotic, and depressed.

Tranquilizers, sedatives, and stimulants are addictive, and in conjunction with alcohol they can be deadly. Persons who take excessive doses of either sedatives or certain tranquilizers for extended periods of time will experience dramatic withdrawal symptoms including convulsions, tremor, abdominal and muscle cramps, vomiting, and sweating.[14]

Alarming information that only recently has come to light is that some patients will experience withdrawal from such drugs as Librium and Valium when they have been taking normal therapeutic doses, with no abuse.[15] These symptoms include tremors, agitation, fear and anxiety, stomach cramps, and sweating. Since these symptoms of withdrawal so closely resemble the anxiety manifestations for which women in particular originally receive these drugs, and since so many millions of women are taking these drugs, they represent a complex problem for counselors.

Sexism in medical practice is rooted in the socialization of women to be passive recipients of care from authoritarian male doctors, plus doctors' socialization which trivializes women's medical problems and fosters attitudes that demean women patients. The results are that many women suffer needlessly from treatable organic problems labeled as psychogenic, experience irreparable damage or death because of ignored symptoms, or unwittingly fall into drug dependence due to doctors' attempts to "help" women adjust through drugs to an uncomfortable sex-typed role.

The implications are clear—it is vital for women to become informed partners in their own medical care. This will involve learning about key medical issues concerning women and developing skills to assert their rights in the sexist dynamics that pervade the health care of women. Useful tools in this task will be information sharing and assertiveness training to assist women in getting information on their own and getting responses they want from professionals. Some authors suggest limiting the practice of women's medicine (obstetrics/gynecology) to women practitioners. At some future date that may be thinkable or possible; at present, however, since 97 percent of all obstetrician/gynecologists are male, women are faced with the art of the possible in dealing with sexism in their medical care.

Notes

1. Linda Bakiel, Susan Daily, and Carolyn Kott Washburne, ed., *Women in Transition: A Feminist Handbook on Separation and Divorce* (New York: Scribners, 1975), p. 392.
2. Boston Women's Health Collective, *Our Bodies Ourselves* (New York: Simon and Schuster, 1976), p. 337.
3. Barbara H. Korsch and Vida F. Negrete, "Doctor-Patient Communication." *Scientific American,* 227 (1972), 66–72.
4. Gena Corea, *The Hidden Malpractice* (New York:Marron Co., 1977), p. 77.
5. Food and Drug Administration, "Alert on DES," *FDA Drug Bulletin,* 8, (1978), p. 3.
6. Mary Howell, "What Medical Schools Teach About Women," *New England Journal of Medicine,* 291 (1974), 304–07.
7. Pauline Bart and Diana Scully, "A Funny Think Happened on the Way to the Orifice," *American Journal of Sociology,* 28 (1973), 1045–50.
8. R. Seidenberg, "Drug Advertising and Perceptions of Mental Illness," *Mental Hygiene,* 55 (1971), 21–31.
9. *Our Bodies Ourselves,* p. 185.
10. Food and Drug Administration, "Estrogens and Endometrial Cancer," *FDA Drug Bulletin,* 6 (1976), 2–3.
11. Annabel Hecht, "Women and Drugs," *FDA Consumer,* October 1978, pp. 7–12.
12. Jody Forman-Sher and Jonica Homiler, "An Overview of the Problem of Combined Drug/Alcohol Dependencies Among Women," paper presented at the International Conference on Alcoholism and Addictions, Zurich, Switzerland, June 1978.
13. Ann H. Clark, *National Consumers League Position on Minor Tranquilizers,* paper presented at the public hearing before the Food and Drug Administration, Rockville, Maryland, March 1978.
14. David Haskell, "Withdrawal of Diazepam," *Journal of the American Medical Association,* 233 (1975), 135.
15. Arthur Rifkin, Frederick Quitkin, and Donald Klein, "Withdrawal Reactions to Diazepam," *Journal of the American Medical Association,* 236 (1976), 2173.

PRO: Women's Health

Developing a New Interdisciplinary Specialty

by Karen Johnson, M.D.

Abstract. This paper argues that medicine is based on a male paradigm that does not permit high-quality comprehensive care for women within existing medical specialities. Suggestions are made to alleviate the shortcomings of the current paradigm by including women. A call for the development of a specialty in women's health is made. Types of resistance to this proposal, stemming from sexism, economics, and alliances to existing specialties, are also discussed. Finally, it is argued that bringing the study and practice of women's health to parity with the understanding and treatment of men must be achieved rapidly and comprehensively using an active and multifaceted approach.

Introduction

No existing medical specialty is devoted exclusively to the comprehensive care of women. Many of us providing health care for women in a variety of existing specialties believe that the absence of such a comprehensively trained specialist is a significant problem in the health care services offered to women. This problem could be solved through the development of an interdisciplinary specialty in women's health.

Medicine as a Paradigm Based upon Experiences with Men

With the exception of physicians in one surgical specialty, obstetrics-gynecology, physicians caring for women base the majority of their diagnoses and interventions on clinical trials and studies with men, often unknowingly. However benevolent the original intentions in excluding women from drug trials and clinical studies, their absence has led to unnecessary morbidity

From *Journal of Women's Health,* Vol. 1, No. 2, 1992. Copyright © 1992 by Mary Ann Liebert, Inc. Reprinted by permission.

and premature mortality. For example, the Baltimore Longitudinal Study on Aging started in 1958 and did not include women for the first 20 years. This omission delayed the discovery of the link among osteoporosis, calcium, estrogen, and progesterone, resulting in the needless suffering and death of hundreds of thousands of women.

More recently the AIDS epidemic has highlighted the serious consequences of assuming that diseases in women manifest with exactly the same signs and symptoms as diseases in men. Until 1991 the Center for Disease Control (CDC) criteria for AIDS was based on men. HIV positive women presenting with cervical cancer, pelvic inflammatory disease, and vaginal thrush were diagnosed much later in the disease process. Not only did these uniquely female diagnoses delay treatment and thus shorten life expectancy compared with men, they often caused undue economic hardship because meeting the CDC criteria was a prerequisite to receiving public assistance available to patients with AIDS.

Other problems are created by the assumption that our experience with men is transferable to women. Although cardiovascular disease is the leading cause of death in women, we would hardly know it based on most of the research in this field. The initial study affirming that aspirin could be used as preventive therapy for coronary disease included more than 22,000 subjects, all male. The Mr. FIT study (Multiple Risk Factor Intervention Trials) identified coronary disease risk factors in 15,000 subjects, again all men. Even when women's risk of cardiovascular disease is assessed, clinical experience and interventions with men may not be applicable to women. Women may present with different symptoms in the office; they often arrive further in the progression of a myocardial infarction in the emergency room; they are more likely to die in the operating room.

Many diseases common in both men and women have a substantially higher incidence in women. It is not entirely clear why. Diseases of the gastrointestinal tract are just one example. Gallstones occur earlier in women and women continue to have a greater prevalence of them throughout their lives. Biliary dyskinesia occurs more often in women. Irritable bowel syndrome and gastroparesis are three times more common in women than men. Women are more susceptible to the hepatotoxic effects of alcohol than men. However, as is often the case in diseases that occur in both genders, clinical investigations have been carried out mostly in men. As a result in caring for women we cannot be confident that our diagnostic techniques and medical interventions are sound.

Health matters that occur exclusively (or primarily) in women such as menstruation, premenstrual symptoms, uterine fibroids, menopause, and breast cancer have received less attention than the patient population (52% of adults) would warrant. This has hindered our ability to offer advice with confidence.

Sometimes relying on the male paradigm is nothing short of ludicrous. Consider the study at Rockefeller University in which researchers were analyzing the effects of obesity on estrogen activity and the tendency to develop breast and uterine cancer. All the subjects were male. Although it is finally a widely held belief that women and men are equal, they are not the same—physiologically or psychologically. Using men as the medical standard from which women diverge is unpardonable.

Crossing Boundaries

Now that the consciousness of medicine has been raised, it has been suggested that improving women's health care can be achieved by making adjustments in the education of physicians within existing specialties. This plan on its own would not address the numerous health concerns experienced by women that do not easily fit into any existing specialty. Consider the woman whose abdominal pain is finally diagnosed as endometriosis. Lacking an interdisciplinary-trained women's health specialist, the recommended interventions are likely to be biased by the specialty training of her provider. A primary care physician may be inclined to prescribe analgesics for pain, whereas a gynecologist leans more toward hormonal or surgical interventions. A psychiatrist or other mental health provider may need to be included to assist with corollary emotional distress or sexual dysfunction. Two or more physicians are required to provide complete care, an inefficient and expensive process.

Many medical problems experienced by women present similar dilemmas. Two additional examples are premenstrual symptoms and domestic violence. Premenstrual symptoms are inadequately defined within the existing paradigm, but they are certainly experienced by many women. Lacking agreement about diagnosis and treatment, specialists tend to interpret symptoms through their own frame of reference. Domestic violence is a major health hazard for American women, but it is overlooked by many physicians. Untrained in a broader understanding of women's health, physicians' impressions are biased by the perspective of their own specialty. When presented with only a small part of the clinical problem, they often fail to piece together the larger diagnostic picture. A woman complaining of insomnia or suffering with a fracture may be treated in an emergency room or family practice center, but never asked directly about physical abuse. Although the lack of a unified approach to premenstrual symptoms can lead to discomfort and distress, the failure to accurately diagnose domestic violence can be life threatening. What is called for in these and many other situations experienced by women is an interdisciplinary approach.

Correcting the Paradigm

Most physicians until recently have been unaware that the practice of medicine is based on a male paradigm. Many of the problems that have arisen because of this have been identified. There is now relative agreement within the medical profession that these problems must be addressed, but we are by no means in agreement as to the method.

Some believe that we have crossed the barriers to the full inclusion of women's health care needs and that we can correct the existing medical paradigm by alterations within current specialties. This belief is at odds with the limited achievements women have made in other areas when analogous omissions were brought to light, as noted in Faludi's *Backlash*.

Representatives from at least three specialties—internal medicine, obstetrics-gynecology, and family practice—have argued that these specialties can adequately meet the comprehensive needs of women patients. I question their assertions. Unless practitioners of these specialties have taken it upon themselves to round out their standard residency training, few are qualified to call themselves women's health specialists in the manner I am arguing is required.

At present most internists have inadequate knowledge of women's reproductive health, extremely limited experience with the psychosocial aspects of women's health care, and a discipline that is built entirely on a male paradigm. Although obstetrics-gynecology training is based upon experiences with women, it is arguable whether it can genuinely be considered a primary care specialty. The training is fundamentally surgical, and the inclusion of a psychosocial perspective is also limited.

Family physicians argue that they are in the best position to offer high-quality comprehensive care for women. This is true within the context of the current medical paradigm. Their interdisciplinary training serves them well in approaching the multiplicity of women's health care concerns. However, the training and practice of family medicine require these physicians to divide their attention among women, men, and children.

Certainly family physicians treat the young as well as the elderly and more than other specialists gain a psychosocial perspective in their training. Nevertheless, this has not negated the need for the specialty of pediatrics or the subspecialty of geriatrics. Pediatricians' focused attention on children and geriatricians' focused attention on the elderly have led to improved health care for the youngest and the oldest of patients. Specialists in women's health will bring similar benefits to all our woman patients—no matter what specialty we practice.

I do agree with colleagues who caution that a specialty in women's health must not be viewed as alleviating the imperative that every existing medical specialty revise its content to include the accurate and respectful treatment of women. However, I do not believe that these efforts will be adequate. Nor do I think that these improvements and the development of a new interdisciplinary specialty are mutually exclusive. They would be complementary.

Placing Women's Health in the Larger Context

The idea of a specialty in women's health is a logical extension of the women's health movement that began in the 1960s. Physicians influenced by this movement began to articulate the need for a specialty in women's health by the 1980s. The recent increased interest in women's health at all levels is gratifying; however, attention to the concerns of women has been inconsistent during this century. It would be a mistake to assume the current flurry of activity in women's health will continue without formalizing the specialty.

Having a medical specialty in women's health could be viewed much like having a room of one's own. Just as departments of women's studies have been instrumental in assuring that women's experiences are accurately represented in the academic community, a specialty in women's health would serve a similar purpose in medicine.

Those who believe it will be sufficient to simply add women's health to existing specialties would be wise to study the history of science, the sociology of knowledge, and the role of values in science if the missed opportunities of other pioneers are to be avoided. Nineteenth century scientists argued that the rigors of a university education would drain energy from women's reproductive organs. These and other socially expedient biases were used to justify the exclusion of women from positions of authority and decision making. Unless health issues are approached from a solid interdisciplinary, pro-woman perspective, I am not confident that current or future physicians will serve women significantly better than their earlier counterparts. We have already seen a great deal of the money targeted for new research in women's health funneled into the existing "old boys" research network. This is worrisome and disappointing to those of us who had hoped for more adventuresome funding and innovative projects. Rest assured, the age-old debate of autonomy versus integration will wage on as we struggle with how to include women's health in medical training. Common sense and experience suggest that we must do both. It is from the power base of a residency in women's health that efforts to mainstream are most likely to be successful. Furthermore, women's health is a separate body of knowledge and deserves to be treated as a legitimate area of inquiry.

Positioning a Women's Health Specialty

There are several possible routes to specialization. Women's health could be a primary care specialty like pediatrics or subspeciality like geriatrics. Alternatively, much like toxicology, it could be a field of study. Entry from any number of specialties would be possible. The positioning of the specialty is less critical than its content. Women's health must be based on research and experience with women, not men.

Those of us interested in fostering the development of an interdisciplinary specialty in women's health have many resources to turn for valuable advice and information. Nursing, a female-dominated profession, has had training programs in women's health for over a decade. Feminist scholars in health psychology and women's studies also have much to offer.

There are already many interesting and active steps being taken within medicine to assure a better response to women's health care needs. Since 1982, hospital-affiliated multidisciplinary women's health centers have offered a closer approximation of an interdisciplinary approach than more conventional group practices. This summer Harvard Medical School held their fifth annual conference on women's health, combining internal medicine, obstetrics-gynecology, and psychiatry. The American Medical Women's Association is preparing a multidisciplinary postgraduate course on the health care needs of women. Fellowships in women's medicine have started to appear at several institutions, and a number of medical schools offer electives in women's health. Nevertheless, a growing number of medical students longing to specialize in women's health express frustration at the lack of a residency program anywhere in the United States. For now, highly motivated trainees are left to customize existing residencies to achieve their goal of specializing in women's health (D. Moran, personal communication).

Resistance

The resistance to this proposal has been intense and is no doubt determined by many factors. Change is almost always anxiety provoking. In this case the anxiety is fu-

eled by forces as divergent as sexism, economics, and alliances to existing specialties.

Treating women with knowledge drawn from research on men is enough of a problem without being compounded by pervasive sexism. This is an issue in patient care that we have hardly begun to address. Sexist behavior ranges from simple patronizing to explicit harassment and abuse. One male obstetrician has suggested that unless male physicians correct their sexist attitudes and behavior, they should not be allowed to provide health care for women.

Unfortunately, sexism is not unique to male physicians. It is embedded in the professionalization of almost every medical student. How else can we interpret the disturbing revelation this year of a graduating medical student that in the anatomy lab female breasts were designated as "waste" and tossed in the trash without careful dissection and examination? This behavior is unconscionable when one in nine American women can expect to develop breast cancer within her lifetime.

Arguments that a specialty in women's health will lead to costly fragmentation and overspecialization do not make sense. It is the current arrangement that causes these problems. Divisions in medicine are arbitrary and based on any number of factors including physician interest, expanding scientific knowledge, and political agendas. Siphoning funds from other critical areas such as AIDS and cancer research will undoubtedly be used as economic scarecrows. At a less conscious level some will be concerned that specialists in women's health will compete more favorably for women patients. Women are the greatest users of health care. Yet another potential financial loss is hard to swallow when physicians are already feeling under siege.

Those of us specializing in the care of women have been cautioned against proposing the development of a new specialty just as medicine is being forced to tighten its belt. The proposal of a new specialty at this time may seem to burden a crumbling system. But it is in this climate that attending to the health care needs of women is even more urgent. Unless we are vigilant about the quality and availability of care for women, it is likely with any of the insurance reforms currently under consideration that health care services for women will be the first to suffer.

Even many well-meaning physicians are unconvinced that a specialty is needed. They believe that theirs is either providing perfectly adequate care for women or that with only modest efforts the quality of care can be raised to acceptable levels. Their identification with their own training interferes with an accurate understanding of the problem.

Framing the Solution

What most opponents fail to appreciate is that women's health is a unique body of knowledge and skills based upon experience with women that cross the boundaries of existing specialties. Women's health care needs are not being met, and cannot be met, within the existing medical paradigm.

The criterion of the American Board of Medical Specialists for a new specialty is that it must "represent a distinct and well-defined field of medical practice" such as "special concerns with problems of patients according to age, sex, organ systems or interaction between patients and their environment." With practice specialties ranging from addiction medicine to undersea medicine, I am hard pressed to understand why a specialty embracing 52% of the adult population is unreasonable or unnecessary.

Conclusion

When it comes to women's health, there are far more questions than answers. Specialists devoted to women's health care in a number of fields are beginning to provide some answers, but the information is fragmented and unknown to physicians who have no particular interest in the field.

It is not only discriminatory, but truly dangerous to fail to bring the study and practice of women's medicine to parity with the understanding and treatment of men rapidly and comprehensively. This can and must be achieved through an active and multifaceted approach. This includes physicians examining their practices and attitudes for social or cultural biases that affect medical care, funding medical research in women's health, and increasing the number of women in positions of authority in teaching, research, and the practice of medicine. The Women's Health Initiative, a multidisciplinary, multiinstitute intervention study to address the major causes of death, disability, and frailty among middle-aged and older women, is an important step, as is the creation of the Office of Research on Women's Health. However, as valuable as these efforts are, they are insufficient. Women deserve no less than children who have specialists in pediatrics and the elderly who have specialists in geriatrics. A new interdisciplinary specialty in women's health is required.

References

A list of references is available in the original source.

CON: Women's Health as a Specialty
A Deceptive Solution

by *Michelle Harrison, M.D.*

Abstract. A proposed call for a new specialty in women's health is an attempt to rectify current inadequacies in the care of women. This paper discusses nineteenth century origins of the current organization of medical specialties in which the male body is the norm and woman becomes "other." Nineteenth century attitudes toward women, with the belief in the biological inferiority of women due to their sexual organs, and the replacement of midwives by physicians, became the basis of this bifurcated system of care in which women require two physicians for their ongoing care. A reorganization of medical specialties is proposed in which: (1) Internal medicine incorporates the primary care aspect of gynecology, as does family medicine; (2) Obstetrics and gynecology remains the surgical and referral specialty that it is; (3) Interdisciplinary research addresses gaps in understanding the role of reproductive events, hormones, and cycles to normal and pathological functioning; (4) Medical students are taught to identify across gender lines; (5) All specialties are examined for the purpose of making them "user friendly" to women; and (6) The medical profession addresses and rectifies past inequities in the conceptual framework about women and their subsequent denial of leadership opportunities. The need for education in women's health is acknowledged, but with the goal of making that need obsolete. A new specialty has the potential to further isolate women's issues from mainstream medicine and to marginalize its practitioners.

The proposition that women's health become a separate specialty derives from the failure of the established medical system to address adequately the health care needs of women. These inadequacies exist in the social, medical, educational, and research aspects of women's health. Even though women consume proportionally more medical services than do men, the basic organization of medical specialization has been based upon a male standard to which woman is the eternal exception. Although the establishment of a separate specialty of women's health may initially seem appealing, it has the potential of further isolating the women's perspective in delivery of health care, while simultaneously marginalizing those practitioners who commit themselves to its practice.

This paper discusses the history of the development of the current system of medicine with its adaptation toward the male body and psyche. A model of health care in which women's bodies are the norm, not the exception, is developed.

Nineteenth Century Attitudes

The current treatment of women has its roots in the history of medicine in America, which in turn reflected the prevailing cultural attitudes toward women. Dr. Charles D. Meigs, Professor of Midwifery and the Diseases of Women and Children at Jefferson Medical College in Philadelphia, in 1838 translated the following from the French physician Velpeau:

> Puberty, or the marriageable age, is announced in girls, as it is in boys, by numerous changes. . . . The young girl becomes more timid and reserved; her form becomes more rounded. . . . Her eyes, which are at once brilliant and languishing, express commingled desires, fears, and tenderness; the sensations she experiences and the sense of her own weakness, are the causes why she no longer dares to approach the companions of her childhood but with a downcast look.

The biological transition from girl to young woman was seen as the causative factor in her change in personality. Biology was deemed destiny, and hers was to be one of fear and weakness.

The nineteenth century saw the development of a sizable population of women who, because of industrialization and urbanization, became part of a middle class in which women's employment outside the home was unnecessary. So, while the vast majority of women throughout the world toiled in fields and factories, bore child after child, then aged and died early, Western Europe and America were creating a new version of woman expressive of new political and economic times. The new version conveniently placed women out of competition with men and created a biological basis for that exclusion. Meigs, in an 1859 collection of his own lectures, wrote, "The sexuality of the woman does in its essence consist in the possession of that peculiar structure called ovarian stroma—her heart, brain, lungs, all her viscera, all indeed that she is, would not make her a female without the primordial central essence—stroma." He continues, "She demands a treatment adapted to the very specialties of her own constitution, as a moral, a sexual, germiferous, gestative, or parturient creature." Women's sexuality then became the heart of the justification of difference, and difference invariably meant lesser.

Laqueur, in *Making Sex: Body and Gender from the Greeks to Freud,* describes the Greek model in which the genders were measured by metaphysical perfection in hierarchical relation to each other. This early model of "one sex" in various states of perfection and imperfection was replaced in the nineteenth century with a model of biological divergence based upon anatomical and physiological incommensurability. What had previously been a variation on a single human body became two distinct sexes, believed to be different in every aspect. The shift had been one of changing from comparing grades of apples to comparing apples and oranges, male and female.

Laqueur argues that the polarities of gender can be understood as polarities of power and that "the competition for power generates new ways of constituting the subject and the social realities within which humans dwell." As if to illustrate Laqueur's point, Dr. Alfred Stille in his presidential address to the American Medical Association in 1871 stated, "If, then, woman is unfitted by nature to become a physician, we should, when we oppose her pretensions, be acquitted of any malicious or even unkindly spirit." Woman had been discovered to be a new species, one conveniently unsuited to compete with men in the profession of medicine.

Nineteenth century medicine developed along two lines simultaneously. The body of medicine treated men and the nonreproductive aspects of women's health. Childbirth and common gynecologic problems were usually left to midwives, in part because of prohibitions against male physicians examining female sexual organs. Women's genitals began to be "observed" by physicians in the mid nineteenth century. With the development of gynecologic surgery, which established gynecology as a recognized field, and the successful effort on the part of medicine to define childbirth as a surgical procedure, female midwives were replaced by male obstetricians and gynecologists.

The lifting of cultural prohibitions against the gynecological examination of women by men opened the way for increasing male knowledge about female reproductive anatomy and physiology. If not for the pursuit of economic and professional power on the part of physicians, there might have been a partnership with the midwives, with benefit to both professions and especially to women as patients. Instead there was the destruction of midwifery and a loss of the ways in which women had for centuries attended to the needs of other women. The midwives' care of women exclusively meant that for midwifery, the female body was the standard, the normal, the regular. With the transfer of care to a male medical profession, in which the standard was the male body, the body without female parts, woman's body became "other." With the destruction of midwifery and the paucity of women physicians, the woman's body with its sexual organs was now a foreign body to the overwhelmingly male medical profession and the exclusively male gynecologic surgeons.

The stage was thus set for the current organization of medicine in which internal medicine attends to the nonreproductive aspects of women's health and the generative-related conditions are relegated to the obstetrician-gynecologist. The woman's body with its sexual and generative functions had been medicalized, even in those processes that can be viewed as normal functions. Because medicine was organized around a male body and because physicians were male, nothing about a woman's menstrual cycle or reproduction was "normal." It was all new. She had to be "managed," an approach to women that has not significantly changed.

Nineteenth century medicine attributed the state of women's mental health to the health of their ovaries. Mental illness (at times defined as the inability to accept culturally defined roles, with symptoms including a desire to run away from home, dislike of a husband, or a refusal to sleep with him) was attributed to the dysfunc-

tion of sexual organs. The reproductive organs became the seat of not just sexual passions but were seen as the cause of insanity. Clitoridectomy was the first operation performed to check woman's mental disorder. Proponents of castration described the benefits of removal of the ovaries: "the moral sense of the patient is elevated . . . she becomes tractable, orderly, industrious, and cleanly." There was apparently some recognition that castration could lead to postoperative insanity, in which case further surgery was recommended, namely removal of the uterus and Fallopian tubes. Clitoridectomy, castration, and hysterectomy were the nineteenth century treatment of uncontrolled female emotions. The operation was successful if the woman "was restored to a placid contentment with her domestic functions."

Normality was defined as male, with sanity therefore being closer to male function than to female function. Barker-Benfield suggests that the identification of female sexuality with madness was a result of the assumption that "man's madness" was the norm within the society and therefore woman's was easier to cure. Female "madness" was also easier to see because to the extent it expressed resistance to stereotypic roles, it stood in sharp contrast to the social and political prohibitions of the society.

Such practices as the nineteenth century surgical treatments to return women to their acceptable "passivity" may seem shocking by contemporary standards. Less obvious are the current ways in which society accommodates male behavior and male "madness." For example, although the current diagnosis of posttraumatic stress disorder describes the woman's reaction to rape, an adequate framework to describe the causative behavior on the part of the male aggressor is lacking. The psychological effects of sexual harassment on the part of the victim can be described, but the language and understanding of perpetrators is wanting.

The long delay in recognizing wife battering and marital rape may be traced to the nineteenth century when, "throughout much of the bourgeois century, all across the Western world, women remained virtual chattels in the hands of their fathers, and later, of their husbands." For the last two centuries it was the women victims of battering and marital rape who were brought for mental health services. Society's acceptance of, and possibly hopelessness about, male violence may prevent perception of these acts as deviant and destructive.

Sex role stereotyping within the mental health field was aptly described by Broverman et al., who described sex biases in interpretation of behavior by clinicians. In their 1970 study, a healthy adult (nonspecified sex) had attributes more like a healthy male than a healthy woman. They found that "clinicians are more likely to suggest that healthy women differ from healthy men by being more submissive, less independent, less adventurous, more easily influenced, less aggressive, less competitive, more excitable in minor crises. . . ."

These findings from 1970 are not unlike the descriptions of Velpeau (quoted above) in 1838 or those describing results of castration. In those intervening 130 years, a civil war was fought, women organized and fought for the right to vote, they organized against alcohol, they entered the professions of medicine and law against great odds, they joined the military for two world wars, and yet the stereotypes prove more resilient than reality. Women's sex and sexuality continued to be perceived as the basis for her inferiority. Physicians had, "turned the stereotype of feminine frailty into a medical principle."

The diagnosis of late luteal phase dysphoric disorder was added to the *Diagnostic and Statistical Manual* of the American Psychiatric Association in 1987. This diagnosis describes a mental disorder whose etiology is the menstrual cycle and whose language includes anger as a symptom of mental illness. Although few would dispute that the menstrual cycle may affect how some women feel, including anger, there is an important distinction between influencing and causing symptoms and behavior.

Men and women are influenced in mood by weather, light, diet, general health, and day of the week, but few would designate those as the determinants of mental illness. However, old beliefs persist, in practitioners and in women. When a contemporary woman visits her gynecologist because she is irritable with her children premenstrually, she is the "medical" expression of the nineteenth century view of women's mental state being controlled by her ovaries. Likewise, her gynecologist is supporting this premise when ovariectomy is the treatment recommended for the woman's mood or behavioral problems. Chemical and surgical castration remain accepted treatments for disorders of mood.

Educating for Women's Health

The establishment of training programs in women's health is a separate issue from the creation of a new specialty. There is an enormous job to be done in educating the medical profession and institutions. Ideally, this would be a task undertaken with the aim of eventual obsolescence. Fellowships are needed in order to teach and to create meaningful research. However, to create a new specialty, to certify those physicians trained to take care of women, would allow the rest of those in medicine to feel absolved of responsibility for addressing the needs of women, and more inclined to leave the sensitive care

of women to those few practitioners who are now the "experts." In reality, only a very small percentage of women (and of a given social class) would have access to this care, and the vast majority of women would continue as they do now with their bifurcated care.

The Call for a Specialty

The problems in contemporary medicine that have brought forth the call for a new specialty in women's health are related to: (1) unexplored and unanswered questions in research and education related to women's health; (2) the ways in which women's health needs are not met; and (3) the bifurcation of routine medical care of women.

Given the shortcomings of the present medical system, the call for a separate specialty is understandable. It comes out of frustration, disappointment, and mistrust. The presence of increasing numbers of women physicians has led to a reassessment as to whether medicine could do a better job in addressing needs of women patients. However, there is no aspect of this new proposed specialty that should not be an integral part of the education and practice of every physician, male or female. Rather, the solutions lie in a reorganization of current medical specialization and a demand for the provision of services that more adequately address the needs of women patients.

Questions for Research and Education

Major gaps exist in the understanding of differences in female physiology and pathology, related, but not restricted, to the menstrual cycle. Because of the "foreign nature" of female bodies to a male medical profession, the menstrual cycle and its effects were for a long time ignored, stigmatized, or left strictly to gynecology. Were all males to menstruate, the interrelated effects of the menstrual cycle on other aspects of a person's health would have been considered essential, even fascinating, areas of study, worthy of the best research and funding. In fact, the vast majority of physicians have never experienced menstruation, looked at sanitary pads, handled tampons, or had cramps. Though it may not be necessary to experience illness in order to understand or treat them, the lack of understanding or familiarity with what is normal may result in a tendency to pathologize the entire process. That deficiency in personal experience may limit one's ability to be comfortable with integrating menstruation into a "normal" body.

On the other side, the fact that women are not defined by their menstrual cycles does not mean that this process is irrelevant. It is clear that many medications react differently over the course of the menstrual cycle, yet this area remains largely unexplored. Pharmacologic research has been done on males in part because the menstrual cycle becomes a confounding factor in analysis of results. However, the drugs are then used on women and those confounding effects become clinical effects—poorly understood because of a paucity of research. The research that is needed is not necessarily on the menstrual cycle itself, but rather interdisciplinary research that looks at the menstrual cycle in relation to heart disease, asthma, seizures, and lupus, areas where it is already clear that gender is relevant. Interdisciplinary and gender-conscious research is needed to look at osteoporosis in relation to nutrition, exercise, vitamins, *and* the menstrual cycle. Current research and understanding of substance abuse lacks any systematic or "systems" study of the effects of the menstrual cycle or of menopause.

The designation of obstetrics and gynecology as *the* women's specialty may have actually isolated the understanding of interrelations between menstruation, pregnancy, and other metabolic processes. And, because of the bifurcation in treatment and approach to women's health, the rest of medicine has tended to leave these questions to obstetrics and gynecology.

There is a consistency to the problems identified in the care of women. The common thread is the lack of integration of women's physiologic and metabolic processes into the body of medicine. As a result, the female body remains somewhat "foreign," something a bit more alien to (primarily male) physicians than a regular (male) body.

The Problem of Shortcomings in the System

The differential attention paid to male versus female patients has been documented. Armitage, Schneiderman and Bass, in a study of physician response to complaints in men and women, speculate that "they might be responding to current stereotypes that regard the male as typically stoic and the female as typically 'hypochondriacal!'" Recent literature has addressed differences in referral patterns for male and female cardiac patients and in their selection for coronary angiography and coronary revascularization. This research attempts to discriminate between bias in the care of women and their different needs because of different courses of specific illness. If there is bias in the care of women cardiac patients, it must be addressed, but it does not warrant the development of separate surgery based upon the "female" heart as opposed to a "male" heart. Whatever differences exist in severity of illness, circulation of coronary arter-

ies, or innervation of conducting muscle, they are all within overlapping variations of both male and female hearts. With the exception of those organs involved in reproduction, the vast majority of human organs are truly androgynous.

The Bifurcation of Medical Care of Women

Internal medicine is founded on the model of a male body, with women as "other." That specialty attends to the medical illnesses of the entire male body and part of the female body, whereas obstetrics and gynecology treats those parts of the body related to reproductive health. The result is that most women during their reproductive years must go to two physicians to get their whole body attended to, or use one and forgo the services of the other.

The archaic nature of this arrangement is nowhere more evident than in the assessment of abdominal disorders. The partitioning of the abdominal cavity into the domain of two specialties reflects the dual origins of internists descending from the regular physicians and ob-gyns replacing midwives. No clear anatomical distinction exists, however, between abdomen and pelvis in a female. The area is a continuous cavity divided by imaginary lines that delineate the boundaries of the specialist's territory rather than anatomical structures. The gastrointestinal tract passes through the pelvis and may adhere to the ovaries; endometrial tissue may migrate to the diaphragm, and yet the woman with abdominal pain must visit two doctors, each of whom only partially examines her and then communicates findings with the other by phone or written report, or through the patient. In a male it would be akin to having initial chest pain evaluated by two different doctors, one for the heart and one for the lungs. One doctor would only listen to heartbeats, the other only to breath sounds. Each would then write reports back to the other as to whether the shortness of breath and pain on deep inspiration were of cardiac or pulmonary origin. The need for two physicians to evaluate abdominal pain in a woman is equally absurd.

It is the organization of medical knowledge and practice that are the problem, not the female body. Whereas internal medicine and ob-gyn fall short of addressing the whole woman, family medicine takes care of the whole woman, but in the context of her family, a social role not a medical condition. The one specialty that teaches care of the whole woman also includes children and men. In other words, either a specialty treats only parts of the woman, or it treats all of her and her family.

Rather than the establishment of a new specialty based upon the care of more than half of all adult patients, the current system, in both its structure and content, must address the needs of women as an integral and legitimate aspect of the practice of medicine within every specialty. There simply is no special training for an orthopedist treating women or a radiologist reading women's films or a cardiologist listening to a woman's heart. There is rather the necessity for all orthopedists, all radiologists, and all cardiologists—indeed, all physicians—to look beyond bias and sex stereotyping, and to view being female as only one aspect of the biological, social, and psychological person.

If all human bodies were female and social structure was based upon some other factor than gender, the thorough knowledge of the body would be the medical standard. For instance, anatomically, the physician would examine the whole body because vaginas would not be alien anatomical parts but rather within the norm. If men had large breasts, they would be included in the routine examination of a person. The same physician who examines for spleens and prostrates would be expected to feel for breast lumps. The internist examining for abdominal pain would also do a pelvic exam as part of the assessment, and at the same time, would also do a Pap if needed. In other words, the female reproductive and sexual parts would be part of the everyday practice of an everyday physician.

Even though childbirth has become a surgical procedure, pregnancy remains a metabolic process with the major risk factors being related to the medical health of the woman. Hypertension and diabetes, normally the domain of internists, in pregnancy becomes the domain of the obstetrician-gynecologist, a highly trained surgeon. The major difficulties of the postpartum period are likewise not surgical. Bleeding may occasionally be a problem, but the physician is more likely to encounter thyroid disease, depression, and questions about medications that might pass into breast milk. These are areas more appropriately addressed by an internist or family physician than by a surgeon.

Marginalization of "Women's Health" Specialists

The entrance of women and minorities into male-dominated fields has more commonly led to what the anthropologists term "ritual contamination" of a field than to an increase in the prestige of the women who enter the profession. A field created for the nonsurgical routine care of women, whose practitioners would invariably be mostly female, would likely become a relatively low-paid, low-status field with little or no opportunities for advancement or access to power within universities or specialty societies. Just recently in this century

women have entered into medicine in significant numbers. However, their continued inability to achieve positions of power makes it likely that "women's health" would become a marginalized area for a few dedicated (probably mostly female) physicians. Meanwhile, the rest of medicine would continue as it is, with both the male body and male psyche the standard of normality and health. And, as long as the standard is male, "other" invariably will mean less.

Women do not need special practitioners. Except for diseases of the male reproductive tract and some rare genetic diseases, there are no illnesses restricted to men only. The basic diseases of man are the diseases of woman. The surgical care of women's reproductive organs would rightfully remain the domain of the obstetrician/gynecologist. Although ob-gyns would like to be designated as the primary care physicians of women, it is more likely that internists or family physicians will retain expertise in pelvic exams rather than ob-gyns adding to their training the routine management of diabetes, hypertension, heart disease, gastric ulcers, pneumonia, and all the other diseases encountered in the routine primary care of women.

Necessary Changes

The changes needed to rectify current shortcomings are broad in scope but necessary if anything except cosmetic changes are to be made. Hospital facilities can be dressed up in pink colors and new labeling, but unless the need for fundamental changes in the structure of medicine are acknowledged and implemented, health for the vast majority of women will go unaltered. The basic deficiencies and biases that exist in the conceptual framework of woman—as a biological, psychological, and social person—will continue to undermine any attempt to put women on an equal medical and professional footing with men. The changes needed are as follows.

1. The current specialty of internal medicine must incorporate the menstrual cycle and reproduction into its conceptual framework. The routine gynecologic care of women must be a part of the practice of internal medicine. Family medicine, while continuing to provide primary care for a woman, must recognize her individual existence separate from the family.

2. Obstetrics and gynecology should remain the specialty for referral of obstetric and gynecologic difficulties.

3. Interdisciplinary research must address gaps in the understanding of female functions and their relationship to normal and pathological conditions.

4. Medical students must be taught to identify with patients across gender lines.

5. All medical specialties must be examined for ways in which they are or are not "user friendly" to women.

6. Organized medicine, including medical schools and professional societies, must begin to actively address and rectify those unfounded assumptions about the biological inferiority of women that have been the basis for exclusion of women from medicine and from positions of leadership and power within medicine.

It is not clear what medicine would look like without the standard of the male body and the concomitant underlying assumptions of a biological basis for female passivity and weakness. However, we have the opportunity to find out. Women as patients and as professionals should not settle for a small corner of medicine as a women's health specialty, however appealing that might be. Women instead need to establish their rightful place and perspective within the body of medicine, a body that has been entirely too male in its conceptual framework as well as its membership. There is no medical imperative for a new specialty. Instead, there is an urgent social and economic imperative to restructure medical specialization and to create a nonadversarial body of knowledge and code of practice, in which gender may represent difference but not "other," and certainly not less.

References

A list of references is available in the original source.

Thinking About Women's Health
The Case for Gender Sensitivity

by Amal J. Khoury, PhD, MPH and
Carol S. Weisman, PhD

The last decade has seen an unprecedented level of public debate and policymaking on women's health, including substantial increases in funding for women's health research on a range of topics. There is growing recognition that women's health is not limited to reproductive health, but includes such conditions as heart disease, lung cancer, and HIV/AIDS, and women's health advocates have drawn attention to how women's health care is affected by some specific access and quality issues. Perhaps not surprisingly, some critics of this trend argue that women are not the most disadvantaged group with respect to health and health care. Members of the men's health advocacy community claim that there are "inequities" between women and men in access to health resources and argue that "men are the at-risk population" requiring more attention. The implication is that the successes of women's health advocates detract attention from men's health.

We contend that a better framework for addressing both women's health and men's health is one that focuses less on gender equity in access to resources and more on gender sensitivity—that is, attention both to gender differences and to gender-specific needs in research, practice, and policy. This approach holds the greatest potential for improving the health of both women and men.

Gender Sensitivity in Research

There are a number of gender differences in health between American women and men that cannot be easily interpreted as favoring one sex or the other. Women in the United States have a longer life expectancy and lower mortality rates than men at all ages. However, women report more disease and disability than men and more time lost from regular activities because of disease and disability, throughout most of the life span. With regard to mental health, women experience higher rates of depression, anxiety, and eating disorders, whereas men have higher rates of substance abuse and antisocial personality disorders.

Reprinted from *Women's Health Issues,* V12(2), by A. J. Khoury and C. S. Weisman, "Thinking about Women's Health: The Case for Gender Sensitivity," pp. 61–65. Copyright © 2002, with permission from Jacobs Institute of Women's Health.

The reasons for these differences are not fully understood. In fact, many of women's health problems are different from men's due to a combination of biological, psychological, and social factors. There are the obvious examples related to reproductive biology (e.g., complications of pregnancy, cancers of the male and female reproductive organs), and there are more subtle examples related to social roles and life circumstances (e.g., women are more likely than men to live in poverty and to be exposed to domestic violence and sexual abuse; men engage in more physical risk-taking). A growing body of scientific knowledge suggests how gender (the sociocultural roles and expectations that attach to the sexes) and not just biological sex affects health problems and approaches to treatment. Even for health problems that women and men share, such as heart disease and HIV/AIDS, differences in disease etiology, presentation, and course have important implications for prevention, diagnosis, treatment, and rehabilitation.

The gender sensitivity frame calls for expanding the knowledge base about how sex and gender affect the health of both women and men, and for designing appropriate interventions based on this knowledge. Research on conditions exclusive to one sex (e.g., ovarian cancer, prostate cancer) clearly is needed. Research on health problems that women and men share needs to move beyond controlling for "sex" in analyses to investigating gender differences in how conditions are experienced by men and women. The gender sensitivity frame also extends to the development of health technologies for diagnosis and treatment, which, until recently, has used mainly male models. It is worth noting that gender sensitivity is particularly needed in developing countries where gender differences in many health conditions remain largely uncharted.

Gender Sensitivity in Health Services

Despite increasing attention to quality-of-care issues, little attention has been paid to how gender is associated with patterns of health care utilization and quality. Adult women consume more outpatient and inpatient health services than adult men, and men are less likely than women to have a regular source of care. In addition, there is evidence of gender dimensions of doctor-patient communication and coordination of services. Scholars in the United States and abroad have called for gender sensitivity in health care delivery as a way of promoting the appropriateness of services, particularly reproductive health services, and services to elderly women and men. The examples below pertain to women's health.

The quality of information exchange between providers and patients affects women's satisfaction with health care, trust in the health care system, and compliance with treatment. The 1998 Commonwealth Fund Survey of Women's Health found that more women than men changed doctors in the past 5 years due to dissatisfaction with the quality of communication. A gender-sensitive approach calls for improving communication by emphasizing provider knowledge of women's health problems, attention to women's concerns, provision of complete information to women (e.g., treatment options, side effects of treatment, steps to avoid problem in the future), and joint decision making. Research is needed to identify ways to improve interpersonal relationships between women and their health providers. For example, one study found that a single question, "What would you really most of all want me to do for you today?" was more effective in eliciting responses from female patients than a series of medically oriented questions about the patient's diagnosis. This question allowed the provider to focus on gender-based problems of the patient, often of emotional origin, rather than on the symptoms of the problems alone.

Service coordination and follow-up has a gender dimension because of the fragmentation in women's primary health care. The reproductive and non-reproductive components of basic well-women care are separate, and mechanisms for coordination among services are often lacking. Many U.S. women use two types of physicians (typically an obstetrician—gynecologist and a family physician or internist) for regular care. Without appropriate communication between providers, this can lead to inefficiencies in the delivery of care, higher costs, undue access burdens on women, and risks to women of both gaps and redundancies in services. A gender-sensitive approach to primary care seeks to integrate the components of care for women using organizational and educational strategies. Organizational strategies include multidisciplinary team approaches to providing primary care and co-location of services in comprehensive primary care women's health centers, such as the clinical centers of the National Centers of Excellence in Women's Health. Educational strategies include innovations in medical education and in residency and fellowship training to increase content in women's health and gender issues.

Gender Sensitivity in Health Policy

Health policies that affect financial and nonfinancial access to health care services often have an important gender component. Gender has been an explicit factor in policy regulating managed care plans: mandating direct access to obstetricians—gynecologists within health plans and minimum hospital stays after childbirth were prominent policy initiatives in the 1990s. The gender issues involved in health insurance policy are more subtle. More men than women are uninsured at any given point in time, largely because Medicaid targets poor pregnant women and parents of young children. In general, women are more dependent than men on publicly financed health insurance (Medicaid and Medicare) and have fewer financial resources with which to pay for care. Initiatives to restructure Medicaid and Medicare therefore have important if unintended consequences for women, and policymaking would benefit from including gender perspectives in decisions about eligibility requirements, covered benefits, and provider reimbursement.

Privately insured women rely more than men on dependent coverage and less on private insurance through their own jobs. Dependent coverage may become more difficult to obtain as premiums increase and employers seek ways to reduce health insurance costs, particularly during our current economic downturn. The consequences for women's insurance coverage could be considerable.

Nonfinancial barriers to care also are related to gender. Factors such as the availability of specific health services in some communities (particularly obstetric services and fertility-control services), the availability of transportation and child care, and the availability of translator and other culturally sensitive services are all important facilitators of care. Because women in our culture are caregivers and have the primary responsibility for the health care of family members, policy initiatives that improve women's capacity to negotiate the health care system will impact the health care of families.

Conclusion

Gender sensitivity in research, practice, and health policy points the way to better health for both women and men. The gender sensitivity frame does not assume that women's health and men's health are in conflict. Instead, it highlights the need to examine sex and gender as variables in biomedical research; to develop health technology based on men's and women's needs and models; to investigate ways to improve the quality of health care for women and men, using gender-based strategies when necessary; and to include gender perspectives in the process of developing and monitoring policy initiatives. Advocates for both women's health and men's health can benefit from this framework and help the nation achieve the goal of eliminating health disparities.

References

A list of references is available in the original source.

Exploring the Biological Contributions to Human Health
Does Sex Matter?

Over the past decade new discoveries in basic human biology have made it increasingly apparent that many normal physiological functions—and, in many cases, pathological functions—are influenced either directly or indirectly by sex-based differences in biology.

This realization, however, has been slow in coming. Considerable attention has focused on differences and similarities between females and males at the *societal* level by researchers evaluating how individual behaviors, lifestyles, and surroundings affect one's biological development and health. Similarly, at the level of the *whole organism* clinicians and applied researchers have investigated the component organs and systems of humans. However, scientists have paid much less attention to the direct study of these differences at the basic *cellular* and

> *Sex* refers to the classification of living things, generally as male or female according to their reproductive organs and functions assigned by chromosomal complement.
>
> *Gender* refers to a person's self-representation as male or female, or how that person is responded to by social institutions based on the individual's gender presentation. Gender is rooted in biology and shaped by environment and experience.

molecular levels. Where data are available, they have often been a by-product of other areas of research. Historically, the research community assumed that beyond the reproductive system, such differences do not exist or are not relevant. Still, scientific evidence of the importance of sex differences throughout the life span abounds.

Although an individual can be characterized initially by the presence of particular reproductive organs, sex differences encompass much more than that. Evidence suggests that the distinct anatomy and physiology that develop as a result of having been dealt two X chromosomes (XX) or an X chromosome and a Y chromosome (XY) at fertilization can have a much broader influence on an individual's health than was previously thought. While it is anatomically obvious why only males develop prostate cancer and only females get ovarian cancer, it is not at all obvious why, for example, females are more likely than males to recover language ability after suffering a left-hemisphere stroke or why females have a far greater risk than males of developing life-threatening ventricular arrhythmias in response to a variety of potassium channel-blocking drugs.

Recent research has shed some light on these puzzles. In the case of stroke, for example, functional magnetic resonance imaging has shown that females rely on both sides of the brain for certain aspects of language, whereas males predominantly rely on the left hemisphere.

Differences in the prevalence and severity of a broad range of diseases, disorders, and conditions exist between the sexes. Investigators are now positioned to move to the next level of study, where the mechanisms and origins of sex differences can be explored.

Two questions at the core of these explorations are: (1) How can information on sex differences be translated into preventative, diagnostic, and therapeutic practice? and (2) How can the new knowledge about and understanding of biological sex differences and similarities most effectively be used to positively affect patient outcomes and improve health and health care?

The Institute of Medicine formed a committee to evaluate and consider the current understanding of sex differences and determinants at the biological level and to identify current and potential barriers to the conduct of research in this area. The committee's report, *Exploring the Biological Contributions to Human Health: Does Sex Matter?* contains findings and recommendations to facilitate scientific endeavors in this area, take advantage of new opportunities in basic and applied research, and fill identified research gaps.

Recurring Themes

Three common recurring messages emerged from the committee's review.

- **Sex matters.** Sex, that is, being male or female, is an important basic human variable that should be considered when designing and analyzing studies in all areas and at all levels of biomedical and health-related research. Differences in health and illness are influenced by individual genetic and physiological constitutions, as well as by an individual's interaction with environmental and experiential factors. The incidence and severity of diseases vary between the sexes and may be related to differences in exposures, routes of entry and the processing of a foreign agent, and cellular responses.

- **The study of sex differences is evolving into a mature science.** There is now sufficient knowledge of the biological basis of sex differences to validate the scientific study of sex differences and to allow the generation of hypotheses. The next step is to move from the descriptive to the experimental and establish the conditions that must be in place to facilitate and encourage the scientific study of the mechanisms and origins of sex differences.

- **Barriers to the advancement of knowledge about sex differences in health and illness exist and must be eliminated.** Scientists conducting research on sex differences are confronted with an array of barriers to progress, including ethical, financial, sociological, and scientific factors.

Every Cell Has a Sex

Rapid advances in molecular biology have revealed the genetic and molecular basis of a number of sex-based differences in health and human disease, some of which are attributed to sexual genotype—XX in the female and XY in the male. Genes on the sex chromosomes can be expressed differently between males and females, because of the presence of either single or double copies of the gene and because of the phenomena of differing meiotic effects, X-chromosome inactivation, and genetic imprinting. The inheritance of either a male or female

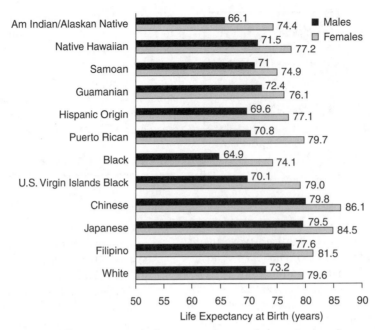

Although actual life expectancy differs among ethnic groups, the consistency in the observation of an advantage for females across ethnic groups is striking.

Source: NCHS and NIH. Data are from 1989 to 1994.

genotype is further influenced by the source (maternal or paternal) of the X chromosome. The relative roles of the sex chromosome genes and their expression explains X-linked disease and is likely to illuminate the reasons for heterogeneous expression of some diseases within and between the sexes.

These findings argue that there are multiple, ubiquitous differences in the basic cellular biochemistry of males and females that can affect an individual's health. Many of these differences do not necessarily arise as a result of differences in the hormonal regime to which males and females are exposed but are a direct result of the genetic differences between the two sexes. Further research should be conducted to determine the functions and effects of X-chromosome- and Y-chromosome-linked genes in somatic cells as well as germ-line cells, determine how genetic sex differences influence other levels of biological organization (cell, organ, organ system, organism), including susceptibility to disease, and develop systems that can identify and distinguish between the effects of genes and the effects of hormones.

Sex Begins in the Womb

Sex differences of importance to health and human disease occur throughout the life span, although their specific expression varies at different stages of life. Some differences originate in events occurring in the intrauter-

ine environment, where developmental processes differentially organize tissues for later activation in the male or female. In the prenatal period, sex determination and differentiation occur in a series of sequential processes governed by genetic and environmental factors. During the prepubertal period, behavioral and hormonal changes manifest the secondary sexual characteristics that reinforce the sexual identity of the individual through adolescence and into adulthood. Hormonal events occurring in puberty lay a framework for biological differences that persist through life and contribute to variable onset and progression of disease in males and females. It is important to study sex differences at all stages of the life cycle, relying on animal models of disease and including sex as a variable in basic and clinical research designs.

Sex Affects Behavior and Perception

Basic genetic and physiological differences, in combination with environmental factors, result in behavioral and cognitive differences between males and females. Sexual differences in the brain, sex-typed behavior and gender identity, and sex differences in cognitive ability should be studied at all points in the lifespan. Hormones play a role in behavioral and cognitive sexual dimorphism, but are not solely responsible. In addition, sex differences in perception of pain have important clinical implications. Research is needed on the natural variations between and within the sexes in behavior, cognition, and perception, with expanded investigation of sex differences in brain organization and function.

Sex Affects Health

Males and females have different patterns of illness and different life spans, raising questions about the relative roles of biology and environment in these disparities. Dissimilar exposures, susceptibilities, and responses to initiating agents, and differences in energy storage and metabolism result in variable responses to pharmacologic agents and the initiation and manifestation of diseases such as obesity, autoimmune disorders, and coronary heart disease, to name a few. Understanding the bases of these sex-based differences are important to developing new approaches to prevention, diagnosis, and treatment.

The Future of Research on Biological Sex Differences

Being male or female is an important fundamental variable that should be considered when designing and analyzing basic and clinical research. Historically, the terms *sex* and *gender* have been loosely, and sometimes inappropriately, used in reporting research results, a situation that should be remedied through further clarification. Conducting studies that account for sex differences might require innovative designs, methods, and model systems, all of which might require additional re-

sources. Studies relying on biological materials would benefit from a determination and disclosure of the sex of origin of the material, and clinical researchers should attempt to identify the endocrine status of research subjects. Longitudinal studies should be designed to allow analysis of data by sex. Once studies are conducted, data regarding sex differences, or the lack thereof, should be readily available in the scientific literature. Interdisciplinary efforts are needed to conduct research on sex differences.

There is a lack of awareness that the consequences of genetics and physiology may be amenable to change. The committee noted that, historically, studies on race, ethnicity, age, nationality, religion, and sex have sometimes led to discriminatory practices. The committee believes, therefore, that these historical practices should be taken into consideration so that they will not be repeated. The past should not limit the future of research but should serve as a guide to its use. Ethical research on the biology of sex differences is essential to the advancement of human health and should not be constrained.

In the report, the committee expresses its expectation that the public, scientific, and policy communities will agree that the understanding of sex differences in health and illness merits serious scientific inquiry in all aspects of biomedical and health-related research. Until the question of sex is routinely asked and the results—positive or negative—are routinely reported, many opportunities to obtain a better understanding of the pathogenesis of disease and to advance human health will surely be missed.

Summary of Barriers to Progress in Research on Sex Differences

Terminology
- There is inconsistent and often confusing use of the terms sex and gender in the scientific literature and popular press.

Research Tools and Resources
- The conduct of research on sex differences and longitudinal research may require more complex studies and additional resources.
- Information on sex differences can be difficult to glean from the published literature.
- Useful information on the sex of origin of cell and tissue culture material is often lacking in the literature.
- There is a lack of data from longitudinal studies encompassing different diseases, disorders, and conditions across the life span.

- There is a lack of consideration of hormonal variability.

Interdisciplinary and Collaborative Research
- The application of federal regulations is not uniform.
- Opportunities for interdisciplinary collaboration have been underused.

Non-Health-Related Implications of Research on Sex Differences in Health
- There is a lack of awareness that the consequences of genetics and physiology may be amenable to change.
- The finding of sex differences can lead to discriminatory practices.

Summary of Major Recommendations

- Promote research on sex at the cellular level.
- Study sex differences from womb to tomb.
- Mine cross-species information.
- Investigate natural variations.
- Expand research on sex differences in brain organization and function.
- Monitor sex differences and similarities in all human disease.
- Clarify use of the terms *sex* and *gender*.
- Support and conduct additional research on sex differences.
- Make sex-specific data more readily available.

- Determine and disclose the sex of origin of biological research materials.
- Conduct and construct longitudinal studies so that the results can be analyzed by sex.
- Identify the endocrine status of research subjects (an important variable that should be considered when possible in analyses).
- Encourage and support interdisciplinary research on sex differences.
- Reduce the potential for discrimination based on identified sex differences.

For More Information . . .

Copies of *Exploring the Biological Contributions to Human Health: Does Sex Matter?* are available for sale from the National Academy Press; call (800) 624-6242

or (202) 334-3313 (in the Washington metropolitan area), or visit the NAP home page at **www.nap.edu.** The full text of this report is available at **http://www.nap.edu/catalog/10028.html**

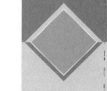

How to Tell Your Doctor a Thing or Two

by Morton Hunt

If you're like most Americans, you've lost a lot of faith in doctors in recent years. In 1966 the Louis Harris survey organization reported that 73 percent of Americans had a great deal of confidence in the medical profession: by 1977 the figure had dropped to 43 percent.

As a result a new kind of patient has appeared—a patient who is questioning and even argumentative, sometimes mistrustful, often balky. This patient goes doctor-shopping, files complaints with medical societies, sues for malpractice. She may join one of the hundreds of new medical-consumer (patient) organizations that defend patients against their own doctors. She—or he—no longer silently listens to the doctor with awe but speaks up, wants to be told everything and to be convinced, and reserves the right to reject the doctor's advice or to ask for a second opinion.

I've been talking to leaders of the medical profession and of medical-consumer groups, and both sides

agree on one thing: Doctors throughout America are seeing the new kind of patient increasingly often in their offices. Although some doctors—including my own—look approvingly on patients of this new breed, the majority view them with disapproval and even hostility. By training, position and tradition, doctors tend to play the role of Wise Patriarch Whose Word is Law, and they expect their patients to be Good Children Who Obey Without Argument. They consider the new breed "difficult," "troublemakers" and—above all—"bad" patients.

But there is growing evidence that nowadays the "bad" patient is a better one, in terms of medical results, than the "good" patient. According to a number of recent research studies, the passive, uncomplaining, unquestioning patient is less likely to get well quickly than the new kind. Or as Eli Glogow, director of the graduate program in health administration at the University of

Reprinted with permission from Bread & Roses, Women's Health Center, Milwaukee, Wisconsin. (Specific date uncertain, probably late 1970s.)

Southern California, succinctly puts it, "the 'bad patient' gets better quicker."

Why? Not because the "bad" patient—whom I'll call the "active" patient— refuses to follow instructions. Indeed, medical journals report that the independent patient is apt to carry out doctors' orders faithfully, once he or she accepts them, while the passive patient is more likely to forget or quietly disobey.

But following instructions is only part of it. What gives the active patient better odds at regaining health quickly or staying healthy is a whole new concept of the patient's role. Essentially it consists of taking responsibility for one's own health care—becoming an adult rather than a child in the doctor-patient relationship. That means finding the best doctor available but getting another opinion if doubtful about a major recommendation; defending oneself against overmedication and unnecessary surgery; and in general acting as the doctor's partner, collaborator and equal.

It is out of necessity that such patients are becoming ever more numerous for there has been a revolution in the nature of medical practice. In recent years the doctor-patient relationship has become coldly impersonal, and not very reassuring to the patient. Here are some of the reasons:

- The number of drugs, tests and special technological procedures has vastly increased. As a result, patients spend more time with nurses and technicians, less time with the doctor himself. Diseases get treated but treatment becomes an assembly-line affair.
- The new technology makes for greater specialization. Specialization makes for higher fees—and so more doctors want to specialize (more than four out of five now do so). In consequence there are fewer general practitioners, and the patient has to wait longer and settle for less time with a G.P. than ever before.
- Specialization also means that the patient is subdivided and parceled out among doctors—the gynecologist, the allergist, and so on—and is to each not a person but a symptom in some part of the body. Many patients get medical care from several doctors but have no one doctor who *cares*. There's the rub. Dr. W. Walter Menninger of the Menninger Foundation, a center of psychiatric research, says that most of the grievances patients have against doctors involve breakdown in the *caring* aspect of the physician-patient relationship, not in the quality of technical care.

One young woman I know worried about menstrual spotting and went to a busy gynecologist who, with little explanation, did a suction extraction of the endometrium (the mucus lining of the uterus). Unprepared for the invasive and painful procedure, she left the office shaken and burst into tears on the sidewalk. Months later she said to him as casually as she could, "Doctor, that last visit was so unpleasant I thought I might never come back"—to which he replied just as casually, "If you ever feel that way again, I think you *shouldn't* come back." Caring? He'd sneer at the word.

- We Americans move about more than ever. We become separated from the doctor who knows us best, and what he or she knows about us is, in most cases, lost or forgotten. Yet you, the patient, have no legal right in most states to make the doctor turn over his records to you. (If you ask, he'll send them to another doctor—but few patients ask.)
- Group practice, growing by leaps and bounds, gives the busy doctor much-needed relief and free time and assures you that someone will be on hand when needed. But the substitute doctor rarely knows your medical history or has time to read through your folder. Unless you can fill in the gaps in this stranger's knowledge of you—and have the courage to do so—you may get indifferent or even hurtful treatment.

One 30-year-old woman went to her medical group when a rash spread over her arms and chest. An overworked doctor who had never seen her before asked her a few questions and concluded—correctly—that it was an allergic reaction; summer sunshine and an antibiotic she'd been taking didn't go well together. He prescribed a form of cortisone to be taken by mouth, and a week later she was in the hospital with a bleeding ulcer. Buried in her folder and unread by the doctor had been notes about a tendency on her part toward ulcers: cortisone treatment brought the condition to an acute state.

- The profit motive has altered the patient-doctor relationship. Profitmaking is an old, respectable incentive to businessmen and professionals alike, but it can easily lead to exploitative and unfair practices. That's why watchdog agencies protect consumers from impersonal big business. But medicine, though it too is now impersonal and big business—doctors' fees total over $26 billion a year—remains virtually unregulated except by itself.

Exploitation by doctors takes many forms. In a study of one group of internists, researchers found that some of the doctors ordered patients to come back for follow-up visits twice as often as others did, even though all were treating the same kinds of patients. Three of four doctors polled by the American Medical

Association this year admit that they now order anywhere from one to several extra tests per patient—not for the patient's benefit but for their own, as protection from potential malpractice suits. But it is the patient who pays—and who is exposed to extra risks.

The most serious conflict between the patient's best interest and the profit motive occurs when the doctor stands to gain the most. A surgeon who will earn many hundreds of dollars from performing an operation is likely to be less objective, when deciding whether to recommend it, than a surgeon who is not involved and therefore impartial. A recent Congressional study indicates that one of every six operations is unnecessary: that's more than 3 million needless operations per year, costing $4 billion and leading to nearly 12,000 postoperative deaths. In some specialties the figures are even higher; various research teams have termed anywhere from a quarter to a half of the 800,000 hysterectomies performed each year "unjustified" or "unnecessary."

Reaction to all this was inevitable. Liberal doctors and medical administrators drafted "bills of rights" for patients, and a few legislators tried to get some of them enacted into state law. Labor unions and veterans' organizations began to fight for "patients' advocates" in clinics and hospitals, to listen to patients' grievances and take their complaints to the authorities. Everywhere the new breed of patient began to appear.

And perhaps most important, medical-consumer organizations sprang up, most of them offshoots of the 1960s consumer movement. Public Citizen, the national organization headed by Ralph Nader, set up the Health Research Group in Washington, D.C. Headed by Sidney M. Wolfe, a dynamic young doctor, it gathers research data and uses them to lobby for stronger Government controls over drug advertising, prescription writing, the use of x-rays; for the patient's right to obtain personal medical records; and for controls over cost and quality of health care in general.

In recent years other medical-consumer groups have been started in many cities by churches, by campus organizations and by women's groups. Some of them, chiefly educational, publish pamphlets, newsletters or books on medical matters, or operate Tel-Med libraries. (You phone, ask to hear a tape on a medical matter that concerns you and get plugged in to a four-to-seven minute cassette at no charge.) Others also offer counseling and advice and make referrals to doctors or clinics. Still others, like Nader's health group, are interested chiefly in bringing pressure to bear on city and state officials to control medical costs and practices and in getting consumer-minded representatives onto the governing boards of hospitals, medical-insurance plans and relevant state agencies.

In the long run it will be these collective efforts that will rebuild the patient-doctor relationship in a new, democratic form. Meanwhile what can you, the individual, do for yourself? A good deal. From my conversations with medical-consumer leaders I have put together a seven-point program for the new-style patient:

1. *Care for yourself as far as possible.* Save the doctor's time and your own—and your money—by doing at home certain things you can learn through community-health projects and self-care courses taught by medical-consumer groups. You can learn to take and record your own blood pressure and that of your husband and children (these days *everyone's* blood pressure is considered important information; the equipment costs as little as $20). You can learn to adjust the dosage of your own or your children's medication, within limits set by the doctor. You can give yourself or others in your family regular injections (allergy shots, for instance), when needed. Professor Lowell S. Levin, of the Yale University School of Medicine, a specialist in public health, says that the time has come for the "rediscovery of the lay function in health," and maintains that the informed patient can become the most important practitioner in the medical-care system.

2. *Keep your own medical records.* Since in most states you can't gain access to doctors' records, ask your doctor for his findings every time you visit him—your pulse, blood pressure, hemoglobin and white-cell count—whatever he checks; and don't settle for "It's fine." You have a moral if not a legal right to precise information. So start a notebook. Keep track of whatever the doctor tells you, plus the dates of illnesses, their symptoms and duration, diagnoses, medications taken and their effects.

   Also ask your doctor for the results of all tests and lab reports. A few doctors already provide such information; others do not but will if you ask; and many others will refuse. If your doctor refuses, you can either accept defeat or look for another doctor. You also can ask any medical-consumer group what the law is in your state; it may support your claims, and if it does, tell the doctor so.

3. *Come to the doctor prepared.* Before your visit, jot down everything you want to tell the doctor. Include the questions you want to ask. It's amazing how things will slip your mind when you're talking to a hurried doctor or when you're spraddled out on an examination table with some unseen gadget making its way into you. Many feminist groups urge patients to take along a friend to hold the list of questions and remind you of things you forget. Most

doctors will ask a third party to leave before an examination, but this is only custom: A.M.A. spokesmen and consumer-group leaders agree that doctors should, and for the most part will, allow a third party to remain if the patient asks them to.

4. *Exercise your right to choose and refuse.* Even with a doctor you believe in—and all the more with one who is new to you—you should take an active part in decisions affecting you. Ask for a detailed explanation of the possible side effects of any recommended drug or procedure. Ask if there are alternate ways to treat your problem. Give due weight to the doctor's preference, but also to your own. It's your body and your life.

If the doctor calls for tests, ask how necessary they are; it's quite in order for you to say you'd like to keep costs down. And ask about risks; it's quite proper for you to say you'd like to avoid any x-rays that are of only marginal value, since it's not the individual exposure that endangers you but an excessive lifetime total of exposures. And it's also your right to say that you prefer to live with your medical problem—or even die of it—rather than submit to a painful, risky treatment if the outcome is highly uncertain.

But if you question the doctor's advice or decline to follow any of his recommendations, won't he be angered? It depends in part on how you put it—and on what kind of person he is. Says Dr. Wolfe, of the Health Research Group, "The doctor who gets huffy when you ask questions or express preferences is a doctor to stay away from. The doctor you should look for is the one who realizes that you have a right to ask questions and to decide what you want to do with your life."

Do you really have a right to refuse any of the doctor's orders? Medical-consumer leaders and A.M.A. officials agree that unless your disease endangers the public welfare, you do have such a right—but that if you exercise it, the doctor may exercise a corresponding right to stop treating you. If you're pregnant or seriously ill or worried, you may be afraid to risk it; you may choke back your questions or objections and play the part of the "good" patient.

But speaking up needn't mean confrontation. Denise Fuge, coordinator of the Women and Health Committee of the New York Chapter of NOW, says patients shouldn't *confront* the doctor, but should seek to *communicate* their fears, wishes and personal values openly and honestly. "Most doctors," she says, "don't know what women are thinking, and they'd like to. They'd respond to the patient much more sensitively if they did."

5. *Get a second opinion.* Before you agree to surgery or any other major procedure, or when some ailment isn't getting better under your doctor's management, tell him that you'd like a second opinion and that you feel sure he wouldn't mind your getting one. He probably will mind, but won't say so or threaten to stop treating you; publicly, most doctors are opposed only to mandatory (legally required) second opinions. Privately, though, many of them feel like Dr. James Sammons, executive vice-president of the A.M.A., who is against them in general.

"I'm opposed to them," he told me, "because the patient's right of choice is lost—he tends to assume the second opinion is more intelligent than the first one." What Dr. Sammons ignores is that the second opinion, though not necessarily more intelligent than the first, is disinterested and hence less subject to unconscious bias. Not all doctors, incidentally, are against second opinions; one quarter of a sample of doctors polled by the magazine *Medical World News* favored them, and the trend is in that direction.

6. *Ask for enough time.* Don't let yourself be rushed. "You're paying for an expensive service," says Maryann Napoli, of New York's Center for Medical Consumers and Health Care Information, "and consultation is part of it. It's important for your mental health as well as your physical health to have your questions fully answered and your doubts resolved."

Denise Fuge, of NOW, recommends that you say something like, "Doctor, I came to you because I've been worried, and I need more time to talk to you. If you're too busy today, please tell me when you can spend more time with me and I'll come back." A women's medical-consumer group in New York, HealthRight, also suggests that you ask the nurse some of your unanswered questions; nurses are often sympathetic and less rushed than the doctor.

But if your doctor regularly allows less time than normal—15 minutes is the national average duration of routine office visits—and doesn't respond to your request for more time, he may be the wrong doctor for you.

7. *Don't let yourself be treated as an inferior.* This is one of the trickiest points, and perhaps one of the most important. Many doctors treat you in ways that put you at a psychological disadvantage. Some gynecologists in particular address patients by their first names even when they scarcely know them; it makes the patient feel a little like a child. Many women resent this; a few fight back. When a gynecologist greeted one woman, whom he had seen only once before, with "What brings you here today, Lillian?" she said sweetly, "I've got galloping

vaginitis again, Bernard." Bernard took the hint. Generally, though, a more formal way of setting the matter straight will work better. For instance: "Doctor, I would much prefer to be called Ms. So-and-so," or, "I really don't like being addressed by my first name."

Similarly, it may make you feel inferior to be undressed and in a gown when you first meet the doctor. If so, tell the nurse you want to speak to him before you undress. This is a delicate matter; the doctor may have set office rules. But Dr. Menninger points out that when you come to exhibit some disease to the doctor, you are apt to feel shame and humiliation, and since such feelings tend to make you a docile patient rather than an active one, it is important to resist anything that intensifies them.

Things will never be what they once were. But the new doctor-patient relationship need not be one of antagonism; it can be one of equality and cooperation. This is what most of the medical-consumer groups, and most active patients are really seeking.

And within the ranks of doctors there are signs of evolution toward a new image of the good doctor—no longer the wise patriarch whose word is law, but a dedi-cated expert who is ready to give you the help you need and the kind of help you choose. Increasingly, medical journals carry articles advocating democratic ways of dealing with patients and favoring patient participation in the making of medical decisions.

Professor Julia Frank, of the Yale University School of Medicine, writing in the *New England Journal of Medicine,* urges doctors everywhere to make the patient "an equal member of the team." An editorial in a recent issue of the *Journal of the American Medical Association,* noting the spread of "participatory democracy" in our society, says, "It is simply no longer possible for the physician to make moral and value decisions for his patients." And Professor Levin, writing in *Public Health Reports,* sounds a call for massive self-reform by the health professions: "The high value placed on the compliant patient must be transferred to the active, even resistant, patient." He predicts the creation of a "new social contract between professionals and lay persons"—a contract from which the doctor will benefit, by sharing responsibility with those he treats.

And it is a contract from which the patient will benefit by gaining self-respect and a sense of control over her own life—and by getting better quicker.

The Gynecologic Exam and the Training of Medical Students

An Opportunity for Health Education

by Judith Schmidt

This article is a personal account written by a senior health education major about her experience as a teaching associate (TA) in training medical students for the gynecological examination. This method of using teaching associates who "teach on their own bodies" has evolved in medical schools across the country in recent years. It is an attempt to counter inadequate medical school preparation in this important area of women's health and to improve the physician-patient relationship in gynecological medicine. Lack of sensitivity to female patients has taken the form of high rates of malpractice litigation in gynecology, a situation which might well be reversed given the improved communication between physician and patient. Medical school teaching staff across the country have now widely accepted the use of teaching associates as the most effective teaching method for this part of the complete physical examination.

One of the ideas emphasized in this approach is that of the "activated patient." An activated patient is one who is fully and equally involved as a participant in the examination process. One projected outcome

From *Health Values,* Vol. 10, No. 2, March/April 1986, pp. 33–36. Copyright © 1986 by Judith Schmidt. Reprinted by permission of the author.

of this approach is greater personal responsibility for one's health such as doing self-breast exams. But the potential of using this approach goes beyond mere "disease prevention" of traditional medical care. It gives female patients a sense of control over what happens to them—both inside and out of a gynecologist's office—and enters a psychological and social health dimension that makes the concept known as "high-level wellness" accessible. In the context of medical intervention by physicians during the gynecological exam, the potential exists to take steps toward the goal of optimal wellness. This article attempts to explore that potential.

"What's it like doing that sort of thing?" curious and sometimes incredulous friends ask. I have just told them about my job. I am a teaching associate (TA) for the instruction of the gynecological examination to first and second-year medical students. As such, I am a "professional patient." I give feedback to these students about their technique and attitude, and most important, about the way they communicate with me as a patient during the gynecological exam.

I respond to my friends' questions by telling them my job is demanding. I experience the same feelings that any woman facing a breast and pelvic exam does, including anxiety and nervousness. But overall, I feel good about doing it. I feel that what I am doing is important.

The next question, "Does it pay well?" The implication is that the only reason for my engaging in such an occupation must be money. "Yes, it does," is my answer. "And well it should! My job takes a good deal of knowledge and ability." Not only does it require knowledge of female sexual and reproductive anatomy, but it means that I must be comfortable discussing my own anatomy with others. It requires good teaching and interpersonal skills, plus a lot of sensitivity about a topic that is emotionally loaded for students and patient alike.

"But money isn't the main reason I do it," I explain. My own experiences with gynecologists have for the most part not been satisfactory. The opportunity to improve this area of women's health through my input into the training of medical students appeals to me. Also, as a student majoring in health education at the same university, I see the potential for patient education and the role physicians might play in this process. As a TA, I feel I have some influence in this direction.

"Does your job take training?"

"Yes it does," I respond, as I visualize our initial training sessions. In these first sessions, we learn right along with the medical students. We all become part of a "learning team" which I can now see is beneficial for reducing anxiety and developing a comfortable working relationship with the students prior to the actual examination.

Just as the medical students do, we watch the Bates videotape, "Female Pelvic Examination." And just as they do, we practice inserting the speculum and examining internal anatomy manually on the plastic Gynny model. As I practice using the speculum on the Gynny model, the idea then seems less scary to me. I wonder, as a health educator, whether offering other women this experience on a Gynny model prior to a pelvic exam might lessen their anxiety, as it has mine.

In these initial training sessions my actual teaching role begins. I am called upon to recall my own feelings during the gynecological exam. The medical students are also encouraged to explore the kinds of feelings that they, as physicians, might experience. How should the physician, for example, handle a situation in the best interests of the patient and him or herself if sexually attracted to the patient prior to the examination? Issues such as these are dealt with in these sessions.

Emphasis in these training sessions is put on the importance of involving the patient during the process of the exam itself. An activated patient who is involved in such a way has some sense of control over what is happening to her during her exam. Again, as a teaching associate I am called upon to describe how being "activated" in this way as a patient allows me to feel less victimized during the gynecological exam.

Part of this initial discussion focuses on empathy. To learn to empathize with female patients, all the students are required to disrobe, drape, and get into the lithotomy position—or into the stirrups, as it is commonly called. Through this first-hand experience, medical students can vividly relate to the feelings of vulnerability shared by their female patients as they lie naked, legs suspended, waiting to be examined—covered only by a thin piece of paper that fails to intercept the cool flow of air over one's usually concealed private anatomy.

After these preliminary training sessions, my difficult work begins. I find that my anxiety soon disappears as I get actively involved in teaching. The students are much more nervous than I am so that relating to them in a calm and confident way has the effect of putting us both at ease.

The nature of the suggestions that I give during the actual examination stresses technique. I might suggest that a student flatten his or her hand while palpating my abdomen. I might help a student identify that fleeting moment when my ovaries roll past. But I do not emphasize the mechanics, as I know these will improve with practice.

The general feedback I give each student in turn afterward about how well he or she communicated with me and attended to my emotional needs is far more important. I begin by reinforcing those things which I like. This might include confirming that the student maintained eye contact with me and watched my face for non-verbal signals indicating discomfort. Or it might mean commending a student's effective use of firm and reassuring touch. Then, I follow with a suggestion for improvement. This might include suggesting to the student that he or she replace specialized medical jargon with common conversational language that the patient can more easily understand.

Occasionally, my job demands that I be assertive. For example, I had to tell a male student that I was uneasy having his groin against my knee, while having my breast examined—under ordinary circumstances a female patient might interpret this in a sexual way. We were both embarrassed, but he expressed appreciation for telling him this.

Only once did I find it necessary to tell a student about poor attitude. "I am uncomfortable with the way you treated me—as if I were a plastic model," I had to say. Fortunately, this is rare as most students are respectful and caring to the extreme.

I am proud of the student who is able to include me actively and equally as a participant. I keep a mental check-list during the exam of the various ways the student might accomplish this. Does the student remember to offer me a mirror? Does he or she offer it in such a way that is *not* just an off-hand question? ("Do you want a mirror?") But rather in a way so that *I*, as patient, understand that it is important and acceptable to know about my own female anatomy. "Would you like to hold a mirror while I examine your pelvic area? That way I can better explain to you what *I* see, and *you* can see everything for yourself?"

There are other check-offs on my mental list. Does the student offer me the option of having my head raised during the pelvic part of the examination to facilitate communication between us? Does the student actively solicit my verbal input; not just telling and explaining, but questioning and encouraging any questions *I*, as patient, might have regarding my anatomy or sexual functioning?

Finally, I consider certain non-verbal aspects of our communication exchange. I consider the student's attitude. Is it flippant or overbearing in any way? Does the student display appropriate respect and a willingness to share power in the interaction that goes on between us? What clues do I get from facial expression, body position and movement that support my assessment?

By assessing the answers to all these questions, I am able to evaluate how well I was activated as an involved and equal participant during the examination. When done effectively, this process allows me to feel in control—not as a passive bystander whose body is "being done to."

At this point, relating the notion of the activated patient to the idea of wellness begins. By actively engaging female patients in the gynecological exam itself, the physician can play an important role in aiding the female patient in knowing and being comfortable with her body. Not only might this have a spin-off effect of encouraging women to practice self-examination and prevention at home (I am an example of one who only began doing regular self-breast exams since beginning this job even though I had long known the appalling statistics about breast cancer), but it might help overcome those culturally programmed negative feelings that many women still have about their bodies and lead to a greater degree of sexual satisfaction.

At the end of the teaching session, it is my time for reinforcement. The students all express their gratitude. They are relieved that doing a procedure that had worried them has turned into a positive learning experience; they give me credit. I accept their thanks and express my hope that they will use what they have learned here to make the experience of the gynecological exam a better one for their patients.

One of my fears when I took this job was how the students would react when we would meet in public after the training sessions. I knew this was inevitable as I am a student on the same campus in a small city. Contrary to my worries, I have not felt the slightest embarrassment. Rather I sense a mutual respect between us resulting from the difficult task we shared together.

This feeling of mutual respect might not be something peculiar to my own particular experience. Perhaps it is a reflection of this kind of interaction between a patient-oriented physician and an activated, involved patient. It is an interaction that is designed to allow the patient to feel more in control and, in so doing, to enhance her self-esteem.

The positive effect of this interaction for the patient and its contribution to her overall health status should not be minimized. Replacing negative feelings that many women still have regarding their sexual-reproductive anatomy with positive ones can enhance a woman's sense of well-being and personal fulfillment. Satisfying such a psychological health need represents a step on that continuum toward that elusive concept known as high level wellness. Entering this psychological and social health dimension goes beyond the purely physical realm of traditional medical care.

Medical intervention by a physician which attempts to accomplish such a task is a concrete way to lessen the gap between disease prevention and that lofty goal of optimal wellness. It is an intervention mutually rewarding to patient and physician alike.

Bibliography

1. DiMatteo R M, Friedman HS: *Social Psychology and Medicine.* Oelgeschlager, West Germany, Gum and Hain, Publishers, Inc., 1982.
2. Miller G D: The gynecological examination as a learning experience. *Journal of the American College Health Association* 1974; 23(2).

Cadavers, Dolls, and Prostitutes
Medical Pedagogy and the Pelvic Rehearsal
by Terri Kapsalis

My first question, as I suspect yours may be, was, "what *kind* of woman lets four or five novice medical students examine her?"—James G. Blythe, M.D.

Fearing the Unknown

In a paper entitled "The First Pelvic Examination: Helping Students Cope with Their Emotional Responses," printed in the *Journal of Medical Education* in 1979, Julius Buchwald, M.D., a psychiatrist, shares his findings after ten years of conducting seminars with medical students starting their training in OB/GYN. He locates six primary fears associated with a first pelvic examination: (1) "hurting the patient"; (2) "being judged inept"; (3) the "inability to recognize pathology"; (4) "sexual arousal"; (5) "finding the examination unpleasant"; and (6) the "disturbance of the doctor-patient relationship" (when a patient reminded them of somebody they knew, e.g., mother or sister).

Because the pelvic exam produces fear and anxiety in medical students, numerous methods have been used to offer them a pelvic exam "rehearsal." This practice performance is meant to help soothe or disavow student fears while allowing them to practice manual skills. The types of practice performances adopted reveal and pro-

mote specific ideas about female bodies and sexuality held by the medical institution. The use of gynecology teaching associates (GTAS), trained lay women who teach students using their own bodies, is a relatively new addition to pelvic exam pedagogy that will be examined at length. Previous to and contemporaneous with this practice, medical schools have cast a variety of characters as subjects of this pelvic exam rehearsal, including actual patients, cadavers, anesthetized women, prostitutes, and plastic manikins such as "Gynny," "Betsi," and "Eva". The ways medical students have been taught to perform pelvic exams illustrate the predicament of the gynecological scenario, a situation in which a practitioner must, by definition, examine women's genitals in a clinical and necessarily nonsexual manner. The array of pedagogical methods used to teach pelvic exams reveals how the medical institution views female bodies, female sexuality, and the treatment of women.

In pelvic exams, physicians-to-be are confronted with both female genital display and manipulation, two highly charged cultural acts. If students have previously engaged in gazing at or touching female genitals, most likely they have done so as a private sexual act (e.g., male students engaging in heterosexual activities and female students masturbating or engaging in lesbian activities). Occasionally there are male or female students who, for a variety of reasons, have had little or no exposure to naked female bodies, and their fears often revolve around a fear of the "unknown," which in the case of women's genitals takes the form of a particularly stigmatized mystery.

Students seem to find it very difficult to consider female genital display and manipulation in the medical context as entirely separate from sexual acts and their accompanying fears. Buchwald's list of fears makes explicit the perceived connection between a pelvic examination and a sexual act. "A fear of the inability to recognize pathology" also reflects a fear of contracting a sexually transmitted disease, an actual worry expressed by some of Buchwald's student doctors. Likewise, "a fear of sexual arousal" makes explicit the connection between the pelvic exam and various sexual acts. Buchwald notes that both men and women are subject to this fear of sexual arousal. "A fear of being judged inept" signals a kind of "performance anxiety," a feeling common in both inexperienced and experienced clinical and sexual performers. "A fear of the disturbance of the doctor-patient relationship" recognizes the existence of a type of "incest taboo" within the pelvic exam scenario. Buchwald shares anecdotes of students feeling sick or uncomfortable if the patient being examined reminded them of their mother or sister. Buchwald's work deviates from most publications dealing with the topic of medical students and pelvic exams. Largely, any acknowledgment of this precarious relationship between pelvic exams and sex acts is relatively private and informal, taking place in conversations between students, residents, and doctors, sometimes leaking into private patient interactions. For example, as a student in the 1960s, a male physician was told by the male OB/GYN resident in charge, "During your first 70 pelvic exams, the only anatomy you'll feel is your own." Cultural attitudes about women and their bodies are not checked at the hospital door. If women are largely marketed as sexualized objects of the gaze, why should a gynecological scenario necessarily produce different meanings?

Rehearsing Pelvics

Teaching medical practices is the act of constructing medical realities. In other words, the student is continuously learning by lecture and example what is right and acceptable and, conversely, what is wrong and unacceptable in medical practice. The intractability of medical

teaching from medical practice is built into the very title of Foucault's *Birth of the Clinic*. The translator's note recognizes the importance of the choice of the word "clinic": "When Foucault speaks of *la clinique,* he is thinking of both clinical medicine and of the teaching hospital so if one wishes to retain the unity of the concept, one is obliged to use the rather odd-sounding clinic." Medical pedagogy, including textbooks (the focus of the following chapter) and experiential learning, is symbiotic with medical practice; the two work together in the formation, transferal, and perpetuation of medical knowledge. With regard to pelvic exams, this medical knowledge has been acquired in a number of ways.

Many medical students have encountered their first performance of a pelvic exam on an actual patient. Oftentimes a group of students on rounds would repeat pelvic exams one after another on a chosen patient while the attending physician watched. If we consider that the pelvic exam is often sexualized by novice practitioners, this pedagogical situation resembles a "gang rape." Many times there is little communication with the woman being examined, nor is her explicit consent necessarily requested. Due to the intimidation of the medical institution, a woman may not resist repeated examination, even if she is adamantly against the use of her body for pedagogical purposes. This actual patient situation is one that Buchwald locates as anxiety provoking for the medical student (he fails to mention the anxiety this may cause the woman being examined). This situation adds to what Buchwald refers to as the student's "fear of being judged inept": "a frequent remark was, 'if the resident sees the way I'm going about it, he'll think I'm stupid.' In some respects what began to evolve was the image of the experienced, wise, worldly, and sexually competent adult (the resident or attending physician) sneering at the floundering explorations of an adolescent (the medical student) who is striving to become a 'man.'" Buchwald's reading of this situation is gendered inasmuch as he compares the pelvic exam to an adolescent male rite of passage. This gendered reading is telling. The medical apparatus, particularly this 1970s version, incorporates specifically gendered male positions of physician and medical student. Even though there are increasing numbers of women medical students, physicians, and medical educators, the structures of this apparatus, specifically the structures of medical pedagogy, are in many instances unchanged or slow in changing and require a female medical student to fit into this masculinized subject position. Her relationship to this ascribed subject position, particularly as a medical student, may be uncomfortable, as she may be split between identifying with the woman pelvic patient (as she herself has most likely undergone such exams) and with her newly forming role as masculinized spectator. As a medical educator, I frequently witness such a split in female medical students. As Laura Mulvey describes, "trans-sex identification is a *habit* that very easily becomes *second nature.* However, this Nature does not sit easily and shifts restlessly in its borrowed transvestite clothes." Although Mulvey is discussing female cinematic spectatorship, her words are applicable to female medical spectatorship as well. While the anxieties located and described by Buchwald as very "male" in nature may be the very same anxieties experienced by a female medical student, these anxieties take on different twists and meanings with female physicians-in-training.

Other than the attending physician, one person within the pelvic equation who might also judge the student as inept or whose presence might distract the student from performing a proper first exam and therefore cause the student anxiety, is the patient herself. Cadavers, anesthetized women, and anthropomorphic pelvic models like the plastic manikins "Gynny," "Betsi," and "Eva" are pelvic exam subjects who, for a variety of reasons, are rendered absent and therefore cannot talk back or have an opinion about the medical student's performance. These female models alleviate anxiety regarding inappropriate patient performance since they cannot possibly act out. The pedagogical use of these models may also have been developed in order to avert other student fears. If the woman's body is anesthetized, dead, or replaced altogether by a plastic model certainly there can be no fear of causing her pain. However, this logic is questionable in the case of the anesthetized patient: How might repeated pelvic exams under anesthetic affect how a woman "feels" both psychologically and physically when she wakens?

More importantly, the legality of this practice is extremely questionable. How many women would actually consent to this practice? Many women are anxious at the thought of a single pelvic exam, let alone multiple exams. Furthermore, the fear of a pelvic exam is often associated with feeling vulnerable and out of control; under anesthetic, a woman is particularly vulnerable and out of control. And yet teaching medical students how to do pelvic exams on anesthetized women appears to be widely practiced, although public discussion of this method outside (and inside) the medical community is relatively scarce. At a 1979 conference sponsored by the Women's Medical Associations of New York City and State, New Jersey, and Connecticut held at Cornell University Medical College, this issue was discussed and found its way into the *New York Times,* where the conference recommendation was quoted: "If examined in the operating room, patients must be told prior to anesthesia that they will be examined by the members of the

operating team, including the medical student." Decades later this recommendation is often unheeded. For example, a surgical nurse I interviewed provided a common scenario: "While doing an exam on a woman who is sedated for a urological procedure, a physician may discover that she has a prolapsed uterus. The student or students observing the procedure will then be invited to perform a bi-manual exam on the woman [inserting two fingers in her vagina while pressing on her abdomen] in order to feel her uterus." I have overheard physicians at a prestigious Chicago medical school encouraging students to "get in surgery as much as possible to get pelvic exam practice." The assumption is that students will not be intimidated by an unconscious woman and that the patient will, in addition, have relaxed abdominal muscles, thus permitting easy palpation of her ovaries and uterus. Many physicians have not heard about such "practicing" and are outraged at the suggestion, maintaining that this is medically sanctioned sexual assault. Some physicians who are aware of the practice dodge the questionable issues, maintaining that for some students it is the only way they will learn.

But what *are* students learning in this scenario? By using anesthetized women, cadavers, or plastic models as pelvic exam subjects students are being taught that a model patient (or patient model) is one who is essentially unconscious or backstage to the performance of the pelvic exam; she should be numb to the exam, providing no feedback and offering no opinions. In the tradition of Sims's experiments, passive and powerless female patients are considered ideal "participants" in the learning process. In addition, students practicing on essentially silent and lifeless models are learning that the manual skills associated with completing a pelvic exam are more important than the fundamental skills needed to interact with the patient—skills that ideally would help the patient relax and participate in the exam.

Perhaps these rehearsal methods are used under the assumption that an anesthetized, dead, or plastic model is unerotic and will thus relieve students of Buchwald's fear #4, "a fear of sexual arousal." And yet the rendering of the object of manipulation or the gaze as passive simply heightens the power differential between examiner and examined that can in effect tap into an altogether different system of erotics. Necrophilia may be coded into a pelvic examination on a cadaver. Similarly, there have been noted cases of sexual abuse when patients are under anesthetic. Likewise, the anthropomorphically named pelvic manikins "Gynny," "Betsi," and "Eva," with their custom orifices for medical penetration, could be recognized as the medical correlates to inflatable sex dolls.

In the late 1970s, numerous medical pedagogues were reexamining what one physician referred to as "the time-honored methods" of pelvic exam pedagogy: students examining anesthetized women, conscious patients, cadavers, or plastic models. The problems with these methods were discussed in a number of articles. The authors of the 1977 article "Professional Patients: An Improved Method of Teaching Breast and Pelvic Examination" in the *Journal of Reproductive Medicine* found that training medical students on actual patients "has many disadvantages, including infringement of patients' rights, inadequate feedback and moral and ethical concerns. Another approach that is widely used is the anesthetized preoperative patient. Again, problems include informed consent, increased cost and/or risk and lack of an interpersonal exchange. The introduction of the 'Gynny' and 'Betsi' models has been an attempt at improvement, but not without drawbacks, which include a lack of personal communication, unreal exposure and difficulty with 'live' correlation." Where was the medical community to find these living models? Some went to what must have seemed a very natural source. In the early 1970s a number of schools, including the University of Washington Medical School and the University of Oklahoma Physician's Associate Program, hired prostitutes to serve as "patient simulators." What other women would accept payment for spreading their legs? Logically, these educators felt that a prostitute would be the most fitting *kind* of woman for the job. In a sense, the patriarchal medical establishment took the position of a rich uncle, paying for his nephew, the medical student, to have his first sexual experience with a prostitute. This gendered suggestion assumes that female medical students are structurally positioned as masculinized "nephew" subjects as well.

Although lip service has been paid to the supposed importance of desexualizing the pelvic patient, in choosing prostitute patient models, medical educators inadvertently situated the exam as a sexualized act. They must have thought that only a prostitute would voluntarily submit to exams repeatedly and for nondiagnostic purposes. Or perhaps the underlying assumption was that a lady *pays* to get examined whereas a whore *gets paid* for the same exam. It may have also been assumed that prostitutes are more accustomed to and have a higher tolerance for vaginal pain than other women and would thus be more fitting practice models for novice students. In choosing to hire prostitutes as patients the boundaries of pornographic and medical practice were collapsed. Within this scenario of a hired prostitute, the student physician was put in the position of a medicalized lover or "john." Certainly Buchwald's fear #3, "a fear of sexual arousal," was confirmed and even encouraged by hiring prostitutes. Buchwald notes that certain students "appeared to project their anxiety by asking, 'what

should I do if the patient starts responding sexually?'" By hiring prostitutes as pelvic patients, the medical establishment not only enforced the trope of the "seductive patient," but also paid for it. "Playing doctor" in this pelvic rehearsal cast with patient prostitutes threatened to translate the pelvic exam into an act of sexualized penetration and bodily consumption.

In many cases when prostitutes were hired, the medical student was led to believe that the woman being examined was a clinical outpatient rather than a prostitute. Thus the prostitute still had a relatively passive position in the training of medical students. In order to properly perform her role as clinical outpatient, she could offer the student little feedback. In addition, the working logic of the medical educators remained relatively opaque inasmuch as the student was not directly learning about the medical establishment's opinion of model patients. And yet these attitudes undoubtedly found their way into medical practice. Years later, students are still told by certain unaware medical faculty that GTAS are prostitutes. Today certain faculty still conclude that no other *kind* of woman would submit her body to multiple exams in exchange for a fee. This points to the importance of understanding the recent history of pelvic pedagogy. Those physicians trained in the 1970s are the same physicians practicing and educating today.

Some physicians found fault with the use of prostitutes as pelvic models. According to the authors of "Utilization of Simulated Patients to Teach the Routine Pelvic Examination," "the employment of prostitute patient simulators is not satisfactory. The prostitutes employed by the PA (Physician's Associate) program were not articulate enough to provide the quality of instructive feedback necessary for an optimal educational experience. Their employment was costly at $25 per hour, and that expense prohibited their extensive and long-term use. Also, and more importantly prostitutes had abnormal findings on examination prior to their utilization." Pathology was not desirable in these model patients: in the pelvic rehearsal, students were not to be distracted by abnormal findings. Rather, the patient simulator needed to be standardized as normal like the plastic model. In addition, the prostitute was expensive. She received market value for her bodily consumption, unlike the income-free corpse, indebted actual patient, and the cut-rate graduate students that the authors of the article hired at $10 per hour. And although prostitutes did offer some student critique (comments such as "poor introduction," "too serious," "too rough," and "forgot to warm the speculum") their language skills were not medically acceptable. What the medical establishment needed was a model who could engage in medicalese, was more cost efficient, and had normal, healthy anatomy. The GTA would be the answer.

The GTA Program

In 1968 at the University of Iowa Medical School's Department of Obstetrics and Gynecology, Dr. Robert Kretzschmar instituted a new method for teaching junior medical students how to perform the pelvic exam. For the pelvic model he used a "simulated patient," first defined in the medical literature as a "person who has been trained to completely simulate a patient or any aspect of a patient's illness depending upon the educational need." Many simulated patients were actresses and actors hired by the medical establishment to realistically portray a patient. Their critical feedback was not traditionally requested. They simply served as a warm body for the practicing student. This stage of Kretzschmar's program was not dissimilar to the other programs that hired prostitutes. Initially, Kretzschmar adhered to this simulated patient model. He hired a nurse for the role of patient. She agreed to repeated exams by medical students; "however, it was necessary to compromise open communication with her, as she was draped at her request in such a way as to remain anonymous." The curtain rose but the nurse's knowledge, thoughts, feelings, and face remained backstage. All that was revealed was the object of the exam: the woman's pelvic region. The logic behind draping the simulated patient presumed that if "only a whore gets paid" for a nondiagnostic exam, perhaps the nurse could avoid whore status by becoming faceless and silent.

In many gynecology textbooks, as will be examined in the following chapter, a similar logic prevails. Photographs picturing women are cropped so that faces are not shown or bands are placed across eyes to maintain the model's anonymity. If the woman's face and eyes are pictured, the photo could enter the realm of pornography; the woman imaged cannot be soliciting or meeting the medical practitioner's gaze, a potentially sexualized act. If the nurse who served as simulated patient was draped to maintain her anonymity she was in effect attempting to desexualize her body for the medical gaze. But is this an effective strategy for the desexualization of the exam? Is a faceless, vulnerable female body less erotic? In addition, although this professional patient model rehearsal did save actual patients from the task of performing the role of pelvic model, it did little to encourage communication between student and patient. Maintaining such anonymity taught the students that it was acceptable and even preferable for them to ignore the woman backstage behind the drape. They were also shown that a modest woman, unlike a prostitute, would need to disassociate her face from her body. And therefore, a modest woman preferred to be treated as though she were anonymous and invisible.

In 1972, Kretzschmar instituted a different program. The new simulated patient, now named the gynecology teaching associate (GTA), would serve as both patient and instructor, stressing the importance of communication skills in addition to teaching the manual skills required to perform a proper pelvic exam. Unlike the nurse clinician who was first hired as a simulated patient in 1968, the GTA would actively teach and offer feedback to medical students, forsaking any anonymity through draping. The GTAS first hired by Kretzschmar were women who were working on or had received advanced degrees in the behavioral sciences but who had no formal medical training. The women had normal, healthy anatomy and were willing to undergo multiple exams. They then received elaborate instruction in female anatomy and physiology, pelvic and breast examination, self-breast-examination and abdominal examination, with an emphasis on normal anatomy. They worked in pairs, one GTA serving as "patient" TA, one as "instructor" TA. They were assigned a small group of medical students and conducted the educational session in an exam room. The "patient" TA received the exam, role-playing as patient and co-instructor, while the "instructor" TA remained alongside the students, helping and instructing them during the exam. After receiving two exams the "patient" TA changed from gown to street clothes and became "instructor" TA, and the "instructor" TA changed from street clothes to gown to become the "patient" TA. The teaching session was then repeated with a new group of medical students, thus assuring that one TA of each pair would not receive all the exams.

Kretzschmar's GTA model provided a radically new way of teaching medical students how to do pelvic and breast exams. No longer was the simulated patient a teaching tool; now she was both teacher and patient. The women's movement undoubtedly influenced this model. In the 1960s and '70s women were demanding better health care and some took matters into their own hands by establishing self-help groups and feminist clinics. In fact, many early GTAS were directly associated with these groups and clinics and believed their new position within the medical establishment as GTA could allow them to bring their alternative knowledge to the heart of the beast.

Kretzschmar received a variety of critical responses from the medical community for his new GTA program. Some were positive, applauding him for his innovative method and his success in avoiding a "men's club" attitude by hiring women as teachers. Some, however, were skeptical at best. They were particularly cautious regarding the GTAS' motives for participating in such a perverse endeavor. The epigraph to this chapter—"What *kind* of woman lets four or five novice medical students examine her?"—was a question asked by many physicians, according to Kretzschmar. Some human subjects committee members who reviewed the GTA concept "felt that women who were willing to participate must be motivated by one or more of several questionable needs, such as desperate financial circumstances (in which case exploiting their need would be unethical). Others fear the women would be exhibitionists or that they would use the pelvic exam to serve some perverse internal sexual gratification (in which case portraying them as normal to medical students would be irresponsible)." Once again, the pelvic exam was compared to a sexual act by the medical establishment. Cultural fears regarding female sexuality and its perversions surface in these objections to the GTA program. Only a nymphomaniac would seek out multiple exams, enjoying repeated penetration with speculums and fingers. Also, poor women might lower themselves to such embodied work out of desperation, thereby aligning the GTA with the prostitute in an explanatory narrative. Furthermore, the committee questioned the psychological stability of the GTA, with the assumption "that women who are emotionally unstable might be attracted to the program, or that undergoing repeated examination might be psychologically harmful." These human subject committee members reveal their nineteenth-century ideas about (white) women: frail female psychological health and sexual health are seen as mutually dependent and delicate partners. If their equilibrium is tipped by the "pleasure" or pain incurred by the excessive sexualized act of multiple pelvic exams, then who knows what horrors will take place.

Unquestionably, teaching female genital display and manipulation has been the cause of a great deal of anxiety. These fears are much more reflective of the medical institution's constructions of the female psyche and female sexuality than of any actual threat to women posed by the role of GTA. One reason the role of GTA could seem threatening to these critics is that they were faced with a new and potentially powerful position for women in the predominantly male medical establishment. Their attempt at pathologizing the GTA could have been propelled by a desire to maintain the status quo: that *normal* women are passive, quiet, disembodied recipients of a hopelessly unpleasant but necessary pelvic exam. For them, perhaps this was the least threatening alternative.

Despite its early critics, Kretzschmar's model has become the pedagogical norm in the vast majority of institutions. Over 90 percent of North American medical schools employ this instructional method, recognized as "excellent" by the Association of Professors of Gynecology and Obstetrics Undergraduate Education Committee. Many GTA programs throughout the country maintain the same basic form as Kretzschmar's 1972 incarnation, though there is some variation. For example,

some schools have GTAS working alone, rather than in pairs; a few schools still hire the more passive live pelvic model or "professional patient" to be used in conjunction with an instructing physician. The use of pelvic manikins, anesthetized women, cadavers, and actual patients continues to supplement some student learning.

Beginning in 1988, I was employed as a GTA by the University of Illinois at Chicago (UIC) medical school. Periodically, I also taught at two other Chicago-area medical schools and in one physician's assistant program. Excepting one institution, all my teaching experiences have followed Kretzschmar's GTA model. For the institution that had not adopted Kretzschmar's model, I worked as a "professional patient." A physician or nurse-midwife served as instructor, and I was hired primarily to model the exam for three students and the instructor. Whenever a clinician-instructor was unable to attend, I volunteered to work as both instructor and model, adopting a variation of Kretzschmar's model.

In discussing the GTA, I will collapse the roles of instructor and patient GTA into a single role. While this is reductive of the complexity of the partner relationship assumed by the instructor and patient GTAS, it may help clarify their common mission. And indeed many schools have collapsed the roles of the two GTAS into a single GTA who is paired with three or four students. After years of teaching, I find this to be a better model. It is impossible for students to position the instructor as silent patient if she is the only educator in the room. When there is a single teacher who also serves as "patient" students are faced with the jarring experience of examining a woman who knows more about gynecological exams than they do.

The Teaching Session

The students enter the exam room, where the GTA wears a patient gown. She is both their teacher and the object of their examination. The GTA explains the purpose of the teaching session. She is a healthy woman with normal anatomy who is there to help the students learn how to perform a proper breast and pelvic exam. Medical students, however, have been indoctrinated into a system that privileges pathology. They have learned that what is normal and healthy is not as interesting as what is abnormal and unhealthy. Some students seem disappointed when they are told that the GTA session is one part of their medical education in which they will not be presented with pathology.

The GTA explains that the patient, performed by herself, is there for a yearly exam. She has no complaints. Rather, they are there to have the experience of examining a normal, healthy woman and thus should offer the "patient" feedback after each part of the exam, letting her know that "everything appears healthy and normal." The GTA emphasizes that no woman can hear the phrase "healthy and normal" too much. For many medical students "healthy" and "normal" are new additions to their medical script. Often, these second- and third-year medical students admit that the GTA session is the first time they have been encouraged to use these words. In a moment that struck me as simultaneously encouraging and tragicomic, one student, upon hearing me discuss the phrase "healthy and normal," pulled a 3×5 notecard and pen out of his pocket. He then said, "Tell me those words again. I want to write them down so I can remember them." In medical pedagogy, pathology is the norm, and normalcy is often viewed as mundane or unremarkable. For a woman in need of her yearly pap smear, the clinician's preoccupation with pathology can have sad consequences, both adding to the woman's anxiety about the possibility of the clinician finding that something is wrong and leaving her with the feeling that something is wrong regardless of actual clinical findings.

During the GTA session, other aspects of the students' scripts are rewritten and relearned. They are taught to use words that are less sexually connotative or awkward. For example, "I am going to *examine* your breasts now" as opposed to "I'm going to *feel* your breasts now." A number of script adjustments are made: "insert" or "place" the speculum as opposed to "stick in"; "healthy and normal" as opposed to "looks great." Changes are encouraged with regard to tool names: "footrests" as opposed to "stirrups"; "bills" rather than "blades" of the speculum.

When I was working as a "professional patient" with a young white woman physician as instructor, she kept referring to the "blades" of the speculum while teaching the students. I explained to her that many people within the medical community were replacing the term "blades" with "bills" because of the obvious violent connotations of the term, especially given that it refers to that part of the speculum placed inside the woman's body. The physician replied, agitated, "Well, we don't say it to the *patient.*" Her assumption was that words that circulate within the medical community do not affect patient care or physician attitudes toward patients as long as those words do not reach the patient's ears. This is naive and faulty thinking, resistant to change, disabling the idea that language does indeed help structure attitudes and practice.

Furthermore, in that scenario *I* was the patient and the word "blade" was being used to refer to the part of an instrument that was to be placed inside *my* body. My thoughts were largely ignored even though I was

hired to perform the role of patient. For the rest of the session, the physician begrudgingly used the word "bills," looking at me and punching the word each time she used it. Weeks later I worked at the same institution with a young white male physician whose language was considerate and carefully chosen and who continually encouraged my feedback and participation within the session. He consistently referred to the "bills" of the speculum of his own accord. By seeking out a patient's opinion and input within both a teaching situation and an actual exam, the clinician is relinquishing a portion of control and offering the patient more power within the exam scenario. As is evident in these two examples, gender does not necessarily determine a clinician's attitudes toward patients or the patient model.

The GTA offers many tips on how the clinician may help the patient feel more powerful and less frightened during an exam. "Talk before touch" is a technique used in the pelvic exam by which the clinician lets the patient know that she or he is about to examine the patient: with the phrase "You'll feel my hand now," the clinician applies the back of her or his hand to the more neutral space of the insides of a patient's thighs. Since the patient cannot *see* where the clinician's hands are, this technique offers her important information about where and when she will be touched.

Eye contact is another important and often ignored part of the pelvic exam. The GTA reminds the student to maintain eye contact with her throughout most parts of the exam. Many women complain that oftentimes clinicians have spoken at their genitals or breasts rather than to them. Eye contact not only offers the clinician another diagnostic tool, since discomfort and pain are often expressed in a patient's face, but it also makes the patient feel as though she is being treated as a person rather than as fragmented parts. In order to facilitate eye contact, the students are taught to raise the table to a 45-degree angle rather than leaving it flat. This has the added benefit of relaxing the woman's abdominal muscles. Specific draping techniques are taught so that the student-clinician cannot hide in front of the drape, ignoring the parts of the woman that reside backstage behind the curtain.

Given that the medical institution routinely segments and dissects bodies for examination, maintaining eye contact with the patient is often difficult for students. Considering the sexual overtones of this particular exam, many students (and practitioners) find it very difficult to meet their patient's gaze. Likewise, there are patients who will not look into their examiner's eyes due to shame or embarrassment or a desire to be "invisible." While this is always a possibility, the GTA asserts that the practitioner must initiate eye contact even if the patient declines the offer, so that the patient at least has a choice of whether to "look back" at the clinician.

Similarly, the GTA encourages students to continuously communicate with the patient, informing her as to what they are doing, how they are doing it, and why they are doing it. For example, the student must show the woman the speculum, holding it high enough so that she can see it (without aiming it at her like a gun), while explaining, "This is a speculum. I will insert this part, the bills, into your vagina, opening them so that I can see your cervix, the neck of your uterus. I do this so that I can take a pap smear, which is a screening test for cervical cancer." Many women have had dozens of pelvic exams without ever having had the opportunity to see a speculum. More often, they hear the clanking of metal as the speculum is snuck out of its drawer and into their vagina.

Clinicians should not use words that patients will not understand, nor should they patronize patients; rather, they should piggyback medical terms with simpler phrases. In addition, students are taught that women should be given verbal instruction when they need to move or undress. For example, the woman should not be handled like a limp doll as a clinician removes her gown for the breast exam; instead the woman should be asked to remove her own gown. This helps her feel a little more in control of her own body and space. Ideally, the pelvic exam can become an educational session and the patient a partner in her own exam.

Lilla Wallis, M.D., an OB/GYN professor at Cornell University Medical School and a strong advocate of the GTA program, promotes this idea of "the patient as partner in the pelvic exam," and in addition encourages the use of many techniques popular within the women's health movement. Wallis adopts what some institutions might consider radical techniques. For instance, she urges clinicians to offer patients a hand mirror so that they might see what is being done to them. The patient is encouraged to look at her own genitals and not feel as though this were a view limited to the practitioner. Wallis also questions the draping of the patient: "This separates the patient from her own body. It suggests that the genitals are a forbidden part of her body that she should modestly ignore. It also isolates the doctor." Instead, she believes that patients should have the choice of whether to be draped or not. She refers to the use of GTAS as "a quiet revolution" in American medical schools, believing that GTA programs will lead to better, more thoughtful care by physicians.

Is the rehearsal with GTAS enough to change medical attitudes about women, female sexuality, and women's bodies? Can the use of GTAS actually affect these attitudes? While I was working as a "professional patient" or "model" at an esteemed Chicago-

area medical school, an interesting sequence of events happened that pointed out to me the vast difference between teaching students as a GTA and serving as a "model." The physician I was to be working with was delayed at a meeting, so I started working with the four medical students. I stressed patient communication, helping the woman relax, "talk before touch," and educating the woman during the exam. The students were responsive, as the vast majority of students are, understanding my explanations for why these techniques were important and making an effort to adopt them as they made their way through the breast and pelvic exam.

I had finished teaching all four students how to do a breast exam and two students had completed pelvic exams, when the physician, a young white man, rushed in, apologizing for being late. He then proceeded to contradict much of what I had taught the students. I argued my points, but he insisted that many women were not interested in explanations or education but just "wanted it to be over with." He taught students a one-handed technique so that only one hand ever got "dirty," leaving the other hand free. He basically ignored my presence, so much so that at one point I had to dislodge his elbow, which was digging into my thigh as he leaned over, bracing himself on me, to see if my cervix was in view. The two remaining students were visibly more nervous than the students who had already had their turns. They were rushed and forgot "talk before touch" in an attempt to incorporate the shortcuts that the physician had taught them.

At the end of the session, he encouraged the students to get into surgery to examine as much pathology as possible: "I have an 18cm uterus I'll be working on. Come by." I pictured this enlarged uterus alone on a surgical table without it's woman-encasement. He assured the students, "The only way you're going to learn what is normal is to see a lot of pathology." I had emphasized the wide variety of what is normal, how vulvas were all different and that students would need to see a lot of normal anatomy to understand what was not normal. After this physician's intrusion, the lone female medical student in the group kept looking at me at each point the physician contradicted me. She smiled at me empathetically, understanding the severity of the emotional and political sabotage I must have been feeling as both an educator and a naked woman "patient." Before the students left, three of the four shook my hand, genuinely thanking me for helping them. The one student who had been resistant to some of the techniques I had taught them was more suspicious. He said to me sternly, "Can I ask you, what are your motivations for doing this?"

The View from the Table

Implicit in the role of the GTA is a fundamental contradiction. On the one hand, she is an educator, more knowledgeable than medical students about pelvic and breast exams although she holds no medical degree. In this sense she is in a position of power, disseminating various truths about the female body and its examination. On the other hand, the GTA is bound to a traditionally vulnerable and powerless lithotomy position: lying on her back, heels in footrests. Oftentimes, her body is viewed as the true learning tool, with her words taking a back seat to this "hands-on" educational experience. In an interview, one GTA expressed her frustration: "Sometimes I feel like it's strange being nice, being like an airline hostess of the body. For example [she points two fingers as stewardesses do at cabin exits], 'Now we're coming to the *mons pubis.*' You have to be nice. I've seen some GTAs who were strong and businesslike about it, and I don't feel comfortable doing that but it's a strain having to be nice." This is a beautiful metaphor for describing the GTA's predicament: She is there to make medical students comfortable as they journey across the female body. Comparing the GTA to an airline hostess highlights the pink-collar service role she performs: she is working for the medical school in a position that only women can fill and she is there to make the students feel less apprehensive and more knowledgeable. The fact that she needs to be "nice" while presenting her own body points to one of the performative aspects of the GTA's role as educator. Like the stewardess, the GTA is costumed with a smile, a well-defined script, and a uniform.

In her book *The Managed Heart: Commercialization of Human Feeling,* Arlie Russell Hochschild connects Marx's factory worker to the flight attendant; both must "mentally detach themselves—the factory worker from his own body and physical labor, and the flight attendant from her own feelings and emotional labor." The case of the GTA becomes an interesting blend of these two types of alienation. She is like the flight attendant in that she manages her own feelings, what the GTA above calls "being nice." She must learn how to deal with the occasional hostile or overtly sexual medical student customer. She is there to make the student's trip through the female body comfortable, safe, and enjoyable. But it is her own body, not the meal tray or the fuselage of the airplane, that she is presenting to the paying customer. In this sense, the GTA is like Marx's factory laborer who uses his own body. She is getting paid for her body's use-value in the production of a trained medical student.

Structurally, with regard to physical labor and the management of feelings, the GTA resides in a position similar to that of a prostitute. Both GTAs and prostitutes sell the use of their body for what may be loosely termed "educational purposes." Both must manage their feelings, acting the part of willing recipient to probing instruments. Medical school history aside, GTAs and prostitutes have a good deal in common. This is perhaps why numerous GTAs have remarked on their husband's or partner's discomfort with their work. Certainly not all GTAs have partners who consider their teaching to be a sexual act and so object to or are threatened by it. But partner discontent is not uncommon. One GTA explains, "My boyfriend had problems with my teaching when I first moved in with him. It didn't bother him before I was living with him. I moved in only a couple of months before we got married and then he started voicing his complaints. . . I think they [significant others] are afraid it's sexual and I think the students are afraid it's sexual. They're afraid about how they're going to react, whether they're going to be aroused, but it's so clinical." Another GTA present at this interview said she had a similar problem in that her boyfriend was "concerned" and "uneasy": "I said to him if you're going to give me $150 to sit with you or have sex with you or whatever, fine, otherwise I'm going to make my money."

GTAs' partners are not the only ones who have been distressed by the GTA role. Some early women's health activists expressed a different kind of uneasiness as they quickly realized the pink-collar nature of the job. When the GTA program was first starting in the 1970S, these feminist health activists participating in the project sensed that they were still expected to mimic a patriarchal medical performance, employing language, techniques, and attitudes that reinforced the established power differential between pelvic exam clinician and female patient. These groups felt that working for a medical school did not allow them enough autonomy to teach what were, for them, important exam techniques. They believed that change within the medical establishment was virtually impossible and encouraged women not to participate in pelvic teaching within medical schools. Of these GTAs, some simply discontinued their work with medical students. Others continued teaching self-motivated medical students who would voluntarily visit feminist self-help clinics for continuing education. These feminist teachers regarded this new experience as highly valuable. As one activist notes: "The rapport experienced by the program participants and the [feminist teaching] nurses had been astounding . . . The result was an exploration with students of such topics as sexuality, abortion, contraception and ambivalent feelings regarding their roles." After refusing the medical institution's version of a proper pelvic exam rehearsal, these health activists composed their own.

In his article about medical students' six fears of pelvic exams, Buchwald accepted student fears without either questioning why young physicians-to-be would have such fears or searching for the cultural attitudes underlying them. Indeed, he might have been employing a Freudian psychoanalytic model that would entirely justify such fears: faced with the abject, castrated vulva, medical students *would* be terrified by the exam. These feminist teachers who rejected the GTA program, however, confronted and questioned student fears, realizing the importance of helping these future caregivers shed deep anxieties and ambivalences regarding female bodies. For years, medical pedagogues blatantly sidestepped these issues by employing teaching methods that would simply ignore or Band-aid student fears: hiring prostitutes would confirm student ideas regarding promiscuous female sexuality and its relationship to the pelvic exam; the use of plastic manikins would soothe student fears of touching real female genitals; while the use of anesthetized women and cadavers would present an unconscious "model" patient. Only with the use of GTAS have medical schools attempted to incorporate women patients' thoughts, feelings, and ideas into pelvic exam teaching. And yet, as these feminist teachers pointed out decades ago and as my experiences have occasionally confirmed, it may be impossible to educate students properly within the medical institution given unacknowledged cultural attitudes about female bodies and female sexuality.

• • •

The pelvic exam is in itself a pedagogical scenario. The woman receiving the exam, despite the political or philosophical orientation of the clinician, is taught attitudes about female bodies. In this respect, the physician is as much a pedagogue as a healer, if the two roles can be separated. In teaching medical students, one is therefore teaching teachers, transferring knowledge, methods, and attitudes to those practitioners who will in turn conduct private tutorials with individual women who seek their care. Thus the methods used to teach medical students how to do pelvic exams significantly structure how these physicians-to-be will educate their future patients. The various ways medical students have been taught to do pelvic exams are intimately related to the medical institution's attitudes toward women and in turn structure how future practitioners perceive and treat their women patients.

The use of GTAS alters the normal pelvic scenario to some degree. Here the "doctor" is being educated by the "patient," a potentially powerful role for the GTA. As an educator, she may critique the student from the patient's perspective (e.g., "Use less pressure," "you're not palpating the ovary there"). One would think that the medical student would not argue with the woman who is experiencing the exam. And yet, because the GTA is not a physician, the student is sometimes skeptical of her expertise, doubting her advice even if it is based on her bodily experience. The very fact that her experience is bodily may serve to deny the importance of her role. Her embodiment of the exam makes her a curious and suspect educator in the eyes of many since she is being *paid* for the use of her body in addition to her teaching skills. Her role continually elicits questions about what *kind* of woman she must be to undergo multiple exams.

In the GTA's educational performance there is no hypothetical signified, no abstract female body; rather the GTA is a fleshy referent with her own shape, anatomical variation, and secretions. At the site of the GTA, medicine, pornography, and prostitution mingle, highlighting medical attitudes regarding female sexuality, vulvar display, and genital manipulation. The teaching session may be a "representation" of a "real" exam, but for the GTA, as well as the medical student, it is simultaneously representation *and* practice.

It is curious, but not surprising, that the medical institution has focused so much attention on the GTA's role. Instead of focusing on what *kind* of woman would allow multiple exams to be performed on her, physicians might be more justified in asking how the medical establishment perceives the proper pelvic model or model patient. Or to turn the question back onto the medical institution itself, one might ask what *kind* of man or woman will *give* multiple exams. Unless there is a continued investigation of the medical structures that construct and reflect attitudes about female bodies and sexuality, the answer to this question might indeed be something to really fear.

References

A list of references is available in the original source.

Women's Health Events of the 20th Century

by Office on Women's Health, U.S. Department of Health and Human Services

1906– The Food and Drug Administration Established: This agency is established by the Pure Food and Drug Act to regulate the safety of foods and medicines, giving women new support in protecting themselves and their families.

1908– Protecting Working Women and Children: The Supreme Court upholds the right of states to ensure the safety of working women and children who had not been included in labor union protection in *Muller vs. Oregon.*

1912– The Federal Children's Bureau Established: One of its first tasks was to write and distribute two public health pamphlets directed at

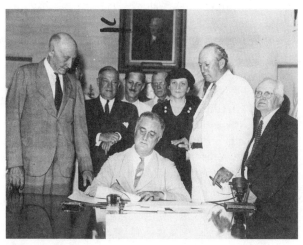

President Franklin D. Roosevelt signing the Social Security Act of 1935. Also shown from left to right: Representative Robert Doughton (D-NC); Senator Robert Wagner (D-NY); Representative John Dingell, Sr. (D-MI); Unknown man in bowtie; Secretary of Labor Frances Perkins; Senator Pat Harrison (D-MS); Congressman David L. Lewis (D-MD). Photo courtesy of the Library of Congress.

women consumers: Prenatal Care and Infant Care. By century's end, women were able to access health information through thousands of self-help books, Internet web sites, and government publications.

1913– The First Public Discussion of the Word Cancer: A Ladies' Home Journal magazine article entitled "What Can We Do About Cancer?" was published. The American Society for the Control of Cancer was formed that same year.

1915– Radical Mastectomy Proven Effective for Breast Cancer: This disfiguring surgery, developed by Dr. William Halstead, became the standard of care for women with breast cancer.

1916– First Birth Control Clinic Opens: Margaret Sanger and her sister Ethyl Byrne opened a birth control clinic in Brooklyn, New York. The authorities shut it down ten days later under the Comstock Law. In those ten days, nearly 500 women came in for help and advice on contraception. The Comstock Law, passed in 1873, defined information on birth control and contraception as obscene and outlawed its distribution.

1921– The Sheppard-Towner Act: This law provided federal funding (with matching state funds) to reduce maternal and infant mortality. It was fiercely opposed by the American Medical Association (AMA), and some members of Congress as too socialistic. Some of the influential pediatricians in the AMA who were in favor of the bill broke off from the organization and created the American Academy of Pediatrics. The law was allowed to lapse in 1929.

1929– Selling Mrs. Consumer Published: This popular book was written by a female home economics and marketing expert, and highlighted women's roles as the primary household consumers.

1933– Sodium Pentathol Introduced as Anesthesia for Childbirth: This drug replaced opiates and other sedatives that had a longer lasting effect on mother and baby, and meant that more women could have pain relief during labor and delivery.

Source: *A Century of Women's Health: 1900–2000* by the U.S. Department of Health and Human Services, Office on Women's Health, 2002.

1935– Title V of the Social Security Act: This maternal and child health legislation authorized grants-in-aid to states to fund maternal, infant, and child health programs, including services for crippled children.

1935– Cure Found for "Childbed" Fever: Sulfanomides were introduced as a cure for puerperal fever, contracted from unsterile conditions during childbirth and a leading cause of maternal death.

1936– *U.S. vs. One Package:* Margaret Sanger and the National Committee for Federal Legislation on Birth Control won a judicial decision (*U.S. vs. One Package*) that exempted doctors from the Comstock Law restrictions on dissemination of contraceptive information.

1938– The Food and Drug Administration's Authority Broadened: The agency was given authority to regulate cosmetics and medical devices.

1942– Planned Parenthood Named: The American Birth Control League changed its name to Planned Parenthood, over the objections of its founder, Margaret Sanger. Planned Parenthood was believed to be a more acceptable name to mainstream America.

1943– Emergency Maternity and Infant Care Program: This program provided free and complete maternity care to the wives and infants of men serving in the four lowest grades of the military during World War II. The program ended in 1949.

1950– The American Cancer Society Begins Promotion of Breast Self-exam: There is still no scientific proof by century's end, that it actually improves breast cancer survival rate.

1953– The Kinsey Report Published: Sexual Behavior in the Human Female was published by researcher Michael Kinsey, as a companion to the 1948 Report, Sexual Behavior in the Human Male. More than 5,500 interviews with women showed that many enjoyed having a sexual life. This provoked widespread controversy, and altered the perception of women's sexuality. Later analyses have questioned much of Kinsey's methodology.

1956– La Leche League Formed: This group was started by seven mothers to promote breastfeeding after it fell out of fashion in the 1920s. It was not until the year 2001 that the U.S. Department of Health and Human Services released its first policy promoting breastfeeding, calling it the best source of infant nutrition.

1956– Dependents Medical Care Act: This program provided Government-sponsored health insurance (CHAMPUS) for the dependents of members of the Armed Forces.

1959– The Barbie Doll Created: This was the first popular doll to be shaped like a woman, with an impossible-to-attain figure. Little girls everywhere loved the doll, but critics claimed it encouraged girls to adopt unhealthy habits to stay unreasonably thin, and set an unrealistic standard of beauty for decades to come.

1960– The FDA Approves the Birth Control Pill: The Pill gave women unprecedented reproductive freedom. The controversy over its approval eventually led to the first package insert that explained the risks and benefits of a medication. By the year 2000, it was still one of the most popular forms of birth control.

1961– Worldwide Alert on Thalidomide: The efforts of a woman scientist, Frances Kelsey, M.D., Ph.D., led the FDA not to approve thalidomide for use in the U.S., saving countless numbers of babies from the severe deformities seen among babies in Europe. Worldwide alarm led to legislation in the United States in 1962 that gave the FDA new authority to require that drugs must be shown to be effective prior to approval, and also required manufacturers to report unexpected harm (adverse events).

1965– Birth Control Made Legal for Married Couples: In *Griswold vs. Connecticut,* the Supreme Court overturned one of the last state laws to prohibit the use of contraceptives by married couples.

1965– Medicaid and Medicare: Medicare was created as a national program to provide federal coverage for health services to individuals aged 65 and over, a population that was disproportionately female. Medicaid was passed as part of President Lyndon Johnson's War on Poverty and provided medical assistance to poor families with dependent children, low-income elderly, the blind, and people with disabilities. It was designed to be administered by each of the 50 states.

1965– Family Planning Funds: As part of the War on Poverty, the Office of Economic Opportunity made available federal funding for family planning for low-income women.

1970– Our Bodies, Ourselves Published: This popular book was produced by the Boston Women's Health Book Collective. It was written by women (not medically trained) to teach other women about their bodies, and it encouraged them to be critical health care consumers.

1970– Medical Schools Sued for Gender Discrimination: In 1965, only 7 percent of medical students in the U.S. were women. The Women's Equity Action League sued most medical schools in the nation to correct this inequity. By the late 1990's nearly half of medical students were women. Still, by the end of the century, only eight U.S. medical schools were headed by women deans.

1970– Title X Family Planning Funding: This law established a federally-funded program nationwide to provide family planning services to low-income women.

1971– The National Cancer Act Passed: This law, signed by President Richard M. Nixon, greatly expanded funding for cancer research.

1972– Title IX Revolutionizes Athletics for Women: Title IX of the Education Amendments of 1972 prohibited sex discrimination in all educational programs receiving federal funding.

1973– *Roe vs. Wade:* While a woman's right to abortion is not explicitly found in the Constitution, and while the practice of abortion was opposed by many Americans, the U.S. Supreme Court held in this landmark case that limiting a woman's right to terminate her pregnancy violated the Due Process clause of the 14th Amendment.

1974– The Food and Drug Administration Outlaws the Dalkon Shield: This brand of intrauterine device was ruled to be unsafe due to increased complications with pregnancies and a higher risk of pelvic inflammatory disease.

1975– National Women's Health Network: This organization was founded to give women a voice in the U.S. health care system.

1976– Hyde Amendment: This amendment banned the use of Medicaid funds for abortion services, unless a woman's life was in danger. The law was broadened in 1994 to allow Medicaid coverage for abortion in cases of rape or incest.

1978– Pregnancy Discrimination Act: This law prohibited sex discrimination in employment on the basis of pregnancy, childbirth, or related medical conditions.

1979– Patricia Harris, an African American, is appointed as the first female Secretary of Health, Education, and Welfare: Later that year, Congress established a separate Department of Education and Harris' department became the Department of Health and Human Services. Harris was a professor at Howard University Law School and a business-woman before her appointment.

1980– Surgeon General's Report on Women and Smoking: This report documented the growing number of women smokers and warned that if the trend was not reversed, smoking related diseases in women will reach epidemic proportions. By century's end, the prophecy was realized. A new Surgeon General's Report on Women and Smoking, written in 2000, revealed that since the release of the 1980 report, three million women had died prematurely from smoking related illnesses.

1981– National Black Women's Health Project: This organization was established by Byllye Avery to improve the health of Black women by providing wellness education and services, health information, and advocacy.

1981– Maternal and Child Health Services Block Grants: This law consolidated programs for maternal, infant, child, and adolescent health at the State level, and transferred funding directly to the states in a block-grant format.

1983– The Public Health Service's Task Force on Women's Health Established: This task force signified a new level of federal commitment to women's health issues.

1983– The Komen Race for the Cure is Established: The Race for the Cure was established by Susan Goodman Komen to raise money for breast cancer research, education, screening and treatment programs. The five-kilometer race began as a single event in Dallas, Texas, and by century's end became a series of more than a hundred races in the U.S. and around the world, with 69,000 runners and walkers, raising three million dollars annually.

1983– Margaret Mary Heckler is named the first Secretary of the Department of Health and Human Services: She served 16 years in the United States House of Representatives as a Republican from Massachusetts. As Secretary, Heckler introduced a system of set rates for Medicare payments to hospitals. She also helped to win Congressional approval of a law that helped ensure payment of court-ordered child support.

1985– Lumpectomy Declared As Effective Breast Cancer Treatment: Studies were released that showed lump removal combined with radiation therapy was as effective a treatment as mastectomy for many breast cancers.

1986– New Policy on Women's Health Research: The National Institutes of Health established a policy to increase participation in women's health research, but in 1990, an Institute of Medicine Report said NIH was not moving quickly enough to implement this policy.

1987– Lung Cancer surpasses breast cancer as the leading cause of cancer death in women.

1989– Women's Health Equity Act: This law, introduced by the Congressional Caucus for Women's Issues, called for an increased focus on women's health through research, services, and prevention activities.

1990– Dr. Antonia Novello is Confirmed as the First Woman Surgeon General of the United States: She is also the first minority to be appointed to this position.

1990– Office of Research on Women's Health is Established: This office was established at the National Institutes of Health to stimulate and serve as a focal point for women's health research. Public hearings and a scientific workshop held at Hunt Valley, Maryland, produced the report "The National Institutes of Health: Opportunities for Research on Women's Health," which served as a blueprint for research at the NIH.

1990– Society for the Advancement of Women's Health Research Founded: This organization's mission was to improve the health of women through research.

1990– Breast and Cervical Cancer Mortality Prevention Act: This Congressional act provided mammograms and pap smears to underserved women (including low-income women, older women, and minority women).

1991– Office on Women's Health Established: The Office on Women's Health was established at the U.S. Department of Health and Human Services during the presidency of George H. W. Bush, to better coordinate women's health activities, programs, and research throughout the U.S. Public Health Service.

1992– Mammography Quality Standards Act: This law was designed to set national standards and a uniform system of quality control for mammography clinics across the country.

1992– Infertility Prevention Act: This Act provided additional funds to establish screening, treatment, counseling, and follow-up services for sexually transmitted diseases that could lead to infertility in women if left undiagnosed and/or untreated.

1993– NIH Revitalization Act: This law required the inclusion of women and members of racial and ethnic minority groups in all federally-funded population-based studies.

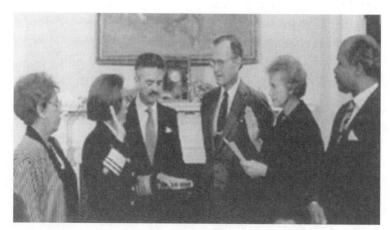

Antonia Coello Novello, M.D. (1944–), the first woman and the first minority to be appointed as Surgeon General of the United States. Pictured, Dr. Novello being sworn in by Justice Sandra Day O'Connor in a ceremony at the White House on March 9, 1990. Also in the photo, President George Bush (center right), Secretary of the Department of Health and Human Services Louis Sullivan (far right), and Dr. Novello's husband and mother. Photo courtesy of the U.S. Department of Health and Human Services, Washington, D.C.

1993– Family and Medical Leave Act: This law provided employees with the right to take up to 12 weeks of unpaid leave during a 12-month period for family or medical reasons without the threat of having to leave their job permanently.

1993– National Action Plan on Breast Cancer (NAPBC) Established: This public-private partnership was established by President William J. Clinton in response to a national petition drive (2.6 million signatures) coordinated by the National Breast Cancer Coalition. Its goal was to establish a comprehensive national plan to address the breast cancer epidemic. After providing leadership and sparking interest on issues from genetic testing to public education and clinical trials, the work of the NAPBC was handed over to private groups and the National Cancer Institute in 2000.

1994– Violence Against Women Act: This Act defined new federal crimes of violence against women and enhanced penalties to combat sexual assault and domestic violence.

1994– Offices of Women's Health established at the Food and Drug Administration and the Centers for Disease Control and Prevention.

1994– BRCA1 and BRCA2 Identified: The DNA sequences of two genetic mutations linked to breast cancer were discovered, leading to the possibility of genetic testing for high risk women.

1994– Women of Childbearing Years Can Participate in Clinical Trials: The FDA issued guidance lifting the ban on inclusion of women with childbearing potential from early clinical studies (Phase 1 and early Phase 2). This ban (which had been in place since 1977) had been a significant barrier to women's participation in clinical trials.

1996– The Personal Responsibility and Work Opportunity Reconciliation Act of 1996: A provision of this bill, Support for Families Transitioning into Job, was designed to help more mothers move into jobs. The law also guaranteed that women on welfare would continue to receive health coverage for their families, including at least one year of transitional Medicaid when they leave welfare for work.

1996– National Centers of Excellence in Women's Health Designated: The DHHS Office on Women's Health designated the first six National Centers of Excellence (CoEs) at academic medical centers around the country. These were model "one-stop-shopping" health programs designed to integrate women's health research, clinical services and public education. By century's end,

there were fifteen CoEs, and three National Community Centers of Excellence in Women's Health, with more planned for the future.

1996– Women's Health in the Medical School Curriculum Published: This first guideline for including women's health issues in medical school curriculum was published by the Office of Research on Women's Health, the Health Resources and Services Administration, and the DHHS Office on Women's Health.

1997– An Agenda for Research on Women's Health in the 21st Century: This document expanded the Hunt Valley vision for women's health research in the broader context of cultural and ethnic origins, geographic location, and socioeconomic strata.

1997– FDA Office of Women's Health Launches "Take Time to Care Campaign": This three year effort reached over 26 million Americans with the message "Use Medicines Wisely." Done in partnership with the National Association of Chain Drug Stores and more than 80 other participating organizations, this campaign targeted the issue of preventing adverse drug reactions and medication errors.

1998– Gender Differences in Susceptibility to Environmental Factors Published: This Institute of Medicine report encouraged more research into how certain factors, such as genetics and hormones, affect susceptibility to environmental influences in health status.

1998– The National Women's Health Information Center (NWHIC) Launched: The DHHS Office on Women's Health launched the first commercial-free combined Web site and toll-free phone number for women's health information. By century's end, NWHIC was receiving more than four million "hits" and several hundred thousand "user sessions" a month.

1999– Contraceptive Coverage in the Federal Employees Health Benefits Program: This law was attached to the 1999 Treasury, Postal Service, and General Government Appropriations Bill to offer contraceptive coverage to women insured through the Federal Employees Health Benefits Program.

1999– Women's Health in the Dental School Curriculum Published: The first women's health curriculum recommendations for dental schools were released by the NIH Office of Research on Women's Health and the Health Resources and Services Administration.

1999– Lesbian Health: Current Assessment and Directions for the Future: This Institute of

Medicine report recommended more research into health issues that might be unique to lesbian women.

2000– The Breast and Cervical Cancer Prevention and Treatment Act: This Congressional Act is designed to enable states to provide treatment services to eligible women through the Medicaid program.

2000– Exploring the Biological Contributions to Human Health: Does Sex Matter?: This Institute of Medicine report was initiated in 2000. It concluded that "every cell has a sex" and that medical research should focus more on sex differences and determinants on the biological level.

The Women's Health Movement in the United States

From Grass-Roots Activism to Professional Agendas

by Sheryl Burt Ruzek, PhD, MPH and Julie Becker, MA, MPH

The grass-roots women's health movement grew rapidly during the 1970s and 1980s, but contracted by the end of that decade. Surviving organizations must now negotiate roles and relationships with newer women's health organizations that burgeoned in the 1990s and that are typically professionalized and disease specific. They differ from grass-roots groups through: 1) their relationships to broader movements for social change; 2) leadership; 3) attitudes toward biomedicine; 4) relationships to corporate sponsors; 5) educational goals; and 6) lay versus professional authority. There is little overlap between women's health advocacy organizations identified by the National Women's Health Network and two Internet search engines. The proliferation of newer organizations dilutes the role of grass-roots groups as information brokers for women in the United States and raises questions about who will speak for women in the electronic age. (*JAMWA.* 1999;54:4–8)

Women's health activists have generated public debate and spearheaded social action in a number of waves throughout US history, waves that Carol Weisman views as part of a women's health "megamovement" that has spanned two centuries. The US women's health movement grew rapidly through the 1970s; broadened its base with women of color and others in the early 1980s; and contracted, was co-opted, and became institutionalized during the late 1980s and 1990s. Surviving grass-roots organizations are now negotiating roles and relationships with newer, more professional women's health support and advocacy organizations. While both older and newer women's health organiza-tions seek improvements in women's health care, their focus and priorities vary.

In this article, we analyze the historical development of the grass-roots women's health movement in the United States, note key contributions, and differentiate surviving movement organizations from the newer, professionalized women's health advocacy groups. Distinguishing between grass-roots and more professional women's health groups becomes particularly important as we move into the global "information age." Because public trust of mainstream medical institutions is eroding, as evidenced by the growth of alternative and complementary medical practices and the increasing distrust of managed care organizations, both grass-roots and professionalized health advocacy groups are likely to play key roles in defining the quality and trustworthiness of health information. Growing calls for accountability and improved patient satisfaction create windows of opportunity for health advocates to use their influence and authority to shape how the quality of health information and services will be defined.

Social Movements and Social Change

The women's health movement's very success makes differentiating surviving grass-roots movement organizations from professionalized ones that are historically, ideologically, and strategically aligned with this episode of activism particularly challenging. For conceptual clarity, it is important to note that social scientists have long distinguished between general social movements and specific social movements. Theorists of social movements are particularly careful to differentiate between grass-roots movements and professionalized movements that emerge from within established institutions. General social movements affect the public's consciousness of many issues and bring about social change in many arenas. The general feminist movement of the 1960s and 1970s spawned dozens of specific movements and hundreds of movement organizations. As specific social movements gain momentum, they, like general social movements, shape public consciousness beyond the smaller world of movement organizations.

It is also crucial not to confuse formally constituted movement organizations with social movements themselves, although these groups represent the active components of a movement. As health activists differentiated themselves within the broader feminist movement and developed an identity as a specific grass-roots feminist movement, they founded organizations such as the Boston Women's Health Book Collective, the Federation of Feminist Women's Health Centers, DES Action, and the National Women's Health Network.

Rise and Development of the Women's Health Movement

More than three decades ago, when access to medical information was restricted almost exclusively to physicians (who were mostly men), laywomen's insistence on access to medical research was truly "revolutionary." Few books on women's health could be found in bookstores, except for books on childbirth. The assumption was simply that physicians were the experts and women were to do as instructed. Breaking open this closed system, laywomen asserted that personal, subjective knowledge of one's own body was a valid source of information and deserved recognition, not scorn.

The women's health movement grew rapidly through the leadership of several grass-roots groups with strong ties to other social change movements, particularly the abortion rights, prepared childbirth, and consumer health movements. As the general feminist movement of the 1960s and 1970s sought equal rights and the full participation of women in all public spheres, many believed that without control over reproduction, all other rights were in jeopardy. Thus in the early years, reproductive issues defined many branches of the movement and shaped group consciousness and social action. Reproductive rights remain central to feminist health agendas worldwide.

Feminist health writers such as Barbara Seaman, Barbara Ehrenreich and Deirdre English, Ellen Frankfort, Gena Corea, Claudia Dreifus, and columnists for prominent feminist newspapers galvanized women to explore their own health, providing critical momentum for the emerging grass-roots movement. The Boston Women's Health Book Collective produced the enormously popular *Our Bodies, Ourselves,* which has gone through numerous US and many other language editions worldwide. The Federation of Feminist Women's Health Centers "invented" and championed gynecological self-help and woman-centered reproductive health services. The National Women's Health Network (NWHN) linked a wide array of local groups to provide a voice for women in Washington. Monitoring legislation, Food and Drug Administration actions, and informing the public about women's health issues continue to be central to this organization's mission. A few nationally prominent groups focused on specific diseases or conditions (eg, DES Action, the Endometriosis Association). Members of pivotal groups and other health activists traveled, spoke, and published widely, and used contacts with the media effectively, becoming spokespeople for the rapidly growing movement.

An important achievement of the women's health movement was transferring women's health from the domain of largely male experts to women themselves. Developing in parallel with self-help medical care movements, consciousness-raising and gynecological self-help became strategies for empowering women to define their own health and create alternative services. Local movement groups in all 50 states were providing gynecological self-help, women-controlled reproductive health clinics, clearinghouses for health information, and referral services and producing their own health educational materials. Advocacy ranged from accompanying individual women seeking medical care to advising and influencing state and local health departments. By the mid-1970s, more than 250 formally identifiable groups provided education, advocacy, and direct service in the United States. Nearly 2,000 informal self-help groups and projects provided additional momentum to the movement (B. Seaman, unpublished data, 1998). Although ideologically committed to being inclusive, the leadership of the women's health movement remained largely white and middle class in North America during the early years. Sterilization abuse mobilized women of color to seek government protection during the 1970s, and groups such as the Committee to End Sterilization Abuse (CESA) were founded.

The women's health movement grew increasingly visible globally, with groups such as ISIS in Geneva creating opportunities for worldwide feminist health activism. By the mid-1970s, there were more than 70 feminist health groups in Canada, Europe, and Australia. Today, there are growing efforts to make connections with feminist health activists worldwide, both in industrialized and developing countries.

As the women's health movement evolved in the United States, the distinct health needs of diverse women emerged, and women of color formed their own movement organizations such as the National Black Women's Health Project, the National Latina Women's Health Organization, the Native American Women's Health Education and Resource Center, and the National Asian Women's Health Organization. Women of color health organizations gained national recognition and developed agendas to protect women against racist sterilization and contraceptive practices; to widen access to medical care for low-income women, including abortions no longer covered by Medicaid; and to focus on diseases and conditions affecting women of color such as lupus, fetal alcohol syndrome, hypertension, obesity, drug addiction, and stress related to racism and poverty that were ignored or misunderstood by largely white movement groups. By the late 1980s, the National Black Women's Health Project had established local chapters with more than 150 self-help groups for African-American women.

Other women added distinct health agendas. Lesbians, rural women, and women with disabilities joined older women's groups and women with specific health concerns to direct attention to their particular needs. Groups such as the Dis-Abled Women's Network, the Older Women's League, and the Lesbian Health Agenda broadened constituencies and issues. With the rise of environmental health concerns, groups such as the Women's Environmental Development Organization (WEDO) built bridges between feminist health activism and other movements for social change.

Like other social movements, the women's health movement has gone through periods of emergence, rapid growth, decline, and institutionalization. Grass-roots feminist health organizations declined in the 1980s, apparently as a result of changes in movement adherents and the social context in which movement groups operated. For example, many founders of movement organizations returned to school, began families, or entered the paid labor force, as have the next generation of women who increasingly juggle careers and families, thus reducing the traditional volunteer labor pool. Much of organized feminism as it evolved both in media imagery and academe, came to be seen as distant or disconnected from ordinary women's lives. The success of single-issue groups, particularly acquired immune deficiency syndrome (AIDS) organizations, to secure funding for direct services, education, and research presented new models for health activism. And the discovery of mainstream health institutions that "marketing to women" could increase profits led to the designation of a wide array of clinical services as "women's health clinics." By the 1990s, women's health services were widespread, although most were now part of larger medical institutions. In a recent national survey of women's health services, most centers founded in the 1960s and 1970s claimed a commitment to a feminist ideology; those founded later or sponsored by hospitals were significantly less likely to report this commitment.

By the end of the 1980s, most alternative feminist health clinics had ceased to exist, and the survivors had broadened their range of services and affiliated with larger health systems. Gynecological self-help has virtually disappeared. The surviving grass-roots movement advocacy and education groups such as the NWHN face declining support from both individuals and foundations as they compete with newer organizations for members and resources. Thus, grass-roots groups contracted internally as they were diluted externally by the growing prominence of both mainstream women's support groups (on a wide array of health issues ranging from alcohol problems to breast cancer) and disease-focused health advocacy groups whose efforts supported the growing federal initiatives for greater equity in women's health research (S.B. Ruzek, unpublished data, 1998).

From Grass-Roots Ideologies to Professional Institutional Agendas

The success of the women's health movement is reflected in the extent to which mainstream organizations and institutions, particularly federal agencies, have incorporated or adopted core ideas and created new opportunities for women's health advocates. By the 1990s, the reform wings of feminism had made significant claims for gender equity in all social institutions. With a growing number of women in Congress, in the biomedical professions, and in health advocacy communities, organizations that had pursued very different paths to improving women's health coalesced around the 1989 General Accounting Office (GAO) report showing that the National Institutes of Health (NIH) had failed to implement its policy of including women in study populations. The GAO report proved to be a catalyst for pressuring Congress and the NIH to take action, and by the end of 1990, the Women's Health Equity Act was passed, and the NIH established the Office of Research on Women's Health. In 1991, the NIH undertook the Women's Health Initiative, the largest project of its kind, seeking data on prevention and treatment of cancer, cardiovascular disease, and osteoporosis. Although grass-roots women's health groups have criticized many aspects of the research and have attempted to rectify perceived problems in consent procedures and inclusion criteria, they have largely supported greater federal funding of biomedical research into women's health. Thus the women's health movement critique of biomedicine and the call for demedicalizing women's health care was reframed into a bipartisan agenda for equity. Scientific and professional interest in women's health burgeoned in the early 1990s. Spurred by growing federal investment in women's health and by the "cold-war dividend" funding of women's research through the Department of Defense, health activists saw opportunities to collaborate with scientists and professionals who were eager to take advantage of these new research priorities.

To maximize the likelihood of obtaining federal funding for research on women's health, scientists and their consumer allies focused on specific diseases. This narrowing of focus was critical for navigating federal funding streams that are tied to specific diseases and organ systems. The new "disease-oriented" organizations reflect the interests of women who expect a high level of professionalism. Facing dual roles as workers outside the home and traditional caretakers inside the home, the highly educated women who support the new single-issue groups may find that their interests lie in organizations that dispense professionally endorsed information, solicit donations, and carry out advocacy efforts on behalf of women. Thus the success of women's entry into the labor force, changes in cultural ethos, and women's own commitment to specialization and professionalism may explain why the narrower, highly professionalized women's health equity organizations attract

women who do not identify either with broader movements for social change or with feminism per se.

AIDS advocacy groups also raised a new standard of effectiveness for health activists. They not only successfully increased funding for education and research, but gained a voice in how these added appropriations from government and foundations would be spent. Thereafter, breast cancer advocates and others (ovarian cancer advocates, Parkinson patients and their families, etc.) adopted many of the AIDS organizations' strategies, albeit with a more professional and less confrontational style. A growing willingness to own illness and become "poster people" for cancer, as people with AIDS have done effectively, put a face on diseases that women privately and pervasively feared. Creating strong alliances between consumers, medical professionals, and researchers, breast cancer advocates rallied behind a specific cause that affected many of them directly or through family and friends. Many local support and advocacy organizations joined larger, well-funded organizations such as the National Breast Cancer Coalition, leaving behind older-style support groups and feminist health organizations with broader agendas.

Using well-established letter-writing and advocacy strategies, breast cancer activists testified at hearings, held press conferences, and took their case to the NIH. In collaboration with growing bipartisan support in Congress and the scientific community, advocates succeeded in increasing federal funding for breast cancer research from $84 million to more than $400 million in 1993. Breast cancer advocates also insisted that survivors be involved in shaping research agendas and educational efforts and aligned themselves more consistently and collaboratively with scientists than some AIDS activists or earlier grass-roots movement leaders had.

The success of breast cancer advocacy quickly created a "disease du jour" climate, where professionals rallied people directly or indirectly affected by particular diseases to lobby for increased funding. Ovarian cancer was the next women's disease to achieve national prominence. While this approach secures more resources for particular groups in the short run, it pits diseases against each other, turning research funding into a "popularity contest" or war of each against all—to be won by the group that can make the most noise or wield the greatest political pressure. A result may be overfunding some diseases without regard for their prevalence, contribution to overall population health, or likelihood of scientific value. In this environment, orphan diseases will join orphan drugs as the unfortunate, but unavoidable downsides of market-driven research and medicine.

Differences of Grass-Roots and Professionalized Women's Health Organizations

In a market-focused society, identifying differences is important for establishing a niche, and like other organizations, movement groups emphasize their unique features. Grass-roots women's health movement groups see themselves as different from what they perceive the more professional, mainstream organizations to be, although these differences are not always clearly articulated. After observing a wide range of groups for three decades, we have found that surviving grass-roots advocacy groups are differentiated from most professionalized, disease-focused groups in the following six ways.

Social Movement Orientation. The founders of many grass-roots feminist groups had ties to progressive or radical social movements that emphasized social justice and social change, to which many remain committed. In contrast, the newer professionalized support and advocacy organizations are typically more narrowly focused on a single disease or health issue, and except for environmentally focused groups such as WEDO, few are integral to broader social movements for social change (although some individual members may have such commitments).

Leadership. Although some women physicians who were critical of medical education, training, and practice were leaders of the grass-roots women's health movement, lay leadership was the norm. The role of physicians relative to others remains a point of contention. In contrast, the professionalized support and advocacy groups formed in the 1990s had a growing pool of women physicians, scientists, and other highly trained professionals to turn to for leadership.

Attitude Toward Biomedicine. A recurring theme in the grass-roots women's health movement has been the demand for "evidence-based medicine," long before this term came into vogue. Major feminist advocacy groups aligned themselves with scientists and physicians who sought to put medical practice on a more scientific basis at a time when it was resisted by many clinicians. Grass-roots health activists were critical of the side effects of inadequately tested drugs and devices, particularly early high-dose oral contraceptives, diethylstilbestrol, and the intrauterine device. They also questioned the number of unnecessary hysterectomies and radical mastectomies performed. In short, consumer groups sought to protect women from unsafe or unnecessary biomedical interven-

tions. The professionalized advocacy groups founded in the 1990s focus more on ensuring women an equitable share of biopsychosocial science and treatment. The growing number of women physicians and scientists also facilitates alliances with women consumers because perceived interests in safety and effectiveness make these relationships seem mutually beneficial.

Relationships with Corporate Sponsors. Older grass-roots advocacy groups remain deeply concerned about the effects of drug and device manufacturers sponsoring journals and organizational activities. In fact, this issue is a pivotal source of strain between grass-roots groups and professionalized women's health organizations. While organizations of women physicians and professionalized advocacy groups rely heavily on corporate sponsorships, older grass-roots groups avoid such relationships on grounds that financial ties affect the willingness of groups to criticize sponsors, promote competitors' products, or address alternative or complementary therapies that might undermine conventional prescribing patterns. Refusing support from corporate sponsors remains a hallmark of grass-roots movement groups, but they struggle financially as a result. Because professionalized groups accept corporate support, they have more resources for education and advocacy.

Goals of Education. Both older and newer women's health organizations share the goal of educating women to improve their own health and make decisions about their own care. A central feature of grass-roots feminst groups, particularly through the 1970s was to demystify medicine and to encourage women to trust their subjective experience of their own health. Having access to larger numbers of women physicians may have reduced the perceived need to demystify medicine, and professionalized organizations appear largely concerned with making their highly educated constituencies aware of medical and scientific information.

Lay Versus Professional Authority. Grass-roots health groups remain committed to substantial lay control over health and healing and to expanding the roles of such nonphysician healers as midwives, nurses, and counseling professionals. They would involve consumers in all aspects of health policy making, not simply transfer legitimate authority from male to female physicians. In professionalized organizations, women physicians become the primary societal experts on women's health matters.

The grass-roots women's health movement organizations leave a legacy of making health an important social concern and educating women to take responsibility for their own health and health care decision making. The movement as a whole has made substantial efforts to influence powerful social institutions—organized medicine, the pharmaceutical industry, and regulatory agencies. In partnership with newer, professionalized equity organizations, health movement activists have taken up mainstream reform efforts that will become increasingly important as medical care is dominated by market forces. Thus the current episode of women's health activism overlaps with, but is, in many ways, different from the activism of the 1960s and 1970s. These distinct episodes of women's health activism need to be differentiated and understood in the specific historical contexts in which they emerged, recognizing the distinct roles that their history may lead them to play in the future.

The Next Challenge: Who Will Speak for Women in the Electronic Age?

The electronic communication technologies foster a climate in which researchers and consumers expect to find information instantaneously and effortlessly. The reliability of information in electronic media is often questionable, however. Until data can be transformed into usable knowledge that can shape human action, the information age will not fulfill its promise. Neither grass-roots women's health movement organizations nor newer professionalized disease agenda groups have adequately grappled with how to communicate with their constituencies effectively. Both types of groups as well as government and mainstream health organizations will have to assess, manage, and distribute what each sees as "reliable" health information. Organizational survival may depend increasingly on teaching both "customers" and staff how to use reliable information effectively.

Because of the role of advocacy groups in health policy making in the United States, how they present themselves and are perceived are important. As electronic media provide all-comers the opportunity to claim organizational status in an increasingly "virtual" world, and the number of groups claiming to speak for women increases, how will the public differentiate among them? As we navigate the uncharted "information age," the ability of the grass-roots women's health movement to remain viable appears somewhat precarious because the technology allows anyone with a computer and minimal skill to "create" an organization with worldwide visibility. Most movement organizations have not moved beyond hard copy resource centers and clearinghouses, in part because they have well-established communication networks that have served them well in the past (S.B. Ruzek, J. Becker, unpublished data, 1998). Newer professionalized advocacy groups are better funded and

more attuned to technological advancements. As electronic communications gain prominence, those who position themselves in this media will be perceived as speaking for women. In an effort to address the complexity of electronic media, the Boston Women's Health Book Collective is including a section on how to assess the adequacy of electronic sources of information in the 1998 edition of *Our Bodies, Ourselves.*

To assess the complexity of the environment in which grass-roots activist groups find themselves at the close of this century, and to determine the array of groups that present themselves as speaking for women, we compared the number of national women's health advocacy organizations easily identified through two worldwide web search strategies with those identified by the National Women's Health Network in 1994 as meeting their criteria: national, women-controlled or a women-controlled project of a larger organization, feminist outlook, mostly consumer controlled, and primarily advocacy, not just engaged in service or education. In an effort to identify organizations that might easily be identified by the public, Yahoo, a common Internet search engine, was used along with Healthfinders, the electronic database that the Department of Health and Human Services unveiled for public use in May 1997. Using the term "women's health organizations," 339 groups were located on the two Internet sources. After coding them for meeting two of the five NWHN criteria (being national and having an advocacy agenda beyond service or education), and removing duplications, 223 women's health advocacy organizations were identified, 46 by the NWHN, 53 by Healthfinders, and 124 by Yahoo.

When we cross-tabulated the data, it became clear that there is little overlap in the women's health advocacy organizations identified by these three sources. Only the Society for the Advancement of Women's Health Research was identified by all three. Six organizations were identified by both the NWHN and DHHS Healthfinders; 9 were identified by both DHHS and Yahoo; and 13 were identified by both NWHN and Yahoo. Thus, "who speaks for women's health" in the electronic age very much depends on where one looks—and how willing one is to sort through hundreds of self-characterized "women's health organizations." In this environment it is unclear how the women's health movement will continue to be perceived as a key information broker in an increasingly complex sea of women's health information.

Grass-roots health movement groups remain important forces for increasing awareness of women's health issues and are viewed as trustworthy sources of information by feminist groups in the United States and worldwide. Newer, professionalized equity organizations, too, face competition from a growing array of institutions that claim expertise in matters of women's health. The challenge for both types of women's health groups will be to differentiate themselves from others whose interests lie more in marketing than in meeting diverse women's health needs. Both types of groups need to be allies for widening access and equity in health care for all women, not just some women, in the next century.

References

A list of references is available in the original source.

Crossing Cultural Borders with "Our Bodies, Ourselves"

by Sally Whelan and Jane Pincus

With just three weeks to go before the Utrecht meeting that would bring together groups from around the world that are translating/adapting *Our Bodies, Ourselves (OBOS)*, the last piece of funding came in, last minute requirements of embassies and visa offices were met, necessary documents produced, and the final hotel rooms booked. I (Sally) sat bolt upright in bed at 5 AM one morning, realizing that if I got on email immediately, I might be able to catch our colleague Codou Bop on-the-spot at her computer in Senegal, or Liana Galstyan in Armenia to find out if wired funds had gotten through. This instant messaging worked splendidly.

It was an honor to attend this exciting meeting; now, the events of the past two months have made us even more keenly aware of the essential need for this kind of global dialogue. The only other large gathering of groups working on translations/adaptations of *Our Bodies, Ourselves* was in 1995 at the Fourth World Conference on Women held in Beijing. This time we arranged to carve out our own time and place.

Kathy Davis, a feminist sociologist at the University of Utrecht, and Marlies Bosch, presently a facilitator of the Tibetan translation project, helped organize and facilitate the meeting. The Federation of Women's Self-help Centers, a coalition of groups funded by the Dutch government, graciously offered us a large, sunlit room. Chantal Soeters, one of Kathy's students, took notes. Seated at tables designed to come together in a comfortable ellipse, twenty-one participants from Japan, Armenia, Poland, Tibet, Senegal, Mexico, Bulgaria, Serbia, the Netherlands, and the U.S. put faces to the voices we had come to know through email and fax over the last several years. For the next three days, women described the dramatic challenges they faced in creating adaptations of *Our Bodies, Ourselves*.

Six New Books

Bulgaria

Kornelia Slavova and Tatyana Kotzeva

The Women's Health Initiative in Bulgaria took the risk of publishing their book in a culture where women's roles have been "re-traditionalized" in the transition from Communism to democracy, and where feminism is seen as a Western, anti-male, anti-family, and pro-lesbian ideology. The *collective* voice of *OBOS* reverberates cynically, as does the idea of *sisterhood,* conjuring up a leftist agenda that smacks of Marxism and Leninism. A straight translation would have been culturally inappropriate.

Over-medicalization is not an issue, as basic needs in health care are not yet met, nor are abortion rights an issue, particularly not a moral one, because abortion is the primary method of birth control. Pro-natalist attitudes make for an especially difficult and charged environment for women experiencing infertility.

Speaking to the societal antipathy towards feminism, the authors recast it within the perspective of gender justice, providing a special chapter about women's issues during the nineteenth and twentieth centuries. Throughout, they emphasized the rights of women in their roles as consumers, patients and citizens. They address their introduction to men as well as women.

After sometimes challenging negotiations, the book was published by a prestigious publisher, Colibri, and came out in July.

Serbia

Stanislava Otasevic and Bobana Macanovic

Much of the Serbian adaptation of *OBOS* was produced in war-torn Serbia. The coordinating group, The Autonomous Women's Center Against Sexual Violence supports and counsels women survivors of male violence.

A team composed of nine women from five groups, spent over a year translating and adapting *OBOS,* publishing it themselves. Stanislava and Bobana proudly brought copies—hot off the press!—to our meeting, with the cover photo of the first ever "Take Back the Night" march in 1995 in Belgrade. Each page contains just one column of text, leaving a lot of space for women to write in their own experiences, for they said "These books will have many owners."

This is the first book available in Serbia on the politics of women's health. In a country that conceals health statistics for military and economic purposes, documentation about women's health takes on a unique power. War has severely affected the health care situation, with long waiting lists, shortage of money and medicines, and general depression. Often Serbian women's bodies have literally been used as weapons for military and political purposes; thus, these women have experienced them as instruments of pain and suffering, not as a functional or pleasurable part of their lives. Material on sexuality takes on a special importance.

As the authors see it, living within a regime that abhorred diversity and had well developed 'mechanisms of hate,' it is essential to underscore the diversity of Serbian women, and they especially have attempted to give visibility to lesbians and women with disabilities.

Recent events have increased substance abuse and the use of anti-depressant drugs, discussed at length in the book. The authors dropped the 'Nutrition' chapter, for it seemed terrible to speak of food when people were starving; 'Women in Motion' was dropped too, for it also lacked relevance, pertinent only to affluent people.

The authors hope that their printer's comment, when they picked up the finished book in June, augurs well for a positive reception of the Serbian *OBOS*. He said: "This book should be given to each daughter by her father." It is a testament to their strength, courage and perseverance that there is any Serbian edition at all.

Armenia

Liana Galstyan

The Armenian adaptation of *OBOS* arrived last month in our mailbox, almost ten years after work on this book began. During the past decade, Armenia endured an earthquake, severe losses in electricity and heating fuel, and paper shortages—some photos from the project's first phase show the translators in a candlelit room wearing gloves. Faced with hardships and logistical problems, the project was stalled until Dr. Mary Khachikian met Judy Norsigian at the Armenian World Medical Congress in Boston during 1996 and agreed to assume coordination of the project. After that point, the vision and dedication of Mary and her colleagues shaped a process and a product that is now beautiful to behold with its multi-colored cover filled with images of Armenian women of all ages.

With a declining birthrate and economic hardship causing serious emigration from the country, the book, with its extensive section on contraception, faced some resistance from some government officials and members of the media even before its actual publication. For some, the legacy of the Armenian genocide also contributes to a pro-natalist sentiment. Still, Liana reported, the authors managed to offer extensive information about birth control. They significantly adapted the infertility section of the book, as STDs cause infertility rates to be very high (28%). The book makes a special attempt to reach young women with chapters on body image and sexuality.

The coordinator of the Armenian Family Health Association plans to organize a series of awareness-raising workshops for women throughout Armenia, including educators, health providers and women in social service agencies. This edition holds special meaning for Judy Norsigian, who is also Armenian and visited Armenia for the first time last year to participate in an Armenian women's conference and to help with completion of the book project.

Senegal

Codou Bop

The present challenge for the authors of the "inspired" African-French edition of *OBOS, Notre Corps,*

Notre Santé is to secure funding for printing and distribution of their already completed manuscript. The book will serve twenty-one francophone countries. With French (the language of colonization) as the necessary working language, it will be distributed for free to schools, health centers and women's groups, and translated into local dialects. The BWHBC is currently seeking donors who may wish to contribute to this endeavor.

Most Africans are being increasingly harmed by a new kind of re-colonization, among them the World Bank's structural adjustment policies, increased debts to the global North, devalued currencies and the privatization of health and education, which used to be free or cost very little.

Women have little or no access to health care, land, jobs, or schooling. False interpretations of the Koran increasingly stand in the way of women's health and rights. Young women rank low in the social hierarchy of power, with 56% married and mother of a baby by age seventeen. In general, women belong to fathers, husbands or uncles. Their role is to take care of others. Since they are not "allowed" to be ill, and there is no such thing as an "unhealthy" woman, women buy over-the-counter medications to ease symptoms enough to carry on with their work.

Some practices are oppressive and harmful: For instance, to be fat is desirable, since thinness is associated with poverty and AIDS. Thus, women are too often encouraged to eat high-fat diets and discouraged from exercising. Fifteen to nineteen year old women are most afflicted by HIV/AIDS (an insidious myth teaches that a man infected with AIDs need to have sex with a virgin to purify himself). Women use bleach to whiten their skin (a result of colonialism), causing skin cancer and kidney problems.

The book emphasizes the cultural, economic, political and religious contexts in which African women live. It empowers a woman by telling her she belongs to herself, and constantly encourages her not to feel guilty taking care of herself. One chapter describes pre-colonial matrilineal societies in which women did have a great deal of power.

Mexico

Ester Shapiro, Alan West, U.S., and Lourdes Ruiz

An extensive cultural adaptation of *OBOS* was produced by approximately twenty Latin American women's health groups spanning the Americas and the Caribbean in collaboration with a Boston-based editorial team of Latinas. Ester, coordinating editor of *NCNV*, discussed some of *NCNV's* departures from *OBOS*, the

tasks faced in adapting a US feminist text (by emphasizing "mutual help" rather than "self-help" and eliminating some of the overtly ideological attitudes, for instance), and how the book's text became a living tool for lively networking and community organizing.

The audience for *NCNV* is huge and very varied. As women worked in coalition across lines of continent and nation, North and South, locally and regionally, they broadened the definition of social change work to emphasize working with men and other social change movements. The "Católicas por el Derecho a Decidir" (Catholics for a Free Choice) prolife/prochoice perspective on abortion within the framework of women's sacred responsibility for preserving life was tremendously important. *NCNV* embodies a participatory health education model, with an emphasis on community building and outreach.

As the only translation/adaptation project based at the BWHBC, *NCNV* has served in many ways as a bridge between *OBOS* and other projects worldwide. Important commonalities arise between *NCNV* and other books.

NCNV redefines feminism within a gender and social justice model, as in the Bulgarian edition. It places great emphasis throughout, as does the francophone African edition, on the need to balance the care of others with the care for one's self. And like the Arabic edition from Egypt, inspired by *OBOS*, but a new book altogether, *NCNV* acknowledges the importance of religion and spirituality in discussions of women's health.

Ester offered her extensive knowledge in networking, media outreach, and promotion and held special sessions with participants whose books are already published, and for whom promotion and community outreach are now a priority. Alan provided an analysis of cross-cultural translations, which always involve the implementation of power relationships via the language used. Translation consists of a constant historic, poetic interaction between the text itself, the language and the culture. Lourdes, developer of CIDHAL's impressive website, discussed the use of electronic media and encouraged us to think about how our books, or sections of books, can be brought into the electronic age.

Japan

Toyoko Nakanishi, Toshiko Honda, and Miho Ogino

Authors of the 1988 Japanese edition of *OBOS*, veterans of the translation/adaptation process, they brought to our circle at Utrecht invaluable experience and knowledge. They also brought, straight from the printer the day before their departure for Utrecht, the first-ever translation of *Sacrificing Ourselves for Love*—a book co-authored by deceased BWHBC founder Esther Rome and Jane Wegsheider Hyman. They chose this book to translate because it deals with dieting, eating disorders, cosmetic surgery, domestic violence, rape, STDs, and HIV/AIDS—all serious problems today in Japanese society. Research carried out in Osaka City reveals that 2 out of 3 women have experienced some kind of violence from their husbands or lovers. In May, 2001, Japan enacted a new law attempting to reduce this violence. The authors working on *SOFL* included information on shelters and counseling services for battered women.

The Japanese women did not face censorship in publishing *OBOS* in the late '80s, even when introducing subjects such as lesbians, masturbation, people with disabilities, or the sexuality of older women. However, the Japanese language itself was a challenge. For traditional characters, such as those for pubic hair ('shameful hair'), they substituted a new, positive language of sexuality.

It was useful to hear how a mostly direct translation of *OBOS* became specifically useful to Japanese women. The authors conducted their own research. They added the responses of over 200 clinics and hospitals to a survey designed to provide information on rates/policies on such things as episiotomy, labor positions, contraception, partners permitted at birth, and abortion services. They substituted information about the Japanese medical system, health insurance system, and Japanese law in pertinent places in the text, as well as the names of foods and drugs available in Japan.

OBOS inspired the formation of many groups that began to meet to discuss and conduct research on the birth control pill, endometriosis, menopause, reproductive technologies, sexual harassment, and domestic violence. Many new books have sprung up based on the information and experiences gathered. As a result of increased interest in and visibility of women's health issues, the atmosphere of shame and secrecy surrounding women's bodies and sexuality has been dispersed to a considerable degree.

Upcoming Projects

Poland

Malgorzata (Gosia) Tarasiewicz

Pending funding, the Network of East West Women—Polska will focus on reaching young women. They envision putting selected portions of *OBOS* on the internet, using popular stars. Already, three women singers have agreed to deliver messages about health and sexuality. The site will be interactive, with room for ques-

tions. Magazines will reach women in rural areas and a short story competition for young women will encourage them to talk about their bodies. In these ways they will collect Polish women's experiences for a booklet.

They anticipate attacks from the Catholic hierarchy and media that will cast them as "perverts." But given that in their country prenatal exams are forbidden, abortions illegal, homophobia extensive, and bribes often required for health services, they are determined to bring about some change. "In two years, when we meet again, we'll tell you our story," said Gosia.

Tibet

Lobsang Dechen with Marlies Bosch, the Netherlands

Five hundred Tibetan Buddhist nuns, their country occupied by the Chinese, live in exile in Dharamsala, India at the Tibetan Nun's Project. Lobsang Dechen, a co-director of the nunnery, attended the Utrecht meeting. Through body awareness workshops held last year, the nuns identified some of the topics most useful to them. In meetings held this fall at the nunnery with Marlies Bosch, co-facilitator of the project from the Netherlands, women selected content from *OBOS* to be used for booklets in Tibetan.

Because most of the nuns are young (seventeen to twenty-two years) and without previous exposure to health information, they may also use parts of Ruth Bell's *Changing Bodies, Changing Lives* (for teens) to enhance body awareness and teach basic health concepts. Dechen hopes that in the future they can make available to Tibetan women living in Tibet the information they have gathered.

The Last Day

Marlise Mensink of MAMA CASH, a women's foundation in the Netherlands

With fundraising a constant reality for all groups, we each spoke about how our groups had raised money for our book projects. Marlise stressed the collaborative aspects of the funder/recipient relationship—funders love to give their money away and 'ideals need money!'—and made amusing, practical suggestions about how raising money can be most effective.

Norma Swenson and Jane Pincus, BWHBC co-founders and *OBOS* co-authors

We presented a brief history of the first *OBOS*, BWHBC's early ideals and activities, and some history of the US Women's Health Movement. We mentioned the times of right-wing censorship of *OBOS*. In the post-meeting evaluations, participants said how important it was for them to hear BWHBC's story. Utrecht gave them a chance to:

> "listen to the extraordinary history of the book in the US; to learn stories and crucial moments in producing and publishing its different editions; I was impressed with the enthusiasm of the women who were struggling for the publication of *OBOS;* I was surprised to find that they faced inspection and religious restriction."

To complete the circle, Norma describes her reaction to the stories of these extraordinary women and their works:

> "As I listened to their stories of truly daunting conditions—war, political opposition, lack of funds, lack of time, inadequate and unreliable technology, and dozens of other obstacles—I was strongly moved. I felt there is really no comparison between what we have gone through to produce *OBOS* over the years, under conditions of peace and relative ease and prosperity, and what so many of them have been going through. What we all seem to have in common is the willingness to pour volunteer time, money and effort into producing these books if necessary and the determination to get this vital information in accessible language into the hands of women who clearly need it. As I have felt many times over the years in many different places across the world, women can and do cross cultural borders powerfully with *OBOS,* and with us. I feel very privileged to have been there."

Upcoming Projects

The BWHBC plans to:

* provide ongoing technical assistance to groups in every stage of the translation/adaptation process;
* complete a translation/adaptation guidelines packet that identifies typical challenges faced by groups around the world and illustrates through first-hand accounts how coordinating groups have resolved problems;
* explore the establishment and coordination of a revolving loan fund program to support translation projects on a temporary basis, ensuring they can bring their projects to fruition and disseminate their books as widely as possible;
* and facilitate communication, through a listserv, among emergent and experienced groups producing *OBOS*.

A million thanks to all who participated in the meeting as well as those who contributed funds—the Global Fund for Women, the MacArthur Foundation, Conservation Food and Health Foundation, and an anonymous donor. Thanks also to Ester Shapiro, who coined the title of the meeting. We appreciate all who have joined with us in this critical global work.

Many thanks for the support we received this year from foundations not already mentioned in this newsletter: Ford Foundation, Packard Foundation, Rockefeller Foundation, Mellon Foundation, Pettus-Crowe Foundation, Educational Foundation of America, Dickler Family Foundation, Harvard Pilgrim Health Care Foundation, and Tufts Health Plan.

Tales Out of Medical School

by Adriane Fugh-Berman, MD

With the growth of the women's health movement and the influx of women into medical school, there has been abundant talk of a new enlightenment among physicians. Last summer, many Americans were shocked when Frances Conley, a neurosurgeon on the faculty of Stanford University's medical school, resigned her position, citing "pervasive sexism." Conley's is a particularly elite and male-dominated subspecialty, but her story is

"Man to Man at Georgetown: Tales Out of Medical School" by Adriane Fugh-Berman. Reprinted by permission from the January 20, 1992 issue of *The Nation.*

not an isolated one. I graduated from the Georgetown University School of Medicine in 1988, and while medical training is a sexist process anywhere, Georgetown built disrespect for women into its curriculum.

A Jesuit school, most recently in the news as the alma mater of William Kennedy Smith, Georgetown has an overwhelmingly white, male and conservative faculty. At a time when women made up one-third of all medical students in the United States, and as many as one-half at some schools, my class was 73 percent male and more than 90 percent white.

The prevailing attitude toward women was demonstrated on the first day of classes by my anatomy instructor, who remarked that our elderly cadaver "must have been a Playboy bunny" before instructing us to cut off her large breasts and toss them into the thirty-gallon trash can marked "cadaver waste." Barely hours into our training, we were already being taught that there was nothing to be learned from examining breasts. Given the fact that one out of nine American women will develop breast cancer in her lifetime, to treat breasts as extraneous tissue seemed an appalling waste of an educational opportunity, as well as a not-so-subtle message about the relative importance of body parts. How many of my classmates now in practice, I wonder, regularly examine the breasts of their female patients?

My classmates learned their lesson of disrespect well. Later in the year one carved a tick-tack-toe on a female cadaver and challenged others to play. Another gave a languorous sigh after dissecting female genitalia, as if he had just had sex. "Guess I should have a cigarette now," he said.

Ghoulish humor is often regarded as a means by which med students overcome fear and anxiety. But it serves a darker purpose as well: Depersonalizing our cadaver was good preparation for depersonalizing our patients later. Further on in my training an ophthalmologist would yell at me when I hesitated to place a small instrument meant to measure eye pressure on a fellow student's cornea because I was afraid it would hurt. "You have to learn to treat patients as lab animals," he snarled at me.

On the first day of an emergency medicine rotation in our senior year, students were asked who had had experience placing a central line (an intravenous line placed into a major vein under the clavicle or in the neck). Most of the male students raised their hands. None of the women did. For me, it was graphic proof of inequity in teaching; the men had had the procedure taught to them, but the women had not. Teaching rounds were often, for women, a spectator sport. One friend told me how she craned her neck to watch a physician teach a minor surgical procedure to a male student; when they were done the physician handed her his dirty gloves to discard. I have seen a male attending physician demonstrate an exam on a patient and then wade through several female medical students to drag forth a male in order to teach it to him. This sort of discrimination was common and quite unconscious: The women just didn't register as medical students to some of the doctors. Female students, for their part, tended (like male ones) to gloss over issues that might divert attention, energy or focus from the all-important goal of getting through their training. "Oh, they're just of the old school," a female classmate remarked to me as if being ignored by our teachers was really rather charming, like having one's hand kissed.

A woman resident was giving a radiology presentation and I felt mesmerized. Why did I feel so connected and involved? It suddenly occurred to me that the female physician was regularly meeting my eyes; most of the male residents and attendings made eye contact only with the men.

"Why are women's brains smaller than men's?" asked a surgeon of a group of male medical students in the doctors' lounge (I was in the room as well, but was apparently invisible). "Because they're missing logic!" Guffaws all around.

Such instances of casual sexism are hardly unique to Georgetown, or indeed to medical schools. But at Georgetown female students also had to contend with outright discrimination of a sort most Americans probably think no longer exists in education. There was one course women were not allowed to take. The elective in sexually transmitted diseases required an interview with the head of the urology department, who was teaching the course. Those applicants with the appropriate genitalia competed for invitations to join the course (a computer was supposed to assign us electives, which we had ranked in order of preference, but that process had been circumvented for this course). Three women who requested an interview were told that the predominantly gay male clinic where the elective was held did not allow women to work there. This was news to the clinic's executive director, who stated that women were employed in all capacities.

The women who wanted to take the course repeatedly tried to meet with the urologist, but he did not return our phone calls. (I had not applied for the course, but became involved as an advocate for the women who wanted to take it.) We figured out his schedule, waylaid him in the hall and insisted that a meeting be set up.

At this meeting, clinic representatives disclosed that a survey had been circulated years before to the clientele in order to ascertain whether women workers would be accepted; 95 percent of the clients voted to welcome women. They were also asked whether it was acceptable to have medical students working at the clinic; more than 90 percent approved. We were then told that these results could not be construed to indicate that clients did not mind women medical students; the clients would naturally have assumed that "medical student" meant "male medical student." Even if that were true, we asked, if 90 percent of clients did not mind medical students and 95 percent did not mind women, couldn't a reasonable person assume that female medical students would be acceptable? No, we were informed. Another study would have to be done.

We raised formal objections to the school. Meanwhile, however, the entire elective process had been postponed by the dispute, and the blame for the delay and confusion was placed on us. The hardest part of the struggle, indeed, was dealing with the indifference of most of our classmates—out of 206, maybe a dozen actively supported us—and with the intense anger of the ten men who had been promised places in the course.

"Just because you can't take this course," one of the men said to me, "why do you want to ruin it for the rest of us?" It seemed incredible to me that I had to argue that women should be allowed to take the same courses as men. The second or third time someone asked me the same question, I suggested that if women were not allowed to participate in the same curriculum as the men, then in the interest of fairness we should get a 50 percent break on our $22,500 annual tuition. My colleague thought that highly unreasonable.

Eventually someone in administration realized that not only were we going to sue the school for discrimination but that we had an open-and-shut case. The elective in sexually transmitted diseases was canceled, and from its ashes arose a new course, taught by the same man, titled "Introduction to Urology." Two women were admitted. When the urologist invited students to take turns working with him in his office, he scheduled the two female students for the same day—one on which only women patients were to be seen (a nifty feat in a urology practice).

The same professor who so valiantly tried to prevent women from learning anything unseemly about sexually transmitted diseases was also in charge of the required course in human sexuality (or, as I liked to call it, he-man sexuality). Only two of the eleven lectures focused on women; of the two lectures on homosexuality, neither mentioned lesbians. The psychiatrist who co-taught the class treated us to one lecture that amounted to an apology for rape: Aggression, even hostility, is normal in sexual relations between a man and a woman, he said, and inhibition of aggression in men can lead to impotence.

We were taught that women do not need orgasms for a satisfactory sex life, although men, of course, do; and that inability to reach orgasm is only a problem for women with "unrealistic expectations." I had heard that particular lecture before in the backseat of a car during high school. The urologist told us of couples who came to him for sex counseling because the woman was not having orgasms; he would reassure them that this is normal and the couple would be relieved. (I would gamble that the female half of the couple was anything but relieved.) We learned that oral sex is primarily a homosexual practice, and that sexual dysfunction in women is often caused by "working." In the women-as-idiots department, we learned that when impotent men are implanted with permanently rigid penile prostheses, four out of five wives can't tell that their husbands have had the surgery.

When dealing with sexually transmitted diseases in which both partners must be treated, we were advised to vary our notification strategy according to marital status. If the patient is a single man, the doctor should write the diagnosis down on a prescription for his partner to bring to her doctor. If the patient is a married man, however, the doctor should contact the wife's gynecologist and arrange to have her treated without knowledge of what she is being treated for. How to notify the male partner of a female patient, married or single, was never revealed.

To be fair, women were not the only subjects of out-moded concepts of sexuality. We also received anachronistic information about men. Premature ejaculation, defined as fewer than ten thrusts(!) was to be treated by having the man think about something unpleasant, or by having the woman painfully squeeze, prick or pinch the penis. Aversive therapies such as these have long been discredited.

Misinformation about sexuality and women's health peppered almost every course (I can't recall any egregious wrongs in biochemistry). Although vasectomy and abortion are among the safest of all surgical procedures, in our lectures vasectomy was presented as fraught with long-term complications and abortion was never mentioned without the words "peritonitis" and "death" in the same sentence. These distortions represented Georgetown's Catholic bent at its worst. (We were not allowed to perform, or even watch abortion procedures in our affiliated hospitals.) On a lighter note, one obstetrician assisting us in the anatomy lab told us that women shouldn't lift heavy weights because their pelvic organs will fall out between their legs.

In our second year, several women in our class started a women's group, which held potlucks and offered presentations and performances: A former midwife talked about her profession, a student demonstrated belly dancing, another discussed dance therapy and one sang selections from *A Chorus Line*. This heavy radical feminist activity created great hostility among our male classmates. Announcements of our meetings were defaced and women in the group began receiving threatening calls at home from someone who claimed to be watching the listener and who would then accurately describe what she was wearing. One woman received obscene notes in her school mailbox, including one that contained a rape threat. I received insulting cards in typed envelopes at my home address; my mother received similar cards at hers.

We took the matter to the dean of student affairs, who told us it was "probably a dental student" and suggested we buy loud whistles to blow into the phone when we received unwanted calls. We demanded that the school attempt to find the perpetrator and expel him. We were told that the school would not expel the student but that counseling would be advised.

The women's group spread the word that we were collecting our own information on possible suspects and that any information on bizarre, aggressive, antisocial or misogynous behavior among the male medical students should be reported to our designated representative. She was inundated with a list of classmates who fit the bill. Finally, angered at the school's indifference, we solicited the help of a prominent woman faculty member. Although she shamed the dean into installing a hidden camera across from the school mailboxes to monitor unusual behavior, no one was ever apprehended.

Georgetown University School of Medicine churns out about 200 physicians a year. Some become good doctors despite their training, but many will pass on the misinformation and demeaning attitudes handed down to them. It is a shame that Georgetown chooses to perpetuate stereotypes and reinforce prejudices rather than help students acquire the up-to-date information and sensitivity that are vital in dealing with AIDS, breast cancer, teen pregnancy and other contemporary epidemics. Female medical students go through an ordeal, but at least it ends with graduation. It is the patients who ultimately suffer the effects of sexist medical education.

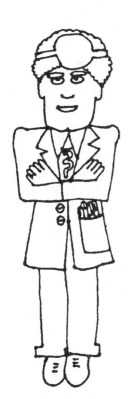

Is Medical School the right choice for *you?*
A SELF-EVALUATION TEST FOR THE PRE-MEDICAL STUDENT
Answer true or false

T   F

☐   ☐   1. Mothers often overreact to the most trivial symptoms in their children.

☐   ☐   2. Mothers are often guilty of denial followed by neglect in not bringing a symptomatic child to the doctor.

☐   ☐   3. Women often imagine breast lumps.

☐   ☐   4. Women should examine their breasts often enough, but not too often*

☐   ☐   5. Informing patients of the side effects of the drugs prescribed for them will cause the patients to experience these side effects in their most virulent form.

☐   ☐   6. Women are sexually excited by gynecological examinations.

☐   ☐   7. Patients never ask the really interesting questions.

☐   ☐   8. A certain amount of physical discomfort is to be expected in anyone over 35, and old people should keep their symptoms to themselves.

☐   ☐   9. No doctor can ever really be guilty of malpractice.

☐   ☐   10. Most people when asked to describe your personality would say, "He's not real warm."

Too often if the lump disappears in a few months; *not often* enough if the lump turns out to be malignant.
ANSWERS: You know who you are.

Women in Medicine

by Rebecca D. C. Perry, MD

Woman, homemaker and caregiver are roles that have been linked since the birth of humanity. Hence, consideration of women physicians and their attempts to combine and balance their roles as doctors, spouses and parents is not a new subject. However, as medical education and delivery methods change, expectations on the part of the public, the profession, and women themselves keep this issue relevant. "Choice" seems to be the watchword of the late 1990s and new millennium, and women are choosing more and more to have it all—profession and family.

Women in medicine in this country have had an interesting evolution. Women have been in medicine since the mid 1800s, and during the latter half of that century there were actually 16 medical schools exclusively for women. Women were accepted into the formerly "male only" schools around the turn of the century, leading to dissolution of the women's schools. Within a decade, however, this admission tolerance disappeared, and even into the 1960s women were faced with quotas when applying to established medical schools. Only in the last 30 years or so have we seen a significant change in admission policies, due in part to increased interest in the profession by women and an increased public demand for female physicians. Now most schools have classes that are 40 percent to 50 percent female. Greater gender disparity among practicing physicians still exists, but this will change in the coming decades as these classes enter the work force.

Trying to balance family and profession begins in medical school—sometimes before—and continues throughout active practice years. This is not unique to the practice of medicine nor to women, but is a challenge that, by nature of the profession, often results in problems for women that are not encountered elsewhere. Attempts to address some of these concerns so that women physicians can successfully integrate their professional and personal lives has necessitated flexibility on the part of schools, residency programs and employers. Paradoxically, these changes have also enhanced the ability of the male physician to more successfully integrate these aspects of his life.

The main challenge has to do with childbearing and childrearing—issues that have not historically been of concern to male physicians because it has long been accepted that a man can easily be physician, husband and father. Such is not a "given" for female physicians, but clearly should be. Changes in expectations and practice styles are allowing easier acceptance of the idea that women can be physicians, wives and mothers.

Maternity leave is an issue that has been addressed by most schools and employers, though there is still some variability in plans. Because of women's biological clocks, this issue often arises during training years or early employment. Hence, women seeking employment should investigate an organization's policies. Furthermore, specialty board requirements can decrease program flexibility because if one is to remain eligible to sit for boards, the amount of resident leave time allowed annually is set. Overall, though, maternity arrangements are available in most situations, and consequently, male physicians often now have paternity benefits as well.

Child care and time for family involvement are generally the most pressing concerns for women with families. And in this age of gender equality, they are major concerns for men as well. It has been an interesting and welcome outcome of gender integration in medical practice that male and female physicians have greater opportunity to be involved with their families than had previously been expected or seen.

Still, women physicians encounter unique problems because of partner choice and lingering traditional role expectations. Over three-fourths of women physicians are married, and over 90 percent of their spouses work outside the home. In comparison, only 45 percent of male physicians' spouses are employed outside the home. About half of women physicians are married to physicians. In contrast, only 10 percent of male physicians are married to physicians. When both marriage partners have unpredictable office hours and nighttime and weekend call coverage, the concerns about adequate family time and child care issues are obviously compounded. Therefore, despite improved representation and the movement toward equality and acceptance for women in the profession, there remain unique concerns for women who choose to "have it all." However, the changing climate of medicine including practice types, patient expectations, and a shift in attitudes about the priority of family has resulted in ever-increasing opportunities to fulfill this goal.

Specialty choice by women physicians has traditionally leaned towards primary care specialties, with almost two-thirds choosing pediatrics, family practice, internal medicine, obstetrics gynecology, and psychiatry. In addition to practices that lend themselves to closer patient relationships, these specialties may have more controllable office hours. And in multi-specialty clinics, more colleagues may be available to share call in primary care specialties than in subspecialties or surgical specialties.

Women physicians are also less likely to work independently than are men and are more likely to be employees of clinics or organizations. The trend toward consolidation of small practices into larger groups has allowed more flexibility regarding practice style for all physicians, and women physicians certainly benefited. The addition of positions such as hospitalists and emergency medicine physicians has also offered opportunities for very fixed and predictable work hours—the ideal for a woman trying to balance family and profession. And in many ways, these types of positions enhance patient care, resulting in a "win-win" situation for physician and patient.

Any change in health care delivery that results in predictable time commitments benefits both women and men physicians. The concern is always what the tradeoff will be for patients—the quality of the doctor-patient rapport and continuity of care. The individual physician must come to terms with these concerns and make choices accordingly. In some instances, the trend toward managed care has already mandated some of these choices for patients and physicians. It remains to be seen whether this is a good or a bad thing.

The fact that 90 percent of working women physicians have employed partners also allows greater flexibility in income requirements, which in turn allows greater flexibility in practice style choices and income disbursement. Women physicians usually are not the sole family supporter so part time and shared practices allow more family time. This usually results in a lower total family income, but this is an acceptable tradeoff for many dual income families. Changing practice structures are conducive to this type of arrangement by offering jobs that have predictable hours. Walk-in clinic popularity is a prime example of patient demand actually serving physician needs in some circumstance. Patients get service when they want, an ever-increasing expectation in this day of consumer demand, and there is a position available for the physician, male or female, who prefers this type of lifestyle and patient relationship. However, both sides lose the intimacy of the established patient-doctor relationship for the sake of time and convenience, and the individual must decide if this is right for him or her. Perhaps as consumers of health care make more demands for convenience at the price of loss of continuity, this type of practice style will become the norm.

Dual incomes also provide extra income for quality child care. In-home care is feasible for these higher but split income families, which makes the choice to work a bit easier for the woman physician. Additionally, many employers are providing child care on site. This includes many health care facilities, which have been at the forefront of this move. Because health facilities often have 24-hour staffing, child care is needed around-the-clock for all employees, thus physicians benefit as well.

As women have claimed their position in the medical profession and no longer see the need to prove themselves, it is becoming more acceptable to seek less demanding clinical situations that make combining work and family easier and more fulfilling. Women physicians certainly continue to choose very busy medical careers and successfully combine them with busy and fulfilling family lives. However, in the absence of a partner in a full time homemaker role, this lifestyle can eventually be exhausting and result in a shortened active professional life by virtue of early retirement or a career change. Thus, women anticipating such a career choice should carefully evaluate and plan for this possibility with respect to retirement plans and benefits. Those women from the medical school classes of 30 years ago are now nearing retirement and may find themselves victims of this problem. Those at the other end of the career timeline would be wise to consider this issue earlier rather than later.

Nonorthodox spousal work arrangements also are becoming both more common and more accepted in society, which has been a plus for women physicians. A small percentage do in fact have homemakers for spouses—men who manage the home and care for the children as a full-time job. With increasing computer technology, many gainfully employed people are working from their homes, enabling them to attend to home activities as part of their workday. This has been a wonderful development for women physicians, whose spouses may choose to work from the home. Not only does it free these women to pursue their careers as they choose, but it allows them to be more comfortable with their choice as the children are with a parent rather than a baby sitter. The mother may miss out on some things but the child doesn't, and that is all important to most parents.

The change in consumer attitude toward the medical profession has been distressing to the physician in many ways. We see the savvy patient becoming more expectant, more questioning and perhaps less respectful of the profession. Perhaps this reflects a trend toward personal respect for the physician from the patient and is a good thing for both the patient and the physician. By demanding the physician to become more human, consumer acceptance of the physician's needs is certainly enhanced. This makes the physician's choices regarding the priority of family more acceptable to the patient because he or she can identify with these needs. The female physician is no longer "wonder woman" but rather just a working mom, and the general populace can identify with that. What may have been perceived a generation ago as "lack of professional dedication" when a female physician wanted to be home to go to her child's school program is now understood as a working mother's reasonable request. When we share experiences, it is much easier for us to accept and understand each other's needs. The tradeoffs here are more potential than absolute. The patient's loss of reverence for the profession of medicine need not mean a loss of respect for the physician as a professional and individual. That is determined by the physician-patient relationship, which is the responsibility of the individual physician to develop and nurture. A trusting relationship of mutual respect is certainly good for both patient and physician—it's good for patient care and allows the physician to expect and have a personal life as fulfilling as any other profession—a major "plus," particularly for the female physician trying to "have it all."

In summary, balancing professional and personal life for the female physician is probably more achievable now than at any time in history and promises to become increasingly more so in the future. Changes in the structure and delivery of medicine will allow for this but perhaps at the price of less patient-doctor intimacy. This has happened without regard to the role of women in medicine but it is something from which women trying to integrate family and profession will benefit. As long as patient care is not compromised, this can work to the benefit of all involved as long as both sides realize that there will be tradeoffs and are willing to accept them.

What Impact Have Women Physicians Had on Women's Health?

by Judith Lorber, PhD

The proportion of women in medicine in the United States is approaching that of men, but women physicians are still the minority in positions of power. Research has shown that women physicians order more preventive tests for women patients, are more attuned to patients' psychosocial needs, and have developed more patient-oriented communication styles than men physicians. Recent organized efforts of women physicians have brought attention to many gender gaps in medical research and practice. If more women move into policy-making positions, especially in education and research, their gender-sensitive perspective could permanently influence the profession as a whole.

Women have been entering medical schools in the United States in greater numbers since the 1960s. In the last decade, women have even outnumbered men in some medical school classes, including at Harvard. As in other countries where the proportion of women physicians is growing, it may be time to assess the impact women physicians have had on US medicine. Has their presence made a difference in women's health care, or have they assimilated men's biases and perspectives? What effect have women physicians' organizations had? What is the future role of women in American medicine?

Is Medicine Turning into Women's Work?

The changing structure of medical practice in countries with medical systems once dominated by men has led to an influx of women into medicine. In the United States before World War II, physicians were usually solo, fee-for-service practitioners with sole authority over their patients. Since 1945, medicine has been subject to more regulation and has been paid for by governments and an expanding insurance industry. As doctors' authority has been diluted and their income decreased, fewer white men have applied to medical school, leaving an occupational niche for women and nonwhite men, similar to what has happened in other desegregating occupations. Despite their increasing numbers, however, women physicians are not equitably represented in medical leadership. They are not usually mentored by senior men physicians for positions of authority in medical schools and research centers, and their rate of promotion in medical schools tends to be slower than that of men.

The structure of work and family life has not allowed women physicians with family responsibilities to add extensive administrative responsibilities or committee work to the time they spend with patients. Women physicians who remain single or enter into childless dual-career marriages could be formidable competitors for men with homemaker wives, but there is still a glass ceiling on how far women can rise in positions of authority.

As a result, the top positions in large medical centers, medical schools, and research centers are still predominantly held by men. These institutions develop medical knowledge, decide what medical students are taught, and determine practice standards for diagnosis and treatment. Because women are underrepresented in high-level positions as chiefs of service in hospitals, deans of medical schools, or directors of large research centers, they have yet to make much impact on the production and dissemination of medical knowledge and standards of practice. I believe that where they themselves are in control—in their own practices—they have made a difference for women patients.

Are Women Physicians Better for Women Patients?

Referral rates for breast and cervical cancer screening seem to depend on the gender of the doctor. Studies including thousands of patients in the United States have found large, statistically significant differences in the rate at which women and men physicians recommend these tests.

Even though coronary heart disease is the major cause of death for women in the United States, they are less likely than men to be routinely tested for cardiovascular symptoms and more likely to suffer unrecognized heart attacks. Women with severe symptoms are not as likely as men with lesser symptoms to be given coronary arteriography, catheterization, or bypass surgery. As a result, they are more likely to die of myocardial infarction than men of the same age, and the postoperative mortality rate for coronary artery bypass surgery has been found to be significantly higher in women than men.

In order to address problems like these, Bernadine Healy, MD, as director of the National Institutes of Health, established an Office of Research on Women's Health and began the Women's Health Initiative. The WHI not only studies the illnesses that affect women alone, but also looks at previously neglected gender differences in illnesses that affect women and men, such as acquired immune deficiency syndrome (AIDS).

Do Women Physicians Have More Caring Practice Styles?

Today, men and women physicians both say they have to understand their patients' daily lives, work and family roles, and emotional needs to adequately treat them for physical illness, but patients claim that women physicians are more "humane." Women physicians may act differently toward patients, or patients may feel they are less intimidating and so can be asked more questions and argued with. Women physicians tend to encourage patients to participate by asking what they expect and think—and by listening to their answers. They talk more to their patients, but, more important, allow patients to talk more as well, especially about personal and family issues. A study that found little difference in verbal communication between men and women physicians also found that women physicians' nonverbal communication styles were more supportive than those of men physicians. In comparing patients' behavior, they found that both men and women patients spoke more to women physicians, and that women patients offered more medical information to women than to men physicians. The women physicians encouraged their women patients' narratives with supportive statements, "uh-huhs," and nodding. In contrast, the women physicians' interactions with men patients, who were usually older than they were, showed evidence of tension and role strain.

In another study, 45 lesbians, half of whom were women of color, were more likely to evaluate men physicians negatively than they were women physicians. These patients wanted knowledge that would enable them to promote and maintain their own health and well-being, and they also appreciated being involved in the diagnosis and decisions about treatment.

The overall thrust of these studies of doctor-patient relationships in the United States, where seeing a woman doctor is a relatively new phenomenon for older patients, is that women physicians present themselves to patients as warm and supportive, which may be at odds with the expected image of authority and competence.

Because so many women physicians are in primary care, patients come to them with all their problems— major and minor illnesses, physical and emotional symptoms. There is a danger, then, that women will become "the de facto psychosocial experts in the care of patients and increasingly assume responsibility for the management of emotionally distressed patients." This expertise can have a backlash; patients may be more dissatisfied with their care if a woman doctor does not live up to their expectations.

Physicians of either gender in office practice generally prefer patients who allow them to carry out their work with a minimum of fuss and who are cooperative, trusting, appreciative, and responsive to treatment. In one study, however, more women than men physicians said they liked their patients. The differences patients perceive between men and women physicians may be a self-fulfilling prophecy. If patients think women physicians are more empathic, the women may cultivate an expressive style to meet patients' expectations. Women physicians may or may not be more attuned to the "whole patient" because they are women, but if patients think they are, they may prefer a woman physician, especially for primary care. Doctors in group practice or clinic settings, however, have a fixed time to spend with patients. They are usually not in a position to structure their delivery of health care to be sensitive to patients unless they are in their own solo or small group practices.

In sum, where they are in control of their work, women physicians have had a positive impact on women's health care through more extensive screening for life-threatening illnesses and through practice styles that are sensitive to patients' social and psychological problems.

Have Women Physicians Transformed Medicine?

In the 1970s in the United States, activists in the feminist health movement established client-run clinics for women patients that stressed education in health matters,

gynecological self-examination, and alternative therapies. Their goal was to take the control of women's bodies out of what they saw as an oppressive medical system. The problem women patients faced, according to the ideas of the feminist health movement, was twofold: men physicians who allowed patients very little control over their own care, and medical research and practices that ignored many of women's needs.

Although the directors of feminist clinics preferred women physicians for their legally required medical backup, they were not trusted any more than men physicians because both had been trained in the masculinist medical curriculum. The activists in the feminist health movement thought that by educating women patients to be more assertive and knowledgeable health consumers, they would put pressure on the medical system to modify the way physicians were taught to practice. The feminist health movement, the influx of women physicians into obstetrics/gynecology, and the presence of mid-wives in hospital settings did change how pelvic examinations were done and made childbirth more participatory and family-oriented. But medicine in general continued to be insensitive to gender issues.

Much of the feminist health movement's critical thrust had been abandoned by the 1990s, but it left a heritage of clinics and managed care centers that offer woman-centered family practices and obstetrics/gynecology, often provided by women physicians. The consumer movement in health care has also enormously strengthened all patients' rights to question their care.

Have these individual assets coalesced into an impact on medicine as a whole?

The greater number of women physicians has tilted the gender balance; women are no longer a minority vulnerable to stereotyping and informal discrimination, but a visible, vocal, and increasingly powerful group. Numbers alone have not made the difference, however. Organizing *as* women professionals and *for* women patients has been equally important. The arguments over whether women physicians should form a separate "interest bloc" and whether women's health should be a separate specialty seem to have evolved into a strategy of wide-ranging woman-centered medicine.

In the last few years, women physicians in the United States have promoted research and held conferences on women's medical needs and insisted that trials of new drugs include women. A workshop held in 1997 called for participatory research based on "women's experience, both of their physiology and of their psychosocial, home, and work environments." Women physicians have called attention to the particular needs of lesbians and women with AIDS and disabilities, and to such human rights issues as female genital mutilation and politically motivated rape.

If women physicians are to make a transformative impact, their specialized knowledge of women's medical needs has to become part of medical school curricula, and their patient-oriented perspective has to be routinely incorporated into teaching and training. In addition, the gender-sensitive perspective developed in women's health care conferences and journals needs to become part of mainstream medical thinking and include men's gender-based risks and traumas as well. Making such an impact takes the authority, prestige, and resources held only by heads of medical institutions. When women are equal to men in these positions as well as in clinical practice, I predict that the differences women have made in their own practices, through their own medical organizations, and in their research and publications will be seen throughout the profession.

References

A list of references is available in the original source.

Confronting the Myths
Can America Halt the Slide Toward Health Care Meltdown?
by Bob LeBow, MD, MPH

Rigoberto sat nervously on the edge of the exam table and broke into tears. A large and reserved 17-year-old, he had asthma and a nasty cough that hadn't improved in two weeks. I was about to prescribe an inhaler and antibiotics. "What's wrong?" I asked. He glanced at his mother. "On our way here, I found out we didn't have money to pay for the visit," he said, wiping his eyes with the back of his hand.

I reassured him that, since we were a community health center, money wasn't a problem. I forewarned our pharmacy to give him the prescriptions without pressing for payment. But after I left the exam room, our collections person entered and politely asked for eight dollars, our "nominal" fee. Mother and son broke into tears of embarrassment and left without the medications.

American health care is once again at a "crossroads," one of several windows of opportunity for change that we have had over the past 90 years. The last "opportunity moment" in American health care—marked by President Clinton's ill-fated and ill-conceived "managed-competition" proposal—ended in 1994 with the collapse of his plan. Since then, we have had a vacuum in leadership and direction. "Market" principles and the pursuit of profit have become the norm for health care. Cost shifting from employers to employees has accelerated, and access to care has become more difficult. The number of uninsured Americans has grown and now, with the economic downturn, is increasing even more.

America's brief "managed-care revolution," with its temporary slowing of some health care costs, is dead. The American public would no longer put up with being exploited and abused by managed-care organizations. As for the uninsured, their situation has only become worse.

As we approach this new crossroads for health care, our system is failing and in imminent danger of collapse or "meltdown." Fortunately, for the moment, the system is still capable of meeting the health care needs of many who find themselves in a crisis. We have wonderful technology. There are thousands of dedicated and caring clinicians and others who try their best to help people in need. But more and more the needs of people are not being met. The number of Americans without adequate access to care is growing. More and more, Americans are delaying care or going without needed services. They show up at a crisis stage in increasingly beleaguered emergency rooms.

Hospitals are overcrowded and understaffed. Over 90 percent of our nursing homes have an inadequate number of nurses. Ambulances circle around waiting for an open spot at an emergency room. Medical errors happen much too frequently. Costs are soaring. Patient expectations are soaring too, as new technologies and drugs become available. Waste abounds as money that could be used for patient care is instead diverted to pay for higher administrative costs that are a result of the increasing (and unnecessary) complexity and "gaming" of our system. Our federal programs, Medicare and Medicaid, are endangered. There is no planning, no vision for the future, as our nonsystem seems to be imploding.

Millions of Americans, the 40+ million without health insurance, have been deprived of their dignity, and we're in danger of losing our dignity as a nation. America is the only developed nation that fails to guarantee access to needed care for all its citizens and the only advanced country that permits someone to go bankrupt because of poor health. Even Americans who have health insurance are increasingly being squeezed or sometimes forced to forego care, as depicted somewhat melodramatically in the recent movie "John Q." A survey done at the end of 2001 showed that 43 percent of Americans with private insurance feared that their family's insurance coverage might be eliminated or reduced in the next year.

Millions of Americans have become "health care beggars." Millions more, including middle-class Americans, are at risk of joining them as beggars in the near future as the cost of health care soars.

Our Poor Performance and Perverse Incentives

Despite our standing as the richest country in the world—and despite our spending nearly twice as much per person on health care than any other country—the overall results have been disappointing, dehumanizing, and at times even abysmal. Our health status indicators rank us near the bottom among the developed countries in such measures as life expectancy and infant mortality. In 2000 the World Health Organization ranked the U.S. health care system at number 37 overall.

Meanwhile, our population grows more obese and sedentary. Substance abuse continues at a high rate.

Failure to deal adequately with mental health has contributed to our burgeoning prison population. And debt from health care is now the second highest reason for personal bankruptcy. The pursuit of profit has assumed primacy over the pursuit of what is best for people.

Why the disconnect? Where have we failed? Does anybody care?

Our health care system—or, more precisely, nonsystem—has evolved into a monster, a disorganized, overly complex creature that robs people of their health, their money and their dignity. Yet the great majority of Americans are unaware—or clueless—of what has happened to America's health care. Blind belief in certain icons of American economic theory—icons that have limited relevance to health care—have helped cause our current dilemma.

Faith in "the market" and competition, stress on "personal responsibility" and individualism, and dislike of government regulation or managed anything have contributed to the creation of a system which turns a blind eye to millions of patients like Rigoberto who "do without." We Americans live in a milieu of purposeful health care ignorance. Merchants of misinformation and myth spend millions of dollars to keep us clueless. By doing so, they limit improvements in our health care system to piecemeal bits of change. Remember Harry and Louise? The bus from Canada? Citizens for a Better Medicare? They're only a few of the scams perpetrated on the American public by the vested interests. By delaying or averting a comprehensive solution, the health care entrepreneurs prolong the time they are able to reap profits from the system. Profits they keep for themselves and their shareholders while my patients, and millions more like them, are forced to become "health care beggars" or "go without."

A large part of our problem stems from the perverse incentives of the system. For much too long, America's health care system has been driven (on the supply side) by self-interest. Instead of commitment to community and cooperation, the overriding ethic of health care in America has become self-interest and the pursuit of profit. The American people have been left out of the equation. Even worse, they have been systematically duped and then blamed for being "overutilizers" by some of the same special-interest groups that misled them. Americans are told to exercise more "personal responsibility," a code word for shifting costs to the consumer. But they have been set up by the health care industry (insurers, drug companies, medical establishment) to have high expectations and to create a demand for expensive goods and services. As for the people who can't afford the expensive services, they don't matter. There are no profits to be made from the poor, unless they can qualify for a government program that will pay their bills.

The Search for a Comprehensive Solution

An interest in universal coverage once again seems to be growing, though it appears to be morphing into a less ambitious goal of "reducing the number" of the uninsured. Some of the factors creating pressure for health care reform include an economic recession, a growing unemployment rate, and the accelerating costs of health care. Health insurance premium rates rose by 11 percent in 2001 and are expected to rise 15 percent in 2002. The events of 9/11 also may have reawakened some sense of community in America as well as a questioning of the axiom that less government is always better. There is also a growing sense of despair from the ever-increasing number of Americans who are hurting from being *under*insured. Including the 40 million uninsured Americans, we are reaching perhaps a critical mass of people, a total of maybe as many as 90 million (not even including Medicare beneficiaries), who need help. With the growing number of people in distress, including many more middle-class Americans, there is bound to be a more strident demand for change.

Groups (such as the insurance industry, the pharmaceutical companies, and some elements of the medical care establishment) with special financial interests in our health care system will likely continue to play games of disinformation to derail significant change. And they will twist the mantra of "personal responsibility" to make people believe that financial barriers to care, like increased deductibles and co-pays, are good for them. They will invoke the "mantra" of "socialized medicine" to attack any increased role for government. Yet government needs to have a role—at the very least in oversight, coordination, and leadership—if we are to fix our failing health care system.

We are hearing increasingly about incremental or "piecemeal" reforms, about vouchers, tax credits, medical savings accounts, and "defined contributions" from employers. There are now a plethora of ideas about how to "cover more Americans." Most of them are complex, and some experts argue that we may have to make our system more complex than it already is. But people who have been working within the system, and who appreciate the abuses and loss of dignity suffered by so many Americans seeking adequate health care, know these "piecemeal" solutions will only prolong the agony and maintain the status quo. And the status quo has become increasingly intolerable as our system heads toward meltdown.

Getting America Clued In

I've written this book in an effort to shed light on the degree of cluelessness that permeates American health care. I have attempted to use my 30 years of experience working within a dysfunctional health system and my efforts as a health care activist to sort out the realities and the myths. I am concerned that the "piecemeal" direction in which we seem to be headed will not help my patients or the millions of other Americans who are likely to join their ranks as "health care beggars." I worry that even friendly allies who advocate for "doing something" will compromise the chances for millions of Americans to get the health care they need. If even a few million Americans are left hanging in limbo, our nation will not have regained its dignity.

I have not included lengthy economic analyses. Instead, I have provided a selective bibliography that readers can refer to for more detailed information. I have tried to concentrate on an analysis of the key issues that we must address to achieve meaningful reform. I have also attempted to provide an ad hoc type of road map for reaching the goal. Some of the principal themes that I address in this book include:

- The high degree of misinformation and myth that has been intentionally used by what I have termed the "modern-day snake oil merchants" to hawk their products and discredit system changes that might limit their influence or profits.
- The twisted "market" model as it has been applied to health care. How, instead of putting the customer first, it has in fact put the patient last.
- How the "personal responsibility" mantra and co-pays/deductibles act as barriers to care and are used to "blame the victims" and shift cost or increase profits.
- How we need to think more in terms of societal or community responsibility.
- A smattering of real patient experiences: misadventures of the uninsured and the underinsured. (All the names have been changed.)
- How Americans have missed the boat on prevention and what we must do about it.
- Affordability, and the poor value we get for our health care investment in America, especially compared to other developed nations.
- What direction do we need to take at this crossroads? How can we arrive at a solution that is really universal and affordable and provides *everyone* with the health care they need?
- The importance of "one risk pool"—and not lip service to "pluralism"—in reaching a universal

coverage that is fair and affordable and does not exclude the sick.

- Some humility in admitting that health care alone cannot give America good health, that it takes a wider approach involving social and economic change, including efforts at prevention, to reach good health.
- That Health Care for All is a key first step in returning dignity to individuals, families, and our nation, and that, without it, we will be unable to resolve the gaping health disparities that we have in America today.

"One Risk Pool"/National Health Insurance

I believe that unless America chooses a solution that incorporates the concept of "one risk pool," such as national health insurance, we will never solve our dilemma. Former Senator Bob Kerry expressed his support for this approach when he testified before the Senate Finance committee in March 2002. He advised against adding a prescription drug benefit to Medicare—"not unless you are prepared to make fundamental changes in the way Americans finance the cost of their health care." He went on to assert:

> "Beginning with a universal entitlement does not mean higher spending or more governmental interference with the choices made by patients or providers. In truth, it could mean a lot less of both. It would mean that we would start thinking about ourselves as a single group of 280 million Americans who are all part of the same health system and who all need to face the challenge of matching our appetite for quality with our capacity to pay."

Perhaps there are solutions other than national health insurance—or its equivalent—for America to achieve universal coverage in a way that is both comprehensive and affordable. It's possible that we could model a solution after approaches adopted by some European countries and express the goal as "assuring universal access to care for all needed medical services." However, as described in the chapters that follow, it is difficult to imagine how there could be a fairer, more efficient approach than "one risk pool" that would truly cover *every* person in America. The type of solution envisaged in this book is embodied in this concept. "One risk pool" is virtually synonymous with what is referred to as a "single-payer" approach, though they are not precisely the same since "one risk pool" refers more to the group of people covered as opposed to a payment mechanism.

Under "one risk pool" everybody in America would be covered in the same health insurance plan. There would be no questions about enrollment or eligibility. Since the largest possible number of people would be "pooled together," there would be economies of scale. There would be no more "cherry-picking," no more excluding of the poor or the sick from access to needed care. No one would go bankrupt because of medical bills. Savings from the elimination of middlemen and other administrative costs would allow every person coverage with a comprehensive package of benefits without increasing our overall spending on health care.

Instead of premiums, co-pays, and deductibles, the plan would be funded through progressive taxation and would have a trust fund specifically devoted to the plan, much like today's Medicare. There would be a larger government role in collecting the taxes and overseeing the plan. But the delivery system would remain predominantly private, as it is today. Each person would be able to choose any provider of services he or she chose, in effect *increasing* choice. "One risk pool" refers to the financing mechanism only, has no direct effect on the delivery system, and does not in any way diminish the role of the private sector in providing health care. It is not socialized medicine. It is a way to minimize administrative costs and create equity.

The general principles that comprise this approach, which would in effect be a form of national health insurance, include the following:

- True universality. Everybody in, nobody out, with one risk pool. No more "cherry-picking," or exclusion of high-risk people from coverage.
- Tax-based financing, like Medicare, in accordance with income, instead of premiums, deductibles, and co-pays. *Not* free care, since everybody pays into the system through taxes.
- Full choice of providers in a delivery system that remains a mix of private and public. *Not* socialized medicine, but national health insurance in the same way Medicare is a national insurance program.
- Elimination of the odd link between employers and health insurance coverage.
- Coverage for all necessary services, including inpatient and outpatient care, emergency care, long-term care, mental health, treatment for substance abuse, prescriptions, and basic dental and eye care with no discrimination by type of illness or ability to pay.
- True integration of public health and preventive services with adequate funding, both on a personal and community basis.

- Continued funding for the special services necessary to serve special population groups; e.g., immigrants, migrant farm workers, and the disabled.
- The practice of medicine based on scientific principles.
- A national trust fund dedicated specifically to health care.
- National planning that allows a high degree of local autonomy. A national health board with regional or state-by-state equivalents.
- Public accountability. Eliminates the "opaque" (hard to fathom) financing practices of the current system.

- Global budgeting, which entails setting priorities, but is flexible enough to support medical education, research, and excellence in medicine.
- Simplified administration with greatly reduced administrative costs, leaving 90-95 percent of health care funds for patient care, prevention, and research.
- Reasonable and equitable reimbursement for health care providers.
- Insurance companies would be allowed to sell policies only for uncovered services.
- Treatment of health as a "public good" instead of as a market commodity.

Scientific Terms Explained

by Adriane Fugh-Berman, MD

Some of the terms you'll come across repeatedly in this book may be unfamiliar to you. It's worth learning them, since they're universally used to explain the results of scientific experiments. and knowing them will not only help you read this book but will stand you in good stead when you read about scientific experiments elsewhere.

Fortunately, scientific terminology isn't hard to learn. That doesn't mean you're going to remember every single term after reading this chapter once. Just let whatever sticks in your mind stick, and ignore the rest. Then, when you encounter a term you're not sure about, refer back to this chapter, or look it up in the index. (I've boldfaced the terms where they're defined in this chapter, to make them easy to find.)

Study is a very broad term that covers almost everything that's looked at objectively. A human participant in a study—that is, one of the people whose responses, reactions or whatever are being studied—is called a **subject.**

A **case study** is a report on one unusual subject by a doctor. Both case studies and stories patients report themselves are called **anecdotal evidence.** Doctors joke that if we see two cases, we say we're seeing something "time after time," and if we see three cases, we call it a

case series. Joking aside, a case series should consist of at least five cases. Case series are useful for indicating that something interesting is going on that may merit more formal study.

A **survey** is a kind of study that reports the results of interviewing people on whom no **intervention** is done. (Compare *trial,* below.) Since nothing new—no new drug, procedure, dietary restriction or whatever—is given to them or done to them, we say surveys are **observational.** Like the three studies cited in the *Introduction,* surveys simply try to discover how common a disease, treatment. condition or behavior is—or what **correlations,** or **associations,** there may be between various diseases, behaviors, etc. (There's a subtle distinction between a *correlation* and an *association* that isn't worth going into here.)

A **positive correlation** means that the more you have of A, the more you have of B. A **negative** (or **inverse**) **correlation** means that the more you have of A, the *less* you have of B. So, for example, there's a positive correlation between a high-fat diet and heart disease (the more fat you eat, the greater your chance of getting heart disease), and a negative correlation between eating broccoli and getting certain cancers (the more broccoli you eat, the smaller your chance of getting these cancers).

Correlations can't prove anything absolutely. For example, just because an increased number of storks in an area coincides with an increased number of births, that doesn't prove that storks bring babies.

How many people have a given condition at a given point in time is called its **prevalence** (for example, the number of color-blind people per 100,000 in the US today, or the number of people who were carrying tuberculosis bacteria on January 1, 1900). How many new cases of a condition occur over a given period of time is called its **incidence** (for example, the number of babies born in a given year who are color-blind, or the number of new TB cases in the last month). The study of prevalence and incidence falls into the field of **epidemiology,** which looks at patterns of disease and the factors that influence those patterns.

A **retrospective study** looks to the past for clues—you start with the disease and try to find out what caused it. For example, retrospective studies found that the prevalence of cigarette smoking among patients with lung cancer was higher than the prevalence of cigarette smoking among people without lung cancer. (Since you can't intervene in the past, all retrospective studies are observational.)

Retrospective studies can be large or small. To improve their quality, the **case-control** method is often used. This means that, when comparing a group with the disease to a group without it, the two groups are matched as closely as possible with regard to factors like age, sex, geographic location or any other variable that might affect the likelihood of getting the disease. The perfect case-control study would be of a group of identical twins where one twin in each pair developed a disease and the other twin in each pair didn't.

A **prospective study** is one in which subjects are followed forward in time instead of backward. Unlike retrospective studies, prospective studies can be either observational or interventional. Two famous prospective trials are the Nurses' Health Study, in which about 100,000 nurses have been answering annual questionnaires since 1976, and the Health Professionals Follow-up Study, in which about 50,000 physicians and other health professionals have been answering annual questionnaires since 1986.

By analyzing their responses, many associations have been discovered, including the positive correlation between hormone replacement therapy and breast cancer (that is, hormone replacement tends to increase one's risk of getting breast cancer) and the negative correlation between vitamin E intake and cardiovascular disease (that is, taking E tends to decrease heart disease risk).

Unlike a survey, a **trial** is a study in which the subjects receive an experimental intervention. Since you can only intervene in the present, not in the past, trials are always prospective. A **clinical trial** is one in which the subjects are human—as opposed to **preclinical trials** that use animals, bacteria, cells, etc.

In a **controlled trial,** at least two groups are compared. The **treated,** or **experimental** group receives the intervention, while the other—called the **control group** or simply the **control**—doesn't. Or different groups may receive different interventions. The groups studied in a trial are also called **arms.**

In a **placebo-controlled** trial, an inactive pill or procedure—the **placebo**—is given to the control group. *Placebo* is Latin for *I will please [you];* placebos got that name because any intervention, including simple attention, tends to make people feel better. Certain conditions, such as headaches, arthritis and hot flashes, are particularly responsive to placebos—as are some individuals.

Overall, the average **placebo effect** is an astonishing 33% (although it can range from much lower to much higher). In other words, an average of a third of the subjects in clinical trials will report significant improvement simply from being given a sugar pill (or some other placebo). So to demonstrate that a treatment works, you have to show that it does significantly better than the placebo that's given to the control group.

A **randomized** trial is one in which subjects are assigned to different groups as randomly as possible—by flipping a coin, or using a random number generator. If the researcher decides which subjects go into which group, or if the subjects assign themselves, intentional or unintentional **bias** can creep in and the groups may no longer be comparable (all the sicker patients might end up in one group, for example).

A **crossover** trial is one in which each patient is in each group at different times. For example, group A starts on drug X, and group B starts on the placebo; then, midway through the trial, the subjects are crossed over to the other arm (group A starts taking the placebo and group B starts taking the drug).

Blinding (sometimes, but less frequently, called **masking**) means that the researchers and/or the subjects don't know which group each subject is in. In a **single-blind** study, the subjects don't know but the researchers do (theoretically, it could also mean that the subjects know and the researchers don't, but there wouldn't be much point to that). Most nonsurgical studies are at least single-blind, since subjects' knowing whether they're getting an experimental treatment or a placebo is obviously likely to affect their responses.

In a **double-blind** study, neither the researchers nor the subjects know which group the subjects are in; all information is coded, and the code isn't broken until the end of the trial. (An exception is made when the difference between the two groups is so pronounced—

everyone in the control group is dying, say, and everyone in the treated group is getting well—that it would be un-ethical to continue to deny the treatment to the controls.)

Double-blinding is important because researchers can give subtle, unconscious cues that can change sub-jects' responses quite independently of the treatment being tested. If the researchers don't know who's getting the treatment and who's getting the placebo, they can't put out those signals.

Saying that a treatment worked in 50% of the sub-jects tested obviously means a lot more if you're talking about 2000 subjects than if you're talking about two. So a good researcher involves statisticians before a trial be-gins in order to determine the **sample size** (the number of subjects) that will be necessary to show that the re-sults are **statistically significant**—that is, unlikely to be due to chance.

Statistical significance isn't black and white; it's a matter of degree—what are the *odds* that this result was due to chance? It's measured by something called the **p value** (the *p* stands for *probability*). P values look like this: <.1, <.05, <.01, etc. (< means *less than*). To trans-late a p value into English, move the decimal point two spaces to the right and say "percent."

A p value of <.01 means that the probability that the results occurred by chance is less than 1%. That's a good study. A p value of <.1 means that the probability that the results occurred by chance is less than 10%. That isn't so great, since it means that there's almost one chance in ten that the results are meaningless. In general, a p value of <.05 is considered statistically significant.

A large sample size helps to control for **confound-ing variables** (also called **confounding factors** or sim-ply **confounders**). For example, a small trial on cardio-vascular disease might happen to have a larger number of smokers in one group than the other. In this case, smoking would be a confounding variable, since it's known to cause cardiovascular disease.

If the sample size is large enough, however, one can assume that known—and unknown—confounders will be evenly distributed between the groups. To see why this is, imagine flipping a coin. If you flip it ten times, there's a reasonable chance it will come up heads 70% of the time (7 heads, 3 tails). If you flip it a thousand times, there's almost no chance it will come up heads 70% of the time (700 heads, 300 tails).

To put all this together—the gold standard for med-ical research is a prospective, randomized, double-blind, placebo-controlled trial with a sample size large enough to produce a p value of <.05 or lower. Many of the stud-ies in this book don't achieve that standard—but then neither do most of the studies behind conventional med-ical therapies. If I limited the studies cited here to ones

that meet that standard, this wouldn't be a book but an article . . . a short article.

Still, it's useful to know what the gold standard is, because everything—including trials of conventional medical therapies—should be held up to it. (Studies that don't meet the standard aren't necessarily wrong, but they're not proof. Future trials should adhere to the gold standard as much as possible.)

There are just a few more terms you should know. A **meta-analysis** is a relatively new kind of study in which you combine the results from a number of selected trials in order to come to some general conclusions. Meta-analyses are usually done when a number of small trials give ambiguous, conflicting or statistically insignificant results. When all of the decent trials are combined, there may be enough subjects in the combined treatment group to reach a statistically significant conclusion.

Let's say we're doing a survey of weights in a tiny village that has just eleven inhabitants. There are five children, who weigh 40, 50, 65, 65 and 65 lbs (the last three are triplets); three women, who weigh 105, 110 and 125 lbs; and three men, who weigh 150, 160 and 840 lbs (this last guy has a hormonal disorder).

If we add up all the weights, we get 1780 lbs; if we divide that by 11, we get 162 lbs. This is the **mean**—it's what we're talking about when we use the word *average* in everyday speech. But it would be very misleading to say that the average person in this village weighs 162 lbs, since all but one of the inhabitants weigh less than that. To deal with situations like this, statisticians have come up with two other kinds of averages—the median and the mode.

The **median** is the value in the middle of the distribution—the one halfway between the bottom and the top. In this particular example, the median—105 lbs—gives a much better idea of the average weight than the mean does.

The **mode** is the value that occurs most frequently; in this example, it would be 65 lbs (the triplets). In some distributions, the mode is a better indication of what's representative than either the mean or the median.

The **FDA** (the Food and Drug Administration, a regulatory agency of the federal government) requires specific kinds of trials on human subjects before it will approve new drugs. (Animal studies and the like have typically been done before these trials take place.) A **Phase I** trial simply tests for safety; it's usually done on healthy volunteers, without a control group.

In a **Phase II** trial, the drug is given to people with the condition or disease to be treated; it supplies some preliminary data on whether the treatment works, and supplements the safety data of the Phase I trial. Phase II trials may or may not use a control group.

A **Phase III** trial assesses efficacy, safety and dosage, compared with standard treatments or a placebo. Phase III trials are usually randomized and controlled.

Phase I, II, and III trials are usually performed as part of an **IND** (an *investigational new drug* application to the FDA). After the Phase III trial is completed, the manufacturer can submit an **NDA** (a *new drug application*) which requests permission to market the drug.

Not routinely required, **Phase IV** studies are done after drugs are approved by the FDA and can be sold to the public. They're randomized trials or surveys that attempt to evaluate longterm benefits and risks.

Finally, **in vitro** (literally, "in glass") refers to studies done in artificial environments like test tubes, and **in vivo** to studies done in living organisms.

Evaluating Online Health Information

by Kiki Zeldes

While the Internet offers a wealth of material on many different aspects of women's health, the quality of the information varies greatly. When you visit a website, it's important to consider the source of the information and to critically view any material you find. Remember that anyone can create a site and put up any content he or she wants. Some sites push dubious medicine, both Western and alternative; some are concerned only with selling you their products; and some sites (as well as research studies) are biased by the drug companies, professional societies, and other advertisers who support them.

Separating questionable or misleading information from accurate and reliable material can sometimes be daunting. Below are some questions to ask to help yourself evaluate the quality of the health information you find.

1. **Who developed and maintains the site?**
   Any good health-related site should make it easy for you to learn who is responsible for the site and its content. Sites are run by government offices, universities, pharmaceutical and other private companies, nonprofit organizations, practitioners, and individuals.

2. **Who pays for the site?**
   It costs money to run a website. Although some sites are labors of love, most have an outside source of funds and this should be clearly presented on the site. How does the site pay for its existence? Does it sell advertising? Does it sell products or services? Is

it sponsored by a drug company? Is it funded through grants or donations? The source of funding can affect what content is presented, how the content is presented, and what the site owners want to accomplish on the site. Try to figure out if the author(s) or site owner(s) has a financial interest or anything else to gain from proposing one particular point of view over another.

3. **Who is the author of the particular material you're reading?**
   The authors and contributors of all content should be clearly identified. Often information posted is collected from other websites or from offline sources. If the person or organization in charge of the site did not create the information, the original source should be clearly labeled.

4. **What is the basis of the information on the site?**
   In addition to identifying who wrote the material you are reading, the evidence that material is based on should be provided. Medical facts and figures should have references, and opinions or advice should be clearly labeled as such and set apart from information that is "evidence-based" (that is, based on research results).

5. **Is the material dated?**
   All content should be dated, so you can tell when the material was written, when it was posted, and when it was last revised.

6. **Does the information sound too good to be true?**
   Be wary of "cures" for incurable diseases. Question sites that credit themselves as the sole source of in-

formation on a topic as well as sites that disrespect other sources of knowledge.

7. **Do sites that ask you for personal information have a privacy policy?**

   Make sure your information won't be shared by others without your permission.

8. **Is there a way to contact the site?**

   There should be a way for you to contact the site owners with problems, feedback, and questions, and someone should respond to your messages in a timely way. If the site hosts chat rooms or other online discussion areas, it should tell visitors what the terms of using this service are. If a site is moderated, you should be able to find out who the moderator is and how he or she was chosen.

Some of the information above was taken from the following sources: *Health Information on the Internet,* an American Association of Retired Persons (AARP) brochure, and *10 Things to Know about Evaluating Medical Resources on the Web,* a brochure from the National Cancer Institute.

Below are some additional resources to help you evaluate the quality of online health information.

Using Health Information on the Internet A well-written, clear and extensive guide to evaluating health information from Canadian Health Network.

The Good, The Bad & The Ugly: or, Why It's a Good Idea to Evaluate Web Sources Evaluation criteria from a New Mexico State University reference librarian.

Health Information on the Internet: How to Get the "Right Stuff" From NOAH, New York Online Access to Health.

How to Evaluate Media Reports about Health Research Fact sheet from Breast Cancer InfoLink.

How to Find Medical Information Tips from the Federal Consumer Information Center.

Taking Charge of Health Information A consumer's guide created by the Center for Risk Analysis at the Harvard School of Public Health.

Tips for Health Consumers: Finding Quality Health Information on the Internet. Online article by the Internet Healthcare Coalition.

The QUICK (Quality Information Checklist) checklist Great resource to help kids evaluate the information they find on the Internet.

WORKSHEET—CHAPTER 1
Women and the Health Care System

1. The 1979 classic article "Sexism in Women's Medical Care" sets the scene for discussions on how sexism impacts women's health and the field of medicine. Using this article, identify at least two things which you feel have improved significantly since 1979 and identify two things which you feel still need to be improved:

have improved since 1979	still need to improve

2. Describe your "best" and "worst" health care experiences. Briefly, identify the behaviors (or other characteristics) which were different for you and the health providers in the two situations. Referring to "How to Tell Your Doctor a Thing or Two," can you identify ways that you were or were not an "active patient" in the two situations?

3. Building on information in several articles, describe how the gynecological exam becomes symbolic of the consumer-health practitioner relationship and identify things every woman should be able to expect as a part of a good gynecological exam.

4. Outline both sides of the debate on the question, "Will increasing the number of women doctors increase the quality of care which women receive as health care consumers?"

yes

no

5. You have been asked to rewrite the article, "Women in Medicine" as an article on "Women in the Health System." You have been asked to be more inclusive in thinking of how race, class, sexual identity, ageism, and disability issues impact on the issue of balancing work and family. Identify several points you would want to make.

6. Choose one article on women's health from a Web-site. Print it out to attach to this worksheet. Evaluate the article based on the guidelines in "Evaluating On-Line Health Information."

7. The Ruzek and Becker article, "The Women's Health Movement in the US," identifies different philosophies and priorities of grass-roots and professionalized women's health organizations. Briefly summarize information from the articles on the chart below and identify your own values/visions on each topic.

Topic	Grass-roots Organizations	Professionalized Organizations	My View
1. Social Movement Orientation			
2. Leadership			
3. Attitude Toward Biomedicine			
4. Relationship With Corporate Sponsors			
5. Goal of Education			
6. Lay versus Professional Authority			

CHAPTER 2

Inequalities and Health

A core part of developing an analysis of women's health issues is working towards an understanding of why "some women have a better chance of being healthy than other women." This involves learning how racism, anti-Semitism, poverty, homophobia, ageism, attitudes towards disabilities, fatphobia, and other forms of oppression: multiply the effects of sexism; impact on women's mental and physical health; affect access to the determinants of health (such as good nutrition, pollution-free environment, housing, education, rewards for employment); influence or determine one's access to the health system; impact the cultural appropriateness of the health system if one has access to it, and whether or not one's group is appropriately and respectfully represented in research on women's health issues. Articles in this chapter are chosen to stimulate dialogue on this complex topic and help us work towards a better understanding of how oppressions impact on health so that working against oppressions and our own ways of perpetuating oppressions can be an ongoing part of our work towards a health care system more appropriate for *all* women (and men). The reader is reminded that this book is planned to complement, rather than overlap with, *The Black Women's Health Book,* which reflects leadership and groundbreaking work by African-American women, and the National Black Women's Health Project specifically, on how racism has impacted women's health.

The first three articles set the tone for how we have tried to work on anti-oppression issues in this book. Audre Lorde's classic articles look at the intersection of *all* forms of oppression and how a basic understanding of power and control issues (who benefits from the inequalities in society and what strategies are used to keep the status quo/the inequalities in place) is fundamental to understanding any and all forms of oppression. It is important to note that while Audre Lorde's life was devoted to educating us about the widest range of oppressions and begging us to look at their intersections rather than looking at a hierarchy of oppressions, Lorde also emphasized that in a racist society, racism plays a dominating role in maintaining power differentials. Ricky Sherover-Marcuse, a Jewish feminist, also devoted her life to anti-oppression work. Her "Unlearning Racism" captures some of the essence of the powerful, life changing Unlearning Racism Workshops which she facilitated around the country, encouraging each of us to take responsibility for starting to unlearn oppressive misinformation that we have learned as a part of our socialization in a racist society. Perhaps her most inspiring work was to stimulate everyone committed to anti-oppression work to look at how we could consciously work at being *allies* for each other and for "each other's issues." Peggy McIntosh's "White Privilege: Unpacking the Invisible Knapsack" has proven to be a non-threatening but effective way to help white people examine ways in which we have privileges in a racist society. Frameworks such as this are essential to help us recognize ways we may benefit (any time a part of us fits Audre Lorde's mythical norm list on page 80) from being on the "more powerful side" of societal inequalities. Readers are encouraged to adopt the white privilege article to develop a list of their own privileges they have as white people, as heterosexuals, as middle class, as abled bodied, or as people educated sufficiently to be reading this text book.

The next five articles present overviews to encourage critical thinking, discussions, and work related to oppressions-as-health issues. Additionally, the excellent new book, *Unequal Health: How Inequality Contributes to Health or Illness,* by Grace Budrys (Rowman and Littlefield, 2003) is highly recommended. "Does Racism Harm Health?" specifically addresses connections between racism and health though frameworks introduced will be also be useful for making connections between other forms of oppression and health. "Health Disparities in the United States" from the American Medical Student Association (AMSA) web-site gives a number of facts related to the problem of health disparities and moves on to identify reasons for disparities and suggestions for action and advocacy for working against inequalities in health care. It is promising to read, "As the future doctors of America, AMSA believes that all physicians-in-training must take a pro-active role in eliminating health disparities."

"Cultural Humility versus Cultural Competence" introduces a profoundly more useful and realistic way to think of our anti-oppression work than to think we are somehow going to "master" a certain body of knowledge and then cross off that off our list of jobs to be done! The article, specifically addressing physician training outcomes for multi-cultural education, helps us think through what will be necessary to meet the above stated AMSA goal. However, the analysis offered is just as relevant to *all* readers of this book studying and working to improve women's health. Slightly paraphrasing Tervalon and Murray-Garciá,

> Cultural humility is proposed as a suitable approach for our anti-oppression work. Cultural humility incorporates a life long commitment to self-evaluation and self-critique, to redressing power imbalances wherever they occur, and to developing mutually beneficial and non-paternalistic partnerships whenever and wherever possible on behalf of individuals and defined populations.

"Minority Women and Advocacy for Women's Health" provides a wealth of health data examined through the lenses of both gender and ethnicity and against the historical background of separate advocacy for women's health and minority health. Serving as an introductory overview to focusing attention on specific issues for particular groups, the "umbrella" article "Health at the Margins" draws attention to commonalities and unique issues of being distanced from the center of power and privileges experienced by women of color, lesbians, women with disabilities, women in poverty, rural women, and women living in the Global South.

In order to recognize the ways that racism and other forms of oppression impact on every health issue, we have tried to include articles by a diverse group of people in many chapters of this book. The next articles in this chapter are intended to highlight, rather than isolate, a few of the many specific issues which are related to racism, anti-Semitism, class, and disability issues. Vanessa Gamble's "Under the Shadow of Tuskegee: African Americans and Health Care" examines the long history of racism in medicine, which results in the fact that many African Americans do not trust the health system. In "Health and Indigenous people," Michael Bird, former President of the American Public Health Association, draws attention to the urgency of improving the health of indigenous people, while also emphasizing that indigenous people have much to offer including, "the importance of the spiritual essence of all people, and our relationships to each other and the environment." The academic paper, "La Sufrida: Contradictions of Acculturation and Gender in Latina Health," is an important reminder of the complexities of studying health status, predictors of health or health behaviors, or disparities in health access for any group of women and why it is crucial to always remember the huge intra-group differences for any group of women. "Expanding Health Options for Asian and Pacific Islander Women" looks at a project especially designed to gauge Asian and Pacific Islander women's awareness of HIV and reproductive health issues to develop peer leadership. "Blazes of Truth" and "JAP: The New Anti-Semitic Code Word" discuss the oppression and meanings of using the term "Jewish American Princess."

"Strained Class Windows" looks at the role of poverty in a woman's life. A major gap in this book is that it is still nearly impossible to find useful data on how class impacts health in the US. Class analysis, building on officially published figures, is core to women's health writing in many other countries, but "the U.S., unlike most industrialized nations, does not regularly collect or publish mortality statistics or other health information by class" ("The Class Gap" by Vincente Navarro in *The Nation,* April 8, 1991, pp. 436–437). Is that a reason for, or a reflection of, Americans' confusion about the role of class in our lives? Class differs from other forms of oppression in a very fundamental way. For other issues, a goal is to celebrate and value our differences and to eliminate *the oppression* related to the issue. With class (poverty), the goal is to *eliminate* that form of difference. As Judith K. Witherow says at the end of her "Strained Class Windows" article, "I would like to see the problems caused by classism worked on continually until all women share equally in the benefits of society."

"Disability and the Medical System" and "Simply Friend or Foe?" give us an overview of some of the health and medical issues for women with disabilities, and through illustrations, offers the abled-bodied ideas for how to be allies to people with disabilities.

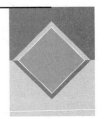

Age, Race, Class, and Sex
*Women Redefining Difference**

by Audre Lorde

Much of western European history conditions us to see human differences in simplistic opposition to each other: dominant/subordinate, good/bad, up/down, superior/inferior. In a society where the good is defined in terms of profit rather than in terms of human need, there must always be some group of people who, through systematized oppression, can be made to feel surplus, to occupy the place of the dehumanized inferior. Within this society, that group is made up of Black and Third World people, working-class people, older people, and women.

As a forty-nine-year-old Black lesbian feminist socialist mother of two, including one boy, and a member of an interracial couple, I usually find myself a part of some group defined as other, deviant, inferior, or just plain wrong. Traditionally, in American society, it is the members of oppressed, objectified groups who are expected to stretch out and bridge the gap between the actualities of our lives and the consciousness of our oppressor. For in order to survive, those of us for whom oppression is as American as apple pie have always had to be watchers, to become familiar with the language and manners of the oppressor, even sometimes adopting them for some illusion of protection. Whenever the need for some pretense of communication arises, those who profit from our oppression call upon us to share our knowledge with them. In other words, it is the responsibility of the oppressed to teach the oppressors their mistakes. I am responsible for educating teachers who dismiss my children's culture in school. Black and Third World people are expected to educate white people as to our humanity. Women are expected to educate men. Lesbians and gay men are expected to educate the heterosexual world. The oppressors maintain their position and evade responsibility for their own actions. There is a constant drain of energy which might be better used in redefining ourselves and devising realistic scenarios for altering the present and constructing the future.

Institutionalized rejection of difference is an absolute necessity in a profit economy which needs outsiders as surplus people. As members of such an economy, we have *all* been programmed to respond to the human differences between us with fear and loathing and to handle that difference in one of three ways: ignore it, and if that is not possible, copy it if we think it is dominant, or destroy it if we think it is subordinate. But we have no patterns for relating across our human differences as equals. As a result, those differences have been misnamed and misused in the service of separation and confusion.

Certainly there are very real differences between us of race, age, and sex. But it is not those differences between us that are separating us. It is rather our refusal to recognize those differences, and to examine the distortions which result from our misnaming them and their effects upon human behavior and expectation.

Racism, the belief in the inherent superiority of one race over all others and thereby the right to dominance. Sexism, the belief in the inherent superiority of one sex over the other and thereby the right to dominance. Ageism. Heterosexism. Elitism, Classism.

It is a lifetime pursuit for each one of us to extract these distortions from our living at the same time as we recognize, reclaim, and define those differences upon which they are imposed. For we have all been raised in a society where those distortions were endemic within our living. Too often, we pour the energy needed for recognizing and exploring difference into pretending those differences are insurmountable barriers, or that they do not exist at all. This results in a voluntary isolation, or false and treacherous connections. Either way, we do not develop tools for using human difference as a springboard for creative change within our lives. We speak not of human difference, but of human deviance.

Reprinted with permission from *Sister Outsider* by Audre Lorde, The Crossing Press, Trumansburg, N.Y., 1984 Copyright 1984 by Audre Lorde.
*Paper delivered at the Copeland Colloquium, Amherst College, April 1980.

Somewhere, on the edge of consciousness, there is what I call a *mythical norm,* which each one of us within our hearts knows "that is not me." In america, this norm is usually defined as white, thin, male, young, heterosexual, christian, and financially secure. It is with this mythical norm that the trappings of power reside within this society. Those of us who stand outside that power often identify one way in which we are different, and we assume that to be the primary cause of all oppression, forgetting other distortions around difference, some of which we ourselves may be practicing. By and large within the women's movement today, white women focus upon their oppression as women and ignore differences of race, sexual preference, class, and age. There is a pretense to a homogeneity of experience covered by the word *sisterhood* that does not in fact exist.

Unacknowledged class differences rob women of each others' energy and creative insight. Recently a women's magazine collective made the decision for one issue to print only prose, saying poetry was a less "rigorous" or "serious" art form. Yet even the form our creativity takes is often a class issue. Of all the art forms, poetry is the most economical. It is the one which is the most secret, which requires the least physical labor, the least material, and the one which can be done between shifts, in the hospital pantry, on the subway, and on scraps of surplus paper. Over the last few years, writing a novel on tight finances, I came to appreciate the enormous differences in the material demands between poetry and prose. As we reclaim our literature, poetry has been the major voice of poor, working class, and Colored women. A room of one's own may be a necessity for writing prose, but so are reams of paper, a typewriter, and plenty of time. The actual requirements to produce the visual arts also help determine, along class lines, whose art is whose. In this day of inflated prices for material, who are our sculptors, our painters, our photographers? When we speak of a broadly based women's culture, we need to be aware of the effect of class and economic differences on the supplies available for producing art.

As we move toward creating a society within which we can each flourish, ageism is another distortion of relationship which interferes without vision. By ignoring the past, we are encouraged to repeat its mistakes. The "generation gap" is an important social tool for any repressive society. If the younger members of a community view the older members as contemptible or suspect or excess, they will never be able to join hands and examine the living memories of the community, nor ask the all important question, "Why?" This gives rise to a historical amnesia that keeps us working to invent the wheel every time we have to go to the store for bread.

We find ourselves having to repeat and relearn the same old lessons over and over that our mothers did because we do not pass on what we have learned, or because we are unable to listen. For instance, how many times has this all been said before? For another, who would have believed that once again our daughters are allowing their bodies to be hampered and purgatoried by girdles and high heels and hobble skirts?

Ignoring the differences of race between women and the implications of those differences presents the most serious threat to the mobilization of women's joint power.

As white women ignore their built-in privilege of whiteness and define *woman* in terms of their own experience alone, then women of Color become "other," the outsider whose experience and tradition is too "alien" to comprehend. An example of this is the signal absence of the experience of women of Color as a resource for women's studies courses. The literature of women of Color is seldom included in women's literature courses and almost never in other literature courses, nor in women's studies as a whole. All too often, the excuse given is that the literatures of women of Color can only be taught by Colored women, or that they are too difficult to understand, or that classes cannot "get into" them because they come out of experiences that are "too different." I have heard this argument presented by white women of otherwise quite clear intelligence, women who seem to have no trouble at all teaching and reviewing work that comes out of the vastly different experiences of Shakespeare, Molière, Dostoyefsky, and Aristophanes. Surely there must be some other explanation.

This is a very complex question, but I believe one of the reasons white women have such difficulty reading Black women's work is because of their reluctance to see Black women as women and different from themselves. To examine Black women's literature effectively requires that we be seen as whole people in our actual complexities—as individuals, as women, as human—rather than as one of those problematic but familiar stereotypes provided in this society in place of genuine images of Black women. And I believe this holds true for the literatures of other women of Color who are not Black.

The literatures of all women of Color recreate the textures of our lives, and many white women are heavily invested in ignoring the real differences. For as long as any difference between us means one of us must be inferior, then the recognition of any difference must be fraught with guilt. To allow women of Color to step out of stereotypes is too guilt provoking, for it threatens the complacency of those women who view oppression only in terms of sex.

Refusing to recognize difference makes it impossible to see the different problems and pitfalls facing us as women.

Thus, in a patriarchal power system where white-skin privilege is a major prop, the entrapments used to neutralize Black women and white women are not the same. For example, it is easy for Black women to be used by the power structure against Black men, not because they are men, but because they are Black. Therefore, for Black women, it is necessary at all times to separate the needs of the oppressor from our own legitimate conflicts within our communities. This same problem does not exist for white women. Black women and men have shared racist oppression and still share it, although in different ways. Out of that shared oppression we have developed joint defenses and joint vulnerabilities to each other that are not duplicated in the white community, with the exception of the relationship between Jewish women and Jewish men.

On the other hand, white women face the pitfall of being seduced into joining the oppressor under the pretense of sharing power. This possibility does not exist in the same way for women of Color. The tokenism that is sometimes extended to us is not an invitation to join power; our racial "otherness" is a visible reality that makes that quite clear. For white women there is a wider range of pretended choices and rewards for identifying with patriarchal power and its tools.

Today, with the defeat of ERA, the tightening economy, and increased conservatism, it is easier once again for white women to believe the dangerous fantasy that if you are good enough, pretty enough, sweet enough, quiet enough, teach the children to behave, hate the right people, and marry the right men, then you will be allowed to co-exist with patriarchy in relative peace, at least until a man needs your job or the neighborhood rapist happens along. And true, unless one lives and loves in the trenches it is difficult to remember that the war against dehumanization is ceaseless.

But Black women and our children know the fabric of our lives is stitched with violence and with hatred, that there is no rest. We do not deal with it only on the picket lines, or in dark midnight alleys, or in the places where we dare to verbalize our resistance. For us, increasingly, violence weaves through the daily tissues of our living—in the supermarket, in the classroom, in the elevator, in the clinic and the schoolyard, from the plumber, the baker, the saleswoman, the bus driver, the bank teller, the waitress who does not serve us.

Some problems we share as women, some we do not. You fear your children will grow up to join the patriarchy and testify against you, we fear our children will be dragged from a car and shot down in the street, and you will turn your backs upon the reasons they are dying.

The threat of difference has been no less blinding to people of Color. Those of us who are Black must see that the reality of our lives and our struggle does not make us immune to the errors of ignoring and misnaming difference. Within Black communities where racism is a living reality, differences among us often seem dangerous and suspect. The need for unity is often misnamed as a need for homogeneity, and a Black feminist vision mistaken for betrayal of our common interests as a people. Because of the continuous battle against racial erasure that Black women and Black men share, some Black women still refuse to recognize that we are also oppressed as women, and that sexual hostility against Black women is practiced not only by the white racist society, but implemented within our Black communities as well. It is a disease striking the heart of Black nationhood, and silence will not make it disappear. Exacerbated by racism and the pressures of powerlessness, violence against Black women and children often becomes a standard within our communities, one by which manliness can be measured. But these women-hating acts are rarely discussed as crimes against Black women.

As a group, women of Color are the lowest paid wage earners in America. We are the primary targets of abortion and sterilization abuse, here and abroad. In certain parts of Africa, small girls are still being sewed shut between their legs to keep them docile and for men's pleasure. This is known as female circumcision, and it is not a cultural affair as the late Jomo Kenyatta insisted, it is a crime against Black women.

Black women's literature is full of the pain of frequent assault, not only by a racist patriarchy, but also by Black men. Yet the necessity for and history of shared battle have made us, Black women, particularly vulnerable to the false accusation that anti-sexist is anti-Black. Meanwhile, womanhating as a recourse of the powerless is sapping strength from Black communities, and our very lives. Rape is on the increase, reported and unreported, and rape is not aggressive sexuality, it is sexualized aggression. As Kalamu ya Salaam, a Black male writer points out, "As long as male domination exists, rape will exist. Only women revolting and men made conscious of their responsibility to fight sexism can collectively stop rape."[1]

Differences between ourselves as Black women are also being misnamed and used to separate us from one another. As a Black lesbian feminist comfortable with the many different ingredients of my identity, and a woman committed to racial and sexual freedom from oppression, I find I am constantly being encouraged to pluck out some one aspect of myself and present this as the meaningful whole, eclipsing or denying the other parts of self. But this is a destructive and fragmenting way to live. My fullest concentration of energy is available to me only when I integrate all the parts of who I am, openly, allowing power from particular sources of my living to flow back and forth freely through all my different selves, without the restrictions of externally imposed definition. Only then can I bring myself and my energies as a whole to the service of those struggles which I embrace as part of my living.

A fear of lesbians, or of being accused of being a lesbian, has led many Black women into testifying against themselves. It has led some of us into destructive alliances, and others into despair and isolation. In the white women's communities, heterosexism is sometimes a result of identifying with the white patriarchy, a rejection of that interdependence between women-identified women which allows the self to be, rather than to be used in the service of men. Sometimes it reflects a die-hard belief in the protective coloration of heterosexual relationships, sometimes a self-hate which all women have to fight against, taught us from birth.

Although elements of these attitudes exist for all women, there are particular resonances of heterosexism and homophobia among Black women. Despite the fact that woman-bonding has a long and honorable history in the African and African-American communities, and despite the knowledge and accomplishments of many strong and creative women-identified Black women in the political, social and cultural fields, heterosexual Black women often tend to ignore or discount the existence and work of Black lesbians. Part of this attitude has come from an understandable terror of Black male attack within the close confines of Black society, where the punishment for any female self-assertion is still to be accused of being a lesbian and therefore unworthy of the attention or support of the scarce Black male. But part of this need to misname and ignore Black lesbians comes from a very real fear that openly women-identified Black women who are no longer dependent upon men for their self-definition may well reorder our whole concept of social relationships.

Black women who once insisted that lesbianism was a white woman's problem now insist that Black lesbians are a threat to Black nationhood, are consorting with the enemy, are basically un-Black. These accusations, coming from the very women to whom we look for deep and real understanding, have served to keep many Black lesbians in hiding, caught between the racism of white women and the homophobia of their sisters. Often, their work has been ignored, trivialized, or misnamed, as with the work of Angelina Grimke, Alice Dunbar-Nelson, Lorraine Hansberry. Yet women-bonded women have always been some part of the power of Black communities, from our unmarried aunts to the amazons of Dahomey.

And it is certainly not Black lesbians who are assaulting women and raping children and grandmothers on the streets of our communities.

Across this country, as in Boston during the spring of 1979 following the unsolved murders of twelve Black women, Black lesbians are spearheading movements against violence against Black women.

What are the particular details within each of our lives that can be scrutinized and altered to help bring about change? How do we redefine difference for all women? It is not our differences which separate women, but our reluctance to recognize those differences and to deal effectively with the distortions which have resulted from the ignoring and misnaming of those differences.

As a tool of social control, women have been encouraged to recognize only one area of human difference as legitimate, those differences which exist between women and men. And we have learned to deal across those differences with the urgency of all oppressed subordinates. All of us have had to learn to live or work or coexist with men, from our fathers on. We have recognized and negotiated these differences, even when this recognition only continued the old dominant/subordinate mode of human relationship, where the oppressed must recognize the masters' difference in order to survive.

But our future survival is predicated upon our ability to relate within equality. As women, we must root out internalized patterns of oppression within ourselves if we are to move beyond the most superficial aspects of social change. Now we must recognize differences among women who are our equals, neither inferior nor superior, and devise ways to use each others' difference to enrich our visions and our joint struggles.

The future of our earth may depend upon the ability of all women to identify and develop new definitions of power and new patterns of relating across difference. The old definitions have not served us, nor the earth that supports us. The old patterns, no matter how cleverly rearranged to imitate progress, still condemn us to cosmetically altered repetitions of the same old exchanges, the same old guilt, hatred, recrimination, lamentation, and suspicion.

For we have, built into all of us, old blueprints of expectation and response, old structures of oppression, and these must be altered at the same time as we alter the living conditions which are a result of those structures. For the master's tools will never dismantle the master's house.

As Paulo Freire shows so well in *The Pedagogy of the Oppressed*,[2] the true focus of revolutionary change is never merely the oppressive situations which we seek to escape, but that piece of the oppressor which is planted deep within each of us, and which knows only the oppressors' tactics, the oppressors' relationships.

Change means growth, and growth can be painful. But we sharpen self-definition by exposing the self in work and struggle together with those whom we define as different from ourselves, although sharing the same goals. For Black and white, old and young, lesbian and heterosexual women alike, this can mean new paths to our survival.

> We have chosen each other
> and the edge of each other battles
> the war is the same
> if we lose

> someday women's blood will congeal
> upon a dead planet
> if we win
> there is no telling
> we seek beyond history
> for a new and more possible meeting.[3]

Notes

1. From "Rape: A Radical Analysis, An African-American Perspective" by Kalamu ya Salaam in *Black Books Bulletin,* vol. 6, no. 4 (1980).
2. Seabury Press, New York, 1970.
3. From "Outlines," unpublished poem.

There Is No Hierarchy of Oppression

by Audre Lorde

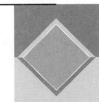

I was born Black, and a woman. I am trying to become the strongest person I can become to live the life I have been given and to help effect change toward a liveable future for this earth and for my children. As a Black, lesbian, feminist, socialist, poet, mother of two including one boy and a member of an interracial couple, I usually find myself part of some group in which the majority defines me as deviant, difficult, inferior, or just plain "wrong."

From my membership in all of these groups I have learned that oppression and the intolerance of difference come in all shapes and sizes and colors and sexualities; and that among those of us who share the goals of liberation and a workable future for our children, there can be no hierarchies of oppression. I have learned that sexism (a belief in the inherent superiority of one sex over all others and thereby its right to dominance) and heterosexism (a belief in the inherent superiority of one pattern of loving over all others and thereby its right to dominance) both arise from the same source as racism—a belief in the inherent superiority of one race over all others and thereby its right to dominance.

"Oh," says a voice from the Black community, "but being Black is NORMAL!" Well, I and many Black people of my age can remember grimly the days when it didn't used to be!

I simply do not believe that one aspect of myself can possibly profit from the oppression of any other part of my identity. I know that my people cannot possibly profit from the oppression of any other group which seeks the right to peaceful existence. Rather, we diminish ourselves by denying to others what we have shed blood to obtain for our children. And those children need to learn that they do not have to become like each other in order to work together for a future they will all share.

The increasing attacks upon lesbians and gay men are only an introduction to the increasing attacks upon all Black people, for wherever oppression manifests itself in this country, Black people are potential victims. And it is a standard of right-wing cynicism to encourage members of oppressed groups to act against each other, and so long as we are divided because of our particular identities we cannot join together in effective political action.

Within the lesbian community I am Black, and within the Black community I am a lesbian. Any attack against Black people is a lesbian and gay issue, because I and thousands of other Black women are part of the lesbian community. Any attack against lesbians and gays is a Black issue, because thousands of lesbians and gay men are Black. There is no hierarchy of oppression.

Reprinted with permission from *Council on Interracial Books for Children Bulletin,* vol. 14, No. 3–4, 1983. (1841 Broadway, Rm. 500, New York, N.Y. 10023)

It is not accidental that the Family Protection Act, which is virulently anti-woman and anti-Black, is also anti-gay. As a Black person I know who my enemies are, and when the Ku Klux Klan goes to court in Detroit to try and force the Board of Education to remove books the Klan believes "hint at homosexuality," then I know I cannot afford the luxury of fighting one form of oppres-sion only. I cannot afford to believe that freedom from intolerance is the right of only one particular group. And I cannot afford to choose between the fronts upon which I must battle these forces of discrimination, wherever they appear to destroy me. And when they appear to destroy me, it will not be long before they appear to destroy you.

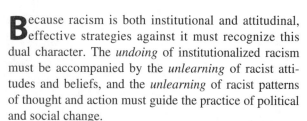

Unlearning Racism

by Ricky Sherover-Marcuse

Because racism is both institutional and attitudinal, effective strategies against it must recognize this dual character. The *undoing* of institutionalized racism must be accompanied by the *unlearning* of racist atti-tudes and beliefs, and the *unlearning* of racist patterns of thought and action must guide the practice of political and social change.

Institutionalized racism can be defined as the sys-tematic mistreatment of people of color (Third World people). Defining racism in this way highlights the fact that racism is not a genetic disease which is inherent in white people, but that it is a form of social oppression which is the result of the institutionalized inequalities in the structure of a given society.

Attitudinal racism can be defined as the set of as-sumptions, feelings, beliefs, and attitudes about people of color and their cultures which are a mixture of *misin-formation* and ignorance. By "misinformation" I mean any assumption or attitude which in any way implies that people of color are less than fully human. Defining attitudinal racism as misinformation about people of color which has been imposed upon white people means that racism is not a moral defect which some (bad) white individuals have, but a social poison which has been given to all of us, albeit in many different forms.

Attitudinal racism and institutional racism feed off each other. The systematic mistreatment of any group of people generates misinformation about them which in turn becomes "explanation" of or justification for their continued mistreatment. As a result, misinformation about the victims of social oppression becomes socially empowered or *socially sanctioned misinformation.* This is what differentiates this sort of misinformation from prejudice. Socially sanctioned misinformation gets recy-cled through the society as a form of conditioning which becomes part of our "ordinary" assumptions, and as a result social oppression is viewed either as "natural" or as the fault of the victims themselves.

For example, the misinformation that people of color are stupid or indifferent to the value of human life becomes the "explanation" as to why there is a higher rate of infant mortality among certain groups in the populations. This "explanation" then justifies the attitude that there is really nothing one can do about in-fant mortality since this problem is basically due to the character or personality structure of the ethnic group involved.

For the past five years I have been doing workshops with groups of white people on "Unlearning Racism". The purpose of these workshops is to help whites to become aware that we have a personal stake in overcoming and un-learning the racist conditioning that was imposed upon us. Having racist beliefs and attitudes is like having a clamp on one's mind. *Unlearning* racism is partly a process of *re-learning* how to get accurate information from and about people of color. This involves *relearning* how to really lis-ten to people of color without making judgments or as-sumptions about what we think they are going to tell us.

When white people become aware of the ways in which *our lives* have been limited and restricted by racism, we become aware of *our interest* in ending this oppression. The most effective action that white people can take against racism will be action which springs not from a sense of guilt or pity, but from our own *knowl-edge* that in working against racism we are moving to-wards our own human liberation.

White Privilege

Unpacking the Invisible Knapsack

by Peggy McIntosh

I was taught to see racism only in individual acts of meanness, not in invisible systems conferring dominance on my group.

Through work to bring materials from Women's Studies into the rest of the curriculum, I have often noticed men's unwillingness to grant that they are overprivileged, even though they may grant that women are disadvantaged. They may say they will work to improve women's status, in the society, the university, or the curriculum, but they can't or won't support the idea of lessening men's. Denials which amount to taboos surround the subject of advantages which men gain from women's disadvantages. These denials protect male privilege from being fully acknowledged, lessened or ended.

Thinking through unacknowledged male privilege as a phenomenon, I realized that since hierarchies in our society are interlocking, there was most likely a phenomenon of white privilege which was similarly denied and protected. As a white person, I realized I had been taught about racism as something which puts others at a disadvantage, but had been taught not to see one of its corollary aspects, white privilege, which puts me at an advantage.

I think whites are carefully taught not to recognize white privilege, as males are taught not to recognize male privilege. So I have begun in an untutored way to ask what it is like to have white privilege. I have come to see white privilege as an invisible package of unearned assets which I can count on cashing in each day, but about which I was 'meant' to remain oblivious. White privilege is like an invisible weightless knapsack of special provisions, maps, passports, codebooks, visas, clothes, tools and blank checks.

Describing white privilege makes one newly accountable. As we in Women's Studies work to reveal male privilege and ask men to give up some of their power, so one who writes about having white privilege must ask, "Having described it, what will I do to lessen or end it?"

After I realized the extent to which men work from a base of unacknowledged privilege, I understood that much of their oppressiveness was unconscious. Then I remembered the frequent charges from women of color that white women whom they encounter are oppressive. I began to understand why we are justly seen as oppressive, even when we don't see ourselves that way. I began to count the ways in which I enjoy unearned skin privilege and have been conditioned into oblivion about its existence.

My schooling gave me no training in seeing myself as an oppressor, as an unfairly advantaged person, or as a participant in a damaged culture. I was taught to see myself as an individual whose moral state depended on her individual moral will. My schooling followed the pattern my colleague Elizabeth Minnich has pointed out: whites are taught to think of their lives as morally neutral, normative, and average, and also ideal, so that when we work to benefit others, this is seen as work which will allow "them" to be more like "us."

I decided to try to work on myself at least by identifying some of the daily effects of white privilege in my life. I have chosen those conditions which I think in my case *attach somewhat more to skin-color privilege* than to class, religion, ethnic status, or geographical location, though of course all these other factors are intricately intertwined. As far as I can see, my African American co-workers, friends and acquaintances with whom I come into daily or frequent contact in this particular time, place, and line of work cannot count on most of these conditions.

Peggy McIntosh is Associate Director of the Wellesley College Center for Research on Women. This essay is excerpted from her working paper, "White Privilege and Male Privilege: A Personal Account of Coming to See Correspondences Through Work in Women's Studies," copyright © 1988 by Peggy McIntosh. Available for $6.00 from address below. The paper includes a longer list of privileges. Permission to excerpt or reprint must be obtained from Peggy McIntosh, Wellesley College Center for Research on Women, Wellesley, MA 02181; (781)283-2520.

1. I can if I wish arrange to be in the company of people of my race most of the time.
2. If I should need to move, I can be pretty sure of renting or purchasing housing in an area which I can afford and in which I would want to live.
3. I can be pretty sure that my neighbors in such a location will be neutral or pleasant to me.
4. I can go shopping alone most of the time, pretty well assured that I will not be followed or harassed.
5. I can turn on the television or open to the front page of the paper and see people of my race widely represented.
6. When I am told about our national heritage or about "civilization," I am shown that people of my color made it what it is.
7. I can be sure that my children will be given curricular materials that testify to the existence of their race.
8. If I want to, I can be pretty sure of finding a publisher for this piece on white privilege.
9. I can go into a music shop and count on finding the music of my race represented, into a supermarket and find the staple foods which fit with my cultural traditions, into a hairdresser's shop and find someone who can cut my hair.
10. Whether I use checks, credit cards, or cash, I can count on my skin color not to work against the appearance of financial reliability.
11. I can arrange to protect my children most of the time from people who might not like them.
12. I can swear, or dress in second hand clothes, or not answer letters, without having people attribute these choices to the bad morals, the poverty, or the illiteracy of my race.
13. I can speak in public to a powerful male group without putting my race on trial.
14. I can do well in a challenging situation without being called a credit to my race.
15. I am never asked to speak for all the people of my racial group.
16. I can remain oblivious of the language and customs of persons of color who constitute the world's majority without feeling in my culture any penalty for such oblivion.
17. I can criticize our government and talk about how much I fear its policies and behavior without being seen as a cultural outsider.
18. I can be pretty sure that if I ask to talk to "the person in charge," I will be facing a person of my race.
19. If a traffic cop pulls me over or if the IRS audits my tax return, I can be sure I haven't been singled out because of my race.
20. I can easily buy posters, postcards, picture books, greeting cards, dolls, toys, and children's magazines featuring people of my race.
21. I can go home from most meetings of organizations I belong to feeling somewhat tied in, rather than isolated, out-of-place, outnumbered, unheard, held at a distance, or feared.
22. I can take a job with an affirmative action employer without having coworkers on the job suspect that I got it because of race.
23. I can choose public accommodation without fearing that people of my race cannot get in or will be mistreated in the places I have chosen.
24. I can be sure that if I need legal or medical help, my race will not work against me.
25. If my day, week, or year is going badly, I need not ask of each negative episode or situation whether it has racial overtones.
26. I can choose blemish cover or bandages in "flesh" color and have them more or less match my skin.

I repeatedly forgot each of the realizations on this list until I wrote it down. For me white privilege has turned out to be an elusive and fugitive subject. The pressure to avoid it is great, for in facing it I must give up the myth of meritocracy. If these things are true, this is not such a free country; one's life is not what one makes it; many doors open for certain people through no virtues of their own.

In unpacking this invisible knapsack of white privilege, I have listed conditions of daily experience which I once took for granted. Nor did I think of any of these perquisites as bad for the holder. I now think that we need a more finely differentiated taxonomy of privilege, for some of these varieties are only what one would want for everyone in a just society, and others give license to be ignorant, oblivious, arrogant and destructive.

I see a pattern running through the matrix of white privilege, a pattern of assumptions which were passed on to me as a white person. There was one main piece of cultural turf; it was my own turf, and I was among those who could control the turf. *My skin color was an asset for any move I was educated to want to make.* I could think of myself as belonging in major ways, and of making social systems work for me. I could freely disparage, fear, neglect, or be oblivious to anything outside of the dominant cultural forms. Being of the main culture, I could also criticize it fairly freely.

In proportion as my racial group was being made confident, comfortable, and oblivious, other groups were likely being made inconfident, uncomfortable, and alienated. Whiteness protected me from many kinds of hostility, distress, and violence, which I was being subtly trained to visit in turn upon people of color.

For this reason, the word "privilege" now seems to me misleading. We usually think of privilege as being a favored state, whether earned or conferred by birth or luck. Yet some of the conditions I have described here work to systematically overempower certain groups. Such privilege simply *confers dominance* because of one's race or sex.

I want, then, to distinguish between earned strength and unearned power conferred systematically. Power from unearned privilege can look like strength when it is in fact permission to escape or to dominate. But not all of the privileges on my list are inevitably damaging. Some, like the expectation that neighbors will be decent to you, or that your race will not count against you in court, should be the norm in a just society. Others, like the privilege to ignore less powerful people, distort the humanity of the holders as well as the ignored groups.

We might at least start by distinguishing between positive advantages which we can work to spread, and negative types of advantages which unless rejected will always reinforce our present hierarchies. For example, the feeling that one belongs within the human circle, as Native Americans say, should not be seen as privilege for a few. Ideally it is an *unearned entitlement.* At present, since only a few have it, it is an *unearned advantage* for them. This paper results from a process of coming to see that some of the power which I originally saw as attendant on being a human being in the U.S. consisted in *unearned advantage* and *conferred dominance.*

I have met very few men who are truly distressed about systemic, unearned male advantage and conferred dominance. And so one question for me and others like me is whether we will be like them, or whether we will get truly distressed, even outraged, about unearned race advantage and conferred dominance and if so, what we will do to lessen them. In any case, we need to do more work in identifying how they actually affect our daily lives. Many, perhaps most, of our white students in the U.S. think that racism doesn't affect them because they are not people of color; they do not see "whiteness" as a racial identity. In addition, since race and sex are not the only advantaging systems at work, we need similarly to examine the daily experience of having age advantage, or ethnic advantage, or physical ability, or advantage related to nationality, religion, or sexual orientation.

Difficulties and dangers surrounding the task of finding parallels are many. Since racism, sexism, and heterosexism are not the same, the advantaging associated with them should not be seen as the same. In addi-

tion, it is hard to disentangle aspects of unearned advantage which rest more on social class, economic class, race, religion, sex and ethnic identity than on other factors. Still, all of the oppressions are interlocking, as the Combahee River Collective Statement of 1977 continues to remind us eloquently.

One factor seems clear about all of the interlocking oppressions. They take both active forms which we can see and embedded forms which as a member of the dominant group one is taught not to see. In my class and place, I did not see myself as a racist because I was taught to recognize racism only in individual acts of meanness by members of my group, never in invisible systems conferring unsought racial dominance on my group from birth.

Disapproving of the systems won't be enough to change them. I was taught to think that racism could end if white individuals changed their attitudes. [But] a "white" skin in the United States opens many doors for whites whether or not we approve of the way dominance has been conferred on us. Individual acts can palliate, but cannot end, these problems.

To redesign social systems we need first to acknowledge their colossal unseen dimensions. The silences and denials surrounding privilege are the key political tool here. They keep the thinking about equality or equity incomplete, protecting unearned advantage and conferred dominance by making these taboo subjects. Most talk by whites about equal opportunity seems to me now to be about equal opportunity to try to get into a position of dominance while denying that *systems* of dominance exist.

It seems to me that obliviousness about white advantage, like obliviousness about male advantage, is kept strongly inculturated in the United States so as to maintain the myth of meritocracy, the myth that democratic choice is equally available to all. Keeping most people unaware that freedom of confident action is there for just a small number of people props up those in power, and serves to keep power in the hands of the same groups that have most of it already.

Though systemic change takes many decades, there are pressing questions for me and I imagine for some others like me if we raise our daily consciousness on the perquisites of being light-skinned. What will we do with such knowledge? As we know from watching men, it is an open question whether we will choose to use unearned advantage to weaken hidden systems of advantage, and whether we will use any of our arbitrarily-awarded power to try to reconstruct power systems on a broader base.

Does Racism Harm Health? Did Child Abuse Exist Before 1962? On Explicit Questions, Critical Science, and Current Controversies

An Ecosocial Perspective

by Nancy Krieger, PhD

Research on racism as a harmful determinant of population health is in its infancy. Explicitly naming a long-standing problem long recognized by those affected, this work has the potential to galvanize inquiry and action, much as the 1962 publication of the Kempe et al. scientific article on the "battered child syndrome" dramatically increased attention to—and prompted new research on—the myriad consequences of child abuse, a known yet neglected social phenomenon. To further work on connections between racism and health, the author addresses 3 interrelated issues: (1) links between racism, biology, and health; (2) methodological controversies over how to study the impact of racism on health; and (3) debates over whether racism or class underlies racial/ethnic disparities in health. (Am J Public Health. 2003:93:194-199)

Did child abuse exist before 1962, when C. Henry Kempe and coauthors published the now classic article "The Battered-Child Syndrome"? Certainly. Did it harm health? Yes, if current research is any guide. Before the Kempe et al. article catapulted the issue onto the mainstream US medical and public health agenda, had anyone previously raised concerns about child abuse? Absolutely. Since the early 1800s, numerous individuals and organizations—many in fields that came to be known as public health, medicine, social work, philanthropy, and criminal justice—had attempted to investigate, raise public awareness about, and ameliorate problems of family violence. Public and scientific attention to the issue, however, waxed and waned in concert with broader societal concerns.

Kempe's article in a prominent scientific journal nevertheless was and remains enormously influential. Why? In part, because it explicitly named—and simultaneously highlighted the health consequences of—a volatile societal problem then hidden from view by dominant beliefs about the sanctity of family life. The unnamable problem, once named, became less nebulous and more tangible, something that could be more rigorously documented, monitored, and analyzed, bolstered

by the belief that—with adequate will and resources—it could ultimately be rectified.

Forty years later, in 2002, we are reaching a similar juncture: the unnamable is again becoming named, and explicit investigation of racism as a harmful determinant of population health is gaining entry into mainstream public health and medical discourse. At issue are the myriad ways in which racism—and other forms of social inequality and discrimination—can adversely affect health across the life course via varied, intertwined economic, environmental, psychosocial, and iatrogenic pathways. The scientific question "Does racism harm health?" prompts a plenitude of hypotheses, each meriting serious scientific attention and resources.

Is it, however, novel to posit that racial/ethnic disparities in health arise from inequitable race relations? Surely not. Are we the first to suggest that health is harmed not only by heinous crimes against humanity, such as slavery, lynching, and genocide, but also by the grinding economic and social realities of what Essed has aptly termed "everyday racism"? Once again, no. In the mid-1800s, leading US abolitionists and physicians, Black and White alike, challenged convention by arguing that the poorer health of the Black relative to the

White population resulted not from innate inferiority but rather White privilege, enforced via slavery in the South and legal racial discrimination in the North.

The Choctaw and Cherokee nations, forcibly evicted from their homelands after the US Congress passed the Indian Removal Act in 1830, likewise understood that their health was being decimated by not only territorial but also cultural dispossession, justified in the name of White supremacy. Concerns about health consequences of racism clearly are not new; to suggest otherwise is to misstate the historical record. Rather, reflecting the historical impact of racial inequality on not only health but also health sciences, the stark reality is that, despite long-standing awareness of the problem, the serious scientific study of racism as a determinant of population health remains in its infancy.

One way to move to the next stage is to consider current conceptual issues in the field, given that scientific knowledge is more often spurred by clarification of our thinking than by technological breakthroughs. In this spirit, I address 3 interrelated issues from the vantage of an epidemiologist guided by an ecosocial perspective: (1) links between racism, biology, and health, including recognition of biological expression of race relations and racialized expressions of biology; (2) methodological controversies over how to study the impact of racism on health; and (3) debates over whether racism or class underlies racial/ethnic disparities in health.

Racism, Biology, and Health

Clarity of terminology is critical for any science. A first step for analyzing the contribution of racism to racial/ethnic disparities in health is being explicit about definitions of racism, race/ethnicity, and the link between these concepts. In essence, both are interdependent expressions of inequitable and institutionalized societal race relations. More specifically, *racism* refers to institutional and individual practices that create and reinforce oppressive systems of race relations whereby people and institutions engaging in discrimination adversely restrict, by judgment and action, the lives of those against whom they discriminate.

Race/ethnicity, in turn, is a social rather than a biological category, referring to social groups, often sharing cultural heritage and ancestry, that are forged by oppressive systems of race relations justified by ideology. One group benefits from dominating other groups and defines itself and others through this domination and the possession of selective and arbitrary physical characteristics (e.g., skin color). Although once trumpeted as scientific "fact," the notion that "race" is a valid, biologi-

cally meaningful a priori category has long been—and continues to be—refuted by work in population genetics, anthropology, and sociology. The fact that we know what "race" we are says more about our society than it does our biology.

Why do these sorts of explicit definitions matter? Because they provide a conceptual foundation for integrating thinking about racism *and* biology as a means of understanding and investigating the impact of racism on health. Both matter. Two diametrically opposed constructs are at issue, constructs that nevertheless are routinely conflated in the scientific literature. The first is *biological expressions of race relations;* the second is *racialized expressions of biology.* The former draws attention to how harmful physical and psychosocial exposures due to racism adversely affect our biology, in ways that ultimately are embodied and manifested in racial/ethnic disparities in health. The latter refers to how arbitrary biological traits are erroneously construed as markers of innate "racial" distinctions.

Consider skin color. The biology of pigmentation and its direct relationship to certain skin-related disorders is real. Whether or not racism existed, people with lighter vs darker skin (i.e., less vs more dispersed melanosomes) would be at higher risk of malignant melanoma, given sufficient exposure to sunlight (and especially bad sunburns before puberty). By contrast, damage resulting from adverse use of skin lightening products, as prompted by the ideology that lighter is better, would constitute a biological expression of race relations.

Skin color, in turn, would become a racialized expression of biology if, absent any evidence, it were treated as a valid marker for other unspecified genetic traits, reflecting a presumption that the biology of "race" equals the biology of gene frequencies. This was the logic of the flawed research agenda egregiously exemplified by the Tuskegee syphilis study, unnaturally intended to determine whether the "natural history" of untreated syphilis in Blacks was the same as that previously observed in Whites, in light of hypothesized differences in their nervous systems.

As Cruickshank has recently pointed out, however, drawing on lessons from the Human Genome Project and systems biology, it is a logical and biological fallacy to assume that gene expression is equivalent to gene frequency. Consider the recent, rapid secular changes in obesity, hypertension, and diabetes among populations of West African descent living in the United Kingdom, the Caribbean, and the United States, as well as in West Africa, to use but one diasporic example. Only changes in gene expression, not gene frequency, can explain the speed of these trends. Even so, myriad epidemiological studies continue to treat "race" as a purely biological (i.e., genetic) variable or seek to explain racial/ethnic disparities in health absent consideration of the effects of racism on health.

By clearly distinguishing between and emphasizing the importance of taking into account both racism and biology, these 2 constructs make clear that we can never study human biology—or behavior—in the abstract. Exemplifying that we instead study people in context is Sapolsky's cautionary tale: If adrenal glands are studied only among cadavers of the poor, long since hypertrophied as a result of excess excretion of cortisol, then—as occurred in the early 20th century—the wealthy will be diagnosed with adrenal deficiency disorder. Simplistic divisions of the social and biological will not suffice. The interpretations we offer of observed average differences in health status across socially delimited groups reflect our theoretical frameworks, not ineluctable facts of nature.

Methodological Controversies

How then, methodologically, can we test the hypothesis that racism harms health? Addressing this scientific question raises several critical questions and controversies. At issue is the need for—and strengths and limitations of—studies that directly and indirectly assess the impact of racism on health, whether employing quantitative or qualitative methods. By direct, I mean health studies explicitly obtaining information on people's self-reported experiences of—and observing people's physiological and psychological responses to—real-life or experimental situations involving racial discrimination. By indirect, I mean studies that investigate racial/ethnic disparities in distributions of deleterious exposures or health outcomes and explicitly infer that racism underlies these disparities. Each approach has its flaws, and both are necessary, addressing questions the other cannot.

Highlighting why both direct and indirect approaches are necessary are 5 key pathways through which racism can harm health, by shaping exposure and vulnerability to the following: (1) economic and social deprivation; (2) toxic substances and hazardous conditions; (3) socially inflicted trauma (mental, physical, and sexual, directly experienced or witnessed, from verbal threats to violent acts); (4) targeted marketing of commodities that can harm health, such as junk food and psychoactive substances (alcohol, tobacco, and other licit and illicit drugs); and (5) inadequate or degrading medical care. Also relevant are health consequences of people's responses to discrimination. These responses—each with its own set of potential health impacts—can range from internalized oppression and harmful use of psychoactive substances to reflective coping, active resistance, and community organizing to end discrimination and promote human rights and social justice.

From this perspective, the direct approach is necessary for investigating pathways pertaining to socially inflicted trauma. There is no substitute. The caveat, well recognized in the enormous body of literature on "stress" and health, is that such research must reckon with not only exposures but perceptions of these exposures, as well as cognitive issues pertaining to memory and disclosure. The scientific task is therefore to understand how various threats to validity can affect investigations relying on self-report data. Potential solutions include the following: research on what constitutes valid self-report measures of racial discrimination; experimental studies (as conducted in the areas of housing and job discrimination) that employ "testers" of the same age, gender, and physical size, equipped with identical resumes but differing in terms of their race/ethnicity; or psychological and criminal justice studies investigating differences in perception of and responses to designated scenarios.

Notably, conduct of such studies requires appraisal of participants' racial/ethnic identity. Recent suggestions, however well intentioned, to "abandon" use of racial/ethnic categories in public health research, on grounds that "race" is not a valid scientific concept, err on 2 accounts. First, such an argument implies that only biological, and not social, variables are "real" and can be studied scientifically. Second, it presumes that the race/ethnicity of persons reporting experiences of racial discrimination is irrelevant, thereby rendering it impossible to distinguish between—or evaluate the health effects of—racial discrimination reported by people of color and that reported by White people.

The indirect approach, in turn, is necessary for most of the other pathways listed, precisely because they involve exposures that extend beyond individual perception. Knowledge of racial discrimination in wages, for example, can be obtained only if one knows what others are paid. Similarly, knowledge of racial inequality in the provision of medical care, above and beyond disrespectful interpersonal interactions, can be obtained only by comparing the types of treatment offered to groups that exhibit equivalent morbidity rates but differ in regard to their race/ethnicity.

Herein lies the rub. A claim recently advanced by some social epidemiologists, notably Cooper and Kaufman, is that we cannot make causal inferences based on studies comparing health outcomes across different racial/ethnic groups. Why? Because, they argue, such studies violate the counterfactual criterion of exchangeability. That is, people who are "exposed" should, in principle, be capable of being "unexposed." Using this logic, their debatable example is that smokers differ from nonsmokers only because they smoke; in principle, the "treatment" of smoking could be randomized.

By contrast, according to Cooper and Kaufman, there is no way a White person could ever be or become a Black person or have the lifetime set of related experiences contingent upon being Black. The exposure of "race" is thus nonexchangeable and also, in their examples, uniform. Because commonly used statistical tests presume exchangeability, they assert that parameter estimates for racial/ethnic contrasts have no valid causal interpretation, including in relation to racial discrimination.

The fallacy of their argument is contained within their counterfactual propositions. Cooper and Kaufman in effect relegate "race" to an intrinsic trait. They confuse the fact that people cannot simply "choose" their race/ethnicity, in that it is conditioned by the racial/ethnic relations of the society into which they are born, with the consequences of experiencing differential— and variable—treatment by virtue of inequitable race relations. The appropriate counterfactual is thus as follows: What would happen if people were randomized to discriminatory treatment, as occurs with racial discrimination? As is often the case in epidemiology, we cannot perform such an experiment to test this hypothesis regarding racial/ethnic disparities in health across the life course and instead must rely on observational studies.

More broadly, the counterfactual contrast is of a world with and without racism. In the latter, people with darker vs lighter skin would in fact be "exchangeable"— as human beings—and thus equally at risk for all ailments other than those directly involving skin color (e.g., melanoma, vitiligo). This contrast, premised upon a common humanity, underlies the "tester" studies alluded to earlier regarding housing and job discrimination. It also underlies inferences made comparing health outcomes across birth cohorts; obviously, someone born in 1910 cannot be "exchanged" with or have the same set of experiences as a person born in 1940 or in 1970. Birth cohort comparisons of both rates of disease and exposures, however, are critical for assessing whether cross-sectional associations—even those derived from randomized clinical trials—can in fact explain secular changes in health.

As with any scientific research, poorly specified counterfactuals are what threaten causal interpretation, and all observational studies—not only those concerned with social determinants of health—must consider carefully their motivating counterfactuals. Even the smokers and nonsmokers of Cooper and Kaufman's example would, after all, violate a strict "exchangeability" criterion, because the fact and process of being a smoker brings with it an array of other correlated exposures and life histories.

Racism or Social Class: The Limits of "Either/Or" Logic

The third and final conceptual controversy builds on the first and second. It is the debate over whether "racism" or "social class" explains racial/ethnic disparities in health and, relatedly, which is causally prior. Typically argued with reference to the Euro-American legacy of colonization and the slave trade, the logical and historical fallacy is to frame this debate as "either/or" rather than as "both/and." As attested to by reams of sociological and historical research, class and race relations are in fact intertwined. Since the global expansion of European power and economies in the mid-15th century and contingent territorial conquest and intercontinental slave trade, people have lived in a world of racialized class relations and class-contingent race relations. It logically follows that racial/ethnic inequalities are shaped and fostered by class inequalities, and vice versa.

The same holds for other types of discrimination that render people socially and economically vulnerable (e.g., discrimination based on gender or sexuality). Translated to health research, it is therefore an empirical question, not a philosophical principle, whether pathways involving economic deprivation and/or noneconomic manifestations of racial discrimination contribute to racial/ethnic disparities in health. Or, put simply, the answer to the crude question "Which matters—race or class?" can be one, the other, neither, or both. This is why we need scientific research: to test competing hypotheses.

Being Explicit about Racism: A Scientific Necessity

In conclusion, recalling the example of child abuse, the point of explicitly naming and scientifically investigating racism as a determinant of population health is to generate valid knowledge to guide actions designed to improve public health. It is not to imply that racism is solely a public health or medical problem or that solutions will come primarily from public health or medical initiatives. Nor is health research required to "prove" that racism is "bad"; it is, by definition, and in many instances it is illegal as well. Rather, the point is that neglecting study of the health impact of racism means that explanations for and interventions to alter population distributions of health, disease, and well-being will be incomplete and potentially misleading, if not outright harmful. Of course, work in this field will, inevitably, be fraught with controversy, because the exposure raises important themes of accountability, agency, and human rights.

That there are legal, political, and economic consequences of attributing disparities in health status to racial discrimination is, however, no more or less germane than it is for research on any other determinant of societal health, whether child abuse, ambient air pollution, tobacco, or food. The canard that research on health consequences of racism is "political" rather than "scientific" is blatantly incorrect: it is in fact political and unscientific to exclude the topic from the domain of legitimate scientific inquiry and discourse. Nor is this insight new: James McCune Smith and John Rock, 2 of the first credentialed African American physicians in the United States, said as much a century and a half ago. Rather, the task at hand is to bring the knowledge and methods available in our generation to the pressing public health problem of persistent racial/ethnic disparities in health.

References

A list of references is available in the original source.

Health Disparities in the United States

What Is the Problem?

Health disparities exist in access, treatment, outcomes, and health status.

Access

- Low-income Americans run the highest risk of being uninsured. In 1999, 42.6 million people lacked health insurance, and the numbers have increased in years since. Among minority groups, Hispanics are the least likely to have health insurance (34.3% uninsured), followed by American Indians and Alaska Natives (27.1% uninsured) based on a 3-year average (1997–1999). Compare this to 21.6% of Blacks, 20.9% of Asians and Pacific Islanders, and 11.6% of white non-Hispanics who lack health insurance.
  Source: Current Population Survey conducted by the U.S. Census Bureau in March 2000

  For more information about access to care, please check out AMSA's Universal Health Care website.

Treatment

- Numerous studies over the past two decades have documented racial and ethnic differences in care for heart conditions. The strongest studies provide credible evidence that African Americans are less likely than whites to receive diagnostic procedures, revascularization procedures and thrombolytic therapy. Eighty-four percent of studies (done from 1984-2001) investigating this idea found racial/ethnic differences in cardiac care for at least one of the minority groups under study.
  Source: Racial/Ethnic Differences in Cardiac Care, The Weight of the Evidence, October 2002
- HIV infection is now the leading cause of death among African Americans between the ages of 25 and 44 and the second leading cause of death among Latinos in this age group. The most telling data showing concerns about adequacy of treatment for minorities come from the HIV Cost and Services Utilization Study that looked at the use of triple drug antiretroviral therapy, a treatment regimen that is very effective in delaying disability and prolonging the life of persons with HIV. African Americans were more than twice as likely as whites to not receive combination drug therapy and 1.5 times more likely to not get preventive treatment for pneumocystic carinii pneumonia (a common, but preventable, infection in people with HIV) than whites. Latinos were 1.5 times more likely than whites to not get combination drug therapy (Shapiro et al, 1999).

Outcomes

- Heart disease is the leading cause of death for all racial and ethnic groups in the United States. In 1999, rates of death from cardiovascular disease were about 30% higher among African American adults than among white adults.

- The incidence of diabetes among American Indians and Alaska Natives is more than twice that of the total population, and the Pima Indians of Arizona have the highest known prevalence of diabetes in the world. The prevalence of diabetes is 70% higher among African Americans and nearly 100% higher among Hispanics than among Caucasian individuals.
Source: HHS Fact Sheet, U.S. Dept of Health and Human Services, Sept. 2002

Health Status

- As recently as 2000, African Americans and Hispanics accounted for roughly 75% of all adult AIDS cases, although they only comprise 25% of the U.S. Population. African American and Hispanics also make up 81% of all pediatric AIDS cases.
Source: HHS Fact Sheet, U.S. Dept. of Health & Human Services, Sept. 2002

- In women, racial and ethnic minority groups are more likely to be overweight or obese than non-Hispanic whites. The same holds true for Mexican-American men vs. non-Hispanic men. This risk factor contributes to the fact that 10.2% of all Hispanic Americans have diabetes.
Source: HHS Fact Sheet, U.S. Dept. of Health & Human Services, Sept. 2002, Health Gap Datastats, OMHRC

What Are the Reasons?

There are many factors that may contribute to racial and ethnic disparities in healthcare. Among the better-controlled studies performed to assess these factors, the vast majority indicated that minorities are less likely than whites to receive needed services, including clinically necessary procedures. Let's look at some of the reasons for this:

- **Operation of Healthcare Systems:** This incorporates the legal and regulatory climate in which healthcare systems operate and includes factors such as cultural or linguistic barriers (e.g. the lack of interpretation services for patients with limited English speaking skills), fragmentation of healthcare systems (which could include the possibility that minorities are disproportionately enrolled in lower-cost health plans that put greater per-patient limits on healthcare spending and available services), and incentives to physicians to limit services. Where minority patients tend to receive care is also important to consider, as they are less likely to access care in a private physician's office, even when insured at the same level as whites). If you ask a physician why the health care system treats people unfairly based on race or ethnic background, you would probably get an answer related to this idea. Fifty-eight percent of physicians attributed the problem to the simple fact that many people from minority groups live in areas where there are fewer doctors or other health providers.

- **Physician Biases and Patient Perceptions:** Medical school does an excellent job of teaching the diagnosis and treatment of clinical disease but fails to prepare future physicians to incorporate psychosocial and cultural factors and overcome personal biases in the care of patients. It is reasonable to assume that the majority of healthcare providers find prejudice morally wrong and at odds with their professional values, but healthcare providers, like other members of society, may not recognize manifestations of prejudice in their own behavior. A study based on actual clinical encounters done by van Ryn and Burke (2000) found that doctors rated black patients as less intelligent, less educated, more likely to abuse drugs and alcohol, more likely to fail to comply with medical advice, more likely to lack social support, and less likely to participate in cardiac rehabilitation than white patients, even after patients' income, education, and personality characteristics were taken into account. These findings suggest that while the relationship between race or ethnicity and treatment decisions is complex, providers' perceptions and attitudes toward patients are often influenced in subtle ways by patient race or ethnicity.

- **Greater clinical uncertainty when interacting with minority patients:** Any degree of uncertainty a physician may have relative to the condition of a patient can contribute to disparities in treatment. In order to make a diagnosis, a doctor must depend on inferences about severity based on what they can see about the illness and on what they observe about the patient (including race, age, gender, and sometimes socioeconomic status). If the information related to the illness is lacking or deemed to be inaccurate, the doctor tends to rely on his observations of the patient (which may include unfair assumptions) to make diagnostic decisions. The consequence is that treatment decisions and patients' needs are potentially less well matched.

The factors listed above were confirmed by patients in focus groups who said that stereotypes, language barriers, lack of respect, improper diagnosis and treatment, and economics were the main reasons for racial and ethnic health disparities.

What Is Being Done and What Can We Do?

Education may be one of the most important tools as part of an overall strategy to eliminate healthcare disparities. Healthcare providers and medical students alike should be aware that racial and ethnic disparities exist in healthcare, often despite providers' best intentions.

Medical Student Action

- Medical schools must begin to address cultural diversity and physician bias if our nation strives to eliminate health disparities. AMSA is piloting cultural competency curricula at Mercer University School of Medicine, University of Massachusetts Medical School, Saint Louis University School of Medicine, and Penn State College of Medicine through the AMSA Foundation's PRIME (Promoting, Reinforcing and Improving Medical Education) project.

  For more info on PRIME or the Culture and Diversity Curriculum Project, check out http://www.amsa. org/programs/prime.cfm.

- The PRIME project was also awarded an initiative through the American Medical Student Association Foundation by the U.S. Department of Health and Human Services, Health Resources and Services Administration, Bureau of Health Professions, Division of Medicine and Dentistry to create a module called Breaking Barriers that focuses on how barriers to health care negatively impact health, and what people in the healthcare field can do to tear down these barriers.

Healthcare Providers

Given that stereotypes, bias, and clinical uncertainty may influence clinicians' diagnostic and treatment decisions, education may be one of the most important tools as part of an overall strategy to eliminate health disparities. Cross-cultural education programs have been developed to enhance health professionals' awareness of how cultural and social factors influence healthcare, while providing methods to obtain, negotiate, and manage this information clinically once it is obtained.

The Breaking Barriers module created by the AMSA Foundation's PRIME project has a link to The Providers Guide to Quality and Culture, an excellent resource for learning how to give culturally competent care to individuals from different racial and ethnic backgrounds. Take the Quality and Culture Quiz to find out how culturally aware you are.

Another great resource: Cultural Competency in Medicine

Notable Sponsors and Advocacy Organizations

- HHS Secretary Tommy Thompson recently announced $85 million in grants to eliminate racial and ethnic health disparities among minority communities "highly affected" by several diseases, including HIV/AIDS, cancer, and diabetes. www.omhrc.gov/healthgap/

- The National Center on Minority Health and Health Disparities (NCMHD) promotes minority health and strives to lead, coordinate, support, and assess the NIH effort to reduce and ultimately eliminate health disparities. They envision an America in which all populations will have an equal opportunity to live long, healthy and productive lives. In accordance with this mission, they recently provided $74.5 million to various institutions, and HHS' Office of Minority Health awarded 65 grants totaling $10.5 million— $4.6 million of which is supported by funds from the Minority AIDS initiative—to support state-based efforts to eliminate health disparities.

  Much of this money will go toward research on minority health disparities, while some will go to community-based projects that will work to reduce "high-risk" behaviors such as tobacco use, physical inactivity or poor eating habits, as well as to improve health care access. Another portion will fund minority health offices in 14 states or go toward supporting the development of "effective and durable" service delivery among community organizations and health departments involved in HIV/AIDS treatment and prevention.

- The Henry J. Kaiser Family Foundation and The Robert Wood Johnson Foundation are also two key players in the fight against health disparities. They are currently undertaking an initiative to raise physician awareness about disparities in medical care, beginning with cardiac care. www.kff.org/ whythedifference

- The Office of Minority Health offers great statistics about health care for minorities.

What Can You Do Right Now?

- *Take the Challenge! Student Action for Zero Health Disparities*(309KB PowerPoint Presentation—download now)
  A slide show that outlines current health disparities with a closer look at the causes and student-driven solutions. (*HTML VERSION*)
- *Advocacy Scorecard*
  We are compiling information about advocacy services available at individual medical schools. How does your school rate? Please have your DEAN fill out our online survey.
- *Share your Experiences*
  Have you witnessed an act of discrimination on the wards? Or a remarkable demonstration of cultural sensitivity in the classroom? Support AMSA's Diversity in Medicine Initiative by adding your experiences to this exciting collection

As the future doctors of America, AMSA believes that all physicians-in-training must take a proactive role in eliminating health disparities. Through self and peer education, innovative curriculum development and local and national policy changes we can make a significant impact to achieve this goal. For questions or more information contact pres@www.amsa.org and visit AMSA's *Advocacy Action Committee.*

of members' stories. View the current results (PDF 143KB).

For More Information

Institute of Medicine Report ("Unequal Treatment")
   Scroll down to the article *Unequal Treatment: Confronting Racial and Ethnic Disparities in Health Care* (March 20, 2002)
Kaiser Family Foundation on Minority Resources
Closing the Gap, U.S. Dept. of Health & Human Services

Cultural Humility versus Cultural Competence: A Critical Distinction in Defining Physician Training Outcomes in Multicultural Education

by Melanie Tervalon, MD, MPH and

Jann Murray-García, MD, MPH

Abstract: Researchers and program developers in medical education presently face the challenge of implementing and evaluating curricula that teach medical students and house staff how to effectively and respectfully deliver health care to the increasingly diverse populations of the United States. Inherent in this challenge is clearly defining educational and training outcomes consistent with this imperative. The traditional notion of competence in clinical training as a detached mastery of a theoretically finite body of knowledge may not be appropriate for this area of physician education. Cultural humility is proposed as a more suitable goal in multicultural medical education. Cultural humility incorporates a lifelong commitment to self-evaluation and self-critique, to redressing the power imbalances in the patient-physician dynamic, and to developing mutually beneficial and nonpaternalistic clinical and advocacy partnerships with communities on behalf of individuals and defined populations.

Melanie Tervalon and Jann Murray-Garcia, *Journal of Health Care for the Poor and Underserved,* Vol. 9, No. 2, copyright 1998 by Journal of Health Care for the Poor and Underserved. Reprinted by Permission of Sage Publications, Inc.

The increasing cultural, racial, and ethnic diversity of the United States compels medical educators to train physicians who will skillfully and respectfully negotiate the implications of this diversity in their clinical practice. Simultaneously, increasing attention is being paid to nonfinancial barriers that operate at the level of the physician/patient dynamic. This dynamic is often compromised by various sociocultural mismatches between patients and providers, including providers' lack of knowledge regarding patients' health beliefs and life experiences, and providers' unintentional and intentional processes of racism, classism, homophobia, and sexism.

Several recent national mandates calling for innovative approaches to multicultural training of physicians have emerged from various sources. The Pew Health Professions Commission, specifically seeking to give direction to health professions education for the twenty-first century, stated that "cultural sensitivity must be a part of the educational experiences that touches the life of every student." The Institute of Medicine defines *optimal primary care* as including "an understanding of the cultural, nutritional and belief systems of patients and communities that may assist or hinder effective health care delivery."

The necessity for multicultural medical education provides researchers and program developers with the challenge of defining and measuring training outcomes and proving that chosen instructional strategies do indeed produce these outcomes. However, in the laudable urgency to implement and evaluate programs that aim to produce cultural competence, one dimension to be avoided is the pitfall of narrowly defining competence in medical training and practice in its traditional sense: an easily demonstrable mastery of a finite body of knowledge, an endpoint evidenced largely by comparative quantitative assessments (i.e., MCATs, pre- and postexams, board certification exams).

Rather, cultural competence in clinical practice is best defined not by a discrete endpoint but as a commitment and active engagement in a lifelong process that individuals enter into on an ongoing basis with patients, communities, colleagues, and with themselves (L. Brown, MPH, Oakland health advocate, personal communication, March 18, 1994). This training outcome, perhaps better described as cultural humility versus cultural competence, actually dovetails several educational initiatives in U.S. physician workforce training as we approach the twenty-first century. It is a process that requires humility as individuals continually engage in self-reflection and self-critique as lifelong learners and reflective practitioners. It is a process that requires humility in how physicians bring into check the power imbalances that exist in the dynamics of physician-patient communication by using patient-focused interviewing and care. And it is a process that requires humility to develop and maintain mutually respectful and dynamic partnerships with communities on behalf of individual patients and communities in the context of community-based clinical and advocacy training models.

Self-reflection and the Lifelong Learner Model

Increasing trainees' knowledge of health beliefs and practices is critically important. For instance, the Cambodian child who comes in with the linear marks of "coining," a Southeast Asian healing practice, should not be mistaken for the victim of parental child abuse.

To be avoided, however, is the false sense of security in one's training evidenced by the following actual case from our experience: An African American nurse is caring for a middle-aged Latina woman several hours after the patient had undergone surgery. A Latino physician on a consult service approached the bedside and, noting the moaning patient, commented to the nurse that the patient appeared to be in a great deal of postoperative pain. The nurse summarily dismissed his perception, informing him that she took a course in nursing school in cross-cultural medicine and "knew" that Hispanic patients overexpress "the pain they are feeling." The Latino physician had a difficult time influencing the perspective of this nurse, who focused on her self-proclaimed cultural expertise.

This nurse's notion of her own expertise actually stereotyped the patient's experience, ignored clues (the moaning) to the patient's present reality, and disregarded the potential resource of a colleague who might (albeit not necessarily) be able to contribute some relevant cultural insight. The equating of cultural competence with simply having completed a past series of training sessions is an inadequate and potentially harmful model of professional development, as evidenced by this case.

In no way are we discounting the value of knowing as much as possible about the health care practices of the communities we serve. Rather, it is imperative that there be a simultaneous process of self-reflection (realistic and ongoing self-appraisal) and commitment to a lifelong learning process. In this way, trainees are ideally flexible and humble enough to let go of the false sense of security that stereotyping brings. They are flexible and humble enough to assess anew the cultural dimensions of the experiences of each patient. And finally, they are flexible and humble enough *to say that they do not know when they truly do not know* and to search for and access resources that might enhance immeasurably the care of the patient as well as their future clinical practice.

In a related manner, an isolated increase in knowledge without a consequent change in attitude and behavior is of questionable value. In fact, existing literature documenting a lack of cultural competence in clinical practice most reflects not a lack of knowledge but rather the need for a change in practitioners' self-awareness and a change in their attitudes toward diverse patients. These data indicate that the prescription of clinical resources from prevention services to potentially life-saving procedures is often differential, dependent on the race or ethnicity of the patient. For example, a study in a university emergency department showed that Latinos were half as likely as white patients to receive analgesia for the same, usually very painful, long-bone fractures, regardless of the linguistic capability or insurance status of the patient. A follow-up study in the same institution showed no difference in physicians' assessment of the level of pain experienced by white and Latino patients experiencing the same, isolated injury. Another study showed that while African Americans are twice as likely to go blind from progressive ophthalmologic diseases such as glaucoma, they are half as likely to receive sight-saving procedures. Such disturbing evidence from the medical profession is a sobering reflection of the parallel reality and tragic costs of racism that persist in American society and that potentially influence every physician.

Clearly, program developers and researchers cannot, in our cultural competency training, simply stimulate a detached, intellectual practice of describing "the other" in the tradition of descriptive medical anthropology. At the heart of this education process should be the provision of intellectual and practical leadership that engages physician trainees in an ongoing, courageous, and honest process of self-critique and self-awareness. Guiding trainees to identify and examine their own patterns of unintentional and intentional racism, classism, and homophobia is essential.

One way to initiate such a constructive process is to have trainees think consciously about their own, often ill-defined and multidimensional cultural identities and backgrounds. In leading trainees into this process of cultivating self-awareness and awareness of the perspectives of others, trainers and program planners have used the following pedagogical approaches with success: small-group discussions; personal journals; availability of constructive professional role models from cultural groups and from the trainee's groups; and videotaping and feedback, including directed introspection of residents' interactions with patients. Recognition and respect for others' cultural priorities and practices is facilitated by such initial and ongoing processes that engender self-knowledge.

At the same time and by the same process of self-reflection, awakening trainees to the incredible position of power physicians potentially hold over all patients, particularly the poor, is critical. Especially in the context of race, ethnicity, class, linguistic capability, and sexual orientation, physicians must be taught to repeatedly identify and remedy the inappropriate exploitation of this power imbalance in the establishment of treatment priorities and health promotion activities.

Again, humility, and not so much the discrete mastery traditionally implied by the static notion of competence, captures most accurately what researchers need to model and hold programs accountable for evaluating in trainees under the broad scope of multicultural training in medical education.

Patient-focused Interviewing and Care

Embodied in the physician who practices cultural humility is the patient-focused or language-focused interviewing process. Studies of patient-physician communication have shown a strong bias on the part of physicians against patient-initiated questions and agendas, with physicians in one study initiating over 90 percent of the questions. Another study demonstrated that although poor and minority patients wanted as much information regarding their conditions as did other patients, they received less information regarding their conditions, less positive or reinforcing speech, and less talk overall.

Patient-focused interviewing uses a less controlling, less authoritative style that signals to the patient that the practitioner values what the patient's agenda and perspectives are, both biomedical and nonbiomedical. With these communication skills, perhaps along with other specifically cross-cultural interaction techniques, physicians potentially create an atmosphere that enables and does not obstruct the patient's telling of his or her own illness or wellness story. This eliminates the need for a complete mastery of every group's health beliefs and other concerns because the patient in the ideal scenario is encouraged to communicate how little or how much culture has to do with that particular clinical encounter.

For example, Ridley describes the uniqueness of a patient by detailing the patient's "conjoint membership in eight cultural roles:" as a Mexican American, male, father, husband, Catholic, mechanic, night-school student, and resident of East Los Angeles. Only the patient is uniquely qualified to help the physician understand the intersection of race, ethnicity, religion, class, and so on in forming his (the patient's) identity and to clarify the relevance and impact of this intersection on the present illness or wellness experience. Relevant and effective prevention, health promotion, and therapeutic strategies can then be developed that take into account the patient's life priorities, health beliefs, and life stressors. Humility is a prerequisite in this process, as the physician relinquishes the role of *expert* to the patient, becoming the *student* of the patient with a conviction and explicit expression of the patient's potential to be a capable and full partner in the therapeutic alliance.

Community-based Care and Advocacy

There is increasing consensus that a substantial portion of physicians' clinical training needs to occur in community sites. It is argued that training needs to happen in arenas where most physicians will eventually practice, away from the university-based, largely tertiary medical center. Part of this training directive includes a population-based approach to health promotion and disease prevention that works toward the optimal health of communities; that is, health in its broadest sense of physical, mental, and social well-being. Evans states that "surely a small part of each physician's responsibility should extend beyond the care of individual patients to the advocacy for changes in the community's policies and practices that influence determinants of health, causes of disease, and the effectiveness of health services."

Competency in advocacy is actually mandated by the American Academy of Pediatrics as a skill to be acquired during pediatric residency. This professional skill is to be taught by way of "structured educational experiences that prepare residents for their future role as advocates for the health of all children . . . with particular attention to underserved populations."

It is hoped that community-based care and advocacy training would go beyond working with community physicians and even beyond training in legislative advocacy to include systematically and methodically immersing trainees in mutually beneficial, nonpaternalistic, and respectful working relationships with community members and organizations. Experiencing with the community the factors at play in defining health priorities, research activities, and community-informed advocacy activities requires that the physician trainee recognize that foci of expertise with regard to health can indeed reside outside of the academic medical center and even outside of the practice of Western medicine. Competence, thus, again becomes best illustrated by humility, as physician trainees learn to identify, believe in, and build on the assets and adaptive strengths of communities and their often disenfranchised members. Requiring ongoing self-reflection and a parallel notion of patient-(community-) focused interactions, the possibility then exists for planning, practice, and advocacy in community health work in which physicians and physician trainees are both effective students of and partners with the community.

Institutional Consistency

The same processes expected to affect change in physician trainees should simultaneously exist in the institutions whose agenda is to develop cultural competence through educational programs. Self-reflection and self-critique at the institutional level is required, encompassing honest, thorough, and ongoing responses to the following questions: What is the demographic profile of the faculty? Is the faculty composition inclusive of members from diverse cultural, racial, ethnic, and sexual orientation backgrounds? Are faculty members required to undergo multicultural training as are the youngest students of the profession? Does the institutional ethos support inclusion and respectful, substantive discussions of the clinical implications of difference? What institutional processes contradict or obstruct the lessons taught and learned in a multicultural curriculum (i.e., if it is taught that practitioners should not use children or other family members as translators, does the institution provide an accessible alternative?)? What is the history of the health care institution with the surrounding community? And what present model of relationship between the institution and the community is seen by trainees?

Time-limited and explicit educational goals are one dimension of demonstrated institutional cultural competence. For instance, developing a written plan of faculty recruitment and/or curricular development to be in place by a designated date could be a point to which the community and/or other external entities hold the institution publicly accountable with regard to issues of race, ethnicity, language, culture, sexual orientation, and class in health care.

Summary of the Challenge to Medical Education Researchers

The emphasis on demonstration of process as opposed to endpoint is not meant to imply that training outcomes in cultural competence programs cannot be measured or monitored. Capturing the characteristic of cultural humility in individuals and institutions is possible, especially with mixed methodologies that use qualitative methods (including participant observation, key informant interviews, trainees' journals, and mechanisms for community feedback) and action research models to complement traditional quantitative assessments (pre- and postknowledge tests, patient and trainee surveys) of program effectiveness. A potentially valuable measure is the documentation of an active, ongoing institutional process that includes training, established recruitment and retention processes, identifiable and funded personnel to facilitate the meeting of program goals, and dynamic feedback loops between the institution and its employees and between the institution and patients and/or other members from the surrounding community.

This is not to say that the measurement of individuals' or institutions' cultural competence is a well-developed area of research. Witness this present discussion on defining training outcomes. Indeed, the definition and measurement of program effectiveness in producing cultural competence is a relatively new arena of inquiry in need of careful and attentive intellectual leadership. Nonetheless, acknowledging the necessity for creativity in a program's development and evaluation stages will help avoid the pitfall of adopting the status quo in documenting clinical competence.

Conclusion

In this critically important dialogue of defining training outcomes, it is proposed that the notion of cultural humility be distinguished from that of cultural competence. Cultural humility incorporates a lifelong commitment to self-evaluation and critique, to redressing the power imbalances in the physician-patient dynamic, and to developing mutually beneficial and non-paternalistic partnerships with communities on behalf of individuals and defined populations.

Acknowledgments

This work was supported by grants from the California Wellness Foundation, the Federal Office of Minority Health (DHHS), the East Bay Neonatology Foundation, and the Bay Area Physicians for Human Rights.

References

A list of references is available in the original source.

Minority Women and Advocacy for Women's Health

by Shiriki K. Kumanyika, PhD, MPH, Christiaan B. Morssink, MA, MPH, and Marion Nestle, PhD, MPH

US minority health issues involve racial/ethnic disparities that affect both women and men. However, women's health advocacy in the United States does not consistently address problems specific to minority women.

The underlying evolution and political strength of the women's health and minority health movements differ profoundly. Women of color comprise only one quarter of women's health movement constituents and are, on average, socioeconomically disadvantaged. Potential alliances may be inhibited by vestiges of historical racial and social divisions that detract from feelings of commonality and mutual support.

Nevertheless, insufficient attention to minority women's issues undermines the legitimacy of the women's health movement and may prevent important advances that can be achieved only when diversity is fully considered.

Women's health advocacy in the United States does not consistently address problems specific to women in ethnic and socioeconomic subgroups. Numerous differences in the health concerns of minority and majority women have been documented. As shown in Table 1, Black women have a shorter life expectancy than White women by 5 years, 50% higher all-cause mortality rates, and death rates from major causes such as heart disease, cerebrovascular disease, and diabetes that are often 2 to 3 times higher than those for White women. Breast cancer incidence is similar for Black and White women, but Black women have higher breast cancer mortality. Among younger and reproductive-aged women, maternal mortality and homicide rates are 4 times higher for Black women than for White women, and the rate of HIV-related deaths is 12 times higher for Black women. The complexity of women's health advocacy emanates, in part, from the fact that the inequities at issue do not carry over into mortality disparities vis-à-vis men. This is generally true across ethnic groups (Table 1). In contrast, minority health advocacy has been organized primarily around attempts to leverage the data that show striking ethnic disparities in mortality. Thus, taking a minority perspective on women's health may "confuse the issue" to the extent that it draws attention to the favored health status of White women relative to Black women or other women of color.

At issue, then, is how to crease awareness of the special health concerns of minority women within the women's health movement and to ensure that the concerns of minority women are incorporated as integral components of the larger women's health agenda. Although some authorities now argue that the minority health perspective must be included in any discussion of the health of women in the United States, the dilemmas that minority women confront in embracing "women's" health may not be generally recognized. In this commentary, we describe these dilemmas. Our objective is to help advocates for both minority health and women's health to serve their constituents.

Emancipation as an Underlying Theme

There are profound differences in the outlook and relative political strength of the women's health and minority health movements, but, as with many social movements, both center around a theme of emancipation. With respect to gender, emancipation issues center around the effect of discrimination against women in patriarchal societies, regardless of class, caste, or other such considerations—namely, "glass ceilings." voting rights, and pay equity in comparison with males, as well as reproductive rights, research equity, and access to and equity in health care.

These gender issues are a rallying point for social or political action among minority women, but minority women also have issues related to race or ethnicity. White women have the luxury of being able to ignore racial biases and are free to focus exclusively (or almost so) on gender problems. In contrast, minority women experience and must simultaneously guard against both racism and sexism. These two forces, although similar in some respects, operate independently.

White women have the advantage of understanding the dominant culture as well as sharing the obligations associated with participation in it. In this sense, the discussion of gender equity among White men and women is a negotiation among *cultural equals*—people who share a common language, norms, and values. Minority women—who have been distanced from the majority culture by history, language, religion, and other factors related to race and ethnicity—do not have the same stake in the majority culture; they enter discussions of equity with an entirely different set of premises. For example, many minority women may perceive White women as having exploited the civil rights movement to achieve their own goals. In addition, middle-class minority women may experience pressure to become assimilated into the dominant culture while also continuing to face reminders of their exclusion from it, which hinders their sense of commonality with White women.

Differing Evolution of Health Advocacy

The evolution of the women's health and minority health movements is depicted schematically in Figure 1 as variations on a general advocacy model. Inequalities or other flaws in health and social systems create specific problems and issues that become focal targets of social movements and that generate advocacy for special funding, special programs, new regulations, or new methods for accomplishing goals. Successful health movements decrease disparities in health status or health services and increase equality of attention to health concerns. However, there are fundamental differences in the character of the women's health and minority health movements.

As shown in Figure 1, the women's health movement evolved as an offshoot of the modern women's rights movement that encompassed the activism in the 1960s, the development of the National Organization for Women, the consciousness-raising groups of the 1970s, and the introduction of academic departments of women's studies into universities. An important milestone was the Roe v Wade decision of 1973, with ensuing legislative struggles over reproductive rights. Such concerns led to increased advocacy for control of more general health

TABLE 1 Gender and Ethnic Comparisons of Selected Health Indicators for US Blacks and Whites

Indicator	Females White	Females Black	Females Black-White Difference or Ratio[c,d]	Males White	Males Black	Males Black-White Difference or Ratio[c,d]	Gender Difference or Ratio[a,b] White Males vs White Females	Gender Difference or Ratio[a,b] Black Males vs Black Females
Life expectancy at birth, 1998[e]	80.0	74.8	-5.2	74.5	67.6	-6.9	-5.5	-7.2
Life expectancy at 65 y, 1998[e]	19.3	17.4	-1.9	16.1	14.3	-1.8	-3.2	-3.1
Years of potential life lost before 75 y, 1998, age adjusted, all causes, per 100,000 population[e]	4751	9283	2.0	8352	16626	2.0	1.8	1.8
All-cause mortality (per 100,000), age adjusted, all ages, 1996–1998[e]	358	549	1.5	576	921	1.6	1.6	1.7
Cause-specific mortality (per 100,000) within age group, 1997[f]								
Homicide, 15–24 y[f]	3.2	13.3	4.2	13.2	113.3	8.6	4.2	8.5
Suicide, 15–24 y[f]	3.7	2.4	0.6	19.5	16.0	0.8	5.3	6.7
Motor vehicle accidents, 15–24 y[f]	18.4	11.3	0.6	39.8	32.7	0.8	2.2	2.9
HIV related, 24–44 y[f]	2.4	29.3	12.2	13.2	76.7	5.8	5.5	2.6
Diseases of the heart, 45–64 y[f]	92.2	224.6	2.4	249.0	455.5	1.8	2.7	2.0
Malignant neoplasms, 45–64 y[f]	213.3	276.6	1.3	247.0	416.8	1.7	1.2	1.5
Breast neoplasms, all ages, age adjusted[g]	19.0	26.2	1.4	...	...	...	...	...
Breast neoplasms, 35–44 y[g]	12.6	23.6	1.9	...	...	...	...	...
Cerebrovascular disease, 45–64 y[f]	19.7	56.3	2.9	25.4	87.9	3.5	1.3	1.6
Diabetes, 45–64 y[f]	17.2	52.9	3.1	21.3	57.3	2.7	1.2	1.1
Maternal mortality (deaths per 100,000 live births), all ages, age adjusted, 1998[e]	4.2	16.1	3.8	...	...	...	...	...
Hypertension (%), 20–74 y, age adjusted, 1988–1994[e]	19.3	33.8	1.8	24.3	34.9	1.4	1.3	1.0
Osteoporosis (%), females ≥50 y, 1988–1991[g]	21.0	10.0	0.5	...	...	...	...	...
Low-birthweight infants (% of live births), 1998[e]	6.5	13.1	2.0	...	...	...	...	...
Cancer incidence (new cases/100,000 population), all ages, age adjusted, 1996[e]								
Lung and bronchus	43.7	47.2	1.1	68.4	101.4	1.5	1.6	2.1
Breast	113.3	100.3	0.9	...	...	...	...	...
Colon and rectum	35.5	41.8	1.2	50.7	50.9	1.0	1.4	1.2

[a] Life expectancy from birth or 65 y is difference in years for males minus years for females.
[b] Indicators other than life expectancy are ratios (males divided by females).
[c] Life expectancy from birth or 65 y is difference in years for Blacks minus years for Whites.
[d] Indicators other than life expectancy are ratios (Black divided by White).
[e] Data are from the National Center for Health Statistics.
[f] Data are from Hoyert et al.
[g] Data are from the Third Nutrition Monitoring Report.

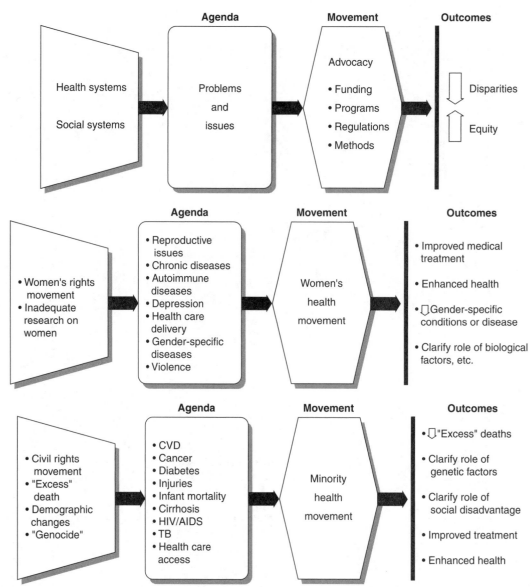

FIGURE 1 Schematic portrayal of the evolution of health advocacy in general (top), in women's health (middle), and in minority health (bottom).

Note: CVD = cardiovascular and cerbravascular disease; TB = tuberculosis.

matters and to greater attention to women's issues in mainstream medical research. Today, the women's health agenda includes conditions that occur throughout the entire life cycle and all types of diseases, as well as more general problems such as depression, lack of health care, and domestic violence. Efforts are made to link this US agenda to global women's health issues. The desired outcomes of successful advocacy for women's health include improvements in medical treatment and decreases in the incidence and prevalence of disease conditions specific to women. An additional goal is to clarify the role of social

factors as determinants of women's health and to avoid the reductionist view that health difference between men and women are entirely biological in origin.

In contrast, the minority health movement evolved as an offshoot of the civil rights struggle that is unique to the sociopolitical history of the United States, and it is equally relevant to both sexes. Current advocacy for minority health is anchored in a 1985 federal task force report documenting "excess deaths" among minority groups compared with the White population. For example, the task force found that among Native Americans and African Americans younger than 45 years, death rates were 47% and 42% higher, respectively, than would be expected on the basis of death rates for Whites. For persons 70 years and younger in these 2 groups, 22% and 42% of deaths, respectively, were "excess deaths." Disparities in some areas were seen to have persisted or worsened even in the presence of societal changes intended to improve the condition of minority groups.

The minority health movement is linked to the history of adversarial relations between the White American majority and people of color. Without regard to gender, these adversarial relations include stigmatization of people with dark skin, legal and de facto segregation and discrimination, and a host of painful historical associations with slavery, the Tuskegee study, involuntary sterilization, and internment in wartime relocation camps. At the extreme, the historic events and patterns of discrimination have led some minority observers to charge that the present situation in health care resembles earlier efforts to achieve the genocide—systematic annihilation—of the African American population; they argue that the poor health care in minority communities is a deliberate effort to encourage the gradual disappearance of an unwanted group. This deep, historically based distrust of the medical establishment and the mainstream society affects both women and men in minority populations.

Recent scientific and policy shifts may further marginalize minority group members from mainstream health advocacy. For example, the genomic revolution has created a climate that appears to favor biological explanations over social explanations for diseases. Although minority group categorizations are not biological designations, research on ethnic differences has a high potential for being misunderstood in such a climate and could well stimulate a new "eugenics" debate in which racial and ethnic health disparities are attributed to biological inferiority rather than to environmentally determined conditions such as poverty. The fear of such a scenario would tend to create closer allegiances within minority groups across gender lines but provoke tension within gender groups across ethnicity lines.

White vs Minority Women: The Numbers Game

Minority women are no less in the minority—numerically, regarding political power, and with respect to the risk of being stereotyped or misunderstood—when the topic is limited to females. The women's health movement draws on *half* the US population for its constituency, but minorities—men and women—make up only about *one fourth* of the US population. The "minority population," however, comprises several subpopulations whose only common characteristic is being "non-White," and women in a specific minority population may constitute as few as 1% (American Indian) or no more than 10% to 12% (Hispanic or African American) of the female population. In contrast, *half* the constituents of the minority health movement or any subset of it would be expected to be women. Thus, in terms of numbers of constituents and relationship to the White majority, the women's health movement is more powerful than the minority health movement, even when the diverse minority populations speak as one voice. For numerical reasons alone, minority women might view the women's health movement as dominated by White women and feel "more equal" when pursuing health advocacy from a minority health perspective. Nonminority women who fail to understand these proportionalities may view minority women who give priority to minority issues (and advocate for both minority men's and women's health) as insufficiently informed about or loyal to women's rights issues. In addition, in the constant competition for funding and access to the national political agenda, attention to women's health issues may appear to dilute the resources that might be available for minority issues. This scenario would be less adversarial if the health issues for all women were the same, but, as we explain, they differ in several important respects.

Addressing Minority Women's Health

Considerations of minority women's health are fraught with vestiges of the historical relations noted earlier, but also with additional issues related to social class. For both minority and majority women, feelings of mutual support may be inhibited by recollections of domestic servitude that reinforce the higher social class basis of the women's health movement as opposed to the minority women's health movement. In addition, stereotypical views about Black women and sexuality may inhibit open discussion of reproductive health issues in interracial advocacy forums. Underlying views of abortion diverge between Black and White women; for example, White women generally perceived abortion as an issue of the right of control over their bodies, whereas many African American women view abortion through the prism of "this country's shameful history of sterilization abuse."

Within women's health, views of minority women's health issues may also be distorted by spurious theories about race-based disease "immunity" and related biases in medical thinking. Clinicians or researchers may deny or understate the potential relevance to minorities of conditions such as coronary heart disease that at one time had lower prevalences among minorities than among Whites. Although myths and misperceptions may be refuted by hard data—for example, those showing disease rates in minority populations that surpass those in the White population—the availability of data does not immediately erase biases from clinical practice and teaching. Even when discussions are relatively free of stereotypes, biases, and competition between causes, health issues for minority women do not always fit well into the generalities applied to women's health overall.

Toward a Unified Perspective

On February 21, 1998, President Clinton announced an initiative committing the nation to the goal of eliminating by 2010 long-standing disparities in health status that affect racial and ethnic minority groups. In light of this initiative, the dilemmas for minority women become even more profound. For women of color, working toward common goals for the benefit of all women, majority as well as minority, requires a suspension of attention to overriding issues of racial bias. This suspension, however, carried a price; it may separate minority women from the support systems that minority communities offer to men and women alike. A focus on gender issues *independent of race,* therefore, requires minority women to choose between racial issues and women's issues and therefore polarizes the debate. For reasons of community support alone, most, if not all, minority women must give priority to struggles against racial and ethnic discrimination. Thus, minority women tend to view women's issues from a perspective that is not shared with *any* other group—White women, White men, or minority men. This isolation may act as a barrier to social action, professional accomplishment, or health behaviors considered appropriate and desirable by majority women.

Can common ground be found on which to forge alliances to integrate gender- and ethnicity-based health advocacy? Could, for example, the women's health movement (re)frame HIV/AIDS, with its potential for vertical transmission to offspring and its higher burden in Black and Hispanic women, as a mainstream women's health issue, even though it might draw resources from health issues more salient for White women? Is it acceptable for policymakers to claim as a breakthrough in *women's* health a pathway first elucidated in *minority* women? For example, systemic lupus erythematosus affects more women than men, but it affects more Black than White women and has a poorer outcome in Black women. Should studies of Black women with lupus take priority in this field? In contrast, osteoporosis affects proportionately more White than minority women, although all women are at higher risk than men. A consideration of *both* lupus and osteoporosis as agenda items for the women's health movement could easily be embraced by a broad coalition of women, but the battle for priorities is likely to prove uneven if resources are limited.

A key question for researchers is how the women's health movement can exploit, in a positive way, the element of diversity as a means to better understand disease causation and progression. That is, ethnic differences in disease occurrence or prognosis may be caused by risk factors with different distributions and different time trends by ethnicity—for example, socioeconomic status variables, reproductive patterns, dietary and physical activity practices, alcohol consumption, occupational exposures to carcinogens, area of residence and migration, and certain gene frequencies. The identification of variables that mediate ethnic differences in disease patterns may lead to new etiologic hypotheses for closer study. Lin and Kelsey give examples of how the study of variation within and across diverse ethnic groups has been applied to the study of breast cancer, osteoporotic fractures, and several other health outcomes and discuss the methodological challenges inherent in this approach.

Minority health and women's health constitute different movements and different venues for action. However, many minority women's issues are also, in some form, issues for women in general. Thus, the goals of action for women's health can be mutually supportive even when the perspectives and strategies of participants vary by race and ethnicity. Health aspects on which minority women diverge from White women should not prevent the development of a shared women's health agenda. Recognition and acceptance of differing agendas among women will go much further in facilitating cooperation than will forcing alliances in which gender is the only permissible variable.

References

A list of references is available in the original source.

Health at the Margins

by Gabrie'l J. Atchison

In this issue, we are asking how different forms of discrimination affect the quality of healthcare that women receive. What are the barriers to women's health? We include information about women of color, lesbians, women with disabilities, women living in poverty, rural women, and women living in the Global South. This article is a brief overview of information about women in different groups, which shows that there are some interesting similarities from group to group. Marginalized women in general seem more likely to die from preventable diseases and health conditions, because they reach professionals too late. They experience higher levels of stress and have less leisure time, which contributes to unique health problems. There is not enough research about the health needs of women at the margins, so healthcare providers cannot help them adequately. Violence is a major health risk in the lives of marginalized women. Poverty and racism are also especially linked to high incidences of HIV infection and AIDS deaths.

Women of Color

African American Women

Black women face stereotyping and discrimination in their healthcare. They are less likely to have health insurance, more likely to face great financial barriers to adequate healthcare, less likely to have information about symptoms, and less likely to have healthcare facilities in their neighborhoods. Due to high levels of stress, African American women are disproportionately represented among the obese in this country and have high rates of hypertension, heart disease, and stroke, three other stress-related conditions. African American women have the highest death rate due to HIV of any racial/ethnic group. There is no research explaining why this is so. AIDS is the leading cause of death for African American women between the ages of 25 and 44. Homicide and violence is the fourth leading cause of death in this group. Maternal mortality is four times higher for African American women than white women, and African Americans have the highest infant mortality rate

of any racial group. Native American women and African American women experience and witness violence more often than other groups of women.

Latinas

Latino families have the highest rates of poverty in the United States; almost 30 percent of Latinas live in poverty. Their healthcare problems are compounded by language barriers, racism, and lack of access to healthcare facilities. Like African American women, Latinas are often diagnosed when it is too late for proper treatment, especially with breast cancer. For undocumented Latinas, there is an additional fear of being reported and deported, so many women do not have access to healthcare at all for themselves or their children. Latinas experience high levels of severe depression, and have the highest prevalence of lifetime depression. For Latinas, the leading causes of death are heart disease, diabetes, and stroke. Diabetes is the second highest cause of death for Latinas between the ages of 55 and 74. Latinas have the second highest death rate due to HIV.

Asian American Women

Like Latinas, the Asian American community is diverse in language, culture, and geographic location. There is not enough information about this diversity, so more research is needed. According to the information that is available, Asian Americans who live in poverty face similar racial discrimination in healthcare, combined with the added burden of language and cultural differences and undocumented immigration status among some communities. Some of the research suggests that Asian American women do not have adequate access to reproductive healthcare providers. Many Asian American women work in factories or in small, family-owned businesses and do not have any access to healthcare. Unsafe and unhealthy work environments also contribute to their health problems.

Native American Women

Native American women face logistic and cultural barriers to obtaining healthcare services. Many Native American women live in rural communities and have limited access to transportation, and there is only a small number of healthcare facilities available to them. In some Native communities, women have traditionally been the healers for other women, so Native American women find going to male doctors uncomfortable. Many women do not seek preventative services. There are high rates of smoking and alcohol and drug addiction in these communities and very few culturally specific recovery programs. Accidents and violence are the most common causes of death among this group of women. Almost one quarter of all Native American women live in poverty. They experience racial discrimination, high unemployment, environmental racism, and poor quality housing; and they often live near toxic waste or other forms of environmental hazards and lack access to safe water.

Immigrant Women of Color

Ten percent of the United States population are immigrants. Of that group, more than half are from Latin America and one quarter is from Asia. Women in these populations experience racism as well as language and cultural barriers to receiving healthcare. The Personal Responsibility Work Opportunity and Reconciliation Act of 1996 restricted immigrant women's access to healthcare services and insurance by allowing states to deny Medicaid benefits to immigrant families. Many immigrants live in poverty and have no access to healthcare.

Lesbians

Little attention is paid to the special health needs of lesbians. There should be more research which takes into account the diversity of lesbian women. Lesbians experience job discrimination and because of this may end up in low-paying jobs or feel forced to stay in the closet about their sexuality. Most lesbians are not covered by their partners' insurance. Lesbians also face a great deal of discrimination trying to receive healthcare, most of which stems from the assumption of heterosexuality by providers. Lack of legal recognition can prevent lesbians from getting financial support when a partner becomes ill or dies. Typically lesbians cannot benefit from life insurance, family leave, workers' compensation, or hospital visitation rights. Lesbian women are also susceptible to hate crimes and violence. Since lesbians are less likely to use contraceptives and may be reluctant to discuss their sexual lives with providers they fear will discriminate against them, they may not have regular gynecological checkups, including preventative services like cervical and breast cancer screenings. There is a lack of information about the health habits of lesbians outside of their sexual behaviors. The issue of domestic violence in lesbian communities is a major health concern. A disproportionate number of youth suicides are young lesbians who cannot find acceptance or approval. Because of ageism and homophobia, the special health needs of the older lesbian community are invisible. There can be safety problems in nursing homes because of homophobia among attendants and other personnel. Healthcare providers are urged to challenge their own assumptions of heterosexuality and those of their colleagues to make healthcare more inclusive of lesbians. Simply using language like "partner" as opposed to "boyfriend" or "husband" would make a difference. Physicians could also change office registration forms, questionnaires, and informational brochures to include information about lesbians.

Women with Disabilities

Women with disabilities face a multitude of barriers to proper healthcare. Some of these barriers include physical inaccessibility of medical offices, limited availability of information, inaccessible public transportation, and inadequate treatment or outright refusals of treatment by healthcare providers. Health maintenance organizations place strict limits on therapeutic, supportive, and home services, which severely limit disabled women's ability to live independently. There are also problems because women are not able to use specialists as primary care providers, and alternative therapies are often not covered. There is a lack of research on disabled women and health, but some of the special concerns for this group are violence and barriers to adequate mental and reproductive healthcare. Disabled women are at high risk for depression and eating disorders, and are often either denied medication or are oversedated. They experience forced sterilization, coerced abortions, and unauthorized hysterectomies. Disabled women and girls are very vulnerable to emotional, physical, and sexual abuse by partners, family members, and care givers, and since they are often not believed when they report this abuse many of these crimes go unreported. Girls with disabilities are almost twice as likely as other girls to be sexually abused and assaulted.

Caring for a Disabled Child

Taking care of a child with a disability demands a great deal of time and can cause a lot of stress. When a women lives in poverty, having a disabled child can be completely overwhelming. Visits with doctors and specialists can be an all-day event, especially if one had to spend a long time on public transportation. This often means missing days from work. Working low-income women most often receive no sympathy from employers for these absences. Low-income women who have to work to provide for the care of their children are often accused by their children's care providers of not loving or attending to their children enough. For developmentally disabled children, the quality of attention they receive in their early years affects the quality of life they will have as adults.

Women Living in Poverty

In the United States and globally, women are disproportionately represented among the people living in poverty. In the United States, health is a commodity, and things like gym memberships, medication, and vacations and leisure time are all too expensive for women living in poverty. Without an adequate income, women cannot afford healthcare, health insurance, safe housing, or nutritious food. Serious illness of a parent or child can result in economic ruin for many poor families. Many of the women and girls in prison are there because they sold drugs or did sex work to support themselves and their children. The lack of public transportation in poor communities makes travel to healthcare facilities difficult. Violence is a major cause of death among poor women and many advocacy groups are pressuring politicians for gun control laws to reduce the level of deaths and serious injuries to women caused by gunshots.

Rural Women

Rural Women are almost non-existent in psychological literature, but we know that rural women experience barriers to healthcare because of isolation, fewer resources, lack of transportation, and lack of access to medical and mental health services, which are often concentrated in cities. Rural women have a higher incidence of anxiety and depression. Often, the only providers in rural areas are from the public health centers. Rural women have to travel far for healthcare, only to see a doctor with less training. Because rural women have less contact with doctors, they have lower levels of preventive care.

Women in the Global South

"The Global South" is a phrase used to describe countries commonly referred to as "developing countries"—the term is meant to bring attention to the relationship between the colonizer and the colonized and to economic privilege and control. The phrase incorporates many different countries and relationships between countries. Women are overrepresented among the poor in the Global South, and women's poverty is destructive to women and children's health in these countries. Women and girls are often the last to eat and thus are often malnourished. Their health problems are considered less important than men's problems. For example, the number of women with HIV in Africa is considerably higher than that of men with the disease, yet men are receiving more care and treatment. Adolescent girls are particularly vulnerable because of lack of information about reproductive health, lack of power in sexual relations, scarcity of reproductive health services, and susceptibility to sexual abuse and violence. It is estimated that women in the Global South work twice as many hours as men. They also work in dangerous, unhealthy environments like sweatshops, the informal economy, and the sex industry. Many women work at paid jobs and still have to provide care for children, men, and the elderly. Poverty combined with high levels of stress exacerbate health problems faced by women.

Under the Shadow of Tuskegee

African Americans and Health Care

by Vanessa Northington Gamble, MD, PhD

Abstract The Tuskegee Syphilis Study continues to cast its long shadow on the contemporary relationship between African Americans and the biomedical community. Numerous reports have argued that the Tuskegee Syphilis Study is the most important reason why many African Americans distrust the institutions of medicine and public health. Such an interpretation neglects a critical historical point: the mistrust predated public revelations about the Tuskegee study. This paper places the syphilis study within a broader historical and social context to demonstrate that several factors have influenced—and continue to influence—African Americans' attitudes toward the biomedical community. (*Am J Public Health.* 1997;87:1773–1778)

Introduction

On May 16, 1997, in a White House ceremony, President Bill Clinton apologized for the Tuskegee Syphilis Study, the 40-year government study (1932 to 1972) in which 399 Black men from Macon County, Alabama, were deliberately denied effective treatment for syphilis in order to document the natural history of the disease. "The legacy of the study at Tuskegee," the president remarked, "has reached far and deep, in ways that hurt our progress and divide our nation. We cannot be one America when a whole segment of our nation has no trust in America." The president's comments underscore that in the 25 years since its public disclosure, the study has moved from being a singular historical event to a powerful metaphor. It has come to symbolize racism in medicine, misconduct in human research, the arrogance of physicians, and government abuse of Black people.

The continuing shadow cast by the Tuskegee Syphilis Study on efforts to improve the health status of Black Americans provided an impetus for the campaign for a presidential apology. Numerous articles, in both the professional and popular press, have pointed out that the study predisposed many African Americans to distrust medical and public health authorities and has led to critically low Black participation in clinical trials and organ donation.

The specter of Tuskegee has also been raised with respect to HIV/AIDS prevention and treatment programs. Health education researchers Dr Stephen B. Thomas and Dr Sandra Crouse Quinn have written extensively on the impact of the Tuskegee Syphilis Study on these programs. They argue that "the legacy of this experiment, with its failure to educate the study participants and treat them adequately, laid the foundation for today's pervasive sense of black distrust of public health authorities." The syphilis study has also been used to explain why many African Americans oppose needle exchange programs. Needle exchange programs provoke the image of the syphilis study and Black fears about genocide. These programs are not viewed as mechanisms to stop the spread of HIV/AIDS but rather as fodder for the drug epidemic that has devastated so many Black neighborhoods. Fears that they will be used as guinea pigs like the men in the syphilis study have also led some African Americans with AIDS to refuse treatment with protease inhibitors.

The Tuskegee Syphilis Study is frequently described as the singular reason behind African-American distrust of the institutions of medicine and public health. Such an interpretation neglects a critic historical point: the mistrust predated public revelations about the Tuskegee study. Furthermore, the narrowness of such a representation places emphasis on a single historical event to explain deeply entrenched and complex attitudes within the Black community. An examination of the syphilis study within a broader historical and social context makes plain that several factors have influenced, and continue to influence, African Americans' attitudes toward the biomedical community.

Black Americans' fears about exploitation by the medical profession date back to the antebellum period and the use of slaves and free Black people as subjects for dissection and medical experimentation. Although physicians also used poor Whites as subjects, they used Black people far more often. During an 1835 trip to the United States, French visitor Harriet Martineau found that Black people lacked the power even to protect the graves of their dead. "In Baltimore the bodies of coloured people exclusively are taken for dissection," she remarked, "because the Whites do not like it, and the coloured people cannot resist." Four years later, abolitionist Theodore Dwight Weld echoed Martineau's sentiment. "Public opinion," he wrote, "would tolerate surgical experiments, operations, processes, performed upon them [slaves], which it would execrate if performed upon their master or other whites." Slaves found themselves as subjects of medical experiments because physicians needed bodies and because the state considered them property and denied them the legal right to refuse to participate.

Two antebellum experiments, one carried out in Georgia and the other in Alabama, illustrate the abuse that some slaves encountered at the hands of physicians. In the first, Georgia physician Thomas Hamilton conducted a series of brutal experiments on a slave to test remedies for heatstroke. The subject of these investigations, Fed, had been loaned to Hamilton as repayment for a debt owed by his owner. Hamilton forced Fed to sit naked on a stool placed on a platform in a pit that had been heated to a high temperature. Only the man's head was above ground. Over a period of 2 to 3 weeks, Hamilton placed Fed in the pit five or six times and gave him various medications to determine which enabled him best to withstand the heat. Each ordeal ended when Fed fainted and had to be revived. But note that Fed was not the only victim in this experiment; its whole purpose was to make it possible for masters to force slaves to work still longer hours on the hottest of days.

In the second experiment, Dr J. Marion Sims, the so-called father of modern gynecology, used three Alabama slave women to develop an operation to repair vesicovaginal fistulas. Between 1845 and 1849, the three slave women on whom Sims operated each underwent up to 30 painful operations. The physician himself described the agony associated with some of the experiments: "The first patient I operated on was Lucy. . . . That was before the days of anesthetics, and the poor girl, on her knees, bore the operation with great heroism

and bravery." This operation was not successful, and Sims later attempted to repair the defect by placing a sponge in the bladder. This experiment, too, ended in failure. He noted:

> The whole urethra and the neck of the bladder were in a high state of inflammation, which came from the foreign substance. It had to come away, and there was nothing to do but to pull it away by main force. Lucy's agony was extreme. She was much prostrated, and I thought that she was going to die; but by irrigating the parts of the bladder she recovered with great rapidity.

Sims finally did perfect his technique and ultimately repaired the fistulas. Only after his experimentation with the slave women proved successful did the physician attempt the procedure, with anesthesia, on White women volunteers.

Exploitation after the Civil War

It is not known to what extent African Americans continued to be used as unwilling subjects for experimentation and dissection in the years after emancipation. However, an examination of African-American folklore at the turn of the century makes it clear that Black people believed that such practices persisted. Folktales are replete with references to night doctors, also called student doctors and Ku Klux doctors. In her book, *Night Riders in Black Folk History,* anthropologist Gladys-Marie Fry writes, "The term 'night doctor' (derived from the fact that victims were sought only at night) applies both to students of medicine, who supposedly stole cadavers from which to learn about body processes, and [to] professional thieves, who sold stolen bodies—living and dead—to physicians for medical research." According to folk belief, these sinister characters would kidnap Black people, usually at night and in urban areas, and take them to hospitals to be killed and used in experiments. An 1889 *Boston Herald* article vividly captured the fears that African Americans in South Carolina had of night doctors. The report read, in part:

> The negroes of Clarendon, Williamsburg, and Sumter counties have for several weeks past been in a state of fear and trembling. They claim that there is a white man, a doctor, who at will can make himself invisible and who then approaches some unsuspecting darkey, and having rendered him or her insensible with chloroform, proceeds to fill up a bucket with the victim's blood, for the purpose of making medicine. After having drained the last drop

of blood from the victim, the body is dumped into some secret place where it is impossible for any person to find it. The colored women are so worked up over this phantom that they will not venture out at night, or in the daytime in any sequestered place.

Fry did not find any documented evidence of the existence of night riders. However, she demonstrated through extensive interviews that many African Americans expressed genuine fears that they would be kidnapped by night doctors and used for medical experimentation. Fry concludes that two factors explain this paradox. She argues that Whites, especially those in the rural South, deliberately spread rumors about night doctors in order to maintain psychological control over Blacks and to discourage their migration to the North so as to maintain a source of cheap labor. In addition, Fry asserts that the experiences of many African Americans as victims of medical experiments during slavery fostered their belief in the existence of night doctors. It should also be added that, given the nation's racial and political climate, Black people recognized their inability to refuse to participate in medical experiments.

Reports about the medical exploitation of Black people in the name of medicine after the end of the Civil War were not restricted to the realm of folklore. Until it was exposed in 1882, a grave robbing ring operated in Philadelphia and provided bodies for the city's medical schools by plundering the graves at a Black cemetery. According to historian David C. Humphrey, southern grave robbers regularly sent bodies of southern Blacks to northern medical schools for use as anatomy cadavers.

During the early 20th century, African-American medical leaders protested the abuse of Black people by the White-dominated medical profession and used their concerns about experimentation to press for the establishment of Black controlled hospitals. Dr Daniel Hale Williams, the founder of Chicago's Provident Hospital (1891), the nation's first Black-controlled hospital, contended that White physicians, especially in the South, frequently used Black patients as guinea pigs. Dr Nathan Francis Mossell, the founder of Philadelphia's Frederick Douglass Memorial Hospital (1895), described the "fears and prejudices" of Black people, especially those from the South, as "almost proverbial." He attributed such attitudes to southern medicine practices in which Black people, "when forced to accept hospital attention, got only the poorest care, being placed in inferior wards set apart for them, suffering the brunt of all that is experimental in treatment, and all this is the sequence of their race variety and abject helplessness." The founders of Black hospitals claimed that only Black physicians possessed the skills required to treat Black patients opti-

mally and that Black hospitals provided these patients with the best possible care.

Fears about the exploitation of African Americans by White physicians played a role in the establishment of a Black veterans hospital in Tuskegee, Ala. In 1923, 9 years before the initiation of the Tuskegee Syphilis Study, racial tensions had erupted in the town over control of the hospital. The federal government had pledged that the facility, an institution designed exclusively for Black patients, would be run by a Black professional staff. But many Whites in the area, including members of the Ku Klux Klan, did not want a Black-operated federal facility in the heart of Dixie, even though it would serve only Black people.

Black Americans sought control of the veterans hospital, in part because they believed that the ex-soldiers would receive the best possible care from Black physicians and nurses, who would be more caring and sympathetic to the veterans' needs. Some Black newspapers even warned that White southerners wanted command of the hospital as part of a racist plot to kill and sterilize African-American men and to establish an "experiment station" for mediocre White physicians. Black physicians did eventually gain the right to operate the hospital, yet this did not stop the hospital from becoming an experiment station for Black men. The veterans hospital was one of the facilities used by the United States Public Health Service in the syphilis study.

During the 1920s and 1930s, Black physicians pushed for additional measures that would battle medical racism and advance their professional needs. Dr Charles Garvin, a prominent Cleveland physician and a member of the editorial board of the Black medical publication *The Journal of the National Medical Association*, urged his colleagues to engage in research in order to protect Black patients. He called for more research on diseases such as tuberculosis and pellagra that allegedly affected African Americans disproportionately or idiosyncratically. Garvin insisted that Black physicians investigate these racial diseases because "heretofore in literature, as in medicine, the Negro has been written about, exploited and experimented upon sometimes not to his physical betterment or to the advancement of science, but the advancement of the Nordic investigator." Moreover, he charged that "in the past, men of other races have for the large part interpreted our diseases, often tinctured with inborn prejudices."

Fears of Genocide

These historical examples clearly demonstrate that African Americans' distrust of the medical profession has a longer history than the public revelations of the

Tuskegee Syphilis Study. There is a collective memory among African Americans about their exploitation by the medical establishment. The Tuskegee Syphilis Study has emerged as the most prominent example of medical racism because it confirms, if not authenticates, long-held and deeply entrenched beliefs within the Black community. To be sure, the Tuskegee Syphilis Study does cast a long shadow. After the study had been exposed, charges surfaced that the experiment was part of a governmental plot to exterminate Black people. Many Black people agreed with the charge that the study represented "nothing less than an official, premeditated policy of genocide." Furthermore, this was not the first or last time that allegations of genocide have been launched against the government and the medical profession. The sickle cell anemia screening programs of the 1970s and birth control programs have also provoked such allegations.

In recent years, links have been made between Tuskegee, AIDS, and genocide. In September 1990, the article "AIDS: Is It Genocide?" appeared in *Essence,* a Black woman's magazine. The author noted "As an increasing number of African-Americans continue to sicken and die and as no cure for AIDS has been found some of us are beginning to think the unthinkable: Could AIDS be a virus that was manufactured to erase large numbers of us? Are they trying to kill us with this disease?" In other words, some members of the Black community see AIDS as part of a conspiracy to exterminate African Americans.

Beliefs about the connection between AIDS and the purposeful destruction of African Americans should not be cavalierly dismissed as bizarre and paranoid. They are held by a significant number of Black people. For example, a 1990 survey conducted by the Southern Christian Leadership Conference found that 35% of the 1056 Black church members who responded believed that AIDS was a form of genocide. A *New York Times*/WCBS TV News poll conducted the same year found that 10% of Black Americans thought that the AIDS virus had been created in a laboratory in order to infect Black people. Another 20% believed that it could be true.

African Americans frequently point to the Tuskegee Syphilis Study as evidence to support their views about genocide, perhaps, in part, because many believe that the men in the study were actually injected with syphilis. Harlon Dalton, a Yale Law School professor and a former member of the National Commission on AIDS, wrote, in a 1989 article titled, "AIDS in Black Face," that "the government [had] purposefully exposed Black men to syphilis." Six years later, Dr Eleanor Walker, a Detroit radiation oncologist, offered an explanation as to why few African Americans become bone marrow donors. "The biggest fear, she claimed, is that they will become victims of some misfeasance, like the Tuskegee incident where Black men were infected with syphilis and left untreated to die from the disease." The January 25, 1996, episode of *New York Undercover,* a Fox Network police drama that is one of the top shows in Black households, also reinforced the rumor that the US Public Health Service physicians injected the men with syphilis. The myth about deliberate infection is not limited to the Black community. On April 8, 1997, news anchor Tom Brokaw, on "NBC Nightly News," announced that the men had been infected by the government.

Folklorist Patricia A. Turner, in her book *I Heard It through the Grapevine: Rumor and Resistance in African-American Culture,* underscores why it is important not to ridicule but to pay attention to these strongly held theories about genocide. She argues that these rumors reveal much about what African Americans believe to be the state of their lives in this country. She contends that such views reflect Black beliefs that White Americans have historically been, and continue to be, ambivalent and perhaps hostile to the existence of Black people. Consequently, African-American attitudes toward biomedical research are not influenced solely by the Tuskegee Syphilis Study. African Americans' opinions about the value White society has attached to their lives should not be discounted. As Reverend Floyd Tompkins of Stanford University Memorial Church has said, "There is a sense in our community, and I think it shall be proved out, that if you are poor or you're a person of color, you were the guinea pig, and you continue to be the guinea pigs, and there is the fundamental belief that Black life is not valued like White life or like any other life in America."

Not Just Paranoia

Lorene Cary, in a cogent essay in *Newsweek,* expands on Reverend Tompkins' point. In an essay titled "Why It's Not Just Paranoia," she writes:

> We Americans continue to value the lives and humanity of some groups more than the lives and humanity of others. That is not paranoia. It is our historical legacy and a present fact; it influences domestic and foreign policy and the daily interaction of millions of Americans. It influences the way we spend our public money and explains how we can read the staggering statistics on Black Americans' infant mortality, youth mortality, mortality in middle and old age, and not be moved to action.

African Americans' beliefs that their lives are devalued by White society also influence their relationships with the medical profession. They perceive, at times correctly, that they are treated differently in the health care system solely because of their race, and such perceptions fuel mistrust of the medical profession. For example, a national telephone survey conducted in 1986 revealed that African Americans were more likely than Whites to report that their physicians did not inquire sufficiently about their pain, did not tell them how long it would take for prescribed medicine to work, did not explain the seriousness of their illness or injury, and did not discuss test and examination findings. A 1994 study published in the *American Journal of Public Health* found that physicians were less likely to give pregnant Black women information about the hazards of smoking and drinking during pregnancy.

The powerful legacy of the Tuskegee Syphilis Study endures, in part, because the racism and disrespect for Black lives that it entailed mirror Black people's contemporary experiences with the medical profession. The anger and frustration that many African Americans feel when they encounter the health care system can be heard in the words of Alicia Georges, a professor of nursing at Lehman College and a former president of the National Black Nurses Association, as she recalled an emergency room experience. "Back a few years ago, I was having excruciating abdominal pain, and I wound up at a hospital in my area," she recalled. "The first thing that they began to ask me was how many sexual partners I'd had. I was married and owned my own house. But immediately, in looking at me, they said, 'Oh, she just has pelvic inflammatory disease.'" Perhaps because of her nursing background, Georges recognized the implications of the questioning. She had come face to face with the stereotype of Black women as sexually promiscuous. Similarly, the following story from the *Los Angeles Times* shows how racism can affect the practice of medicine:

> When Althea Alexander broke her arm, the attending resident at Los Angeles County-USC Medical Center told her to "hold your arm like you usually hold your can of beer on Saturday night." Alexander who is Black, exploded. "What are you talking about? Do you think I'm a welfare mother?" The White resident shrugged: "Well aren't you?" Turned out she was an administrator at USC medical school.

This example graphically illustrates that health care providers are not immune to the beliefs and misconceptions of the wider community. They carry with them stereotypes about various groups of people.

Beyond Tuskegee

There is also a growing body of medical research that vividly illustrates why discussions of the relationship of African Americans and the medical profession must go be-

yond the Tuskegee Syphilis Study. These studies demonstrate racial inequities in access to particular technologies and raise critical questions about the role of racism in medical decision making. For example, in 1989 *The Journal of the American Medical Association* published a report that demonstrated racial inequities in the treatment of heart disease. In this study, White and Black patients had similar rates of hospitalization for chest pain, but the White patients were one third more likely to undergo coronary angiography and more than twice as likely to be treated with bypass surgery or angioplasty. The racial disparities persisted even after adjustments were made for differences in income. Three years later, another study appearing in that journal reinforced these findings. It revealed that older Black patients on Medicare received coronary artery bypass grafts only about a fourth as often as comparable White patients. Disparities were greatest in the rural South, where White patients had the surgery seven times as often as Black patients. Medical factors did not fully explain the differences. This study suggests that an already-existing national health insurance program does not solve the access problems of African Americans. Additional studies have confirmed the persistence of such inequities.

Why the racial disparities? Possible explanations include health problems that precluded the use of procedures, patient unwillingness to accept medical advice or to undergo surgery, and differences in severity of illness. However, the role of racial bias cannot be discounted, as the American Medical Association's Council on Ethical and Judicial Affairs has recognized. In a 1990 report on Black-White disparities in health care, the council asserted:

> Because racial disparities may be occurring despite the lack of any intent or purposeful efforts to treat patients differently on the basis of race, physicians should examine their own practices to ensure that inappropriate considerations do not affect their clinical judgment. In addition, the profession should help increase the awareness of its members of racial disparities in medical treatment decisions by engaging in open and broad discussions about the issue. Such discussions should take place as part of the medical school curriculum, in medical journals, at professional conferences, and as part of professional peer review activities.

The council's recommendation is a strong acknowledgment that racism can influence the practice of medicine.

After the public disclosures of the Tuskegee Syphilis Study, Congress passed the National Research Act of 1974. This act, established to protect subjects in human experimentation, mandates institutional review board approval of all federally funded research with human subjects. However, recent revelations about a measles vaccine study financed by the Centers for Disease Control and Prevention (CDC) demonstrate the inadequacies of these safeguards and illustrate why African Americans' historically based fears of medical research persist. In 1989, in the midst of a measles epidemic in Los Angeles, the CDC, in collaboration with Kaiser Permanente and the Los Angeles County Health Department, began a study to test whether the experimental Edmonston-Zagreb vaccine could be used to immunize children too young for the standard Moraten vaccine. By 1991, approximately 900 infants, mostly Black and Latino, had received the vaccine without difficulties. (Apparently, one infant died for reasons not related to the inoculations.) But the infants' parents had not been informed that the vaccine was not licensed in the United States or that it had been associated with an increase in death rates in Africa. The 1996 disclosure of the study prompted charges of medical racism and of the continued exploitation of minority communities by medical professionals.

The Tuskegee Syphilis Study continues to cast its shadow over the lives of African Americans. For many Black people, it has come to represent the racism that pervades American institutions and the disdain in which Black lives are often held. But despite its significance, it cannot be the only prism we use to examine the relationship of African Americans with the medical and public health communities. The problem we must face is not just the shadow of Tuskegee but the shadow of racism that so profoundly affects the lives and beliefs of all people in this country.

References

A list of references is available in the original source.

Health and Indigenous People: Recommendations for the Next Generation

by Michael E. Bird, MSW, MPH

We are the first people of this land. . . . We are Indigenous peoples throughout this land and all over the planet we call Mother Earth.

For American Indians, the reality is that the founding fathers of the United States (none of them Indians), in order to establish a more perfect union that provided them with life, liberty, and the pursuit of happiness, displaced a people who had occupied this continent for thousands of years and denied those people their lives, liberty, and happiness. It is a fact.

Disparity, Dispossession, and Health Inequalities

In 1970, President Richard Nixon delivered the following statement in a message to Congress:

> The first Americans—the Indians—are the most deprived and most isolated minority group in our nation. On virtually every scale of measurement—employment, income, education, health—the condition of the Indian people ranks at the bottom. This condition is the heritage of centuries of injustice. From the time of their first contact with European settlers, the American Indians have been oppressed and brutalized, deprived of their ancestral lands, and denied the opportunity to control their own destiny.[1]

Last year at the 129th annual meeting of the American Public Health Association, we created a plenary session on indigenous health. This session provided an opportunity for indigenous people to speak to the issues that affect the health of the native peoples of Hawaii, Central America, Canada, Alaska, and the continental

From *The American Journal of Public Health,* Vol. 92, No. 9, September by Michael E. Bird. Copyright © 2002 by American Public Health Association. Reprinted by permission.

United States. We shared our experiences as individuals and as indigenous people from a variety of settings. We learned more about our similarities and differences. And what we gained was a sense of network, of a community brought closer by the threat of the power of ignorance and hate, and by the unacceptability of despair and disparity.

In my mind, disparity and dispossession go hand in hand. The massive dispossession that removed native people from their ancestral lands—not to mention the genocide and cultural eradication that followed—can hardly be imagined by most people. This story is not unique to American Indians. It is all too familiar for Native Hawaiians, Australian Aborigines, the Maori of New Zealand, and tribes throughout Central and South America. It may even apply to the Irish of Northern Ireland.

Wherever there has been dispossession, we see in the dispossessed populations significant damage in health, in educational levels, and in social well-being. And dispossession of one's land is not the only form of dispossession. Native peoples have been dispossessed of their labor, language, culture, and religious beliefs as well. We are only beginning to comprehend the consequences of what occurred long ago and still continues throughout the world. What is most important, though, is that we raise the collective awareness in this country to the level of undeniable truth: dispossession is at the root of health disparities.

Indian Health Services data show that American Indians and Alaska Natives have the worst health status of any group in this country. In 1993, their infant mortality rates were higher and life expectancy lower than those of the general population. American Indian and Alaska Native people are dying at younger ages than the rest of the nation. The leading causes of death among American Indians and Alaska Natives are heart disease and cancer, but in the area of behavioral health, these peoples' death rates are significantly higher as well: death from alcoholism, 579% higher; unintentional injury, 21% higher; suicide, 70% higher; and homicide, 41% higher. The diabetes mortality rate is 231% higher among American Indians and Alaska Natives than in the US population as a whole. Unfortunately, some of the highest rates of diabetes in the world are found in American Indian communities.

United We Stand

The most interesting result of the 2001 plenary session on indigenous health was how remarkably similar the historical experience has been for all indigenous populations. Another similarity was the description across the board of the relatively healthy nature of indigenous populations prior to contact, and the healthy living conditions that are universally described by historians and the first explorers. Clearly, the stories and the statistics bear witness to a certain pathology.

Indigenous peoples have given so much of themselves. And they offer the world even more at a time when the United States is struggling: The importance of the spiritual essence of all people, and our relationships to each other and the environment. Respect for all living things, and for human beings' place in the web of life. The importance and recognition of the role of spirituality in health. The concept of the well-being of all vs the benefit of few. The value of family and family wellness. The importance of balance in one's life and life choices. The village concept. The concept of mind, body, and spirit, and the importance of this concept to the health of individuals and communities. Generosity and reciprocity. An indigenous world view that predates the "alternative" Western view that has yet to prove its long-term sustainability and viability.

Indigenous people know the meaning of personal responsibility—but in a different, non-Western context. The concept is much broader, more humane and functional. If I am responsible only to myself, that kind of personal responsibility can be selfish and self-serving. It does not recognize the symbiotic nature of relationships that are important on this shrinking planet. Personal responsibility for indigenous people recognizes relationships and connections to others (family, tribe, community, world community). If I am to do well, then others must also do well. I am not isolated in thought, deed, or action. All are related and interconnected. I am personally responsible; I am my brother's keeper!

Improving the Health of Indigenous Peoples

Improving the health of indigenous peoples will require an effort beyond the indigenous community, from all individuals and institutions in public health. Our task is to reach and educate those people and organizations, and all branches of the federal, state, and local governments. We must help them understand who we are and how we have been affected. We must assume that this is a doable task, to bring together the data and the political process with wisdom and heart.

As a means to that end, we can put our energy into supporting and encouraging students from indigenous communities to enter the field of public health. Scholarship programs do exist, but many, many more could be established. Mentoring programs that create helpful relationships between students and those of us already in the field will ensure that the next generation continues to explore developments in health care while at the same time honoring traditional values and beliefs.

And we must maintain our commitments within our indigenous communities to be supportive of each other. Together, we are strong and capable. We are not the sum of our disparities. We will enter the broad arena as brothers and sisters on our way to building positive health and greater visibility for all of us.

But if justice on this earth can be imagined, so can a practical way to achieve it. Provided, that is, we are willing to reconcile ourselves to achieve it. Provided, that is, we are willing to reconcile ourselves to each other, and to historical truth.[2]

References

1. Message from the President of the United States transmitting recommendations for Indian policy 91st Cong. 2nd sess (July 8, 1970; H Doc 91-363).
2. Bothwell ARX. We live on their land: implications of long-ago takings of Native American Indian property. Annual Survey of International and Comparative Law (Golden Gate University School of Law). 2000:6:175.

La Sufrida

Contradictions of Acculturation and Gender in Latina Health

by Denise A. Segura and Adela de la Torre

Research in women's health has recently uncovered significant disparities in access and health status among ethnic women and women of color. For Latina and Chicana/Mexicana women, acculturation, as one of the most important predictive factors in both health access and health status measures, tends to frame empirical research and inform health policy. What is problematic in these empirical models, however, is the assumption that acculturation is a static process that can be captured and measured by specific attributes such as language, ancestry, behaviors, and attitudinal preferences. Overreliance on assumptions of static acculturation objectifies the immigrant woman subject by denying her power in the decision-making process. This results in descriptive attributes becoming "objective" criteria that predict good or bad health outcomes.

This paper challenges the static modeling design used in empirical studies of Chicana/Mexicana women's health that depict these women as objects who acquiesce to the environment rather than subjects who transform their environments. After reviewing the standard models that predict "good health outcomes" based on lower rates of acculturation, we will juxtapose these findings with more recent qualitative studies of Mexican immigrant women that illustrate how women reinvent their cultural identities within the process of migration, wherein class and gender locations are problematized. By examining the dynamic nature of Chicana/Mexicana cultural identity as part of the larger process of cultural identity reconstruction in the United States, we propose an alternative model to understand this group's observed health behaviors. We argue that the health behaviors examined empirically and accounted for within the aegis of a static acculturation model may mask a critical renegotiation of gender position for recent Mexican immigrant women. The items typically used to measure cultural identity and acculturation in much of the health services research form at best crude measures of immigrant status for specific Latina/o subpopulations but provide little understanding of the fluid and contradictory nature of cultural identity across immigrant categories. This understanding is essential if we are to provide more effective health policy and services to this group.

A major conclusion of this study is the need to reformulate current acculturation scales to incorporate the dynamism of cultural identity and cultural transformation of immigrant Mexican women as processes rather than outcomes. Furthermore, we argue that the current popular trend of promoting the "good" health behaviors of recent Mexican immigrants should be challenged as ignoring the cultural contradictions that exist and are often rooted in patriarchal family structures.

La Sufrida

La Sufrida, the long-suffering, self-effacing, ever-present self-sacrificing mother-image is present in many Chicano/Mexicano households. *La sufrida* is a virginal archetype that maintains and reproduces Chicano/Mexicano culture. She is the woman who will not eat so her children and husband can eat. She is the woman who will not adorn her face or body, the woman whose happiness is integrally bound to her family's well-being. As Gloria Anzaldua states, "The welfare of the family, the community, and tribe is more important than the welfare of the individual. The individual exists first as kin . . . and last as self" (1987:18).

Today we begin to deconstruct this culturally heroic icon of Chicano/Mexicano womanhood and family ideology. We contend that the ideological "presence" of the self-sacrificing Chicana/Mexicana martyr-mother within Chicano/Mexicano family research lays a foundation for much of the way health care services and delivery are constructed. This stereotype interjects itself into acculturation frameworks, obscuring the complexity of gender as a social construction among Chicanas/Mexicans in favor of a static moment in a population's history and culture. We argue that deconstructing the image of *la sufrida* is essential both to retire stereotypes and to identify transformative elements of Chicano/Mexicano culture that might be accessed to improve the health care situation of this population. Ultimately, we propose the development of theoretical and policy approaches that analyze gender strategies among Chicanas/Mexicanas in order to develop (among other things) more effective intervention strategies.

Deconstructing *la sufrida* begins by understanding real and perceived differences between Chicanas/Mexicanas and other American women. Socioeconomically and culturally, these differences include language, ideological configurations, preferred behaviors, customs, and so on. How "difference" is represented and evaluated, however, has profound implication for Chicana/Mexicana health treatment and policy development. Here we present just a few portrayals of "difference" from the academic and popular presses:

The difference between Anglo and Mexican-American women may be related to the fact that Mexican Americans have more positive views of housewives than Anglos. (Hurtado 1995:45)

Some of the hottest new imports from Latin America—to replace "intimidating and materialistic American women"—are marriage-minded Latin ladies . . . from good families where respect for husband and marriage are taught at an early age. (*Hispanic Link Weekly Report* 1989)

The women's movement has opened opportunities, she says, but it hasn't shown the Latina how to be whole. From 9 to 5, she sees herself as a career woman, from 5 to 8 as a mother; from 8 to 11 as a wife. (Alvarado 1991)

In summary, the stereotyped Mexican-American family has a high regard for authority, an adherence to tradition a philosophy of acceptance and resignation, and a religious orientation. (Padilla 1971:67)

These excerpts speak to the popular image of *la chicana* or *la mexicana* as family-centered, marriage-minded, and respectful. This one-dimensional Chicana/Mexicana *la sufrida* stereotype encompasses an idealized set of characteristics associated with "traditional" Chicano/Mexicano culture. The image of *la sufrida* wearing a black dress, entering the church to kneel reverently at the feet of the Virgen de Guadalupe to light a candle with money she has scraped together by denying herself any number of unnamed diversions or pleasures, and praying for her family is a picture reified in film (those few that have Latinas in them), novels, or calendars. The stereotype of the "good" Chicana/Mexicana as sacred and holy, self-sacrificing, familistic, and fatalistic frames much of the literature accessed by health care professionals today. Most important, these stereotypes have operated within acculturation models developed in the social sciences to explain behavioral differences between Anglo women and Chicanas/Mexicanas.

Acculturation Models Used in Health

Research that examines health behaviors of Mexican-origin women increasingly focus on the role of acculturation and health care outcomes. Typically these applied behavioral models attempt to explain why women of more recent immigrant origins are more likely than native-born and more acculturated Chicana/Mexicana women to exhibit health behaviors that are "protective factors" for these women and their families. This particular finding has gained prominence in part by countering the conventional wisdom on the primacy of socioeconomic factors in determining health outcomes. In the case of Chicanas/Mexicanas the more recent immigrants, despite their horrendous poverty and lack of access to health care, continue to have good birth outcomes, have low rates of alcohol and tobacco consumption, and maintain sexually monogamous lifestyles more often than their more acculturated counterparts. The effects of an evolutionary, linear acculturation process on health behaviors suggests negative impacts; Markides et al. (1990) argue that acculturation and alcohol consumption are positively related to younger stressors that affect Hispanic women's decisions to consume alcohol. Research on single mothers (Stroup-Benham, Trevifio, and Trevifio 1990) illustrates the economic stress among less-educated Mexican-American women. However, it is noted that the influence of acculturation on consumption is very complex and depends on variations such as age, sex, and type of measure of alcohol consumption.

Indeed, several studies on alcohol consumption indicate that multiple incomes combined with the restructuring of the family unit, increases the probability of alcohol consumption for these women. Acculturation, therefore, cannot explain why single female heads of household consume more alcohol than women in dual-female-headed households or women in dual-parent households. As Stroup-Benham and her colleagues argue, the stressors associated with being a single female head of household may be better indicators of health behaviors than acculturation.

Other studies that focus on the effects of acculturation on health seek to explain illicit drug use. Amaro et al. (1990) suggests that acculturation into U.S. society, as reflected by language use, is related to higher rates of illicit drug use. In this model, acculturation was measured simply by identifying the respondent's place of birth and language use, without attempting to access the social and economic context.

Underlying these static models of acculturation are psychometric constructs that assume the key cultural attributes of Mexican-origin women are defined by descriptors such as English-language fluency, ethnic identity, values, ideology, and cultural customs (Cuellar, Harris, and Jasso 1980). In the highly regarded Cuellar Acculturation Rating Scale, substantial explanatory power is derived from the language component. Yet Cuellar admits that "obviously, the 20 items contained in [the scale] do not tap all of the components of acculturation. It is acknowledged that perhaps the more important constructs of acculturation may not even be measured by this scale" (Cuellar, Harris, and Jasso 1980:209). Despite this caveat from the author himself, the acculturation scale is nonetheless used as a critical predictor for health behaviors among Mexicana/Chicana women, even though it captures at best only the immigrant status of these women, much as a snapshot fixed in time. Since few studies acknowledge the limitation inherent in the use of such fixed acculturation scales, they subsequently tend to reify the knowledge acquired from these discrete scales. Worse, overreliance on these scales obscures an appreciation of acculturation as a dynamic and continuous process that cannot possibly be captured by models that rely on discrete variables. Nonetheless, tacit acceptance of this discrete variable permeates the health behavior literature on Chicana/Mexicana women.

The following chart illustrates the use of acculturation scales as a predictor of health behaviors.

Author	Acculturation Index	Acculturation Var. Design (Yes)	Acculturation Var. Design (No)
Mainous 1979	Self-concept as a variable	Relation between self-concept and accult.	
Cuellar, Harris, and Jasso 1990	Defines accult. model (multidimensional)	Relation between host culture and accult.	
Markides et al. 1990	Accult. stress model and accult. model	Relation between health risk behaviors and accult.	
Stroup-Benham, Trevifio, and Trevifio 1990	Sociocultural	Relation between drinking behavior and accult.	
Mainous III 1989	Self-concept as a variable	Relation between self-concept and accult.	
Olmedo and Padilla 1978	Sociocultural	Relation between sociocultural factors and accult.	

(continued)

Author	Acculturation Index	Acculturation Var. Design (Yes)	Acculturation Var. Design (No)
Olmedo 1979	Diachronic and synchronic		
Rodriguez 1983	Sociocultural		
Scribner and Dwyer 1989	Sociocultural		No variable design mentioned
Ginzberg 1991	Socioeconomic		No variable design mentioned
Marin et al.1993	Research infrastructure		No variable design mentioned
Moore and Hepworth 1994	Socioeconomic		Acculturation was not a predictor

The first six examples demonstrate empirical research in which the acculturation variable design was utilized, while the remaining six either did not mention a variable design or concluded that acculturation was not found to be a predictor.

In the first example, Mainous (1979) investigated self-concept in relation to acculturation. An acculturation variable design was applied in which the respondent's self-concept as an insider or an outsider to his/her native culture was examined. Results indicated that the respondent's self-concept was an important element in determining their level of acculturation. Cuellar, Harris, and Jasso (1990) also utilized an acculturation scale in which the study measured the amount of acculturation to the host culture the subject had adopted. The study attempted to attain a holistic picture of the acculturation process through developing a gauge to calibrate the amount of acculturation that had taken place. Thus, acculturation was based on a multidimensional approach.

The subsequent application of an acculturation design was measured by Markides et al. (1990) in which acculturation influences were examined in relation to the health risk behavior of Mexican-Americans (consisting of health service utilization, cigarette smoking, alcohol consumption, and diet). In relation to alcohol and acculturation, for example, the author found a positive correlation.

In the case of Stroup-Benham, Trevifio, and Trevifio (1990), the consumption of alcohol was found to be influenced by the level of acculturation the participant had attained over his or her lifetime. In the example of Olmedo and Padilla (1978), acculturation was affected by sociocultural characteristics. Subjects who were exposed to the host culture for a longer period of time were expected to rate higher on the acculturation scale.

In the final example in which acculturation was focused on, Mainous (1989) reexamined the relation between self-concept and the respondent's level of accul-turation. Results similar to those of the previous study in 1979 were found—self-concept appeared to influence the measurement of acculturation.

Half of the twelve articles that examine health behaviors and outcomes for Latina/Chicana/Mexicana women identify acculturation as having a significant impact on the health and well-being of these women and/or their children. That is, Latina/Chicana/Mexicana women who are less acculturated have better health outcomes. The immediate policy implication of these findings is that acculturation is bad for your health. The focus, therefore, in this kind of research is to identify the moment when acculturation becomes disadvantageous to health behaviors. But this linear model obscures the complexity of both acculturation and health behaviors. Moreover, it diminishes Chicana/Mexicana agency.

Revisioning Culture and Gender Identity for Mexican Immigrant Women

Research on Chicana/Mexicana health behaviors often assumes that their actions are best understood within the context of a unique set of ethnic and cultural traditions. To ascertain the degree of adherence to Chicano/Mexicano culture, many researchers (as we have seen) rely on acculturation scales. However, the multidimensional process of acculturation is all too often reduced to the simplest measurable component, that is, Spanish-language use. Although language loyalty may be a good indicator of immigrant status, its utility for understanding acculturations is limited. If we think of acculturation as a process of acquiring knowledge to enhance one's ability to survive and prosper in a new society, clearly Spanish-language use can be viewed as one item in a woman's knowledge reservoir, as opposed to a "barrier" to a full social participation. The local opportunity structure and lack of human capital are also important. Spanish, as the "home" of a woman's expressions of self and the means through which she interprets reality and opportunity, cannot be underestimated as a source of strength, survival, and betterment as she explores her changing environment in interaction with others. As a proxy for acculturation, however, it is limited, especially when we consider differences among Chicanas/Mexicanas that flow from their class, gender roles, sexual orientation, and immigrant status.

Instead of relying conceptually and methodologically on acculturation we might delve into what Renato Rosaldo calls the "cultural borderlands" and move beyond cataloguing shared patterns and meanings to problematize survival tools and social expressions among women (Rosaldo 1989:26-38). If we accept the premise that culture is not just a system of shared patterns and behaviors but includes continuous performance and conflicting ideologies, then it is vital to reject reductionism in models of acculturation inasmuch as they render invisible critical components of Chicana/Mexicana identities.

Recent scholarship reveals important differences between U.S.-born women of Mexican descent and women raised in Mexico who now reside in the United States. Socioeconomically, Mexicana immigrants' educational levels are lower (fifth or sixth grade, on average) than those of U.S.-born Chicanas (tenth or eleventh grade, on average); their language use varies; and their employment is distinct (e.g., more Mexicanas labor in blue-collar occupations, whereas Chicanas tend to work in white-collar jobs) (Ortiz 1995). If we consider sexual and fertility behaviors, foreign-born Latinas and Mexicanas tend to be more sexually conservative regarding the number of sexual partners and age at first intercourse as well as more likely to have planned their pregnancies and be married or living with a partner (Becerra and De Anda 1987; Rapkin and Erickson 1990). Foreign-born Latinas are also less likely to have knowledge of or experience with birth control and are more likely to begin their prenatal care later in pregnancy or eschew it altogether (Becerra and De Anda 1987; Rapkin and Erickson 1990). Other research argues that birth outcomes are more favorable for Mexican-born women residing in the United States vis-à-vis U.S.-born women of Mexican descent (Guendelman et al. 1990). This research lends additional support to the theory that an inverse relationship between acculturation and good health among Mexican women exists, caused by a more protective lifestyle among less-acculturated women, regardless of socioeconomic status or age. This study notes possible measurement error, since foreign-born Mexicana women are prone to a reporting bias. For example, Mexico-born women are less likely to receive a pregnancy examination which can result in lower reporting of miscarriages and induced abortions.

Underreporting of medical problems and conditions can easily skew research directions and distort the effect of acculturation. The National Latina Health Organization states, "Latinos are less likely to receive preventive or regular health care than other Americans." Moreover, a "larger percent of Latinas than white women had never heard of or received a Pap smear, breast exam, or mammogram. Almost twice as many Latinas as white women had never heard of breast exams and nearly three times as many had never heard of mammograms" (National Latina Health Organization 1996). Thus, underreporting may contribute to the development of a false image of better health among less acculturated Mexicana women. This possibility argues for the need for research studies to carefully delineate acculturation effects from those that may be more closely aligned to income and education.

Other evidence contradicts acculturation theses concerning patterns of educational attainment and social mobility among women and men of Mexican descent. Third-generation Chicanos tend to be overrepresented among low educational achievers than their first- and second-generation counterparts (Hayes-Bautista, Schink, and Chapa 1988; Chapa and Valencia 1993). Similarly, mobility patterns in general rise markedly for the second generation (children of adult immigrants) and either stabilize or move downward with the third generation. These socioeconomic realities must contextualize an understanding of the process of culture and identity among Chicanas and Mexicanas today.

Feminist-based research on Chicana and Mexicana women emphasizes the dynamism within their cultural adaptation and identity formation. Immigrant women experience continuous shifts in cultural identity formation as renegotiation of gender roles occurs with changes in their economic or family status. Until recently, much of the research on Mexicano migration was male-certified and documented the economics of immigration. In this literature, examinations of Mexicana women and immigration were anchored within the family nexus. That is, Mexicana women typically were viewed as migratory appendages to the breadwinner Mexicano man. Recent research contests this view and asserts that often Mexicana women have their own reasons for emigrating that sometimes include reuniting with an absent husband, but at other times reflect motivations to escape abusive spouses, seek a freer environment to express one's sexuality (Arguelles and Rivero 1993), and/or gain a better life (Hondagneu-Sotelo 1994). Whether the reason is to reunite the family or to enact individualistic needs, Mexicana women's innovation in immigration is only now becoming visible to researchers and policy makers.

As members of a racial-ethnic minority whose political, economic, and cultural uniqueness has been historically undermined and devalued, Chicanas have maintained and affirmed a distinct set of values and behavior that emphasize familism, *compadrazgo,* and a collectivist orientation (Griswold de Castillo 1979; Segura and Pierce 1993). Research on Chicanas is shifting to emphasize both an analysis of gender role attitudes and behaviors as well as the contradictions posed by contestation and agency within families and their communities. For example, the existence of alternative mothering models within Chicano communities that utilize women in the kinship network to provide physical and affective care for children and emotional and economic support for parents (Segura and Pierce 1993) offers insight into potential health care intervention strategies. Pesquera's study of professional, blue-collar, and white-collar Chicana workers explores women's recasting of traditional cultural values to reconcile the "competing urgencies" of family and paid employment. She finds a positive relationship between women's class locations and economic contributions to the household vis-à-vis their spouses and their ability to successfully renegotiate the household division of labor (Pesquera 1993:181). The creativity of Chicanas to reinvent culturally prescribed traditional motherhood by renegotiating parenting with partners is finding voice in other feminist scholarship (Lamphere, Zavela, and Gonzales 1993). This research illustrates that gender roles are dynamic and subject to renegotiation as part of the process of facilitating the economic survival of the household and a woman's own sense of self.

The complexity of gender in Mexicano households intersects with economic opportunity. Recent research on Mexicano immigrants observes that with employment, women often assert themselves more directly in family decision-making. In some cases, as Hondagneu-Sotelo shows (1994), patriarchal authority is hotly contested. In other cases, patriarchal control is subverted covertly and bolstered by the relative economic strength of the woman (Segura 1994). The contradictory pressures of migration on "Traditional gender roles and practices" is also highlighted in de la Torre's study of Mexican agricultural migrants (1992). De la Torre found that the pressures of paid employment required these women to shift away from the traditional practice of breast-feeding infants and toward bottle-feeding. This renegotiation of traditional health practices exemplifies how migrant women can (and do) adapt their behavior to accommodate both the economic and health needs of their families as they cross new employment boundaries.

Conclusion

So what does all this mean? Chicanas and Mexicana migrant women often desire to affirm traditional practices and values. These preferences are often ideological and subject to change. In the case of Chicanas, the local context—the contradictions of race-ethnicity in inner cities and suburbs, where expressions of cultural heritage constantly shift and vary by class—is critical to explore, rather than "measure" by a static acculturation measuring stick. For Mexicanas, affirmation of traditional practices and values reverberates with the pressures of migration and settlement. Thus, what is "traditional" is adaptation and innovation, both of which flow from Mexicana/Chicana agency.

Acknowledgments

Adela de la Torre would like to acknowledge graduate assistant Arli Eicher for her help in completing this paper.

References

A list of references is available in the original source.

Expanding Health Options for Asian and Pacific Islander Women

by collective members of Massachusetts Asian AIDS Prevention Project
Edited by Ramani Sripada-Vaz and Sue Lowcock

Women of Asian and Pacific Islander (API) descent are often a forgotten group when it comes to access to health care and education. It is a difficult enough task to begin to dismantle the myth that APIs are a "model minority," that we are all academic and economic achievers with no health problems. API women are further marginalized when it comes to gaining culturally and linguistically appropriate reproductive health and HIV/AIDS information. Little research has been done to this date to determine the level of HIV awareness, risk factors for HIV transmission and accessibility of health services for women of API descent living in the United States.

According to the 1990 census, Asians made up 2.4 percent of the population in Massachusetts, with the Chinese community being the largest (37.5 percent), followed by Asian Indian (19 percent), Vietnamese (10.4 percent) and Cambodian (9 percent) populations. Though Boston had the largest Asian population in 1990, Lowell had the largest concentration of Asians, of which 56.3 percent were Cambodian. API women make up approximately half of the state's Asian population.

The Massachusetts Asian AIDS Prevention Project (MAAPP), a nonprofit organization established in 1995 to prevent the spread of HIV among APIs in Massachusetts, initiated the Women's Needs Assessment Project to focus on prevention of HIV. We targeted four separate groups of API women: Chinese, Vietnamese, Cambodian and Bangladeshi. This project was done in collaboration with South Asian Women for Action, South Cove Community Health Center, Refugee and Immigrant Health Program (Massachusetts Department of Public Health), and Vietnamese and Cambodian community-based individuals.

First, a knowledge questionnaire specific to women was developed and translated into four languages: Chinese, Vietnamese, Khmer and Bengali. Next, a list of focus group questions were designed to elicit ideas, behaviors and attitudes related to HIV, general reproductive health and access to health information. The participants and facilitators were also asked for suggestions about the best strategies for reaching API women.

All four focus groups were held from September to November 1996, with a total of 34 women attending. The majority of the women were from lower-income backgrounds and spoke some English. The following is a snapshot of what happened during one of the sessions:

A small group of women gathered together on a Sunday evening in October, and between cups of tea and occasional bursts of giggles, they chatted about how they feel HIV can affect their lives. Because of cultural and religious values, they had difficulty discussing premarital and extramarital sex. It was also difficult to talk about the critical subject of safer sex because their religions prohibit contraception. The women felt that they are not at risk for HIV because they do not engage in "sexual misconduct." In a social context, where the male partner is always perceived as dominant, many of the women felt the need for an outside third party to intervene in order for safer sex and condom-use to happen, since sex is not always negotiable within a marriage without the help of a medical, legal or familial authority figure.

Gaps in knowledge were common in all four ethnic groups, particularly regarding the transmission of HIV. Some misconceptions that were presented include:

- AIDS is a disease that only affects those who live in big cities and have multiple partners.
- Only anal sex transmits HIV.
- Nothing can be done to prevent a baby from getting infected during pregnancy/delivery.
- When people are married, there is no need to practice safer sex.
- Keeping in good physical shape is the best way to keep from getting AIDS.

- A shower after sex reduces the risk of getting AIDS.
- Withdrawal by a man before orgasm prevents transmission of HIV.

These results have implications for the need to tailor HIV-prevention materials to be more woman-specific, taking into account basic transmission facts. In addition to these knowledge indicators, focus group discussions also identified key themes surrounding behaviors and attitudes. Some of these include:

- Poor knowledge of family planning methods and prevention of sexually transmitted disease, including condom use.
- Difficulty negotiating contraception with partners because of taboos around talking about sex and gender inequity.
- Reliance on personal physicians for health information. Emphasis on belief that HIV is transmitted only if there is "sexual misconduct."
- Homophobia and lack of familiarity with sexual diversity. Low self-perception of risk because the women were not "promiscuous." Fear of and stigmatization of people with HIV at workplaces. Fear of and stigmatization of children with HIV at their children's schools.

While discussion of these and other taboo topics was difficult for focus group participants, we did find that women were able to talk about sexuality, HIV/AIDS and gender issues. Such discussion was possible because the issues were raised in a safe, peer-supported environment, within the context of broader women's health issues. The ideas and recommendations that came from the focus group discussions, and which will be presented to other community members, form the basis for future advocacy efforts by MAAPP with providers and institutions serving API women.

MAAPP is currently organizing a Women's Advisory Group for our upcoming Women's Health Leadership Initiative, which aims to promote and expand API women's reproductive health options and knowledge through a process empowering women to learn about their reproductive health, discover their own bodies, and enhance their self esteem. We will encourage API women to educate their peers and become advocates for improved culturally competent and linguistically accessible reproductive health services.

The National Asian Women's Health Organization (NAWHO) advocates on a national level for such services, and has created an API women's health agenda. MAAPP is truly grateful for the opportunity to work with national organizations such as NAWHO because it is often difficult to work on the local and state level when policies are also being made on a national level. If you or anyone you know is interested in participating in MAAPP's women's program please call Ramani Sripada-Vaz at (617)262-2900.

Blazes of Truth

by Susan Schnur

When I was 12 years old, my parents sent me off to Camp Ramah in the Poconos. That June, I was a dull kid in an undershirt from Trenton, New Jersey, outfitted in lime-green, mix-and-match irregulars from E. J. Korvette's. By the end of August, though—exposed as I was, for two months, to suburban Philadelphia's finest pre-adolescent fashion cognoscenti—I had contracted that dread disease: *"JAP* itis."*

Symptoms included not only the perfection of an elaborate, all-day, triple-sink procedure for dyeing white wool bobby socks to the requisite shade of dirty white (we called it oyster), but also my sudden, ignominious realization that the discount "Beatlemania" record my mother had bought for me the previous spring was not, after all, sung by the real group.

This article was originally published in *Lilith,* the independent Jewish women's quarterly; subscriptions are $16.00 per year, from *Lilith,* 250 West 57th Street, New York, NY 10107. It is being reprinted here by permission.
*The term JAP refers to Jewish American Princess.

I'm not even sure that the term *JAP* existed yet back then (I don't think it did), but, in any case, by October I was—more or less—cured. I put the general themes of entitlement, of materialism, of canonized motifs (in those days, Lord and Taylor was the label of choice rather than Bloomingdale's) at the back of my mental medicine chest for the next two decades.

It wasn't until six months ago, actually—while teaching a course at Colgate University called "Contemporary Issues of Jewish Existence"—that I again gave the subject of *JAPs* a moment's pause.

A unit on *JAPs* was decidedly *not* on my course syllabus (I taught the standards: Holocaust—Faith—Immigration—Assimilation—Varieties of Religious Experience—Humor—Israel—Women). But my students, as it turned out, were obsessed with *JAPs.*

Week after week, in personal journals that they were keeping for me, they talked *JAPs:* the stereotypes, dating them, hating them, not *being* them, *JAP* graffiti, *JAP* competitiveness, *JAPs* who gave them the willies back home in Scarsdale over spring break.

I had been raised on moron jokes; *they* had been raised on JAP jokes. ("What does a *JAP* do with her asshole in the morning? Dresses him up and sends him to work.")

Little by little, I came to realize that the *JAP* theme was by no means a one-note samba. It was kaleidoscopic and self-revealing; the students plugged it into a whole range of Jewish issues. I began to encourage them to look at their throwaway *JAP* comments with a measure of scrutiny.

The first, and most striking, ostinato in the students' journals was the dissociative one. As one Jewish student framed it, "There are so many *JAPs* in this class, it makes me sick." (An astonishing number of students were desperate to let me know this.)

Since over one-third of the class was not Jewish (the enrollment was 30), and since there was no one in the class that I would have identified sartorially as a *JAP,* this was an interesting fillip.

"That's funny," I started commenting back in these students' journals. "The other students think *you're* a *JAP.*"

Eventually, one Jewish student wrote, "Maybe when I talk about *JAPs* and that whole negative thing, it's a way for me to get 'permission' to assimilate."

Another wondered why he feels "like every *JAP* on campus somehow implicates me. That's a very 'minority culture' reflex, isn't it? Why am I so hung up on how everyone else perceives Jews?"

Some students perceived the *JAP* phenomenon, interestingly, as a developmental phase in American Judaism—a phase in which one parades both one's success and one's entitlement. "When my best girlfriend

from childhood was bat mitzvahed," wrote one student after reading *A Bintel Brief* and *World of Our Fathers,* "her grandmother gave her a '*JAP*-in-training' diamond-chip necklace. It's like the grandmother was saying, "When I was your age, I had to sew plackets in a Lower East Side sweatshop. So you girls be *JAPs.* Take whatever you can and be proud of it."

A Black student mentioned—during a talk about the socialization of Jewish women—that Jewish women, like their Black counterparts, are encouraged to be extremely competent, but then are double-bound with the message that their competence must *only* be used for frivolous purposes. (Like Goldie Hawn, in *Private Benjamin,* scolding her upholsterer with impressive assertiveness: "I specifically said—the ottoman in mushroom!," or informing her superior officer that she refused to go to Guam because "my hair will frizz.") "Minority women are warned not to be a real threat to anyone," the student explained, "That's how *JAPs* evolve."

Another theme of the students touched on their perception that Jews are sometimes discriminated against not because they are *less* endowed than others, but because they are more endowed (smarter, richer, more "connected"). *JAPs,* then, become, in the words of an Irish Catholic student who was doing reading on theology and the theme of chosenness, "the 'chosen of the chosen'. Unlike Irish Catholics who have been discriminated against because we seem 'un-chosen'," she mused, "people hate *JAPs* because they seem to have everything: money, confidence, style."

Of course, it's probably unnecessary for me to point out that the most prolific *JAP* references had to do with the venerable old feud—the Jewish War-Between-The-Sexes.

One pre-law Jewish male in the class (who was under a lot of pressure and had developed colitis during that semester) stated point-blank that he did not date Jewish women. I was shocked by the number of 20-year-old, seemingly fully-assimilated Jewish males who were right up there with Alexander Portnoy on this subject.

Several students responded to his comment in their journals. "He's angry at *JAPs,*" one woman wrote, "because they get to be needy and dependent, whereas the expectations on him are really high."

Another student related the experience of two friends of hers at SUNY Binghamton: "Someone spray-painted the word *JAP* on their dormitory door," she recounted. "But now I wonder—which one of the girls was being called a *JAP?* The one with the dozen Benetton sweaters, or the one who'd gotten 750 on her L-SATs?" The question being, of course, which is ultimately more threatening . . . the demanding woman or the self-sufficient one?

JAP: The New Antisemitic Code Word

by Francine Klagsbrun

Isn't it odd that the term *JAP*, referring to a spoiled, self-indulgent woman, should be so widely used at a time when women are working outside their homes in unprecedented numbers, struggling to balance their home lives and their work lives to give as much of themselves as they can to everybody—their husbands, their kids, their bosses?

Jewish women, like women throughout society, are trying to find their own paths, their own voices. And, along with other changes that have taken place, they have been finding themselves Jewishly. And yet we hear the term *JAP* being used, perhaps almost more now than ever before. Why?

The new found, or rather newly accepted, drive of women for achievement in many arenas threatens many men. What better put-down of the strong woman than to label her a "Princess"? She is not being attacked as a competitor—that would be too close to home. No—she's called a princess, and that label diminishes her, negating her ambition and her success.

One may note, and rightly so, that there are materialistic Jewish women—and men too. But are Jews the only people guilty of excesses in spending? Why should the word "Jewish" be used pejoratively to describe behavior we don't approve of?

I think the answer is that there is an underlying antisemitic message in that label. Loudness is somehow "Jewish." Vulgarity is somehow "Jewish." All the old stereotypes of Jews come into play in the use of the term *JAP*. In this day, polite Christian society would not *openly* make anti-Jewish slurs. But *JAP* is O.K. *JAP* is a kind of code word. It's a way of symbolically winking, poking with an elbow, and saying, "well you know how Jews are—so materialistic and pushy."

What is interesting is that this code word can be used in connection with *women*—the Jewish American *Princess*—and nobody protests its intrinsic antisemitism.

This article was originally published in LILITH, the independent Jewish women's quarterly; subscriptions are $16.00 per year, from LILITH, 250 West 57th Street, New York, NY 10107. It is being reprinted here by permission

An Hispanic woman in the class talked about what she called "the dialectic of prejudice"—that is, the contradictory nature of racist or sexist slurs as being, in itself, a diagnostic of irrational bias. "A JAP is portrayed as both frigid and nymphomaniacal," she wrote. "She's put down both because of her haughty strut that says, 'I'm independent', and because of her *kvetching* that says, 'I'm dependent'."

A twist on this theme was provided by a Jewish woman who commented, "Whatever Jewish men call us—cold, hot, leech, bitch—it's all the same thing: They're afraid they can't live up to our standards."

A psych major in the class took a different tack. "It's not that the Jewish male really believes Jewish women are terrible, rather that he simply wants majority culture males to believe it. It's like when territorial animals urinate on a tree," she explained. "It's a minority male's possessive instinct. Like a sign that says, 'Robert Redfords—stay away!'"

Finally, several Jewish students framed their relations with one another in the context of Jewish family systems. "Lashing out at Jewish women—calling them all *JAPs* or refusing to marry them—is a way to get back at the entire high-expectation, high-pressure Jewish family," stated one student in response to a film I showed in class called "Parenting and Ethnicity." "You can lash out by becoming an academic failure," he went on, "or you can become a doctor—which is less self-destructive—and then simply refuse to marry a Jewish woman."

Towards the end of the term, a feminist friend pointed out to me something I had not considered: that the characterizations of *JAPs* and Yuppies are often identical—the difference being, of course, that a Yuppie designation is still generally taken as neutral or even positive, whereas there is hardly one of us left—I don't think—who would compete for the label of *JAP*.

All in all, I trust that the larger lessons in all of these *JAP* ruminations have not been lost on my students. For example: Why has it become socially sanctioned to use a *Jewish* designation *(JAP)* for a description that fits as many Christians as Jews? Or why—along the same lines—is it okay to use a *female* designation (again, *JAP*) for a description that fits as many men as women? Or sensing what we now sense, shouldn't we refuse any truck altogether with the term *JAP?*

Strained Class Windows

by Judith K. Witherow

You People   Every time I hear those ignoble words used, I know it isn't going to be good. They will always make me mentally and physically cringe.

When you hear those words from birth on, as part of your name, you know which rung of the ladder you're standing on.

"You People should have indoor plumbing. How can you stand that outhouse?" "You People need to have electricity and running water." "Your house looks so small. How many of You People sleep in one bed?" (I shared a bed with two sisters, and, in the winter, our body heat was probably the only thing that kept us from freezing to death.) "Why don't You People paint your house?"

Gee, poverty makes you so damned dumb that none of these things ever occur to you. Someone pointing them out is like a giant wake-up slap on the forehead.

We could have painted any bare wood shack we ever lived in seven different colors, and it wouldn't have changed a thing. Oh, people would have said, "You People are so gaudy," but that is how much tangible difference it would have made. There would have been less money for food and other survival necessities, but what the hell, it might have made us easier to look at. That's what it is all about, isn't it? Looks?

Not the kind of looks where someone is rolling their eyes while they are "trying" to talk to you. This habit is the twin of "You People," and you just want to haul out a piece of tape and hold their eyes still so they can clearly see what you are saying.

I'm 49 years old, and I still don't have this class thing figured out. For that matter, I don't know for sure whether classism or racism is worse. Most times I can't even figure out why I'm being treated the way I am.

I honestly thought I could be objective writing this article, but the deeper I dig into old buried familial grief graves, the more angry and sad I become. If this weren't so God awful important, I'd throw the dirt back on, but how are we ever going to change anything unless all sides are totally truthful?

As a poor, mixed blood Native American, raised in the northern Appalachians, I invite you into my life and reveal to you the sights, tastes, smells, and life-limiting experiences that you might not have been privy to.

I keep wanting to say I know all the big words I'm using. It's very important to me that you know I'm not being pretentious, that these are no one else's words but mine. If that is classism in reverse, I will readily say I am sorry. My partner, Sue, helps me proofread but that is the extent of the input. Sometimes people assume someone of my background could not be literate. I can't tell you how many times someone has asked me if I actually wrote a particular article.

I hear the same thing from many family members, but for a different reason. The first time I showed my mother a poem I had written, she asked if I really knew all those words, or did I find them in a dictionary? Often I get quizzed about an article I've written. Someone will say, "Did that really happen?" It's like, "Judith, you'll be in deep, deep trouble if you put a lie in print." Right. The nonfiction police will bust my butt.

The printed word has always been cause for heated discussion in my family. They don't believe anyone would print something that isn't true. This includes *The National Enquirer.* I've learned that the older generation can survive easier without the ugly truths at this late date, so I concentrate on working with the younger ones. The truth doesn't always set you free. It bruises and bleeds like no other injury ever could, but pain can open the gates to gain.

I graduated from high school and made my family very proud. Looking back, I can see I was purposely kept at lower class levels even though I had good grades. No one ever mentioned scholarships or college to me. (As a result, I earned a living as a textile factory worker, waitress, and housekeeper.) I believe you get weeded out of the further education track at an early age. It's not the grades that count. It's your family's potential that is measured by the class yardstick. (You People would just take up a space that could be used by someone really serious.) Some very fine minds get lost this way. Yes, you could go to college at a later date, but by then life has had so many whacks at you that it rarely leaves you with the time or confidence to try it. Survival often means feeding the belly before the brain. The deprivation of either causes lifelong pain. There is only so much humiliation you can cram into a child before you effectively crowd her out of the system.

My father quit school in third grade to help raise his brothers and sisters. He was self-educated and gave me an abiding love of the written word. My mother made it to the eighth grade. Her one clothing outfit for school was the top of a dress for a blouse and the bottom of a man's overcoat for a skirt. She never stopped grieving for her lost chance. She often spoke of her proudest moment as winning a poetry recital before she had to quit school.

When my father was in his seventies and dying of cancer, he asked me to cover for him because he had told the nurse a lie. I thought she must have asked him about smoking or drinking. He said, "She asked me how far I had went in school. I thought fifth grade sounded much better so I told her that. You back me up, kid." I asked him why he didn't just say he had graduated? He looked like someone had pulled a gun on him. "Jesus, girl, you can't say anything like that." I tried to explain to him it was a bullshit question, but he was having none of it.

You see, after many years of subjugation, you become your own overseer. To this day, I see my nieces and nephews trash each other before the rest of society gets a chance. I understand the dynamic perfectly. If you make fun of or hurt each other, then the second time around it doesn't hurt as much. You have already been prepared. When you depersonalize pain and suffering, you can ignore it. Only when a human face is superimposed on poverty will this barbaric practice end.

The first house I remember us living in contained three small rooms. (The next tenants used it as a chicken coop.) My father had to walk stooped over because the ceilings were about five feet high. He was six foot tall. There was no water or electricity, of course. The creek out back served as a washing machine, a refrigerator, and a bathtub.

We never lived in a place that had screen doors or screens in the windows. This allowed everything, including snakes, to come and go at will.

We learned at an early age to pound on the floor before getting out of bed. This was so you didn't accidentally step on a rat and get bitten. Why the hell do rats always overrun the poor? I can tell you it is not for the food. Maybe it's just easier access.

When it snowed in the mountains, it would drift in through all the cracks that weren't full of paper or rags. We had very few blankets, so coats, rugs, or clothes helped to keep us warm. The roof had so many holes that we didn't have enough pots or pans to catch all the rain that trickled through. Too bad we didn't have one of those glass ceilings I hear so much about. I'll bet those suckers could keep you dry, warm, and in your place.

This basically describes all the houses we grew up in. Each move was a little better than the last. When I was five, we moved to a house that had electricity. At age 14, we moved to a house that had both water and electricity. We never acquired a place with screens or one that wasn't overrun with rats. Yes, we set traps. Yes, we put out poison. Many times my brother and I would sit in the basement with a .22 rifle and pick them off when they popped their heads out.

People many times equate poverty with laziness. We always worked. Dad worked at a sawmill and as a lumberjack. Later on, he became a carpenter. He never missed work, and he never received any benefits.

My dad, a good-looking, proud man, came from a long line of alcoholics, as did my mother, but only he succumbed to it. It still follows the male lineage on both sides of the family. Twice while growing up, I heard people use my dad's name as a synonym for drunk. If the alcohol colored and clouded the ugliness and made it bearable, I can understand and forgive that. Yes, I'm sure the cheap wine he drank took material and mental tolls on all of us, but it was an illness he fought all of his life.

One time Dad committed himself to an alcohol rehabilitation institution. Mom had to apply for welfare and sign a non-support order that she was told would never be served. It was protocol. (It was the only time she applied for benefits.) On the day of Dad's release after two months of treatment, the police came and took him away in handcuffs because of the nonsupport warrant. On the way home from jail, he stopped and bought a bottle of wine. It caused a breach in my parents' relationship that never healed. None of us had ever been in any trouble with the law. The law was something you feared with all of your being. It still is for us older ones.

Mom worked as a housekeeper for several families. I was ashamed of her for doing that. When high school girls whose homes Mom cleaned would tell me in a loud voice at school what a wonderful job Mom did, I wanted to die. On the other hand, to Mom's dying day, she would brag about what a good job she had done and how pleased her employers were.

She also did waitress and factory work and thought it was a great honor that she had never been fired from any job. Me, I just wanted to shake her when she would start these raps and say, "Of course, they didn't fire you. You were every shit-working boss's dream. You never complained, and you left a piece of your heart and health everywhere you worked." Of course, I never said it out loud to her.

She looked at me in total amazement whenever I tried to say that perhaps things weren't as cut and dried as they appeared. She was the dearest, kindest woman I have ever known. I will never stop missing her truly honest compassion. May she rest in peace. I doubt I ever will.

Work. That's all we ever knew from childhood up. You name it, and we sold it or did it. We picked and sold strawberries, blackberries, elderberries, and blueberries. We sold Rosebud salve by the gross. Remember those tacky cardboard mottos that said "HOME SWEET HOME?" Sold them. Countless packs of seeds also sold door to door. Lawnmowing, gardening, babysitting, etc.

One of the hardest jobs was picking princess pine. It's used to make funeral and Christmas wreaths, etc. You find it growing wild in the wintertime. It looks like wispy little pine trees. You get paid six cents a pound for it. Believe me, it takes more back-breaking work than you can ever imagine to fill a burlap sack with it. Digging through the snow in search of it without the benefit of gloves or boots is something you wouldn't wish on anyone. We would miss school to help with this. Whoever was the youngest at the time would be placed in a hurriedly fashioned lean-to for shelter from the elements. Another young one would stay nearby and keep the fire going while the rest of us picked.

Our favorite spot, one where you weren't walking forever to find the pine, was on a state game reserve. One time, after picking all day, we dragged our sacks up to the dirt road where Dad was to meet us. Instead of Dad, we were met by a game warden. He made us dump out all of our piney. He said he had been watching us

work all day long, and he wanted to teach us a lesson. Granddad and the rest of us were scared, but Mom told us it would be all right.

Later that night we went back and picked it all up by the light of the moon. Mom said that it was too much work picking something growing wild—that should be yours for free—only to have it wasted by someone who didn't know the first thing about nature.

Because of background and lifestyle, our family is riddled with disease and disability. The water we drank wherever we lived came out of mountains that had been strip-mined for coal. This same water would flow down the river and kill all of the fish and other living organisms.

The little town of 400 where we were raised is now full of cancer, multiple sclerosis, and many other diseases. I had cancer and had a section of my right foot removed. I have multiple sclerosis as do other members of my family. It is uncommon to have so many cases in such a small region. It's not contagious, so what is the common denominator?

We moved from the mountains in 1964, but apparently not in time. All of us have arthritis. Most have several of the following: high blood pressure, diabetes, emphysema, vitiligo, learning disabilities, heart and lung disease, sarcoidosis, eczema, kidney or liver disease or alcoholism.

I wish there had been free lunch programs back then. I know our health problems due to malnutrition could have been avoided. When I hear anyone go into a diatribe about all You People wanting handouts, I go a bit crazy. My main memory of my childhood is always being hungry. Oh sure, we gardened, hunted, and fished, but it was never enough to feed eight or more people at one time.

Does society still not get it? An unhealthy child will be an even more unhealthy adult. A sick, uneducated adult will not be able to work and contribute like a healthy educated one can. This dynamic will cost from the cradle to the coffin if it is not interrupted. Unlimited resources that are now being spent to make war all over the globe could be redirected to save the same amount of people.

My hope is that after all of the articles on class are printed in this issue, they will not just be read and then forgotten. If more people aren't willing to work to help us change our destiny, the loss will soon be insurmountable. I would like to see the problems caused by classism worked on continually until all women share equally the benefits of society.

Disability and the Medical System

by the Boston Women's Health Book Collective

Women with disabilities constantly struggle to find health care workers who are sensitive to their needs. For nondisabled women, experiences such as childbirth tend to raise awareness of abuses in the medical system. But women with disabilities, particularly those raised with a disability or with very severe medical difficulties, constantly encounter patronizing attitudes and ignorance by health care practitioners, damaging their sense of independence and well-being, and seriously reducing the quality of care.

The overlap of sexism with discrimination against people with disabilities restricts employment, education, and participation in the community for the approximately 30 million U.S. women with disabilities, who are among the most frequent consumers of medical services. While not all disabled people need medical treatment, such non-medical services as Social Security benefits, wheelchair transportation, and personal care attendant benefits require "certification as disabled" by a doctor.

Yet physicians get little, if any, training about or exposure to people with disabilities. A woman with cerebral palsy reported going to the doctor for an ear infection; he told her he'd never met a person with CP and spent 20 minutes asking her probing questions unrelated to her ear. When another woman visited a dermatologist because of a blister from her brace, he became visibly alarmed to find a woman in a wheelchair in the examining room. On the other hand, some doctors only meet disabled people who are in medical crisis, and disability is viewed solely as a dysfunction; medical schools offer virtually no training in the social and political issues of disability, let alone the impact of sexism, racism, or homophobia on women with disabilities.

The recent passage of the Americans with Disabilities Act of 1990, which has sweeping provisions for accessibility of facilities and services, signals the growing political strength of disabled people. But the medical system lags behind in recognizing disabled women as adults, capable of independent, self-directed lives. For example, if a disabled woman questions a doctor's recommendation, the response is often brutal; a blind diabetic woman who questioned her doctor's prescription was told, "You are hardly in a position to decide. If you'd followed your doctor's advice, you probably wouldn't be blind."

Disabled women, often displayed with little or no clothing in front of groups of medical students, are beginning to communicate their feelings of violation and humiliation. Doctors justify this kind of objectification—bordering on abuse—as necessary to teach students; they are baffled that disabled women have begun to protest.

One of the most pervasive myths is that disabled women are not sexual beings capable of sexual relationships and motherhood. A woman with spina bifida asked her gynecologist for birth control and was asked, "What for? What would you do with it?" The medical system has lagged in addressing the reproductive health needs of women with various kinds of disabilities. By far, most of the medical research on the topic focuses on male reproduction and sexual function.

Medical benefits are another quagmire of inequity. Women with disabilities must fight harder than men to justify their need for benefits since women may not have "worked" in the Social Security system enough to qualify for Medicare. Often only the most sophisticated self-advocates who have access to legal advice can obtain their rights in the system. Others become discouraged by the vast bureaucratic requirements and give up.

With the increasing competition and privatization in the health care industry, hospitals are under pressure to be profitable. Screening technologies such as genetic testing, and extensive investigation into family medical histories, are being used increasingly to identify patients who may be poor financial risks. This strategy, called "skimming," often used by insurance companies to disqualify policyholders, hits women the hardest.

Another area of concern is personal care attendant services, which would allow severely disabled people to

Preventing Doctor Abuse

1. Remember: you are in charge of your care; regard the doctor and other health workers as consultants who are employed by you.
2. Don't accept inappropriate or hurtful interaction. If confronting your doctor is hard, role playing first with friends may help you assert yourself.
3. Take a friend with you to take notes and provide support. Make sure the doctor knows that the friend or interpreter, if you use one, is not your guardian and that all communication should be directed to you.
4. To find a good doctor, ask women you trust; avoid the phone book or other listings. Call first to ask if the doctor has experience with your disability; ask about wheelchair or other accessibility.
5. Ask your general practitioner to find out about a specialist's experience with disabled people before referring you for an appointment.
6. Get a new doctor if you feel frightened, threatened, abused, or not respected as a capable adult; if your friend isn't allowed in the examination room without an acceptable reason; if the doctor isn't understandable and willing to learn from you about disabled people.
7. If you like your physician, tell her or him why. Refer others to that doctor.—M.S.

live in the community outside of institutions; obtaining such services is the new priority of the Denver-based activist organization Americans with Disabilities for Attendant Programs Today (ADAPT), which led the successful fight for wheelchair-accessible transportation.

Women with disabilities have few resources to challenge abuses; many are just now gaining the confidence to speak out, and their organizations have only begun to identify the nature of the mistreatment. As a group, disabled women tend to be poor, unemployed, and unlikely to pursue malpractice litigation; pro bono legal services are needed to support the legal rights of this emerging constituency.

We must assist disabled women in becoming more assertive, understanding their legal rights, and exploring medical alternatives, so that all of us can function as informed consumers of medical services.

For more information contact: ADAPT, (303) 733-9324; Disability Rights Education and Defense Fund, (202) 986-0375; Project on Women and Disability, (617) 277-5617. Also, the following books are available: *Past Due: A Story of Disability, Pregnancy and Birth,* by Anne Finger (Seal Press, $10.95); *Women with Disabilities: Essays in Psychology, Culture and Politics,* edited by Michelle Fine and Adrienne Asch (Temple University Press, $35); and *With Wings: An Anthology of Literature by and About Women with Disabilities,* edited by Marsha Saxton and Florence Howe (The Feminist Press, $12.95)—Marsha Saxton

Simply . . .Friend or Foe?

from New Internationalist

The able-bodied can be allies of disabled people—or they can be patronizing oppressors. Here are a few ways in which non-disabled readers can be friends instead of foes.

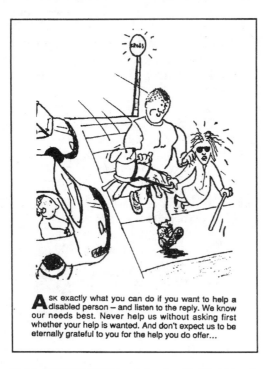

ASK exactly what you can do if you want to help a disabled person — and listen to the reply. We know our needs best. Never help us without asking first whether your help is wanted. And don't expect us to be eternally grateful to you for the help you do offer...

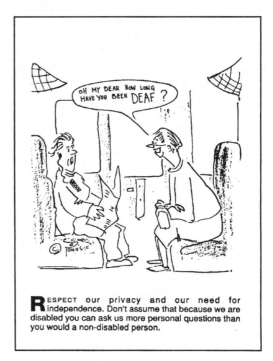

RESPECT our privacy and our need for independence. Don't assume that because we are disabled you can ask us more personal questions than you would a non-disabled person.

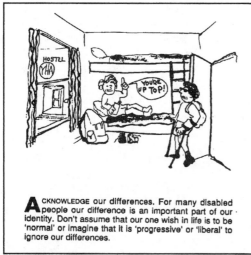

ACKNOWLEDGE our differences. For many disabled people our difference is an important part of our identity. Don't assume that our one wish in life is to be 'normal' or imagine that it is 'progressive' or 'liberal' to ignore our differences.

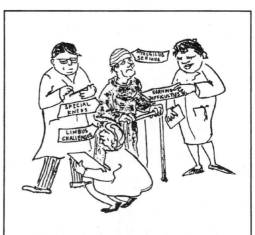

THINK about the way society creates barriers for us. Take account of the social and economic context in which we experience our medical condition. But don't reduce us to our medical conditions. Why should it matter to you what our condition is called?

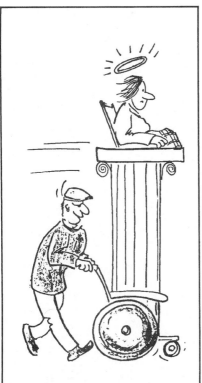

Challenge patronizing attitudes towards us. We want your empathy not your pity. Putting us on a pedestal or telling us how 'wonderful' and 'heroic' we are does not help. This attitude often conceals the judgment that having an impairment is intolerabale — which is very undermining for us.

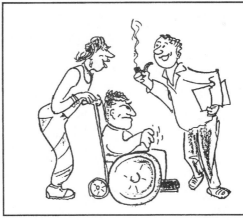

RECOGNIZE our existence. A gaze can express recognition and warmth. Talk to us directly. Neither stare at us — nor immediately look away either. And never talk about us as if we weren't there.

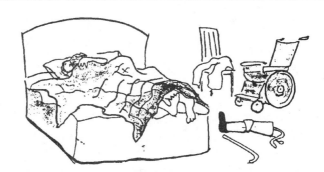

REALIZE that we are sexual beings, with the same wishes, needs and desire for fulfilling relationships as non-disabled people. Don't assume that we will never have children. And if a disabled person has a non-disabled lover don't jump to the conclusion that the latter is either a saint or has an ulterior motive.

APPRECIATE the contribution that we make to society in the fields of work, politics and culture. We engage in these activities for the same reasons as you do — but we may have some different insights to offer. Don't assume that we are passive — or that our activities are a form of 'therapy' to take our mind off our disability. Most disabled people are financially hard up and so we may have a greater need to earn a living than you.

This section is inspired by *Pride Against Prejudice* **by Jenny Morris and produced in conjunction with Claire King and Beverly Ashton. The cartoons are by Tony Meredith.**

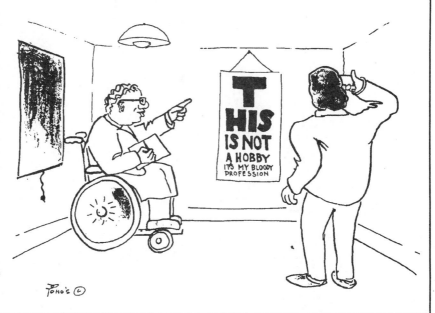

WORKSHEET—CHAPTER 2
Inequalities and Health

Although this chart of oppressions deserves much discussion and different people may choose to express this differently, this chart may be useful in answering questions on this worksheet.

Mythical norm (Non-target)	Oppressions	Targets
White people	Racism	People of color
Men	Sexism	Women, transgender
Young (not too young)	Ageism	Old/very young
Heterosexual	Homophobia	Gays, lesbians, bisexuals
Able-bodied	Ableism	People with disabilities
Christian	Anti-Semitism (Religious Narrowness)	Jews, Muslims Other religious groups
Thin	Fatphobia	Fat people
Middle class	Classism	Poor people

The term "mythical norm" comes from Audre Lorde's writings, particularly in *Sister Outsider*.
Ricky Sherover-Marcuse used the terms "non-target" and "target" groups in her Unlearning Racism Workshops.

1. Identify two ways that you think that your sex, race, or family income have influenced your interactions with health care providers or your access to the health care system.

2. Based on the oppressions chart above, identify one "mythical norm" (or non-target) group you are in. Describe the age and situation in which you first became aware that you had certain privileges or power because you belonged to this group.

3. Rewrite the "White Privilege: Unpacking the Invisible Knapsack" article to demonstrate ways you have (or understand) privilege in an unequal society. If you are a white person, identify ways that white privilege is *presently* a part of your life. If you are a person of color, rewrite the white privilege article to demonstrate ways you experience privilege because of your class, sexual identity, college education or because you do not have a disability.

4. Based on the oppressions chart above, identify one "target" group to which you belong. Identify ways in which you think belonging to this target group is similar and different from belonging to another target group. (Be specific about which two target groups you are comparing.)

5. Having identified a target group you are in, describe ways in which you feel you may have internalized society's negative messages about this group.

6. List ways that in your daily life you could or do interrupt sexist, racist, anti-Semitic, ageist, or homophobic incidents or behaviors.

7. You are helping plan a women's health course. Choose two different women's health topics. Suggest specific ideas of how you could plan to make sure that anti-oppression issues are central to the material covered for these topics.

CHAPTER 3

Gender Roles, Sex, and Marketing

Most introductory women's studies courses devote some class time to a discussion of gender roles. Many of the inequalities in our society are reinforced through the perpetuation of gender roles and through the arguments that these roles are somehow biologically determined and inevitable. (We use the term *gender* roles to emphasize that these roles are socially and culturally constructed, not biologically determined sex roles.) Gender role stereotyping plays a part in every issue discussed in this book and has an impact on women's roles as health care consumers and providers. This chapter brings together a number of themes related to the health ramifications of narrowly defined gender roles, narrow definitions of "males" or "females" as absolutes, the marketing of images of women and health and the marketing of products to women and their practitioners.

The first article, Leslie Doyal's "Hazards of Hearth and Home," gives an excellent global overview of women's health issues in the context of women's roles in different societies, exploring, among other issues, both the physical and psychological hazards of housework, the stress of caretaking and "emotional housework," and the impact of economic inequalities on women's health. Complementing Doyle's analysis of the health of women related to their roles at home, Jeanne Mager Stellman's "Perspectives on Women's Occupational Health" examines the same issues related to women's work outside the home. The key theme that women are often unable to take care of their own health because they are so busy taking care of others emerges in both articles whether the discussion is of women's paid or unpaid work.

"Male and Female Hormones Revisited" critiques the common use of the terms "male hormones" and "female hormones" and how this terminology reflects and perpetuates misunderstandings about the role of hormones vs. socialization in determining male and female similarities and differences. Many women and men find it liberating, or at least interesting, to learn that women and men are much more alike biologically than most of have been led to believe and that many differences between girls and boys, women and men, are more socially constructed than biologically determined. Of course, in a society where both females and males were equally valued, it would not particularly matter what was biological or social/cultural in origin. However, in a society in which what is identified as "masculine" is valued/rewarded more than what is labeled "feminine" (for example, see "If Men Could Menstruate," and "Mental Health Issues") demystifying biological vs. societal roles of sex/gender differences is an important political issue and biological determinism (the attempt to explain complex human behaviors by simplistic biological explanations) has been used as a very powerful tool to maintain the status quo and inequalities.

Feminists and others working for social change have certainly questioned rigid sex role socialization. Similarly, transsexuals and transgendered people have questioned our narrow definitions of "male" and "female" as absolutes and moved (some of) us toward thinking about what more fluid definitions of sex and gender would mean. "Intersexuals: Exploding the Binary Sex System" looks very specifically at how at least 1 of every 2000 people would benefit from living in a society in which the definitions of "male" vs. "female" were less rigid and where the medical establishment was not given the power to mutilate the bodies of children who do not easily fit into the male/female sex system. This article introduces us to the Intersex Society of North America (ISNA) and the issues they are raising about the routine practice of doctors' performing major surgery on young children. But it also raises much more fundamental questions about whether we can even envision a society in which new parents could be told, "Your child is intersexual, in other words, neither a boy nor a girl. There are resources available to help you raise your child in a healthy way. Go home and love your child as you would any other." (For a discussion of the challenges for trans and intersex people to live safely, read "Trans and Intersex Survivors of Domestic Violence" in Chapter 6, p. 281.)

In a more academic article on the same topic, Cheryl Chase, a founder of the ISNA interviewed for the "Intersexuals: Exploding the Binary Sex System," challenges feminists and the medical system to recognize our double standards in ignoring or encouraging the issue of intersex genital mutilation in the US but critiquing female genital mutilation in Africa. In her thought provoking chapter, " 'Cultural Practice' or 'Reconstructive Surgery'? US Genital Cutting, the Intersex Movement, and Medical Double Standards," from the excellent book *Genital Cutting and Transnational Sisterhood,* edited by Stanlie M. James and Claire C. Robertson, Chase states that:

> Examining the way that first-world feminists and mainstream media treat African practices and comparing that treatment with their response to intersex genital mutilation (IGM) in North America exposes some of the complex interactions between ideologies of race, gender, colonialism, and science that effectively silence and render invisible intersex experience in first-world contexts.

She concludes,

> I suggest that intersex people have had such difficulty generating mainstream feminist support not only because of the racist and colonialist frameworks. . .but also because intersexuality undermines the stability of the category "woman" that undergirds much first-world feminist discourse.

The remaining articles in this chapter explore images and narrow definitions of women and health from the viewpoint of how they are manipulated to sell us ideologies and products, including many products which are not only not needed but are also dangerous. Now that drug companies are allowed to advertise their products directly to consumers (without FDA approval for ads before they are used), understanding the power of ads and learning to critique ads are essential components of consumer health literacy. While most consumers are totally unaware of how much they are influenced by ads, studies have shown that one-third of patients have asked their health care practitioners about medication they have seen advertised and 15% of patients admit they would consider changing physicians if they were not given a prescription for a medicine they saw advertised (*The Truth About Hormone Replacement Therapy,* 2002, by the National Women's Health Network, p.14).

The unhealthy narrow definition of health itself is examined in the "Picture of Health" through the lens of how health is represented in photographs in health textbooks. In images very similar to those seen in advertising, those portrayed as "healthy" exclude large segments of the population, leaving a group of young, white, thin, and physically abled to represent health. Health is presented in these images as a commodity that many will not be able to acquire, in other words, a privilege, not a right.

The articles "Treating Disease with a Famous Face" and "Manufacturing Need, Manufacturing 'Knowledge' " expose some of the techniques used to market products and the need for products to both consumers and clinicians. In powerful examples of resistance, the American Medical Student Association's Pharm Free Campaign demonstrates how medical students are organizing against the influence drug companies have on their medical education, and the excellent Center for Medical Consumers' *Health Facts* provides two different sets of guidelines for consumers on what to look for in drug ads and how to read drug ads.

Hazards of Hearth and Home

by Lesley Doyal

Synopsis—Women's health cannot be understood simply in terms of their biological characteristics. Improved theoretical analysis and more effective political action both require an exploration of the causal links between women's daily lives and their experiences of health, illness and disability. Recent research relating to these issues is explored in two linked articles: "The Hazards of Hearth and Home" and "Waged Work and Women's Well Being" (Vol. 13 No. 6).

Domestic work varies around the world but it universally involves low status, lack of economic power, and extensive social and emotional responsibilities. The implications of this labour for women's health are explored in this first article through an examination of the physical and psychological hazards of housework, the impact of caring on women's well-being, the stresses of emotional housework, inequalities in the allocation of household resources, the social and economic context of the ageing process in women, and the effects of domestic violence. These issues are placed in the context of the feminisation of poverty and differences between women in the developed countries and the Third World are explored.

Introduction

Women's health has traditionally been understood in terms of their reproductive systems. Thus, doctors locate women's problems in the specialist areas of gynaecology and obstetrics and assume that this takes care of those health problems peculiar to the female sex. Even women's overrepresentation among those diagnosed as suffering from certain types of mental illness is frequently explained by reference to some ill-defined biological nature, related, however obscurely, to their reproductive characteristics.

The reductionist model of health and illness that lies behind these practices has come under increasing attack in recent years. Research has shown that social and economic factors such as class, race, and country of residence are crucially important in mediating the biological processes underlying disease, death, and disability in both sexes. People do not become sick or remain healthy simply because of their genetic inheritance and their accidental contact with disease causing agents. The causal processes involved are much broader, encompassing living and working conditions, access to basic necessities, power and autonomy, and the quality of human relationships.

Feminists have taken this analysis a step further, using these ideas to explore the particular health problems experienced by women. While most women have a longer life expectancy than men from the same social group as themselves, they report more ill health and distress than men, use primary care and hospital services more than men, and suffer more long-term disability. The nature and severity of women's health problems obviously vary according to race, class, and economic status, but this overall gender difference remains remarkably constant. Researchers are now beginning to explore the reasons for this, linking women's patterns of morbidity and mortality to the nature of gender divisions in society and particularly to the continuing inequalities between the sexes. Findings from this new research are used to explore the links between women's health and two main areas of activity in their lives—domestic labour and waged work.

Domestic Labour in a Global Context

Women have traditionally been responsible for most of the work done in the domestic sphere. However, very little is known officially about the nature of household work or the conditions under which it is performed. While there have been periodic panics about women's capacity to look after their families'—and therefore the nation's—health, the impact of their domestic work on

Reprinted from *Women's Studies International Forum*, Vol. 13, No. 5, by Lesley Doyal, "Hazards of Hearth and Home," pp. 501–517, © 1990, with permission of Elsevier.

women's own well-being has rarely been a cause for concern. Indeed the role(s) of housewife and mother have generally been seen as healthy, despite considerable evidence to the contrary. So what is the nature of this work that most women spend so much of their time performing?

Their domestic responsibilities involve women in a complex web of activities that are often difficult to disentangle. For most, the central threads consist of care of a husband (or male partner), care of children and other dependents, and housework. Although the balance of these responsibilities will vary during the life cycle, these basic jobs form the core of women's domestic work in most societies. Not surprisingly, the nature and volume of this labour and the circumstances under which it is carried out have profound effects on women's physical and mental health.

In the developed countries, the common stereotype of the housewife is of a consumer who does a relatively small amount of low status, unskilled work, much of which involves spending money earned by a man. The reality, however, is very different. In the first place, most domestic work is done not by full-time housewives, but by women who are also engaged in some combination of paid and unpaid work outside the home. This pattern now applies in the majority of countries around the world—rich and poor, socialist and capitalist. In the second place, domestic work involves many (often unrecognized) skills and much effort. Indeed, most women with children (with the exception of the very affluent) spend their lives in continuous activity, putting together what the Italian feminist Laura Balbo has called "survival strategies" for themselves and their families (Balbo, 1987, p. 45).

But despite its obvious social utility, women's domestic work is unpaid—a fact which demeans it, and sets it apart from most other work done by adults. This inevitably has psychological significance for women, lowering their self-esteem and minimizing their sense of their own worth. It also affects them in more material ways, by reinforcing their economic dependence on others. Although many mothers with young children are now in paid employment, few can earn enough to support themselves and their families while continuing to do unpaid domestic work. Hence, most are forced, along with full-time housewives, into economic dependence on a male wage earner. Others have to rely not on an individual man but on the state to provide for their basic needs. In either case, economic dependence seriously limits women's autonomy and inhibits their control over their own lives and their health.

At the same time, women also have to take responsibility for those who are dependent on them for emotional and physical sustenance. Most of their daily work involves women in the servicing of others (Kickbusch, 1981). Put in more romantic terms, women's work consists of care of their "loved ones." This care can range from washing a partner's clothes through cooking a child's dinner to comforting a teenager worried about spots or cleaning up after the dog has been sick. It is distinguished from the same work in a laundry, cafe, or health centre because it is done for love rather than money. That is to say, women are expected to care *about* other people as well as caring *for* them (Graham, 1984). Thus, many women bear the double burden of their own economic dependence on a man or the state along with the dependency of their families on them for physical and psychological survival.

So far we have been talking in general terms about the elements of domestic work as it is performed by women in most countries around the world. The recognition of these basic similarities is important in reminding us that whatever the circumstances, patriarchal societies give women ultimate responsibility for the well-being of their families, often at considerable cost to their own health. However, this responsibility will have different implications according to the socioeconomic circumstances in which it has to be fulfilled. This point is most clearly illustrated through contrasting the lot of the majority of women in the industrialized countries with those in the Third World.

Housework and childcare are not the same in Birmingham, England or Birmingham, Alabama, as they are in the slums of Sao Paolo or the rural wastes of the Sahel. The most obvious difference is the level of material resources to which a woman has access to meet her family's needs. As we shall see, poverty itself is a major factor influencing the impact that a woman's domestic work has on her health, and most Third World women are very poor by comparison with those in Britain or the United States. But taking the analysis one stage further, we also need to recognize that the nature of domestic work itself is very different in the Third World.

Women in the rich countries work out their survival strategies through their own and often a partner's negotiations with the labour market and/or the state. This will often be difficult, time-consuming and exhausting, and the impact on the health of poor women should not be underestimated as they cobble together wages, benefits, subsidies, or rebates to underwrite the purchase of their necessities. However, even these options are not available to millions of women in the Third World. They have little or no money to spend in the cash economy and welfare services are not available to fill the gap. As a result, they have to weave their patchwork of survival through the direct production of their own and their family's needs. Many are engaged in subsistence agriculture, growing and then processing the food they are not rich enough to buy. Fuel is collected in the form of firewood rather than purchased from a gas or electricity supply company and water is collected from a local source rather than flowing to the house through pipes. Thus, the physical burdens of their domestic labour are very much greater and this is clearly reflected in their experiences of morbidity and mortality. These international variations will be explored in more detail as we look at the different aspects of women's domestic work and its impact on their health.

The Hazards of Housework

Throughout the world, women perform many millions of hours of housework every day—most of it unacknowledged and barely visible. In the developed countries it is widely assumed that technological innovation has led to a reduction in the hours spent on housework. However, there is little evidence to support this belief. The introduction of basic services, such as running water and gas and electricity, along with the later development of vacuum cleaners, washing machines, and other domestic appliances certainly ameliorated the hard physical labour that characterized the lives of so many workingclass women in the 19th and early 20th centuries (Oren, 1974; Pember Reeves, 1980; Llewellyn Davies, 1978; Spring Rice, 1981). However, there was little reduction in the number of hours worked (Vanek, 1974; Meissner et al., 1988). Nor is there evidence that women's greater participation in waged work has led to a more equal division of domestic labour. Instead, women have retained the moral responsibility for ensuring that all domestic work is done, whether they are employed outside the home or not. They must organize it and worry about it, even if they do not do everything themselves, with inevitable effects on their health.

Despite (or sometimes because of) the development of modern technology, housework can still be physically and mentally exhausting, especially when conditions are difficult. Domestic accidents are a common hazard, especially for older women, and are more likely to happen when the fabric of the home is substandard. An old and dilapidated house will be more difficult to keep clean and will often threaten the safety of women and children. Since they have to spend more time than men indoors, women are more affected by defects, such as condensation and dampness which can aggravate respiratory disorders, as well as increasing the physical burden of housework. Looking after a home and its inhabitants can also bring the worker into contact with a wide range of toxic chemicals that are largely unregulated and have often been inadequately tested (Dowie et al., 1982; Rosenberg, 1984). Most of these are domestic products of various kinds such as cleaning fluids, bleaches, detergents, insecticides, and pesticides that are commonly used in the home and garden. It has been estimated that the average household in the United States contains some 250 chemicals that could send a child to hospital (Rosenberg, 1984).

There is also growing evidence that in the course of their housework women may be put at risk by hazardous chemicals encountered by their partners at their place of work. Research has shown that they can be endangered by asbestos fibers and radiation brought home on their husband's clothes or on his person. It also seems likely that some cases of cervical cancer may be caused by substances to which the man is occupationally exposed, which are then passed on to the women during intercourse (Robinson, 1981). Thus, the domestic workplace is not necessarily free from the chemical hazards of the industrial setting. Toxic substances do not become safe simply because they cross the threshold of the home and more research is needed to identify these dangers, as well as more effective regulation to control them.

However, it is the psychological hazards of housework which have attracted most attention, at least in the developed countries. To understand the reasons for this we need to look more closely at the nature of the work itself, at its social and economic status, and at the conditions under which it is performed. We can then explore the effects these have on women's sense of themselves, their control over their lives, and their potential for growth.

In Ann Oakley's study of full-time British housewives, most saw the main advantage of their job as the negative one of freedom from the constraints of employment (Oakley 1974). Few were positively happy with their work, with 70% expressing themselves 'dissatisfied' overall (Oakley, 1974). The women described most of their household tasks as monotonous, boring, and repetitive. Interestingly, it is these very characteristics of unskilled labour that occupational psychologists have shown to be most stressful in the context of male waged work. Although they are not formally controlled by a boss, most women doing housework experience very powerful pressures, both from other people and from inside their own heads. Ann Oakley asked one of the women in her study whether she found housework monotonous. Sally Jordan replied:

> Well, I suppose I do really, because it's the same thing every day. You can't sort of say, "I'm not going to do it," because you've got to do it. Take preparing a meal: it's got to be done, because if you didn't do it, the children wouldn't eat. I suppose you get so used to it, you do it automatically. When I'm doing housework, half the time I don't know what I'm thinking about. I'm sort of there, and I'm not there. Like when I'm doing the washing—I'm at the sink with my hands in water, and I drift off. I daydream when I'm doing anything really—I'm always going off in a trance, I don't hear people when they talk to me. (Oakley, 1976, p. 147)

Thus, women are able to get little job satisfaction from routine housework and this is exacerbated by their lack of social and economic status (Berk, 1980). Most adults are paid for their work, and lack of such rewards limits self-esteem and gives a sense of worthlessness. Moreover, housework tends to be noticed only when it has *not* been done, giving women little opportunity for positive reinforcement, even of a nonmaterial kind.

These negative feelings are reinforced by the circumstances under which domestic labour is carried out. Housework is paradoxical in that it is usually done at home in isolation from most other adults, but when combined with childcare it also offers little opportunity for solitude. Despite widespread social and economic change, women continue to do almost all their household tasks in individual nuclear family units, with modern architectural styles often reinforcing this separation. However, the housewife may also find that her time is not her own. She will have to respond to the needs of others, may find very little time or energy to do things for herself, and rarely has physical space of her own. Under these circumstances, the demands on women are often high, and the real possibilities for control are low—again a situation clearly identified as stressful in the context of waged work (Karasek, 1979).

An additional feature of domestic work which can pose a threat to women's health is its open-endedness. Just as there are no absolute goals or standards, so there is no obvious end to the working day. For men and older children, home is perceived as a place of rest and recovery from the stresses and strains of real work done in the world outside. However, for most women the home is also a workplace and remains so for most of their waking hours. Many find it difficult to separate work and leisure; indeed those with young children are never really off duty, and their working hours can even extend to periods of sleep.

Not surprisingly, surveys in the developed countries have shown that women indulge in fewer leisure activities than men. The hobbies and pastimes they mention tend to be domestic or home-based (listening to records or tapes, watching TV, reading, needlework and knitting, crafts and cooking) and they are frequently combined with ironing or child care (Deem, 1986). Relatively few are able to have outside interests, and active participation in sport is rare indeed. The reasons for this are closely related to women's family situation: lack of material resources, reluctance of men to allow them out alone, and the difficulty of getting someone else to look after the children, as well as the male-domination of many leisure and sporting facilities. This lack of leisure in general, and sport in particular, has obvious implications for women's physical and mental health:

> . . . the notion of "wellbeing" is closely tied up with opportunities for leisure. The fewer opportunities women have for leisure, the less the chance that they will see themselves as enjoying such wellbeing, which includes more than feeling healthy and/or fit and implies a sense of confidence about and enjoyment of life in general, which is difficult if that life consists mainly of being stressed, overworked, tense and continually feeling tired as well as having a poor body image. (Deem, 1986, p. 425)

Ultimately, the most damaging aspect of housework for women's mental health may be the lack of opportunity it offers for personal development. Some women do get a great deal of satisfaction from tasks done in and for their households, and develop considerable skills in the process. However, the structure of the job offers no opportunity for growth or advancement and few chances of wider social recognition for achievement. Of course, women do learn to deal creatively with challenges and crises throughout their lives. Indeed many individuals and families would not have survived without their tenacity, problem-solving abilities, and sheer hard work. However, those tasks are rarely of their own choosing and may offer little in the way of increased personal autonomy.

Why then do so many women go on doing housework under these conditions with so little complaint? One reason is their early socialisation which means that many have extreme difficulty in expressing any dissatisfaction they may have with housework. To do so may be to threaten their identity as a good wife and loving mother.

The power of this repression is reflected in what Jessie Bernard has called the "paradox of the happy marriage." During her classic investigation of male and female perceptions of marriage, men expressed a considerable degree of dissatisfaction, but appeared to have relatively good mental health as measured by a questionnaire. Women, on the other hand, were more likely to say they were happily married but exhibited much poorer mental health (Bernard, 1972). This contradiction was especially acute among full-time housewives, many of whom simultaneously expressed high levels of satisfaction with marriage, as well as serious psychiatric symptoms. Indeed Bernard describes what she calls the "housewife syndrome" consisting of nervousness, fainting, insomnia, trembling hands, nightmares, dizziness, heart palpitations, and other anxiety symptoms. She concluded that "the housewife syndrome is far from a figment of anyone's imagination" (p. 47) and that "being a housewife makes women sick" (p. 48).

But it is depression above all, that seems to be an occupational hazard among fulltime housewives, especially those with young children. Both clinical experience and community research have shown that many women staying at home experience intense frustration, which is usually expressed in feelings of emptiness, sadness and worthlessness (Brown & Harris, 1978; Nairne & Smith, 1984). Too often these feelings go unacknowledged; women are said to be "like that" and the front door closes on a great deal of misery and distress. George Brown and Tirril Harris working in South London found that one-third of a random sample of workingclass women with children under six who were fulltime caregivers were suffering from what could be classified as "clinical depression." However, few had sought medical help. When women do take emotional problems to their doctors they are usually offered a chemical solution. In reality, however, it is the nature of women's domestic labour, their relationships with other people and their dependent status that makes them more likely than any other group to experience depression and anxiety, but less likely to confront the real reasons for their frustrations and dissatisfactions.

Who Cares for the Caregivers?

As well as doing the housework the majority of women also care for dependents. The intensity of this work varies over the lifecycle and some women never do it at all. However the vast majority become mothers at least once in their lives—in Britain the figure is now about 80%. This can be immensely rewarding and for many women motherhood is the most important and creative aspect of their lives. However, the reality of day to day childcare can also be both physically and emotionally demanding, especially under difficult circumstances (Graham & McKee, 1980; Richman, 1976; Boulton, 1983). For first-time mothers in particular, the responsibility of a tiny baby can be very onerous and nights without sleep exhausting and demoralizing.

Despite the lip service paid to motherhood as a social duty and a valued activity, few researchers have explored the reality of childcare from a woman's perspective. In an attempt to fill this gap, the British sociologist Mary Boulton recently carried out a series of in-depth interviews with young mothers (Boulton, 1983). Her intention was to disentangle women's feelings about the daily labour of childcare from their love for their children or their response to the status of motherhood itself. Almost two-thirds of women in the study experienced a strong sense of meaning, value, and significance in looking after their children. This is clearly important because a purpose in life is central to a feeling of well-being. However over one third did not feel this way (Boulton, 1983). Moreover, some 60% of her middle-class respondents and 44% of those who were working class found looking after children to be predominantly an irritating experience. Thus, the majority did not find childcare "naturally rewarding." Yet this was their fulltime work.

Many of the women referred to stress in their lives and identified a number of factors contributing to it. The lack of boundaries to their role meant that they were always trying to create structures and find themselves physical and mental space. They complained that childcare interfered with other activities, especially housework, and that children often undid what had just been achieved. For some women, childcare was isolating and limited them to relationships with other women in a similar position. Many also pointed out that children greatly curtailed their freedom of action because there was so much effort and anxiety involved in taking them out.

Overall, about 50% of Mary Boulton's sample said they were wholly content with their lives as mothers, about one-fifth were wholly discontented, while about one-quarter were in between. That is to say they accepted the situation, but wished it could be different. Significantly however, many of those who reported themselves satisfied also stated that their experiences of childcare were negative. This suggests that, as we saw in the context of housework, many women may simply accept situations over which they have no control, living much of their lives vicariously through others, with inevitable effects on their own well-being.

As well as caring for healthy children, women also look after dependent adults and chronically sick children. Again, precise information is difficult to obtain because this domesticated nursing is one of the most invisible of all forms of labour. In the British context, estimates suggest that at least 1.4 million people (out of a total population of just over 60 million) act as principal caregivers to adults and children with disabilities severe enough to warrant support in daily living tasks

(Green, 1988). The vast majority of these are women. Some 15% of all British women of working age care for dependents over and above their normal family duties and many of them are also in paid employment (Martin & Roberts, 1984). Moreover, the need for such care is rising as the number of elderly and disabled people in the population increases. Indeed, the community care policies now fashionable in much of the industrialized world are based on the implicit assumption that women will continue with these unpaid labours (Osterbusch et al., 1987; Finch, 1984; Finch & Groves, 1983). Yet there is evidence that they may not be conducive to the promotion of women's own well-being.

The daily grind of caring has been well documented in a number of research studies (Equal Opportunities Commission, 1982; Finch & Groves, 1983; Briggs & Oliver, 1985). Caring for adults can be especially demanding both physically and psychologically. Much of the strain comes from the nature of the job itself—long hours, nightly disturbances and sometimes the trying behaviour of the person being cared for or the inability to hold a serious conversation. Stress is also caused by the conditions of caring, particularly the isolation that often results when the person cannot be taken out and no substitute care is available. Above all, caring for adults can cause emotional problems that do not arise in caring for normal children. The daughter who cares for a parent and the wife who cares for a husband may have to negotiate new relationships under difficult circumstances, often with very little support. One British woman looking after her husband has described her experiences in the following terms:

> The tiredness associated with looking after someone disabled was the hardest thing for me to adjust to . . . the tiredness is, of course, due to different causes for each caregiver, but the exhaustive effect is the same—for me, the tiredness comes from the physical exertion of caring for someone with severe multiple sclerosis, and from the mental stress of seeing the person you love best in the world suffering from such a disease. (Briggs & Oliver, 1985, p. 39)

Under these circumstances, women's own health will often suffer. This is especially true for women on what has been called the caring tricycle—the lifetime of responsibility which begins with care of children, continues into middle age with care of an aging parent, and ends with responsibility for a frail partner.

Doing Emotional Housework

Some of the more subtle aspects of women's domestic labour can be summarized as emotional housework. This is the least visible part of their work and consists of activities designed to ensure the happiness and emotional wellbeing of other family members—managing social relationships within the home to keep the old man happy and the kids quiet. While this labour is rarely perceived as such by women or their families, it is often a major burden. Arlie Hochschild has vividly described the processes involved:

> The emotion work of enhancing the status and wellbeing of others is a form of what Ivan Illich has called "shadow labour": an unseen effort which, like housework, does not quite count as labour but is nevertheless crucial in getting things done. As with doing housework the trick is to erase any evidence of effort, to offer only the clean house and the welcoming smile. (Hochschild, 1983)

But who is looking after women's needs while they smile for others? Sadly, the answer for many is no one. The traditional division of labour in the family means that women frequently do not receive the emotional sustenance they might have expected from their nearest and dearest. While adult daughters may provide support, this is rarely true of grown-up sons and male partners.

Luise Eichenbaum and Susie Orbach have written extensively on this problem from their experiences as feminist psychotherapists (Orbach & Eichenbaum, 1984; Eichenbaum & Orbach, 1985). They make the important point that the social stereotype of the clinging, passive female leaning on a strong and independent man is usually the reverse of the truth. Most men, they say, are looked after by women all their lives, from their mothers and other female relatives through female teachers to their wives or female partners in adulthood. A girl, on the other hand, is brought up to assume that she will marry a man and provide nurturance, care, and emotional support for him and his children. While she is expected to *appear* "dependent, incompetent and somewhat fragile," the internal reality is rather different:

> . . . behind this outward facade is someone who, whatever the inner state, will have to deal with the emotional problems met in family relationships, a person who knows that others will expect to rely and lean on her, a person who fears that she will never really be able to depend on others or never feels content about her dependency. (Eichenbaum & Orbach, 1985, p. 21)

Thus, many adult women cannot fulfill their own basic need for nurturance and emotional fulfillment, despite—or because of—their position at the hub of what is widely regarded as the most caring institution in modern society.

These insights derived from the psychoanalytic tradition are consonant with women's own accounts of their situation, as reported in a number of recent studies. Agnes Miles, a British sociologist, recently carried out in-depth interviews with some 65 women and men diagnosed as suffering from depression. About half of the women blamed their depression on an unhappy marriage, whereas most men referred to work and health problems (Miles, 1988). When asked about the support they had received, only 24 out of 65 women named their male partner as their main confidante and not all of these were satisfied with the quality of the relationship:

> (Iris, 24, no children). "There is only my husband. I wish there was someone else. Mostly I keep my thoughts to myself. I hoard my thoughts, then I get upset and tell my husband because there is nobody else. I usually regret it afterwards. He is part of the trouble, but who else can I talk to?"
>
> (Bridget, 29, two children 4 and 7). "I wish I had more people, I wish I had a woman friend. My husband is there but he doesn't want to talk, not like women talk to each other. He doesn't understand. He just says, don't bother me with nonsense." (Miles, 1988, pp. 94–95)

Many of the women in Miles' sample also expressed their fear of putting too much of a burden on other people. They were afraid that what little help was available would be withdrawn and, even more fundamentally, saw themselves as unworthy of support. Interestingly, the men in Miles' sample did not report the same problems in getting support from their wives. As Miles expressed it, "both took for granted that this was the natural order of things" (p. 113).

Susannah Ginsberg and George Brown uncovered a similar pattern in their study of women in the North London suburb of Islington. Again they were interviewing women who would be clinically diagnosed as a case of depression, in an attempt to see how relatives, friends, and doctors responded to their problems. This research repeated the now-common finding that signs of depression in women (such as inexplicable crying) are often given little attention since they are regarded as normal for women, especially when they are young mothers or menopausal (Ginsberg & Brown, 1982). Three quarters of those interviewed (27/37) who were living with their husbands felt that he had given little or no support. Mrs. Thomas, for instance, commented as follows:

> "I told my husband how depressed I've been feeling. He just sits in silence. If he could just talk things out and suggest something—but he doesn't."
>
> "Has he suggested you should go to the doctor?"
>
> "No, he doesn't realize anything is wrong. He doesn't notice that I haven't been getting on with things." (Ginsberg & Brown, 1982, p. 93)

Three quarters of the women (34/45) also felt they received little or no support from their mother or other relatives such as sister, or friends. The majority (32/37) who were living with their husbands said they did try to talk about their depression but most were unsuccessful. The majority of husbands apparently responded with such comments as "You're imagining it all," "Stop being silly," or "You mustn't talk like that, there's the baby" (Ginsberg & Brown, 1982, p. 95).

It seems, then, that women's domestic labour, especially their role in caring for others, is not always conducive to their own good health. Their mental well-being in particular will often be put at risk, and adequate support is not available when they are in need. As we shall see, this is especially true in the context of material poverty.

The Feminisation of Poverty

Women have always been overrepresented among the world's poor and recent years have seen a worsening of their situation (Scott, 1984). Although impoverished women are to be found in all countries, the majority live in underdeveloped parts of the world and it is here that the rigours of domestic work are at their most severe (Buvinic, Lycette, & McGreavey, 1983). Of course, men in the Third World are also poor, but it is women who must manage the consequences of poverty for the whole family. This often means performing physically heavier work and working longer hours than men (Dankelman & Davidson, 1988; Momsen & Townsend, 1987; Sen & Grown, 1988). In Tanzania, for instance, a recent study showed that women work an average of 3069 hours a year compared with 1829 hours for men (Taylor, 1985). Similarly, women in the Gambia spend 159 days a year on farmwork compared to men's 103 days (Mair, 1984). Moving to Asia, a study conducted in several rural villages in Kaunataka showed that the labour of women and children together contributed almost 70% of the total human energy expended on village work, even when strictly domestic tasks such as sweeping, washing clothes and childcare were excluded (Kishwar & Vanita, 1984).

Thus, women in the Third World bear a heavy weight of domestic responsibilities. Moreover, their material poverty and, for many, the exhaustion of frequent childbearing, add to their burdens. While climate, culture, and conditions vary between countries, these women are united by their poverty and the harshness of the social, economic, and physical environment in which they carry out their labours. As we shall see, this daily struggle is reflected in their general state of health and well-being.

In the richer parts of the world, most housewives can take for granted the existence of a constant supply of clean water. However, there are millions of women from rural areas of Bangladesh to the crowded barrios of Latin America who must face the daily task of acquiring enough water to meet the needs of their families. This is a physically demanding job which in rural areas will often mean a lengthy journey, but it is very rarely done by men.

Water is needed not just for drinking, but for sanitation and waste disposal, washing, childcare, vegetable growing, and food processing and also for economic uses such as keeping animals, irrigating crops, and brewing beer (Dankelman & Davidson, 1988). All this has to be fetched by women—usually on their heads because few have access to a vehicle of any kind or even a donkey (Wijk-Sijbesma, 1983). Many walk miles every day to a stream, well, or pond for a few pots of water. In urban areas, women depend on public taps which will usually mean long waits and no privacy for bathing. In many slums even public taps are not available, so that women face a long journey or the payment of a high price to a street vendor for water of dubious quality (Dankelman & Davidson, 1988).

Under these circumstances, water will have to be consumed sparingly, making other domestic tasks more difficult. Moreover, insufficient or polluted water will often result in illness, adding to the woman's burden. It is generally assumed that some 80% of all diseases in Third World countries are water-related. Diarrhoea, for instance, is a major cause of death among young children and is closely correlated with the absence of a clean water supply. Women themselves suffer additional problems caused by lack of adequate sanitation because religious and moral prohibitions mean they often have to wait until dark to avoid being seen in the act of defecation. This can lead to constipation and strain on the bladder and also exposes them to the risk of assault (Dietrich, 1986).

As well as supplying water, many Third World women are also responsible for ensuring an adequate amount of fuel for cooking, boiling water, and heating and lighting the house. Again, this very arduous task is rarely done by men and is a significant factor in the endemic exhaustion of many rural women. Throughout the world women are carrying loads of up to 35 kilograms, distances as much as 10 kilometers from home. This weight exceeds the legal allowance for women carrying heavy loads in an industrial setting in many countries. The distance women have to travel varies depending on where they live, and the time taken can be as much as three or four hours per day. In some areas including the Sahel, Gambia, and parts of India, the journeys can be even longer and deforestation means that they are increasing (Agarwal, 1986). As supplies of firewood diminish, women and children are having to spend even more time on collection. In parts of Bihar, for instance,

where seven to eight years ago poor women could get enough wood at 1.5 to 2 kilometers, they now have to trek 8 to 10 kilometers every day (Agarwal, 1986).

This growing shortage of fuel has meant that cooking has now become more labour-intensive and traditional methods have to be adapted to conserve energy. In some places the traditional wood fuel has been replaced by substances, such as cattle dung and crop residues. These biomass fuels are less convenient for cooking; the fire has to be stoked continuously and the smoke is even more dangerous than woodsmoke (WHO, 1984). Emissions from biomass fuels are major sources of air pollution in the home, and studies have shown that cooks inhale more smoke and pollutants than the inhabitants of the dirtiest cities. In one study quoted by WHO, a female cook was said to inhale an amount of benzopyrene (a known carcinogen) equivalent to 20 packs of cigarettes a day. Chronic carbon monoxide poisoning has also been reported (Dankelman & Davidson, 1988). Pollution of this kind has been identified as a causal factor in the high level of respiratory and eye disease found among Third World women. It can also cause acute bronchitis and pneumonia, as well as nasopharyngeal cancer among those exposed from early infancy (WHO, 1984).

As well as ensuring supplies of water and fuel, many Third World women are also directly involved in the production of food for their families (Dixon-Mueller, 1985). They grow a variety of crops either for immediate consumption or to be sold or bartered in the village or local market, and raise poultry or small animals. When food is scarce or there is a drought, they may have to scour the countryside for edible matter such as the roots and leaves of plants. This raw food then has to be processed, often by laborious and lengthy methods. These processes will vary between cultures and climates, but Madhu Kishwar's account of Indian peasant women gives some indication of the quantity of work involved:

> Grain or pulses to be consumed have to be hard-cleaned, little pebbles or pieces of dirt hand-sifted or painstakingly removed, one by one before the cooking of every meal. Many women have to hand-pound the paddy or grind the wheat two or three days a week in order to make it consumable. The paddy first has to be boiled and dried in the sun before it is husked. To husk 20 pounds of paddy, two women can easily spend two to three hours, and it takes much longer if a woman has to do it alone. . . . Thus, cooking even the most simple and basic foods commonly used in the diet of ordinary families is very exhausting. (Kishwar & Vanita, 1984, p. 4)

These accounts make it clear that the domestic labour of most Third World women is extremely hard.

The work is physically strenuous and the hours are long, leaving many millions exhausted, undernourished, and vulnerable to premature death. Moreover, most are involved in frequent childbearing, resulting in levels of debility which can only be guessed at, since morbidity data for rural women are rare, and mortality data crude and uninformative.

While some of the worst living and working conditions are suffered by women in the Third World, this should not blind us to the fact that there are also many women in the developed countries who suffer the ill effects of both absolute and relative poverty on their health (Gelpi, Hartsock, Novack, & Strober, 1983; Glendinning & Millar, 1987; Scott, 1984). In the United States, the richest country in the world, almost two-thirds of impoverished adults are women. This overrepresentation of women among the poor must be explained by reference to the sexual division of labour in the wider society. Women are confined to a secondary status in the labour market, yet their work in the home is not financially rewarded. State welfare benefits mirror this low earning capacity, thus perpetuating a lifetime of economic dependence and poverty for many working-class women. In Britain, for instance, working women make up over two-thirds of the 8 million people whose wages are below the poverty line. Similarly, some two-thirds of all elderly people live in poverty and six million of this nine million are women. Female-headed families, too, represent a significant group in poverty. Thus, many women in rich as well as poor countries suffer the ill-effects of poverty.

The ill health women experience as a result of deprivation is often compounded by the allocation of resources within the family. Research has shown that even in households where the aggregate income is above the poverty line, women may not have enough to meet their own needs. This is because the division of income and wealth between individuals is often unequal (Glendinning & Millar, 1987; Land, 1983; Pahl, 1980). Women tend to get (or take) less both because of their economic dependence and lack of power, but also because of their concern for other family members. Thus, women are more likely than men to be poor when living alone, they may be poor members in nonpoor households, or they may be the poorest in a poor household. In all cases, their health will be at risk.

Bread for the Breadwinner?

We can illustrate these inequalities in the allocation of household resources by looking at gender differences in nutrition. Although women are usually responsible for the purchase and preparation of food and often its production too, many do not have the power to determine distribution between family members, and their own health may suffer as a consequence. Adequate nutrition is a basic human need which cannot always be met for the entire household in conditions of poverty. Research in many countries around the world has shown that when the family income is too low, it is women who are especially prone to nutritional deficiency. Under these circumstances, food is often the only item of expenditure that can be manipulated to make ends meet and it is usually women who go short to ensure that the needs of the children and the breadwinner are met (Oren, 1974).

Yet women themselves have particular nutritional needs, which often go unrecognized or ignored. Menstruation, pregnancy, and lactation all increase women's need for protein and iron. This is difficult to measure precisely, but it has been estimated that pregnant women need 350 extra Calories per day, while those feeding their babies need another 550 Calories, as well as three times the normal intake of calcium and double the amount of vitamin A (Protein-Calorie Advisory Group, 1977). Research in both the developed countries and the Third World has shown that many women do not get enough of the right food to meet these needs.

A study carried out by the London-based Maternity Alliance in 1984 showed that despite the existence of the British welfare state some women are still not able to feed themselves adequately during pregnancy. The average cost of the diet recommended for pregnant women by the Department of Health in 1988 was £15.88. This represented nearly half the weekly benefit payable to a single person and a third of that for a couple (Durward, 1988). As a result, the many pregnant women on supplementary benefit could not afford to eat what was officially defined as necessary to sustain their own health and that of their unborn children.

In the Third World, the nutritional problems of poor women are, of course, much greater. The combination of lack of food and, in some countries, severe discrimination against women, results in serious undernutrition for many mothers and daughters (World Health Organization, 1986). According to the Protein-Calorie Advisory Group of the United Nations (PAG), there are definite indications of maldistribution of food at the family level in many parts of Africa with women getting the least even in pregnancy (Protein-Calorie Advisory Group, 1977). In some cultures, it is common for boys to be breastfed considerably longer than girls and for girl children to be fed less well than boys, thus reducing their chances of surviving infancy. Adult men often sit down to eat before their women and children, who get what remains (Leghorn & Roodkowsky, 1977; Carloni, 1981;

Maher, 1981). Thus, food which is itself in scarce supply is distributed according to the prestige of family members rather than their nutritional needs. As a result, many women become anemic, especially during pregnancy, due to a lack of basic nutrients. Estimates suggest that in the Third World as many as half of nonpregnant women and two-thirds of pregnant women are anemic due to iron deficiency and folate and vitamin B12 deficiency combined with parasitic infections (WHO, 1979).

The authors of a recent study in Bangladesh set out to determine whether or not the very poor health record of women in that country could be explained by inequalities in the allocation of food and medical care (Chen, Huq, & d'Souza, 1981). The results were startling. Fourteen and four-tenths percent of female children in the sample were found to be severely malnourished, compared with 5.1% of males. This appeared to be directly related to food intake because dietary surveys showed that per capita male food intake considerably exceeded that of females at all ages. Overall, males averaged 1,927 calories per capita compared with 1,599 calories for females. The male excess was as high as 29% during the childbearing years of 15 to 44. These differences remained even when the data were adjusted for body weight, pregnancy, lactation, and activity levels, indicating that they must be seen as a relevant factor in explaining women's excess mortality.

In concluding, the authors of the study make the important point that these gender inequalities in life and death should not be seen as merely the response to scarcity. Indeed, they were found in rich as well as poor families, reflecting the fundamental inferiority of women's position in a profoundly patriarchal society. Of course, the reasons for male preference are a complicated mixture of the material as well as the ideological—girls cannot earn as much to help the family budget, have to be given a dowry, and are not able to support their parents during old age. But all too often the end result is serious damage to the health of girls, with many of those who survive to adulthood passing on their debility to future generations.

Older Women: The Invisible Majority

So far we have talked mainly about the impact of domestic tasks on the health of women in their childbearing years. However, in the developed countries, at least, it is older women who are most often confined to the home and who form the largest single group living in poverty. Even those who are not materially deprived frequently face serious health problems, yet these go largely unnoticed in societies that prioritize youth, vitality, and innovation. A combination of ageism and sexism means that older women are all too often marginalised sexually, socially, and economically in ways that threaten their well-being.

Older women are now the fastest growing group in poverty in the United States and Britain. In the United States, one-fifth of women aged 65 and over are below the poverty line, and women are twice as likely as men to experience poverty in old age. The single elderly are poorest of all and are predominantly female—three-fifths of women over 65 are alone compared with only a quarter of men. This reflects both the age difference of most couples at marriage and women's longer life expectancy. Older women from ethnic minorities suffer disproportionately from the effects of poverty. Forty-two percent of aged black women are in absolute poverty and a staggering 82% in near poverty, according to the 1980 U.S. Census. A similar situation prevails in Britain, with two-fifths of elderly women (38%) living on or below the poverty line, compared with 25% of men; two-thirds of all older British women are on the margins of poverty (Walker, 1987).

The poverty of older women stems directly from their lifelong economic dependency on men, the nature of their domestic responsibilities, and the existence of a dual labour market. Those women who do not engage in waged work are never able to earn state benefit in their own right. Hence, dependency in their early and middle years is carried over into old age. Even those who do work outside the home are often unable to build up a reasonable income for themselves in retirement. Many worked in low paid jobs without pension provision. Moreover, their working lives are usually disrupted by childrearing and sometimes caring for elderly parents, giving them little opportunity to build up a reasonable contributions record. Most, therefore, remain dependent on men, who usually die first, leaving them with only a minimal state pension to rely on. As a result, many experience health problems either caused or exacerbated by inadequate living conditions, insufficient heating, and lack of a nutritionally balanced diet.

Of course, not all the health problems older women face can be related directly to poverty. Many also suffer the psychological problems associated with retirement from work. Almost no research has been carried out on this topic because it has generally been assumed either that women do not work outside the home or that they are not deeply attached to their jobs (Fennell, Phillipson, & Evers, 1988). Thus, women appear only as shadowy wives in studies of men's retirement problems. Yet the few accounts we have from older women themselves suggest that the tensions are very similar for both sexes, and are likely to result in similar health problems (Ford &

Sinclair, 1987). Most older women also have to cope with the denial of their sexuality at the same time as the physical and psychological distancing of their children.

Very few studies have investigated the health problems of older women, and routine medical statistics tell us little about their well-being. However, we know that in both the United Kingdom and the United States, elderly women are much more likely than men to be disabled. Twice as many British women in the over-65 age group are severely or very severely disabled compared with men of the same age, while the figure is five times greater in the 75-plus age group (Harris, Cox, & Smith, 1971). Women suffer three times as much arthritis as men and osteoporosis is also a significant cause of reduced female mobility. Mental health problems are even more difficult to identify and measure, but older women appear to continue the excess identified in younger age groups, with higher rates of depression and dementia than their male counterparts. Alan Walker comments on the basis of British data that older women are "more likely than men to suffer from psychological problems such as loneliness or anxiety and to have lower levels of morale and life satisfaction" (Walker, 1987).

Overall, women seem to suffer longer periods of chronic ill health than men, but their deaths are rarely caused by the same disease(s) that disabled them in life. Men, on the other hand, tend to have shorter periods of disability and to die from the problems that have bothered them while they are alive (Verbrugge, 1985). Interestingly many older women seem to play down their ill health, either because of low expectations—"You can't expect much at my age"—or shame at being unable to manage any more (Fennell et al., 1988, p. 109). However, others seem to welcome illness as liberating them from a lifetime of caring for others, especially when their dependents are no longer alive (Herzlich, 1973). In any case, too many remain behind closed doors, struggling to look after themselves with little material or emotional support.

The situation of older women in underdeveloped countries is obviously different in several ways. In the first place, relatively few survive to old age at all, and those who do are often severely debilitated by frequent childbearing and hard physical labour. Second, they are more likely than women in the developed countries to be supported and looked after within the extended family. Indeed in many societies older women occupy important social roles—grandmother, mother, or mother in law, performer of religious or magical rites, senior wife— which offer more status than those of younger men. Those societies where women are required to be attached to a male adult usually have mechanisms to ensure that widows are not left alone. In India, for instance, remar-

riage is not encouraged among high-caste Hindu women and a son will be expected to support his mother while in some African societies, a widow is inherited by her husband's brother. Thus, older women in many parts of the Third World are less likely to suffer the isolation and invisibility of those in the developed countries, and in some cultures their status is even enhanced.

However, this is by no means always the case. Childless widows in particular often find themselves without social or financial security. Moreover, there is growing evidence that in many countries the breakdown of the traditional family-support system with industrialization and urbanization is increasing the vulnerability of divorced and widowed women (Youssef & Hetler, 1983). In parts of India, the expectation that a widowed daughter-in-law will be absorbed into her husband's family is no longer always adhered to. Instead, widows often return to their own families or set up (often very poor) households. Similar findings of lack of support for widows have been reported from Africa, from Upper Volta, Morocco, Zambia, and Swaziland (Youssef & Hetler, 1983). Thus, the problems of older women in the industrialized countries are increasingly being felt by those in the Third World as modernization removes their traditional sources of emotional and material sustenance, and therefore their access to reasonable health.

The Home as Haven?

Despite the dangers discussed above, it is a common myth that the home is a haven, offering protection from the dangers of the world outside. Indeed, many women are afraid to go out at night, staying behind closed doors to ensure their safety. The reality, however, is very different, as I explore in this final section.

It is clear that both the fear and the reality of domestic violence constitute a major threat to women's health. The use of physical force in the home is relatively common and most of it is inflicted on women by men (Dobash & Dobash, 1980). Precise estimates are difficult to achieve because so many victims are reluctant to reveal their private suffering. Indeed, the authors of a major British study suggest that only 2% of such assaults are reported to the police (Dobash & Dobash 1980). However, a number of studies designed to reveal the extent of this hidden violence have given broadly similar findings for the United States and Britain. A large-scale national study carried out by Murray Straus and his colleagues in the United States reported that over 12% of the married women interviewed had suffered severe violence at some point in their marriage, while a total of 28% had experienced physical violence of some kind (Straus et al., 1980). A British study involved interviews with all the women living in seven neighbouring streets in inner Leeds. About one-fifth of those interviewed had been the victims of violent attacks in their homes during the previous year (Hanmer & Saunders, 1984).

There is evidence of domestic violence in most countries around the world. In India, in particular, the uncovering of this abuse and its elimination has been a major focus of the new feminist movement (Mies, 1986). Urban and rural women, working class and middle class are all potential victims of domestic violence and Mies argues that their suffering has increased as the process of modernization gets under way. The most dramatic and widely publicized cases include the so-called dowry murders, in which women have been abused and eventually murdered because their husband and often his family are not satisfied with the money and goods she brought to the marriage. Many are deliberately burnt to death, but a cooking accident is blamed. Others commit suicide because the pressures on them are too great (Mies, 1986; Kishwar & Vanita, 1984).

Thus, the evidence demonstrates that a significant proportion of the women who live with men have the quality of their lives diminished by domestic violence. Moreover, this experience is shared by those in different social groups and societies, uniting women across class and racial divides. All women are potentially at risk from male violence, but paradoxically it is wives or co-habitees who get the worst treatment. Moreover, it is often their domestic work that provides the immediate excuse for a battering—a meal not ready on the table, a shirt not ironed, the house not clean enough, too much money spent on food, or a bout of "nagging." The physical damage caused is often severe, necessitating medical treatment or hospitalization. In the Dobashes' study of the survivors of violence, nearly 80% reported visiting the doctor at least once during their marriage for injuries inflicted by their husbands. Nearly 40% said they had sought medical care on five or more occasions and many felt their husbands had prevented them from getting medical help when they needed it. Another study of women in British refuges found that 73% had put up with violence for three or more years. Thirty percent had suffered life threatening attacks or had been hospitalized for serious injuries such as fractured bones (Binney, Harkell, & Nixon, 1981).

As well as the physical damage, it is clear that domestic violence is a major cause of psychological stress and trauma. Sixty-eight percent of the British women in refuges said that mental cruelty was one of the reasons they left home (Binney et al., 1981). Many victims are emotionally debilitated by anxiety about the next attack and feel shocked, upset, angry, and bitter at what is hap-

pening to them. Sadly, many feel guilty and blame themselves:

> I actually thought if I only learned to cook better or keep a cleaner house everything would be OK. . . . It took me five years to get over the shame and embarrassment of being beaten. I figured there had to be something wrong with me. (Dobash & Dobash, 1980, p. 119)

The authors of a recent study in North London found that women who had been battered were twice as likely to be depressed and had lower self-esteem than those who had not received such treatment (Andrews & Brown, 1988). Years of violence often leave women in a situation where alternatives are difficult to visualize. The socially constructed dependencies that they already experience are exacerbated by physical intimidation and violence. Moreover, attempts to get help from social workers, police, and other authorities too often lead to further humiliation and rejection (Stark, Flitcraft, & Frazier, 1979).

Thus, women become double victims of the batterer and the social agencies who too often assign the blame to women and resist any intervention in the private lives of man and wife. Indeed, one American writer has used the term *learned helplessness* to describe the condition in which so many battered women

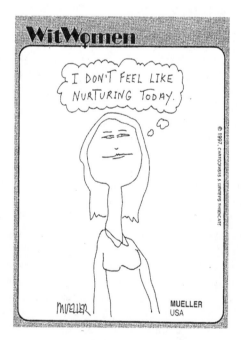

Mueller, Cartoonists & Writers Syndicate/cartoonweb.com.

find themselves (Walker, 1979). Constrained by lack of confidence, isolation, fear, and lack of money, too many are forced to remain for lengthy periods in relationships that threaten their health and sometimes even their lives.

Conclusion

Thus, research findings accord with some women's own subjective experience in associating many of their health problems with their domestic responsibilities. Women's traditional duties are not always good for their health, given the circumstances of inequality and sometimes deprivation under which they often have to be carried out. Not surprisingly perhaps, there is growing evidence that despite their subordination in the labour market, women sometimes improve their health by working outside the home. I explore the implications of this in Part Two.

References

A list of references is available in the original source.

Perspectives on Women's Occupational Health

by Jeanne Mager Stellman, PhD

This commentary provides a brief history of the development of the field of women's occupational health and safety. It discusses the broadening of the field from one with a reproductive health focus to one that considers women in their many roles and varied stages of life. Much of this widening of focus was contemporaneous with the growth of the women's movement. The paper emphasizes that the work burden borne by employed women in general includes responsibilities for homemaking and caregiving in addition to paid employment. Possible implications of these multiple roles are discussed, as are the major social, physical, biological, and chemical hazards encountered in traditional female employment. A research agenda for overcoming some of the research and policy barriers to a complete understanding of women's occupational health burden and to development of preventive policies is proposed.

Several publications and events in the late 1970s and early 1980s marked the beginning of the idea that women's occupational health was a neglected issue and was worth exploring in its own right. Three decades earlier Baetjer had written her classic text on women workers, based on her work for the armed services, which had coped with thousands of women working in wartime industries. When Baetjer studied "Rosie the Riveters," she found that women could do just about anything that needed to be done—particularly if machines and equipment were better suited for them. She presciently noted that better ergonomic design would improve the health and productivity of men, too. Her work, however, did not spark a movement because at the end of World War II all the Rosies were unceremoniously ousted from their industrial jobs. Those who remained in gainful employment were relegated to traditional women's jobs, which were then universally viewed as "safe." (We should also note that Alice Hamilton, widely considered to be the "mother" of occupational medicine in the United States, was also concerned with women and girls on the job and was a valiant crusader on their behalf.)

From *Journal of the American Medical Women's Association,* Spring 2000, Vol. 55, No. 2 by Jeanne Mager Stellman. Copyright © 2000 by the American Medical Women's Association. Reprinted by permission.

The 1970s and 1980s were years of great change for women. The following is a nonexhaustive list of important landmarks in the development of women's occupational health as a field. Chavkin, Hricko, Hunt, and Stellman wrote or edited monographs about the health of women on the job. Small amounts of money were found by feminist visionaries to fund some of the work. In 1979 the Women's Occupational Health Resource Center was established and began more than a decade of publishing, educating, and training on topics relevant to the health of women workers.

In more recent years, Messing, in particular, has pioneered in studies and writing that have concentrated on fundamental methodological issues in women's occupational health research (or the lack thereof). Several signal scientific symposia were organized; the National Cancer Institute's conference on women and cancer, for example, resulted in a multi-issue series in the *Journal of Occupational Medicine*. Women's occupational health is now being integrated into women's health in general, as in the latest edition of Goldman and Hatch.

One important aspect of the development of women's occupational health as a distinct subject is the struggle to define women's occupational health as more than reproductive health. There has been a rebellion against the concept of "permanently pregnant until proven otherwise," while keeping in mind that not very much is known about the relationship between women's reproductive health and working conditions. One of the earliest efforts was instigated by Clara Schiffer and written by Vilma Hunt, two "highly persistent women." Schiffer, then an official in the Department of Health, Education and Welfare, somehow found the funds for Hunt to compile a report on reproductive health of women workers. The report was an instant bestseller; it created an idea, and, indeed, led to a movement. Hunt's report brought reproductive hazards to the attention of the National Institute for Occupational Safety and Health and led the way to the publication of guidelines on the employment of women during pregnancy—a very radical notion indeed!

The concept that women's occupational health issues begin and end at the uterus dominated labor legislation for the better part of this century and led to such employment practices as "fetal protection policies," wherein all fertile women were banned from jobs and workplaces with potential exposure to toxins, while men were permitted to work in these environments. These policies galvanized opposition in the feminist and labor communities and eventually led to the landmark unanimous US Supreme Court decision in *UAW v Johnson Controls,* in which the Court declared fetal protection policies invalid. The Court stated that fetal protection policies failed to protect the reproductive health of men, who could also be affected by such hazards, and contradicted laws prohibiting employment discrimination on the basis of pregnancy. The ideas that male reproduction is not invulnerable and that women were more than reproductive vessels and had control over their reproductive choices in the workplace had reached officialdom. They were the law of the land.

Despite the struggle to establish an identity for women's occupational health issues, I believe we need to examine whether "women's" occupational health as a distinct subject should exist. Are there data demonstrating that women develop different occupational diseases or suffer different injuries than men? The answer is a brief but unsatisfactory yes and no. The answer is brief because we have few data. It is yes because women have different work experiences and exposures than men and no because in those industries where men and women have similar exposures, no studies have demonstrated that they develop different diseases.

The question is extremely difficult to answer quantitatively because, as Messing and others have described in detail, men and women have very different employment patterns, so accurate gender-based extrapolations are challenging; the full health and safety implications of the multiple role issue, discussed below, are not understood; little research has been devoted to comparative rate studies; and research into the health and safety hazards of female-dominated industries is still sparse.

Why is this so? Part of the neglect arises from the general neglect of occupational health and safety as a subject for research. Extremely small budgets, few specialists, and much political opposition to prevention (such as in the attempt to develop an Occupational Safety and Health Administration standard on ergonomics) characterize this field. And the notion that traditional white-collar women's jobs are safe is still dominant.

Women's Work Burden

Women are the majority of the adult population, and the rate of women's employment outside the home and the number of years they remain on the job continue to rise. The steep trend of increased gainful employment was somewhat slowed during the recession of 1990, but according to the Bureau of Labor Statistics, the upward trend appears to have resumed in 1994.

Women work in a narrower range of industries than men, even within the same professional sector. In the health care industry, which is the largest in the United States, the proportion of women in the health-diagnosing professions is low, but the proportion of female nurses, therapists, and aides is high. Women work in textiles, in small machine operations, and on assembly lines. In the blue-collar industries, women are clustered into operator, fabricator, and laborer job titles, while men occupy the entire spectrum of jobs. Even in the same industry and job title, men and women may actually perform different tasks.

Although the wage differential between men and women has been narrowing, an extremely wide gap still exists, particularly for women who do not hold high-paying, professional jobs. Women workers also have, on average, much less pension and medical care coverage than men, partly because more women than men do not follow continual full-time employment trajectories. They have gaps in their careers in order to raise their children, care for other dependents, and carry out household chores. Part-time work, in general, is lower paid and comes with fewer fringe benefits.

Of course, the very concept of career gaps helps perpetuate the myth that somehow there are two kinds of work: the "real" work of paid employment and "women's work," which is all the other, unpaid labor still carried out primarily by women. Economists have imposed an artificial dichotomy between real work and women's work—a dichotomy that is particularly inappropriate in those less developed countries where traditional women's work does provide the means by which the society more or less survives.

More women with very young and school-age children split their lives between paid employment and unpaid mothering-household tasks in America than in any other nation. There is a certain irony in this because American women have the least societal support to assist them in meeting their multiple role obligations (eg, child care, paid maternity leave, child support supplements, assured health care).

From an occupational health perspective, the important question is whether the juggling of these multiple roles exacts a toll on women's health. Collins et al have recently summarized mental health issues related to women's workplace health. They have noted that although employed women enjoy better health overall, when assessed by both objective and subjective measures, not all women experience health benefits from work. Studies focused on job satisfaction and job fit have demonstrated that multiple roles can be health enhancing when there is a good "fit" between worker and job and the roles are wanted, but they can have negative effects if they are not. There is remarkably little evidence of a gender interaction with workplace stress factors and physical health outcomes. Indeed, it has been found that such other factors as poorly designed workstations, monotonous repetitive work, and ill-fitting protective equipment are more likely to be associated with physical health effects than are any presumed inherent female characteristics.

Key Problem Areas

In addition to stress on the job and stress that arises from juggling multiple roles, other key conditions and exposures are particularly relevant to women workers. These include musculoskeletal disorders, exposure to toxic agents, infections, and accidents, including violence on the job.

Many women experience repetitive strain injuries, such as carpal tunnel syndrome, at a rate that far exceeds that of men. Many people associate carpal tunnel syndrome with the data entry keyboard, the computer mouse, and clerical occupations, but the operating of machinery on assembly lines and in tending retail stores accounted for most of the musculoskeletal distress reported in workers' compensation claims in 1995. Half of all workers who suffered from carpal tunnel syndrome missed at least 30 days of work, while the majority of workers suffering lacerations and cuts returned in less than 10 days. (One must interpret these data carefully; some of the differences in recorded rates could be because women in industrial jobs are more likely to file claims or have diseases reported to authorities than women in clerical occupations.)

Silverstein et al found that women's jobs involve more repetitive motion than men's, and many also involve more static effort. Since, on average, a female worker will be smaller than a male, working heights, hand tools, and foot pedals may require her to work in awkward positions since they will have been designed for the larger male. Recent years have seen the development of more equipment that is suitable for women, but the toll of damage to the carpal tunnel noted above indicates that much more needs to be done.

Several studies have found an association between awkward working postures, extensive standing, increased physical loads, and preterm deliveries.

Many female-dominated industries carry a risk of infection. Health care, with its exposure to blood-borne and other patient-staff transmitted pathogens, is an obvious example. Child care workers, school teachers, social workers, and other caregivers are also at risk. The most important infectious diseases include hepatitis (A, B, C, D, non A-E), varicella, tuberculosis, measles, mumps, rubella, human immunodeficiency virus, Epstein-Barr virus, and cytomegaly virus. Unfortunately, good data on prevalence by occupation are not available.

The overall burden of occupational cancer and other diseases related to toxic exposures to women workers is not known. Health care workers, again, have among the greatest potential for exposure to carcinogens (x-rays, ethylene oxide, dichloromethane, and ethyl acrylate, for example). Other hazards include cadmium oxide and lead used in making ceramics, pottery, and bricks (refractories), all female-intensive occupations. Artists and craftsworkers could also be at risk from these exposures. Dry cleaning and laundries and electrical appliances and electronics industries are noteworthy for their potential exposures to such chlorinated solvents as chloroform and 1, 2-dichloroethane and tetrachloroethylene. Many of these establishments are small, and their employees may not be provided with adequate ventilation or protective equipment and may not have their illnesses and injuries reported.

Environmental tobacco smoke can be an occupational health hazard for women employed in hotel and food service establishments.

Exposure to alkylating agents, lead, mercury, DDT, lindane, toxaphene, polychlorinated byphenyls, polybrominated biphenyls, and cadmium have been associated with altered menses. These agents have also lead to ovarian atrophy, as has azathioprine, and 2, 4-D exposure has lead to infertility in women.

Women suffered approximately one-third of all lost worktime incidents (667 200) reported in 1995. Nursing and personal care facilities are one of the high-rate industries for lost worktime illnesses and injuries. Nursing homes ranked first for overexertion (3.2 lost worktime cases per 100 workers), with a rate more than quadruple the national rate. Nurses' aides, orderlies, and attendants accounted for more than 40% of the total reported cases. Handling patients was the primary cause of overexertion. Falls, violence, and being struck by objects are other major causes of incidents in the nursing home industry. Waitresses, maids, assemblers in factories, sales workers in miscellaneous commodities, cashiers, packaging machine operators, and stock and inventory clerks, all in female-intensive occupations, reported significant injury rates.

Homicide is the leading cause of occupational mortality among American workers and accounted for about 40% of all female deaths on the job between 1992 and 1996. About 16% of female deaths on the job are actually attributable to domestic violence that spilled over into the workplace (in comparison to about 1% of male deaths). Two-thirds of all the homicides occurred in the retail and service industries. Robbery was the primary motive.

Future Agenda

There are great differences in the social circumstances that surround the lives of men and women. Caregiving responsibilities, ability to earn income, pensions, access to health care, and social support systems differ widely by gender. The employment trends and the organization of work are different. Analysis of the female-dominated work environment and female-dominated social responsibilities is comparatively neglected. Paid employment, career development and all its associated benefits are a natural and expected part of every woman's life. At the same time that these sex differences continue to exist, the world of work itself is continually changing. The organization of work, the number of years of work during one's lifetime, the degree of automation, and the physical demands are continually evolving. Such sex differences are probably of far greater importance with respect to occupational health than are the differences in hormone levels, body fat content, or physical stature that most people focus on in research and policy deliberations.

I recently proposed a research agenda for the future that included the obvious need to carry out research and develop policies with respect to gender-based social differences, particularly in relationship to the changing world of work. Such research should include the systematic definition of the actual conditions under which women labor in the home and at the workplace; it should measure the physical environment and document tasks and loads. We desperately need to modify the various record-keeping and surveillance systems that exist so that the full range of women's labor is counted. We need to develop adequate outcome measures that go beyond frank morbidity and mortality for assessing the health and well-being of women workers. We need to do a much better job of counting the morbidity and mortality that does exist and relating it to workplace conditions, where appropriate. We might look to methods being developed for outcomes research in health services for examples of assessment of the quality of life.

The information gained from such a research agenda could help ensure continued equalization of opportunity between the sexes and further recognition that women's work is neither "safe" nor necessarily special.

References

A list of references is available in the original source.

Male and Female Hormones Revisited

by Mariamne H. Whatley

In 1985 a chapter I wrote, "Male and Female Hormones: Misinterpretations of Biology in School Health and Sex Education," in which I examined in detail problems with both content and language in health and sexuality texts, was published in *Women, Biology, and Public Policy* (edited by Virginia Sapiro, Sage Yearbooks in Public Policy Studies, vol 10). Since then there have been a lot of changes in health education, sexuality education, and general knowledge about women's health and biology. However, when I reread the chapter to see how out-of-date it was, I was interested to find that the main points I made then are still very relevant.

One of central examples I presented was of the common use of the terms "male hormones" and "female hormones" to refer to androgens and estrogens respectively. By using this terminology, educators imply that men and women have two very different sets of hormones, which naturally could be seen as affecting development, behavior, and abilities, and could serve as the basis for believing incorrectly that there are biologically-determined sex roles, rather than culturally and socially influenced gender roles. In fact, men and women share the same hormones, but they appear in varying amounts. The average man will have higher levels of androgens than the average woman and the average woman will have higher levels of estrogen than the average man. However, just by looking at hormone levels a scientist could not determine with certainty whether an individual were male or female, because there is so much variation across individuals, across the lifespan, at different parts of the menstrual cycle for women, and even at different times of the day (Men's levels of androgens may vary more in a day than a woman's estrogen levels do over a month). There are a number of reasons, therefore, why it is scientifically inaccurate to refer to male hormones and female hormones:

1. Both males and females produce both androgens and estrogens.
2. The adrenal glands and the gonads (ovaries, testes) produce both hormones in both sexes.
3. Both males and females need both androgens and estrogens for normal development.
4. Both hormones increase in both males and females at puberty.
5. Androgens and estrogens are steroids which are very similar in structure and can be interconverted (changed from one to the other) in our bodies.
6. Knowing hormone levels alone is not enough to determine whether an individual is biologically male or female.

In spite of these facts, much sexuality and puberty education material still refers to estrogens and androgens as very distinctly female or male. For example, in discussing female puberty, only estrogen will be discussed as a factor in changes in development, leaving out the fact that androgens do play a role in the development of girls, as well as of boys, in such changes as muscle growth, hair distribution, acne, and libido (sex drive). If androgen is presented as only a *male* hormone, then muscle development in girls is seen as abnormal. Boys on the other hand also normally produce estrogen, which sometimes reaches high levels at puberty, causing changes that may be seen as "female," such as temporary breast enlargement (gynecomastia) or more fat distribution on the hips. A boy with gynecomastia will undoubtedly feel uncomfortable no matter how sensitively the topic is handled, but it certainly won't help if he and his peers have all learned that breast enlargement is caused by estrogen, the *female* hormone. On the other hand, if the message is that all boys and men produce estrogens but that the levels can fluctuate, especially during puberty, and cause temporary breast enlargement, that boy might at least have some assurance that he is "normal."

At the other end of the reproductive cycle, there are often discussions of hormones in relationship to aging. Information on menopause may present postmenopausal women as becoming more "male" as their estrogen decreases and androgen becomes proportionately higher. Such changes may have to do with loss of breast size

Printed by permission of the author, 1999.

and density, growth of facial hair, and redistribution of body fat, so there is less on hips and thighs and more in the abdomen. Because her whole life, a woman has been told that she has "female hormones," the menopause literature which presents menopause as a total lack of estrogen or an "estrogen deficiency disease" is giving the message that the factor that makes her female is gone. She is, therefore, not really female any longer. When Robert Wilson wrote the book *Feminine Forever,* which extolled the virtues of exogenous estrogen to counter the effects of menopause, much of his focus was on the loss of estrogen as causing a loss in femininity and sexuality. While there has been much criticism of his work and, in recent years, there has been a decrease in the negative descriptions of menopause, these views do still persist. Discussing the fact that estrogen does not disappear after menopause and that androgens are actually converted to estrogens in fat and muscle cells can help give women a clearer view of what the real hormonal changes are. Also recognizing that their whole lives, they have gone through changing balances of hormones places menopause more in the context of ongoing biological processes rather than a new, completely different stage. Before puberty, girls and boys have very similar levels of hormones and the low estrogen in girls is certainly not considered an "estrogen deficiency disease" that needs to be treated with "estrogen replacement."

There are other implications of viewing estrogens and androgens as distinct hormones not shared by the sexes. If hormones are believed to have certain effects on behavior or abilities, then the association of a hormone with only one sex will imply biological limitations. For example, some scientists believe that androgen levels cause changes in aggression. There has been a long debate about this which includes such key opposing arguments as: the fact that behavior and environment can themselves alter hormone levels, so a high level of androgen may be a *result* of being in an aggressive position rather than a *cause* of it; the definition of aggression as very loose, ranging from rough and tumble play in primates to success in business and politics. If it were accepted that androgen levels cause aggression and aggression were loosely defined as meaning being able to compete in a highly competitive field, such as business or politics, then women would be seen as unable to compete in these areas. And, of course, women who are as aggressive (or assertive) as men may be seen as not really normal women. While we hope most people have discarded these outdated views, the basic misunderstanding of biology seeps into many discussions of women's abilities in general and in discussions of specific women. When someone refers to a woman as "ballsy," it may be seen as a compliment for her being a gutsy woman ready to take on challenges, but is also a backhanded compliment because it also implies she is not fully a woman, figuratively possessing testes—the major producer of androgens.

A discussion of changing the language which is used to describe hormones may seem trivial, as did attention to changing the generic male (e.g., mankind). However, a view of the world underlies choices we make in language and a change in language—however small—can cause a shift in perception. Just as we now refer to firefighters and police officers rather than firemen and policemen, to represent more accurately the status of women in the workforce, so must we also clean up our scientific language to reflect scientific reality, which is so often distorted and misrepresented.

Intersexuals

Exploding the Binary Sex System

by Kim Klausner

I sat in a restaurant in the Castro section of San Francisco waiting to meet Cheryl Chase, founder of the Intersex Society of North America (ISNA). A lone woman entered the eatery and it soon became clear that this was the person I was waiting for. After settling ourselves at a table I did my best with innocuous small talk, hoping to find a connection with this person I would soon be interviewing. "So, you were born in New York City?" I ventured. Cheryl looked at me oddly and replied, "No, why?" I scratched my head and mentioned that I had seen a reference to her being operated on as an infant at a prestigious New York City hospital. She matter-of-factly said, "I wasn't born in New York; I was mutilated there."

Cheryl's response took my breath away, and well it should have. I gazed at this courageous woman and saw someone who was determined to transform an intensely personal experience into far reaching political action. As we ate, she willingly revealed intimate details about her life and body to me, a stranger, with the hope that I would join her effort to change oppressive medical practices and the assumptions behind them. Her particular experience is important to know only insofar as it can be used to illustrate larger social relations. During our lunch I was alternately struck by two processes that seemed to underlie all that Cheryl talked about: 1) that the personal is the political and 2) that the medical profession embodies the prevailing cultural assumptions about sex, biology, and gender and uses its authority to enforce particular power relations.

Before I get too far along with *my* thoughts, however, let me share a little about what ISNA is, mostly in the words of the organization itself. ISNA is "a peer support, education, and advocacy group founded and operated by and for intersexuals, individuals born with anatomy or physiology which differs from cultural ideals of male and female." Intersexuals, sometimes called hermaphrodites, are a physically diverse group of people, with bodies that are not easily categorized in our either/or male/female sex system. According to doctors, intersexuals are females born with clitorises that the doctors consider too long and males born with penises that are deemed too short. In a certain sense, the medical establishment hardly recognizes the integrity of the category "intersexual," preferring to dismiss intersexuals as deficient males or females. One of ISNA's first goals is to redefine the terms of their very existence.

The concept of intersexuality confronts the dominant cultural conception of "sex anatomy as a dichotomy: humans come in two sexes, conceived of as so different as to be nearly different species." ISNA challenges this view with the assertion that "anatomic sex differentiation occurs on a male/female continuum with several dimensions."

(If your eyes glaze over at the mention of chromosomes and you can't quite remember, or never knew, what gonads are, feel free to skip the next two paragraphs.) ISNA continues its explanation of intersexuality with, "Genetic sex, or the organization of the 'sex chromosomes,' is commonly thought to be isomorphic to some idea of 'true sex.' However, something like 1/500 of the population have a karyotype [that is, chromosomal arrangement] other than XX (most females) or XY (most males)." As an example, ISNA points to women athletes subject to genetic testing. In recent years, women Olympic athletes have had to undergo genetic tests, and as a result a number of them have been disqualified as 'not women,' after winning. These women, of course are not men—they, like many other intersexuals, have atypical karotypes (though one gave birth to a healthy child after having been barred from competition).

The genitals of intersexual people vary along the male-female continuum. As is pointed out in ISNA literature:

Intersexual genitals may look nearly female, with a large clitoris, or with some degree of posterior labial

From *Sojourner,* January 1997, Vol. 22, No. 5, pp. 7–8. Copyright © by Kim Klausner. Reprinted by permission.

Author's note: If you want to know more about inersexuality or ISNA, contact the organization by e-mail (info@isna.org or cchase@isna.org), at their web site (http://www.isna.org), or by snailmail at P.O. Box 31791, San Francisco, CA 94131.

fusion. They may look nearly male, with a small penis, or with hypospadias [a condition where the urethra opens on the under surface of the penis]. They may be truly "right in the middle," with a phallus that can be considered either a large clitoris or a small penis, with a structure that might be a split, empty scrotum, or outer labia, and with a small vagina that opens into the urethra rather than into the perineum.

Internal reproductive organs may be partially developed or discordant with external genitals. For instance, there are people whose genitals have the same appearance as most females, but inside have testes and no uterus or ovaries. Some people have combined gonads, that is, ovo-testes. Some people who have male-appearing genitals have a uterus, ovaries, and tubes.

To summarize, ISNA asserts that medical science has effectively promoted the "objective fact" that there are but two sexes, male and female, and that people are either one or the other. If truth be told, and it is, thanks to ISNA, people can be virtually all male, all female, or some of both (though, the popular concept of two sets of genitals—male and female—is not possible). It should be noted that we're just talking biology here; this doesn't even attempt to address questions about the social construction of gender or how children are raised to be boys or girls.

ISNA wants the immediate end to practices that arise from the medical model established in the 1950s that asserts that "children with visibly intersexual anatomy cannot develop into healthy adults." They want to stop emergency sex assignment and reinforcement of sex assignment with early genital surgery, which often causes serious sexual dysfunction. They also want an end to the dishonesty of health care providers who, in their discussions with parents and intersexuals, cover up the true status of the intersex child. ISNA does not, however, oppose using medical technology when it is necessary. "For instance," Chase explains, "some children are born with ambiguous genitals because of adrenal hyperplasia, which can be life threatening. Doctors should treat those aspects of this condition that affect the health and comfort of the child, such as preventing him or her from going into salt shock."

When an infant is born with genitals that don't conform to our idea of either male or female, ISNA wants doctors to be honest and not say, as they currently do, "Well, we can't determine what sex your child is by looking at it, but we can perform tests that will tell us, and then we can alter its genitals so it looks more like the sex it is." Rather, they'd prefer that new parents be told, "Your child is intersexual, in other words, neither a boy nor a girl. There are resources available to help you raise your child in a healthy way. Go home and love this child as you would any other." Chase succinctly sums it up with "we want an end to harmful and medically unnecessary cosmetic surgery, secrecy, and lying."

Obviously, this approach requires a radical rearrangement of our society. At the least, we need some new pronouns since "it" hardly describes a new baby. What ISNA is advocating is so profoundly disorienting that I've even had feminist friends roll their eyes at me and say, "So what, these people want to dismantle our society's concept of the male-female dichotomy? Good luck!" Or "How many people does this affect anyway? I mean, shouldn't we be dealing with issues like racism or poverty, things that affect much larger groups of people?" The number of people born intersexual is not huge, although it is probably greater than you imagine (1 out of every 2,000 births).

Accepting ISNA's claims means recovering the authority we have given to the medical establishment to assign and enforce sex roles. Most people hardly give the concept that sexes are assigned by society a thought. It is something that is determined by biology; if an infant has a penis, then it is a boy. It sounds simple enough. But transgendered people, who don't fit neatly into male or female categories, know that the medical establishment closely guards its prerogative to enforce sex roles. In most parts of the United States, transpeople have to feign a mental disorder to obtain an operation that is forced on intersexual children. In both cases the medical profession assumes the role of sex judge. Doctors tell the parents of the intersexual infant, "Based on the evidence, this is a girl, even though part of her anatomy looks almost male," while telling the person who wants to take hormones in the hopes of uncovering a body that more closely resembles their identity, "I will not prescribe these drugs unless you prove to me that you think you're really a (wo)man (and straight, too)."

If we are to honor the experience of many transsexuals, we must admit it is possible to be a female born with a penis or a male born with a vagina. We feel compelled to identify newborns as male or female, but maybe we should wait and let the kid decide whether s/he is male, female, or both. Chase points out that it's only been in the past 50 years or so that the medical profession has arbitrated these questions. For centuries, intersexuals navigated without the "help" of the sex judges. In some cultures, intersexuals were ignored, in some they were accorded high status, and in others they were reviled.

Feminists have long advocated that gender is culturally constructed. Well, why not sex? Somehow, the material nature of genitals, internal organs, and even hormones coursing through our bloodstreams lends credence to the medically or biologically based construction of sex. You cannot be fooled by something you can actually see or touch. Intersexuals and transpeople are starting to tell us otherwise. Sex cannot always be easily articulated in morphological terms and the diversity of anatomical differences among humans arrays us along a sex spectrum, not into two mutually exclusive categories.

The argument that sex is not biologically determined challenges decades of feminist theory and practice. If it is no longer clear that there are two distinct sexes, a theory resting on these two categories of existence becomes unstable. How can men oppress women if the boundaries between each group are permeable? Or if we no longer know who fits in each category? For these reasons, some feminists have found transpeople and intersexuals threatening. But do intersexuals alter the paradigm?

Unfortunately, oppressive relations can flourish without immutable, biologically based categories. The existence of mixed-race people has not brought an end to racism. While some Black civil rights organizations may fear that the institutionalization of mixed-race categories on the census will dilute their political power, I doubt that any of them think that the disappearance of mixed-race people from their statistical ranks will cause racism to crumble. And a person with parents of different races still faces racist prejudice and discrimination as s/he walks through life. In the case of men and women, perhaps imagining a sex continuum makes gender more important than sex. And this raises the question of the connection between gender and sex. The more I think about it, the more unsure I am that things are as they seem. But of course, many queer people have known this with their bodies and minds since they were young children.

Having the medical establishment (aided and abetted by the legal system) in charge of defining what the sexes are and how individual people fit into this schema provides reassurance—at least to those who have faith in the medical-judicial system—that sex assignment is not done on an arbitrary or capricious basis. It is, after all, scientifically proven. But what happens when people's experiences deviate from the accepted medical facts? Intersexual bodies are mutilated to maintain the current paradigm, just as gay people are institutionalized, women are called hysterical, and transpeople are thwarted in their efforts to realize themselves.

Here you might ask, "Why wouldn't a parent want to take advantage of the amazing medical techniques we have available to help her newborn child adjust to the world as it is? Wouldn't it be cruel to the child to force it to lead a life of being different?" The intersexuals connected with ISNA are saying simply and clearly they would rather be "different" than mutilated. Further, they want to help change our conception of normal so they won't have to feel out of place. Since an intersexual person knows, at some level, that s/he is different, the only thing surgical alteration seems to accomplish is the mental well-being of doctors,

parents, and others who are more concerned with the intersexual's body than their mental well-being. In fact, the doctor's or parents' peace of mind is sometimes obtained at a monumental price: intersexuals report both sexual dysfunction and profound feelings of being unacceptable.

(It is certainly possible that some intersexuals are happy that they were altered. But they are the only ones who know. There have been no long-term studies on the effects of surgery on intersexual infants. The medical profession seems remarkably uninterested in knowing about the lives of intersexual adults. Perhaps if you are in this situation you will share your feelings with other *Sojourner* readers.)

This professionally sanctioned violation of a human body not only causes physical trauma but is also accompanied by a tremendous sense of shame about one's body. When an intersexual is born, a life of secrecy begins. It starts in the labor and delivery room. One can feel the palpable discomfort of the medical staff when they are unable to quickly answer the question, "is it a girl or a boy?" The intersexual teen is generally not told the truth about what has been done to his/her body, which magnifies an already difficult period of transition. And many intersexual people eventually carry the secret themselves as they hide their status from lovers.

When Cheryl Chase was born, the doctors told her parents that their child was a boy. When their son was a year old, a medical expert informed them, "This child is not really a boy. We will fix the problem by removing what looks like a penis but we suggest that you move to another city and start over again, telling people you have a daughter." Her parents renamed her Cheryl and did exactly that. Does the shame and secrecy sound similar to that experienced by the child of alcoholics or one who is sexually abused?

At 40, Cheryl still feels the painful reverberations of how the medical profession and her family treated her as someone born intersexual. Of this experience, she says simply, "It destroyed my whole family; we are scattered to the winds." From her mother who was given tranquilizers in response to her concerns about her infant's body, to her father who lay on his deathbed telling Cheryl that she was "bad from the day you were born," to her sisters who do not want biological children of their own, to her aunt who was unable to support Cheryl in her quest for the truth out of "loyalty" to her sister, there have been no winners here.

ISNA provides ample material from which to analyze power relations, particularly the way that science, as it is embedded in our particular culture, helps maintain a sexist hierarchy. For me, as someone who fits quite easily into a binary sex system, intersexual liberation is somewhat of an intellectual issue, removed from my day-to-day identity experience. At the same time, I recognize that this movement is led by people whose very core identities and bodies are at stake. As a political activist, I am incredibly rejuvenated by being a witness to this movement. There is something very powerful about a group of people who fuse the intensely personal with the theoretical to create change. I can take this concentrated sense of mission to other political work I do.

The process by which ISNA formed echoes the women's movement of the late '60s. A severe emotional breakdown provoked Chase to start asking questions about how her body came to be. In the course of her investigation, she found other people who had had similar experiences. Last summer, a group of ten intersexual people met for a weekend in Northern California. I happened to meet two of these people shortly after their gathering. They shared a small pile of photographs taken during the weekend. The photos show a bunch of people hanging out in a nice place, nothing remarkable at all. The photos, though, stimulated these two women to recount parts of the weekend, and it soon became clear how potent it had been. The simple act of coming together to share experiences was what they needed to name an oppressive force. Speaking the unspoken is at once both personal and political. In this case, collective action arises from the recognition that one's individual life is not an isolated experience. Cheryl says of her work with ISNA, "If I wasn't doing this, I'd be dead now." Cheryl and other ISNA members are providing an opportunity for other intersexuals, who may be confused or despairing, to continue their healing among those who know the pain from first hand experience. And in doing so, they will change the world.

I am a lesbian parent of two sons. (Or at least I'm assuming they're male, until they tell me otherwise.) When my oldest child was born eight years ago, a lot of people thought that it was unfair to bring a child into the world to face the anticipated harassment he would receive as the son of lesbians. As a parent, it is painful to think that my children will face prejudice (and they will never face discrimination based on their skin color, language learned at home, or income level). I didn't send my son to be raised by a straight couple; instead, I've tried to do what I can to reduce negative attitudes about lesbians. I am lucky that I live in a community that supports me in doing this. It certainly would have been harder and more isolating to take this approach in other parts of the country (even 50 miles from here). But not impossible. Some people are willing to take risks in the hopes that oppressive attitudes or power structures will change. As feminists, what can we do to help parents of intersexual children accept their children as they are and fight to change a world that says they should be changed?

"Cultural Practice" or "Reconstructive Surgery"? U.S. Genital Cutting, the Intersex Movement, and Medical Double Standards

by Cheryl Chase

One of the forms of power that maintains gender boundaries in the United States is the surgical "correction" of infants whose genitals are deemed by medical professionals to be socially unacceptable. Media and scholarly discourses on "female genital mutilation," however, have not engaged these surgeries, instead serving up only representations of African women. These discourses continue a long tradition of making Africans into the "others," suggesting that ethnocentrism is a key factor in the sometimes purposeful maintenance of ignorance about contemporary U.S. genital surgeries. This essay will describe how Americans participate in the production of normatively sexed bodies from those born intersexed, the consequences of such genital surgeries for those subjected to them, the efforts of intersex people to organize to eliminate pediatric genital surgeries and how those efforts have been treated by many feminists, and the double standard regarding representations of genital cutting, depending upon who is cutting and where in the world the cutting is done.

"New Law Bans Genital Cutting in United States" read the headline on the front page of the *New York Times.* The law seems clear enough: "Whoever knowingly circumcises, excises, or infibulates the whole or any part of the labia majora or labia minor or clitoris of another person who has not attained the age of eighteen years shall be fined under this title or imprisoned not more than five years, or both." Yet this law was not intended and has not been interpreted to protect the approximately five children per day in the United States who are subjected to excision of part or all of their clitoris and inner labia simply because doctors believe their clitoris is too big.

Sexual anatomies, genitals in particular, come in many sizes and shapes. U.S. doctors label children whose sexual anatomies differ significantly from the cultural ideal "intersexuals" or "hermaphrodites" (a misleading term because these children are born with intermediate genitals, not two sets). Medical practice today holds that possession of a large clitoris, or a small penis, or a penis that has the urethra placed other than at its tip is a "psychosocial emergency." The child would not be accepted by the mother, would be teased by peers, and would not be able to develop into an emotionally healthy adult. The medical solution to this psychosocial problem is surgery—before the child reaches three months of age or even before the newborn is discharged from the hospital. Although parental emotional distress and rejection of the child and peer harassment are cited as the primary justifications for cosmetic genital surgery, there has never been an investigation of nonsurgical means—such as professional counseling or peer support—to address these issues.

The federal Law to Ban Female Genital Mutilation notwithstanding, girls born with large clitorises are today routinely "normalized" by excising parts of the clitoris and burying the remainder deep within the genital region. And boys with small penises? Current medical practice holds that intersex children "can be raised successfully as members of either sex if the process begins before 2½ years." Because surgeons cannot create a large penis from a small one, the policy is to remove testes and raise these children as girls. This is accomplished by "carv[ing] a large phallus down into a cli-

toris, creat[ing] a vagina using a piece of [the child's] colon," marveled a science writer who spoke only to physicians and parents, not to any of the intersex people subjected to this miracle technology. Efforts to create or extend a penile urethra in boys whose urethra exits other than at the tip of the penis—a condition called hypospadias—frequently lead to multiple surgeries, each compounding the harm. Heart-rending stories of physical and emotional carnage are related by victims of these surgeries in "Growing up in the Surgical Maelstrom" and, with black humor, in "Take Charge: A Guide to Home Catheterization."

"Reconstructive" surgeries for intersex infant genitals first came into wide-spread practice in the 1950s. Because intersexuality was treated as shameful and physicians actively discouraged open discussion by their patients—indeed, recommended lying to parents and to adult intersex patients—until recently most victims of these interventions suffered alone in shame and silence.

By 1993 the accomplishments of a progression of social justice movements—civil rights, feminism, gay and lesbian, bisexual and transgender—helped make it possible for intersex people to speak out. Initially, physicians scoffed at their assertions that intersexuality was not shameful and that medically unnecessary genital surgeries were mutilating and should be halted. One surgeon from Johns Hopkins, the institution primarily responsible for developing the current medical model, dismissed intersex patient-advocates as "zealots." Others cited the technological imperative. Doctors "don't really have a choice" about whether or not to perform surgery insists George Szasz.

By 1997 the intersex movement had gathered enough strength to visit Congress and ask that the Law to Ban Female Genital Mutilation be enforced to protect children not only against practices imported from other cultures but also against this uniquely American medicalized form of mutilation. Their work won coverage in the *New York Times* and on *Dateline NBC,* and by the following year the *Urology Times* was reporting a small but growing "new tidal wave of opinion" from physicians and sex researchers supporting the activists. Sad to report, the struggle of intersex activists against American medicalized genital mutilation has yet to attract significant support or even notice from feminists and journalists who express outrage over African genital cutting.

Hermaphrodites: Medical Authority and Cultural Invisibility

Many people familiar with the ideas that gender is a phenomenon not adequately described by male/female dimorphism and that the interpretation of physical sex differences is culturally constructed remain surprised to learn how variable sexual anatomy is. Although the male/female binary is constructed as natural and therefore presumably immutable, the phenomenon of intersexuality offers clear evidence that physical sex is not binary. Intersexuality therefore furnishes an opportunity to deploy "the natural" strategically as a means for disrupting heteronormative systems of sex/gender/sexuality. The concept of bodily sex, in popular usage, refers to multiple characteristics, including karyotype (organization of sex chromosomes); gonadal differentiation (e.g., ovarian or testicular); genital morphology; configuration of internal reproductive organs; and pubertal sex characteristics such as breasts and facial hair. These characteristics are assumed and expected to be concordant in each individual—either all-male or all-female.

Because medicine intervenes quickly in intersex births to change the infant's body, the phenomenon of intersexuality has been, until recently, largely unknown outside specialized medical practices. General public awareness of intersex bodies slowly vanished in modern Western European societies as medicine gradually appropriated to itself the authority to interpret—and eventually manage—the much older category of "hermaphroditism." Victorian medical taxonomy began to efface hermaphroditism as a legitimated status by settling on gonadal histology as the arbiter of "true sex." The Victorian taxonomy (still in use by medical specialists) required both ovarian and testicular tissue types, microscopically confirmed, to be present in a "true hermaphrodite." Conveniently, given the limitations of Victorian surgery and anesthesia, such confirmation was impossible in a living patient. All other anomalies were reclassified as "pseudo-hermaphroditisms" masking a "true sex" determined by the gonads.

With advances in anesthesia, surgery, embryology, and endocrinology, however, twentieth-century medicine moved from merely labeling intersexed bodies to the far more invasive practice of "fixing" them—altering their physical appearance to conform with a diagnosed true sex. The techniques and protocols for physically transforming intersexed bodies were developed primarily at Johns Hopkins University in Baltimore during the 1920s and 1930s under the guidance of urologist Hugh Hampton Young. "Only during the last few years," Young enthused in the preface to his pioneering textbook *Genital Abnormalities,* have we begun "to get somewhere near the explanation of the marvels of anatomic abnormality that may be portrayed by these amazing individuals. But the surgery of the hermaphrodite has remained a terra incognito." The "sad state of these unfortunates" prompted Young to devise "a great variety of surgical procedures" by which he attempted to normalize the their bodily appearances to the greatest extent possible.

Quite a few of Young's patients resisted his efforts. Emma T., a "'snappy' young negro woman with a good figure" and a large clitoris, had married a man but found her passion only with women. Emma refused surgery to "be made into a man" because removal of her vagina would mean the loss of her "meal ticket" (i.e., her husband). By the 1950s, the principle of rapid postnatal detection and intervention for intersex infants had been developed at Johns Hopkins, with the stated goal of completing surgery early enough so the child would have no memory of it. One wonders whether the insistence on early intervention was not at least partly motivated by the resistance offered by adult intersex people to "normalization" through surgery. Frightened parents of ambiguously sexed infants were much more open to suggestions of normalizing surgery than were intersex adults, and the infants themselves could, of course, offer no resistance whatsoever.

Most of the theoretical foundations justifying these interventions are attributable to psychologist John Money, a sex researcher invited to Johns Hopkins by Lawson Wilkins, founder of pediatric endocrinology. Wilkins's numerous students subsequently carried these protocols from Hopkins to hospitals throughout the United States and abroad. In 1998 Suzanne Kessler noted that Money's ideas enjoyed a "consensus of approval rarely encountered in science." But the revelation in 2000 that Money had grossly misrepresented and mishandled the famous "John/Joan" case (in which an infant was castrated and raised as a girl after his penis was destroyed in a circumcision accident) sent Money's stock into a steep decline.

In keeping with the Hopkins model, the birth of an intersex infant is today deemed a "psychosocial emergency" that propels a multi-disciplinary team of intersex specialists into action. Significantly, they are surgeons and endocrinologists rather than psychologists, bioethicists, intersex peer support organizations, or parents of intersex children. The team examines the infant and chooses either male or female as a "sex of assignment," then informs the parents that this is the child's *true* sex. Medical technology, including surgery and hormones, is then used to make the child's body conform as closely as possible to the assigned sex.

Current protocols for choosing a sex are based on phallus size: to qualify for male assignment the child must posses a penis at least one inch long; clitorises may not exceed three-eighths inch. Infants with genital appendages in the forbidden zone of three-eighths to one inch are assigned female and the phallus trimmed to an acceptable size. The only exception to this sorting rule is that even a hypothetical possibility of female fertility must be preserved by assigning the infant as female, disregarding masculine genitals and a phallus longer than one inch.

The sort of deviation from sex norms exhibited by intersex people is so highly stigmatized that emotional harm due to likely parental rejection and community stigmatization of the intersex child provides physicians with their most compelling argument to justify medically unnecessary surgical interventions. Intersex status is considered to be so incompatible with emotional health that misrepresentation, concealment of facts, and outright lying (both to parents and later to the intersex person) are unabashedly advocated in professional medical literature.

The Impact of "Reconstructive" Surgeries

The insistence on two clearly distinguished sexes has calamitous personal consequences for the many individuals who arrive in the world with sexual anatomy that fails to be easily distinguished as male or female, who are labeled "intersexuals" or "hermaphrodites" by modern medical discourse. About one in one hundred births exhibits some anomaly in sex differentiation, and about one in two thousand is different enough to render problematic the question, Is it a boy or a girl? Since the early 1960s, nearly every medium-sized or larger city in the United States has had at least one hospital with a standing team of medical experts who intervene in these cases to "assign"—through drastic surgical means—a male or female status to intersex infants. The fact that this system for enforcing the boundaries of the categories "male" and "female" existed for so long without drawing criticism or scrutiny from any quarters is an indication of the extreme discomfort that sexual ambiguity excites in our culture. Pediatric genital surgeries literalize what many might otherwise consider a purely theoretical operation—the attempted production of normatively sexed bodies and gendered subjects through constitutive acts of violence. Since the early 1990s, however, intersex people have begun to politicize intersex subjectivity, thus transforming intensely personal experiences of violation into collective opposition to the medical regulation of bodies that queers the foundations of heteronormative gender identifications and sexual orientations.

This system of hushing up the fact of intersex births and using technology to normalize intersex bodies has caused profound emotional and physical harm to intersex people and their families. The harm begins when the birth is treated as a medical crisis, and the consequences of that initial treatment ripple out ever afterward. The emotional impact of this treatment is so devastating that until the middle of the 1990s people whose lives have been touched by intersexuality maintained silence about their ordeal. As recently as 1993, no one publicly disputed surgeon Milton Edgerton when he wrote that in forty years of clitoral surgery on children "*not one has complained of loss of sensation, even when the entire clitoris was removed*" (emphasis in the original).

The tragic irony in all this is that while intersexual anatomy occasionally indicates an underlying medical problem such as adrenal disorder, ambiguous genitals are, in and of themselves, neither painful nor harmful to health. The often debilitating pediatric genital surgeries are entirely cosmetic in function. Surgery is essentially a destructive process. It can remove tissue and to a limited extent relocate it, but it cannot create new structures. This technical limitation, taken together with the framing of the feminine as a condition of lack, leads physicians to assign 90 percent of anatomically ambiguous infants as female by excising genital tissue. Surgeons justify female assignment because "you can make a hole, but you can't build a pole." Heroic efforts shore up a tenuous masculine status for the one-tenth assigned male, who are subjected to multiple operations—twenty-two in one case—with the goal of straightening the penis and constructing a urethra to enable standing urinary posture. For some, the surgeries end only when the child grows old enough to resist.

Children assigned female are subjected to surgery that removes the troubling hypertrophic (i.e., large) clitoris. This is the same tissue that would have been a troubling micropenis (i.e., small penis) had the child been assigned male. Through the 1960s, feminizing pediatric genital surgery was openly labeled "clitoridectomy" and was compared favorably to the African practices that have now become the focus of such intense scrutiny. As three Harvard surgeons noted, "Evidence that the clitoris is not essential for normal coitus may be gained from certain sociological data. For instance, it is the custom of a number of African tribes to excise the clitoris and other parts of the external genitals. Yet normal sexual function is observed in these females." Authors Robert E. Gross, Judson Randolph, and John F. Crigler apparently understand normal female sexual function only as passive penetration and fertility. A modified operation that removes most of the clitoris and relocates a bit of its tip is variously (and euphemistically) called clitoroplasty, clitoral reduction, or clitoral recession and described as a simple cosmetic procedure in order to differentiate it from the now-infamous clitoridectomy. The operation, however, is far from benign.

Johns Hopkins surgeons Joseph E. Oesterling, John P. Gearhart, and Robert D. Jeffs have described their technique. They make an incision around the clitoris, at the corona, then dissect the skin away from its underside. Next they dissect the skin away from the upper side and remove as much of the clitoral shaft as necessary to create an "appropriate size clitoris." Then they place stitches from the pubic area along both sides of the entire length of what remains of the clitoris; when they tighten these stitches, the tissue folds, like pleats in a skirt, and recesses into a concealed position behind the pubic mound. If they think the result still "too large," they further reduce the tip of the clitoris by cutting away a pie-shaped wedge.

For many intersex people, this sort of arcane, dehumanized medical literature, illustrated with close-ups of genital surgery and naked children with blacked-out eyes, is the only available version of *Our Bodies, Ourselves*. Thus, even as fierce arguments over gender identity, gender role development, and social construction of gender rage in psychology, feminism, and queer theory, we have literally delegated to medicine the authority to police the boundaries of male and female, leaving intersex people to recover as best they can, alone and silent, from violent normalization.

My own case, as it turns out, was not unusual. I was born with ambiguous genitals. A doctor specializing in intersexuality deliberated for three days—and sedated my mother each time she asked what was wrong with her baby—before concluding that I was male, with micropenis, complete hypospadias, undescended testes, and a strange extra opening behind the urethra. A male birth certificate was completed for me, and my parents began raising me as a boy. When I was a year and a half old, my parents consulted a different set of intersex experts, who admitted me to a hospital for "sex determination." "Determine" is a remarkably apt word in this context, meaning both to *ascertain* by investigation and to *cause* to come to a resolution. It perfectly describes the two-level process whereby science produces through a series of masked operations what it claims merely to observe. Doctors told my parents that a thorough medical investigation, including exploratory surgery, would be necessary to determine (that is, ascertain) what my "true sex" was. They judged my genital appendage to be inadequate as a penis: too short to effectively mark masculine status or to penetrate females. As a female, however, I would be penetrable and potentially fertile. My anatomy having now been re-labeled as vagina, urethra, labia, and outsized clitoris, my sex was next determined (in the second sense) by amputating my genital appendage—clitoridectomy. Following doctors' orders, my parents then changed my name; combed their house to eliminate all traces of my existence as a boy (photographs, birthday cards, etc.); engaged a lawyer to change my birth certificate; moved to a different town; instructed extended family members to no longer refer to me as a boy; and never told anyone else—including me—just what had happened. My intersexuality and change of sex were the family's dirty little secrets.

At age eight, I was returned to the hospital for abdominal surgery that trimmed away the testicular portion of my gonads, each of which was partly ovarian and partly testicular in character. No explanation was given to me then for the long hospital stay or the abdominal surgery, nor for the regular hospital visits afterward in which doctors photographed my genitals and inserted fingers and instruments into my vagina and anus. These visits ceased as soon as I began to menstruate. At the time of the sex change, doctors had assured my parents that their once-son/now-daughter would grow into a woman who could have a normal sex life and babies. With the confirmation of menstruation, my parents apparently concluded that that prediction had borne out and their ordeal was behind them. For me, the worst part of the nightmare was just beginning.

As an adolescent, I became aware that I had no clitoris or inner labia and was unable to experience orgasm. By the end of my teens, I began to research in medical libraries, trying to discover what might have happened to me. When I finally determined to obtain my personal medical records, it took three years to overcome the obstruction of the doctors whom I asked for help. When I did obtain a scant three pages from my medical files, I learned for the first time that I was a "true hermaphrodite" who had been my parents' son for a year and a half, with a name that was unfamiliar to me. The records also documented my clitoridectomy. This was the middle 1970s, when I was in my early twenties. I had come to identify myself as lesbian at a time when lesbianism and a biologically based gender essentialism were virtually synonymous. Men were rapists who caused war and environmental destruction; women were loving beings who would heal the earth; lesbians were a superior form of being uncontaminated by "men's energy." In such a world, how could I tell anyone that I had actually possessed the dreaded "phallus"? I was an impostor, not really a woman but rather a monstrous and mythical creature. And because my hermaphroditism and long-buried boyhood were the history that underlay the clitoridectomy, I could never speak openly about that either, or about my consequent inability to orgasm. I was so traumatized by discovering the circumstances that produced my embodiment that I could not speak of these matters with anyone.

Nearly fifteen years later, in my middle thirties, I suffered an emotional meltdown. In the eyes of the world I was a highly successful businesswoman, a principal in an international high-tech company. To myself, I was a freak, incapable of loving or being loved, filled with shame about my status as a hermaphrodite, about the imagined appearance of my genitals before surgery (I thought "true hermaphrodite" meant that I had been born with a penis), and about my sexual dysfunction. Unable to make peace with these facts about myself, I finally sought help from a professional therapist, only to find my experience denied. She reacted to each revelation about my history and predicament with some version of "no it's not" or "so what?" I'd say, "I'm not really a woman." She would say, "Of course you are. You look female." I'd say, "My complete withdrawal from sexuality has destroyed every relationship I've ever entered." She would say, "Everybody has their ups and downs." I tried another therapist and met with a similar response. Increasingly desperate, I confided my story to several friends who shrank away in embarrassed silence. I was in emotional agony and found myself utterly alone, with no possible way out. I decided to kill myself.

Confronting suicide as a real possibility proved to be my personal epiphany. In contemplating my own death, I fantasized killing myself quite messily and dramatically in the office of the surgeon who had sliced out my clitoris, forcibly confronting him with the horror he had imposed on my life. But in acknowledging that desire to put my pain to some use, not to waste my life completely, I turned a crucial corner, finding a way to direct my rage productively out into the world rather than aim it destructively at myself. My breakdown became my breakthrough, and I vowed that, whatever it took, I would heal myself. Still, I had no conceptual framework for developing a more positive self-consciousness. I knew only that I felt mutilated, not fully woman, less than fully human even, but I was determined to heal. I struggled for weeks in emotional chaos, unable to eat or sleep or work. I could not accept my image of a hermaphroditic body any more than I could accept the butchered one left me by the surgeons. Thoughts of myself as a Frankenstein patchwork alternated with longings for escape by death, only to be followed by outrage, anger, and determination to survive. I could not accept that it was just or right or good to treat any person as I had been treated—my sex changed, my genitals cut up, my experience silenced and rendered invisible. I bore a private hell within me, wretchedly alone in my condition without even my tormentors for company. Finally, I began to envision myself standing in a driving rain storm but with clear skies and a rainbow visible in the distance. I was still in agony, still alone, but I was beginning to see the painful process in which I was caught up in terms of revitalization and rebirth, a means of investing my life with a new sense of authenticity possessing vast potentials for further transformation. Since then I have seen this experience described by other intersex and transsexual activists.

I slowly developed a newly politicized and critically aware form of self-understanding. I had been the kind of lesbian who at times had a girlfriend but who had never really participated in the life of a lesbian community. I felt almost completely isolated from gay politics, feminism, and queer and gender theory. I did possess the rudimentary knowledge that the gay civil rights movement had gathered momentum only when it could effectively deny that homosexuality was sick or inferior and assert to the contrary that "gay is good." As impossible as it then seemed, I pledged similarly to affirm that "intersex is good" and that the body I was born with was not sick or shameful, only different. I vowed to embrace the sense of being "not a woman" that I had initially been so terrified to discover.

I began a search for community that brought me to San Francisco in the fall of 1992 on the theory that people living in the "queer Mecca" would have the most conceptually sophisticated, socially tolerant, and politically astute analysis of sexed and gendered embodiment. I found what I was looking for, in part because my arrival in the Bay Area corresponded with the rather sudden emergence of an energetic transgender political movement. At the same time, a vigorous new wave of gender scholarship had emerged in the academy. In this context, Morgan Holmes could analyze her own clitoridectomy for her master's thesis and have her study taken seriously as academic work. Openly transsexual scholars, including Susan Stryker and Sandy Stone, were visible in responsible academic positions at major universities.

Into this heady atmosphere, I brought my own experience. I started telling my story to everyone I met. Before long I learned of six other intersex people—including two who had been fortunate enough to escape medical attention. Realizing that intersexuality, rather than being extremely rare, must be relatively common, I decided to create a support network. Soon I was receiving several letters per week from intersex people throughout the United States and Canada and a few from further afield. Although details varied, the letters gave a remarkably coherent picture of the emotional consequences of medical intervention:

> All the things my body might have grown to do, all the possibilities, went down the hall with my amputated clitoris to the pathology department. The rest of me went to the recovery room—I'm still recovering.
> —Morgan Holmes

> I am horrified by what has been done to me and by the conspiracy of silence and lies. I am filled with grief and rage, but also relief finally to believe that maybe I am not the only one.
> —Angela Moreno

As soon as I saw the title *Hermaphrodites with Attitude* I cried aloud for sheer joy. . . . Finally I can say, 'I'm hermaphrodite, I'm intersex, I'm transgender, I'm queer and damn proud,' as tears of joy and belonging stream down my face.

    —Lee

Doctors never consulted me. . . .[T]he idea of asking for my opinion about having my penis surgically altered apparently never occurred to them. . . . Far too many people allow social stigma to cloud their judgment. It's OK to be different.

    —Randy

I pray that I will have the means to repay, in some measure, the American Urological Association for all that it has done for my benefit. I am having some trouble, though, in connecting the timing mechanism to the fuse.

    —Thomas

Toward Social Justice

The peer support network that I formed grew into the Intersex Society of North America (ISNA). ISNA's long-term and fundamental goal is to change the way intersex infants are treated. We advocate that surgery not be performed on children born with ambiguous genitals unless there is a medical reason (to prevent physical pain or illness) and that parents be given the conceptual tools and emotional support to accept their children's physical differences. We also advocate that children be raised either as boys or girls, according to which designation seems likely to offer the child the greatest future sense of comfort. Advocating gender assignment without resorting to normalizing surgery is a radical position given that it requires the willful disruption of the assumed concordance between body shape and gender category. However, this is the only position that prevents irreversible physical damage to the intersex person's body, that preserves the intersex person's agency regarding their own flesh, and that recognizes genital sensation and erotic functioning to be at least as important as reproductive capacity. If an intersex child or adult decides to change gender or to undergo surgical or hormonal alteration of his/her body, that decision should also be fully respected and facilitated. The key point is that intersex subjects should not be violated for the comfort and convenience of others.

One part of reaching ISNA's long-term goal has been to document the emotional and physical carnage resulting from medical interventions. As a rapidly growing literature (see the bibliography on our Web-site, <http://www.isna.org>) makes abundantly clear, the medical management of intersexuality has changed shockingly little in the more than forty years since my first surgery—doctors still cut up children's genitals and still perpetuate invisibility and silence around intersex lives. Kessler expresses surprise that "in spite of the thousands of genital operations performed every year, there are no meta-analyses from within the medical community on levels of success." Surgeons admit to not knowing whether their former patients are "silent and happy or silent and unhappy." There is no research effort to improve erotic functioning for adult intersex people whose genitals have been cut, nor are there psychotherapists who specialize in working with adult intersex clients trying to heal from the trauma of medical intervention. To provide a counterpoint to the mountains of professional medical literature that neglect intersex experience and to begin compiling an ethnographic account of that experience, ISNA has worked to make public the lives of intersex people through our own publications (including our video, Hermaphrodites Speak!) and by working with scholars and the popular media.

ISNA's presence has begun to be effective. It has helped politicize the growing number of intersex organizations as well as intersex identities themselves. When I first began organizing ISNA, I met leaders of the Turner's Syndrome Society, the oldest known support group focusing on atypical sexual differentiation founded in 1987. (Turner's Syndrome is defined by an XO genetic karyotype that results in a female body morphology with nonfunctioning ovaries, extremely short stature, and, variably, a variety of other visible physical differences still described in the medical literature with such stigmatizing labels as "web-necked" and "fish-mouthed.") Each of these women told me what a profound, life-changing experience it had been simply to meet another person like herself. I was inspired by their accomplishments (they are a national organization serving thousands of members) but wanted ISNA to have a different focus—less willing to think of intersexuality as a pathology or disability, more interested in challenging the medicalization of sexual difference entirely, and more interested in politicizing a pan-intersexual revolt across the divisions of particular etiologies in order to destabilize the heteronormative assumptions that underlie the violence directed at our bodies.

Public Discourse on Pediatric Genital Surgeries

Because the politicized intersex community is still quite young, and most intersex people remain too burdened by the crippling emotional consequences of what has been done to them to come out publicly, ISNA has deliberately cultivated a network of non-intersexed advocates who command a measure of social legitimacy and can speak in contexts where uninterpreted intersex voices will not be heard. Because there is a strong impulse to discount what intersex people have to say about themselves (as if we are too close to the issues to offer objective opinions), this sort of sympathetic representation has been welcome—especially in helping intersex people reframe intersexuality in nonmedical terms. Some gender theory scholars, feminist critics of science, medical historians, and anthropologists have been quick to understand and support intersex activism. Feminist biologist and science studies scholar Anne Fausto-Sterling—who wrote, years before ISNA came into existence, about intersexuality in relation to intellectually suspect scientific practices that perpetuate masculinist constructs of gender—became an early ISNA ally. Likewise, social psychologist Suzanne Kessler wrote a brilliant ethnography of surgeons who specialize in treating intersex. After speaking with a number of the normalized "products" of these medical programs, she, too, became a strong supporter of intersex activism. Historian of science Alice Dreger, whose work focuses not only on hermaphroditism but also on other forms of atypical embodiment that become subject to destructively normalizing medical interventions (as in her discussion of conjoined twins in "Limits of Individuality"), has been especially supportive. Fausto-Sterling, Kessler, and Dreger have each written books that analyze the medical treatment of intersexuality as being culturally motivated and criticize it as often harmful to its ostensible patients.

Allies who help contest the medicalization of intersexuality have been especially important, because ISNA initially found direct, nonconfrontational interactions with medical specialists who determine policy on the treatment of intersex infants and actually carry out the surgeries to be both difficult and ineffective. Joycelyn Elders, the Clinton administration's first surgeon general, is a pediatric endocrinologist with many years of experience in managing intersex infants. In spite of a generally feminist approach to health care and frequent overtures from ISNA, she rejected the concerns of intersex people themselves.

Surgeon Richard Schlussel, at a pediatric plastic surgery symposium (which had rejected ISNA's offer to provide a patients' panel) at Mount Sinai Medical Center in New York City in 1996 proclaimed, "The parents of children with ambiguous genitals are more grateful to the surgeon than any—more grateful even than parents whose children's lives have been saved through open heart surgery."

Another pediatrician remarked in an Internet discussion on intersexuality, "I think this whole issue is preposterous. . . . To suggest that [medical decisions about the treatment of intersex] are somehow cruel or arbitrary is insulting, ignorant and misguided. . . . To

spread the claims that [ISNA] is making is just plain wrong, and I hope that this [on-line group of doctors] will not blindly accept them." Yet another physician participating in that same chat, in a marvelous example of the degree to which practitioners of science can be blind to their complicity in constructing the objects they study, asked what was for him obviously a rhetorical question: "Who is the enemy? I really don't think it's the medical establishment. Since when did we establish the male/female hegemony?" Johns Hopkins surgeon Gearhart, quoted in a New York Times article on ISNA, summarily dismissed us as "zealots," but professional meetings in the fields of pediatrics, urology, genital plastic surgery, and endocrinology are abuzz with anxious and defensive discussion of intersex activism. In response to a 1996 protest by Hermaphrodites with Attitude at the American Academy of Pediatrics annual meeting, that organization felt compelled to hold a press conference and issue a statement: "The Academy is deeply concerned about the emotional, cognitive, and body image development of intersexuals, and believes that successful early genital surgery minimizes these issues." The academy refused, however, to speak with intersex people picketing its meeting.

The roots of resistance in the medical establishment to the truth-claims of intersex people run deep. Not only does ISNA's existence imply a critique of the normativistic biases couched within most scientific practice but it also advocates a treatment protocol for intersex infants that disrupts conventional understandings of the relationship between bodies and genders. On a level more personally threatening to medical practitioners, ISNA's position implies that they have—unwittingly at best and through willful denial at worst—spent their careers inflicting a profound harm from which their patients will never fully recover. ISNA's position threatens to destroy the foundational assumptions motivating an entire medical subspecialty, thus jeopardizing their continued ability to perform what surgeons find to be technically fascinating work. Science writer Melissa Hendricks notes that Gearhart is known to colleagues as an "artist" who can "carve a large phallus down into a clitoris" with consummate skill. Given these deep and mutually reinforcing reasons for opposing ISNA's position, it is hardly surprising that medical intersex specialists have, for the most part, turned a deaf ear toward us.

Thus, the most important aspect of our current activities is the struggle to change public perceptions. By using the mass media, the Internet, and our growing network of allies and sympathizers to make the general public aware of the frequency of intersexuality and of the intense suffering that medical treatment has caused, we seek to create an environment in which many parents will have already heard about the intersex movement when their intersex child is born. Such informed parents have proved better able to resist medical pressure for unnecessary genital surgery and secrecy and to find their way to a peer-support group and counseling rather than to a surgical theater.

The Double Standard: First-World Feminism, African Clitoridectomy and Intersex Genital Mutilation, and the Media

African practices that remove the clitoris and other parts of female genitals have lately been a target of intense media coverage and feminist activism in the United States and other industrialized Western societies, and the euphemism *female circumcision* has been largely supplanted by the politicized term *female genital mutilation* (FGM). Analogous medical (rather than folk) operations performed on intersex people in the United States have not been the focus of similar attention—indeed, attempts to link the two forms of genital cutting have met with multiform resistance. Examining the way that first-world feminists and mainstream media treat African practices and comparing that treatment with their response to intersex genital mutilation (IGM) in North America exposes some of the complex interactions between ideologies of race, gender, colonialism, and science that effectively silence and render invisible intersex experience in first-world contexts. Cutting intersex genitals becomes yet another hidden mechanism for imposing normalcy upon unruly flesh, a means of containing the potential anarchy of desires and identifications within oppressive heteronormative structures.

In 1994 the *New England Journal of Medicine* paired an article on the physical harm resulting from African genital cutting with an editorial denouncing clitoridectomy as a violation of human rights but declined to run a reply drafted by University of California at Berkeley medical anthropologist Lawrence Cohen and two ISNA members detailing the harm caused by medicalized American clitoridectomies. In response to growing media attention, Congress passed the Federal Prohibition of Female Genital Mutilation Act in October 1996. That act specifically exempted from prohibition medicalized clitoridectomies of the sort performed to "correct" intersex bodies. The bill's principal author, feminist Congresswoman Pat Schroeder, ignored multiple letters from ISNA members and Brown University professor of medical science Anne Fausto-Sterling asking her to recast the bill's language. "New Law Bans Genital Cutting," the *New York Times* proclaimed and refused to address documentation from

ISNA and Michigan State University professor Alice Dreger pointing out that genital cutting continues to be standard medical practice in the United States.

The *Boston Globe's* syndicated columnist Ellen Goodman has been one of the few journalists covering African genital cutting to make any response to ISNA overtures. "I must admit I was not aware of this situation," she wrote to me in 1994. "I admire your courage." She continued, however, to discuss African genital cutting in her column without mentioning similar American practices. Ironically, Goodman is based in Boston, a Mecca of sorts after Johns Hopkins for the surgical management of intersex children, with prominent specialists operating at Harvard, Massachusetts General Hospital, and Boston Children's Hospital. An October 1995 Goodman column on genital cutting was promisingly entitled "We Don't Want to Believe It Happens Here" but discussed only practices imported to the United States by immigrants from third-world countries.

While anti-excision African immigrant women within the United States have been receptive to the claims made by intersex opponents to medicalized clitoridectomies, first-world feminists and organizations working on African genital cutting have totally ignored us. Only two of the many anti-genital-cutting activist groups contacted have bothered to respond to repeated overtures from intersex activists. Fran Hosken, who since 1982 has regularly published a catalog of statistics on female genital cutting worldwide, wrote me a terse note saying that "we are not concerned with biological exceptions."

Forward International, a London-based, anti-female-genital-cutting organization, replied to German intersex activist Heike Spreitzer that her letter of inquiry was "most interesting" but they could not help because their work focuses only on genital cutting "that is performed as harmful cultural or traditional practice on young girls."

As Forward International's reply to Spreitzer demonstrates, many first-world, anti-FGM activists seemingly consider Africans to have "harmful cultural or traditional practices," whereas we in the modern industrialized West presumably have something better. We have science, and science is linked to the meta-narratives of enlightenment, progress, and truth. Genital cutting is condoned to the extent that it supports these cultural self-conceptions.

Robin Morgan and Gloria Steinem set the tone for much of the first-world feminist analysis of African genital cutting with their pathbreaking article in the March 1980 issue of *Ms.* magazine, "The International Crime of Genital Mutilation." A disclaimer atop the first page warns, "These words are painful to read.

They describe facts of life as far away as our most fearful imagination—and as close as any denial of women's sexual freedom." For *Ms.* readers, whom the editors apparently imagine are more likely to experience the pain of genital mutilation between the covers of their magazine than between their own thighs, clitoridectomy is presented as a fact of foreign life whose principal relevance to their readership is that it exemplifies a loss of "freedom," that most cherished possession of liberal Western subjects. One-half of the article's first page is filled with a photograph of an African girl seated on the ground, her legs held open by the arm of an unseen woman to her right. To her left is the disembodied hand of the midwife, holding the razor blade with which she has just performed a ritual clitoridectomy. The girl's face is a mask of pain, her mouth open, her eyes bulging.

In some twenty years of coverage, Western images of African practices have changed little although they have found their way into more mainstream publications. "Americans made a horrifying discovery this year," the January 1997 issue of *Life* soberly informed readers. The two-page photo spread shows a Kenyan girl held from behind, a hand clamped over her mouth, her face contorted in pain as unseen hands cut her genitals. Interestingly, the girl in this photo is adolescent, her breasts are shown, covered with rivulets of sweat, and there is a definite air of sensuality in the presentation. The 1996 Pulitzer prize for feature photography went to yet another portrayal of a Kenyan clitoridectomy. And, in the wake of Fauziya Kassindja's successful bid for asylum in the United States after fleeing clitoridectomy in Togo, the number of related images from her country skyrocketed. One wonders if Western photojournalists in search of sensational clitoridectomy photos do not represent a veritable tourism boom for a country the size of West Virginia.

These representations manifest a profound act of "othering" African clitoridectomy that contributes to the silence surrounding similar medicalized practices in the "modern," industrialized West. "Their" genital cutting is barbaric ritual; "ours" is scientific. Theirs disfigures; ours normalizes the deviant. The colonialist implications of these representations of genital cutting are even more glaringly obvious when contemporaneous images of intersex surgeries are juxtaposed with images of African practices. Medical books describing how to perform clitoral surgery on intersex children are almost always illustrated with extreme genital close-ups, disconnecting the genitals not only from the individual intersexed person but also from the body itself. Full body shots always have the subject's eyes blacked out. Why is it considered necessary—or at least polite—to black out the eyes of American girls but not the eyes of the African girls used to illustrate Steinem's "International Crime" or *Life*'s more recent "Ritual Agony"? I suspect one reason is that a Western reader is likely to identify with an American but not an African girl. Blacking out the American girl's eyes allows the reader to remain safely on this side of the camera.

First-world feminist discourse locates clitoridectomy not only elsewhere in African but also "elsewhen." An *Atlantic Monthly* article on African clitoridectomy, for example, asserted that the "American medical profession stopped performing clitoridectomies decades ago," and the magazine declined to publish a letter from ISNA contradicting that claim. Academic publications are as prone to this attitude as the popular press. Feminist Martha Nussbaum, in a discussion of judging other cultures, acknowledges, "If two abuses are morally the same and we have better local information about one and are better placed politically to do something about it, that one seems to be a sensible choice to focus on in our actions here and now." But then she counter-factually locates U.S. genital surgeries solely in the past: "As recently as the 1940s, [genital surgeries] were performed by U.S. and British doctors to treat female 'problems' such as masturbation and lesbianism." By collaborating in the silence about intersex genital surgeries, Nussbaum excuses first-world feminists from any obligation to challenge their own cultural practices as rigorously as they do that of others.

In the influential *Deviant Bodies* anthology, visual artist Susan Jahoda's "Theatres of Madness" juxtaposes nineteenth- and twentieth-century material depicting "the conceptual interdependence of sexuality, reproduction, family life, and 'female disorders.'" To represent twentieth-century medical clitoridectomy practices, Jahoda quotes a 1980 letter to the editor of *Ms.* magazine prompted by the Steinem and Morgan article. The writer, a nurse's aid in a geriatric home, says she had been puzzled by the strange scars she saw on the genitals of five of the forty women in her care: "Then I read your article. . . . My God! Why? Who decided to deny them orgasm? Who made them go through such a procedure? I want to know. Was it fashionable? Or was it to correct 'a condition?' I'd Like to know what this so-called civilized country used as its criteria for such a procedure. And how widespread is it here in the United States?"

While Jahoda's selection of this letter does raise the issue of medicalized American clitoridectomies, it again safely locates the cutting in the past, as something experienced a long time ago by women now in their later states of life. Significantly, Jahoda literally passes over an excellent opportunity to comment on the continuing practice of clitoridectomy in the contemporary United States.

Two months earlier, in the April 1980 issue of *Ms.*, noted feminist biologists Patricia Farnes (a medical doctor) and Ruth Hubbard also replied to Morgan and Steinem:

> We want to draw the attention of your readers to the practice of clitoridectomy not only in the Third World . . . but right here in the Untied States, where it is used as part of a procedure to "repair" by "plastic surgery" so-called genital ambiguities. Few people realize that this procedure has routinely involved removal of the entire clitoris and its nerve supply—in other words, total clitoridectomy. . . . In a lengthy article, [Johns Hopkins intersex expert John] Money and two colleagues write, "There has been no evidence of a deleterious effect of clitoridectomy. None of the women experienced in genital practices reported a loss of orgasm after clitoridectomy." The article also advises that "a three-year old girl about to be clitoridectomized . . . should be well informed that the doctors *will make her look like all other girls and women*" (our emphasis), which is not unlike what North African girls are often told about their clitoridectomies. . . . But to date, neither Money nor his critics have investigated the effect of clitoridectomies on the girls' development. Yet one would surely expect this to affect their psychosexual development and their feelings of identity as young women.

Although Farnes and Hubbard's prescient feminist exposé of medicalized clitoridectomies in the contemporary United States sank without a trace, there has been a veritable explosion of work like Nussbaum's and Jahoda's that keeps "domestic" clitoridectomy at a safe distance. Such conceptualizations of clitoridectomy's cultural remoteness—both geographically and temporally—allow feminist outrage to be diverted into potentially colonialist meddling in the social affairs of others while hampering work for social justice at home.

Conclusion

Feminism represents itself as being interested in unmasking the silence that surrounds violence against women and in providing tools to understand the personal as political. Most medical intersex management is a form of violence based on a sexist devaluing of female pain and female sexuality: Doctors consider the prospect of growing up male with a small penis to be a worse alternative than living as a female without a clitoris, ovaries, or sexual gratification. Medical intervention literally transforms transgressive bodies into ones that can

safely be labeled female and subjected to the many forms of social control with which women must contend. Why then have most feminists failed to engage the issue of medical abuse of intersex people?

I suggest that intersex people have had such difficulty generating mainstream feminist support not only because of the racist and colonialist frameworks that situate clitoridectomy as a practice foreign to proper subjects within the first world but also because intersexuality undermines the stability of the category "woman" that undergirds much first-world feminist discourse. We call into question the assumed relation between genders and bodies and demonstrate how some bodies do not fit easily into male/female dichotomies. We embody viscerally the truth of Judith Butler's dictum that "sex," the concept that accomplishes the materialization and naturalization of culturally constructed gender differences, has really been "gender all along." By refusing to remain silenced, we queer the foundations upon which depend not only the medical management of bodies but also widely shared feminist assumptions of properly embodied female subjectivity.

In 1990 Suzanne Kessler noted, "[T]he possibilities for real societal transformations would be unlimited [if physicians and scientists specializing in the management of gender could recognize that] finally, and always, people construct gender as well as the social systems that are grounded in gender-based concepts. . . . Accepting genital ambiguity as a natural option would require that physicians also acknowledge that genital ambiguity is 'corrected' not because it is threatening to the infant's life but because it is threatening to the infant's culture."

To the extent that we are not normatively female or normatively women, we are not the proper subjects of feminist concern. Western feminism has represented African genital cutting as primitive, irrational, harmful, and deserving of condemnation. The Western medical community has represented its genital cutting as modern scientific, healing, and above reproach. When will Western feminists realize that their failure to examine either of these claims "others" African women and allows the violent medical oppression of intersex people to continue unimpeded?

References

A list of references is available in the original source.

The Picture of Health
How Textbook Photographs Construct Health

by Mariamne H. Whatley

Photographs in textbooks may serve the roles of breaking up a long text, emphasizing or clarifying information in the text, attracting the buyer (the professor, teacher, or administrator who selects texts), and engaging the reader. But photographs cannot be dismissed merely as either decorative additions or straightforward illustrations of the text. Photographs are often far more memorable than the passages they illustrate and, because they are seen as objective representations of reality, rather than artists' constructions (Barthes, 1977), may have more impact than drawings or other forms of artwork. In textbooks, photographs can carry connotations, intentional or not, never stated in the text. The selection of photographs for a text is not a neutral process that simply involves being "realistic" or "objective"; selection must take into account issues such as audience expectations and dominant meanings in a given cultural/historical context (Whatley, 1988). In order to understand the ideological work of a textbook, a critique of the photographs is as crucial as a critique of the text itself.

Using ideological analysis to identify patterns of inclusion and exclusion, I examined photographs in the seven best-selling, college-level personal health textbooks. This chapter presents the results of that research. In the first part of the analysis, I examined the photographs that represent "health," describing who and what is "healthy," according to these representations. In the second part of the analysis, I determined where those excluded from the definition of health are represented in the approximately 1,100 remaining photographs in the texts.

Selling Health in Textbooks

Generally, textbook authors do not select specific photographs but may give publishers general descriptions of the type of photographs they wish to have included (for example, a scene showing urban crowding, a woman in a nontraditional job). Due to the great expense involved, new photographs are not usually taken specifically for texts. Instead publishers hire photo researchers to find appropriate photographs, drawing on already existing photographic collections. The result is that the choice of photographs depends on what is already available, and what is available depends to some extent on what has been requested in the past. In fact, because the same sources of photographs may be used by a number of different publishers, identical photographs may appear in competing books. Although authors may have visions of their books' "artwork," the reality may be limited by the selection already on the market. In addition, editors and publishers make decisions about what "artwork" will sell or is considered appropriate, sometimes overruling the authors' choices.

Photographs, especially cover-photos and special color sections, are considered features that sell textbooks, but they also can work as part of another selling process. Textbooks, in many cases, sell the reader a system of belief. An economics text, for example, may "sell" capitalism, and a science text may "sell" the scientific method, both of which help support dominant ideologies. Health textbooks may be even more invested in this selling process because, in addition to convincing readers to "believe" in health, their "success" depends on the readers' adoption of very specific personal behavioral programs to attain health. Health textbooks hold up the ideals of "total wellness" or "holistic fitness" as goals we can attain by exercising, eating right, reducing stress, and avoiding drugs. The readers' belief in health and their ability to attain it by specific behaviors is seen by many health educators as necessary to relevant educational goals; the belief in a clearly marked pathway to health is also part of a process of the commodification of health.

In North America and Western Europe, health is currently a very marketable commodity. This can be seen in its most exaggerated form in the United States in the proliferation of "health" clubs, in the trend among hospitals and clinics to attract a healthy clientele by advertising their abilities to make healthy people healthier (Worcester & Whatley, 1988), and in the advertisements that link a wide range of products, such as high fiber cereals and calcium rich antacids, to health. In a recent article in a medical journal, a physician examined this commercialization of health:

> Health is industrialized and commercialized in a fashion that enhances many people's dissatisfaction with their health. Advertisers, manufacturers, advocacy groups, and proprietary health care corporations promote the myth that good health can be purchased; they market products and services that purport to deliver the consumer into the promised land of wellness. (Barsky, 1988, p. 415)

Photographs in health textbooks can play a role in this selling of health similar to that played by visual images in advertising a product in the popular media. According to Berger (1972), the role of advertising or publicity is to

> make the spectator marginally dissatisfied with his present way of life. Not with the way of life of society, but with his own place within it. It suggests that if he buys what it is offering, his life will become better. It offers him an improved alternative to what he is. (p. 142)

The ideal of the healthy person and the healthy lifestyle can be seen as the "improved alternative" to what we are. It can be assumed that most of us will be dissatisfied with ourselves when measured against that ideal, just as most women are dissatisfied with their body shapes and sizes when compared with ideal media representations.

In effective advertising campaigns the visual image is designed to provoke powerful audience responses. In health textbooks the visual representation of "health" is calculated to sell, and it is likely to have a greater impact on the reader than discussions about lengthened life expectancy, reduction in chronic illness, or enhanced cardiovascular fitness. The image of health, not health itself, may be what most people strive for. In the attempt to look healthy, many sacrifice health. For example, people go through very unhealthy practices to lose "extra" weight that is in itself not unhealthy; being slim, however, is a basic component of the *appearance* of health. A recent survey found that people who eat healthy foods do so for their appearance and *not* for their health. "Tanning parlors" have become common features of health and fitness centers, though tanning in itself is unhealthy. As with being slim, having a good tan contributes to the appearance of what is currently defined as health.

The use of color photographs is particularly effective in selling the healthy image, for, as Berger (1972) points out, both oil painting and color photography "use similar highly tactile means to play upon the spectator's sense of acquiring the *real* thing which the image shows" (p. 141). The recent improvement in quality and the increase in number of color photographs in textbooks provide an opportunity to sell the image of health even more effectively than black and white photographs could.

Selection of Textbooks

Rather than trying to examine all college-level personal health (as opposed to community health) textbooks, I selected the best-selling ones, since those would have the widest impact. Based on the sales figures provided by the publisher of one popular text, I selected seven texts published from 1985 to 1988. Sales of these textbooks ranged from approximately 15,000 to 50,000 for each edition. (Complete bibliographic information on these textbooks is provided in the Appendix. Author-date information for these textbooks refer to the Appendix, rather than the chapter references.) Obviously, the sales figures depend on the number of years a specific edition has been in print. For one text (Insel & Roth, 1988), I examined the newest edition (for which there could be no sales figures), based on the fact that its previous editions had high sales. A paper on the readability of personal health textbooks (Overman, Mimms, & Harris, 1987), using a similar selection process, examined the seven top-selling textbooks for the 1984–85 school year, plus three other random titles. Their list has an overlap with mine of only four texts, which may be due to a number of factors, including differences in editions and changing sales figures.

Analysis I: Healthy-Image Photographs

The first step in my analysis was a close examination of the photographs that I saw as representing "health," the images intended to show who is healthy and illustrate the healthy lifestyle. These included photographs used on covers, opposite title pages, and as openers to units or chapters on wellness or health (as opposed to specific topics such as nutrition, drugs, and mental health). While other pictures throughout the texts may represent healthy individuals, the ones selected, by their placement in conjunction with the book title or chapter title, can be seen as clearly connoting "health." I will refer to these as healthy-image photographs. I included in this analysis only photographs in which there were people. While an apple on a cover conveys a message about health, I was interested only in the question of who is healthy.

A total of 18 different photographs fit my criteria for representing health. I have eliminated three of these from discussion: the cover from Insel and Roth (1988) showing flowers and, from Dinitiman and Greenberg (1986), both the cover photograph of apples and the health unit opener of a movie still from the *Wizard of Oz.* (This textbook uses movie stills as openers for all chapters; this moves the photograph away from its perceived "objective" status toward that of an obvious construction.)

There are a number of points of similarity in the 15 remaining photographs. In several photographs (windsurfing, hang gliding), it is hard to determine race, but all individuals whose faces can clearly be seen are white. Except for those who cannot be seen clearly and for several of the eight skydivers in a health unit opener, all are young. No one in these photographs is fat or has any identifiable physical disability. Sports dominate the activities, which, with the exception of rhythmic gymnastics and volleyball played in a gym, are outdoor activities in nonurban settings. Five of these involve beaches or open water. All the activities are leisure activities, with no evidence of work. While it is impossible to say anything definitive about class from these photographs, several of the activities are expensive (hang gliding, skydiving, windsurfing), and others may take money and/or sufficient time off from work to get to places where they can be done (beaches, biking in countryside); these suggest middle-class activities, whether the actual individuals are middle class or not. In several photographs (windsurfing, hang gliding, swimming) it is hard to determine gender. However, excluding these and the large group of male runners in a cross-country race, the overall balance is 23 males to 18 females, so it does seem that there is an attempt to show women both as healthy individuals and in active roles.

How Health Is Portrayed

A detailed analysis of three photographs can provide insight into how these text photographs construct health. The first is a color photograph of a volleyball game on a beach from the back cover of *Understanding Your Health* (Payne & Hahn, 1986). As with most of these images of health, the setting is outdoors, clearly at a distance from urban life. The steep rock walls that serve as a backdrop to the volleyball game additionally isolate the natural beach setting from the invasion of cars[1] and other symbols of "man-made" environmental destruction and ill health. The volleyball players appear to have escaped into a protected idyllic setting of sun, sand, and, we assume, water. They also have clearly escaped from work, since they are engaged in a common leisure activity associated with picnics and holidays. None of them appears to be contemplating the beauty of the natural setting, but merely using it as a location for a game that could go on anywhere in which there is room to set up a net.

The photograph is framed in such a way that the whole net and area of the "court" are not included, so that some players may also not be visible. On one side of the net are three women and a man, on the other two women and a man. While this is not necessarily a representation of heterosexual interactions, it can be read that way. Two players are the focus of the picture, with the other five essentially out of the action. The woman who has just hit the ball, with her back toward the camera, has her arms outstretched, her legs slightly spread, and one foot partly off the ground. The man who is waiting for the ball is crouched slightly, looking expectantly upward. Her body is partially superimposed on his, her leg crossed over his. This is essentially an interaction between one man and one woman. It would not work the same way if the key players were both female or both male, since part of the "healthiness" of this image appears to be the heterosexual interaction. For heterosexual men, this scene might be viewed as ideal—a great male-female ratio on an isolated beach; perhaps this is their reward for having arrived at the end of this book— this photograph is on the *back* cover—attaining their goal of health.

All the volleyball players are white, young, and slim. The woman farthest left in the frame appears slightly heavier than the others; she is the only woman wearing a shirt, rather than a bikini top, and is also wearing shorts. Besides being an outsider in terms of weight, dress, and location in the frame, she is the only woman who clearly has short hair (three have long hair tied back in ponytails, one cannot be seen completely). Perhaps she can move "inside" by losing weight and changing her image. As viewers, we are just a few steps beyond the end of the court and are also outsiders. As with pick-up games, there is room for observers to enter the game—if they are deemed acceptable by the other players. By achieving health, perhaps the observer can step into the game, among the young, white, slim, heterosexual, and physically active. But if the definition of health includes young, white, slim, heterosexual, and physically active, many observers are relegated permanently to the outside.

If this photograph serves as an invitation to join in the lifestyle of the young and healthy, the second photograph, facing the title page of another book, serves the same function, with the additional written message provided by the title of the book—*An Invitation to Health* (Hales & Williams, 1986). The photograph is of six bicycle riders, three women and three men, resting astride their bicycles. This photograph is in black and white, so it is perhaps not as seductive as the sunny color of the first cover. However, the people in this photograph are all smiling directly at the viewer (rather than just leaving a space in back where the viewer could join in). Two of the women, in the middle and the right, have poses and smiles that could be described as flirtatious. They are taking a break from their riding, so it is an opportune moment to join the fun of being healthy.

As with the volleyball players, all the bicycle riders are young, slim, white, and apparently fit. Another similarity is the amount of skin that is exposed. Playing volleyball on the beach and riding bikes in warm weather are activities for which shorts and short-sleeved shirts are preferable to sweatpants and sweatshirts. The choice of these types of activities to represent health results in photographs in which legs and arms are not covered. Appearing healthy apparently involves no need to cover up unsightly flab, "cellulite," or stretch marks. A healthy body is a body that can be revealed.

The bikers are in a fairly isolated, rural setting. While they are clearly on the road, it appears to be a rural, relatively untraveled road. Two cars can be seen far in the distance, and there may also be a house in the distance on the right side of the frame. Otherwise, the landscape is dominated by hills, trees, and grass, the setting and the activity clearly distance the bike riders both from urban life and from work.

In a third photograph, a health unit chapter opener (Levy, Dignan, & Shirreffs, 1987), we can see a possible beginning to alternative images of health. The players in this volleyball game are still slim, young, and apparently white. However, the setting is a gym, which could be urban, suburban, or rural. While four players are wearing shorts, one woman is wearing sweatpants; there are T-shirts rather than bikini tops, and gym socks rather than bare legs. The impression is that they are there to play a hard game of volleyball rather than to bask in the sun and each other's gaze. Two men are going for the ball from opposite sides, while a woman facing the net is clearly ready to move. Compared with the other volleyball scene, this photograph gives more of a sense of action, of actual physical exertion, as well as a sense of real people, rather than models.

It is interesting to imagine how healthy the volleyball players and bike riders actually are, underneath the appearance of health. The outdoor groups, especially the beach group, are susceptible to skin cancer from overexposure to the sun. Cycling is a healthy aerobic sport, though it can be hard on the knees and back. It is particularly surprising, however, to find that the bikers represented in a health text are not wearing helmets, thus modeling behavior that is considered very risky. Compared with biking, volleyball is the kind of weekend activity that sends the enthusiastic untrained player home with pulled muscles, jammed fingers, and not much of a useful workout. The question also arises as to how the particularly thin women on the beach achieved their weight—by unhealthy weight-loss diets, by anorexia, by purging? The glowing image of health may have little to do with the reality.

Similarities to Advertising

Shortly after I began the research for this chapter, I was startled, while waiting for a movie to begin, to see a soft drink advertisement from which almost any still could have been substituted for a healthy-image photograph I had examined. There were the same thin, young, white men and women frolicking on the beach, playing volleyball, and windsurfing. They were clearly occupying the same territory: a never-never land of eternal sunshine, eternal youth, and eternal leisure. Given my argument that these textbook photographs are selling health, the similarities between soft drink advertising images and textbook healthy images are not surprising. They are appealing to the same groups of people, and they are both attempting to create an association between a desirable lifestyle and their product. You can enjoy this fun in the sun if you are part of the "Pepsi generation" or think "Coke is it" or follow the textbook's path to health. These can be considered one variant of the lifestyle format in advertising, as described by Leiss, Kline, and Jhally (1986).

> Here the activity invoked in text or image becomes the central cue for relating the person, product, and setting codes. Lifestyle ads commonly depict a variety of leisure activities (entertaining, going out, holidaying, relaxing). Implicit in each of these activities, however, is the placing of the product within a consumption style by its link to an activity. (p. 210)

Even a naive critic of advertising could point out that drinking a carbonated beverage could not possibly help anyone attain this lifestyle; on the other hand, it might be easier to accept that the same lifestyle is a result of achieving health. However, the association between health and this leisure lifestyle is as much a construction as that created in the soft drink ads. Following all the advice in these textbooks as to diet, exercise, coping with stress, and attaining a healthy sexuality will not help anyone achieve this sun-and-fun fantasy lifestyle any more than drinking Coke or Pepsi would.

These healthy-image photographs borrow directly from popular images of ideal lifestyles already very familiar to viewers through advertising[2] and clearly reflect the current marketing of health. The result is that health is being sold with as much connection to real life and real people's needs as liquor ads that suggest major lifestyle changes associated with changing one's brand of scotch.

Analysis II: Where Are the Excluded?

For each textbook, the next step was to write brief descriptions of all other photographs in the books, totaling approximately 1,100. The results of the analysis of the healthy image photographs suggested a focus on specific aspects of the description of the individuals and activities in examining the remaining 1,100 photographs. The areas I selected for discussion are those in which "health" is linked to specific lifestyles or factors that determine social position/power in our society. I described the setting, the activity, and a number of observable points about the people, including gender, race, age, physical ability/disability, and weight. These photographs were all listed by chapter and when appropriate, by particular topic in that chapter. For example, a chapter on mental health might have images of positive mental health and also images representing problems such as severe depression or stress. These descriptions of photographs were used to establish whether there were images with characteristics not found in the healthy images and, if so, the context in which these characteristics were present. For example, finding no urban representations among the healthy images, I identified topic headings under which I did find photographs of urban settings.

White, young, thin, physically abled, middle-class people in the healthy images represent the mythical norm with whom the audience is supposed to identify. This not only creates difficulties in identification for whose who do not meet these criteria, but also creates a limiting and limited definition of health. I examined the photographs that did not fit the healthy-image definition to find the invisible—those absent from the healthy images: people of color, people with physical disabilities, fat people, and old people. I also attempted to identify two other absences— the urban setting and work environment. Because there were no obvious gender discrepancies in the healthy images, I did not examine gender as a separate category.

People of Color

After going through the remaining photographs, it was clear that there had been an attempt to include photographs of people of color in a variety of settings, but no obvious patterns emerged. In a previous paper, I examined representations of African-Americans in sexuality texts, finding that positive attempts at being nonracist could be undermined by the patterns of photographs in textbooks that, for example, draw on stereotypes and myths of "dangerous" black sexuality (Whatley, 1988). Rather than reviewing all the representations of people of color in these health textbooks, I will simply repeat what I pointed out earlier—that there is a strong and clear *absence* of photographs of people of color in the healthy-images category. People of color may appear as healthy people elsewhere in the text, but not on covers, title pages, and chapter openers. If publishers wanted to correct this situation, they could simply substitute group photographs that show some diversity for the current all-white covers and title pages.

People with Disabilities

From the healthy-image photographs, it is apparent that people with visible physical disabilities are excluded from the definition of healthy. Therefore, I examined the contexts in which people with disabilities appear in the other photographs. Out of the approximately 1,100 photos, only 9 show people with physical disabilities, with 2 of these showing isolated body parts only (arthritic hands and knees). One shows an old woman being pushed in a wheelchair, while the six remaining photographs all are "positive" images: a number of men playing wheelchair basketball, a man in a wheelchair doing carpentry, a woman walking with her arm around a man in a wheelchair, a man with an amputated leg walking across Canada, children with cancer (which can be seen both as a disease and a disability) at a camp (these last two both in a cancer chapter), and a wheelchair racer. However, three of these six are from one textbook (Payne & Hahn, 1986), and two are from another (Levy, Dignan, & Shirreffs, 1987), so the inclusion of these few positive images is over-shadowed by the fact that three books show absolutely none. In addition, none of these positive images are of women, and the only disabilities represented are those in which an individual uses a wheelchair or has cancer.

This absence of representation of disabled people, particularly women, clearly reflects the invisibility of the physically disabled in our society.

> It would be easy to blame the media for creating and maintaining many of the stereotypes with which the disabled still have to live. But the media only reflect attitudes that already exist in a body-beautiful society that tends to either ignore or ostracize people who don't measure up to the norm. This state of "invisibility" is particularly true for disabled women. (Israel & McPherson, 1983, pp. 4–15)

In a society that values the constructed image of health over health itself, a person with a disability does not fit the definition of healthy. In addition, since the person with a disability may be seen as representing a "failure" of modern medicine and health care

(Matthews, 1983), there is no place for her or him in a book that promises people that they can attain health. The common attitude that disability and health are incompatible was expressed in its extreme by a faculty member who questioned the affirmative action statement in a position description for a health education faculty member; he wanted to know if encouraging "handicapped" people to apply was appropriate for a *health* education position.

Looking at the issue of health education and disabilities, it should be clear that it is easier for able-bodied people to be healthy, so more energy should be put into helping people with disabilities maximize their health. Able-bodied people often have more access to exercise, to rewarding work (economically[3] as well as emotionally), to leisure activities, and to health care facilities. Health care practitioners receive very little training about health issues relating to disability (self-care, sexual health), though they may receive information about specific pathologies, such as multiple sclerosis or muscular dystrophy. The inability to see, hear, or walk need not be the impairments to health they often are considered in our society. Health education is an obvious place to begin to change the societal attitudes toward disability that can help lead to poor physical and emotional health for disabled people. Health textbooks could present possibilities for change by showing ways that both disabled and able-bodied people can maximize health, and this could be done in both the text and the photographs. For example, one of those color chapter openers could include people with disabilities as healthy people. This might mean changing some of the representative "healthy" activities, such as windsurfing. While there are people with disabilities who participate in challenging and risky physical activities, there is no need for pressure to achieve *beyond* what would be expected of the able-bodied.[4] Showing a range of healthy activities that might be more accessible to both the physically disabled and the less physically active able-bodied would be appropriate.

Fat People

There are no fat people in the healthy-image photographs. Some people who agree with the rest of my analysis may here respond, "Of course not!" because there is a common assumption in our society that being thin is healthy and that any weight gain reduces health. In fact, evidence shows that being overweight (but not obese) is *not unhealthy*. In many cases, being very fat is a lot healthier than the ways people are encouraged to attempt to reduce weight—from extreme low-calorie diets, some of which are fatal, to stomach stapling and

other surgeries (Norsigian, 1986). In addition, dieting does not work for 99 percent of dieters, with 95 percent ending up heavier than before they started. Repeated dieting stresses the heart, as well as other organs (Norsigian, 1986). Our national obsession with thinness is certainly one factor leading to an unhealthy range of eating behaviors, including, but not limited to, bulimia and anorexia. While health textbooks warn against dangerous diets and "eating disorders," and encourage safe, sensible weight-loss diets, they do nothing to counter the image of thin as healthy.

Defining which people are "fat" in photographs is obviously problematic. In doing so, I am giving my subjective interpretation of what I see as society's definition of ideal weight. The photographs I have identified as "fat" are of people who by common societal definitions would be seen as "needing to lose weight." In the United States most women are dissatisfied with their own body weight, so are more likely to place themselves in the "need to lose weight" category than to give that label to someone else of the same size.

Not counting people who were part of a crowd scene, I found 14 photographs that clearly showed people who were fat. One appeared in a chapter on the health care system with a caption referring to "lack of preventive maintenance leading to medical problems" (Carroll & Miller, 1986, p. 471), one in a chapter on drinking, and one under cardiovascular problems. The remaining 11 appeared in chapters on weight control or diet and nutrition. Of the 11, one was the "before" of "before and after" weight-loss photographs. One showed a woman walking briskly as part of a "fat-management program" (Mullen, Gold, Belcastro, & McDermott, 1986, p. 125); that was the most positive of the images. Most of the photographs were of people doing nothing but being fat or adding to that fat (eating or cooking). Three of the photographs showed women with children, referring by caption or topic heading to causes of obesity, either genetic or environmental. Only 3 of the 11 photographs were of men. In these photographs, it seems we are not being shown a person or an activity, but a disease—a disease called obesity that we all might "catch" if we don't carefully follow the prescriptions for health. Fat people's excess weight is seen as their fault for not following these prescriptions. This failure results from a lack of either willpower or restraint, as implied by the photographs that show fat people eating and thus both draw on and lend support to the myth that fat people eat too much. The only health problem of fat people is seen as their weight; if that were changed, all other problems would presumably disappear. As pointed out earlier, the health problems of losing excess weight, particularly in the yo-yo pattern of weight loss/gain, may be greater than those created by the extra weight. In addition, the emotional and mental health problems caused by our society's fatphobia may be more serious than the physical problems (Worcester, 1988). These texts strongly reinforce fatphobia by validating it with health "science."

Health educators who consciously work against racism and sexism should carefully reevaluate how our attitudes help perpetuate discrimination against all groups. As Nancy Worcester (1988) points out,

> The animosity towards fat people is such a fundamental part of our society, that people who have consciously worked on their other prejudices have not questioned their attitude towards body weight. People who would not think of laughing at a sexist or racist joke ridicule and make comments about fat people without recognizing that they are simply perpetuating another set of attitudes which negatively affect a whole group of people. (p. 234)

An alternative approach would be to recognize that people would be healthier if less pressure were put on them to lose weight. Fat people can benefit from exercise, if it is accessible and appropriate (low impact aerobics, for example), without the goal needing to be weight loss (Sternhell, 1985). Photographs of "not thin" people, involved in a variety of activities, could be scattered throughout the text, and the pictures of those labeled obese could be eliminated completely. We all know what an obese person looks like; we do not need to have that person held up as a symbol of both unhealthiness and lack of moral character.

Old People

The healthy-image photographs show people who appeared to be predominantly in their teens and twenties, which is the age group toward which these college texts would be geared. Rather subjectively, as with the issue of weight, I will describe as old[5] those who appear to be about 65 or older. Obviously I probably judged incorrectly on some photographs, but since the representations seem to be skewed toward the young or the old, with the middle-aged not so prominent, my task was relatively easy. I identified 84 photographs that contained people I classified as old. Of these, 52 appeared in chapters specifically on aging or growing older, 10 appeared in chapters on death and dying, and the remaining 22 were distributed in a wide range of topics. Of these 22, several still focused on the issue of age. For example, a photograph of an old heterosexual couple in a chapter entitled "Courtship and Marriage" is captioned, "While some people change partners repeatedly, many others spend their lifetime with a single spouse" (Carroll & Miller, 1986, p. 271). One text showed a similar photo

and caption of a heterosexual couple, but also included an old gay male couple on the next page (Levy, Dignan, & Shirreffs, 1987). This represents an important step in terms of deghettoization of gay and lesbian images, and a broadening of views about sexuality and aging. Two photos showed old people as "non-traditional students;" another depicted a man running after recovering from a stroke; and yet another featured George Burns as a representative of someone who has lived a long life. In others of the 22, the age is incidental, as in a man painting (mental health), people shopping in an open market (nutrition), people walking (fitness), a man smoking.

As the societally stereotyped *appearance* of health diminishes, as occurs with aging, it is assumed that health unavoidably diminishes. In fact, while there is some inevitable biological decline with age, many health problems can be averted by good nutrition, exercise, and preventive health care. Many of the health problems of aging have economic, rather than biological, causes, such as lack of appropriate health insurance coverage (Sidel, 1986). In a society that is afraid to face aging, people may not be able to accept that they will experience the effects of aging that they so carefully avoid (if they are lucky enough to live that long). In addition, as with disability, the people who may need to do more to maintain health are those being most ignored.

It is significant that these texts have sections on aging, which contain many positive images, but it is also crucial that health be seen as something that can be attained and maintained by people of all ages. The attempt to include representations of aging in these books must be expanded so that people of all ages are seen to be able to be healthy—a state now seemingly, in those images of health, to be enjoyed only by the young.

Urban Setting

The healthy-image photographs showing outdoor scenes are situated at the beach or in other nonurban settings; it is possible some were set in city parks, but there are no urban markers in the photographs. Bike riding, running, kicking a soccer ball, playing volleyball can all be done in urban settings, though the hang gliding and sky diving would obviously be difficult. Considering the high percentage of the U.S. population that lives in cities (and the numbers of those that cannot easily get out), it seems that urban settings should be represented in the texts. Of the 28 other photographs I identified as clearly having urban settings, I could see only 4 as positive. Two of these showed outdoor vegetable/fruit markets, one showed bike riding as a way of both reducing pollution and getting exercise in the city, and one showed a family playing ball together. Of the rest, 9 appeared in chapters on the environment, with negative images of urban decay, smog, and crowded streets; 10 were in chapters on mental health or stress, showing scenes representing loneliness, stress, or anger, such as a crowded subway or a potential fight on a street corner. Drinking and drug chapters had two urban scenes: "skid row" alcoholics and an apparently drunk man unconscious on the street. There were also three urban scenes in sexuality chapters—two of streets with marquees for sex shows and one showing a "man 'flashing' Central Park" (Payne & Hahn, 1986, p. 348).

There is a clear message that it is unhealthy to live in the city. While this is partly true—that is, the city may have increased pollution of various kinds, specific stresses, less access to certain forms of exercise, and other problems—there are healthy ways to live in a city. One of the roles of health education should be to help us recognize healthier options within the limits imposed on us by economic or other factors. Rather than conveying the message that urban dwelling inevitably condemns people to ill health (unless they can afford to get away periodically to the beach or the mountains), scenes showing health within the city could be presented.

Options for positive images include scenes of outdoor activities in what are clearly city parks, people enjoying cultural events found more easily in cities, gardening in a vacant lot, or a neighborhood block party. Urban settings are excellent for representing walking as a healthy activity. City dwellers are more likely to walk to work, to shopping, and to social activities than are suburbanites, many of whom habitually drive. Urban walking can be presented as free, accessible, and healthy in terms of exercise, stress reduction, and reducing pollution. More indoor activities could be shown so that the external environment is not seen as a determinant of "healthy" activity. These might give a sense of the possibilities for health within what otherwise might appear to be a very dirty, dangerous, stressful place to be.

Work and Leisure

The healthy-image photographs I analyzed were all associated with leisure activities, so I tried to establish how these texts represent work in relationship to health. For this analysis, all photographs of health care workers were excluded, since these are used predominantly to illustrate health or medical issues. Of the 16 other photographs showing people at work, 4 were related to discussions of sex roles and women doing nontraditional work (phone "lineman," lawyer). This seems part of a positive trend in textbooks to reduce sexism. An obvious next step would be to show women in nontraditional work

roles without commenting on them, as is done with a number of photographs of women as doctors. Six of the photographs of work accompany discussions of stress. Besides stress, there are no illustrations of health hazards at work except for one photograph of a farm worker being sprayed with pesticides. Three positive references to work show someone working at a computer (illustrating self-development), a man in a wheelchair doing carpentry, and an old man continuing to work.

Overall, the number of photographs representing work seems low, considering the amount of time we put into work during our lifetime. Blue-collar work is represented by trash collectors in an environmental health section, police officers in a weight control chapter, firefighters under stress, a construction worker in the opener for a stress chapter, the farm worker mentioned above, and women in nontraditional work. Blue-collar work is seen in terms of neither potential health hazards beyond stress nor the positive health aspects of working. The strongest connection between health and work presented involves the stress of white-collar jobs (symbolized by a man at a desk talking on the phone). The message seems to be that health is not affected by work, unless it is emotionally stressful.

The photographs in this book seem to be aimed at middle-class students who assume they will become white-collar workers or professionals who can afford leisure activities, both in terms of time and money. Those who work in obviously physically dangerous jobs, such as construction work, or in jobs that have stress as only one of many health hazards, are rarely portrayed. These people are also likely not to be able to afford recreation such as hang gliding (and also might not need the stimulus of physical risk taking if their job is physically risky in itself). These photographs serve to compartmentalize work as if it were not part of life and not relevant to health.

Rather than selecting photographs that reinforce the work-leisure split and the alienation of the worker from work, editors could include photographs that show the health rewards of work and the real health risks of a wide variety of work. For example, a photograph of a group of workers talking on a lunch break could be captioned, "Many people find strong support networks among their co-workers." Another photograph could be of a union meeting, illustrating that work-related stress is reduced when we have more control over the conditions of our work. In addition the mental health benefits of a rewarding job might be emphasized, perhaps in contrast with the stress of unemployment. Health risks, and ways to minimize them, could be illustrated with photographs ranging from typists using video display terminals to mine workers. A very important addition would be inclusion in the healthy-image photographs of some representation of work.

Conclusion

The definition of health that emerges from an examination of the healthy-image photographs is very narrow. The healthy person is young, slim, white, physically abled, physically active, and, apparently, comfortable financially. Since these books are trying to "sell" their image of health to college students, the photographs presumably can be seen as representing people whom the students would wish to become. Some students, however, cannot or may not wish to become part of this vision of the healthy person. For example, students of color may feel alienated by this all-white vision. What may be most problematic is that in defining the healthy person, these photographs also define *who can become healthy*. By this definition many are excluded from the potential for health: people who are physically disabled, no longer young, not slim (unless they can lose weight, even if in unhealthy ways), urban dwellers, poor people, and people of color. For various social, economic, and political reasons, these may be among the least healthy groups in the United States, but the potential for health is there if the health care and health education systems do not disenfranchise them.

The healthy-image photographs represent the healthy lifestyle, not in the sense of the lifestyle that will help someone attain health, but the white, middle-class, heterosexual, leisure, active lifestyle that is the reward of attaining health. These glowing images imitate common advertising representations. An ice chest of beer would not be out of place next to the volleyball players on the beach, and a soft drink slogan would fit well with the windsurfers or sky divers. It must be remembered, however, that while college students may be the market for beer, soft drinks, and "health," they are not the market for textbooks. Obviously, the biggest single factor affecting a student's purchase of a text is whether it is required. The decision may also be based on how much reading in the book is assigned, whether exam questions will be drawn from the text, its potential future usefulness, or its resale value.

The market for textbooks is the faculty who make text selections for courses (Coser, Kadushin, & Powell, 1982). While the photographs may be designed to create in students a desire for health, they are also there to sell health educators the book. Therefore, health educators should take some time examining the representations in these texts, while questioning their own definitions of who is healthy and who can become healthy. Do they actually wish to imply that access to health is limited to young, white, slim, middle-class, physically abled, and physically active people? If health educators are committed to increasing the potential for health for *all* people, then the focus should not be directed primarily at those for whom health is most easily attained and maintained. Rethinking the images that represent health may help restructure health educators' goals.

It is an interesting exercise to try to envision alternative healthy-image photographs. Here is one of my choices for a cover photograph: An old woman of color, sitting on a chair with a book in her lap, is looking out at a small garden that has been reclaimed from an urban backlot.

Acknowledgments   I would like to thank Nancy Worcester, Julie D'Acci, Sally Lesher, and Elizabeth Ellsworth for their critical readings of this chapter and their valuable suggestions.

Notes

1. Cars appear in health textbook photographs primarily in the context of either environmental concerns or the stresses of modern life.
2. Occasionally, photographs used were actually taken for advertising purposes. For example, in a chapter on exercise there is a full-page color photograph of a runner with the credit "Photo by Jerry LaRocca for Nike" (Insel & Roth, 1988, p. 316).
3. Examining the wages of disabled women can give a sense of the potential economic problems: "The 1981 Census revealed that disabled women earn less than 24 cents for each dollar earned by nondisabled men; black disabled women earn 12 cents for each dollar. Disabled women earn approximately 52 percent of what nondisabled women earn" (Saxton & Howe, 1987, p xii).
4. "Supercrip" is a term sometimes used among people with disabilities to describe people with disabilities who go beyond what would be expected of those with no disabilities. It should not be necessary to be a one-legged ski champion or a blind physician to prove that people with disabilities deserve the opportunities available to the able-bodied. By emphasizing the individual "heroes," the focus shifts away from societal barriers and obstacles to individual responsibility to excel.
5. I am using "old" rather than "older" for two reasons that have been identified by many writing about ageism. "Older" seems a euphemism that attempts to lessen the impact of discussing someone's age, along with such terms as senior citizen or golden ager. The second point is the simple question: "Older than whom?"

References

A list of references is available in the original source.

Appendix: Textbooks Examined for This Chapter

Carroll, C., & Miller, D. (1986). *Health: The science of human adaptation* (4th ed.). Dubuque, IA: Wm. C. Brown.

Dintiman, G. B., & Greenberg, J. (1986). *Health through discovery* (3rd ed.). New York: Random House.

Hales, D. R., & Williams, B. K. (1986). *An invitation to health: Your personal responsibility* (3rd ed.). Menlo Park, CA: Benjamin/Cummings Publishing Company.

Insel, P. M., & Roth, W. T. (1988). *Core concepts in health* (5th ed.). Mountain View, CA: Mayfield Publishing.

Levy, M. R., Dignan, M., & Shirreffs, J. H. (1987). *Life and health.* (5th ed.). New York: Random House.

Mullen, K. D., Gold, R. S., Belcastro, P. A., & McDermott, R. J. (1986). *Connections for health.* Dubuque, IA: Wm. C. Brown.

Payne, W. A., & Hahn, D. B. (1986). *Understanding your health,* St. Louis: Times Mirror/Mosby.

Treating Disease with a Famous Face

by Alex Kuczynski

A publicist from a big agency with corporate clients called on a hunch.

"This might be a long shot," she said. "But this is the hot new disease."

Everybody who is anybody has I.B.S., she said, rattling off names: a comedian, an actress, a celebrity couple. Even John F. Kennedy, whose diagnosis was just made, posthumously.

And I.B.S. stands for?

"Irritable bowel syndrome," the publicist said. Lynda Carter—an actress perhaps best remembered as Wonder Woman in the 1970's—was to be the new celebrity spokeswoman for the syndrome.

And so a few days later, there was Ms. Carter, addressing a luncheon at a Midtown Manhattan hotel about, well, constipation. "Sometimes people go two, three, four days, without. . . ." she said, then squeezed a toothy, anxious smile onto her face.

An expectant silence followed. Ms. Carter, who as a superheroine wore golden wristlets that magically deflected bullets, coughed and sallied forth.

"I mean, if Bob Dole can talk about his penis. . . ." she added, sounding helpful.

She was right, of course. In America, there is scarcely any disorder, no matter how lowly, that has not had its image enhanced thanks to a celebrity spokesman. Anemia and its cures have been championed by Danny Glover, rheumatoid arthritis by Kathleen Turner and bladder control by Debbie Reynolds. Rare syndromes have found spokesmen in Ben Affleck (ataxia-telangiectasia) and Rob Lowe (febrile neutropenia).

The public does not always understand that many of these celebrity champions are paid players in the marketing strategies of pharmaceutical companies, who pull the strings to make them dance before the public and news media. Ms. Carter is on the payroll of the Novartis Pharmaceuticals Corporation, which markets an I.B.S. drug. Mr. Dole, of course, was hired by the maker of Viagra.

While attaching a celebrity to a disease can motivate sufferers to seek treatment or lead to more research financing, the arrangements are ethically complicated, medical experts say. Last summer, CNN and ABC adopted polices to assure that viewers are told of celebrities' ties to drug companies after stars like Ms. Turner and Lauren Bacall spoke of their ailments on news programs without mentioning they were paid.

Despite the networks' bearing down, the practice continues and the relationship between stars and sickness has evolved further, affecting both the public's perceptions of treatment and financing for research. Dr. Arthur Caplan, the director of the Center for Bioethics at the University of Pennsylvania, said the relationship between celebrities and disease has become so cozy that he is now supervising a study of the impact on drug sales and public health.

The celebrity-disease partnership is a natural, if undesirable, signal of the continuing transformation of health care from a profession run by doctors and scientists to one run by marketers, he said.

"We have handed it off to the M.B.A.'s, who in positioning competing companies say, "Hey I remember that marketing class I took at Wharton; I bet we can get a leg up with a celebrity,'" Dr. Caplan said. "If Swifty Lazar had called up pharmaceutical companies 20 years ago and said: 'Hey, I've got a stable of celebrities; want some?' the pharmaceutical companies would have looked at him as if he were completely insane."

If Swifty Lazar, the legendary Hollywood talent agent, were alive today, he might be Barry M. Greenberg, the chairman of Celebrity Connection, a Los Angeles firm that specializes in hooking up Hollywood stars with pharmaceutical companies. Mr. Greenberg maintained that any celebrity, no matter how famous, is available to endorse a drug for almost any disease, no matter how unpleasant, for a price.

"The joke around here is, 'If someone is willing to pay off the debt of the Vatican Bank, I can get the pope to do a commercial for them,'" he said.

Amy Doner Schachtel, the president of Premier Entertainment Consulting, which competes with Mr. Greenberg's firm, arranged the marriage between Ms. Carter and Novartis.

She would not say how much Ms. Carter was paid, but fees for similar alliances can range from tens of thousands of dollars to $1 million, said Ms. Doner Schachtel, who has helped arrange paid deals for Mr. Lowe and Mr. Glover.

"Sometimes they are paid for a one-day appearance and sometimes they are paid for 20 days over the course of a year," Ms. Doner Schachtel said. "So the fees obviously vary."

Ms. Doner Schachtel, who has been linking celebrities with drug companies since 1996, maintains a database of stars and diseases. In the case of Ms. Carter, she spent months calling agents before finding a celebrity with a suitable connection to irritable bowel syndrome; Ms. Carter's mother has I.B.S.

During Ms. Carter's New York luncheon, attended mostly by members of the press, she said at least three times, "I am not promoting any specific drug."

But it was a problematic notion. Although Ms. Carter did not mention a drug by name, she discussed a specific kind of I.B.S.—I.B.S. with constipation in women patients—for which the only drug on the market, Zelnorm, is made by Novartis. (I.B.S. is defined by gastroenterologists as a collection of symptoms that includes abdominal discomfort, like bloating and gas, with either diarrhea or constipation, or an alternation of the two.)

Gregory Baird, the vice president for communications of Novartis, saw nothing wrong in the use of celebrities to market health care. "In the end, I think we're better if we can still find the Lynda Carters of the world who can say, 'Women, here is permission to talk about what you have,'" he said.

Dr. Lawrence J. Brandt, the chief of gastroenterology at Montefiore Medical Center, said that Zelnorm relieves symptoms of constipation-predominant I.B.S., but that it should be prescribed only for women. Too few men were included in the clinical trials to determine its effectiveness, he said, adding, "It's a good drug."

Celebrity affiliation can, at times, attract much needed attention. Katie Couric, the co-host of "Today," has helped to raise about $20 million for colon cancer research since the death of her husband, Jay Monahan, in 1998. She has done so without remuneration from a corporate partner.

However, even when stars are not paid, their association with a medical condition might not always be in the public's best interest, said Jeff Stier, the associate director of the American Council on Science and Health, a nonprofit organization that studies public health and financing issues. Mr. Stier pointed out that Julia Roberts testified in May before the House Subcommittee on Labor, Health and Human Services Appropriations about Rett syndrome, a developmental disorder that occurs most often in infant girls, leaving them unable to control their movements. Ms. Roberts, who was invited to testify by Representative Steny H. Hoyer of Maryland, had befriended a young girl who suffered from the disease and later died.

The actress asked the subcommittee for $15 million for the National Institutes of Health for research, five times current financing. The institute's decision has been delayed until January, said Kathryn Kissam, a spokeswoman for the International Rett Syndrome Association.

While Ms. Roberts may have brought attention to a rare disease—and donations from CNN and C-Span viewers who might not have otherwise heard of Rett syndrome—the money might have been better directed to a more common illness, Mr. Stier said.

"My underlying view is that when celebrities give of their time, that is always a good thing," he said. "However, I am concerned that all too often, because of the way our political system and our society work, that celebrities sometimes play too great a role in directing limited resources for public health."

Dr. Caplan, the medical ethicist, is supervising a study of celebrities' impact on research financing and consumer drug use.

Celebrities, he said, often want to raise money for so-called orphan diseases. "And that is wonderful," he said. "But the science may not yet be there to treat a certain form of Alzheimer's in quite the same way it is there to treat, say, diarrhea in third-world Africa."

"You could save a lot of lives with simple vaccinations, with oral rehydration in Africa," he continued. "But the celebrity fund-raisers don't care. It is not wrong to raise that money. But someone on the political or foundation or even university side ought to say, 'Thank you, Mr. Celebrity, and you ought to give us a little discretion.'"

Ms. Doner Schachtel said: "People can be skeptical of the celebrity angle. But the reality is that Americans listen to celebrities, not the medical expert who is unknown to them. How else are you going to get the word out so effectively on public health issues?"

Yet there is always the risk that celebrities' endorsements will backfire. Two years ago, Ms. Doner Schachtel found an earlier spokeswoman for I.B.S., Camille Grammer, the wife of Kelsey Grammer of "Frasier."

Appearing on "Today" two years ago with his wife and discussing her I.B.S. condition, Mr. Grammer said,

"We can't basically make a lot of plans because you never know when an episode might come on."

At the time, the Grammers were being paid by Glaxo Wellcome as part of a public awareness campaign. Later that year, the company brought out an I.B.S. drug, Lotronex. But it was withdrawn from the market in November 2000 after being linked to severe gastrointestinal side effects and patient deaths.

Last month, the drug's maker, now GlaxoSmithKline, reintroduced Lotronex, which is specifically for women with diarrhea-predominant I.B.S., with restrictions.

Ramona DuBose, a spokeswoman for the company, said that the Grammers had been paid by the company, but that they were not recommending any drug treatments at the time. "Theirs was an effort to raise public awareness," Ms. DuBose said.

And as long as bowels are irritable, it appears that there will always be a celebrity to spearhead the cause. No disease has a stigma so severe that it cannot be overcome by compensation, said Mr. Greenberg of Celebrity Connection.

"There are some things that are yucky and problematic, like eczema and seborrhea," he said. "But there are other things that we thought were taboos that our former presidential candidate waded right into. And celebrities will do anything if the price is right." He paused thoughtfully, then added: "Do you know any celebrities? Some of them are poor."

Mr. Greenberg said he could only think of one disease that would be difficult to pair with an eager celebrity.

"I don't think we'll see genital warts in my lifetime," Mr. Greenberg said.

Manufacturing Need, Manufacturing "Knowledge"

by the National Women's Health Network Writing Group (Adriane Fugh-Berman, M.D., Cynthia Pearson, Amy Allina, Jane Zones, Ph.D., Nancy Worcester, Ph.D., Mariamne Whatley, Ph.D., and Charlea Massion, M.D.)

Several major medical journals recently announced a jointly created policy to refuse to publish research sponsored by pharmaceutical companies unless the researchers involved were guaranteed scientific independence.[1] While laudable, such a move addresses only a tiny part of a pervasive problem: pharmaceutical companies influence almost every piece of information available to doctors and consumers. Consumers may be totally unaware of the diverse ways that their health care providers have been influenced by pharmaceutical companies and medical device manufacturers; practitioners themselves may not be aware of how their ideas and "education" on drug treatments have been manipulated by the companies that sell these products.

Ersatz or Co-opted Consumer Groups

Ads are reinforced by educational campaigns that appear to be independent but are also paid for—and influenced by—the same companies. Companies seek out—or even invent—nonprofit groups and offer them money to do specific educational campaigns that they believe will help sell their products. These decoy organizations produce and distribute educational materials under their own name, and consumers can't tell who wrote the text or who paid for it. One example is a series of fact sheets on women's health produced by the Coalition of Labor Union Women and paid for by Eli Lilly. The fact sheets cover a range of health issues including menopause, cancer, osteoporosis and heart attack. It's surely no coincidence that Eli Lilly's drug Evista has been promoted (often misleadingly) as having potential uses for all of those health problems.

Sometimes these fact sheets are accurate and well balanced, and sometimes they are simply thinly disguised advertisements. What matters is that a health issue is raised as a concern that appears to be coming from an independent group concerned only with promoting women's health, rather than a corporation bent on making a profit. This is a particularly pernicious strategy because it undermines consumer trust in groups that were created to work for the public interest.

The NWHN surveyed women's health organizations, including disease-specific organizations (such as the Arthritis Foundation and the American Heart Association) that influence policy for substantial segments of the female population. Fifty-one of 80 groups that were approached responded. Ten of 17 professionalized women's health organizations (run by clinicians or researchers) acknowledged financial support from companies that provide services or products to their constituencies. The National Alliance of Breast Cancer Organizations (NABCO), for example, lists over 50 sponsors in its annual report; Bristol Myers Squibb, a major manufacturer of chemotherapy drugs, contributed over $100,000 to NABCO in 1996. Five professionalized organizations accepted no corporate donations, and two receive money from industries that do not have a direct financial interest in their issues.

Grassroots organizations (consumer-run) were less likely to accept industry donations; 19 of 31 (61.3%) grassroots organizations received no money from industry, and four (13%) accepted non-compromising corporate donations. Three provided no financial information, and five (16.3%) (four of them disease-specific) accepted donations from companies whose business interests intersect with the health issues of their constituencies.

News Stories

When you opened up your Sunday paper and read in a *Parade* magazine cover story that supermodel Lauren Hutton calls estrogen her favorite beauty secret, did you know that she is a paid spokesperson for Wyeth Ayerst, manufacturer of the biggest-selling estrogen (and in fact biggest-selling drug)? This is just one example of the ways that drug companies spend money to influence consumer opinions about their products.

Drug companies are working to influence every source of consumer health information, including the actual news. In addition to traditional press releases and press conferences announcing the results of new studies

or the launch of new products, companies now produce what look like actual news stories in the form of video news releases and sample articles, which television and radio stations, newspapers and magazines can broadcast or print directly. This tactic is very effective. In one survey, every one of more than 100 television news stations surveyed had used some part of a video news release. While responsible journalists will not use the company-sponsored materials without putting them in the context of a fuller story, they are still putting the company's materials, and importantly the product name, in the news and into the minds of their viewers and readers. When Pfizer launched Viagra, more than 210 million viewers saw some part of the company's video news release.

Even when reporters decide on their own that a new study is worth covering as news, they don't always do a good job of covering the story in a way that's useful for women. Reporters may take the company's promotional materials at face value, presenting beneficial findings in the most positive light and down-playing or ignoring entirely any potential risks. For example, a study that reviewed 70 news stories about positive new findings about Merck's osteoporosis drug Fosamax found that barely 50 percent mentioned adverse effects, and 70 percent quoted experts or studies with a financial tie to the company (only a third pointed this out to the viewer or reader).[2]

Websites

Websites have quickly become a critical source of health information for consumers. Like any other information source, information on the Web is subject to influence by corporate advertising efforts. For example, *womensorganizations.org,* a website that presents itself as a source of information on important women's health issues sponsored by a coalition of national women's groups, is paid for in part by a grant from Eli Lilly. Even though the Web is a new source of information, women need to be aware that it is just as subject to influence as any other and in some cases is more so since regulatory oversight procedures have not yet been established.

New Drug Campaigns

When a new drug is launched, pharmaceutical companies often mount an all-out assault on all these fronts. The goal of these efforts is to make sure that consumers hear about the new drug as often as possible, and always in the most positive terms possible. The more control the companies have over consumer information sources, the better they like it.

Before Merck launched a campaign for its osteoporosis drug Fosamax, it gave a large grant to a leading consumer group for older women with the explicit understanding that the grant would be used to "educate" older women with the message that they should worry about osteoporosis. Merck obviously hoped that this investment would raise the level of women's concern about the strength of their bones. To reinforce this concern, Merck began running direct-to-consumer ads featuring frail older women in pain contrasted with vivacious, active seniors in control of their lives, and used text to imply that medication was needed to prevent disability.

Next, Merck took this newly created fear and concern on the part of older women and translated it into action. They began marketing bone density testing, first by making it more available, then by making it more affordable.[3] Even before Fosamax was approved, Merck purchased a small company that manufactured bone density testing equipment and expanded its production, so that many more bone density machines were available.[4] Merck also gave the National Osteoporosis Foundation a large grant to promote a toll-free number through which consumers motivated by supposedly independent educational campaigns could find the location of nearby bone density screening.

And because bone density screening isn't cheap, Merck added a final piece to its campaign, a public policy initiative to persuade the federal government to pay for bone density screening tests through Medicare. This component of the campaign was replicated at the state level targeting private insurers.

Having successfully frightened women into worrying about bone strength and to get that strength measured, Merck had created the perfect environment to sell its product. Every component of its campaign contributed to sales of Fosamax, the only non-hormonal drug approved at the time for osteoporosis prevention. Yet, the vast majority of women affected by Merck's effort would never know the true motivation for that information, much less who paid for it.

This article is excerpted from *The Truth about Hormone Replacement Therapy: How to Break Free from the Medical Myths of Menopause* (National Women's Health Network, Prima Publishers, Rosedale, California, 2002). $15.95, $10.95 for Network members. Available in bookstores and on the Network's website *(www .womenshealthnetwork.org).*

References

1. Okie S. *Washington Post,* August 5, 2001, A1.
2. Moynihan R, Bero L, Ross-Degnan D et al. "Coverage by the news media of the benefits and risk of medications." *New England Journal of Medicine* 1999; 342(22):1645-50.
3. Tanouye E. "Merck's osteoporosis warnings pave the way for its new drug." *Wall Street Journal,* July 28, 1995.
4. Sherwood L. Presentation to FDA Radiological Devices Panel meeting, May 17, 1999.

AMSA's PharmFree Campaign

The pharmaceutical industry has ramped up its spending on marketing dramatically over the past few years. In 2000, according to IMS Health, the pharmaceutical industry spent $13 billion, more than 10 cents of every prescription dollar, on marketing and promotion to health providers contributing to the astronomical prescription costs our patients must bear.

On the wards, we are often expected to attend pharmaceutical company sponsored "educational" conferences. Research has shown that these conferences are associated with learning and disseminating inaccurate information, and with inappropriate prescribing.

AMSA PharmFree Timeline

Jan 2002: *Excerpt from President's Column*

March 2002: *AMSA House of Delegates passes groundbreaking no free lunch association policy*

April 2002: *AMSA President and Executive Board draft Model Oath and launch Revitalizing Professionalism Campaign*

There Is No Such Thing as a Free Lunch

As medical students, we must advocate for better professionalism training and in particular resist the penetration of medical education by the pharmaceutical industry. To this end, we would like to announce the AMSA Pharm-Free Campaign to educate and train our members to professionally and ethically interact with the pharmaceutical industry.

The Rx Industry and Persephone

Persephone was the beautiful daughter of the ancient Greek goddess Demeter. As the story goes, Hades, Lord of the Underworld, kidnapped her and brought her to his lair in Hell, guarded by Cerberus, the three-headed dog. While she was in captivity, she wisely refused the gifts and jewelry Hades lavished upon her to win her favor; but out of hunger, she said yes to six pomegranate seeds. When she was liberated and returned to her mother, Hades protested and pointed out that she had accepted the seeds. Though she was a cheap date, she had let him pay for dinner and thus she "owed him something." To repay her debt, she was required to live with Hades as his wife in the realm of the dead for six months out of the year, and she was forever dubbed "Queen of the Underworld."

It's hard to blame Persephone, the poor thing. And you may even identify with her on days when you feel like a prisoner in the hospital, wandering through the halls of an Underworld you still can't believe you willingly entered. You are starving, but there is no one to liberate you. You must go to the noon conference; your attending and your team are waiting for you and would notice your absence. You arrive at the noon conference and there at the gate is Celebrex, a three-headed dog, and his master, Steven, a smiling drug representative

from Pennsylvania. You peek through the gate and see the greatest wonders that Hades has to offer-a delicious meal complete with brownies. Steven holds something out to you; it's the key to the Underworld, in the shape of a pen bearing the name of his dog. "Why not?" you ask yourself.

There are those who say there has been no new information in the world since 800 B.C. There have been numerous studies done to prove what the ancient Greeks knew all along—"There is no such thing as a free pomegranate seed." Since we can't defend our positions with ancient wisdom alone, I encourage you to visit www.nofreelunch.org. After clicking on "Required Reading," you will find studies that demonstrate that accepting gifts and hospitality from pharmaceutical companies affects prescribing patterns to the benefit of the drug company (because you prescribe more expensive drugs than you would otherwise) and often to the detriment of the patient.

The drug industry tells us that the cost of their drugs is high and rising because they spend so much on research and development (R&D). The truth is that the actual amount spent on promotion is much higher than the amount spent on R&D. Rising drug costs are responsible for a good portion of the increase in health-care spending in the United States. There is a correlation between the rising costs and the money spent on promotion: Just four categories of drugs accounted for 31 percent of the $42.7 billion increase in drug costs form 1993 to 1998. These include seven of the 10 drugs most heavily advertised to consumers in 1998.

I encourage you to take the pledge on the "No Free Lunch" Web site. I know it's not easy, but it will liberate you and your patients from the Underworld. If you have already taken from Hades, no worries-you can still participate in the Pen Amnesty Program, as directed by the site. I also encourage you to come to AMSA's 52nd Annual Convention during March in Houston, Texas, where, among other exciting opportunities, you can meet Dr. Bob Goodman, the internist behind the "No Free Lunch" campaign (see p. 33 for more information about the convention). Good luck! See you all in Houston!

Those Omnipresent Prescription Drug Ads
What to Look Out For

Turn on the TV, pick up a magazine, pass a bus shelter. You're bombarded with prescription drug advertising. Keep the following in mind the next time you think a prescription drug ad appears convincing:

- Ads are not about educating the public; they're about marketing a product. Anyone trying to sell you something isn't going to give you the most balanced picture of the product's effectiveness and risks.

- You are being sold the newest—and therefore, the most expensive—drug of its kind. New is not necessarily better. Pharmaceutical companies need only prove that their drug is better than a placebo; they are not required to prove that it is any better than older, less expensive drugs for the same condition.

  Taking a new medication on a long-term basis is like going into uncharted territory. Most drug trials last only a few months, at best. It takes years and a broader level of usage than usually found in clinical trials before adverse interactions and rare side effects can be identified.

- Notice how unusual it is for an ad to tell you what percentage of people showed improvement taking the drug during clinical trials. This is because many of the most heavily promoted drugs are only moderately effective.

- Much of the advertising dollar goes to "me too" drugs, designed to cut into the market share of a competing blockbuster medication. Think Zoloft and Prozac, Vioxx and Celebrex, Pepsi and Coke.

- If an ad tells you that a drug cuts your risk by 50%, always ask "50% of what?" Daily aspirin cuts the risk of heart attack by 50%. Look carefully at the study results, you might find that halving the risk is less than meets the eye. For example, a five-year study showed that heart attacks occurred in 1% of the participants taking aspirin, as compared with 2% of those taking the placebo.

- Be aware that an ad's graphics alone can be misleading. No one looks sick in these ads. You'll see men with AIDS hiking up mountains and elderly people with osteoarthritis running around with their grandchildren. One might get the impression that a cure has been found for AIDS, osteoarthritis, and chronic pain in general.

- The next time you see an ad featuring a happy woman walking along the beach, be on the alert for a weight loss drug. Notice that the drug's efficacy is contingent upon cutting calories and regular exercise.

- Ads need not be pre-screened for accuracy by the Food and Drug Administration (FDA), though drug manufacturers may voluntarily submit ad copy to the agency beforehand.

- The FDA has issued over 90 warning letters to drug companies about misleading ads in the last year alone. You can learn the names of the offending companies and why the FDA acted by visiting the agency's web site (www.fda.gov), click on drugs, and continue to "Warning Letters and Notice of Violation Letters."

- Once the FDA has been alerted that a pharmaceutical company is running a misleading ad, it takes the agency about six months to verify the charge. Then, the offending company is allowed another six months grace period before retracting the ad. Drug companies usually change their ads yearly anyway.

- A drug company incurs no penalty for having run a misleading ad. In rare circumstances, the company may be required to run a corrective ad.

- The few studies exploring the effect of pharmaceutical promotional activities aimed at physicians show that they can be seriously misled. If they can be fooled, why not us?

- Don't take a drug without reading about it first. Ask for the labeling information from the pharmacist. Go to the local library and consult *The Physicians' Desk Reference.* And for your home library, buy *The Essential Guide to Prescription Drugs 2001* by James J. Rybacki, Pharm.D, and James W. Long, MD, and *Worst Pills, Best Pills* by Sidney M. Wolfe, MD, Larry D. Sasich, Pharm.D, Rose-Ellen Hope, R.Ph, and Public Citizen's Health Research Group.

How to Read a Drug Ad

Fear mongering is the subtext of many of the prescription drugs ads you see on TV and in print. These ads might just as well come out and say: OK, you're healthy now, but any time in the near future you can die from a heart attack, cancer, or hip fracture. The surest route to high profits is the expensive drug that must be taken daily for years, preferably for life, out of fear of a disease that might create symptoms 10, 20, 30 years down the road.

Many of the ads play on fears of aging. Middle-aged people (with the necessary drug-coverage) are the natural targets. It helps to read these ads skeptically because many are riddled with half-truths. Here are some representative examples of the different approaches to advertising prescription drugs to the public. All are bound by the rules of the Food and Drug Administration (FDA).

Sell Fear of the Disease

"Osteoporosis—Could you be at Risk" This is the headline of the current ad campaign sponsored by Eli Lilly, which does not mention its osteoporosis drug, Evista (generic name: raloxifene). Anytime the drug *and* its purpose appears in an ad, then the side effects and adverse reactions must also be included. But Eli Lilly's ad illustrates another option in drug advertising. Instead of identifying its drug, a company can choose to sell the dangers of a given disease, in this case, osteoporosis. Ads like this one must list an 800 number that will generate a free packet of information and your name on the company's mailing list for life.

"Up to half of women over age 50 will break a bone due to osteoporosis in their lifetime. And the risk increases when menopause ends," warns the Eli Lilly ad, which features a fiftyish woman. The statement is true, but choosing the age of 50 as the cut-off is guaranteed to instill fear. The following statements are not found in the ad, but they are also true: A woman's odds of having an osteoporosis-related hip fracture between the ages of 50 and 70 are low. Half of all hip fractures in women occur after the age of 80.

Years ago, the diagnosis of osteoporosis was made only after the person experienced a fracture due to thinning bones. Now, the definition of osteoporosis has changed to simply mean low bone mass. In other words, what was once a risk factor for fracture is now a disease. Susan M. Love, MD, author of *Dr. Susan Love's Hormone Book,* writes that the panel of experts that changed the definition of osteoporosis was funded in part by pharmaceutical companies.

Sell a Test

"See how beautiful 60 can look? See how invisible osteoporosis can be?" This is the headline for Merck's ad, featuring an older woman. It's a good example of the indirect approach to selling drugs: Encourage people to go for testing and invariably you will create many new customers for your drug. Several years ago, Merck announced that it had entered a financial agreement with a major bone density measurement equipment company, in order to get these expensive machines into as many doctor offices as possible.

Merck does not mention its osteoporosis drug, Fosamax, in this ad which simply advises, *"Ask your doctor if a bone density test is right for you."* It almost comes across as a public service announcement. To prompt the hesitant women into action, Merck adds, ominously, *"The fact is, if you're 60 or older, there's a nearly 1 in 2 chance you have osteoporosis."* Yes, this statement is probably true given the above, expanded redefinition of the "disease." However, there is a debate among osteoporosis researchers about the value of measuring bone density because the test can't predict who will eventually have a fracture. Some evidence indicates that bone turnover may be more relevant, but there is no available test for it.

Name the Drug . . . and Its Side Effects

HIGH CHOLESTEROL ISN'T JUST A NUMBER IT'S A WARNING. The message screams out from Bristol-Myers Squibb's ad for its cholesterol-lowering drug, Pravachol (generic name: pravastatin sodium). This represents the type of ad that identifies the drug and its purpose ("protect your heart"), so it must also list side effects and adverse reactions. In the case of a print ad, the side effects appear in tiny type on the next page. Surveys show that few people read the fine print, and this includes doctors.

The ad emphasizes the Pravachol's safety because a competing cholesterol-lowering drug, Baycol, was withdrawn last summer after it caused 31 deaths. The ad attempts to get the people who just went off Baycol to: *"Ask your doctor to tell you more about high cholesterol, the risk of heart attack, and if Pravachol is right for you."*

The safety claims in this ad are: *"Pravachol is no more likely to cause side effects than a placebo (sugar pill) in landmark clinical studies."* Well, yes, that's true, but only the people who turn the page and read the fine print will learn that this refers solely to the FDA-required trials that lasted only four months. Most people who take cholesterol drugs do so indefinitely, and the fine print has 16 lines of side effects experienced by drug-treated people in the longer trials that lasted five to six years.

The long list of side effects was attributed to the entire class of "statin" drugs, which includes Pravachol (pravastatin) and Baycol (cervistatin), Mevacor (lovastatin), and Zocor (simvastatin). The 31 deaths attributed to Baycol were due to a rare condition called rhabdomyolysis, which causes a breakdown of muscle tissue. All statin drugs have this rare risk, according to *The Medical Letter* (9/10/01), a physician publication with no drug advertising.

Name the Drug, But Not the Condition

This is the strangest approach to drug advertising because it mentions the name of a drug but not what it's for. This type of ad circumvents the FDA-requirement of listing side effects once the drug's purpose is identified. It is best exemplified by Schering-Plough Corporation's ads for Claritin, a drug for seasonal allergies. They usually feature a close-up of a young woman's face against a bright blue sky and often some flowers in the background. The message is simply: "Ask your doctor about Claritin."

Claritin stands as a testament to the power of advertising and as a classic example why a drug doesn't have to be any good to become a big seller. Schering-Plough spent a record $136.8 million advertising Claritin directly to consumers in 1999 alone. It paid off. Claritin is the most profitable antihistamine of all time, with annual sales of more than $2 billion, according to *The New York Times*. A month's supply costs about $85.

Claritin is no more effective than older, cheaper antihistamines. Its much-touted advantage is the lack of drowsiness that comes with other antihistamines. Two FDA-required trials showed that Claritin is better than a placebo, but not much better. At 10-milligram doses, Claritin was only 11% more effective than a placebo. Taken at higher, more effective doses, the drug causes drowsiness.

End-Run Around the FDA

TV ads are generally bound by rules similar to those of print ads. In 1997, however, the FDA relaxed the rules for broadcast advertising where it concerns side effects. From that year on, only the major side effects had to be mentioned in radio and TV ads that name the drug and its purpose. This accounts for the massive increase in TV ads for prescription drugs.

But some major side effects can be a major turn-off, and that has led to some creative bending of the FDA rules. And this is best illustrated by Roche's ads for Xenical, a weight-loss drug. How many people would run out and ask their doctors for Xenical after hearing that anal leakage is a common side effect?

Roche has found a way to avoid this information with its two-part TV commercials for Xenical. The first ad does not mention Xenical; it simply shows quick images of a baby growing up to be a heavy-set women while describing excess weight as unhealthy. The second ad names the drug but not the condition, using the same background music and images. By separating the two ads with brief unrelated commercials, Roche has circumvented FDA rules about describing side effects. The ads appeared early this year, and thus far, no warning letter to Roche from the FDA has appeared on the agency's Web site.

What to Consider When Reading a Drug Ad

- Many ads leave the impression that everyone who takes the drug will benefit from it. You will want to know how effective the drug has been proven to be in terms of, say, reducing heart attacks, fractures, or cancer recurrences, etc. Rarely, will a drug ad ever provide this crucial information. Consult the *Physicians' Desk Reference,* which is available at most community libraries. It can also be purchased at most chain bookstores. The book is difficult to read, but it is the only readily available source of data concerning what has been proven in drug trials and how long the trials lasted.
- Avoid taking any newly approved drug when there is an alternative. The pre-approval studies required by the FDA usually last only a few months and do

not include enough participants to uncover rare side effects. In the last decade, a number of prescription drugs have been withdrawn within five years of becoming available due to life-threatening side effects. This has led many consumer advocates to advise people to wait at least five years from the date of release before taking any new drug. This also allows time for follow-up studies to determine whether the new drug is truly an improvement over the older versions of the same medication.

- These ads are increasing the cost of health care for everyone. The 50 most-advertised prescription medicines contributed significantly last year to the increase in the country's spending on drugs, according a new report. It also found that these 50 drugs accounted for almost half of the $20.8 billion increase in drug spending last year. The report was prepared by the National Institute for Health Care Management, a nonprofit research foundation. Only the drugs still under patent, and therefore expensive, are advertised directly to the public.

- Drug ads are not checked by the FDA for accuracy beforehand, though drug companies are free to do so voluntarily. This occurs infrequently. Instead, the ads are pulled only after complaints are made and verified. This usually takes about six months, and the drug company is given several additional months grace period. Companies whose ads are judged to be misleading will receive a warning letter that is published on the FDA Web site. Offending drug companies incur no penalty for misleading the public. They are merely told to withdraw the ad. Many drug companies change their ads every six to 12 months anyway. On rare occasions, a company may be required to run a corrective ad.

- Go to the FDA's Web site (www.fda.gov). You will find a wealth of information about drugs, as well as dietary supplements (herbs and vitamins). On the home page alone, you can go to "Safety Alerts" and see the latest recalls; "Product approvals" for information about the new drug approvals; "How to Report a Problem to the FDA;" and "Drug Information" for standard labeling facts, such as side effects, purpose, warnings for specific drugs.

WORKSHEET — CHAPTER 3
Gender Roles, Sex, and Marketing

1. Demonstrate that you have an understanding of the differences between biologically determined sex differences and socially/culturally determined gender differences by filling in one or more examples on this table:

	Male/Masculine	**Female/Feminine**
Biologically determined sex differences		
Socially/culturally influenced gender differences		

2. For characteristics listed on this chart (and for others you think to add) identify whether that characteristic is more associated (accepted or expected) for one gender or the other and whether *in general* that characteristic is valued or devalued by society.

	Associated with women more than men	**Associated with men more than women**	**Valued**	**Devalued**	**Comments**
passive					
aggressive					
independent					
dependent					
stable					
easily excitable					
strong					
weak					
competitive					
non competitive					
always knows answer					
OK not to know answer					
cares ~ things more than people					
cares ~ people more than things					
earning $ very important					

	Associated with women more than men	Associated with men more than women	Valued	Devalued	Comments
other things more important than $					
hides emotions					
shows emotions					
other					
other					
other					

3. Because gender roles are socially/culturally influenced, what is considered masculine or feminine may change from one historical moment to another or from one country to another. Can you think of an example of this?

4. In what ways is it as dangerous for women to say "Women are more nurturing than men" as it is for people to say that "Men are better at certain things"?

5. A long time peace activist has said, "A prerequisite for being president of the USA should be that a person has to be a mother before they can be president." Describe your reaction to this statement and problems with such statements.

6. Check below which strategies you think are likely to help improve the role of women in society.

_____ Trying to eliminate differences between sexes/genders
_____ Trying to make men more like women
_____ Trying to make women more like men
_____ Making it possible for both men and women to explore both masculine and feminine sides of themselves
_____ Trying to make society value a much wider range of characteristics and behaviors

Briefly comment on why you made the choices you made:

7. Compare the messages girls and boys in your family received about "appropriate" and "inappropriate" behavior for their sex. When were girls praised for feminine behavior? for masculine behavior? Were boys ever praised for feminine behavior?

8. Many people observe that there is more social acceptance for girls acting like tomboys than there is for boys demonstrating "sweet", "sensitive", "doesn't like to fight" behaviors. Explain why this might be.

9. The authors of articles on intersex people want doctors to say to parents of babies with genitals that don't conform to male or female, "Your child is intersexual, in other words, neither a boy nor a girl. There are resources available to help you raise your child in a healthy way. Go home and love your child as you would any other." Identify ways a community and parents could be educated to better prepare for intersex individuals and think of very practical suggestions (i.e., single stall, gender neutral bathrooms) to make life easier for intersex people.

10. After reading "The Picture of Health," describe alternative healthy image photographs which you would like to include if you were designing a health textbook.

11. Collect several drug ads or ads related to health issues aimed at women as consumers from popular women's magazines. Compare what you find with the issues raised in articles in this chapter.

12. Collect several ads about women's health issues/products from medical journals aimed at health practitioners. What messages/stereotypes do the ads give to practitioners about women as consumers?

13. **Male and female physical fitness:** If average untrained college-age men and women are tested for physical fitness, the men are likely to appear to be more fit, particularly in the area of strength. These results fit with the assumption that many make that women naturally have less physical potential than men. However, exercise physiologists find very different results. For example, men tend to have greater strength in both upper (back, arms, shoulders) and lower body, but when the measurement is adjusted relative to body weight, the differences in lower body strength disappear. When untrained men and women begin to do weight-training, the women often progress much faster because they are farther below their potential. Androgens are needed for muscle proliferation, so the fact that the average woman has lower levels of androgens than the average man means there is some limit on her muscle bulk. However, this does not mean much in terms of strength limitation since women can increase greatly in strength without "bulking" (muscles increasing in size). Right now we have no idea what the strength capability of women is since women are so undertrained in terms of strength.

Women have a great capacity for developing endurance. Leading women marathoners can beat all but the best male runners and would, in fact, have won many past Olympic men's marathons with their current times. Women do even better in relation to men in ultra marathons (50 to 100 miles). Women hold many long-distance swimming records and compete directly with men.

When boys and girls are tested for physical performance, they are matched up to ages 10 to 12. In fact, girls are often faster than their male classmates in elementary school. After age 12, boys increase in strength and cardio-vascular fitness more than girls. Exercise physiologists believe these differences may be social rather than biological in origin. It is not hormones that make women weaker but social and cultural processes.

a. Untrained males and females show little difference in lower body strength but larger differences in upper body strength. Show how this situation might arise by examining the activities from early childhood through adulthood that males and females might engage in that are likely to develop upper or lower body strength.

b. Differences in physical performance between males and females generally first appear around puberty. What are the changes in physical activity around puberty that might affect this? What are social and cultural messages that may limit girls' activities at puberty? Compare your own forms of exercise before and after puberty.

c. How does the definition of woman as "weaker" limit women's lives? Examine such issues as work, recreation, and safety. Who benefits from the definition of women as weaker?

CHAPTER 4

Menstruation

We begin this chapter with the classic, "If Men Could Menstruate" by Gloria Steinem. Besides demonstrating that feminists *do* have a sense of humor, this enjoyable, popular article really sets the framework for this chapter. Indeed, it is often the first article discussed in our women's health courses because it so perfectly sets a theme to be addressed throughout the semester: when there are inequalities in a society, everything associated with the valued group will be valued and anything connected with the less valued group will be less valued.

The normal physiological process of menstruation has been defined and redefined by male "experts" throughout history. It has been labeled a disability or illness, as a barrier to higher education for women, as a weakness that justified keeping middle-class women from working outside the home (working class women were expected to continue their work). Later, menstrual cramps were identified as psychogenic in origin, brought on by the fear of femininity or sexuality. Now hormonal fluctuations are blamed for a wide range of symptoms premenstrually, from acne and water retention to depression, homicidal behavior, and self-mutilation. Readers interested in more background on the changing meanings of menstruation are referred to two articles which appeared in earlier editions of this book: "Women, Menstruation, and Nineteenth Century Medicine" by Vern Bullough and Martha Voght, in the excellent *Women's Health in America* edited by Judith Walzer Leavitt, puts the changing definitions and meanings of menstruation within their historical contexts, while at the same time addressing a recurring theme in medical history—"the reluctance of physicians to accept new scientific findings"—and Louise Lander's thought-provoking *Images of Bleeding: Menstruation as Ideology* examines what the social sciences say about the meaning of menstruation, concluding that the meanings will always change because menstruation will always be one aspect of what it means to be a woman in a given cultural and historical context.

An entire volume (Volume 46, numbers 1 and 2, January 2002) of the journal *Sex Roles* is devoted to new research on menstruation which was presented at a 2001 conference of the Society for Menstrual Cycle Research (SMCR). Yes, there is an entire organization devoted to the study of menstruation and menstruation-related issues! SMCR is an excellent example of the changing face of science as more women have opportunities to become scientists and as women—as both scientists and activists—ask for different types of questions to be pursued in scientific research (See SMCR web-site: *www.pop.psu.edu/smcr*).

"Blood and Milk: Constructions of Female Bodily Fluids in Western Society" (see Chapter 11, p. 511) provides a theoretical overview of how the meanings of menstruation/menstrual blood are constructed in Western societies. The voices of women describing their own socialization and experiences of menarche come through in the article "Menarche and the (Hetero) Sexualization of the Female Body" as Janet Lee summarizes 40 narratives about menarche from women ages 18-80. She concludes, "While women internalize negative scripts with the bleeding female body, they also respond with consciousness and resistance: . . . What is crucial here is that this juncture, menarche, is a site where girls become women and gender relations are reproduced. Such relations are about power and its absence; power to define the body and live in it with dignity and safety: power to move through the world with credibility and respect. May this be our futures."

"Female Adolescence: Puberty and Growing Up" describes the history of the discovery that the average weight of girls (whether they mature early or late) at menarche is approximately 103 pounds because a critical, minimum amount of body fat is required before the body is capable of reproduction. This chapter could stimulate discussions on important issues related to what it means that young women's age of menarche and potential pregnancy is so related to body fat composition (the average age of menarche today is 12.6-12.8 years compared to 14.7 years in 1880). Rose Frisch's book, *Female Fertility and the Body Fat Connection,* from which this chapter is taken, provides fascinating, thought-provoking information on body fat as a crucial factor in determining a woman's fertility. In addition, the reader is treated to one woman's personal story of the rewards of being a scientist.

The economics of menstruation is a useful reminder of an overall theme in women's health: there is a huge market and much money to be made any time a company can sell something to groups of healthy women. The worksheet on menstrual products requires the calculation of the financial costs of menstruation related products for one woman in her lifetime. Any reader who multiplies that figure by the number of menstruating women will see the dollar signs which tempt companies to get a piece of the menstruation product market. Since women went "off the rag" and began using disposable menstruation products, there has been a large profitable business in tampons, napkins, and pads. While these are products most women want to keep on the market, the competition and profit motives sometimes mean that consumer health and safety receive minimal attention. The most obvious example was the Rely super absorbent tampon, marketed by Proctor and Gamble, which was associated with toxic shock syndrome deaths in the late 1970's and 1980. Now that toxic shock syndrome (TSS) is no longer in the headlines and in women's magazines, we are concerned that young women (TSS mainly strikes menstruating women under age 30 using tampons) are not learning what they need to know to protect themselves from products (high absorbency products) or circumstances (leaving a tampon in for many hours) which increase risks of TSS. "Don't Just Go With the Flow," from *Teen Voices,* is an excellent example of the type of women's health information which should be available to all women, not just the young women lucky enough to subscribe to this magazine which works to be an alternative ("Because you're more than just a pretty face." Web-site = teenvoices.com) to mainstream teen magazines. This article manages to critique the menstrual products available in most grocery stores and pharmacies, introduce a range of menstrual products which are safer for women's bodies and the environment, encourage a campaign to get natural feminine hygiene products more widely distributed, give a "herstory" of menstrual products, provide information on toxic shock syndrome, and introduce readers to web-sites on natural menstruation products.

When any product will be marketed to large numbers of healthy women, safety standards for that product must be extremely high. We end this chapter with a favorite classic, "The Selling of Premenstrual Syndrome" by Andrea Eagan, which both introduces the topic of premenstrual syndrome (see also Chapter 5) and provides an analysis for critiquing the increasing number of products which are getting to the market and hyped to women and their practitioners (see articles on advertising in Chapter 3 and articles on hormone replacement therapy in Chapter 12) before their long term safety has been studied/proven. This article uses PMS to symbolize the "double-edged sword" women and women's health activists face more generally when we ask that women's health issues be taken seriously: we want good scientific research and health system response to the health issues which affect us, but we do not want these issues to be medicalized or used against women. The words of Andrea Eagan seem as urgent today as they were when they were written in 1983:

> To suddenly discover that thousands of women are rushing to get an untested drug to cure a suspected but entirely unproven hormone deficiency . . . is a little shocking . . . I'm ashamed to see women flocking to use an untested substance about which there is substantial suspicion, whose mode of action is not known, to treat a condition whose very cause is a mystery.

These 1983 words bring us full circle to new examples of the concept that meanings of menstruation will always change because menstruation is always one aspect of what it means to be a woman in changing cultural and historical contexts. In articles alarmingly similar to Eagan's classic PMS article, the next chapter explores the marketing of mood altering drugs for the treatment of Premenstrual Dysphoric Disorder which has not even been proven to exist. With Seasonale (the new packaging of birth control pills so that women have "menstruation" just 4 times a year) being brought onto the market just as this book goes to press, readers are encouraged to watch how the marketing of Seasonale represents society's views of menstruation . . . and women.

If Men Could Menstruate—
A Political Fantasy

by Gloria Steinem

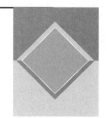

A white minority of the world has spent centuries conning us into thinking that a white skin makes people superior—even though the only thing it really does is make them more subject to ultraviolet rays and to wrinkles. Male human beings have built whole cultures around the idea that penis-envy is "natural" to women—though having such an unprotected organ might be said to make men vulnerable, and the power to give birth makes womb-envy at least as logical.

In short, the characteristics of the powerful, whatever they may be, are thought to be better than the characteristics of the powerless—and logic has nothing to do with it.

What would happen, for instance, if suddenly, magically, men could menstruate and women could not?

The answer is clear—menstruation would become an enviable, boast-worthy, masculine event:

Men would brag about how long and how much.

Boys would mark the onset of menses, that longed for proof of manhood, with religious ritual and stag parties.

Congress would fund a National Institute of Dysmenorrhea to help stamp out monthly discomforts.

Sanitary supplies would be federally funded and free. (Of course, some men would still pay for the prestige of commercial brands such as John Wayne Tampons, Muhammad Ali's Rope-a-dope Pads, Joe Namath Jock Shields—"For Those Light Bachelor Days," and Robert "Baretta" Blake Maxi-Pads.)

Military men, right-wing politicians, and religious fundamentalists would cite menstruation ("*men*struation") as proof that only men could serve in the Army ("you have to give blood to take blood"), occupy political office ("can women be aggressive without that steadfast cycle governed by the planet Mars?"), be priests and ministers ("how could a woman give her blood for our sins?"), or rabbis ("without the monthly loss of impurities, women remain unclean").

Male radicals, left wing politicians, mystics, however, would insist that women are equal, just different, and that any woman could enter their ranks if only she were willing to self-inflict a major wound every month ("you *must* give blood for the revolution"), recognize the pre-eminence of menstrual issues, or subordinate her selfness to all men in their Cycle of Enlightenment.

Street guys would brag ("I'm a three-pad man") or answer praise from a buddy ("Man, you lookin good!") by giving fives and saying, "Yeah, man, I'm on the rag!"

TV shows would treat the subject at length. ("Happy Days": Richie and Potsie try to convince Fonzie that he is still "The Fonz," though he has missed two periods in a row.) So would newspapers. (SHARK SCARE THREATENS MENSTRUATING MEN. JUDGE CITES MONTHLY STRESS IN PARDONING RAPIST.) And movies. (Newman and Redford in "Blood Brothers"!)

Men would convince women that intercourse was *more* pleasurable at "that time of the month." Lesbians would be said to fear blood and therefore life itself—though probably only because they needed a good menstruating man.

Of course, male intellectuals would offer the most moral and logical arguments. How could a woman master any discipline that demanded a sense of time, space, mathematics, or measurement, for instance, without that in-built gift for measuring the cycles of the moon and planets—and thus for measuring anything at all? In the rarefied fields of philosophy and religion, could women compensate for missing the rhythm of the universe? Or for their lack of symbolic death-and-resurrection every month?

Liberal males in every field would try to be kind: the fact that "these people" have no gift for measuring life or connecting to the universe, the liberals would explain, should be punishment enough.

And how would women be trained to react? One can imagine traditional women agreeing to all these arguments with a staunch and smiling masochism. ("The

ERA would force housewives to wound themselves every month": Phyllis Schlafly. "Your husband's blood is as sacred as that of Jesus—and so sexy, too!": Marabel Morgan.) Reformers and Queen Bees would try to imitate men, and *pretend* to have a monthly cycle. All feminists would explain endlessly that men, too, needed to be liberated from the false idea of Martian aggressiveness, just as women needed to escape the bonds of menses-envy. Radical feminists would add that the op-

pression of the nonmenstrual was the pattern for all other oppressions ("Vampires were our first freedom fighters!") Cultural feminists would develop a bloodless imagery in art and literature. Socialist feminists would insist that only under capitalism would men be able to monopolize menstrual blood. . . .

In fact, if men could menstruate, the power justifications could probably go on forever.

If we let them.

Menarche and the (Hetero) Sexualization of the Female Body

by Janet Lee

Menarche—or a woman's first menstrual period—is a central aspect of body politics. Through explorations of oral and written narratives, I suggest that girls' subjective sense of themselves as maturing women at menarche develops simultaneously with a process of sexualization whereby young women experience themselves as sexualized, and their bodies are produced as sexual objects. While women internalize negative scripts associated with the bleeding female body, they also respond with consciousness and resistance.

In high school I wanted to be a beatnik. I too wanted to go on the road, but I could never figure out what would happen if, travelling in Mexico in 1958, I got my period. Were you supposed to carry a supply of Kotex with you? How many could you carry? If you took all you needed, there wouldn't be any room for all those nice jugs of wine in Jack Kerouac's car. The only beatnik I know who even considered this question was Diana diPrima in Memoirs of a Beatnik. She describes her first big orgy, the one with the works, including Allen Ginsburg. As she takes a deep breath and decided to plunge in, so to speak, she pulls out

her Tampax and flings it across the room where somehow it gets irretrievably lost. A grand moment, that. Do I hear you thinking, How gross? Or, How irrelevant? Gross, yes: irrelevant, no. And that's the point. Having to worry about the gross mess becomes a part of life from puberty on. (Dimen, 1986)

Menstruation is a biological act fraught with cultural implications, helping to produce the body and women as cultural entities. The body is a "text" of culture; it is a symbolic form upon which the norms and

Janet Lee, *Gender and Society,* Vol. 8, No. 3. Copyright © 1994. Reprinted by permission of Sage Publications, Inc.

AUTHOR'S NOTE: *This article and ongoing project have been funded by the Oregon Council for the Humanities, a fellowship at the Center for the Humanities at Oregon State University, and by grants from the Research Office and the College of Liberal Arts at Oregon State University. I would especially like to thank my research assistants, Alida Benthin, Jennifer Sasser-Coen, Sindy Mau, and Tamara Schaub, for their help with interviewing, as well as all the women who so graciously shared their memories of menarche.*

practices of society are inscribed. Male desire and policy have been scripted onto the female body at the same time that "woman" has been overdetermined and over-represented in contemporary art, social science and politics, as well as scientific and medical discourses. In this article I share stories of the body in an analysis of the menarche (or first period) experiences of ordinary women who participated in an ongoing oral and written history project. It is primarily through the body that women are inserted, and insert themselves, into the hierarchical ordering of the sexual.

I explore menarche as a central aspect of body politics since it is loaded with the ambivalence associated with being a woman in Western society today. Menarche represents the entrance into womanhood in a society that devalues women through cultural scripts associated with the body. Overwhelmingly, messages associated with menarche in a wide range of cultural and historical contexts are ambivalent. Even those women who have reflected on this experience with positive thoughts and memories have been found to articulate its negative and shameful aspects. To talk of menstruation in contemporary Western culture is to articulate its secretive, emotionally laden, and shame filled aspects.

Within patriarchal and heterosexist societies menarche simultaneously signifies both emerging sexual availability and reproductive potential. While I do not suggest that sexuality and reproduction must be, or have always been, conflated, to focus on menarche is unavoidably to deal with both. In terms of sexuality, the process of sexualization whereby women experience themselves as sexualized in current Western society is a thoroughly heterosexual one; the use of sexuality as a generic term implying heterosexuality illustrates the normalizing powers of language. Sexualization implies heterosexualization, meaning that women are taught to live and discipline their bodies in accordance with the prescriptions of heterosexuality, experiencing themselves as sexual objects for heterosexual male viewing, pleasure, and also as mothers of men's children. As Thorne suggests: "it is during the transition from 'child' to 'teen' that girls start negotiating the forces of adult femininity, a set of structures and meanings that more fully inscribe their subordination on the basis of gender." I emphasize that menarche symbolizes this process, and must therefore be framed within the discourses of the heterosexual, emphasizing its importance in the relationship between reproduction and sexuality generally.

While women's bodies are produced discursively within misogynist societies, women's everyday experiences negotiating adolescence are concretely lived in ways that not only internalize and maintain such discourses, but also actively resist them through appropria-

tion and/or the integration of more positive discourses of the body. While, as Smith suggests, women are always located in a particular configuration of the everyday, "the standpoint of women never leaves the actual," this "actual" involves the negotiation of subject positions through discourse and from which women as subjects emerge. Women's thoughts and behavior are grounded in these particular discursive spaces at the same time that their agency to comply with and resist such discourses is recognized. Attention to the discursive formation of the body does not remove agency from the human subject; instead, it problematizes human behavior and emphasizes how individuals negotiate identities and subject positions. Narratives of women's memories of menarche highlight this interactive nature of discourse and agency; when women remember their first menses, their memories are framed by many competing discourses, having become subjects through the sifting and making meaning out of their experiences.

My methodological focus is phenomenological. I explore the meanings women attribute to menarche, what they think and feel, and the significance of this event as represented in what they say and write. I analyzed forty narratives (twenty-eight oral and twelve written narratives), listening and reading for interpretations of menarche embedded within the everyday, lived experience of women. Written narratives were collected when women could not be interviewed in person, but agreed to share written accounts of their menarche. The oral history interviews were conducted either in women's homes or in an office or seminar room, and sometimes in a public space, although the latter occurred rarely. With participants' consent, a tape recorder was used and interviews were then transcribed. Participants were also asked if they wanted to use a pseudonym; most chose to do this, though some preferred to use their real names. Participants were volunteers who had agreed to participate as word of the project spread through presentations made in classes, flyers in a local physician's office, and through contact with colleagues, students, and friends and the Extended Education Office at Oregon State University.

This local sample was Eurocentric, including thirty white women, three Jews, two African Americans, one biracial woman, three Asian Americans, two Mexican Americans, and three women each from Nepal, Malaysia, and Iran. Since three-quarters of the participants were white, reflecting the general lack of racial and ethnic diversity in Oregon, where this study was done, I must emphasize its limitations and the dangers of overgeneralization. The age range spanned from 18 to 80 years. Five women identified themselves as lesbians and three as bisexuals, although none said they identified as such during early adolescence. Nineteen of the participants are working class and twenty-one are middle class, all residing in the Willammette Valley and south and central Oregon.

I suggest here that menarche is an important time when young women become inserted and insert themselves into the dominant patterns of sexuality. As a crucial signifier of reproductive potential and thus embodied womanhood, menarche becomes intertwined with sexuality. Certain orifices and their secretions take on sexual significance and menarche marks a simultaneous entry into adult womanhood and adult female sexualization. I will share excerpts from the narratives to illustrate themes associated with female sexualization at menarche, exploring the ways these women relate to the female body and menstrual blood. I focus on issues of contamination and alienation, and the relationship between menarche, boys, and developing bodies. Finally, I will discuss issues of consciousness and resistance, exploring ways women have coped with menarche in their everyday lives.

Contaminating Bodies

Historically and cross-culturally, menstrual blood has been considered both magical and poisonous, and menstrual taboos have structured and restricted women's lives. Since women are associated with the body, earth, and nature, and men with the abstract powers of reason, women's bodies connote words like *earthy, fleshy,* and *smelly,* reminding humans of their mortality and vulnerability. Dorothy Dinnerstein captures this in her discussion of the deep-seated cultural perceptions of the female body as corrupting, contaminating, unclean, and sinful. On the one hand, woman is associated with life, while on the other, her bleeding and oozing body is met with disgust, reminiscent of earthly vulnerabilities. Male bodies are not so symbolically marked with such connotations; men are more easily able to imagine their bodies free of such constraints, and they are allowed to project their fears and hatred onto women's flesh. Cultural contexts provide mythologies and images of disgust for women's bleeding that are deeply internalized into the psyche, encouraging women to hate their bodies and men to hate things they recognize as feminine in themselves.

Repeatedly, women in this study stated that their monthly bleeding made them feel ambivalent about their bodies, menarche being clouded by negativity. Almost half of the sample specifically mentioned "the curse" as a term they and others had used to describe menstruation. Edith, a 66-year-old mother and grandmother emphasized the gloom associated with menarche:

It's so long ago . . . I guess it was mid-winter, and waking after dozing to sleep, briefly, having had a "funny" tummy ache—to a sticky, nasty uncomfortable feeling between my legs; slightly smelly too, if I really think deeply, ugh. . . . There was this dark, clammy, gloominess and sort of "dread" accompanying it.

Others also stated that their first menstrual blood made them feel dirty and unclean, ashamed and fearful. Bertha, a Jewish woman in her forties, remembered her menarche as similar to "a feeling I used to feel when I was young and wet my pants. . . . It was a feeling of having soiled myself." Such feelings affect women's sense of self and worth, establishing female bodies and sexuality as bad and corrupting. These memories of shame and embarrassment were shared by Northstar, a Chinese American woman in her late twenties who grew up in Taiwan:

I feel I have a big diaper. I feel everyone can see me . . . Very embarrassed. . . . I know sometimes when I went to my uncle's house that sometimes my aunt would forbid my uncle to take garbage out because she said that we have "women's mess" inside so men cannot carry the garbage out because there are women's pads inside.

With similar sentiment, a white working-class woman in her thirties named Anna wrote that she was "mortified," and felt she needed to hide her shame and embarrassment:

When I first started menstruating (the very first time) I had experienced incredible stomach pains the night before. I stayed in bed all night and was the first one up in the morning. I went to the bathroom and lo and behold there was blood. I felt mortified because I knew what had happened. I felt incredibly ashamed and didn't tell anyone for a year (I used tissue paper). Now I was like my mother, a woman who had a bad smelly part of her. This, for the most part, is also how men see menstruation, as something filthy belonging to a woman that makes them mentally unstable

The disdain associated with menstrual blood encouraged many women to go to great lengths to hide such evidence of their contamination from the potentially disapproving gaze of others. There was overwhelming evidence of women's fears of showing evidence of wearing pads or staining garments or sheets. Three-quarters of all women in the sample specifically shared a story of the embarrassment associated with staining, or a fear that it might happen to them. This illustrates how the bulge or stain becomes a visible emblem of their contamination and shame, announcing their "condition" for all to see. It also symbolizes a lapse in women's task of maintaining the taboo, concealing the evidence and preventing the embarrassment of others (Laws 1990). Seventy-four-year-old Laverne shared the following:

> A problem with menstruating at that time was the napkin pads. They were made out of absorbent cotton with a cotton mesh cover (no shields). They soaked through easily and you often stained your underwear. I always worried that my skirt might be stained and would sometimes wear my coat in school all day long. At Girls High, it was the custom for the Seniors to wear all white every Friday. When I was a Junior, I happened to notice that one of the Seniors was wearing a thin white skirt which showed the outline of her sanitary pad so when I had my Senior skirt made I bought rather heavy material and had a double panel put in the back.

Women tended to see themselves as becoming more visible at the same time that they felt the pressure to conceal evidence of menstruation. Many women talked about wearing baggy clothes or coats to hide evidence of menstruation. Other research has also reported such findings, with women sharing feelings of being afraid of being found out with a strong desire to hide any traces of their period. One study found that it was only after several menstrual periods that girls would share their experiences with anyone other than their mothers. Similar results were found here, with several women using tissue and toilet paper for months, or hiding soiled underwear at the back of drawers and closets.

The most intense and poignant stories of contamination came from childhood survivors of violence. Of the 10 women who shared experiences of incest or child sexual abuse, all connected the violation of their bodies to menarche as a contaminating experience and said that they felt their bodies were dirty and shameful. Hannah, a young, white lesbian, spoke poignantly of the way her feelings about her contaminated body as a survivor coincided with her feelings about her menstrual flow:

> The abuse made me feel awful. It colored everything, so much of what I did, how I felt about my body and my self-esteem. . . . I felt really dirty and you know because I was on my period, and I would cramp more and I just felt dirty, I felt icky, I felt horrible, like people could smell me and I just felt subhuman. . . . I felt kind of shameful to be around men and I don't want to be around people and I don't want people to know at all. . . . I hated the feeling of flowing, I hated just that warm feeling whenever. . . . I felt as if it was something dirty, something horrible coming out and I wanted to not flow as much as possible and if I got really active I would flow more and I didn't want to flow. I just wanted it to stop.

Child sexual abuse survivors' words illustrate the way the vulnerabilities associated with women's emerging sexuality (and in these cases, the exploitation of what these little girls' bodies signified in the context of a society that exploits female sexuality) become integrated so that the body becomes and is experienced by girls as something acted upon, used, and soiled.

Alienated Bodies

Many of the women interviewed experienced menarche as something that was happening *to* them, as something outside of themselves and frequently referred to as "it," giving an illusion of a self that was fragmented. Overwhelmingly, women used the passive voice to describe menarche. Examples include: "I couldn't believe it was happening to me," "we called it 'the visitor,'" "I got it when I was fourteen," "I remember exactly when it started," "this monthly event," and (my favorite) "when it came I was at home."

Karin, a 22-year-old white woman, shared the following:

> I mean she [her sister] had no problem with it. I don't know if she was happy about it because she was on good terms with it. . . . I guess I'm not really in control of it because I just felt like it happened to me, I didn't ask for it, it just suddenly happened.

Similarly, Barbara, a 19-year-old lesbian, also clearly illustrates this sense of bodily alienation: "It was unknown and I really didn't understand it and it was something I couldn't control so it seemed kind of abstract and not within me."

With their passive construction and imagery, these quotes suggest a fragmentation between self and body, a sense of menarche as something a woman has to cope with, adjust to, and manage. Menarche is something that seems to appear from outside, invading the self. Such findings were also reported by Martin, who wrote of the women she interviewed as seeing menstruation as something that happened *to* them, rather than seeing the process as being a part *of* them. While she explained this in terms of the medicalization of the female body and the way a scientifically based society produces images of human bodies as machines, I suggest that there is more at work here, since many women framed menarche as happening "to them" in the context of their emerging understandings of sexuality. Charlotte, a white bisexual mother in her late thirties, shared her feelings about this fragmentation and lack of control, illustrating how menarche is intimately connected to feelings about sexual alienation and objectification (the "it" is her first period):

> When it came, I was a high school exchange student in Europe, staying with the family of a friend. I felt like I was out of control, that something was happening to me that I couldn't stop. I bled terribly all over the sheets and was horribly embarrassed telling my friend's aunt (especially since I didn't know the right words, menstruation is hardly one of the common vocabulary words you have to learn). I remember distinctly being embarrassed because this blood seemed like an emblem of my sexuality, like somehow it indicated that I might run out and have sex, yet really I felt like it was all happening to someone else, not me, like I was watching myself in a movie and now was this sexual being.

The passive, indirect, fragmented language of menarche and menstruation is about sexual objectification and alienation. This sense of bodily alienation is entwined with women's object status in patriarchal societies that allow men subjectivity but construct femininity as a mirror through which men see themselves as human. Adolescence and the journey from girlhood to womanhood involve forms of self-silencing whereby girls become preoccupied with how they are perceived by others. Femininity means moving from assertive actor to developing woman, learning to respond to the word indirectly through the filter of relationships. Women are encouraged to accommodate male needs, understand themselves as others see them, and feel pleasure through their own bodily objectification, especially being looked at and identified as objects of male desire. Again, the voice of a survivor, this time Susan, is especially poignant in illustrating this objectification:

> Becoming a woman kind of opened the avenues which I think I unconsciously kind of knew that men would start looking at me more which was, I think, a little bit scary in a sense. I mean I was confused, I think I wanted to be accepted by the male gender, but yet with this experience [incest] it was a frightening thing because, it wasn't even me, it was like my body, and it was happening to my body. . . . It was no longer my mind or who I was, I mean it was like I was nothing. But yet my body was something, a sex object or something and I couldn't have said it. I didn't think that my body was like a sex object. I mean I couldn't clarify what was a

norm, but, to look back now, that is what it was, my body was a sex object and the menstruation process was, just defined it that much more that I was a woman. . . . You know what I am saying? Because I related to the menstrual cycle, I connected it directly with all this. . . . So there is a connection there, one part of me, I wanted to be that woman for the opposite sex, because it was kind of like expected of me, you know, that I be pleasing to look at and starting that menstrual cycle was my direct link with that, wow, I am a woman. But then there is a bad incident that I don't think had a lot of negative influence on that, but yet it must have somehow, you know, been buried there.

Anxious Bodies

Adolescence is a difficult and vulnerable time when girls focus attention on their bodies in the context of a culture that demands perfect female bodies. In a study that asked pre- and postmenarcheal girls to draw pictures of women, Koff found that girls who had experienced menarche drew considerably more sexually differentiated bodies. She writes about how girls come to experience themselves as more sexually mature at menarche: "It appears that regardless of the actual physical changes that are taking place, the girl at menarche anticipates and experiences a reorganization of her body image in the direction of greater sexual maturity and feminine differentiation."

For many women, the increasing focus on their bodies was associated with painful cramps or even severe dysmenorrhea or painful periods. For example, Mehra, a young Iranian woman, spoke of how she noticed her body more at this time: "Yes, I felt like I paid more attention to my body, how it looked, felt, but also about where the pain comes from. . . . I would focus on that because of the pain." Some, like Laurence, a 20-year-old Malaysian student, started tuning into their body at menarche, becoming more self-conscious generally: "Yes, I guess mentally I became more aware of my body and what you would say 'the journey to womanhood,' yeah, and I became more self-conscious when I had my period. . . . I did become more self-conscious."

Others, like Robin, a young, lesbian biracial woman, were aware that other people treated their bodies differently, and felt that this contributed to their interpretations of menarche:

> Then they [her brothers] started becoming critical of the way I dressed, and my hair and the way I spoke . . . And criticizing and saying you need to go over that way and you need to start wearing

skirts and you need to start doing your hair, and you need to care about what you look like and not talk like this or that. So, I think there was a definite change in how they saw me. . . . I think it did set inside their heads "she is woman, I mean she is not a boy. Yeah, she is different, other."

For most women, anxieties about their developing bodies at menarche concerned the way these bodies looked and might be interpreted by others, rather than how they looked or felt to themselves. Breast development seemed especially fraught with such anxiety. When recounting their first period stories, many women described their feelings toward their breasts, emphasizing how menarche is so often framed within the discourse of the sexual. Although enlarging breasts and hips are visual representations of femaleness, they are also highly constituted in our culture as objects of male desire (to be gazed at) and contribute to the experience of menarche as connected to the process of sexualization. As Haug et al. suggest, "female breasts are never innocent." The excerpt below from Madeleine, a white woman in her thirties, illustrates the anxiety and self-consciousness associated with the developing body at menarche; a body that is being increasingly viewed as sexual, and, given the patriarchal context, a body that is becoming increasingly objectified.

> I remember when I was in 6th grade and this boy called me "stuffy," in other words he was accusing me of stuffing my bra, because I wore a sweater that was, you know, more fitted than the day before and I was developing very early as a 6th grader and I didn't like my body at all, in fact I had a breast reduction when I was in 10th grade. . . . But so, I had a lot of hang-ups about that and they were very painful to me and so it just, my boobs were just so big that, I mean, I am still busty and I mean, they are huge and I was a small person and they got in my way (long laugh) and I really hated them. . . . I just remember feeling that I was going to grow up and the only thing that I would be good for was something like a Playboy bunny or something really you know . . . disgusting or just to be a housewife which was like a fate worse than death. . . . So, I guess that maybe that's why I felt so angry about my period because I associated it with these feelings about my boobs, you know.

At menarche, women say that their physical bodies are becoming problematic; women report that their breasts are too small or too big, hips tend to become enemy sites and there is the overwhelming fear of fat. These reports spanned generations as Florence, an 80-year-old Jewish woman, remembered feeling "ugly and fat," just as did 18-year-old Marie, who, when asked how she felt about her body, responded: "I had a really low self-esteem about my physical appearance and stuff . . . It was pretty heavy dislike." Ambivalence is a good word to describe the feeling that many women report since, while many felt okay about their developing bodies (especially in the context of competition with female friends and the relief from the embarrassment that goes along with being undeveloped—of not "measuring up," so to speak), these were accompanied by strong negative experiences of self-consciousness and embarrassment, and the internalization of ambivalence about women's flesh and sexuality. The relationship here between menarche and sexuality is illustrated by several women who commented that friends of theirs whose bodies had developed early were somehow seen as promiscuous, even though they were just young girls with no active sexual relationships. The use of the term "precocious puberty" in the literature to describe girls with early puberty and onset of menarche is also an example of this issue. Robin shares the following:

> Oh, there was one person I knew who had it before any of us you know . . . this is really terrible, but I think that I thought that she was just a little more ahead of us sexually. I am positive the woman wasn't sexual, but I knew that was a part of getting older, and I knew that getting older meant having sex, and I think seeing someone else with their period made me feel that they were a lot further ahead than I was. . . . I am sure they probably weren't having sex, I don't know, but I saw them as more promiscuous.

Bodies and Boys

Women also make a clear association between menarche and changing relationships with boys through the language of the body. Many were distressed that their camaraderie with boys dissipated. They felt they could no longer be "one of the boys" or their friendships became infused with the sexual tensions of early adolescence and its budding compulsory heterosexuality. Barbara, a strong athlete during adolescence, illustrates this:

> Yeah, I think it was in the sense that it [her menarche] separated me from the boys, and so I felt like I was going to have to dress up and just drop sports by the wayside because now it was like some way of being notified that well, you have had your fun as a tomboy but it is time to really do what you are "supposed" to do.

Women worried about what boys might think, if boys noticed them, if they didn't. Sixty-two-year-old Rowena remembered distinctly how her behavior changed. She wrote, "I began to 'be careful' at school, to not act 'too smart' although I continued to get straight A's. That was stupid."

Women remembered being embarrassed around boys, and especially remembered the teasing and crude comments about menstruation. Urmila, in her twenties and raised in Nepal, shared her memories of such teasing:

> Maybe the [boys] don't understand it, so the only way of doing it is by laughing, making fun . . . they just laugh, making it feel for the girls that they do know, so it sort of makes them dominant and makes the girls feel like "oh, my goodness, I have done something wrong."

Women reported that they learned early that they must hide all evidence of menstruation from boys and men, brothers and fathers. This set up a self-consciousness for girls who were used to playing with boys. Crystal, a young, white, bisexual woman, summed this best: "When I didn't have my period I didn't mind playing with the guys, but when I did, I was afraid someone would see me, like something might leak through or things like that."

In terms of potential sexual relationships with boys, the risk of pregnancy that sets in at menarche influences family dynamics. Research suggests that parents tend to see their daughter's emerging sexuality as more problematic than their son's, with early sexual maturation being associated with greater independence and achievement from parents for boys, and to a lesser extent for girls. Hill and Holmbeck found that menarche was accompanied by intense family turmoil for a large number of the girls in their sample, with daughters reporting more parental control in the first six months after menarche than at any other time. The comments of Elizabeth, a white woman in her forties who grew up in a Catholic home with thirteen brothers and sister, is illustrative of this:

> When I hit my adolescent years our relationship [with her mother] really split because my mother all of a sudden was very suspicious of everything I did. . . . I still remember her just all of a sudden, a suspicion about me, maybe I was becoming sexual.

In predictable ways the double standard of sexual conduct plays itself out as boys are encouraged to sow their wild oats and girls are chastised for similar behavior, resulting in closer monitoring. "I was told by my mother that I was a lady now, so that I had to act like one, and not play with the boys anymore," recalled Darlene, a white working-class woman in her forties. She followed this statement with:

> I started to cry, I said "I'm not ready to be a lady and I like playing with the boys." I guessed the reason I couldn't play with them anymore is that they would smell me too and know my horrible secret. I felt dirty, humiliated and angry.

Finally, the remarks of 77-year-old Greta, a widow and retired teacher, illustrate the responsibilities of potential sexual relations that girls have to assume at menarche:

> During the "curse" as we termed it, I was concerned about odor and spotting. My mother made it clear that now necking and petting could have serious results if we went "all the way"—which could happen if emotions got out of hand.

Consciousness and Resistance

To study menarche is to study the female body as it is contextualized through the sociopolitical constructs of specific societies. In this study, the words that women used to describe menarche are those that symbolize the relationship of women to their bodies in a misogynist society: fear, shame, embarrassment, humiliation, preoccupation, mess, hassle, and so on; however, running through these stories are also tales of consciousness, agency, and resistance. Women are not merely acted upon, nor are they merely powerless pawns embedded in the discursive struggles that determine existence. While these discourses do frame the body, the woman in the body does resist, as Martin has suggested. Women show their resistance to the destructive and alienating discourses associated with menarche through insight and analysis, through telling their stories, and through the many ways that women have learned to cope. Some spoke of increasing solidarity with girls, of using menstruation as a way to manipulate and get their way; many spoke of having done or having a desire to do things differently when their own daughters start to menstruate. It is to these forms of consciousness and resistance that I now turn.

Telling the Story

Since this project involved participants who were volunteers, the women's voices I share here are all those who wanted to have the opportunity to tell their stories. Usually, when the tape had been switched off and women were leaving, they would comment on the benefits of speaking about something that they had never really spoken of in any public way before, something that was an important experience in their lives, but which the society in which they lived, as well as academia, has tended to ignore. "I don't know if it's making any real sense, but it is starting to make more sense to me when I talk about it" was a comment often heard.

For many, the telling of their stories took the form of ongoing analysis and commentary on those experiences, speaking or writing with insight into body politics and the effects of those politics on women's everyday lives. Kay, a white mother and student in her thirties, wrote the following, nicely illustrating this consciousness and insightful analysis:

> First, in fifth or sixth grade, at my elementary school, we were separated from the boys and shown a film about menstruation. Next we were given a packet which contained some kind of feminine hygiene products and propaganda. We considered this whole affair hilarious, embarrassing and yet it took the place of what could be considered a puberty ritual for us girls. We never knew what the boys talked about or what they were told about us, reproductively, etc. But I always somehow felt that they had been given some important secret that day, that we, as girls, were not privy to, and that this was just some kind of weird, divisive act on the part of the administration to distract and codify us. I suppose that sounds like a true paranoid at work, or perhaps hindsight talking, eh? But it's true I did feel that way. . . . I also believe that most of what I experienced, or did not experience, were [sic] consistent with much of the cultural conditioning that women receive from the media and the medical establishment.

Many women revealed a form of resistance in the contradictory voices used to tell their stories. Women moved between the anxious, hesitant and fearful disclosure complete with multiple "umms" and "you knows" to the staging of their stories as a series of adventures, gaining control over the experience and framing it in hindsight as ridiculous. In so doing, they claimed control over events, appropriating them and defusing the pain and anguish. This emphasizes the sometimes contradictory ways gender is negotiated, discourses of resistance being crucial components of this negotiation. Virginia, a 38-year-old white student, illustrates this as she jokes about the story of her first period, laughing and describing the event as a funny experience:

> So I was 10 years old and didn't understand any of it. In fact I misunderstood most of it. What I remember about it from the book was that somehow the menstrual blood came out on the outside of your lower abdomen somehow like it seeped through your skin! (Laugh) . . . and so here's the book telling me that these napkins don't show and I'm holding them up to my stomach and saying yeah, right (laugh), that is going to show, you can't tell me that is not going to show. . . . So I told my mother and it was like "oh," she did seem rather pleased but it wasn't like the kind of pleased where if I got a really good grade or you know, gotten the solo in the school play (laugh). . . . She pulls out the Kotex kit and that is when I begin to connect, this is what it is, it doesn't come out of your stomach!

Hannah, an incest survivor, spoke very poignantly about her first menses. Despite her sadness she tells funny stories of menarche, her humor helping her gain control over he pain:

> I saw blood in my underwear and it was like I just sat on the toilet (laugh) and I am like "mom." She comes in and she was like, "What? Well honey, congratulations, you are a little lady now." I am like, "Say what?!!" I was cramping really bad and I was given medication. It was to get me regulated. . . . I remember lying on the floor and my mom, she used to have bad cramps because she had a tipped uterus, so my grandfather used to buy her a pint of alcohol because they didn't have medication then, and she would drink it and she would pass out and she would be out for a day, so my mom gave me some brandy because she thought it would solve it! (Laugh) Well, after I had the brandy I just started to york it, I was throwing up left and right, so it seems like after that time every period I ever had I would throw up!

Acceptance, Coping, and Appropriation

For some women, especially those at midlife and beyond, there was a general sense of acceptance or resignation to the politics of menarche that was apparent in the narratives. I had never thought of this as a form of resistance until I read Emily Martin's discussion of acceptance, lament, and nonaction as a way of responding to women's reproductive restrictions; yet these ways of coping and surviving are important, and they also subvert the masculinist idea of resistance as oppositional action and behavior. When asked about the specifics of their menarche, many women responded with such comments as "people didn't talk about such things back then," "it was just something I had to endure," "that's the way it was back then." The comments of Alex, an 80-year-old white woman, were typical:

> And in those days we didn't have the sanitary napkins we have today, or even now the Tampax and so on, but you always had that laundry to do. That was just not very pleasant, but it was a thing you did. I mean, that was the way it went.

This acceptance did not always take the form of resignation. Many women, such as Yvonne, an African American woman in her thirties, were angry that they had had to endure certain experiences. "I was pissed" was among Yvonne's comments. Some tempered their frustrations with observations such as "Well, that's just the way it was then you see." The important point is that these were survival and coping mechanisms.

Louis, age 73, talked about the hardships associated with menstruation before the onset of disposable sanitary supplies. She remembers being in a tight spot with no menstrual cloths: "I had a jack knife and I cut up one of my blankets for pads and used those." Women of all ages reported using toiled paper, tissue, and underwear to help them hide their bleeding and cope with their first menses. Some hid evidence, some threw it away, some washed it out when no one was around. Many worked out ways to avoid going to a grocery store where they might be recognized, and others modified their clothes and activities to avoid embarrassment.

Many women told stories of using menstruation as a way to manipulate and have some control over situations. A Mexican American woman in her thirties was not alone in sharing how she avoided showers in school by telling the teacher she had her period, and also telling her boyfriend the same to avoid sexual contact. Greta spoke for many as she wrote:

> As far as school was concerned—during Physical Education, we were benched for three days. CLUB members [those girls who had already started their periods] often considered this a plus as we were not required to wear gym attire.

Bonding and Solidarity

Some women found that the experience of menarche helped girls identify and bond with each other, providing support and solidarity. Amy, an African American student and mother, told how she had pretended to have her period for several months before she actually experienced it in order to feel accepted by her friends. She said: "I was happy because I didn't have to lie anymore, now I was one of the girls. . . . It was important for me to be accepted as one of the group, it was a significant event for that reason." Greta, almost 40 years Amy's senior, talked bout how friends who had "joined the Club" were closer and held in a higher regard by other girls. For many women, then, first menses was an ambivalent time; it was framed by negativity, but at the same time, symbolic of maturation, it brought status. This was usually acted out in the context of sisters and peers, where girls wanted very much to be included in the group. As Thorne suggests, the "popular" girls set the stage; if they were perceived as having started their period, then this development was seen as desirable. Since this status is intertwined with their sexual status, it is complex: girls do not want to start too soon and be seen as too advanced or promiscuous, but they do not want to start last and be branded a less mature child. Timing is definitely of the essence.

The importance such a personal event held within girls' groups was illustrated by Robin, who reported that she was obsessed with the idea of starting her period and looked forward to the drama of it all: "Blood would run down your leg and you would have to run out of class!" She was not daunted by this thought and said, "I wanted very much for it to begin at school. . . . Just for the attention I guess. . . . It was a social thing. All my friends were going to get their period and I wanted to be social."

While most girls suffered the embarrassment of menarche alone, some reported how friends had supported and helped them. Laurence, a young Malaysian woman, spoke of the support and solidarity received from friends when she started her period while away at boarding school:

> It was during choir practice, we were just singing and I felt something weird and so a girl said "you have a little stain on your skirt." The girls' side of the choir was really restless and the guys had no idea what was happening. A bunch of girls, about three of them my close friends, escorted me to the bathroom and everything happened, they got me the pads, told me what to do, everything.

Others also talked and wrote about friends and older sisters who helped them figure out what was happening to their bodies, as well as helped them access and use menstrual products. Karin emphasized how she felt closer to her friends after she started her period:

> I think it kind of brought me closer to girls in a certain way because when you talk about things that are

personal it really kind of strengthens your friend-ships I think, and I think it makes it a very intimate friendship. So I realize that [with] some of my girl-friends I was really closer, I felt very close to them.

Changing the Scripts

For many women, the framing of womanhood at menar-che occurred within the context of the complex dynamic of their relationship with their mothers. Scholars have suggested (and the data here certainly support this) that since girls rely on their mothers at menarche, they report either increased conflict or closeness, depending on the relationship and communication patterns before puberty. Mothers often socialize their daughters into the same re-strictions associated with femininity that they have en-dured, ensuring that their daughters will fit into society and maintaining a shared compliance in the develop-ment of a submissive femininity and gendered sexual identity. Girls may grow to resent their mothers for their role in this at the same time that they may fear becom-ing what they perceive their mothers have become; how-ever, there is much evidence here to suggest that these patterns are being disrupted. Many of the women who had negative experiences with their mothers at menar-che also said that they would never want that to happen to their own daughter, and several went on to tell stories of positive experiences of menarche with adolescent children. Nonetheless, several women also emphasized that even though they had prepared their children and made it a positive experience, their daughters still felt some shame and embarrassment. The values of the cul-ture are strong; children are not raised in a vacuum and quickly internalize the negative messages associated with menstruation.

Judy, a Japanese American in her twenties, shared her desire for a better experience for any future daughters:

If I have daughters of my own in the future, I will tell them more positive things about periods, such as that it's not something you should be ashamed of or something dirty. I would make sure that they'll have some knowledge about menstruation before it starts because, when my period started, I didn't have any knowledge why women have [a] period or how it starts or anything.

Ann, a white mother of two daughters and a grand-mother, spoke with regret that she acted very much like her own mother and was not able to give information and help her daughters feel good about their first menses. She is, however, committed to undoing this piece of family history with her granddaughter:

My mother neglected telling me and I neglected telling my girls and I wouldn't want that to happen to my granddaughter . . . Because I wouldn't want it to come from an outside source like from girls at school. I feel that my daughter really should do this, but like I said, if she doesn't I am prepared to do it for her.

Conclusion

Although women's bodies have been the object of dero-gation and admiration, women themselves have not had the power to control how their bodies might look, act, and feel. Menarche is an event that symbolizes both re-productive and sexual potential and centers attention on the body. Since "woman" is overrepresented through the practices and values of sexuality, menarche takes on loaded meanings that have consequences for women and their everyday lives, scripting relations of power into the discourses and practices that surround women's bodies. The women who participated in the study remembered menarche as an important experience and, for most, this experience provoked anxiety, reminding them of their contaminating natures and encouraging them to hide evi-dence of their bleeding, while focusing attention on the sexualized body and changing relationships with others. Bodies are contextualized in a society that devalues and trivializes women; however, while adult women have in-ternalized the stigma and shame associated with having bodies that bleed and all that this entails in terms of re-strictions on body, mind, and soul, they have responded as active agents, and have resisted these discourses through a variety of means. They continue to resist them as they reminisce about their first menses, viewing their experiences retrospectively, framing and reframing them, hoping to neutralize the pain, perhaps taking back their power.

Menarche is a physiological happening, framed by the biomedical metaphors of current scientific knowl-edge, yet also a gendered sexualized happening, a transi-tion to womanhood as objectified other. What is crucial here is that this juncture, menarche, is a site where girls become women and gender relations are reproduced. Such relations are about power and its absence; power to define the body and live in it with dignity and safety; power to move through the world with credibility and respect. May this be in our futures.

References

A list of references is available in the original source.

Female Adolescence
Puberty and Growing Up
by Rose E. Frisch

You may never have heard of the adolescent "growth spurt"—a sudden, rapid growth first in height, then in weight—but if you are grown up, you have had it. A girl's growth spurt always occurs before menarche. In well-nourished populations like that of the United States, girls experience the spurt beginning at about age 9; boys experience it at about age 11.

Some researchers and the media use the word *puberty* to include all the physical changes that happen around and during the time of the growth spurt. Puberty is a rather fuzzy term that can denote the years of rapid adolescent growth, the appearance of secondary sex characteristics such as breast development and pubic hair, and menarche. Instead of using the category "puberty," I will refer separately to the adolescent growth spurt, the first "growing up" event that lasts for about three years; the development of secondary sex characteristics; and menarche, which follows the spurt.

Together with Roger Revelle (former director of the Harvard Center for Population Studies, where I conduct my research), I spent several years in the late 1960s and early 1970s learning about the weight changes that occur in girls during the adolescent growth spurt. (I'll tell you why shortly.) In that phase of the research, we made a new and important finding: menarche was closely related to a "critical" body weight. We were totally surprised at the connection to body weight. I soon found by reading about other species, however, that girls are just like other mammals, including monkeys and apes, in that sexual maturity is more closely related to body weight than to chronological age.

How did we ever come to research something so crude as kilograms of body weight? (A kilogram is equivalent to 2.2 pounds.) I was trained as a geneticist, and Roger was a well-known oceanographer; neither of us had been interested in body weights. We were inspired to look into adolescence and sexual maturation by our studies of body weight that had nothing to do with either topic—a good way to discover something new in science. At the time we were working on a Harvard project to calculate future world food needs. To estimate calorie requirements, you first have to know the body weights of the population you are planning to feed, so I collected body weight data for females and males of all ages, from birth to age 65 and older, from many developing countries.

An Unexpected Finding

Collecting all those body weights was somewhat boring, so I looked for the age of the largest yearly gain in weight of girls in various populations of developing countries. I knew that this "peak weight gain" always took place before menarche, and I was curious to know at just what age it took place. (Age of menarche was not reported.) For example, I found that Pakistani girls had their largest weight gain at age 13. I could infer, then, that menarche would occur for these girls sometime after that age, probably at 14 or 15.

But then something quite intriguing turned up. Within a generally undernourished population like Pakistan, poor rural girls experienced this peak weight gain at a later age (14) than did better-nourished urban girls (12). This finding agreed with previously published reports showing that poorly nourished girls had their growth spurt and menarche later than did well-nourished girls. What was unexpected was that the rural and urban girls had the *same average weight* at the time of the peak weight gain, although they peaked at different ages. Did the weight itself mean something? If so, what did it represent?

I decided to pursue this interesting discovery. I repaired to the library and began reading the literature on body size at all stages of a girl's sexual maturation. I

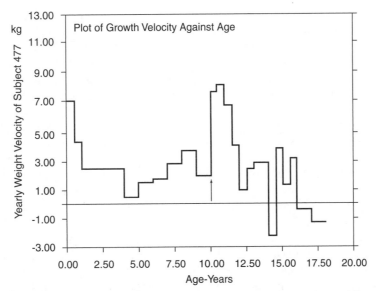

FIGURE 3   The amount of body weight gained each year (in the vertical axis, the weight gain is measured in kilograms; one kilogram equals 2.2 pounds), from birth to age 18, of one girl in the Denver study. The arrow shows the initiation of the adolescent growth spurt in weight at age 10. The rapid rise in weight gain is the spurt, which occurs before menarche, the first menstrual cycle. This girl, a rapid grower, had menarche at age 12.3. As the diagram shows, weight gain slows before menarche.

From R. E. Frisch, "The Critical Weight at Menarche and the Initiation of the Adolescent Growth Spurt, and the Control of Puberty," in *Control of the Onset of Puberty,* ed. M. M. Grumbach, G. D. Grave, and F. E. Mayer (New York: John Wiley & Sons, 1974), 404.

found many research papers, but most of them focused on height rather than weight. When I inquired among anthropologists and pediatricians about the reason for the lack of detailed research on body weight, I was told that body weight was so variable that it was not worth studying in relation to sexual maturation. But as newcomers to the subject, neither Roger nor I had any such prejudice, so we did look at body weight.

Analyzing Growth Data: The Girls' Spurt

To use the most accurate growth data, we relied on longitudinal growth studies in which the same girls were measured regularly as they grew up. In the studies we analyzed, the height and weight of each girl was measured every six months from birth to age 18, and her age of menarche was recorded. There were three such studies of girls and boys in the United States, one in Berkeley (California), one in Boston, and one in Denver. In all three, the subjects were well nourished and middle class.[1] The studies were completed in 1940-1950. We needed all three studies to get a large enough sample because there is always a great deal of variability in human growth.

Figure 3 shows the annual weight gain of one of the girls from birth to age 18. (I plotted similar curves of height and weight gain for each of the 181 girls in the studies.) This girl was a rapid grower and an early maturer. The arrow in the diagram indicates when her growth spurt in weight began at age 10; that sudden, rapid rise in weight gain is "the spurt." The girl's fastest growth in weight occurred at age 12. As you can see in the diagram, menarche occurs after weight gain starts to slow down; in this girl, menarche occurred at 12 years and 4 months (12.3 years). The average age of menarche of the 181 girls was 12 years and 10 months (12.8 years).

What starts that rapid acceleration in growth before menarche? Researchers are still not sure of the control mechanisms, but two things are certain: every normal adolescent girl and boy has the growth spurt before maturing sexually, and adolescents starting the growth spurt eat, eat, and eat; it's hard to keep enough food in stock. Then, after the peak gain in weight, both weight gain and food intake decrease. Little is known about what controls the reduction in food intake. In fact, we still don't know why human beings have an adolescent growth spurt at all. Why not idle along at the same growth rate until menarche?

All mammals seem to have a growth spurt before sexual maturation, but we don't know why this happens, either. One possible reason for the growth spurt in humans is that the rapid growth for girls is accompanied by a large increase in stored, easily mobilized energy—body fat—useful for successful reproduction.

Timing of the "Spurt" and Menarche

In the studies we analyzed, girls began the adolescent growth spurt at 9.5 years of age on average. Menarche occurred about three years after the start of the spurt, at 12.8 years. Many teachers and parents are still surprised at these early ages. Girls experienced the fastest growth in height at 11.5 years of age on average, and their peak weight gain occurred about six months later, at age 12. However, there is a lot of variability around these average ages; this variability is measured statistically by the *standard deviation* (often abbreviated as SD).

In our study, the standard deviation of the ages for each of these adolescent events was about one year. For example, the average age of menarche was 12.8 years with a standard deviation of one year. This means that two-thirds of the girls had menarche between the ages of 11.8 (the average age, 12.8, minus one year) and 13.8 (the average age, plus one year).

Growth rates are so variable because how quickly or slowly you grow at all ages is controlled genetically; you inherit your growth rate. But growth rate can also be affected by environmental factors such as the quality and quantity of food you eat and the amount of energy you expend. Two girls in the same family who eat the same food and have the same environment can grow at very different rates, one fast and one slow. The genetically fast grower will mature sexually before the slow grower does. However, the fast grower will mature later if she diets to become super slim or if she runs twenty miles a week. And the slow grower will mature even later if she changes her life style similarly. Nutrition and energy outputs interact with the genetic control.

Weight at Menarche

Pediatricians conduct growth studies of healthy, normal children, like the studies I analyzed, to establish standards of height and weight for girls and boys at each age. Then they are able to assess whether a girl or boy is growing normally.

Oddly, even though the age of menarche was noted precisely for each of the girls in the growth studies we analyzed, apparently no one had ever asked the simple question, what is the height and weight of girls at menar-

che? After we determined the average height and weight, we especially wanted to know whether early and late menarcheal girls had the same weight at menarche. This was easy to find out because we had each girl's exact age of menarche and her height and weight at every age up to 18. It just took time to gather the data for 181 girls.

We were excited by the answers. For all the girls, the average weight at menarche was 103 pounds (47 kg), and the average age of menarche was 12 years and 10 months (12.8 years). And eureka! Similar to our earlier results on peak weight gain, the early- and the late-maturing girls had the *same* average weight, 103 pounds (47 kg), whether they were younger than 12.8 years or older than 12.8 years at menarche. In 1970 Roger and I published this unexpected result in *Science* magazine, with some speculations as to what it could mean. The reaction to our article was usually incredulity: how could body weight matter? A good question that I set out to answer.

It was already known that height at menarche differed for early and late maturers. The average height for all girls at menarche was 62 inches (158 cm), but late-maturing girls were on average taller at menarche than the earlier maturers. I could now explain why many researchers reported that early maturers had more weight for height than did late maturers: average weights at menarche of early and late maturers are the same, but early maturers are shorter at menarche than late maturers.

When I reported these menarcheal height and weight results and their possible significance at a conference of pediatricians, I was greeted at first with dead silence. Then I was asked, "What is your background, Dr. Frisch?" (the tone of voice implying, how come are you here?). "I have my doctoral degree in genetics," I replied. "And who is Roger Revelle?" someone asked, mispronouncing "Revelle" to rhyme with "jelly." "Oh, Roger is an oceanographer," I answered, "and the director of the Population Center, where I work." More silence. No one apparently thought our new findings on weight at menarche mattered, and my presence was considered one of those aberrations that can happen at a conference. The response didn't trouble me. I had presented my message, and the doctors were polite.

I had been invited to speak at the conference by Dr. Thomas E. Cone Jr., then of Children's Hospital in Boston. Dr. Cone had read our published papers on the weight of girls and the adolescent spurt, including menarche. He was an expert on children's growth, and he found our results provocative and interesting. There were other doctors who also thought, as we did, that we were on to something, and they encouraged us to continue. But soon I learned that clinical doctors and researchers in any field, be it pediatrics, gynecology, or anthropology, are often uninterested in new ides. Some scientists are even hostile to them, especially if the ideas come from a researcher they've never heard of who works in an unrelated discipline (like me). A famous biochemist at Harvard Medical School once asked me, perhaps overly pessimistically, "How do you think new ideas advance, Dr. Frisch?" "I'm not too sure," I replied, thinking of some of my recent experiences. "Funeral by funeral is the answer," he said.

Overall, I had an exciting time pursuing this research. I found that when I had good questions to ask, I could call or write experts in a field, and most would respond generously with answers and advice. In fact, that is how I met some of my co-investigators and mentors. I also followed the sage advice I read in a scientist's memoir (I can't remember whose): choose the experts in a field whom you respect most for knowledge and advice, and ignore the reactions of everybody else.

Earlier Menarche: Girls "Grow Up" Faster

Even before being able to predict menarche for an individual girl, I could explain the well-known but unexplained fact that menarche had occurred progressively earlier during the past one hundred years. As I found, historical studies showed that the average weight at menarche of girls in the United States was the same in the past as it is now, 103 pounds (47 kg). What happened about a century ago was that girls began to grow more quickly in both height and weight because of improved nutrition and a decrease in childhood disease. They became larger sooner and therefore reached the average weight at menarche at an earlier age.

As shown in figure 4 below, the average age of menarche in Europe has become earlier by two to three months per decade over the past century and a half. In the mid-1800s, for example, menarche occurred as late as age 17 in Scandinavia; one hundred years later, the average age had declined to about 14.5. In the United States, the average age of menarche was 14.7 in 1880 and declined to age 14 by 1900. Thereafter menarche occurred earlier by about three months per decade until 1945, when it leveled off at age 12.6 to 12.8.

Since the average age of menarche was 15.5 or 16 a century and a half ago, doctors then defined precocious puberty (abnormally early menarche) as menarche at age 11 or 12. Those ages are now close to the present average age of menarche, 12.6 to 12.8. Doctors now define precocious puberty as menarche at age 8 or 9.

I once heard an eminent anthropologist predict that menarche would become earlier and earlier, so eventually menarche might occur at age 6. First graders! What a thought! It cannot be so.

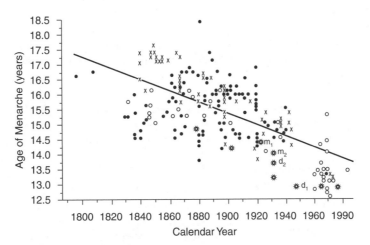

FIGURE 4   Mean (average) or median (middle of the distribution) age of menarche (years) as a function of calendar year from 1790 to 1980. The symbols refer to England (⊙); France (●); Germany (⊗); Holland (□); Scandinavia (Denmark, Finland, Norway, and Sweden) (x); Belgium, Czechoslovakia, Hungary, Italy, Poland (rural), Romania (urban and rural), Russia, Spain, and Switzerland (all labeled ○); and the United States (✳) (U.S. data not included in the regression line). The age of menarche has already leveled off in some European countries as it has in the United States (see U.S. data and text).

Reprinted from G. Wyshak and R. E. Frisch, "Evidence for a Secular Trend in Age of Menarche," *New England Journal of Medicine* 306 (1982): 1033.

Age of Menarche Now Leveled Off

Because menarche is a measure of how quickly girls grow, when girls' growth rates level off, the average age of menarche also levels off. As shown in the figure above, this is what has happened in the United States. Twelve-year-old girls have been the same average height and weight for more than fifty years. They have had good nutrition, and they no longer contract many of the childhood diseases that might slow their growth. Therefore, the average age of menarche has remained the same for the past fifty years as well.

Parents are apparently just becoming aware that the age of menarche is earlier now than it was a century ago. Puberty has become a popular subject in the media, and journalists often consult me to find out the facts. Confusion reigns about the timing of the "first menses," as one interviewer hesitantly described it. In summary, menarche is earlier today than in 1890 and 1900 for girls in the United States, but the trend to an earlier age of menarche has stabilized at 12.6 to 12.8 years.

Factors Delaying the Age of Menarche

Confirming the connection between the age of menarche and how rapidly or slowly girls grow in a particular population, any factor that slows weight growth before or after birth delays the age of menarche. Menarche occurs later in twins than in single-born children, for example, because twins grow more slowly. Malnutrition and undernutrition, both widespread among children in developing countries, delay menarche. Chronic childhood diseases in the United States, such as juvenile diabetes, sickle cell anemia, and cystic fibrosis, also slow growth and delay menarche. High altitude delays menarche by slowing the rate of weight growth both before and after birth; some of the latest average ages of menarche in the world, 17 and 18, occur in poorly nourished girls living at high altitudes in Peru and New Guinea. Then there are the athletes and dancers, who, as we found, fit the same model by undereating and overexercising, thus delaying menarche to the age of 15, 16, 17 or even 20.

A Mile High: Later Menarche of Denver Girls

Girls from Denver provide a particularly good example of how the natural environment can affect growth rate and thus the age of menarche. In the studies we analyzed, Denver girls were well nourished and middle class, as were the Berkeley and Boston girls. But Denver girls had menarche later, at an average age of 13, compared to 12.8 years for the two other groups. Although small, this difference was statistically significant. I couldn't figure out the reason for it until I read that at high altitudes growth in the uterus is slowed, resulting in lighter birth weights for both girls and boys.

But Denver is only a mile above sea level; would that be enough to affect birth weight? Indeed it is. When I added up the birth weights of the girls from Denver, they were 200 grams (7 oz) lighter on average than the birth weights of the girls in the sea-level cities of Berkley and Boston. Birth weights of the boys from Denver averaged 400 grams (14 oz) lighter than the birth weights of the sea-level boys. (Note that boys showed a bigger difference in birth weight than girls. Boys are more sensitive to "environmental insults"—under-nutrition, toxic substances, radiation, and high altitude. No one yet knows why this is so, but the effect of altitude on birth weight is a clear example of the phenomenon.)

How does altitude affect birth weight? The air has less oxygen at high altitudes, and therefore the fetus grows more slowly in the uterus. Consequently, high-altitude newborns weigh less than sea-level babies. But do the high-altitude babies eventually catch up? To find out, I compared the height and weight at every age of the Denver girls and the Berkeley girls, and I discovered that the Denver girls did not catch up in weight. Denver girls weighed less at every age than Berkeley girls, even though both groups of girls were similar in height at every age. Interestingly, during the adolescent spurt, the Denver girls gained the same amount of height (8.7 in; 22.1 cm) and the same amount of weight (37 lb; 17kg) as did the Berkeley girls. It was the growth in weight up to the beginning of the spurt that was slowed. This suggests that the rapid growth during the spurt is controlled independently from the growth before the spurt.

Faster Growth, Earlier Menarche

It is clear that, in general, any environmental—or genetic—factor that slows weight growth also delays menarche. Conversely, any factor that speeds up weight growth, such as ample food and fatty food, is associated with earlier menarche. For example, obese girls have menarche earlier than the average age unless their obesity is associated with pathology.

Individual girls have menarche at all different weights, though. What connects the slow or fast growth rates with the age of menarche? I had no explanation. But I did have an idea as to why body weight at the time of the first menstrual cycle could matter.

Body weight at menarche is close to adult body weight. Remember, for maintenance of the species it is a smart strategy to connect body weight and menarche. The survival of a newborn depends on the infant's birth weight, and the infant's birth weight is correlated with the mother's prepregnancy weight and her weight gain during pregnancy.

What Is the Clue in Body Weight?

What did body weight represent? What was the connection between body weight and sexual maturation? When I discussed these questions with Dr. J. M. Tanner, an expert on adolescent growth at the Institute of Child Health in London, he suggested that I consult the work of Gordon C. Kennedy of Cambridge University. I still recall the excitement of reading Kennedy's papers. He was one of the few researchers who combined the two fields of nutrition and reproduction. Kennedy had found that he could delay sexual maturation (called *estrus* in nonprimate mammals) in rats indefinitely by underfeeding them.

Kennedy stated, "Everybody knows you 'grow up' before you mature sexually." But then he asked the important question, "How do you define being 'grown up'?" (Roger used to say, "In the navy, they said if you are big enough, you are old enough." Kennedy was more precise.)

Based on his research connecting body weight, food intake, and puberty in rats, Kennedy proposed that the signal the brain receives indicating that a female is grown up enough to reproduce successfully is related to the amount of fat stored in the body. Kennedy also proposed that there is a "lipostat," some sort of internal measurement of body fat that is perceived by the hypothalamus, the part of the brain that controls food intake and reproduction. I was so inspired by Kennedy's work that I wrote him to ask if I might visit him; I had the good fortune to visit him twice. I came away from our discussions convinced that a lipostat was somehow involved in female sexual maturation. I decided to follow this "fatness" clue based on the idea that a critical, minimum amount of body fat is necessary for reproduction.

After reading the human and animal body composition literature for about two years (the data for humans were very difficult to follow because at that time there were no direct measures of human body fat), I found that I could indeed predict a minimum weight for height necessary for menarche or regular menstrual cycles from a fatness indicator. I was cheered by this result; when you can predict, nature is telling you something.

I am writing this about three decades after Kennedy published his lipostat idea and more than twenty-five years after my controversial 1974 *Science* article. In 1995, I opened the July issue of *Science* and read of Jeffrey Friedman's cloning of the "obese" gene at Rockefeller University and of the strong evidence for a lipostat. Freidman and other researchers reported that body fat cells produced a protein hormone called leptin (from *leptos,* the Greek word for "thin"). Leptin is perceived by special cells, called receptors, in the hypothalamus. Kennedy's paper of three decades earlier was the first publication cited in the references section of Friedman's article.

After reading Friedman's *Science* article, I sent him some of my articles on body fat, menarche, and ovulation. I also mentioned that I had visited Gordon Kennedy twice. Not long after that I was amazed to receive a call from Friedman. First he asked me about Gordon Kennedy. Then he said, "I thought you would be interested to know that you can make an infertile mouse fertile by injecting leptin," indicating that indeed leptin, and thus body fat, has a role in reproduction. (Dr. Farid Chehab of the University of California Medical Center in San Francisco published this result in *Science* in 1997: prepubertal mice—mice without fat—became pubertal after the injection of leptin.)

I was present when Friedman delivered three lectures on leptin at Harvard Medical School in 1996, and he mentioned my research on the critical-fatness connection to menarche and ovulation. During the question period following one of the lectures, a man asked, "What about weight loss in men? Does it affect their reproductive ability?" "I don't know," replied Friedman. "Does anyone in the audience know?" Silence reigned in the well-filled, sizable amphitheater. I raised my hand. "I do," I said.

"As men lose weight, the first thing to go is libido—as in bulls. Then, as testosterone levels fall further, there is a loss of prostate fluid; then sperm motility and mobility are affected. Then, with an extreme, 25 percent weight loss (the men look like skeletons), sperm production is also affected. Weight gain reverses all of these effects." I was quite surprised that facts known three decades ago were new to this large medical audience, but then, this is a molecular, DNA age.

A Paradox of Population Growth

A question may have occurred to you as you read about a direct link between nutrition and fertility. If undernourishment decreases fertility, how do we explain the rapid population growth of undernourished populations in developing countries? Fertility rates in many developing countries (6 to 7 children per couple) are actually far *below* the maximum human fertility (11 to 12 children per couple) found in well-nourished, noncontracepting populations. Populations of many developing countries are growing rapidly because death rates have decreased (thanks to modern public health measures) while fertility rates have remained the same.

Not to Neglect the Boys

My research focused on girls, but I did compare some of the adolescent events for boys who were in the same longitudinal growth studies.

Boys in the United States begin their rapid growth in height and weight simultaneously, at about age 11 on average, two years later than girls. In developing countries and historically, boys experience the spurt three years later than girls. The rapid growth continues for about three years in boys, as it does in girls, and it decelerates before *genarche,* the boys' equivalent of menarche, at about age 14.6 to 14.8. Genarche is not precisely timed because there is not a clear endpoint for boys such as the first menstrual cycle for girls. Nocturnal emissions usually begin at this time, but this event is not easy to document.

John Crawford, a pediatric endocrinologist then at Massachusetts General Hospital, suggested a possibly more precise endpoint when he urged me to study boys in detail in addition to girls. Crawford noted that apocrine sweat, which has an odor, appears at the time of genarche, so one could determine the timing of genarche by smelling the underarm sweat of boys. I declined the opportunity, and as far as I know, no one else has leaped to do it.

Why do boys start their rapid growth later, and therefore reach sexual maturation later, than girls? One possible reason may be that when girls have menarche, regular ovulatory cycles do not begin immediately. There are often irregular, anovulatory periods. Boys do not have this period of relative infertility; once they are sexually mature, sperm production is at the adult level. Later maturation for boys would therefore be an advantage for successful reproductive outcome—useful in the past, but not now! Whatever the reason, the later growth spurt for boys means that during elementary school there is a period when girls are bigger than boys at the same age. I have been amazed at the large number of men (including my husband) who remembered this time, even thirty or forty years later.

Notes

1. It is important to compare persons of similar socioeconomic backgrounds, as studies have shown that age of growth and maturation differ by social class. See H. P. Bowditch, *Eighth Annual Report* (Boston: Massachusetts State Board of Health, 1877); V. Kiil, *Skrifter utgitt av det Norske Videnskaps-Akademi i Oslo 2,* no. 1 (1939). Kiil's data, collected from different social classes and geographic regions in Norway over 100 years, show "an undoubted connection between the age of the individual at the time sexual maturity commenced and the social conditions under which that person lives" (p. 145).

Don't Just Go with the Flow

Did you ever stop to think about the feminine product(s) you use during your special time of the month? Is it the same product your mom or friends introduced to you when you first got your period? Disposable, bleached pads and tampons you find in the grocery store or local pharmacy . . . that's about all that's out there in period world, right? Wrong! There's a whole other world of menstrual products to choose from. And it doesn't stop there! There are menstrual products out there that are not only safer for our bodies, but will make the environment happy too!

Read on to find out more about these fabulous alternatives, why they're not in stores near you (and how you can get them there).

Words to Know

Shelving or "Slotting" fees: payments product manufacturers must make to retailers to be able to sell their items on store shelves. They range from hundreds to thousands of dollars per item based on the items' placement on shelves. [Eye level costs more.]

Food cooperatives: locally owned stores run by community members that usually offere a wide variety of products and environmentally safe options like recyclable bags and food in bulk.

Natural health food stores: markets or specialty shops offering a variety of natural and organic foods and healthcare products.

Have You Heard of Any of These?

That's right, there are menstrual products you can buy that are safer for you and the environment. There are products actually out there that are chlorine-bleached-rayon-free. Chlorine-bleached rayon is currently found in menstrual products sold in big stores across the country. These two ingredients together are said to make dioxin, which according to a 1994 U.S. Environmental Protection Agency EPA study is found to be cancerous [an estimated 100 of the roughly 1,400 daily cancer deaths in the U.S. are said to be caused by dioxin]. Differences in opinion still surround whether the levels of dioxin found in pads and tampons are high enough to be of any risk to you. But why add any risk, and why contribute to environmental harm?

Start Your Own Campaign!

The sooner we speak out, the sooner change will happen! Tear out this letter, sign your name, get your friends to sign it, and walk it over to your nearby grocery store or pharmacy. Demand that all your menstrual product choices be on the shelves of your grocery store!

Why Aren't They Sold in Most Stores?

Teen Voices asked GladRags, Natracare, and Organic Essentials (three companies that sell a variety of natural menstrual products) why their menstrual products aren't sold

---

To Whom It May Concern,

I shop at your store regularly and I am bothered that you fail to carry any natural feminine hygiene products. I can't believe you're leaving so many of us to have to travel miles out of our way to natural food stores to buy products we should be able to buy on your shelves.

I am well aware that most of these natural feminine hygiene products are produced by small companies that cannot afford high shelving costs like the major brands—but what about the health of your customers? Perhaps your store might consider reducing fees for shelf space for these companies until their sales go up, or help them to advertise their products in your store.

I think you should be more than willing to provide all of us with all our menstrual choices. After all, I'm sure you have women in your lives and care about their health and choices.

Sincerely,

---

in most major grocery stores or pharmacies. Here's what they had to say. Do you want to do something about it?

GladRags

"Alternative feminine hygiene products are not yet sold in most stores because the customers aren't interested in or ready for them. [In particular], I don't think department store shoppers are ready for reusable menstrual alternatives; they are used to disposable products because that's what they see on TV and in magazines.

Women are also seldom actually comfortable with menstruating. Unfortunately few women view their bleeding as a positive empowering experience and don't want to touch or see it happen. When women learn to like menstruating, they will most likely switch to washable pads or healthy options."—Carmen de la Cruz, General Manager

Brenda Mallory founded GladRags in 1992 in Portland, Oregon. She got the idea from the cloth diapers she used for her baby daughter Emma. She first thought she would be making cloth pads from home on her own sewing machine, but orders got too big and now GladRags is sold nationally in natural food stores, food co-operatives, and by its catalog and Web site.

Natracare

"In Canada, the Northwest, and other parts of the U.S., Natracare is sold in some grocery stores. Grocery stores usually ask for a lot of money for products to be placed [on their shelves], and because we're a small company, we don't have the resources to pay these high fees. It's not until the demand [from] women and young women actually going into stores and asking for it that they would actually get it [there]."—Susan Carskadon, Manager in North America.

In Great Britain in 1989, a British national network aired a program on the effects of dioxin pollution and its influences on women's menstrual products. After its airing, many women began boycotting the disposable, bleached pads and tampons they had been using to demand change. Susie Hewson then developed Natracare for the women of Great Britain. It then spread throughout Europe, New Zealand, Canada, and the Sultanate of Oman in the Middle East. Natracare made its way to the U.S. in 1993.

Organic Essentials

"The reason you cannot find Organic Essentials in other major retail stores and discount stores is simply because of lack of education and demand. We believe that every

Not in the Majors

Menstrual Product	How does it work?	Pro-you	Not good for you	Environment friendly?
Bleached with Chlorine-free methods, Cotton Pad	• Disposable. • Can attach to your under wear with its sticky back.	• No harmful dyes. • Dioxin-free	• Harmful pesticides may have been used to grow cotton. • Usually found only in natural health food stores or on the web. • More expensive.	• Better for the environment than commercial pads, but still not too great. • Environment is OK, but could be happier.
Cloth Pad	•Reusable. • Can wrap around your underwear with the help of its buttons or clips.	• It's cheaper. You can just buy one or two and you're set for months.	• Need to wash. • Usually found only in natural health food stores and co-ops.	• Environment is very happy.
Organic Tampon	• Disposable, 100% compressed cotton grown without the use of pesticides or chemical fertilizers. Unbleached and undyed.	• Dioxin-free	• Usually found only in natural health food stores, in co-ops, or on the Web. • More expensive.	• Environment is OK, but could be a bit happier.
Menstrual Cup	• Reusable, flexible rubber cup [usually made out of natural gum rubber] that you insert inside your vagina.	• Dioxin-free • Very cheap. One is enough to have.	• A sink is needed to rinse it out. • Usually have to order through a mail catalog, may be available in certain natural health food stores, in co-ops, or on the Web.	• Environment couldn't be happier!
Sponge	• Reusable, natural sponge found in the ocean!, with a string attached to it.	• Dioxin-free • Cheaper. Can just buy one or two and you're set for months.	• Need to boil it to clean. • Usually have to order through a mail catalog, may be available in certain natural health food stores or on the Web.	• Environment very happy!

Source: "EPA Links Dioxin to Cancer," *The Washington Post,* 17 May 2000: "The Trouble With Tampons," *Vegetarian Times,* July 1996.

In the Majors

Menstrual Product	How does it work?	Pro-you	Not good for you	Environment friendly?
"Common Pad" (Bleached, Dry-weave Pad)	• Disposable. • Can attach to your underwear with its sticky backing.	• Can be thrown right away after use. • Can be found in almost all convenience stores, grocery stores, and some public bathrooms.	• Has pesticides and dyes. • Dry-weave portion of pad is often made out of plastic. • Some contain dioxins.	• No Way!
"Common Tampon" (Bleached Tampon)	• Disposable compressed cotton mixtures that you insert into your vagina.	• Can be thrown away after use. • Can be found in almost all convenience stores, grocery stores, and some public bathrooms.	• Could have pesticides and dyes or could be bleached. • Dioxin risk.	• Very bad for the environment.
Lubricated Tampon	• Disposable tampons with a wet film on them to make inserting them more comfortable.	• The film is sterile and kills the bacteria that cause T.S.S.	• Lubrication could disrupt the body's natural lubrication.	• No Way!

family had their cotton farm certified organic by the Texas Department of Agriculture in 1991.

The Herstory of Our Monthly Visitor

Julia Steinberg, 19
Newton, Massachusetts

So what did women do back in the day about their periods?

• 15th century Egyptian women used tampons too! But their tampons were made of soft papyrus [a tall, grassy plant found on the shores of the Nile River that ancient civilizations used to make paper].

• For centuries, women all over the globe who lived by the sea used natural sponges to absorb their periods.

• Native American women made pads from buffalo and deer skins, cattail down, moss, and even tree bark!

• 19th century American women were really "on the rag" when they got their periods. They did use old rags!

Check Out These Sites
For more info on how and where to get natural menstrual products for yourself, visit these sites for listings and links:
www.critpath.org/tracy/healthy.html
www.borntolove.com/d-list.shtml
www.bloodsisters.org

Check These Books Out!
A Girl's Story by Toni Cade Bambara
The Vagina Monologues by Eve Ensler
Quilting: Poems 1987–1990
See "poem in praise of menstruation," "poem to my uterus," and "to my last period."
by Lucille Clifton

• By 1886, disposable towels were invented in the U.S. but couldn't be marketed because menstruation was considered immoral [evil]! Instead, women wore menstrual pad belts that sometimes even had suspenders.

- In 1922, hundreds of American women bought "sanitary bloomers" [diaper-like undies] from Sears Robuck & Co. catalogue

- While bandaging up patients during World War I, French nurses discovered gauze materials were much better for absorbing periods than cloth diapers.

- With the increased number of working women during the 1920s and 1930s in the U.S., companies began manufacturing the first "tampons" to meet the demand for comfortable period protection.

- During the 1970s, the self-adhesive pads we know today were invented and put on the market, "Beltless freedom."

- By the 1980's women were buying snap-on flannel pads with removable fillers.

- Today, over 50 brands of menstrual products are on the market in the U.S., and are a half billion dollar industry! Products like thong panty pads are even on the market–talk about women refusing to let menstruation into their everyday lives!

Source: Red Flower: Rethinking Menstruation *by Dena Taylor*

The Lowdown on T.S.S.

While on the topic of menstrual products, if you're a tampon user, stories of Toxic Shock Syndrome may have come up once or twice in conversation. Here's the quick lowdown: T.S.S. is caused from the bacteria Staphylococcus aureus. It has been reported that most cases of this bacteria entering the body and spreading its toxins have been through tampon use. Some health experts believe that tampons may produce small cuts along our vaginal walls that can allow this bacteria to enter our bodies. Others believe that the menstrual blood left within or behind tampons may permit the bacteria to grow.

Symptoms of T.S.S.

These symptoms can occur suddenly and may be confused with illnesses like the flu or measles. If you suffer from any of these during your time of the month while wearing a tampon, remove it right away. This can stop the bacteria from growing in 80% of cases. Also see your doctor right away.

- Fever greater than 101 degrees F
- Low blood pressure that may cause you to faint
- Vomiting
- Diarrhea
- Aching muscles
- Sunburn-like rash that results in severe peeling in 1-2 weeks

Easy Ways to Prevent T.S.S.
- Change your tampons every 4 to 5 hours
- Wash your hands before inserting tampons
- Try alternating between tampons and pads, or other alternatives
- Try not to wear tampons while you sleep

Source: Women's Health Interactive; Calgary Regional Health Authority

The Selling of Premenstrual Syndrome

Who Profits from Marketing PMS "The Disease of the 80s"?

by Andrea Eagan

In the summer of 1961, I was working as a laboratory assistant at a major pharmaceutical firm. Seminars were regularly given on recent scientific developments, and that summer, one of them, on the oral contraceptive, was given by an associate of Dr. Gregory Pincus, who was instrumental in the development of the Pill. As a rule, only the scientists went to the seminars. But for this one, every woman in the place—receptionists and bottle washers, technicians and cleaners—showed up. Oral contraception sounded like a miracle, a dream come true.

During the discussion, someone asked whether the drug was safe. Yes, we were assured, it was perfectly safe. It had been thoroughly tested in Puerto Rico, and besides, you were only adjusting the proportions of naturally occurring substances in the body, putting in a little estrogen and progesterone to fool the body into thinking that it was "just a little bit pregnant." The Food and Drug Administration had approved the sale of the birth-control pill in the United States the year before. News of it was everywhere. Women flocked to their doctors to get it. The dream, we now know, was much too good to be true. But we learned that only after years of using the Pill, after we had already become a generation of guinea pigs.

Since then, and because of similar experiences with DES and with estrogen replacement therapy (ERT), because of the work of the women's health movement and of health activists like Barbara Seaman, we have presumably learned something: we have become cautious about medical miracles and scientific breakthroughs. To suddenly discover, then, that thousands of women are rushing to get an untested drug to cure a suspected but entirely unproved hormone deficiency which manifests itself as a condition with a startling variety of symptoms—known by the catchall name premenstrual syndrome (PMS)—is a little shocking.

Often when a drug suddenly makes the news, or when a new "disease" for which there is a patented cure is discovered, it is fairly easy to find the public relations work of the drug manufacturers behind the story. As just one example, estrogen replacement therapy for the symptoms of menopause had been around since the 1940s. But in 1966, a Brooklyn physician by the name of Robert Wilson wrote a book called *Feminine Forever,* which extolled the benefits of ERT in preventing what the author called "living decay." Wilson went on TV and radio, was interviewed for scores of articles. He claimed that *lifelong* ERT, starting well before menopause, would prevent or cure more than 20 different conditions, ranging from backaches to insomnia and irritability. Wilson ran an operation called the Wilson Research Foundation that put out information to the media and received grants from drug companies. Among those contributing to the Wilson Foundation was Ayerst Laboratories, the largest manufacturer of the estrogen used in the treatment of menopause symptoms. Ayerst also funded a group called the Information Center on the Mature Woman, from which regular information bulletins were sent to the media.

Many doctors had misgivings about ERT (the link between estrogen and cancer had been reported since the 1930s), but the information that the public received about ERT was almost entirely positive. One of the few warnings against ERT appeared in *Ms.* in December, 1972. Three years later, in 1975, a study was published in the *New England Journal of Medicine* reporting that estrogen users had a five to 14 times greater incidence of uterine cancer than did nonusers. This was news, and it made the papers. (*The New England Journal,* like several other prestigious medical journals, sends out advance issues to some news services, which is why the networks all have the same story on the same day.)

Women, needless to say, were concerned about ERT. Many simply stopped taking the drug, and sales of Premarin (the brand name of Ayerst's ERT preparation, which accounted for 80 percent of the market) dropped.

Soon after this, Ayerst received a memo on media strategy from Hill & Knowlton, its public relations firm. This memo, the sort that is supposed to be absolutely confidential, became public when someone sent a copy to the New York women's newspaper, *Majority Report.* *MR* published the entire memo under the headline, "New Discovery: Public Relations Cures Cancer." The first part of the plan was to take the spotlight off estrogen and refocus it on menopause. The "estrogen message," said the memo, "can be effectively conveyed by discreet references to 'products that your doctor may prescribe.'" Articles on menopause were to be placed in major women's magazines. Information was also to be fed to syndicated women's page columnists, general magazines and prominent science writers and editors.

The second part of Hill & Knowlton's plan was to counter anticipated negative publicity. A list of potentially damaging events—research reports (one was expected from the Mayo Clinic), FDA announcements, lawsuits—was given. News releases were to be prepared in *advance* of the "damaging commentary . . . in as much detail as possible." When this memo became public (Jack Anderson picked it up after *MR's* publication), Ayerst denied any intention of following its recommendations, but the memo actually outlines the kinds of steps some drug manufacturers take to bring their products to the attention of the public and to counteract criticism.

The same story, with only minor changes, can be told for a number of other drugs, so when I began seeing articles about PMS and progesterone treatment, I immediately had some questions. Why was PMS suddenly "news"? What do we really know about progesterone? And who are the advocates of this treatment?

PMS stories began appearing rather suddenly about two years ago, after two Englishwomen claimed PMS as a mitigating factor in their defense against murder charges. When the stories about these cases appeared, many American women who suffer from cyclical problems naturally became interested in finding out all they could about the condition.

PMS itself is not news. It was first mentioned in the medical literature in the 1930s, and women presumably had it before then. Estimates on the numbers of women affected by PMS vary wildly. Some claim that as many as 80 percent are affected while others place estimates at only 20 percent. Similarly, doctors' opinions vary on the number and type of symptoms that may indicate PMS. They cite from 20 up to 150 physical and psychological symptoms, ranging from bloating to rage. The key to

recognizing PMS and differentiating it from anything else that might cause some or all of a woman's symptoms is timing. The symptoms appear at some point after ovulation (around mid-cycle) and disappear at the beginning of the menstrual period. (It should not be confused with dysmenorrhea or menstrual discomfort, about which much is known, and for which several effective, safe treatments have been developed.)

While PMS is now generally acknowledged to be a physical, as well as a psychological disorder, there is little agreement on what causes it or how it should be treated. There are at least half a dozen theories as to its cause—ranging from an alteration in the way that the body uses glucose to excessive estrogen levels—none of which have been convincingly demonstrated.

One of the most vocal proponents of PMS treatment is Katharina Dalton, a British physician who has been treating the condition for more than 30 years. Dalton believes that PMS results from a deficiency of progesterone, a hormone that is normally present at high levels during the second half of the menstrual cycle and during pregnancy. Her treatment, and that of her followers, relies on the administration of progesterone during the premenstrual phase of the cycle.

Progesterone is not absorbed effectively when taken by mouth. Powdered progesterone, derived from yams or soybeans, can be dissolved in oil and given in a deep, painful muscular injection. Or the powder can be absorbed from vaginal or rectal suppositories, a more popular form. (In this country the Upjohn Company is the major manufacturer of progesterone, which they sell only in bulk to pharmacies where pharmacists then package it for sale. Upjohn makes no recommendation for the use of progesterone and is conducting no tests on the product.)

Although she promotes the progesterone treatment, Dalton has no direct evidence of a hormone deficiency in PMS sufferers. Because progesterone is secreted cyclically in irregular bursts, and testing of blood levels of progesterone is complicated and expensive, studies have been unable to show conclusively that women with PMS symptoms have lower levels of progesterone than other women. Dalton's evidence is indirect: the symptoms of PMS are relieved by the administration of progesterone.

Upon learning about Dalton's diagnosis-and-cure, many women concluded that they had the symptoms she was talking about. But when they asked their doctors for progesterone treatment, they generally got nowhere. Progesterone is not approved by the FDA for treatment of PMS (the only approved uses are for treating cessation of menstrual flow and abnormal uterine bleeding due to hormone imbalance); there is *nothing* in the medical literature showing clearly what causes PMS; and there has never been a well-designed, controlled study here or in England of the effect of progesterone on PMS.

Despite some doctors' reluctance to prescribe progesterone, self-help groups began springing up, and special clinics were established to treat PMS. Women who had any of the reported symptoms (cyclical or not) headed en masse for the clinics or flew thousands of miles to doctors whose willingness to prescribe progesterone had become known through the PMS network. And a few pharmacists began putting up progesterone powder in suppository form and doing a thriving business.

How did PMS suddenly become the rage, or what one New York gynecologist called "the hypoglycemia of the 1980s"? At least part of the publicity can be traced to an enterprising young man named James Hovey. He is reported to have claimed he had a B.A. in public health from UCLA despite the fact that, aside from extension courses, he had been there less than a year. (UCLA does not even have a B.A. program in public health.) He met Katharina Dalton in Holland several years ago at a conference on the biological basis of violent behavior. Returning to the United States, he worked with a Boston physician who opened the first PMS clinic in Lynnfield. A few months later, Hovey left the clinic. He then started The National Center for Premenstrual Syndrome and Menstrual Distress in New York City, Boston, Memphis, and Los Angeles—each with a local doctor as medical director.

For $265 (paid in advance), you got three visits. The initial visit consisted of a physical exam and interview, and a lengthy questionnaire on symptoms. During the second visit, the clinic dispensed advice on diet and vitamins, and reviewed a monthly record the patient was asked to keep. On the third visit, if symptoms still persisted, most patients received a prescription for progesterone.

Last year, James Hovey's wife Donna, a nurse who was working in his New York clinic, told me that they were participating in an FDA-approved study of progesterone, in conjunction with a doctor from the University of Tennessee. In fact, to date the FDA has approved only one study on progesterone treatment of PMS, which is conducted at the National Institute of Child Health and Human Development, an organization unrelated to James Hovey.

Similar contradictions and misrepresentations, as well as Hovey's lack of qualifications to be conducting research or running a medical facility, were exposed by two journalists last year. Marilyn Webb in the *Village Voice* and Jennifer Allen in *New York* magazine both dug into the operation of the clinic and Hovey's past to reveal him as a former Army medical corpsman turned entrepreneur. Hovey left New York and gave up his interest in the New York and Boston clinics. He is currently running a nationwide PMS referral service out of New Hampshire.

In a recent interview, Hovey said that the clinic business is too time-consuming, and that he is getting out. His "only interest is research" he says. He was associated with two scientists who applied to the FDA for permission to do progesterone studies but who were rejected because the FDA considered the doses of progesterone to be too high. At last report, Hovey still headed H and K Pharmaceuticals, a company founded in 1981 for the manufacture of progesterone suppositories, and it is as a supplier that his name has appeared on FDA applications.

Hovey's involvement in PMS treatment seems to have centered on the commercial opportunities. Others, such as Virginia Cassara, became interested in PMS for more personal reasons.

Cassara, a social worker from Wisconsin, went to England in 1979 to be treated by Dalton for severe PMS. The treatment was successful and Cassara returned to spread the good news. She invited Katharina Dalton to Wisconsin to speak and notified the press. Though only one article appeared, it brought women "out of the closet," Cassara says. Cassara began counseling and speaking, selling Dalton's books and other literature. Her national group, PMS Action, now has an annual budget of $650,000, 17 paid staff members, and 40 volunteers. Cassara spends most of her time traveling and speaking.

Cassara's argument is compelling, at least initially. She describes the misery of PMS sufferers, and the variety of ineffective medical treatments they have been subjected to in their search for relief. For anyone who is sensitive to women's health issues, it is a familiar tale: a condition that afflicts perhaps millions of women has never been studied; a treatment that gives relief is ignored. Women, says Cassara, are pushed into diet and exercise regimens that are difficult to maintain and don't always work. One valid solution, she feels, lies in progesterone.

According to FDA spokesperson Roger Eastep, Phase I studies—those that determine how much a particular substance is absorbed by the body and how it works—have yet to be done for progesterone. But in the meantime, more and more doctors are prescribing the hormone for PMS.

Dr. Michelle Harrison, a gynecologist practicing in Cambridge, Massachusetts, and a spokesperson for the National Women's Health Network, is one physician who does prescribe progesterone to some women, with mixed feelings. "I've seen it dramatically temper women's reactions," she says. "For those women whose lives are shattered by PMS, who've made repeated suicide attempts or who are unable to keep a job, you have to do something. But I have a very frightening consent form that they have to sign before I'll give progesterone to them." Harrison also stresses that a lot of PMS is iatrogenic; that is, it is caused by medical treatment. It often appears for the first time after a woman has stopped taking birth-control pills, after tubal ligation or even after a hysterectomy, in which the ovaries have been removed.

When doctors do prescribe progesterone, their ideas of the appropriate dosage can vary from 50 to 2,400 mg. per day. For some women, dosages at the lower end of the scale do not bring relief from their symptoms. It has also been reported by women taking progesterone and in medical literature that the effect of a particular dose diminishes after a few months. Some women are symptom-free as long as they are taking the drug, but the symptoms reappear as soon as they stop, regardless of where they are in the menstrual cycle.

For all these reasons, some women are taking much higher doses than their doctors prescribe. Michelle Harrison had heard of women taking 2,400 mg. per day; Dalton had heard about 3,000; Cassara knows women who take 4,000. Because PMS symptoms tend to occur when progesterone is not being taken, some women take it every day, instead of only during the premenstrual phase. Some bleed all the time; others don't menstruate at all. Vaginal and rectal swelling are common. Animal studies have shown increased rates of breast tumors and cervical cancer. Marilyn Webb, a reporter who began taking progesterone while working on a story about PMS, developed chest pains after several months. She asked all the doctors she interviewed whether any of their patients had experienced chest pains. Every one said that she or he had at least one patient who had.

Reminding her of the history of the Pill, of DES, and of ERT, I asked Virginia Cassara whether she was concerned about the long-term effects of progesterone on women. "I guess I don't think there could be anything worse than serious PMS," she responded. "Even cancer?" I asked. "Absolutely. Even cancer." Later, she said, "I think it's paternalistic of the FDA to make those choices for us, to tell us what we can and cannot put in our bodies. Women with PMS are competent beings, capable of making their own choices."

I don't have severe PMS, and I don't think I fully understand the desperation of women who do and who see help at last within reach. But given our limited understanding of how progesterone works, I do not understand why women like Cassara are echoing drug company complaints of overregulation by the FDA. I'm alarmed to see women flocking to use an untested substance about which there is substantial suspicion, whose mode of action is not known, to treat a condition whose very cause is a mystery. And I fear that, somewhere down the line, we will finally learn all about progesterone treatment and it won't be what we wanted to know.

One doctor, who refused to be quoted by name, cheerfully assured me that progesterone was safe. "Even if a woman is taking 1,600 milligrams per day, the amount of circulating progesterone is still only a quarter of what is normally circulating during pregnancy." And I couldn't help but think of the doctor at the seminar more than 20 years ago: "Of course it's safe. It's just like being a little bit pregnant."

The Vitamin Cure

Diet and vitamin therapies are, according to many doctors, effective in the large majority of PMS cases. Michelle Harrison has found that most of her patients will respond to a hypoglycemia diet: whole grains, no caffeine, lots of water, no sugar, frequent small meals. To this, she adds up to 800 mg. per day of vitamin B6 during the premenstrual phase. Harrison has written a clear and useful 50-page booklet, *Self-Help for Premenstrual Syndrome* ($4.50, plus $1.50 postage and handling, from Matrix Press, Box 740M, Cambridge, Massachusetts 02238), which includes charts for keeping track of symptoms and lots of good advice about diagnosis and treatment, as well as a look at the social and political questions raised by PMS.

Dr. Marcia Storch (author of *How To Relieve Cramps and Other Menstrual Problems*, Workman Publishing, $3.95) and her associate, Dr. Shelley Kolton, believe that reducing salt intake helps to curb water retention and headaches that result from it. They also prescribe 300 to 500 mg. daily of vitamin B_6. Kolton says that this therapy is effective in about 80 percent of all cases, though it may take several months for the treatment to work. (Storch and Kolton do not recommend progesterone because of safety concerns.)—A.E.

WORKSHEET—CHAPTER 4
Menstruation

This worksheet must be optional. Some parts of this worksheet are designed for women who go through reproductive cycles. Women who do not have reproductive cycle and men may or may not want to interview women with reproductive cycles about the personal questions asked in 1 and 3.

1. **Your menstrual cycle.** Observe changes your body goes through during a menstrual cycle. Here are a few things you may want to note. You may think of others you would find interesting to record (cravings, water retention, etc.). See if you can identify when you are ovulating/have ovulated. If you are on oral contraceptives, how will your observations differ from those of women not on synthetic hormones?

   Temperature: Record body temperature (by mouth is fine) first thing in the morning before you get up, before you have anything to drink or smoke. You are more likely to note changes if you have a fairly regular schedule and use a very accurate thermometer.

   Mucus (secreted by the cervical glands): Observe changes in mucus. Choose your own words to describe what you feel. Words like much, some, scant, clear and watery like egg-whites, and sticky are sometimes useful. Remember that contraceptive gels, foams, and semen in the vagina will mask much of what you might notice about mucus.

   Breasts: Fuller, less full, lumpier, tender, "What I think of as `normal,' " and sore may be words useful to describe breast changes.

Date	Temperature	Mucus	Breasts	Other Observations
1				
2				
3				
4				
5				
6				
7				
8				
9				
10				
11				
12				
13				
14				
15				
16				
17				
18				
19				
20				
21				
22				
23				
24				
25				
26				
27				
28				
29				
30				
31				
32				
33				
34				
35				

2. **Menstruation Products.** Calculate how much you or an "average" woman spends on menstruation products in a lifetime. (These calculations can be based on today's prices.) Check current prices for one or two brands of tampons, napkins, or other "menstruation hygiene products." Estimate how much of this product is used for each menstrual cycle. (A woman with a heavy flow will use many more than a woman with a light flow.) For your calculations you will need to figure how many years a woman will menstruate (age of menopause - age of menarche), and how many times a year a woman menstruates. Show your work. (For a very accurate estimation, you would want to think about how pregnancies, lactation, choice of contraception and menstrual changes at different ages would influence your calculations, but you do not need to do this for this question.)

3. **Premenstrual syndrome.** The publicity about premenstrual syndrome (PMS) and advertising for drugs promising a medical-fix for PMS have worked to make women and men regard the premenstrual days as "the bad time of the month" for women.

   a. If a few days are regarded as the relatively "bad" days, then other parts of the cycle must be viewed as relatively "good." Identify "good" things you associate with different parts of your cycle. (These might include such things as times of high energy, times when you require less sleep, times when you most enjoy how your body feels, times when you especially enjoy exercising, times when you find it easy to resist sweet or salty foods, times when you especially enjoy your sexuality.)

   b. Some women identify very positive things about premenstrual days. For many women this is a time when they are most creative, their dreaming is most vivid, they are the most sexually aroused, they find it easiest to "justify" taking time for themselves, they feel most in touch with things in their life which need changing. Identify positive things you, your friends, or your mother notice about premenstrual days.

4. Compare your own or (other) women's stories about menarche with the experiences described in "Menarche and the (Hetero) Sexualization of the Female Body." Describe how you learned about menarche/menstruation and compare this to how you wish you had learned about it.

5. Think about ways in which menarche/menstruation could be introduced to young people as a positive part of women's and men's lives.

    a. Suggest one or more ways to introduce menarche/menstruation as positive to young women.

    b. Suggest one or more ways to introduce menarche/menstruation as positive to young men.

6. **Seasonale.** Collect ads, articles, or friends' comments about Seasonale (the new packaging of contraceptive pills so that women have periods just once a season). What patterns do you see in these messages about attitudes toward menstruation and concerns about the safety of new products on the market which have not been extensively studied?

CHAPTER 5
Women and Mental Health

Many formerly battered women who have been close to death with life threatening physical injuries have said the physical violence had less impact on them than day to day psychological/emotional abuse they survived. Many women with chronic fatigue syndrome so severe that taking a shower became a major goal have said that the worst part of their condition was that people (including doctors) would not believe they were ill and had said that their condition was "all in their heads." Mental and physical health issues have so much impact on each other that in many cases it may be misleading to try to make a distinction and in other cases it can be very dangerous to confuse mental and physical ramifications of a situation. Readers will notice that mental health components are central to every women's health topic.

"Women and Mental Health," by Marian Murphy, provides an overview of definitions of mental health, gender differences in patterns of mental ill health, women and depression, women and mental health services, and positive suggestions for change. This classic article identifies that women's ill health (particularly depression) is very obviously related to the fact that women find themselves in depressing situations. Being active agents to change those situations goes against how women/girls are socialized and the types of activities which are accepted as "suitably feminine" in a world where healthy females are defined as being submissive, dependent, easily influenced and not competitive.

Going into more depth on the same themes, Fiona Rummery provides specific examples of how femininity is socially constructed. She explains that what "is generally regarded as the women's role happens to coincide with what is regarded as mentally unhealthy" so that "whether women comply with or rebel against traditional precepts of femininity, we risk being labeled as 'dysfunctional'." The dilemma then is that mental health services also reflect the values of society, so that a woman's mental health issues get her labeled and treated (often medicalized) as having an individual problem unrelated to the social context of the oppression of trying to "adjust/accept" an inferior role in life. (The article on postpartum depression, in Chapter 11, p. 495, describes another women's mental health issue which is often ignored or individualized, but needs serious research on how it relates to wider social issues.)

The good news is that the availability of feminist therapy, women's self-help groups, and other resources specifically support women to explore and confront the social and cultural contexts of what is making them unhealthy. Now that women who choose to be in therapy have identified that they want counseling which relates to their socialization in a sexist society, consumers need to be alerted to the trend for some therapists to market themselves as "feminist therapists" even if their therapy techniques are fairly traditional. Both Murphy and Rummery describe guiding philosophies a woman seeking feminist therapy should be able to expect. Although Rummery's article focuses on survivors of child sexual assault, it is included in this chapter because it so well presents feminist theory and practice addressing the core social context of women's mental ill health.

"Co-dependency: A Feminist Critique" looks at how the co-dependency label gets put on many of the same behaviors which our society encourages as positive for women and then, "because co-dependency so accurately describes what many of us experience in our lives, we blame ourselves for the behaviors." Bette Tallen's thought provoking article looks at how the concept of co-dependency depoliticizes feminism (or any other movement by people who fight against sexism and racism) but also appeals to many women.

Mood altering drugs are prescribed for women twice as often as for men. There are certainly many times when mood altering drugs are beneficial to women, particularly for short periods of time in conjunction with therapy. However, the overall pattern of high prescription rates for women is of concern and is symbolic of how often women are told directly or indirectly that their problems are "all in their heads." Just as Greaves identifies (in Chapter 7, p. 303) that many women use cigarettes as a way to cope with their lives, mood altering drugs have often been a physician's way of calming a woman down without addressing the real life issues which are upsetting her. The problems of such a pattern are particularly well documented for battered women when mood altering drugs do nothing to stop her abuser's violence but may actually increase her danger by making her miss warning signs of escalating violence, reinforce what her batterer told her about "it's all in your head/you are crazy," and also become the tools with which to commit suicide. The next three articles approach the issues of the over-selling and over-prescribing of mood altering drugs from very different directions but all use Prozac or "born again Prozac," Sarafem, as core topics of discussion. This is not meant to be a critique of Prozac/Sarafem per se, but instead this product is the teaching tool to help us examine dangerous patterns of the over-use of a wide range of mood-altering drugs.

In an excellent *New York Times Magazine* article (October 1, 2000, pp. 17-18, not reprinted here), "Female Troubles" which first exposed how Eli Lilly was repackaging Prozac as a pink-and-lavender capsule to market for premenstrual syndrome, Peter D. Kramer, author of *Listening to Prozac,* observes and asks,

> If drugs are carriers of cultural values, Sarafem looks like a harbinger of change. Women are the primary users of drugs that alter mood. At mid-century, Miltown and Valium were infamous for helping housewives cope, if sluggishly, in settings where discomfort may have been in order. By contrast, at Century's end, when women's place had moved from home to office, the drugs of the moment were the ones that seemed to confer energy and resilience—Prozac and its peers. . . . What does it mean that, as the start of a new century, a drug so many women say has caused them to be less retiring, more confident is being repackaged as a "mother's little helper?"

"Prozac Up at UW" provides glimpses at several important issues related to mood-altering drugs and the use of mental health services through trends at the University of Wisconsin-Madison. Observing that the ratio of students using the University clinic is 60:40 females:males, a psychiatrist estimates that UW-Madison reflects what is seen nationally with approximately 13% of students having mood disorders and depression being the most common. There has been a drastic increase in the number of students using counseling services with approximately 30% of these students being prescribed psychotropic drugs. This brief article introduces several huge topics. What does it mean that "depression is becoming more acceptable as an illness"? While it is a much needed change to think that mental health issues are not stigmatized, is that the "good news"? Or do we see more people actually needing to cope with depressing situations and lives, while effective marketing gets more people labeled as needing drugs to fix them? One more important red flag in this article is the excellent strong statement, "Most college students respond best to anti-depressants when combined with psychotherapy . . . Only in rare cases do campus psychiatrists prescribe drugs without requiring counseling." With an increasing number of insurance plans pushing mood altering medication with no or little counseling and many people unable to get insurance coverage for good counseling, how many people get the chance to improve their mental health with the optimal amount of therapy?

The Center for Medical Consumer's *Health Facts* does a consistent excellent job of informing consumers about critical issues. Their July, 2001, "Born-Again Prozac: Not Worth the Extra Cost" warns consumers that Prozac repackaged as either Sarafem or Prozac Weekly is going to cost them much more for exactly the same drug. This article describes how easily companies can get around the laws intended to encourage cheaper generic equivalents to brand-name drugs once a patent expires. Repackaging a drug, either for a new use or in a new dosage form, allows the companies to continue to enjoy very high profits protected by patents for the supposedly "new" product.

"You, Too, Can Hold a Congressional Hearing" describes how anyone can learn to use political processes to become an activist for women's health. This article traces the steps it took for a group of women, representing many women's health organizations, to alert congressional members to the problems of Sarafem being approved for the treatment of Premenstrual Dysphoric Disorder (PMDD) both because it was simply a way for the drug company to get around the fact that the patent was running out and, most importantly, that there is no evidence that PMDD exists. Using this specific example, this hearing was able to address the broader issues of the dangers of direct to consumer advertising and "the entirely unregulated nature of psychiatric diagnosis." Europe is ahead of the US in not allowing Sarafem to be marketed for PMDD because PMDD is not a proven condition.

Women and Mental Health

by Marian Murphy

What We Mean by Mental Health

Mental health, as opposed to mere absence of mental illness is a complex and often controversial subject. What defines mental health? Who defines it? In terms of women, notions of mental health carry an added burden of value judgments and traditional beliefs. It is my view that mental health is a concept that needs constant redefinition in the light of new knowledge and, within the framework of this discussion, mental health refers not simply to the absence of symptoms or problems but to the presence in a woman of *well-being* and *growth* and the ability of a woman to solve problems in a reality-based way.

A healthy and growing person can be described as moving towards increased acceptance of and openness to herself and others; increased self-support and self-esteem; growing capacity to give and receive love; increased intellectual competence and creativity; greater freshness of perception and richness of feelings (both joy and pain); a more aware, autonomous, and caring value system; a growing sense of closeness to the natural world; a greater frequency of moments of transcendence; a growing enjoyment of living in her present experience. Using this kind of standard, most people live in a state of permanent mental ill health. At the very least, it is estimated that on average we each fulfil less than 10 per cent of our potential for this kind of growth. The extreme forms of this general ill health are reflected in the increasing numbers of people using psychiatric and counselling services and increasing rates of suicide, alcohol/drug abuse and crime.

In the case of women, this situation is compounded by the very standards used to define mental health/illness. There are differing standards of mental health for women than for men among mental health professionals. An often-cited study carried out by Broverman and colleagues (1970) showed that a double standard is employed when assessing the mental health of women and men. Behaviour that was regarded as healthy for an adult, sex unspecified, and thus viewed from an ideal absolute standpoint, was identical to behaviour considered healthy for men, but not for women. This finding that psychiatrists, psychologists and social workers ascribe male-valued stereotypic traits more often to healthy men than to healthy women conceals a powerful, negative assessment of women in general. For instance, these professionals were more likely to suggest that healthy women differ from healthy men by being more submissive; less independent; more easily influenced; more excitable in minor crises; less competitive. Such a combination of traits is a most unusual way of describing any mature, healthy individual.

Another important factor here is the notion of health itself that is used by many professionals working in health services, i.e., an adjustment notion of health. This would suggest that one of the most important factors involved in mental health is adjustment to one's environment. This, together with the existence of different norms of female and male behaviour, also leads to different standards of mental health for women and men. Thus for women to be healthy from an adjustment viewpoint, we must adjust to and accept the behavioural norms for our sex, even though these behaviours are generally less valued socially and are considered less healthy for the generalised competent, mature adult. Acceptance of this adjustment notion of health places women in the difficult position of having to decide whether to exhibit those positive characteristics considered desirable for men and adults such as assertiveness and ambition, thus calling our 'femininity' into question; or to behave in the prescribed 'feminine' manner, accept second-class adult status and possibly live a lie to boot. This strongly suggests that mental health professionals should be concerned that the influence of sex-role stereotypes on their professional activities actually reinforces social and psychological conflict.

Thus, before we even get to the point of looking at the different mental health statistics of women and men, we can begin to consider the possible effects of this double standard of health. A possible implication is that (a) behaviours and feelings exhibited by women and considered 'normal' for us, (e.g., low self-esteem, feelings of depression) and thus not requiring treatment, would be seen as 'symptoms' in men and would be treated;

Reprinted with permission from *Personally Speaking* ed. Liz Steiner Scott, Attic Press Dublin, Ireland 1985.

(b) women exhibiting behaviour which did not conform to these female stereotypes (non-nurturing, lack of interest in childbearing) would be considered 'abnormal' and in need of psychiatric treatment. There is much evidence that this is in fact the case. There are, therefore, numerous implications for both sexes, in the way in which they view themselves and how they should deal with life problems and also in the kinds of treatment they receive from the mental health and medical professions.

Differences in Patterns of Mental Ill Health

The worldwide picture is that the majority of clients for mental health services are women. In North America, for example, women comprise 60–75 percent of clients. In Canada, it has consistently been demonstrated that women receive more prescriptions for all drugs than men and this difference is even more noticeable in the case of psychotropic (mood-changing) drugs, with between 67–72 per cent of these drugs going to women. In Britain, 12 per cent of women take tranquillisers daily for a month or more each year. Although there are no statistics for Ireland, doctors' reports would suggest an equally high level of usage of tranquillisers by women. Women have consistently higher levels of medical consultations than men, both with general practitioners and specialist consultants. What is even more striking than these overall rates of usage of mental health services, which, after all can sometimes be dismissed as differences in help-seeking patterns and willingness to talk about distress etc., is the different patterns of illness displayed by women and men.

In community studies in Britain and the USA where people who have not sought help at all are studied, women consistently report more distress, anxiety and depression. In diagnostic terms, doctors are treating large numbers of women with such clinical conditions as hysteria, eating disorders such as anorexia nervosa (under eating) and bulimia (binge eating) and, most particularly, depression. The incidence of depression in women (matched only by rates of alcoholism in men in Ireland) illustrates the internalised way in which women deal with problems, whereas it appears that men cope by externalising their frustrations. As depression is the most prevalent mental illness among women and has been extensively studied, it may be useful to spend some time on it here.

Women and Depression

Is there something inherent in being a woman that predisposes us to developing an emotional illness? There are a number of possible answers to this question.

Firstly, it is suggested that the incidence of depression is actually more equally divided between women and men but that each sex expresses it differently. It is suggested that men often develop mechanisms such as excessive drinking, or have outbursts of violence. Many treated alcoholics do have symptoms of depression so it would not be unreasonable to infer that men may use alcohol to hide their symptoms of depression. For others, chronic alcohol abuse and the cause and effect factors have not yet been sorted out and, although it is possible to speculate that there are large numbers of depressed men in the community who are simply not visible because of the masking effects of alcoholism, there is no evidence that this is the case.

The differing ratios of depressive ill health in women and men is often accounted for by the fact that women perceive, acknowledge, report and seek help for stress and its related symptoms more readily than men. However, recent studies have shown that women do not experience or report more stressful events than do men nor do we evaluate the standard lists of life events (death of a spouse, separation, change in jobs, etc.) as having greater impact than do men. We must, therefore, conclude that women do actually experience more frequent and more severe symptoms of depression than men.

Could women's depression be accounted for by biological factors? While there is now some evidence to suggest that there is a genetic factor operating in depression, the samples that have been studied are few and there is insufficient evidence to draw conclusions about the way depression is transmitted or to explain the sex differences. Similarly, while there is good evidence that premenstrual tension (PMT) increases rates of depression, it is not a major cause. Also, the amount of female depression that is attributable to the possible effects of oral contraceptives is extremely small indeed. There is excellent evidence that the period following childbirth does induce an increase in depression. However, contrary to widely held views, there is now evidence to show that the menopause has virtually no effect in increasing depression rates. While, therefore, some portion of the sex differences in depression, probably during the child-bearing years, may be explained by reference to biological and hormonal factors, it is not sufficient to account for the consistently large differences.

Sociologists, psychologists, feminists and others concerned with women have become increasingly occupied with explaining why more of us become depressed. The conventional belief is that our long-standing disadvantaged social status causes women to become depressed. The persistence of social status discrimination for women therefore is proposed to explain the greater numbers of us suffering from depression. One extensive study on depression in women suggests that there are two main reasons why we become depressed. This study holds that many women find their situations depressing because of the real social discrimination we experience in our everyday lives; this makes it difficult for us to achieve control by direct action and self-assertion, further contributing to our psychological distress. Such discrimination leads to legal and economic helplessness, dependency on others, chronically low self-esteem, low aspirations and ultimately clinical depression. The second reason why women become depressed is that our socialisation discourages assertiveness. Young women learn to be helpless while we are growing up and thus develop a limited ability to respond when under stress. Instead of learning to act out in frustration or anger as young men do, young women internalise these feelings and become depressed.

Attempts to test these hypotheses have focused on the different rates of mental illness among married and unmarried women.

If these hypotheses are correct, marriage should be of greater disadvantage to women than to men, and since married women are more likely to embody or find themselves in the traditional stereotyped role, they should, therefore, have higher rates of depression. In one study it was found that the higher overall rates of many mental illnesses for women are largely accounted for by higher rates for married women. In every other marital status category, single, divorced and widowed women have lower rates of mental illness. It concludes that being married has a protective effect for males but a detrimental effect for women. Similar conclusions have been reached by researchers in several different countries.

This study and others attribute the disadvantage of the married women to several factors: role restrictions (most men occupy two roles and therefore have two sources of gratification whereas many women have only one); the low prestige of housekeeping and its frustrating effect for many women; the unstructured role of 'housewife', allowing time for brooding and the fact that even if a married woman works, her position is usually less favourable than a working man's.

There are, of course, other important intervening factors such as family size and financial resources. Other researchers have examined the relationship between psychological stress and subsequent affective disorders. They found that working-class married women with young children living at home had the highest rates of depression. Subject to equivalent levels of stress, working-class women were five times more likely than middle-class women to become depressed. Four factors were found to contribute to this class difference: loss of a mother in childhood; three or more children under the age of fourteen living at home; absence of an intimate and confiding relationship with partner; lack of full- or part-time employment outside the home. The first three factors were more frequent among working-class women. Employment outside the home, it was suggested, provided some protection by alleviating boredom, increasing self-esteem, improving economic circumstances and increasing social contact.

From these studies, it can be concluded that the excess of depressive symptoms in women is not entirely due to biological factors inherent in being female, but is contributed to by the conflicts generated by the traditional female role, and the isolation that this role may bring.

The Mental Health Services: How Women Use Them and How Women Are Treated by Them

Given that more women than men experience symptoms of depression and other mental ill health, how is this manifested when we look at the mental health services? To begin with, as already noted, rates of consultation are higher. The usual avenue to the health services is through contact with general practitioners. In this country general practitioners say that at least 25 percent of the consultations are due to psychological factors and that they have neither the training, the time nor the resources to provide appropriate treatment. Moreover, many problems which result from a way of life or a particular difficulty or habit have come to be regarded as diseases rather than problems. Some women's problems which may actually be social, economic, ethical or legal, may be misidentified or wrongly regarded as psychiatric disturbances.

However, there have been few attempts by any western governments to introduce professionals with other than medical training into the first line of contact with people suffering from these kinds of problems and similarly, no attempts have been made to implement programmes of primary prevention and mental health education. The most likely form of treatment, therefore, that a woman will receive for a variety of these problems, is medical, in the form of mood-changing drugs. In fact doctors are more likely to offer tranquillisers to us than to men who present the same complaints, specifically complaints which involve the client being: unhappy, crying, depressed, nervous, worried, restless and tense. For these kinds of complaints men are more likely to receive more physical therapies, laboratory tests and referrals to specialists. Here again the double standard is apparent.

A major contributing factor to this scenario is women ourselves who, in fact, frequently request our doctors to prescribe drug treatment for such symptoms. It has been suggested that this comes about as a result of women's view of our situation, a view which society teaches us. Women have learned to see our resentment and despair about our place in the social structure, as an individual problem, an emotional disorder. Women are trained to invalidate our own experiences, understanding and feelings and to look to men to tell us how to view ourselves. Ideas, concepts, images and vocabularies available to women to think about our experiences have been formulated from the male viewpoint by universities, professionals, industries and other organisations. These are reinforced by images of women in the media: women's magazines, women's novels, women as depicted in advertisements, children's stories and much more. These views are supported by the findings of a Vancouver study that questioned groups of women about their understanding of the uses of minor tranquillisers. Women felt that tranquillisers were sometimes needed to help them cope; coping, for them, meant the management of their roles as housewife and mother. In retrospect, some women expressed doubts about the role of illness that they had accepted and wondered about other options. One woman said: 'I feel that, essentially, when a doctor prescribes a pill for me, it's to put him out of my misery'. Another commented that a prescription for babysitters would have been more useful than a prescription for tranquillisers.

When we look at the training attitudes and practices of doctors and psychiatrists, we see even more blatant examples of sex-bias in treatment. In 1974 a study highlighted the process by which medical schools teach demeaning and derogatory attitudes to women, both as patients and as students. Physicians are taught that women's illnesses are not worth understanding, are unimportant and are of emotional origin. The woman 'patient' is objectified and made fun of. These assumptions about women are part of the very fabric of our society—this appears to be borne out by several studies in the USA on the amount of sex-bias and sex-role stereotyping involved in psychotherapeutic practice. In July 1974, responding to requests by the American Psychological Association Committee on Women in Psychology, a task force was established to look at this whole area. The task force identified four general areas affecting women as clients. The first of these was in the area of support for traditional sex roles. Here the therapists assumed that resolving of problems and self-fulfillment for women come from marriage or perfecting the role of wife without any recognition of women's other potential roles in society. The second general area

was the above-mentioned bias in the medical profession's expectations and devaluation of women. This was exemplified in practice by the use of theoretical terms and concepts (e.g., masochism), to ignore or condone violence towards and victimisation of women; and by the use of demeaning labels such as manipulative, hysterical, etc. when describing female patients. The third general area was the sexist use of psychoanalytic concepts, e.g. labelling assertiveness and ambition with the Freudian concept of penis envy. The fourth area of discrimination identified was the therapist's response to women as sex objects, e.g., heavily weighing physical appearance in the selection of patients or having a double standard for male and female sexual activities and even going as far as seducing female clients.

In view of these findings the American Psychological Association subsequently advocated a whole range of educational efforts to overcome these appalling practices and injustices. There is little evidence to show that these findings have had any effect on the practice of many psychiatrists. In fact, the realisation that 'feminine' characteristics can, in fact, be seen as those of any oppressed group of people tends to be astounding to the psychiatrist.

It is obvious then that the three interacting sets of factors briefly discussed here (a) the medical and mental health systems and the process of medicalisation; (b) the mental health professionals and their attitudes and theoretical backgrounds and (c) the woman and her socialisation; perpetuate a situation which predisposes women to mental, and particularly depressive, illness. Women's problems are treated only as psychological problems, without any prospect of addressing and dealing with the root causes.

Where Do Women Go from Here?

Internationally, the future for our mental health is bleak. In Ireland, as everywhere, additional stress factors such as high unemployment rates and the consequent lack of access to work outside the home for many women, interact with a traditionally male medical and psychiatric culture emanating from a society that clings stubbornly to a view of woman as homemaker and mother. Realisation of the need for a new medical model is appearing, however, and the supposed scientific basis of psychiatry has been greatly criticised. Psychiatrists are beginning to see sexism as a barrier to our understanding of the family and to acknowledge that 'much patriarchal rhetoric has masqueraded as theory.'

Theoretical and practical alternatives are emerging that approach women's problems in ways that are more closely connected with our life experiences. Worldwide, feminist therapy is developing to such a degree that it has been suggested that it has some of the characteristics of a school of psychotherapy. The increased equality of client and therapist, the main focus on environmental interpretations, the movement away from sex-role prescriptions are the features of this new therapy. In Ireland some alternatives to traditional psychotherapy are available but only in urban centres. Women's self-help groups and consciousness-raising groups can be particularly useful here. Women in groups can come to realise that cultural values we have accepted unquestioningly such as maternal success, complete devotion of self to motherhood, and consumerism, as a major source of our tensions and dissatisfactions. Researchers have found that consciousness-raising groups provide a forum in which mildly depressed women with low self-esteem can explore our feelings about ourselves and our life situations. Obviously, participation in such groups is not a substitute for psychotherapy for those women whose problems are long-standing and severe. However, they can provide a useful starting point for women who are beginning to take more personal responsibility for the quality of our lives.

A range of other resources has also begun to emerge which provide support and reduce the isolation of women in extended families. These include family and community resource centres which often provide mother and child clubs, pre-school and day-care facilities, discussion and personal development groups, employment counselling, assertiveness training and legal clinics. 'Return to work' courses, creches in a variety of educational facilities and opportunities for women to come together to work at co-operative ventures are playing a vital role in preventing the development of further mental illness among women. In Ireland, there are few counselling centres which provide education and treatment that is not sex biased, but beginnings are being made.

For women undergoing particular crises, facilities such as rape crisis centres supply practical help, enabling us to confront our anger and avoid chronic and disabling shame and embarrassment. Advice is also available on possible legal action and its implications. Transition houses provide shelter for battered women and their children and have served to alert the community to the enormity of this problem.

Notwithstanding these developments, a great deal still needs to be done. Generally, we need to be more aware of the factors leading to stress and mental ill health. Preventive programmes should be established to help people discover and use their own coping mechanisms and recognise the value of yoga, relaxation techniques, akido, a balanced lifestyle, and other alternatives to the traditional medical response to mental illness.

Caution must be exercised by women anxious to develop alternatives outside the traditional framework of 'the home'. They should not swing to the opposite extreme and create new kinds of 'career' and other pressures that can equally cause an imbalance—to behave like men under stress is not a solution. The ideal would be to redistribute nurturing and work roles between women and men allowing for more balanced lifestyles for all. It is also vital that the new kinds of services already discussed at some length be encouraged and recognised as viable sources of help for women who have hitherto all too often been seen as in need of psychiatric treatment.

Finally, it is imperative that those working in the mental health professions be encouraged, both at pre- and post-qualifying levels, to employ the following guidelines in their dealings with women and that we in turn begin to seek and insist upon a service that embodies the following principles: (1) an equal relationship with shared responsibility between counsellor and client; (2) provision of help in differentiating between the politics of the sexist social structure and those problems over which, realistically, we have personal control; (3) provision of help in exploring our personal strength and how we can use it constructively in personal, work and political relationships; (4) provision of help in confronting unexpressed anger in order to combat depression and to make choices about how to use our anger constructively; (5) provision for helping women to redefine ourselves apart from our relationships to men, children and home including exploration of fears about parental role changes; (6) encouragement to women to nurture ourselves as well as caring for others, thereby raising self-confidence and self-esteem; (7) encouragement of the development of a range of skills to increase women's competence and productivity. This may include assertiveness training, economic and career skills and advice on how to reeducate family and friends who resist change. Although not every counselling situation with women will necessarily incorporate all of these principles they provide a basis for mental health professionals as well as a standard which can be used by women to evaluate the treatment we receive. Women clients, no less than men, have a right to mental health services that are sex-fair, competent and ethical.

Conclusion

Moving from an 'ideal-type' definition of mental health, through some of the examples of ill health in women, and how these are currently treated, I have arrived at suggestions which I believe would help to promote better levels of mental health in women. These suggestions

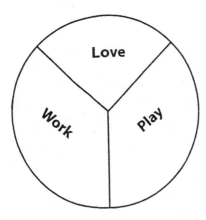

are underlined by a view of people and their psychological needs which I, together with others, working in the mental health services, hold. This view presupposes that mental health involves a balance between three basic areas of life (see diagram): love, based on self-acceptance and self-esteem; work, providing opportunities for a sense of achievement, recognition and status; play, allowing for relaxation and forgetting of self and other preoccupations.

Traditionally, women have loved and worked, men have worked and played. This imbalance has impoverished the lives of both sexes. Ironically, now that some men are beginning to learn to feel and show emotions, affection in relationships is being awarded a status it did not enjoy when found predominantly among women. Women, however, must not only achieve recognition status for the work we do, we must also learn to look after our own needs for relaxation, play and satisfying work and above all for a sense of self that is not defined for us either by society or by our relationships with others. For each individual woman this means maximising existing opportunities for looking at and, if necessary, reordering her lifestyle. For members of the health profession, it means reorganising and eliminating sex-biased practices.

For the community as a whole, it not only means making a commitment to programmes of prevention in the mental health field, but also rejecting the rigid adherence to the stereotypical division of roles, responsibilities and acceptable behaviours between women and men.

It has been because of the growth of feminist thinking and 'psychotherapy' that changes and reanalysis of women and mental health have begun to take place. This development must be guided and supported. It is important for women to recognise our own strengths and contributions in this field and to look to each other for the shared experience and discussion which will allow greater control and responsibilities in our lives.

Questions for Discussion

1. Do you think that the family as we know it is to blame for a considerable amount of mental ill health in women? Discuss.
2. Some women become depressed after childbirth. Why? What other events in women's lives might be the cause of their depression?
3. From your own experience, how does the medical profession treat women as clients? How might you change that attitude?
4. Is it in women's 'nature' to be more prone to mental ill health, especially depression, than men? Discuss.
5. If you have ever taken tranquillisers for any length of time, can you assess how they affected you? Did they help? How? Was it difficult to stop taking them?
6. In what ways can women's groups be a positive force for mental health?
7. If you were in need of professional help, where would you go? Can you think of any alternatives to professional help that might be of use?

References

A list of references is available in the original source.

Mad Women or Mad Society

Towards a Feminist Practice with Women Survivors of Child Sexual Assault

by Fiona Rummery

This chapter examines an aspect of structural violence as embodied in traditional psychiatric labels of mental ill health. Although this discussion revolves around the issues of child sexual assault (which is constituted by physical violation) it does not focus on the interpersonal aspects of such abuse. Rather, it explores the subtler abuse which often informs the framework of societal institutions, such as medicine. When considering violence against women, it is usually overt and direct experiences of violence which are highlighted. It is arguable that women's experiences of systemic violence when seeking assistance are as worthy of detailed assessment. As Irwin and Thorpe argue in the opening chapter in this collection, systemic violence plays a crucial role in allowing interpersonal violence to continue, partly through the processes of silencing and discrediting, as this chapter details.

This chapter considers the question of what it is about a feminist counselling practice that differentiates it from other, more traditional modes of working. It will thus utilise an illustrative discussion of an issue which arose for me whilst working as a sexual assault counsellor. This involved working with an incest survivor who had an extensive history with the psychiatric profession, and my subsequent investigation into this area. As such, this chapter encompasses discussions of the issues involved in child sexual assault generally; women and notions of madness and the way these intersect with constructions of femininity; as well as ideas about working as a feminist practitioner. This is not an exhaustive discussion but rather exists as an exploration of some of the more subtle ways in which we, as workers, must always consider and reconsider the theoretical underpinnings of any practice, as well as constantly analyzing the practical implications of any theoretical formulation.

Child Sexual Assault

Misconceptions, fear and denial surround the issue of child sexual assault, as its existence problematises popular ideas about the fundamental institution of the family. In most cases of child sexual assault the perpetrator is known to the child, and the abuse continues over some time (Waldby 1985). The dominant cultural discourses which attempt to deal with child sexual assault form a powerful and ubiquitous part of the social fabric. More importantly (and confusingly) they are bizarrely contradictory in their nature:

> It doesn't happen; it only happens to poor families; it doesn't happen to THIS family; men do it when their wives are frigid or otherwise unavailable; children are naturally seductive; it doesn't do any harm; it damages for life. (Linnell & Cora 1993, 24)

The sexual assault of children usually involves progressive intrusion over a long period of time, with gradual coercion or co-option of the child, and with disclosure not occurring until some time after the abuse has ended (Cashmore & Bussey 1988). Child sexual assault is a particularly silenced experience; still commonly eliciting responses of disbelief and stigmatisation. It is also a particularly silencing experience in that the intensity and intimacy of violation often leads women to such a state of depression, self-hatred and/or distrust that they are unable or reluctant to talk about it (Stanko 1985; Ward 1984). Much of the early literature on child sexual assault documented the ravages of abuse, focussing on the tragedy of supposedly ruined lives. More recently the focus has shifted towards the process of recovery, with the aid of appropriate intervention. Incest survivors need to be provided with appropriate supportive services that allow them to actively and consciously confront the legacy of their abusive history.

One of the issues that I experienced when I began working with incest survivors, was that a high number had some psychiatric history or diagnosis. Approximately seventy percent of the clients I had seen had been categorised with Borderline Personality Disorder, or as Manic Depressive or as having psychotic episodes and as a result had been hospitalised or prescribed medication. When I questioned these women as to the details of the exact nature of the causes of their depression—or psychotic episodes—I was again surprised by the manner in which the symptoms manifested by these women seemed to me to be normal reactions to abusive situations. This led me to do some reading into women and psychiatry so that I could better understand theoretically the unease I felt intuitively to such psychiatric labelling of women's distress. Moreover, I wanted to incorporate this unease more effectively into my practice.

Women and Madness

The history of the connections between women and madness has been examined by a number of feminist writers in the last twenty years. These have ranged from historians (such as Matthews 1984) through to psychiatrists and social workers (such as Penfold & Walker 1983) and to philosophers (Russell, 1986, 1995). They have examined the manner in which what is defined as 'madness' has changed over time according to context. In addition, they have exposed the manner in which the mental health profession has been used as a mechanism of social control, inextricably intertwined with notions of what constitutes 'femininity'.

The 'science' of mental health will be treated in this discussion as an elastic and value-driven social science. Whilst I acknowledge that some women may be genuinely suffering from psychiatric illnesses, there are also many whose emotions, responses and 'symptoms' are unnecessarily deemed 'sick' within a psychiatric framework. It is this process of pathologising women's behaviour with which this paper is most concerned.

Phyllis Chesler says of her interviews with sixty women aged 17–70 with regard to their experiences in both private therapy and mental asylums: 'Most were simply unhappy and self-destructive in typically (and approved) female ways. Their experiences made it very clear to me that help-seeking or help-needing behaviour is not particularly valued or understood in our culture' (Chesler 1973, XXII).

Central to the definition of what constitutes madness then, is the manner in which femininity is socially constructed. Caplan like Chesler, asserts that: 'A misog-

ynist society has created a myriad of situations that make women unhappy. And then that same society uses the myth of women's masochism to blame the women themselves for their misery' (Caplan 1985, 9).

The traditional 'psychology of women' correlates closely with the 'characteristics of oppression' (Penfold & Walker 1983). Women's sane, average, even self-preserving responses to situations of abuse or oppression are often used as evidence of their own lack of mental health.

Debra

I want at this point to introduce a case example in order to highlight some of the issues referred to throughout. Whilst I am loathe to do this in some senses—as it easily becomes voyeuristic and simplistically condenses a woman's struggle and life—it elucidates my point at different stages of this discussion more effectively than any abstract discussion of 'women' can.

Debra was a woman whom I saw for counselling after she referred herself to the sexual assault service. It was largely through my contact with her that I undertook this research into women and psychiatry. She was thirty-four at the time and had a nine-year-old daughter. She was chronically and sadistically sexually abused by a male family member from the age of approximately eight until sixteen. She has had extensive contact with the psychiatric profession, has had a variety of diagnoses and been prescribed nearly every type of medication. Her first contact with psychiatrists was at age eight when she attempted suicide. After hospitalisation she was labelled 'depressed' and given Valium and sleeping tablets for a number of years.

Her first psychotic episode occurred after the birth of her daughter, at which time she was placed in a psychiatric institution for some months. Since then, intrusive flashbacks of the sexual abuse she had experienced as a child have increased and intensified. She regularly had bouts of depression, suicidal feelings and tendencies as well as repeated psychotic episodes during which time she was hospitalised. She had been prescribed a plethora of drugs, none of which alleviate either the psychotic episodes or her flashbacks. Debra sought counselling at the sexual assault service as her flashbacks had further intensified since the time her daughter turned eight, and she felt strongly that there were things about the sexual assault which she needed to resolve.

Although Debra had a history of extensive contact with health professionals, at no time was she asked about her childhood. Even at age eight, and during her adolescence when Debra was medicated and hospitalised a number of times, the safety and stability of her family life was not questioned. The psychiatrists she saw did not ask her whether she had any ideas about what might be causing her distress. Rather, the manifestations of her emotional distress in response to abuse were treated as symptoms of an illness which could be cured by psychiatric intervention, such as medication.

It became clear to me quite early on that the messages which I was giving Debra directly contradicted those of her psychiatrist, whom she was still seeing. The things that he said to her are best encapsulated in the following examples:

You have no control over this.

You don't know what you need, I know what's *best for you.*

Just do as I say and take the medication.

The sexual assault is not *particularly relevant.* You must not indulge in self-pity and dwell on it. Put it out of your mind, it is in the past now.

You are psychotic and manic depressive. There is nothing you can do about it. You must learn to live with your mental illness.

The work that I undertook with Debra, some of which will be described here, focussed upon validating both her feelings and memories, believing her, and giving her control over the counselling relationship. This approach stems from the belief that the core experiences of child sexual assault are disempowerment and disconnection from self and others. Recovery, therefore, is based primarily upon the empowerment of the incest survivor and the creation of new relationships which are non-abusive. 'No intervention that takes power away from the Survivor can possibly foster her recovery, regardless of how much it appears to be in her best interest' (Herman 1992, 133).

The way in which Debra's psychotic episodes were dealt with by psychiatrists provides an illuminating illustration of the manner in which women's distress is pathologised rather than validated. When I questioned Debra as to the exact nature of her psychotic episodes, these were revealed (over some time) to be a series of extremely distressing memory flashbacks. To label these 'psychotic' effectively removes them from her reality, thereby denying her the opportunity of integration. Whilst these memories were extremely distressing and often bizarre in nature, it was only through exploring them fully that Debra was able to become less afraid of them. As one survivor of childhood sexual abuse wrote: 'I've looked memories in the face and smelled their breath. They can't hurt me any more' (Bass & Davis 1988, 70).

The validation that her terror of flashbacks was an expression of the terror she had felt at the time of the abuse enabled Debra to remove these from the realm of paranoia. By extension, she was then able to turn fear into (justifiable) rage toward a perpetrator who could do such cruel things to a child. This change was in direct contrast to her previous self-blame and confusion about feeling crazy due to her mood hallucinations. The process of remembering and mourning has been well-documented by feminist practitioners as a crucial stage in recovery from childhood trauma of any kind, as it is only through knowing what happened that women can begin to heal and recover from the damage done to them (Herman 1992, 155).

The Problems with Categorisation

A major part of the construction of femininity is the emphasis which is placed upon serving others. This is exemplified in the importance which is accorded to motherhood and women's roles in providing for children. This role, however, has gradually become devalued in western society, so women are ensnared within the paradox of being both glorified and trapped within an oppressive definition of what they should be. At its extreme, some feminist commentators have argued that concepts of femininity and madness are actually interchangeable.

Numerous psychological studies have pointed out that what in the west is generally regarded as the woman's role happens to coincide with what is regarded as mentally unhealthy (Russell 1986, 86; Russell 1995). *The Diagnostic and Statistical Manual of Mental Disorders* (DSM-IIIR), created by the American Psychiatric Association, lists symptoms of all psychiatric disorders and is considered to be the essential reference for those working in Mental Health in the western world. Whilst the length of this chapter prevents greater exposition, it is useful to compare the set of criteria for certain diagnoses, particularly those which are most often assigned to women.

Kaplan (cited in Russell 1986, 82–90) undertook a comparison of the DSM-III description of Histrionic Personality Disorder (which is far more frequently diagnosed in women than in men) with the findings of Broverman's (1972, in Russell) research into what constitutes a mentally healthy woman. The criteria for a diagnosis of Histrionic Personality Disorder are 'self-dramatization, for example exaggerated expression of emotions, overreaction to minor events' (Spitzer & Williams 1987). Remarkably similar is the woman deemed mentally healthy in Broverman's research 'being more emotional and more excitable in minor crises' (as cited in Russell 1986, 82–90).

This comparison illustrates the paradox in which women are placed, in that what are described as healthy feminine attributes can equally be seen as symptoms of psychiatric disorders. Thus, through assumptions about appropriate sex roles on the part of practitioners, a woman who is 'successfully' fulfilling the feminine role by 'revealing emotional responsibility, naivete, dependency and childishness' (Lerner & Wolowitz as cited in Russell 1986, 88) can be very easily diagnosed and labelled. The example used here is by no means the only one. A woman conforming to the female role can also be deemed to have a 'dependent personality disorder', or 'avoidant personality disorder'. These definitions also include a high level of ambiguity, allowing for much interpretation on the part of the practitioner.

Whether women comply with or rebel against traditional precepts of femininity, we risk being labelled 'dysfunctional'. As the above examples reveal, compliance with femininity is not necessarily the safer option, as it can imply any variety of mental disorders; but rebellion against it can be seen as signifying aggressiveness, lack of gender identity, and social maladjustment. The 'catch-22' inherent in this paradox is treacherous for women.

Constructing Reality

The dominant group in any society controls the meaning of what is valid information. For women and other subordinate groups, the version of the world which has been sanctioned as reality does not address their lived experience . . . (Penfold & Walker 1983, 56)

When there is a disjunction between the world as women experience it and the terms given them to understand the experience, women often have little alternative but to feel 'crazy'. Labels of mental ill-health thus create and authorise ways in which women can conceptualise their unhappiness and despair, in a societally acceptable manner. In struggling against this, rather than treating Debra's symptoms as hers alone, a feminist approach seeks to normalise these by placing them within a context. Whilst this does not necessarily alter the feelings she experiences, it does alleviate accompanying feelings of isolation and fault. For example, when I pointed out to Debra that many women experience an increase in intensity and number of memory flashbacks after the birth of a child, or when a daughter reaches the age that they were when the abuse began, she was relieved, and we were able to explore what a daughter's vulnerability might mean to her. I would stress again that this does not necessarily relieve the distress experienced during these flashback episodes, but rather that the panic of feeling 'crazy' and out of control during and afterwards is alleviated. Thus, Debra was able to view her symp-

toms as having a cause, rather than being something intrinsic to her as an individual which she needed to 'learn to live with'. It is important to remember that women's symptoms are real. Although this chapter criticises the fact that these symptoms are seen to constitute an identifiable (or classifiable) mental illness, this does not negate the fact that the symptoms as experienced by individual women can be intense and overpowering. Thus, the theoretical underpinnings of one's practice are revealed in the manner in which one defines women's distress. The psychiatrists who saw Debra acknowledged her distress, as did I. It is the framework in which we interpreted this that differed dramatically.

Mental Illness as Social Control

The institution of psychiatry presents itself as healing, benign and compassionate while obscuring its function as part of the apparatus through which society is ordered. (Penfold & Walker 1983, 244)

Depressed or subservient women serve a social function in that they are unlikely to question their subordinate gender roles nor challenge broader social structures. This is exemplified by Miles (1988) in her discussion of the role of housewife:

The stresses inherent in domestic work and the role of the housewife can lead to neurosis which in its turn is likely to make her even more home-centered and thus vulnerable to further stress . . . [T]he home can become . . . a setting which, by its peculiar strains, 'drives her mad' yet which provides asylum from the impossible demands of the world outside with which she feels that she can no longer cope. (Miles 1988, 7)

If one accepts the premise that the construction of mental health reflects a social ordering of gender, one must then ask what purpose the pathologising of women's behaviour serves. To medicate Debra meant that she remained socially compliant. To label her as crazy enabled both professionals and her family to dismiss those disclosures she did make about the child sexual assault as imagined or exaggerated. This silenced her more effectively than any terror she may have felt.

Jordanova (1981, 106) expands upon this idea, by examining depression within the paradigm of an 'illness'. She compares those illnesses from which men most commonly suffer, with those of women, highlighting how rarely women are allowed to take on the 'sick role': a role which provides relief from day-to-day burdens of work. This is not to negate the underlying framework which operates to posit the female condition as continuously or innately 'sick'. Rather, my point is that men are given societal access to a 'legitimate' sick role. Jordanova effectively contrasts a woman who is depressed and on medication but still expected to perform familial duties, with the more 'serious' illnesses which lead to time spent in bed, relaxation, holidays, and time off work for men. Again, Debra had been medicated and encouraged to 'cope'. For ten years her ability to care for her child and elderly relatives (including her and her partner's grandparents) domestically was actively rewarded, and the time that she spent in hospital frowned upon as indulgent. At no point was she offered the space, time or care to understand and deal with the cause of her distress.

Strategies for a Feminist Practice

Practicing from a feminist perspective will involve a variety of methodological approaches depending upon the context in which one is working. Thus, I do not intend to discuss method, but rather the underlying ideals informing a feminist approach. The ideal is to empower clients to challenge both external power structures and their own internalised oppression. This is necessary because both external and internal oppression can be equally debilitating and disempowering in the manner in which they are personally experienced (Fook 1990, 30).

A feminist approach cannot be a set of 'how-to's' which can be easily adopted. A feminist framework is flexible and evolving, and involves as much an analysis of one's self, as that of the women with whom one is working. This is not to simplify feminism, nor to unify all feminist counsellors into the one category. I acknowledge the diversities within the existing definitions of feminism (and women) and the way in which these manifest in work practices. In order to establish and maintain a feminist practice, the worker must firstly be a feminist. This is in some senses stating the obvious, but I would reiterate that undertaking counselling in a feminist manner is not simply a job or framework which can be utilised and then discarded. Feminist practice is also not merely client-focused. Rather, it extends into all areas of work, examining and analysing the structures in which one is working and in the dynamics between staff members. An example which is pertinent is that of working within a psychiatric institution. In such an environment, one's feminist perspective would be of crucial motivation when interacting with other staff members in the organisation, particularly doctors, and others in positions of power in the hierarchy—in challenging the established frameworks in which they think and label people and which influence their practice.

A feminist approach values collective rather than hierarchical structures and seeks to deconstruct the 'expert worker'—'client in need of help' dynamic, favoring instead empowerment of clients. This is particularly pertinent to a discussion on working with incest survivors. Working from a feminist perspective in essence allows women to be the expert of their own lives. This structuring of one's practices, so that the client is more than merely a recipient, allows the space for them to control the relationship. This is crucial as Herman points out, 'The first principle of recovery is the empowerment of the Survivor. Others may offer advice, support, assistance, affection and care, but not cure' (Herman 1992, 133).

A feminist focus upon validating women's experiences is paramount—indicating to them that they have been listened to, heard, and believed, as this so rarely occurs elsewhere. This again is particularly pertinent to working with victims of sexual assault whose experiences of abuse may have been denied, trivialised or ignored—as in Debra's situation. The silence surrounding sexual assault makes it incredibly difficult for women to speak of their experiences; thus it is not possible to underestimate the impact on a personal level of a worker hearing and believing a woman's disclosure. Working with Debra involved providing constant reassurance that I did believe her memories and that I did not think that she was lying. At times, her fear of having spoken the abuse was palpable. This again reinforces the transformative power of merely disclosing the abusive experiences. It has been stressed that as workers we should never lose sight of the terror of disclosure, adding that on many occasions it is actually as if the perpetrator were in the room: 'The terror is as though the patient and therapist convene in the presence of yet another person. The third image is of the victimiser, who . . . demanded silence and whose command is now being broken' (Herman 1992, 137).

This also highlights the importance of the manner in which the counsellor perceives of change. The worker should not view change simply as a change in behaviour, but rather expand this to create an environment in which it is recognised that change does not have to be structural or large to be of importance. The emphasis is therefore shifted so that an apparently slight change in awareness is valued and its ability to facilitate considerable difference in a woman's life is acknowledged. For Debra this type of change in awareness allowed her to begin to redefine her self and formulate a differing self-image from that previously provided to her. The creation of a new manner in which to perceive her self and her life allowed her to reinterpret her own life experience (Linnell & Cora 1993, 36). This new-found ability to resist the dominant discourse of her experience facilitates the potential for both social and personal empowerment. Goldstein comments that the personal narrative has been the way in which women have attempted (often privately and without recognition) to link up their lived experiences and feelings in the face of social definitions: 'The use of this method is most instructive for social work because it reveals how personal and social change may be spurred by the kind of consciousness raising that occurs when people explore their own stories' (Goldstein 1990, 40).

Another essential feature of a feminist practice is that the worker's values are stated, and there is no pretence at objectivity or impartiality: 'The consciousness of oppression has implications for alternative approaches such as those developed in self-help groups, women's studies, political action and consciousness raising' (Penfold & Walker 1983, Xl).

In my practice, in order to challenge dominant constructions of power and knowledge, I take an overtly non-neutral position. This is achieved through providing the woman with the space, opportunity and information which is necessary for her to begin to consider her own experiences in the light of the broader cultural and social context. An example of this involves providing women with knowledge of the incidence of child sexual assault (as well as common reactions and experiences as detailed previously). This broader context allows the woman's perspective to encompass her own experience as well as the knowledge of a complex social dynamic. It is then possible to provide questions and possibilities which facilitate the reframing of personal experience within the context of this new knowledge (Linnell & Cora 1993, 34). Whilst this mode of working could be accused of not being 'impartial' enough by traditional practitioners, it is important to differentiate here between making one's political and social ideologies clear without rupturing the boundaries of the counselling relationship, and importing the worker's own emotional personal agenda into the working relationship. Herman provides a poignant explanation of the difference between the technical neutrality of the practitioner as opposed to what she calls moral neutrality: 'Working with victimised people requires a committed moral stand. The therapist is called upon to bear witness to a crime. She must affirm a position of solidarity with the victim' (Herman 1992, 135).

She further extends this notion to explain that it does not necessitate a simplicity which assumes that the victim can do no wrong and asserts that rather it involves an understanding of the fundamental injustice of the child sexual assault and the victim's subsequent need for 'a resolution that restores some sense of social justice' (Herman 1992, 135).

If we see that the depression of women speaks their lived experiences and represents a feminised manner of calling for some kind of understanding, then 'a detailed examination is called for which concerns itself not just

with which women in the population get depressed, but how and why' (Jordanova 1981, 106–07).

Social analysis does not necessarily help those women who feel unable to cope with their day-to-day existence. Knowledge that their 'illness' is part of broader structural problems, and attributable to their social situation does not automatically endow them with feelings of joy and liberation. Whilst this is an important long-term aim, it does little to alleviate the suffering women individually experience. It 'highlights the immediacy of the problem for women, and the need to think in terms of immediate action, not just the distant solutions implied in abstract analysis' (Jordanova 1981, 105).

If counselling is about negotiating an adjustment between client and environment (Fook 1990), then the treatment undertaken for women deemed 'mentally unhealthy' has largely sought to adapt them to their environment. A feminist approach, however, would necessitate an examination of the societal factors which have led to the level of emotional distress present. Essentially then, public and private struggles are as inextricably linked as are theory and practice. Most importantly, neither partner in either equation should be treated as superior as each is crucial to the other.

Conclusion

It is necessary for a feminist practice to examine the oppression of women in both private and public, individual and institutional, structural contexts. Although this chapter has utilised the example of parts of one woman's story, as stated earlier this is representative of the experiences of many of the women with whom I have worked. The process of labelling these women when they exhibit intense emotional distress as 'disordered' or 'sick', effectively silences their disclosures of abuse. To accept that there are extremely cruel and sadistic acts perpetrated against children within our society is confronting and difficult. The manner in which social institutions and scientific discourse interact with the ideologies of patriarchy, needs to be exposed, and such interactions condemned for the manner in which they subjugate women.

Labels of mental illness do not exist in a social vacuum. To deny the importance of an individual's abusive childhood is to abdicate the responsibility that we all have for the impact of our actions on others. Such denial contributes to the continuation of such abuse. Links between madness as a social construction, and madness as a subjective experience (or as a 'sane' response to abusive or oppressive experiences) need to be explored. Further, the label of 'madness' when applied to women needs to be viewed with utter skepticism before being accepted as an appropriate diagnosis.

References available in original source.

Co-dependency
A Feminist Critique
by Bette S. Tallen

Thanks to Elliott, Donna Langston, Mara, Rosemary Curb for comments and suggestions although only I am responsible for the opinions expressed here.

I live in a community where co-dependency is big business, where women have had in-hospital treatment for it, where many belong to Co-dependents Anonymous, where therapists advertise in the women's community as specialists in co-dependent treatment. Many women have described themselves to me as co-dependent. This behavior is neither new nor unique. In 1989 when I worked in a Women's Studies Department in a state university in southern Minnesota, we offered a one-credit workshop on co-dependency, we were so flooded by student demand for the course that we had to schedule a second section. This was in a community of less than 40,000 people. Moreover, the more I talk to other women around the country the more I realize none of this behavior is all that unusual. Books on co-dependency are best sellers, not only in feminist bookstores but on national best-seller lists. Women-only and lesbian-only co-dependent groups abound. Treatment centers for women advertise in newspapers as well as on TV.

In short, co-dependency is an idea whose time has come. Sharon Wegscheider-Cruise defines co-dependents as "all persons who (1) are in a love or marriage relationship with an alcoholic, (2) have one or more alcoholic parents or grandparents, or (3) grew up in an emotionally repressive family." (Wegscheider-Cruise, as quoted in Anne Wilson Schaef, *Co-Dependence: Misunderstood—Mistreated,* p.14.) Feminists and non-feminists alike embrace the concept of co-dependency to describe a phenomena that, according to Wegscheider-Cruise affects 96% of the population. *(Ibid.)*

Startlingly few critiques of the concept of co-dependency have emerged from our lesbian and feminist communities. We have no sustained analysis of the history of the term and have had little or no discussion of the political implications of using it as a method of understanding women's lives. Recently, I heard a woman describe another woman who is dying

of cancer as only sick because she was co-dependent (cancer being one of several fatal diseases that co-dependency "causes," at least according to Anne Wilson Schaef [*Co-Dependence,* p.8.]). I was enraged, both as a cancer survivor and as a teacher of courses on women and health, I know only too well about the environmental and political issues that are critical to any discussion of cancer. African-American women and men suffer from and die from cancer in far greater numbers than do white people. Women continue to die from such drugs as DES. Are we all co-dependent? Or are we all suffering from a system that systematically targets certain groups as expendable? In short, what do we as women gain from explaining aspects of our lives as stemming from co-dependency?

Who is a co-dependent person? Who gets to say? Who has the appropriate credentials and skill to label

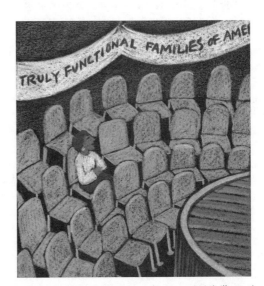

From Sojourner: The Women's Forum, (January, 1990). Illustration © 1990 by Linda Bourke.

someone as co-dependent? The list of symptoms of co-dependency sounds like a catalogue of our lives. Anne Wilson Schaef, for example, lists the following as characteristics of co-dependency: dishonesty, not dealing with feelings in a healthy way, control, confusion, thinking disorders, perfectionism, external referencing, dependency issues, fear, rigidity, judgmentalism, depression, inferiority/grandiosity, self-centeredness, loss of personal morality, stasis and negativism. (*Co-Dependence*, pp. 42–43.) Who hasn't experienced these feelings? John and Linda Friel argue,

> Is it not true that almost everyone had some form of dysfunction in their childhood that could lead to co-dependent symptoms? And if everyone has "it," does it not lose its conceptual and diagnostic meaning. . . . The [DSM-III-R] always describes symptoms, but asks us to look at length and severity of symptoms . . . before we make a definite diagnosis. (*Adult Children: The Secrets of Dysfunctional Families*, p.161)

Since apparently only the "experts" can label co-dependents and since all of us potentially suffer from "it," we are all forced to seek their "expert" advice, treatment, and workshops in order to "get well," or opinion to determine if we are sick in the first place.

Co-dependency as a concept emerged during the late 70's from the therapy community. Melody Beattie suggests that the term emerged simultaneously from several treatment centers in Minnesota. (*Co-dependent No More*, p. 29.) With the concept of co-dependency the therapeutic community attempts to co-opt both the feminist movement and the Twelve Step movement represented by Alcoholics Anonymous.

Alcoholics Anonymous, one of the most successful grassroots movements of our time, was founded in 1935 by two upper-middle-class white males, Bill Wilson and Dr. Robert Smith. It has literally saved the lives of thousands of men and women who would have otherwise died because of their drinking. Much is quite admirable about Alcoholics Anonymous, its offshoot organizations, and the Twelve Steps themselves. However, feminists and lesbians need to examine the roots of AA, et. al. We must also make distinctions between those groups that are under the AA umbrella (such as Al-Anon and Alateen) and are therefore governed by AA's Traditions and those that are not (such as Co-dependents Anonymous). Alcoholics Anonymous attempts to combine the medical knowledge of alcoholism with the pragmatism of William James ("Keep on coming back! It works!") and a form of Christian fundamentalism which is peculiarly American ("Let Go. Let God.")* The founders of AA believed in scaring the alcoholic by hit-

ting "him" (in its early days AA did not admit women) with the medical facts about *his* "disease." Only when the alcoholic had sunk as low as possible, would *he* be amenable to treatment. Underlying the Twelve Step approach to the treatment of alcoholism is a conversion experience, being "born again," after one hits rock bottom. This can involve either a religious experience, as traditionally understood (belief in a patriarchal God) or can also mean an immersion in a community (the community of those recovering) or any number of possibilities in-between. AA historian, Ernest Kurtz, describes it as a, "*salvation* attained through a *conversion,* the precondition of which was the act of *surrender.*" (Ernest Kurtz, *Not-God: A History of Alcoholics Anonymous*, p.182.) Critical to this conversion is not only an understanding of the Twelve Steps but also its grounding in the Twelve Traditions of Alcoholics Anonymous.

The Twelve Traditions are the governing principles of AA, they express many of the principles of first century Christian anarchism on which AA was based. They were designed to keep AA a grassroots, member-focused organization. Not only do the Traditions distance the organization from experts and from treatment approaches, but they also address the forms of self-aggrandizement and endorsement that are seen at the core of alcoholic behavior. They fully explain the Anonymous part of the AA name. Twelve Step groups not under the AA umbrella are not bound by the Traditions. And it is precisely these traditions, to my mind the most positive features of AA, that are getting lost in the Recovery Industry.

It does not take a particularly astute observer of American life to realize how big the Recovery Industry is, judging from its numerous publications, workshops, treatment centers, best-selling books, etc. Its big names are major media stars: their words and ideas come at us from all directions. We are literally bombarded with their messages. And what they have done to the Twelve Step movement is most interesting indeed.

Recently a friend and I visited one of the largest treatment centers for women in southern Minnesota, we were both suitably impressed by the presentation. It was slick, the brochures impeccable, the grounds immaculate, and of course, the facility spacious and inviting (providing the patient was not on medicaid or public assistance, they treat only those with adequate insurance or cash). Critical to the center's treatment program is its inpatient Twelve Step groups. In fact, one of the therapists mentioned that because the center was not given enough time and money from insurance companies to provide truly adequate de-tox (e.g., for some addicted to prescription medications it could take months to bring them safely off the drug but most insurance plans pay only for no more than thirty days in-hospital treatment), groups (along with individual counseling) were the primary treatment. When I questioned the head psychiatrist about requiring patients to attend Twelve Step meetings, since required attendance is antithetical to AA practice, she replied, "Yes, that is a problem," and changed the subject. Questions about how the therapists (many of whom were neither recovering substance abusers nor self-identified co-dependents) could participate in recovery groups were met with the same gracious stonewall of polite avoidance. The presence of therapists as experts, qualified only by training and not by experience, in such meetings, and the compulsory attendance contradict the Traditions and practices of AA (e.g., therapists cannot remain anonymous in group meetings when they see the same clients in individual counseling). Further, this takes place, not in a grassroots setting accessible to all who need help, but in an expensive facility which is enormously profitable. One of the therapists frankly admitted that she had never even heard of the Twelve Traditions. She stated that the only reason the hospital had started the women's unit was because they knew it would make money. And lots of money it makes.

Co-dependency and its treatment lie at the heart of how the Recovery Industry seeks to manipulate and control women. Ostensibly the concept arises out of the Al-Anon movement, the group started by Lois Wilson and Anne Smith that was initially composed of wives of men in AA. Al-Anon was founded on the concept that those who lived with alcoholics were affected by alcohol in some of the same ways as the alcoholic. However, at no time during its founding or since, was it held that alcohol affected the spouse physically, as it affected the alcoholic. The behaviors of the alcoholic were the primary issues. Enabling behaviors of the significant other were not seen as a disease or an addiction, but as a stumbling block to the alcoholic's recovery. The current concept of co-dependency varies from this quite significantly.

First, and perhaps most important, co-dependency is seen as a disease, a progressive, definable disease, with an inevitable outcome, and which, if not treated will result in death. Schaef even argues that, left untreated, the co-dependent will likely die before the addict. (*Co-Dependence,* p. 6.) There is the implication that co-dependency may actually be a more serious condition than addiction to a substance. Co-dependency is characterized as an addiction that produces significant physical symptoms, which some experts believe occur before the co-dependent becomes involved with the substance abuser. As the Friels argue, "[W]e are stating clearly that we do not believe that people become co-dependent because they have been living with an addict. Rather we are stating that they are in a relation-

ship with an addict *because* they are co-dependent." (*Adult Children,* p.157.) The difference between the stance taken by the Recovery Industry and that of Al-Anon is huge. People in Al-Anon, are encouraged to create a healthy distance between themselves and the behaviors of the alcoholic, but they are not viewed as being ill prior to the relationship. Feminists and others who have critiqued Al-Anon say it too often focuses only on the alcoholic and not enough on the significant other.

Second, almost all the behaviors ascribed to co-dependents are traditionally seen as feminine behaviors in this society. How the experts on co-dependency handle this, I believe, underlies much of how the co-dependent movement itself seeks to de-politicize feminism. Melody Beattie, for example, describes the characteristics of co-dependent behavior as low self-worth, repression, obsession, controlling, denial, dependency, poor communication, weak boundaries, lack of trust, anger, and sex problems. (*Co-dependent No More,* pp. 35–47.) These behaviors form feminine identity in American culture. Growing up female means identifying ourselves as weaker, less-worthy, dependent on men, etc., in order to survive. If we resist these messages, we are penalized for our anger and lack of trust.

Because co-dependency so accurately describes what many of us experience in our lives, we blame ourselves for the behavior. In an introductory women's studies class I taught, a student talked about how much she learned from the book *Women Who Love Too Much* and how it helped her understand her feelings about her ex-husband, who battered her. I made an off-handed comment that perhaps the best book would not be on women who love too much but one on men who hit too much. In her journal, she wrote about how my comment "blew her away;" she never thought she could hold him responsible for his own behavior. Co-dependency, thus teaches us that femininity is a pathology, and we blame ourselves for self-destructive feminine behavior, letting men evade any real responsibility for their violent and abusive behavior. The Friels state, "If someone tried to make love to me when I said I didn't want to, this would be an individual boundary invasion." (*Adult Children,* p. 58.) I would call that rape. (They consider incest the result of "weak intergenerational boundaries," p. 60.) Redefining rape as weak boundaries on the part of both victim and perpetrator blames the victim.

Critical to co-dependency analysis is the view that you cannot control the behavior of the addicted person. Although obviously it is true that no one can control anyone else's behavior, the extension of the argument is that a co-dependent cannot even criticize the behavior of the addicted person; rather they are taught to focus exclusively on their own health. Anne Wilson Schaef states that responsibility should no longer imply any kind of obligation, but rather should only be seen as the ability to respond, to explain one's own behavior. She writes, "responsibility is the *ability to respond*. In the Addictive System responsibility involves *accountability and blame*." (*When Society Becomes an Addict,* p. 42.) In this view, women's responsibility is to look at their own behavior: they can neither blame nor hold men accountable for violent and abusive behavior. Sexism, and by extension, any system of oppression, becomes only the problem of the victim; the perpetrator can no longer be held responsible.

Third, the therapy community de-politicizes feminism by insisting that the root cause of co-dependent behavior is being raised in a dysfunctional family. The concept of dysfunctional family is based on the idea that it is possible to have a warm, loving, close nuclear family within the context of racist, capitalist, heteropatriarchy. It betrays the fundamental feminist insight that the patriarchal family itself is the primary institution in the oppression of women. As Simone de Beauvoir states, "Since the oppression of women has its cause in the will to perpetuate the family and to keep the patrimony intact, woman escapes complete dependency to the degree in which she escapes from the family." (*The Second Sex,* p. 82.) Not only does the concept of dysfunctional family ignore the sexism and heterosexism involved in the reality of family life, but it also renders invisible the racism and classism inevitably underlying the "warm, loving, family" conceived of by family therapists and psychologists. It creates, in Audre Lorde's term, a "mythical norm:" a standard by which we all judge ourselves to be wanting. ("Age, Race, Class and Sex: Women Redefining Difference," in *Sister Outsider,* p. 116.) The fantasy of the "functional" family imagines a well-employed father, and perhaps now, an equally well-employed mother, and children, able-bodied and well-adapted to society's definition of their race, class and gender. Families, such as the single-parent African-American family or gay and lesbian families, are seen as dysfunctional by definition and are therefore dismissed without any understanding of how those families may function far better for their members than the white, middle-class, "ideal" family. As Donna Langston has pointed out to me, many of the characteristics of co-dependent behavior, when seen in a working-class context, are actually critical aspects of survival skills. To learn to depend on others is what enables poor and working-class people to survive. To work only on healing the pain from having been raised in a "dysfunctional" family, holds out the hope that it is possible to achieve a fundamentally healthy family in this society without challenging the basic institutions of capitalism,

heterosexism, sexism, racism, and classism that produced the patriarchal family in the first place. When we, as feminists, work on our issues of childhood abuse and neglect, part of the purpose is healing our own pain, but we also must seek to understand the political context that makes such abuse widespread, accepted, and an everyday occurrence, and fight collectively to stop it. The lack of any racial or class analysis in any of the literature on co-dependency underlines the white, middle-class nature of its roots in the therapy community and reinforces my belief that it represents an attempt to de-politicize feminism. Co-dependency adherents argue that we can get "well" without fundamentally altering the very institutions that created the situation in the first place. Beattie goes so far as to argue, that a preoccupation with injustice is a further proof of addiction. (*Co-dependent No More,* p.33.)

Why then is the concept of co-dependency so attractive to so many feminists and lesbians? A primary reason, in my view, is that co-dependency theory so accurately describes the reality of many of our lives. We feel powerless and unhappy. We live in a woman-hating culture where we pay a high price for resisting internalizing messages of feminine weakness and unworthiness. We are taught to depend on men for our survival. Co-dependency treatment offers hope that we can achieve our own private health. It allows those privileged by race, class, or sexual identity, among others to avoid looking at our privileged statuses. Co-dependency theory feeds on our complacency: we are no more responsible for behavior oppressive to others than any man is for his behavior to women. It teaches us that only we are responsible for our fate, that social activism and discontent are merely further symptoms of our "disease." When white women are confronted by women of color about their racism, they can now claim that racism is another symptom of their addiction, and their major task is to "get well." White people are not racist because they are sick, they are racist because they benefit from a system of racial superiority, they are privileged.

Co-dependency offers a relatively safe haven for those who can afford treatment. Its theory addresses many of the same concerns that we as feminists address, but without asking us to pay the high personal price of challenge and criticism. How many times have we felt judged wrongly or trashed in feminist groups without being given adequate space to explain? Co-dependency treatment offers a context of personal support that is all too often missing in our communities.

Co-dependency provides another way to resist the messages of femininity without fundamentally questioning the values of the racist, capitalist, heteropatriarchy we live with. We can get well, are encouraged to resist on a personal level, without ever really having to examine what made us "ill" in the first place. Therefore as we get "better," millions of other women will continue to be born into a culture that is misogynist to the core. Co-dependency theory offers a way to achieve a personal peace without examining the cost of that peace to others.

Note

*For a more detailed discussion of the history and roots of AA see my paper, "Twelve-Step Programs: A Lesbian-Feminist Analysis," in *NWSA Journal,* Summer 1990.

References

Melody Beattie, *Co-dependent No More.* New York: Harper/Hazelden, 1987.

Simone de Beauvoir, *The Second Sex.* New York: Bantam, 1961.

John Friel and Linda Friel, *Adult Children: The Secrets of Dysfunctional Families.* Pompano Beach, Florida: Heath Communications, 1988.

Ernest Kurtz, *Not-God: A History of Alcoholics Anonymous.* Center City, Minn.: Hazelden, 1979.

Audre Lorde, *Sister Outsider.* Trumansburg, N.Y.: Crossing, 1984.

Anne Wilson Schaef, *Co-Dependence: Misunderstood—Mistreated.* Minneapolis: Winston,1986.

Anne Wilson Schaef, *When Society Becomes an Addict.* San Francisco: Harper & Row, 1987.

Prozac Use Up at UW

by Amy Zarlenga

UW–Madison health providers are seeing a steady rise in use of anti-depressants on campus with 30 percent of students who go to counseling clinics now on some form of mood-altering medication.

Dr. Eric Heiligenstein, a psychiatrist at Counseling and Consultation Services and a clinical assistant professor in the UW Medical School, estimated about 12 percent of all UW students have mood disorders, and depression is the most common. National surveys of college-age students show the same figure.

About 30 percent of students seen by health counselors take psychotropic medication, and anti-depressants comprise the bulk of them, Heiligenstein said. The most often prescribed anti-depressants are Prozac and its chemically similar cousins, Paxil and Zoloft.

The number of students using counseling services has dramatically increased by almost 50 percent since 1993 and has forced the number of full-time employees to double, from nine to 20 today. About 12,000 visits were made to campus counselors last year, Heiligenstein said, and much of this is caused by increases in the number of depression cases.

• • •

Julie's story: Julie started taking Prozac, an anti-depressant hailed since its creation as a miracle drug for depression, when she was a UW-Madison freshman and had been feeling different than her usual self.

I was always tired, and I would just cry forever," said Julie, who went to the University of Wisconsin-Madison's Counseling and Consultation Services to get help. There, she was prescribed the drug and worked with a psychotherapist by talking out many of the problems she didn't even know she had.

And cases like Julie's are on the upswing, Heiligenstein said.

Julie soon found out some of her closest friends were taking anti-depressants for the same reason. And today—three years later—she's still taking the drug and claims that without it she'd have flunked out of school and would be living with her parents again.

Anti-depressants stimulate the brain to increase it's production of serotonin, a chemical that is at low levels in people with depression.

Although anti-depressants are most often used to treat the illness for which they were created, they can be used to treat a variety of mental and physical illnesses or ailments, Heiligenstein said, including anxiety, migraine headaches, compulsive behaviors, smoking addiction, and attention deficit hyperactivity disorder.

Prozac was introduced 10 years ago by Eli Lilly & Co. Since then, more than 27 million people, 17 million of whom are Americans, have used the drug.

• • •

Counseling: Most college students respond best to anti-depressants when combined with psychotherapy, Heiligenstein said. Only in rare cases do campus psychiatrists prescribe the drugs without requiring counseling.

"Students come in asking for anti-depressants, and we don't explicitly say this, but we're not waiters or waitresses in a restaurant where people order what they want," he said. "If they want prescriptions alone, we will point them in the right direction, because there are lots of doctors in Madison who will do it that way. But we won't."

Students who go to counseling services have a brief meeting with a therapist or psychiatrist within 24 hours of their request. Staff assess the patients' greatest needs and set up a one-hour appointment for them to meet again.

After the one-hour visit, decisions are made on what route of therapy to take with a patient. Some require medications and therapy, but therapy alone could work for others.

The ratio of females to males seen at the clinic is about 60 percent to 40 percent, respectively. Heiligenstein attributes this to females historically being higher consumers of health care.

Some students are coming to UW already on anti-depressants from doctors in their hometowns, Heiligenstein said.

"I'm getting a lot more calls than I've ever had from parents who have a son or daughter with depression coming to the university and want to make sure we will see them," he said. "We even get calls from the students' doctors. It's a big trend I'm seeing."

The danger involved, however, is some students come to campus unprepared. They run out of pills or only keep contact with their doctor at home for refills. Discontinuing anti-depressants too quickly can result in a depression relapse, Heiligenstein said, and students who simply take the drugs forget the importance of therapy.

• • •

Adolescents' Use Up: The number of adolescents taking antidepressants is also on the rise, leading to more UW students coming into the university with depression, said Sharon Foster, associate professor and assistant clinical professor of pediatrics.

"More adolescents are facing harder situations now than like those 20 years ago," she said. "There's a lot more risk out there now with drugs and alcohol."

Depression is becoming more acceptable as an illness and not a weakness in society, Foster said. The debate continues in current research about how well antidepressants work on young people, but children as young as 5 are taking them, she said.

The UW drinking culture is distracting for students taking anti-depressants, Heiligenstein said. Because alcohol is a depressant, it can wear down the anti-depressant's effect.

"I've often been asked if it's safe to drink with these drugs by students, and we're really careful about this," he said. "I don't feel comfortable giving the blanket statement of 'nothing will happen' because you never know. But I do tell them they won't get better if they keep drinking."

People who take tricyclic anti-depressants—some of the older drugs that include Imipramine, Nortriptyline and Doxepin—can have "horrendous" depressive effects if they drink alcohol, Heiligenstein said. He said the clinic uses the newer anti-depressants partly because employees know many UW students drink.

Julie said that despite an occasional headache and being a little more tired than before taking Prozac, she believes the drug has helped divert her from drinking and keeps her on a schedule.

"I don't really credit the drug itself," she said. "My roommate is the one who woke me up and told me to get help—but it has definitely helped me."

Heiligenstein said the best way to stop taking anti-depressants is to very gradually lower the dosage. The process can take months or even years for people who relapse into depression. But long-term effects of anti-depressants are not dangerous because the drugs are not addictive, he said.

Born-Again Prozac
Not Worth the Extra Cost

Does it make any difference to you whether your pills are purple, purple/pink, or green? Prozac, Eli Lilly's bestselling antidepressant, will soon go off patent; and once that happens the purple versions could cost you about 50% more for exactly the same drug. That's pretty much what it boils down to, though Eli Lilly has mounted an expensive advertising campaign to make you think otherwise about its "new" drug called Sarafem

Except for the color, Sarafem is just a repackaged version of Prozac. It was approved by the Food and Drug Administration (FDA) for the treatment of pre-menstrual dysphoric disorder, a condition that many people think is nonexistent. It has been defined as a "depressed or labile mood, anxiety, irritability, anger and other symptoms, limited to the two weeks before menses." Eli Lilly's ads for Sarafem have left many women irritated and angry, as they are depicted snapping at moments of everyday minor frustrations.

Another retread called Prozac Weekly is now available. It's a once-a-week 90 mg dose. Prozac Weekly and Sarafem are classic examples of how easily companies can get around the laws intended to encourage cheaper generic equivalents to brand-name drugs once a patent expires. Repackaging a drug, either for a new use or in a new dosage form, allows the companies to continue to enjoy unconscionably high profits protected by patents for the "new" product.

Prozac Weekly has been approved by the FDA for "maintenance treatment of depression in people who have responded to daily Prozac." Whether the higher cost of the 90 mg version offers any advantage is arguable. Concerns about the consequences of forgetting to take a daily dose can be laid to rest by understanding how Prozac works. The drug belongs to a class of antidepressants called selective serotonin reuptake inhibitors (SSRIs), which also includes Zoloft, Celexa, and Paxil. Prozac has the longest half-life (the time it takes for half a given dose to be excreted from the body) of any SSRI. Its 4-6 day half-life means that there's no risk in occasionally forgetting a pill.

"The special coating for gradual release of the drug is probably unnecessary in most cases," wrote Michael Craig Miller, MD in *The Harvard Mental Health Letter*. "After fluoxetine [Prozac] has reached a certain level in the blood, most people can take a full week's dose at once without any discomfort or harmful effects."

Oddly enough, when a patent expires and generic competition is introduced, the cost of a brand-name drug tends to go up, according to *Consumer Reports*, which speculates that this could be due to the advertising encouraging brand-name loyalty and the notion that the higher the price, the better the product.

You, Too, Can Hold a Congressional Briefing: The SMCR Goes to Washington About "Premenstrual Dysphoric Disorder" and Sarafem

by Paula J. Caplan, PhD

On February 22, 2002, a Congressional briefing was held on the topic, "Women, Drugs, and 'Premenstrual Dysphoric Disorder': What is Behind the Pathologizing of Mood Changes?" This is the story of how it came to happen and where we go from here.

I was ecstatic when Dr. Joan Chrisler invited me to the Society for Menstrual Cycle Research conference in June, 2001, to coordinate a session to "strategize about what to do about 'Premenstrual Dysphoric Disorder' and Sarafem." That session was the first step on the way to a Congressional briefing, though the latter had not yet entered our minds.

In Avon, Connecticut, the workshop drew many women who were passionately concerned about the topic. I know sometimes I come on like a Mack truck, and I'm not what you'd call a great facilitator, not much good at helping to find solutions the group will like. I had the feeling that my own suggestions, such as demonstrating in front of Eli Lilly's headquarters or the FDA, were not capturing people's imagination, but I hadn't a clue how to get people to say what they wanted.

In walked Joan Chrisler, who listened for a bit and then proposed that we draft a resolution for the SMCR business meeting, and we did that and then headed for the business meeting. Given the absence of evidence that PMDD exists, as well as the common negative effects of Prozac/Sarafem, we proposed that the FDA reconsider its approval of that drug to treat "PMDD", and until that is done, to enjoin Lilly from doing direct-to-consumer advertising (DTCA) about it.

The vote was strongly in favor of the resolution, perhaps helped by the knowledge that the National Women's Health Network (NWHN) was mounting a major campaign about DTCA, and Dr. Diana Taylor, Joan Chrisler, and I were chosen to do follow-through. I still loved the idea of a demonstration, which would include presenting to the FDA head a large scroll with the resolution calligraphied on it. Diana lives on the West Coast, but Joan and I are both New Englanders and met in the summer of 2001 to brainstorm about the next steps to take. Joan noted that the FDA had no head, and as I write this George W. Bush still has not appointed its new Commissioner. We wanted to do something at the time of the Women's Health Conference, then scheduled for October, so people attending the conference could join us.

For more than two decades I had wanted to have a Congressional hearing about the whole enterprise of psychiatric diagnosis, because it is totally unregulated. We had no idea how or if we could arrange for a congressional hearing by October, but we came up with a couple of other ideas. One was to address the Congressional Women's Caucus, even briefly, to inform them about the existence of "PMDD" and Sarafem and alert them to our concerns. Another was to try to hold a Congressional briefing on the subject—not that we knew the first thing about how one makes a Congressional briefing happen. Joan wisely pointed out that, if we aimed to do either or both of those, it might be prudent to defer the FDA action for a while. We also planned to ask other organizations besides the SMCR and NWHN to support our efforts.

After September 11, the national Women's Health conference was postponed to late February. In late September, visiting my daughter's alma mater, Washington College of Law at American University, I ran into Professor Jamin Raskin and told him about our work. He urged me to race up to a lecture hall, where Congresswoman Jan Schakowsky had just given a talk, and tell her he had sent me. Raskin's immediate and serious response to the mention of our aim to have a Congressional briefing was another crucial event. Had he laughed at that aim, it would have been harder to keep trying. I spoke briefly with Schakowsky, a progressive Democrat. She expressed interest in the subject and asked me to follow up with a letter providing her more detail. I did that but received no reply. I learned that it is important to keep phoning, faxing, or emailing because aides are overworked. They may not respond to an initial contact because your issue is not on their Representative's or Senator's legislative agenda, which will not change until after the next election.

Knowing I was going to D.C. right after Thanksgiving, I started making phone calls and requesting meetings with the health and/or women's issues legislative aides in a number of offices. The first was with Schakowsky's Chief of Staff, and with the help of Professor Raskin, I scheduled a talk with two aides for Congresswoman Connie Morella. The first time I entered a Congressional Office Building, I was surprised to find tears in my eyes. As an antiwar protester from 30 years ago, and again now, I would not have expected to be so moved; but it took my breath away to be in a place where an ordinary citizen, could just walk in (through the security machines), feel as though I had a right to be there, and feel that this was where the powerful ideals of democracy live . . . even if only in some of its occupants. Whether sitting in a beautiful inner office with Schakowsky's Chief or leaning on a hallway window ledge with Morella's aides because their office was crowded, I was spurred on to contact aides in other offices because those first ones listened carefully, made good comments, and suggested other leads. I learned quickly that the aides are the ones to ask to see, not the Senators and Congresspeople, who primarily meet with their constituents and colleagues. It struck me that what I was doing was lobbying, and I had no idea how to do it right. Over time, my shyness and sense of being an impostor lessened, but only a little.

In early December, I returned to D.C. to meet with aides in six more legislators' offices. The aides do the research and propose positions to their legislators. On the visit, I saw my Rhode Island Representative, Patrick Kennedy, on the sidewalk and told him I wanted to speak with someone in his office. He gave me the name of the appropriate aide, and saying that the Congressman had told me to call made it easy to get an appointment. Having spread the word about our campaign to friends

of friends, I obtained appointments to meet with aides in still more offices but also made cold calls, asking for brief appointments.

As a lifelong Democrat, I had tended to assume that it would be a waste of time to talk to Republicans, but Morella is an outspoken advocate of progressive causes, and aides from both parties were positive about our concerns about the PMDD and Sarafem story.

I had assumed I'd have about 10 minutes to make our case and ask for support, but many aides gave me half an hour or more from their packed schedules. I explained that there was no evidence that "PMDD" exists and that Eli Lilly, Inc., had worked with the authors of the American Psychiatric Association's *Diagnostic and Statistical Manual of Mental Disorders* to convey the impression that "PMDD" is a real entity and is ameliorated by Prozac, an Eli Lilly product. I explained that Lilly's patent on Prozac was about to expire, but getting the FDA to approve it to treat "PMDD" enabled them to apply for a patent extension, ensuring them additional millions, if not billions, of dollars in future sales. I also said that Lilly had created a pink-and-purple version of Prozac, specially named Sarafem to appeal to women and had mounted a DTCA campaign. Further, I told them that the "PMDD" and Sarafem matter was of concern in and of itself and also was an example of three other major concerns:

1. DTCA advertising of drugs in general;
2. The entirely unregulated nature of psychiatric diagnosis:
3. The fact that, because so many *DSM* categories have not been scientifically shown even to be real entities, anyone assigning a patient an unvalidated diagnosis and then selecting treatment on the basis of that diagnosis is actually subjecting the patient to experimental treatment without their knowledge or consent. I said that many professionals using these labels have no idea that the *DSM* is based on little science.

I found out that Congresswoman Juanita Millender-McDonald was a co-chair of the Congressional Women's Caucus and met with Rae Nicholl, a New Zealander doing a fellowship in her office. Nicholl is an ardent feminist who immediately understood our concerns. My mother and grandmother had always told me that the way to make things happen is to go straight to the top, so—pretending I knew this was an appropriate request but really fearing that things were never done this way—I tried to sound matter-of-fact and asked if we could have ten minutes to address a meeting of the Congressional Women's Caucus. That request was never granted. Back in Rhode Island, well into January, I continued to phone legislative offices and ask to speak to their aides for women's and/or health issues. Often, I got to speak with them. I also contacted members of various women's groups, including the National Organization of Women, to request support. One such aide was Cindy Pelligrini, Chief of Staff and Legislative Director for New York Congresswoman Louise Slaughter, with whom I spoke briefly and to whom I then immediately sent a two-page fax presenting our concerns.

We never found out when the Women's Caucus would meet, but Rae Nicholl told me about a luncheon conference on women's health that was scheduled for January 30, sponsored by Women's Policy, Inc. Going to the latter's website, I learned that Women's Policy, Inc., "is a nonprofit, nonpartisan organization whose mission is to provide nonpartisan public policy research, legislative analysis, and information services to policymakers, the press, and the public on issues important to women and families. It was established in 1995 after the [Republican] House of Representatives voted to abolish . . . the congressional Caucus for Women's Issues. Following the January 1995 vote, the Congresswomen reorganized themselves into a Members' organization by the same name, to continue their bipartisan advocacy on behalf of women. With the encouragement of the Congresswomen, two former staff members of the Caucus started WPI." A phone call to Women's Policy, Inc., saying that Rae Nicholl had suggested I attend the luncheon garnered me an invitation. At the luncheon, I distributed a one-page description of our concerns. The same day, I also met with aides in two more offices, and I received a message from Cindy Pelligrini, saying that Congresswomen Slaughter would be glad to sponsor a briefing and would reserve a room in a House Office Building for us. Thus, we learned we had been wrong to assume we would first have to address the Congressional Women's Caucus in order to begin to garner enough support to find a sponsor for a briefing. (I don't know whether there is any way to have a Congressional briefing other than having a Representative or Senator sponsor it and book the room.) The national conference on Women's Health had been rescheduled for February 21-23, so we chose February 22 for the briefing.

It turns out that the people on the Hill who seem the most supportive and communicate with you the most are not necessarily the ones who will help you make things happen. It had taken only one telephone call and a fax to Cindy Pelligrini to get us a sponsor and a room. I had wrongly assumed that we needed to drum up support from several legislators in order to hold a briefing, but Pelligrini said that Congresswoman Slaughter never minds doing things on her own, a statement that I found both moving and inspiring.

In a three-way call among Joan Chrisler, NWHN Program and Policy Director Amy Allina, and me, and

consulting with Judy Norsigian from the Boston Women's Health Book Collective (BWHBC), we chose the title of the briefing, and Allina designed an invitation. Between Amy and Judy, a list was compiled of the fax numbers for many Representatives and Senators, as well as U.S. legislators who serve on committees or subcommittees relevant to our topic, and NWHN interns Meg Rose and Christine Plummer helped fax them the invitations. At Pelligrini's suggestion, we sent out our invitation, and then the Congresswoman sent her colleagues a letter of her own.

Diana Taylor worked diligently to garner support from other groups, and ultimately the following groups were listed as members of the coalition temporarily created to work on this set of issues: The National Women's Health Network, The Boston Women's Health Book Collective, The Society for Menstrual Cycle Research, The Association for Women in Psychology, the National Association of Hispanic Nurses, The Women's Health Initiative, The Center for Medical Consumers, DES Action, The Working Group on Women and Health Protection, Breast Cancer Action, Prevention First, and The Massachusetts Breast Cancer Coalition. As of this writing, other groups are deciding whether to add their support for the next phase of the work.

The 90-minute briefing was held in beautiful, red-walled Room 1539 in the Longworth House Office Building and was attended by about 25 people—far more than we had dreamed would come—mostly legislative aides or people from government agencies or nongovernmental organizations. The view out the large windows behind the speakers' table was of the Capitol building. Cindy Pelligrini gave a brief welcoming speech and a strong statement of Congresswoman Slaughter's concerns about women's health. Joan Chrisler then spoke on behalf of the SMCR about "Prozac, Patents and Profits—What is PMDD?" Amy Allina spoke for the NWHN about. "Selling Sarafem: Direct to Consumer Advertising," and I spoke on behalf of the Association for Women in Psychology about "Psychiatric Diagnosis: Little Science and No Regulation." We made recommendations for action, including the following:

1. To begin to educate the people of this country about these concerns by appropriating funding for public service announcements, educational pamphlets, and materials about these matters for use in schools, colleges, universities, programs where mental health professionals are trained, and law schools.
2. To propose legislation holding publishers of diagnostic manuals in the mental health field to a standard of full disclosure of the quantity and quality of research behind the diagnostic labels in their books.

3. To propose healthcare legislation requiring professionals who assign diagnostic labels in the mental health field to be well-informed about the quantity and quality of research behind those labels.

4. To propose legislation that will improve the guidelines used by the Food and Drug Administration in assessing research before new drugs and new uses for existing drugs are approved. The guidelines would need to include powerful safeguards to ensure that FDA committees hear from people other than those who have the most to gain from drug approvals.

5. Because there is so much misinformation and disinformation and so little critical thinking about psychiatric diagnosis, to create a forum in which the variety and extent of problems can be presented and as many solutions as possible put forward. For that reason, it is important to schedule Congressional Hearings about the whole enterprise of psychiatric diagnosis.

Following the briefing, many attendees came up to ask questions, and a young woman on a Congressional fellowship to work on women's health until the late summer offered to assist in trying to implement some of the recommendations. A short summary of the briefing was sent to Congresswoman Slaughter. We are now gathering information about other important legislators and aides to whom we should speak about proposing legislation or, as a beginning, proposing House or Senate resolutions, which are much easier to pass than legislation. After the briefing, and exploring legislative routes to change, we have come to understand, even more deeply than before, how much the Congress is hamstrung by their fear of alienating the pharmaceutical companies, who donate huge sums to the campaigns of both Republicans and Democrats. We are also investigating which offices of the Executive Branch of the federal government, particularly Health and Human Services and the Justice Department, are charged with relevant tasks, although the Bush government has shown little interest in increasing regulation. Another possibility we have discussed is trying to persuade one or more state governments to do pilot projects, such as for recommendation #1 or #3.

We know that change takes a long time, but at the June, 2001, SMCR conference, who would have thought that less than nine months later, a large number of women's groups would have come together and had a Congressional briefing? The process of educating and galvanizing support from legislators is well under way, and we are committed to taking the next steps.

If you want to help, you can contact your Congresspeople and Senators and ask them to support any initiatives about these matters. If you would like to send them the information sheet we distributed before the briefing, as well as the post-briefing summary, you will find them on the SMCR website. If you have any ideas for action or any time, ranging from ten minutes on a single occasion to a half-hour a week for several weeks, and you want to help, please get in touch with me at Paula_Caplan@Brown.edu. There is much to be done, and there are tasks of all degrees of involvement and lengths of time required to make them happen.

The briefing was taped recorded, and a copy of the audiocassette can be obtained by sending a $10 check made out to Paula Caplan at 95 Slater Ave.; Providence RI.

Tell Us About Your Activism . . .

No Longer in Whispers

by Karen Milstein

A consumer is not just someone who buys products in our society. I am called a "consumer" because I receive mental health services. For quite some time I have worked as an activist in the mental health field in Madison, Wisconsin. I work to help consumers fight stigma and empower ourselves. This is an uphill fight against strong "phobic" forces around mental illness: societal stigma and self-stigma.

I wear many hats in this city. All of the places I work—for pay or as a volunteer—offer services to persons struggling with mental illness. The struggle is personal. It's where I've been, it's what I know, and helping others helps me. I work for pay at a consumer-run arts-and computer-organization that provides classes for other consumers, ranging from oils to clay to writing. I am also both a part-time weekend staff worker as well as member of a "clubhouse," a place where people with mental illness rejoin the workforce. Finally, this fall I will be working also part-time as a "crisis aide," helping other consumers with various tasks in their lives through our local mental health agency. Wearing these many hats, my life is devoted to encouraging people with mental illness to further their dreams and ambitions.

The vision I work towards is helping people with mental illness to live lives of quality and be granted respect and dignity in our society. So many of the people I know and work with are gentle and highly creative. I also envision giving them a chance to have a life with more promise than hours of loneliness and boredom resulting from living on disability. Granted, I would probably be on the streets without the government support I have had. But it took great creativity to keep my mind alive before I found the local clubhouse, and my present jobs that now fill my time. Life without a respectable full-time job can be an empty, barren life, especially if you have few friends and are revolving through the hospital doors. The agencies I work for rebuild the dignity and pride lost after years of mental distress and hopelessness. So often when one "outs" one's self as a "person with mental illness" one is immediately given less respect and accord. This is certainly an injustice.

For me, activism is making a voice and acting up in the name of injustices done to one because of an aspect of one's identity. I can never forget where I've been and must always strive to go further. "Recovery" is a key word in the mental health field. Helping others find recovery is part of activism. "Thriving" is a word I heard at a workshop last fall in Chicago. "Thriving" is going beyond simply recovery. I hope to help others—and myself—thrive after our oftentimes desperate struggles with mental illness. Mental health problems can be among the most devastating to hit an individual, ripping away one's identity. I hope my efforts in the jobs I occupy make a difference in people's lives, helping them to find new avenues to venture down and finding pride in experiences that are looked down upon in this society, i.e. having been psychotic or hospitalized. At the agencies where I work we are able to talk openly about our experiences with mental distress. This a moving force for consumers. I envision a society in which this can happen. I try to encourage dialogue so the public can learn what mental illness is really about.

These are the things I do: for others, for my own sanity.

WORKSHEET—CHAPTER 5
Women and Mental Health

1. Stress is defined as the non-specific response of the body to demands made on it. These demands can be physical or emotional. The response is non-specific in the sense that, no matter whether the stressor (cause of stress) is seemingly negative or positive, the body responds the same way physiologically. On scales that measure stress of life events, marriage, graduation, and promotion get high stress ratings, along with break-up of a relationship, death in the family, and a jail sentence. If we cannot find ways to manage stress, there can be many possible long term health consequences, such as high blood pressure and high cholesterol (both of which increase the risk of heart disease), lowered resistance to infectious diseases, more migraines if prone to them, various disturbances of the digestive system (including ulcers and colitis), and sleep problems.

   a. List ways you know your body responds to stress.

   b. List several stressors in your life.

   c. List several ways you cope with or manage stress.

   d. If any of your answers to question c have potential negative consequences, identify an alternative positive approach. For example, some people deal with stress by shopping, but a shopping spree can create more stress when the bills have to be paid. Others turn to alcohol or binge eating. What are "healthy" alternatives to these strategies?

   e. Do women and men experience different stressors? Are there differences in the way women and men may choose to or be able to deal with stress? Compare your answer to Marian Murphy's statement, "it appears that men cope by externalizing their frustrations."

2. Mental health is said to be related to a balance of work, play, and love in our lives.

   a. How do these elements balance out in your life?

   b. Thinking through the roles that women and men play in this society, and by rereading the articles "Hazards of Hearth and Home" and "Women's Occupational Health" in Chapter 3, think of whether there are differences for women and men in trying to maintain a balance in their lives. If so, describe some specific differences.

3. What does it mean that mental health professionals give similar definitions for healthy adults and healthy men but describe healthy women as more submissive, less independent, more easily influenced, less competitive?

   a. Does this mean "the only mentally healthy women are the ones who adjust to a world where women are considered inferior?"

   b. Does questioning sexism mean that someone is mentally unhealthy?

4. "Prozac Use Up at UW" reports that many young people are on antidepressants in high school and that this problem is increasing. Identify factors which you think may be related to this.

5. If you are lucky enough to have health insurance, look at your health insurance policy to see what mental health coverage you have. If you wanted or needed counseling, how much counseling would your insurance cover? Can you imagine a situation in which you or a loved one would end up resorting to using mood altering medication without appropriate or sufficient accompanying therapy?

CHAPTER 6

Intimate Partner Violence and Health

Many women define violence—both their actual experiences with violence and their fear of violence—as their number one health issue. "More women are injured in their homes by their spouses or male partners each year than by accidents or illness" (See Ritchie and Kanuha's article). Violence is certainly an issue which affects both women's mental and physical health. In fact, the level of violence a woman has experienced has been found to be a very powerful predictor of her use of medical services, more predictive than demographic variables, other life stressors, self-perceived health, or injurious health habits (I. Schwartz, *American Journal of Preventive Medicine,* 1991, 7(6), pp. 363–373). Many women who have suffered severe physical pain and life threatening injuries from violence have said that the emotional and psychological bruises from abuse take years or decades longer to heal than the physical injuries.

Violence manifests itself in girls' (and boys') and women's lives in many different forms including child abuse, incest, dating violence, sexual harassment, stalking, pornography, sexual assault, date rape, domestic violence, and elder abuse. Although each specific form of violence may be unique in its consequences and the knowledge needed to recognize it, respond to it, and prevent it, all forms of violence (against women) can be defined as issues of power and control where one person or a group takes power and control over another individual or group. Instead of examining the many forms of violence against women, this chapter concentrates specifically on a range of approaches to understanding and addressing the complexities of intimate partner violence. It is expected that readers will draw on these approaches to develop a similar analysis of other forms of violence against women. (Men also get terribly hurt by violence, but men are predominately hurt by strangers, in contrast to women being primarily hurt by people they know and love/have loved. As this chapter concentrates on the health ramifications of intimate partner violence for women, it does not address the important ways that men get hurt by living in a violent society nor examine messages which support violence and unhealthy aggression as signs of masculinity.)

Organizing against violence against women has been some of the most visible and successful work of modern women's movements. For the last three decades, women in all parts of the US and the world have been putting much time, energy, and resources into rape crisis centers, domestic violence programs, incest survivors' groups, and "coordinated community responses" to violence against women. A sophisticated analysis has been developed to show how the abuse of individual women by individual men reflects and is perpetrated by the dominance of men over women in a sexist society. Although social change work is always slower than we imagine, in some ways, the violence against women movements have had an almost "revolutionary" impact on the legal system, the criminal justice system, and the general public's awareness that this is a serious issue. This chapter includes examples of the excellent information which is now produced and distributed by activist groups working to end violence in women's lives.

The continuum of family violence chart demonstrates the relationship of subtle forms of physical, verbal/emotional, and sexual abuse, which society all too often tolerates or condones, to the forms more obviously recognized as serious and deadly. The more subtle forms can themselves have serious consequences and invariably lead to other means of control. It is important to understand that this continuum, an important teaching tool, would look different for different women. While being screamed at would be terribly hurtful for many women, others would be more hurt by "the silent treatment." Abusers usually pay enormous attention to details and *choose* to use the tactics most effective in controlling their partner specifically.

The power and control wheel (developed by battered women and formerly battered women to describe abuse in their lives) is a key tool for educating people that domestic violence is not "just about hitting" but is about an ongoing pattern where one person controls many or all aspects of another person's life. The power and control wheel reminds us that domestic violence is not about an "anger management problem" or "losing control"; it is about *choosing* to *use control.* The cleverest abusers may never get "caught" leaving physical injuries or breaking the law because they so effectively control their partners through the children, by controlling finances, playing mind games, and/or isolating them from their support systems. In contrast to the power and control wheel, the equality wheel (also developed by battered and formerly battered women) serves as an inspiring model of what we want to work for in creating healthy relationships, striving to equalize, rather than use or abuse, power.

Many college women learn about battered women as if domestic violence is something that might happen to them in the future, with too little acknowledgment that at least 1 in 4 young women experience power and control dynamics in dating relationships. An important new study (*American Journal of Public Health,* Volume 93, 2003, pp. 1104-1109) describes "88% of women reporting at least one incident of physical or sexual victimization between adolescence and their fourth year of college when victimization was defined broadly." It seems high school girls and college women are better at identifying one time sexual assault by a stranger than identifying ongoing power and control (including sexual control) in dating relationships. "A More Hidden Crime: Adolescent Battered Women" shows that the ramifications of intimate partner abuse may be even more serious for adolescent than adult women, but that there are far fewer resources or options available to young women.

The next articles and resources in this chapter specifically address the issue of the health system's response to violence against women. Although women who were victims/survivors of violence have long identified violence as a major health issue and have been aware of how violence impacted on their mental and physical health, the health system has been notoriously poor at addressing violence issues and has often played a dangerous role in revictimizing survivors of violence. As articles in this chapter demonstrate, as a result of much activism, professional training, and national attention to medical standards and protocols, health care practitioners are increasingly aware of the health ramifications of violence and their responsibilities. In "The Unique Role Health Workers Can Play in Recognizing and Responding to Battered Women," I (Nancy Worcester) outline the key issues I teach health practitioners about the crucial roles they should play in routinely screening and appropriately responding to domestic violence.

Building on the analysis of the battered women's movement as demonstrated in the power and control and equality wheels, Amanda Cosgrove and Dr. Kevin Fullin (founders of Wisconsin's first hospital-based domestic violence program in Kenosha) developed similar "Medical Power and Control" and "Medical Advocacy/Empowerment" wheels which health workers can use to determine whether their responses to victims/survivors abuse their power (medical power and control) or whether they are using their positions to advocate for women and help them end the violence in their lives.

Violence against women affects women in *all* communities. Although activists have long been careful to emphasize this fact, more attention has been paid recently to going beyond the rhetoric to explore the unique issues faced by different groups of women. There is enormous pressure on women in some communities to hide the violence in their lives. In such communities, a woman may feel even more isolated and hopeless than in a community where violence is acknowledged. Battered women's programs see only a tiny percentage of all the women affected by violence and domestic violence service providers are increasingly aware that they do a better job of serving some groups of women than others. For example, even though many women with disabilities, older women, and lesbians are hurt by domestic violence, disproportionately few victims/survivors in these groups make contact with domestic violence programs. Urgent attention needs to be paid to the unique barriers different women face in trying to end the violence in their lives. The next four articles in this chapter address this issue from different perspectives, in relation to specific groups of people. It is hoped that these articles will stimulate the reader to think about particular barriers to ending violence which other women (not included in these articles) face.

Beth E. Richie and Valli Kanuha's crucial article, "Battered Women of Color in Public Health Care Systems: Racism, Sexism, and Violence" synthesizes many of the key issues in this book specifically as they relate to violence in women's lives and what is needed for an appropriate public health system response. This article very clearly articulates the urgency "to integrate an understanding of violence against women with other forms of oppression (such as racism, classism, ageism) in addition to sexism" and highlights how "women of color have actively and creatively challenged the discriminatory, institutional practices of health care and crisis intervention services." "Anishinabe Values/Social Law Regarding Wife Battering" helps us see that "wife battering among the Ojibwe people emerged as a result of dissolution of traditional lifeways, including spirituality, the structure of government, laws, economics, relationships, values, beliefs, morals, and philosophy that were in place in the pre-reservation era." The article by Diana Courvant and Loree Cook-Daniels, "Trans and Intersex Survivors of Domestic Violence: Defining Terms, Barriers, and Responsibilities" (which includes a very useful definition of terms) helps us think through the barriers to living safely for many trans and intersex people. Gender-segregated services, a fundamental issue for domestic violence programs and important to many survivors, is a major obstacle for this group of survivors. The authors outline many suggestions for how to improve services for trans and intersex survivors.

The excellent article, "Ruling the Exceptions: Same Sex Battering and Domestic Violence Theory" obviously addresses the important issue of violence in lesbian and gay relationships, but also goes deeper to stimulate our broader analysis of intimate partner violence. Similar to the Richie and Kanuha article emphasizing that an analysis of other forms of oppressions must be integrated with sexism for an understanding of violence against women, this article by Gregory Merrill challenges gender-based domestic violence theory to explore "the many dimensions of power and explain(s) the phenomenon of domestic violence as it occurs in all relationship configurations." Three conditions for battering are identified as "learning to abuse; having the opportunity to abuse; and choosing to abuse." It becomes evident how violence is connected to privilege and oppression when one thinks about how society gives very clear messages about who has "the opportunity to abuse without suffering negative consequences:"

> . . . would-be abusive individuals must perceive that they can "get away with it." Because of the pervasiveness of cultural sexism, homophobia, racism, classism, anti-Semitism, ageism, and ableism, some groups are empowered with privileges at the expense of others. For the battered heterosexual woman, the cultural context of sexism and other forms of oppressions which may affect her (such as racism in the instance of a woman of color), as enforced by friends, family members, hospital workers, mental health providers, and the criminal justice system, contribute to an environment in which her abusive partner can batter her without intervention or consequence. Likewise, homophobia, heterosexism, and other forms of oppressions operate in the same way to isolate the battered person in a same-sex relationship, permitting the violence to continue. While the social phenomenon of prejudice does not cause battering, it does create an opportune environment that supports abusive behavior by its refusal to challenge it.

The final article in this chapter is a work-in-progress addressing the controversial topic of women's use of force. Much media attention has recently focused on "violent women" and "mean girls" but nearly all information on this topic has been from an anti-woman, backlash perspective or by people inappropriately misusing a gender-neutral approach. "Women's Use of Force," reflecting work of the Wisconsin Coalition Against Domestic Violence's Education and Emerging Issues Committee, summarizes much of the present thinking of the battered women's movement as captured through a series of recent statewide and national think-tanks and workshops on this topic:

> The challenge is to take violence by women seriously without losing sight of the fact that the patterns of male and female violence within adult intimate relationships are usually very different, often happen within different contexts, and generally have different consequences and that both violence itself and the barriers to ending violence are related to societal inequalities.

Continuum of Family Violence
from Alaska Dept. of Public Safety

PHYSICAL

pushing   punching   slapping   kicking   throwing objects   choking   using weapons   homicide/suicide   **DEATH**

VERBAL EMOTIONAL

name calling   criticizing   "you're no good"   ignoring   yelling   isolation   humiliation   **SUICIDE**

SEXUAL

unwanted touching   sexual name calling   unfaithfulness   false accusations   forced sex   hurtful sex   **RAPE**

Without some kind of help, the violence usually gets worse. The end result can be death.

Power and Control Wheel

by the Domestic Abuse Intervention Project, Duluth MN

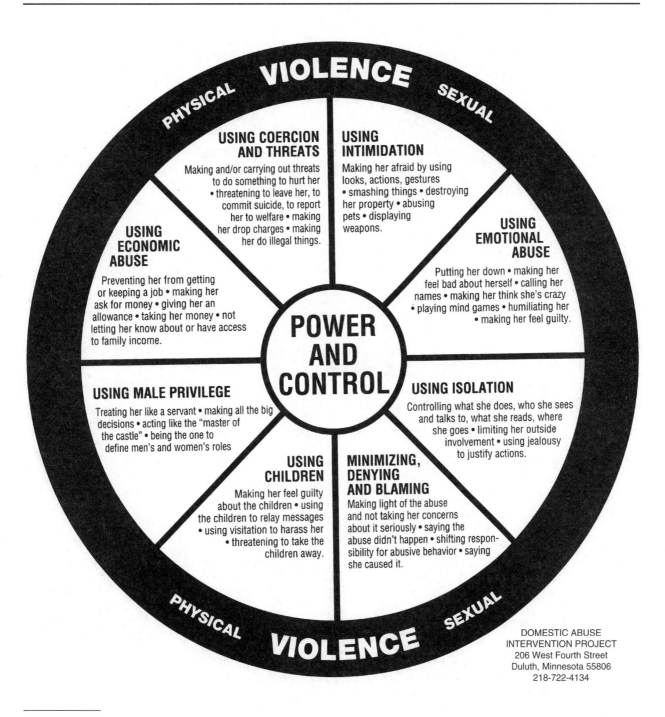

VIOLENCE

PHYSICAL · SEXUAL

USING COERCION AND THREATS
Making and/or carrying out threats to do something to hurt her • threatening to leave her, to commit suicide, to report her to welfare • making her drop charges • making her do illegal things.

USING INTIMIDATION
Making her afraid by using looks, actions, gestures • smashing things • destroying her property • abusing pets • displaying weapons.

USING EMOTIONAL ABUSE
Putting her down • making her feel bad about herself • calling her names • making her think she's crazy • playing mind games • humiliating her • making her feel guilty.

USING ECONOMIC ABUSE
Preventing her from getting or keeping a job • making her ask for money • giving her an allowance • taking her money • not letting her know about or have access to family income.

POWER AND CONTROL

USING MALE PRIVILEGE
Treating her like a servant • making all the big decisions • acting like the "master of the castle" • being the one to define men's and women's roles

USING ISOLATION
Controlling what she does, who she sees and talks to, what she reads, where she goes • limiting her outside involvement • using jealousy to justify actions.

USING CHILDREN
Making her feel guilty about the children • using the children to relay messages • using visitation to harass her • threatening to take the children away.

MINIMIZING, DENYING AND BLAMING
Making light of the abuse and not taking her concerns about it seriously • saying the abuse didn't happen • shifting responsibility for abusive behavior • saying she caused it.

PHYSICAL · SEXUAL

VIOLENCE

DOMESTIC ABUSE INTERVENTION PROJECT
206 West Fourth Street
Duluth, Minnesota 55806
218-722-4134

Equality Wheel

by the Domestic Abuse Intervention Project, Duluth, MN

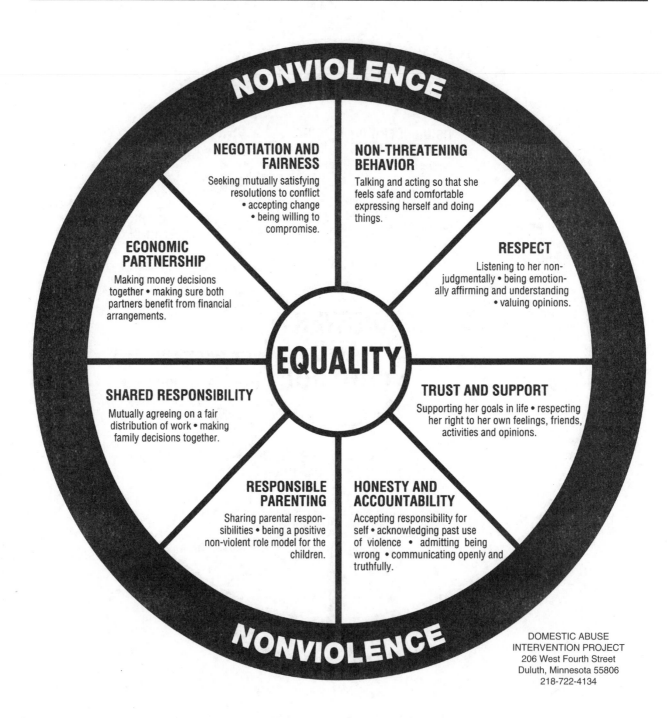

NONVIOLENCE

NEGOTIATION AND FAIRNESS
Seeking mutually satisfying resolutions to conflict • accepting change • being willing to compromise.

NON-THREATENING BEHAVIOR
Talking and acting so that she feels safe and comfortable expressing herself and doing things.

ECONOMIC PARTNERSHIP
Making money decisions together • making sure both partners benefit from financial arrangements.

RESPECT
Listening to her non-judgmentally • being emotionally affirming and understanding • valuing opinions.

EQUALITY

SHARED RESPONSIBILITY
Mutually agreeing on a fair distribution of work • making family decisions together.

TRUST AND SUPPORT
Supporting her goals in life • respecting her right to her own feelings, friends, activities and opinions.

RESPONSIBLE PARENTING
Sharing parental responsibilities • being a positive non-violent role model for the children.

HONESTY AND ACCOUNTABILITY
Accepting responsibility for self • acknowledging past use of violence • admitting being wrong • communicating openly and truthfully.

NONVIOLENCE

DOMESTIC ABUSE
INTERVENTION PROJECT
206 West Fourth Street
Duluth, Minnesota 55806
218-722-4134

A More Hidden Crime

Adolescent Battered Women

by Nancy Worcester

Domestic violence has often been referred to as our nation's most hidden crime. However, after 15 years of activism and the establishment of more than 1000 battered women's shelter programs around the country, the battered women's movement has made many people and community services aware of the fact that huge numbers of women are entrapped in relationships of ongoing abuse of power, control, and physical coercion. The FBI estimates that a woman is battered every 15–18 seconds in this country and that approximately one of every three women experiences some physical violence in her long-term relationship(s). The pervasiveness of the violence may be best represented by the statement that one of every five women probably experiences five or more serious battering incidents each year.

Just as there is finally a public consciousness of the magnitude of the problem of women being battered, we are discovering an even more hidden, perhaps even more prevalent crime—violence against adolescent women. It turns out that most of the understanding of the dynamics of power and control in intimate relationships gained from the battered women's movement applies as much to adolescent women in dating relationships as it does to adult women. Tragically, the ramifications of violence for younger women are often exaggerated by a number of factors, but there are far fewer resources and options available to adolescent than adult women who are trying to end the violence in their lives.

Working to prevent violence in young people's lives must be a highest priority for any of us committed to creating a better world for the next generation and to helping young women maximize on their full potential. The isolation and lowered self-esteem which are so often a *consequence* of violence will have exaggerated ramifications for a young woman if they cause her to limit or eliminate skill-building, career opportunities or educational opportunities which could affect the rest of her life. (It is important to emphasize that the isolation, lowered self-esteem, and unhealthy coping mechanisms which are often observed in abused women are predictable *consequences* of violence and are not the *cause* of the violence. Confusing a consequence of violence with a cause can lead to dangerous, victim-blaming misunderstandings of the violence.)

If a woman is experiencing violence in her dating relationship(s), it will almost certainly be related to many other issues in her life. Anyone working with adolescents will benefit from seeing the connections between violence and the issues they already address. Why she is not always able to show up for study group, why she "had to go" to a concert instead of studying the night before an important exam, why she is no longer best friends with "the nice girl who seemed to have such a positive influence on her" or why she "suddenly" started dressing in a way which always or never shows off her figure may be explained by knowing that a young woman is in a relationship where someone else is taking control over almost all aspects of her life. Health educators need to recognize that many women are beaten up if they try to insist that male partners wear a condom or abstain from sexual activity. Because battering so often starts or accelerates during pregnancy and because sexual assault and other forms of violence are so intimately connected, anyone who works with adolescent pregnancy or sexual assault issues needs to be aware of the connections.

Ironically, many women learn about motherhood and battering at exactly the same time. Retrospective studies show that 25% of battered women experienced their first physical abuse during a pregnancy and that 40–60% of battered women were abused during a pregnancy or during pregnancies. The consequences are a much higher rate of miscarriage, stillbirth, premature delivery, and low birth weight infants in battered than non-battered women. The problem may be even more exaggerated in pregnant teens.

A study looking specifically at physical abuse during teen pregnancy found that 26% of pregnant teens reported they were involved with a man who physically hurt them and 40–60% said that the battering had begun or escalated since their boyfriends knew they were pregnant. This study also provides an urgent reminder that services are not addressing the issue of violence for adolescent women: 65% of pregnant teens had not talked to anyone about the abuse.

Looking at the continuum of violence issues (The Power and Control and Equality Wheels by the Duluth Domestic Abuse Intervention Project (see pp. 259 & 260) and the Continuum of Family Violence Chart (see p. 258), by the Alaska Dept. of Public Safety are particularly useful), it becomes apparent how a range of forms of violence—physical, verbal, emotional, and sexual—are used by abusers to dominate their partners. The more subtle forms of sexual violence (unwanted touching, sexual name calling, unfaithfulness or threat of unfaithfulness, saying "no one else will ever love you", false accusations) are clearly emotionally as well as sexually controlling. These need to be identified as "violence issues" which are related to, and can escalate into, unwanted sex, unprotected sex, hurtful sex and other forms of sexual assault. Sexual violence is often the expression of violence which is the most painful for a woman to discuss. Emotional abuse is almost always present if there are other forms of abuse in a relationship but a clever abuser may achieve sufficient control by emotional abuse without ever resorting to other forms. Women consistently say that emotional abuse is the hardest form to identify (Is this really happening? Is this abuse? Am I making too much of this?) but recognize it as the form of abuse which has the most impact on their lives and their view of themselves. Many women who have been in life-threatening situations say, "The physical battering was nothing compared to the daily emotional abuse." Helping young women see the interconnectedness of verbal, emotional, physical, and sexual power and control issues may be the most useful information in empowering them to end *all* forms of violence in their lives.

By the time adolescents start experimenting with their own dating relationships, they have been bombarded with messages that violence against women is tolerated and even encouraged and that dominance, aggression, and abuse of power and control are appropriate masculine behaviors which are rewarded by society. Today's young people have been exposed to a tolerance and perpetuation of male violence which is unique to this generation. They grew up in the era when the average child was watching 24 hours of television a week with children's programming averaging 15.5 violent acts per hour. By the time they reach 18, the average US adolescent has witnessed approximately 26,000 murders, in their own homes, via the tv screen.

The role of television in sex-role socialization and the perpetuation of male violence has been grossly exaggerated for today's young people because changes in federal regulations, in the early 1980s, allowed the sale of toys directly connected to tv shows, removed regulations limiting the amount of advertising allowed on children's programming, and ruled that product-based shows were legal. The result was a totally new integration of the tv and toy industries. By 1986 all of the ten best selling toys had shows connected with them and by 1988, 80% of children's tv programming was produced by toy companies. Parallel marketing promoted definitions of masculinity and femininity as clearly defined as the distinct lines of boys' toys vs. girls' toys. Because of the new integration of tv and toys, today's young people did not learn to explore their own creativity or imagination in healthy ways but instead learned to "act out their scripts" as dominant and competitive *or* caring, helpless, and concentrating on appearance, either as GI Joe or Ghostbusters vs. Barbie or My Little Pony.

With electronic video games, an even newer and unstudied phenomena, young people get to act out and be rewarded for playing their violent roles. The direct participation in "performing" the violence of video games is predicted to magnify whatever effect more passive tv viewing has on one's acceptance or perpetuation of violence. In a violence promoting and accepting culture, it is not surprising to find that *most* video games are very violent (a sampling of 120 machines in three arcades in Madison, Wisconsin, found that more than 70 involved either hand-to-hand combat or shooting to kill enemies) and that the most popular games in an arcade are the most violent.

Consequently, *unlearning* the tolerance of violence and *learning* how to achieve violence-free, equal relationships are skills which are now as crucial to *teach* young people as reading, writing, math and the use of computers. The way people learn, in their earliest experimentation, to be in intimate relationships can set the pattern for what they expect in future relationships. It is a time when the highest standards should be set! Adolescents need to see models of healthy, equal, violence-free relationships, in order to aim for that in their own lives and *to be able to model that for their peers.*

At this stage, many teens do not have the knowledge or skills to prevent or react against violence in their own lives or in their friends' lives. In fact, exactly the opposite is much more likely. Many young women have said that even when they have told friends they were being hurt by their boyfriends, the response was that they were lucky to have boyfriends. There is enormous peer pressure not to break up. Many teens regard violence as a normal part of dating and have no idea they deserve better. Extreme possessiveness, jealousy, dominance, and not being "allowed" to break up get wrongly identified as desirable, positive signs of caring, love and commitment, rather than strong warning signs that they are in an unhealthy, potentially dangerous relationship.

Figuring out what to expect in relationships may be particularly confusing for anyone who grew up in a home where there was violence. Many young men only see abusing males (in reality and in the media) as role models. Many young women who told their mother about being hurt by their boyfriend, have heard, "you have to learn to take the bad and the good in a relationship to make it work."

Many teens who have grown up in violent homes face the difficulty of trying to figure out how they want to be in their own young adult relationships while they are still learning (or not learning) to cope with being affected by the violence with which they grew up. The battered women's movement has very effectively identified that when a woman is battered, the children are almost always affected by the violence. Seventy-five percent of women who are battered in this country have children living at home. Children in homes where domestic violence occurs are physically abused or seriously neglected at a rate 1500% higher than the national average in the general population. Even witnessing domestic violence can have a tremendous impact on young people and may result in symptoms very similar to those seen in people who have been abused. Helping these young people learn healthy relationship skills can be particularly challenging as many teens do not recognize the impact the violence in their homes has had on them and many teens do not want to talk about witnessing or experiencing abuse.

Particularly crucial to how we help young people learn relationship skills *and* acknowledge that violence in their lives may have already influenced their attitudes and behaviors is how we address the impact of the "intergenerational transmission of violence." There is a confusing body of work which examines how the cycle of violence can be passed on through the generations. We now know the old "dad beats mom, mom beats the children, and the children beat the pets" picture was much too simplistic and inaccurate. Increasingly, it is being shown that the person beating mom may also be the one beating the children and protecting the mother is often the best way to protect the children. Although research is inconsistent in documenting the rates of intergenerational transmission of violence, there is a consistent trend which shows that boys who witness domestic violence as children are more likely to batter their female partners as adults than are men from non-violent homes.

How we use this information can be a key factor in determining whether we help break the intergenerational transmission of violence or actually contribute to its perpetuation. Too much of the literature deals with this data as if were inevitable. Central to breaking the pattern is addressing and researching a different set of questions. *If* 30% of boys who witness violence become abusers, the question must be asked, "What can we learn from the 70% who witness violence but do not become abusers?" What factors help young people who have witnessed violence learn to resist violent behavior? Young people from violent homes who have experienced the ugliness of violence and have learned to value non-violent relationships can be exactly the people most committed to breaking the cycle of violence and can be incredibly effective peer leaders.

Most important, young people must *never* learn that violence is inevitable. Many dating violence resources (including some of the materials I highly recommend on other aspects) include information on the intergenerational transmission of violence without making it clear that the cycle can be broken. Information on warning signs of potential abusers almost always include "boys who grew up in violent homes." What does it feel like to see that information if you are a young man who witnessed violence at home? We must make certain that none of our materials or our messages ever contribute towards a young man feeling that he is destined to be violent.

Studies on dating violence consistently show that many teens in violent relationships have not talked to *any* adults about the violence in their lives. We need to start identifying the barriers which have made us so ineffective on this issue and acknowledge that we are only starting to have the language and tools for opening a dialogue on dating violence.

The good news is that a wide range of excellent resources, curricula, and videos have been produced on dating violence issues and violence-free relationships in recent years. It's a very exciting stage to be working on this issue because no one needs to "start from scratch." However, work needs to be done to make the excellent resources and services available to, and appropriate for, many more teens. Few of the resources address the issue in a way that has any meaning for lesbian, gay or bisexual teens or for young people of color. Many of the materials seem to have the underlying assumption that children grow up in homes where there is one male and one female adult. Special issues for teens with disabilities need to be addressed because of both the high rate of sexual assault of people with disabilities and the complexities of dating which arise from the myth that people with disabilities are "asexual." The obsession with body image and a very narrow definition of attractiveness can also be particularly cruel and abusive in adolescence.

"You deserve to be treated with respect."

"You are not alone if someone is hurting you. There are excellent resources to help you end the violence in your life."

These messages which we have been giving adult battered women for the last 15 years are now the same messages we have to give to much younger women.

References

A list of references is available in the original source.

The Unique Role Health Workers Can Play in Recognizing and Responding to Battered Women

by Nancy Worcester

"**B**attering appears to be the single most common cause of injury to women—more common than automobile accidents, muggings and rapes combined."

Many women identify violence in their lives, and their fear of violence, as the number one health issue they face. For health workers responding to battering, it is important to remember that battering is *much* more than the physical injuries. Violence serves as an excellent reminder that mental and physical health issues cannot be separated. For a woman being abused, physical violence is but one of the tools that her abuser uses to have power and control over many, or all, aspects of her life. Many formerly battered women who have even suffered life-threatening injuries say that the physical violence was nothing compared to the psychological and emotional abuse they endured.

Now that many states have mandatory arrest laws, battered women have been quick to remind us that stopping abuse in a home is much more complex than simply stopping the hitting. Women have noted that a result of abuser counselling can be that abusers learn they can no longer get away with hitting their partners. However, unless larger issues of power and control are also ad-

dressed, the abuser may learn to shift to psychological/emotional forms of abuse and the woman continues to be battered even if she is no longer physically injured.

A wide range of chronic health issues including headaches, backaches, sleep disorders, anxiety, abdominal complaints, eating disorders, depression and chronic pain are particularly common in battered women and are clearly related to the stress of living in a violent relationship.

You See Battered Women Everyday

The FBI estimates that a woman is beaten every 15–18 seconds in this country. Violence affects women of all social groups, ages, races, rural and urban environments, and affects both rich and poor and both heterosexual and lesbian women. Many health workers and health workers' partners live with violence as a part of their lives.

Battered women regularly call upon the health system even though health workers have a poor record of identifying them. Studies have shown that abused women have more health problems than non-abused women, so those who trust the health system and have insurance probably seek health care at disproportionately high rates. Studies have shown that 22–35 percent of all women who use emergency room services are battered women and because the same women may need to return time and time again, almost half of all injuries presented by women in emergency rooms may be a result of abuse.

Although health workers do not regularly ask about battering during pregnancy, it is more common than and has as serious consequences (increased rates of miscarriage, stillbirth, low birth weight babies, and risk of homicide) as the conditions routinely tested for in prenatal care. Retrospective studies of battered women have found that 40–60 percent were abused during pregnancy; 25 percent of battered women say they were beaten for the first time during a pregnancy. The problems may be even more exaggerated in pregnant teenagers. One study found that 26 percent of pregnant teens were currently in a relationship with a man who was abusive; many stated that the abuse had started when they discovered they were pregnant. Most alarming, 65 percent of the battered teens had not talked to *anyone* about the violence in their lives.

Health Workers Can Play a Key Role

Many battered women would like to tell someone about the violence in their lives and would greatly benefit from knowing that their situation is not unusual and that there are a range of excellent resources available to them. Understanding common patterns of domestic violence makes it obvious that health workers who do recognize battered women and empower them to explore their options can play a key role in helping women end the violence in their lives.

Isolation

Isolation is a primary weapon that one person can use to gain control over another person's life. Battered women describe how abusers gradually isolate them from their other social/emotional support networks so that eventually the abuser is the main person in the abused woman's life giving her information about her own value. Messages like "No one else will ever love you" and "You deserve to be beaten" become very powerful when a woman is not hearing any other messages. Understanding that isolation is a *consequence* (*not* a cause) of battering can help health workers recognize that what they say to battered women can be extremely important. Health workers aware of power imbalances in health worker-patient relationships can see why this can be exaggerated when the patient is an abused woman. A health worker who implies that the woman is "the problem" will reinforce the messages she gets at home; the health worker who says "You don't deserve to be hit" will be giving a crucial, different message.

The Cycle of Violence

The cycle of violence is a pattern that many battered women start to recognize in their lives. The battering incident seldom comes from "nowhere," but is the expected "explosion" from a period of increasing tension. Women describe the stress of living in the tension-building stage, the waiting for the straw that will finally provoke the battering, as so awful that some women remember when even a severe battering was almost a welcome "release" from the unbearable tension.

Particularly in the early years of abusive relationships, the battering incident is often immediately followed by a good stage which some women call the "honeymoon stage." The honeymoon stage is the wonderful stage we *all* want in relationships. Understanding the importance of the honeymoon stage in battering relationships can help us understand the complexities of these (and all!) relationships. This is the stage at which abusers say (and think they mean) that they are very sorry and it will never happen again. This is the stage when loving sex, extravagant presents, and a renewing of dreams and life long plans/goals can be very enticing.

If the battering is severe enough to cause injuries, the health worker, particularly emergency service providers, may see the woman immediately after the battering and before the "honeymoon stage." This is a key time to make sure the woman knows her options and resources, because she may be the most open to exploring alternatives to staying in a violent relationship. Once the "honeymoon stage" begins, the woman may be "hooked" into another cycle, convinced that if only she tries harder the violence will end.

Escalation

Unless there is intervention (and a sincere commitment from the abuser to learn totally new ways of communicating in the relationship), battering relationships tend to escalate over a period of time. The battering incidents become more frequent and often increase in severity. (Battered women describe the "honeymoon stage" as being less of a "hook" in long-term battering relationships than are the enormous social and economic pressures which keep them in relationships they know are unhealthy.) Because battered women may be seeing health workers long before they turn to other services, good medical records with clear notes, and even photographs, of injuries and chronic health problems that may be related to domestic violence are essential. These can help health workers who will see the records in the future, and the battered woman herself, to see the emerging pattern.

Revictimizing the Battered Woman

Even though health workers are not good at identifying battered women, studies have found that health workers do treat battered women differently than non-battered women and that the treatment actually contributes to the consequences of battering.

Unless there is an understanding of battering, a woman who calls upon the health system regularly, with a range of symptoms and injuries, may be seen as a frustrating patient by health workers who pride themselves on being able to diagnose and treat specific conditions. Only 5-10 percent of battered women in emergency services are identified as such by physicians on their records. Instead, the ground-breaking work on this by Stark, Flitcraft and Frazier, found that medical records included the labels "neurotic," "hysteric," "hypochondriac" or "a well-known patient with multiple vague complaints" for one in four battered women compared to one in 50 non-battered women. One in four battered women were given pain medications and/or minor tranquilizers compared to one in ten non-battered women. This "treatment" has the same effect as paying fire fighters to *push* people back into burning homes! Medication and victimizing labels reinforce the woman's feeling that she is the problem and may contribute to depression, drug and alcohol abuse, and the high rate of suicide attempts seen as a consequence of battering.

Hospital Protocols Now Required

Effective January 1, 1992, all accredited hospitals are required to have protocols in place describing how they respond to battered women and how health professionals are trained on this issue. This is the ideal time for health workers and battered women's advocates to work together to make sure that protocols serve to empower battered women. There are over 1,000 programs in the U.S. specifically serving battered women. These "experts" can help a woman with the legal, safety, housing and support services she needs.

Empowering Battered Women

Excellent resources are now available for health workers spelling out specific ways to identify and respond to battered women and to help them end the violence in their lives. Responding more appropriately to battered women does not necessarily mean more work for the health care provider. It means *starting* to ask about violence ("Since so many women are hurt by their partners, we ask every patient with injuries like yours whether they've ever been hit/kicked/hurt by their partner.") and documenting it, making sure safety issues are addressed for a woman before she returns to the situation that caused the mental or physical injuries, giving women information about community resources, and *stopping* treating abused women by providing only labels and tranquilizers.

Battered women must be empowered to make their *own* decisions at their *own* pace. Outside intervention,

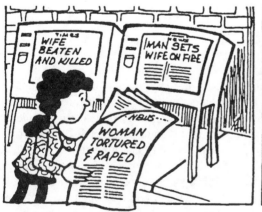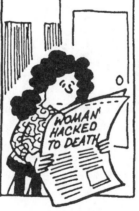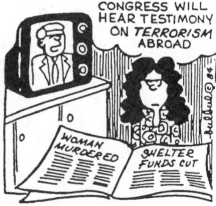

Reprinted with permission from bulbul, Feminist Connection, Madison, WI. December, 1984.

certain behaviors, or trying to leave at the "wrong" time can escalate the violence. Thirty percent of women murdered in this country are killed by the men they had loved. Most of these murders occur when women are trying to get out of a relationship. Understanding the complexities of *leaving* battering relationships is central to serving battered women's needs.

Health workers will seldom know the impact of their responses to battered women. Saying "You don't deserve to be treated like this" or "Here is a list of community resources" may be the advice that saves more lives and does more for the mental health of patients than do other more "medical" skills.

References

A list of references is available in the original source.

Medical Power and Control Wheel and Medical Advocacy Wheel

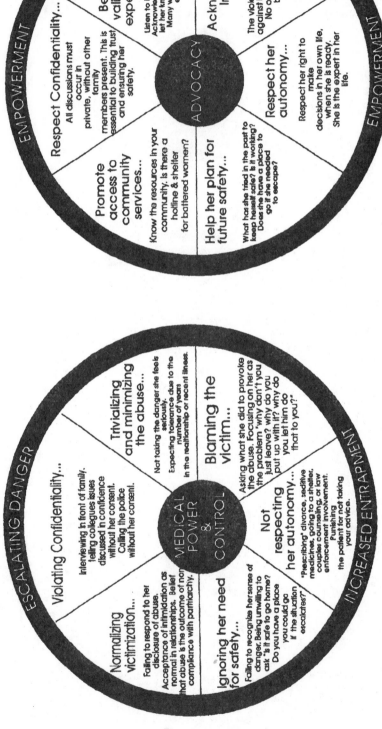

"The Medical Power and Control Wheel"

"The Empowerment Wheel"

Based on the "Power and Control Wheel" and the "Equality Wheel" by the Domestic Abuse Intervention Project. Developed by the Domestic Violence Project, Inc., 3556 7th Avenue, Kenosha, WI 53140, (414)656-8502. Reprinted by permission.

Battered Women of Color in Public Health Care Systems

Racism, Sexism, and Violence

by Beth E. Richie and Valli Kanuha

Introduction

The problems of rape, battering, and other forms of violence against women have existed throughout history. Only recently have these experiences, traditionally accepted as natural events in the course of women's lives, received significant attention as major social problems. For many years there was a tendency for both human service providers and public policy research to focus only on the individual lives of women, children, and men who are damaged or lost due to domestic violence. This narrow focus on individual victims and perpetrators involved in domestic violence rather than on an examination of the role social institutions play in the maintenance of violence against women represents one of the major gaps in our analysis of this pervasive social issue. Paradoxically, the very institutions which have been constructed for the protection and care of the public good—such as the criminal justice system, religious organizations, hospitals, and health care agencies—have long sanctioned disparate and unequal attention to women in society. Only through a critique of these historically patriarchal and often sexist institutions will we comprehend domestic violence as more than individual acts of violence by perpetrators against victims.

Another equally problematic gap in contemporary analysis and study of violence against women exists with regard to race and ethnicity, i.e., how individual and institutional racism affects the lives of women of color who are battered. With a few notable exceptions, there is a very little research on the ways that traditional responses of societal institutions to violence against women are complicated by racism and, therefore, how battered women of color are systematically at a disadvantage when seeking help in most domestic violence situations. The result is that battered women who are African-American, Latina, Asian/Pacific Islander, East Indian, Native-American, and members of other communities of color are vulnerable to abuse not only from their partners, but from insensitive, ineffective institutions as well.

This chapter will address an important factor which is often ignored in our understanding and analysis of domestic violence. While our increasing knowledge of battered women is usually applied in the context that "all women are vulnerable to male violence," the emphasis of this discussion will be on those differential social, economic, and cultural circumstances that render women of color, in particular, vulnerable to male violence at both individual and institutional levels. In addition, this article will focus specifically on the experiences of battered women of color within the health care system, including hospitals, clinics, and public health agencies. As will be described in later sections, many women of color rely significantly on public health institutions not only for ongoing preventive health care and crisis intervention services, but, more importantly, as a viable access point for other services and institutions, e.g., public welfare, housing assistance, legal advice, and so on. Thus the emphasis of this chapter is on the relationship between health care institutions and battered women of color, although similar critiques could be made about the inadequate response of other public institutions (such as religious organizations or the criminal justice system) to battered women of color. Finally, this essay will discuss some effective strategies and programs which address the unique and complex issues affecting women of color who are battered.

Balancing Our Multiple Loyalties: Special Considerations for Women of Color and Victims of Domestic Violence

In order to understand the special circumstances and tensions experienced by battered women of color it is important to understand the interface of gender inequality, sexism, and racism as they affect women both in their racial/ethnic communities and in society at large. Because of the powerful effects of a violent relationship, many battered women are required, either overtly or covertly, to balance the often conflicting needs and expectations of their batterers, their communities, and the larger society. These conflicting expectations, rules, and loyalties often compromise the strategies which are available to liberate women of color from violent relationships. This discussion will serve as a foundation for examining the compound effects of oppression which many women of color face even prior to entering the health care system for medical treatment of and protection from domestic violence.

Communities of color in this country have historically been devastated by discriminatory and repressive political, social, and economic policies. It is commonplace to associate high infant mortality, school drop-out rates, criminality, drug abuse, and most other indices of social dysfunction with African-American, Latino, Native-American, and other non-European ethnic groups. Even among the "model minorities," Asians and Pacific Islanders, groups of new immigrants as well as their assimilated relatives have shown increased rates of HIV and AIDS, mental health problems, and other negative co-factors which are in part attributable to their status as non-majority (nonwhite) people in the United States.

Most everyone, from historians to social scientists to politicians, whether conservative or radical, considers racism to be a significant, if not the primary, cause of this disproportionate level of social deterioration among communities of color. While the dynamics of racism have often been studied from a macro-perspective, comparing the effects of race discrimination on particular ethnic groups vis-à-vis society at large, the differential effects of racism on women versus men of color has not been given due attention. In order to adequately understand any analysis of the combined effects of racism, sexism, and battering, a consideration of gender-based tension within communities of men and women of color, separate from and related to the predominant white society, is required.

There are many stereotypes about women of color which affect not only our understanding of them as women, but particularly our analysis of and sensitivity to

them with regard to domestic violence. For example, many portrayals of women of color espouse their inherent strengths as historical, matriarchal heads of households. While this stereotype of women of color as super home-makers, responsible family managers, and unselfish nurturers may be undisputed, such attributions do not mean that all (or most) women of color are therefore empowered and supported in their various family roles or have positions of leadership within their ethnic communities. Many women of color with whom we work state that they face the burden either of having to be overly competent and successful or having to avoid the too-often painful reality of becoming "just another one of those horror stories or pitiful statistics on the front page of the newspaper." For women of color who are experiencing domestic violence, the implicit community and societal expectation to be strong and continue to care for themselves and their families results in their denying not only the actual existence of battering in their lives, but the extent and nature of that abuse. For example, one Korean woman who was repeatedly punched around her head and face by her husband reported that she used cosmetics extensively each day when she went to Mass with her husband, in order to assure protection of her own, as well as her husband's, dignity among their church and neighborhood friends. When she went to work as a typist in a white business, she was especially careful not to disclose evidence of her abuse, in order to protect both herself and her husband from her co-workers' judgments that "there was something wrong with Korean people."

While public policy makers are concerned about the rapidly escalating crime rate in this country, many leaders in cities predominated by communities of color are becoming increasingly concerned about the profile of those convicted for crimes, i.e., young boys and men of color. The predominance of men of color in correctional facilities (close to 90 percent of the penal population in some cities) has polarized everyone, from scholars to community leaders to policy makers. While most mainstream legislators and public health officials are reluctant to discuss it publicly, there is a rising belief that men of color are inherently problematic and socially deviant. More progressive analysts have ascribed criminal behavior among nonwhite males to historically racist social conditions that are reinforced by criminal, legal, and penal systems which disproportionately arrest and convict men of color at least in part because of their skin color.

There are no equally concerned dialogues about how women of color continue to be victims of crime more often than white women and about the disparate treatment they receive from not only racist, but sexist social systems. An African-American woman who works with battered women as a court advocate states unequivocally that battered women of color are usually treated less respectfully by prosecutors and judges than the white women with whom she works. In addition, when this same court advocate has raised this disparity with her African-American brothers and male friends in her community, she is often derided as being "one of those white women's libbers" who has betrayed "her own" by working on a problem like domestic violence, which will further stigmatize and destroy the men of color who are charged with battering. Unfortunately, this dialectic of the comparable oppression of women and men of color has resulted in a troubling silence about the needs of women of color and led to counterproductive discussions between women and men of color about the meaning and significance of domestic violence, specifically, and sexism in general.

For a battered woman of color who experiences violence at the hands of a man of color from her own ethnic group, a complex and troublesome dynamic is established that is both enhanced and compromised by the woman's relationship to her community. She is battered by another member of her ethnic community, whose culture is vulnerable to historical misunderstanding and extinction by society at large. For the battered woman, this means that she may be discriminated against in her attempt to secure services *while at the same time* feeling protective of her batterer, who might also be unjustly treated by such social institutions as the police and the judicial system. Most battered women of color are acutely aware of how the police routinely brutalize men of color, how hospitals and social services discriminate against men of color, and the ways men of color are more readily labeled deviant than white men. In one Midwestern city, anecdotal reports from court and police monitors have shown that men of color awaiting arraignment for domestic violence charges frequently arrive in court with bruises supposedly inflicted by police officers. One Indian woman stated that when she saw her husband in court the morning after a battering incident, he looked just as bad as she did, with black eyes and bruises about his face. Feeling pity for him, she refused to testify, and upon release he told her of being beaten by police while being transported between the jail and the court house. Although the existence of police brutality is unfortunately not a new phenomenon, it is certainly compromised and complicated in the context of domestic violence, especially for men and women of color who are seeking help from this already devastating problem. For battered women of color, seeking help for the abuse they are experiencing always requires a tenuous balance between care for and loyalty to themselves, their batterers, and their communities.

The situation is further complicated by the fact that communities of color have needed to prioritize the pressing social, economic, and health problems which have historically plagued their people and neighborhoods. Because of sexism, the particular concerns of women typically do not emerge at the top of the list. The values of family stability, community self-determination, and protection of one's racial and ethnic culture are often seen as incompatible with addressing the needs of battered women within communities of color. Most of us who have worked in the domestic violence movement are well aware of the gross misconceptions that battering is just a woman's issue or that domestic violence in communities of color is not as serious as other problems. The most dangerous consequence, for battered women of color, however, is that they are often entrapped by these misconceptions and misguided loyalties and thus remain in the confines of violent and abusive households.

While credit for a broad-based societal response to the problem of violence against women must be given to the feminist movement and its successful grassroots organizing in the mid-1970s, another process of "split loyalties" has emerged, compromising the analysis regarding battered women of color. Those women of color who identify themselves as activists, feminists, and organizers within the battered women's movement often face an additional barrier among their feminist peers when raising issues related to the particular dynamics of domestic violence and race/ethnicity. Many white feminists and the organizations they have created become very threatened when women of color, with their concomitant expanded analysis of battering and racism, have moved into leadership roles. Many women of color in the violence against women movement have challenged the long-standing belief of many white feminists that sexism is the primary, if not the only, cause of women's oppression. In a reform movement which has had such a significant impact on the values, behaviors, and subsequent policies regarding women and violence, the reluctance or inability to integrate an understanding of violence against women with other forms of oppression (such as racism, classism, ageism) in addition to sexism has been disappointing. A more significant concern, though, is the effect of limited analysis on women and children of color who are seeking refuge and safety from both hostile partners and social institutions outside the battered women's movement.

In summary, our understanding of women of color who are battered must be considered against the political, social, and cultural backdrop of their racial and ethnic communities; within the framework of institutional responses that are historically based in racism and other prejudices; and against the background of the feminist agenda, which has been primarily responsible for galvanizing all of the above to address this pervasive social issue. It is in this context that we turn to an examination of the particular influence, concerns, and barriers of the health care system in dealing with battered women of color.

Battered Women of Color: Health Problems and Health Care

Women who are battered are often seriously hurt; their physical and psychological injuries are life-threatening and long-lasting. In one-third of all battering incidents, a weapon is used, and 40 percent result in the need for emergency medical attention. Research suggests that one-third of all adult female suicide attempts can be associated with battering, and 25 percent of all female homicide victims die at the hands of their husbands or boyfriends. More women are injured in their homes by their spouses or male partners each year than by accidents or illnesses.

It is not surprising, therefore, that most battered women report their first attempt to seek help is from a health care institution, even before contacting the police. This is especially true in communities of color, where police response is likely to be sporadic, at best. Yet research indicates that of those battered women using the emergency room for acute treatment of injuries related to an abusive incident, only one in ten was identified as battered. Similar findings have been cited for women using ambulatory care settings. A random sample of women seeking health maintenance visits at neighborhood health clinics revealed that 33 percent were battered women and less than 10 percent received safety information or counseling for domestic violence. The following story of Yolanda (a pseudonym) illustrates the role of health facilities in the lives of battered women.

> Yolanda is a forty-six-year old who received primary health care from a neighborhood health clinic. She uses the services of the walk-in clinic two or more times each month, complaining of discomfort, sleeplessness and fatigue. Yolanda never mentions that her boyfriend abuses her, but her clinic visits correspond directly with the pattern of his alcohol binges. The staff of the clinic know about her boyfriend's mistreatment, because he sometimes comes to the clinic drunk and will threaten her if she does not leave with him.

For Yolanda, the clinic symbolizes a safe, public place of refuge. From her experience, she knows it is legitimate to seek assistance when one is sick, and she trusts health authorities to take care of her needs. Health providers

lose an important opportunity for intervention when they do not offer assistance to Yolanda, especially since they have clear evidence that her boyfriend is violent toward her. She, in turn, feels that the violence must be hidden and that it is a source of shame, since her health care providers do not acknowledge it or offer to help.

For many battered women of color, the unresponsiveness of most health care institutions is symbolic of the overall reality of social disenfranchisement and deterioration in poor, nonwhite communities across the United States. While lack of quality, affordable housing is a major problem for many people of color, the majority of the homeless are women of color and their children. The drug epidemic, particularly crack and heroin use, has had a significant impact on violence against women. There is growing anecdotal evidence to suggest that battered women are often forced to use drugs as part of the pattern of their abuse, yet there is a serious lack of treatment programs for women, particularly poor women with children. The spread of HIV and AIDS among many women of color has been compounded by the HIV infection rate among children of HIV-positive mothers. Many women with HIV report that negotiating for safer sex or clean needles is difficult when they are controlled by violent, coercive partners.

With regard to women and the social problems of drugs, homelessness, and AIDS, most public health officials have been quick to label women as the criminals, rather than the victims of a society that is disintegrating before our very eyes. When we add to the above the battering, rape, and psychological abuse of those same women who are homeless, drug addicted, and HIV-positive, it is clear that the health care system can be either a vehicle for assistance or a significant barrier for women who are seeking protection from a myriad of health and social problems.

The experience of Ana illustrates the interrelatedness that can occur between domestic violence, drug use, HIV infection, and the chronic and acute need for health care. Ana's husband was an injection drug user who had battered her severely throughout their ten-year marriage. He had been very ill for a period of months and had tested seropositive for HIV. Ana was already pregnant when her husband was tested, but he insisted that she carry through with the pregnancy. She was battered twice in the four months since she had gotten pregnant, and after one incident she was unable to get out of bed for two days. Her husband Daniel reportedly was concerned about the baby and took her to the emergency room of their local hospital. During the triage interview, the ER (Emergency Room) nurse noticed the tension between Ana and Daniel but was uncomfortable addressing it. The nurse later reported that she did not want to offend them by suggesting that they appeared to be having "marriage problems" because they were Hispanic, and she understood that Hispanics were embarrassed about discussing such matters with health professionals. After being admitted for observation, Ana began to complain of increased pains in her abdomen. After five days in the hospital, Ana hemorrhaged and lost her baby. At that time, she discovered that she had been tested for HIV and was seropositive. She returned home to a distraught and angry husband, who blamed the baby's death on her. She was beaten again and returned to the ER once more.

Ana's case illustrates one of the most troubling examples of the interface between health care and violence against women. With the longstanding lack of adequate and accessible prenatal care for poor women of color, pregnant women of color who are battered are especially vulnerable. Research indicates that 20 percent of all women who are battered experience the first incident during pregnancy. The situation for pregnant battered women is further complicated by the troubling legal trend to hold women accountable for any damage inflicted upon a fetus in utero. If a pregnant woman is battered and the fetus is harmed, she may be criminally liable for not leaving the abusive relationship. Not surprisingly, in most recent "fetal death" cases across the country, the women who are most severely punished are women of color.

As the health care system has labored under increased social and economical stress, specialized programs for women and for certain communities have also been curtailed. For battered women of color this trend has specific and dangerous affects. With a steady increase in immigrants from Central America, South America, and the Caribbean, battered women who do not have legal status in this country are destined to remain invisible and underserved. Because of their undocumented status and other significant barriers, (such as language and cultural differences), many battered women of color are denied assistance by the same organizations established to protect them, e.g., public welfare, legal advocacy, and health clinics. One battered women's program specifically targeted to serve Caribbean women and their children reports that battered women who must use hospital services for their injuries often have to borrow Medicaid cards from other women in order to conceal their undocumented status. Staff from this same program describe the difficulty that one undocumented woman had even getting out of the house, much less to the hospital, as her batterer was rightfully suspicious that reports of his criminal behavior would also jeopardize *his* illegal status.

Most hospital-based crisis intervention programs do not have multi-lingual or multi-cultural staff who are trained in and sensitive to the special issues of women of color. For example, reliance on translators to communicate with non-English speaking women effectively compromises the confidentiality and protection of battered women who are immigrants, from small ethnic communities, or who must use their own family members as translators to describe painful and private incidents of violence in the home. There are numerous stories of women of color receiving insensitive treatment by health care staff who attribute domestic violent to stereotypes such as "I've heard you Latins have hot tempers" or "Asian women are so passive, it really explains why they get beaten by their husbands."

Finally, if a battered woman of color is also a lesbian, differently abled, or from any other group that is already stigmatized, her access to quality care from health providers may be further compromised. One battered lesbian who was an African American described a physician who was continually incredulous about her claims that a "pretty girl like her" would be beaten by her female lover. In fact, she stopped going to the hospital for emergency attention, even though she had no other health insurance, because she was angry at such homophobic treatment and therefore became increasingly reluctant to use the services of that hospital.

As long as health care institutions continue to be the primary, and usually first, access points for battered women of color, we must require them to institute ongoing training, education, and specialized programs, and to hire culturally knowledgeable staff to address the particular needs of this special group of women.

The Response of Women of Color

Despite the philosophical and political contradictions and the practical barriers described in the previous sections, women of color have actively and creatively challenged the discriminatory, institutional practices of health care and crisis intervention services. Against extremely difficult economic, cultural, and political odds, battered women of color and their advocates have initiated a broad-based response to violence against women in communities of color. Aspects of this response will be summarized in the remainder of the chapter.

One of the most significant developments in response to domestic violence in communities of color has been the creation of grassroots crisis intervention services by and for women of color. The majority of these programs have been organized autonomously from white women, privileging the analysis and experience of women of color by assuming the cultural, historical, and linguistic norms of Asian/Pacific Island, Latin, African-American, Native-American and other nonwhite cultures. Typically located in neighborhoods and communities of color, these programs have a strong emphasis on community organization and public education. While many of these programs struggle for financial support and recognition from mainstream public health agencies and feminist organizations, they endure in great part because they are grounded in a community-based approach to problem solving.

The Violence Intervention Program for Latina women and their children in the community of East Harlem and the Asian Womens' Center in Chinatown are good examples of community-based programs in New York City. Refugee Women In Development (REFWID), in Washington, D. C., has a domestic violence component, as does Arco Iris, a retreat center for Native-American women and other women of color who have experienced violence in Arkansas. In Minnesota, women of color have created a statewide battered women's coalition called Black, Indian, Hispanic and Asian Women In Action (BIHA). In California, California Women Of Color Against Domestic Violence organizes and published a newsletter, "Out Loud," and women of color from seven southern states have created The Southeast Women Of Color Task Force Against Domestic Violence. Nationally, the members of the Women Of Color Task Force of the National Coalition Against Domestic Violence have provided national leadership training and technical assistance on the issues of battering and women of color, and their task force has served as a model for the development of programs for battered women of color across the country.

In addition to providing crisis intervention and emergency shelter services to battered women, these community-based programs and statewide coalitions for women of color are involved in raising the issue of battering within other contexts of social justice efforts. Representatives of grassroots battered women's programs are often in leadership roles on such issues as reproductive freedom, immigration policy, lesbian rights, criminal justice reform, homelessness, AIDS policy, and other issues that affect women of color. The National Black Women's Health Project in Atlanta is a good example of this.

Finally, in the past several years there has been a proliferation of literature on violence against women by scholars and activists who are women of color. Seal Press's New Leaf Series published Evelyn C. White's *Chain, Chain Change: For Black Women Dealing With Physical And Emotional Abuse* and Myrna Zambrano's *Mejor Sola Que Mal Acompanada.* Another good example of analysis by and for battered women of color is a publication by the Center For Domestic And Sexual Violence in Seattle, *The Speaking Profits Us: Violence Against Women Of Color,* a collection of papers edited by Mary Violet Burns. Kitchen Table, Women of Color Press in Albany, New York, has been a leader in publishing writing by women of color, addressing the issue of violence against women in the Freedom Organizing pamphlet series and in many other works.

By providing direct crisis intervention services, educating communities of color, advocating on broader feminist and social justice issues and publishing culturally relevant resources, Asian/Pacific Islanders, Latinas, Native-Americans, African Americans, Caribbeans, and other women of color have demonstrated a strong commitment to addressing violence against women. Our contributions have significantly enhanced both the conventional research on battered women and the progressive work of the battered women's movement, challenging the accepted analysis that violence against women has equivalent effects on all women. We must continue to develop community-based programs that are culturally relevant and responsive to the complexity of experiences faced by women of color, including inadequate health care, unemployment, homelessness, a failing educational system, and violence. Equally important, we must continue to work within our own cultures to challenge those traditions, assumptions, and values that reinforce male domination and ignore women's needs. In so doing, the struggle to end violence against women of color will include individual liberation as well as social reform. For us, the most compelling motivation for continuing this effort comes from the courage, commitment, and endurance that battered women of color have shown in their personal and collective struggles. On a daily basis they persist in defying the limits that violence, sexism, and racism impose on their lives. Our response must be to let their stories challenge and inspire us—women of color, battered women, white women, and men alike—to work actively to end individual and institutional violence against women.

Note

The women described in this essay are referred to anonymously or by pseudonyms to protect their safety and privacy. Their stories are both composites and individual accounts of women with whom the authors have worked.

References

A list of references is available in the original source.

Anishinabe Values/Social Laws Regarding Wife Battering

from Indigenous Woman

In pre-reservation life, there were explicit social laws to deal with the rare occurrence of wife battering. The Ojibwe term used to identify a wife batterer is "Metat-tiggwa Ish" meaning "he who fights his wife always," implying that he is irrational, petty, and jealous. Once a man battered his wife, she was free to make him leave her lodge if they lived among her people. He'd leave her lodge and from then on be known as a man whose wife had broken the household because of abuse. From then on, he could never "marry" again. When a "married" woman was abused by her husband, her brothers were obligated by social law to retaliate against him by not speaking to him, beating him or even killing him. If the couple lived among the man's relatives, his parents were obligated to get her away and return her to her people.

In a situation in which a household had been broken because of abuse, it was not known as a divorced family as it is today. It was viewed as a broken household and the woman was viewed as having self-respect in leaving the destructive relationship behind. In a broken household, the sons could go with the father, the daughters with the mother.

A man who battered his wife was considered irrational and thus could no longer lead a war party, a hunt or participate in either. He could not be trusted to behave properly and thus may bring harm to the other men involved. The wife batterer could no longer own a pipe. If he somehow did, no one would smoke it with him. He was thought of as contrary to Anishinabe law and lost many privileges of life and many roles in Ojibwe society and the societies within.

A man who killed his wife was considered as not Ojibwe anymore. He had broken a primary law of Anishinabe Society, that is an Ojibwe NEVER kills another Ojibwe. He became an enemy of the people. His name would never be spoken again. He would cease to exist.

The children of this household would be given to another family so they would not be known as coming from a man who did not exist, and so they would not be known as the offspring of such a person.

The People: "The Relatives Living Together"

In pre-reservation Ojibwe society beliefs such as the preceding were handed down by ALL the people to the coming generations. For a clan/group to live in unity and cooperation, it was necessary for all to live according to the same beliefs, laws, and values. When people living together do not share the same beliefs, laws and values, there will be confusion as to what is considered proper behavior; individuals will not have a foundation from which to guide their behavior.

Reservation Ojibwe Society

The perspective can be taken that the daily occurrence of wife battering among the Ojibwe people emerged as a result of the dissolution of traditional lifeways, including spirituality, the structures of government, laws, economics, relationships, values, beliefs, morals, and philosophy that were in place in the pre-reservation era, prior to the coming of the white man.

Wife battering, as we have seen, was neither accepted nor tolerated among the Anishinabe people until after the freedom to live Ojibwe was subdued. Wife battering emerged simultaneously with the disintegration of Ojibwe ways of life and the beginning use of alcohol. The behavior of the Ojibwe people under the influence of alcohol is often totally contrary to Anishinabe values. It is especially contrary to the self discipline previously necessary to the development of Ojibwe character.

There is no single philosophy among the people in today's society regarding the social illness of wife battering. Many have forgotten or DID NOT RECEIVE THE TEACHINGS of the social laws surrounding it. In the old Ojibwe society, society itself was responsible for what took place within it; today that is not so. What is the evidence of that statement? The harmful, destructive, traumatic cycle of domestic violence that is befalling the Anishinabe Children of the Nation.

Today we have lost a lot of the traditions, values, ways of life, laws, language, teachings of the Elders, respect, humility as Anishinabe people because of the European mentality we have accepted. For the Anishinabe people to survive as a Nation, together we must turn back the pages of time. We must face reality, do an evaluation of ourselves as a people—why we were created to live in harmony with one another as Anishinabe people and to live in harmony with the Creator's creation.

Ruling the Exceptions
Same-Sex Battering and Domestic Violence Theory
by Gregory S. Merrill

Summary. This paper examines the challenges presented to current gender-based domestic violence theory by the existence of same-sex domestic violence. Charging that dominant theory is heterosexist and ignores the experience of battered lesbians and gay men, Island and Letellier have argued that domestic violence is not a gender issue and advocate a psychological framework that emphasizes batterer treatment. Examining the theoretical conflicts, this paper attempts to demonstrate that sociopolitical and psychological theories can be successfully integrated into a social-psychological model. Such a model, developed by Zemsky and Gilbert, Poorman, and Simmons, is explored and critiqued as an excellent beginning. By integrating psychological principles and sociological concepts, this theory explores the many dimensions of power and explains the phenomenon of domestic violence as it occurs in all relationship configurations. Suggestions for further theoretical considerations and research are made. *[Article copies available from The Haworth Document Delivery Service: 1-800-342-9678.]*

One would hope that this article could begin without the assertion and lengthy accompanying arguments that same-sex domestic violence is a serious problem. Most of the authors who have written about this phenomenon make explicit reference to the degree of resistance to accepting the frequency and severity of its occurrence. In addition to the outright refusal of the lesbian, gay, and bisexual communities to organize around this issue, current domestic violence theory contributes to denial of the problem by failing to recognize and explain same-sex domestic violence. In this paper, I will explore current theory, particularly the tension between feminist sociopolitical theory and the psychological theory proposed by gay male theorists Island and Letellier. I intend to demonstrate that the two theories are not mutually exclusive and can be meaningfully integrated into a social-psychological theory. This integrated theory, while in its early stage of development, has the potential to explain domestic violence as it occurs in all relationship configurations.

Overview of Current Feminist Sociopolitical Theory

To begin to understand the development of theory about domestic violence, we must examine the social and historical context in which it developed. Prior to the rise of the modern women's movement, the existing research and theories minimized domestic violence and, one way or another, blamed the victim. In the late 1960s and early 1970s, feminism flourishing in this country helped to change this minimization through its primary tenet, the personal is political. This tenet called upon women to examine the conditions of their lives, the roles assigned to them (and also made unavailable to them) in families, the workplace, and society in general, vis-à-vis men. Through consciousness-raising groups and efforts, women began to discover the many insidious ways by which they are made second-class citizens, subordinate to men. In particular, women who had experienced men's emotional, physical, and/or sexual abuse began to share their experiences with one another and, as a result, no longer saw battering as an individual problem. Women organized and politicized around the issue of domestic violence, defining it as a crime against women, and therefore, a women's issue.

Using the feminist lens, activists, researchers, and professionals devoted considerable energy to developing a feminist analysis of domestic violence. They determined that violence, the threat thereof, ascribed family roles, and limited economic opportunity acted together to further gender-based oppression. When looking for the root of domestic violence, feminists saw cultural misogyny and sexism. Del Martin convincingly argued that domestic violence is the logical, if brutal, extreme of sexist gender-role socialization. If a culture socializes its men to be brave, dominant, aggressive, and strong, and its women to be passive, placating, dependent, and obedient, and oppresses any attempts at androgyny or "transgendering," then that culture has effectively trained its men and women for bipolar abuser and victim roles, respectively. Men learn that it is permissible to use violence and that they are expected to be in charge of "their" women and children; women learn to accept that their role is one of a subordinate and a caretaker. According to this analysis, domestic violence is a gender-based phenomenon, a socially-based illness used as a tool of the patriarchy to keep women down.

Despite cultural sexism and the resistance of those who persist in believing that victims have some responsibility for the violence, this gender-based theory has become the most commonly accepted explanation for domestic violence among academicians, the domestic violence movement, and lay people. It has won widespread support because it coherently explains the phenomenon in a way which intuitively makes sense. While there is dissent, a substantial body of research supports feminist contentions. Coleman notes that most studies conducted about battering conclude that it is a significant problem that is almost always perpetrated by men against women.

While this theory is inarguably an important starting place, it leaves many questions unanswered and makes many experiences invisible. For example, as Island and Letellier point out, gender-based theory fails to explain why some heterosexual men batter their partners and others do not. Feminists of color also have argued legitimately that the theory does not reflect their experiences.[1]

With few exceptions, most authors have not attempted to integrate the phenomenon of same-sex partner abuse into feminist domestic violence theory. Indeed, it is not easy to do so without contributing to one of the four most popular misconceptions about same-sex partner abuse: (1) an outbreak of gay male domestic violence is logical (because all or most men are prone to violence), but lesbian domestic violence does not occur (because women are not); (2) same-sex partner abuse is not as severe as when a woman is battered by a man; (3) because the partners are of the same gender, it is mutual abuse, with each perpetrating and receiving "equally"; and (4) the perpetrator must be the "man" or the "butch" and the victim must be the "woman" or the "femme" in emulation of heterosexual relationships. Although the body of research on same-sex domestic violence is limited, Coleman, Kelly and Warshafsky, and Renzetti effectively confront and refute the above misconceptions.

Robert Geffner, editor of the *Family Violence and Sexual Assault Bulletin,* expresses a common sentiment when he makes the following statement: "We need to learn more about this [same-sex domestic] violence and be willing to modify our theories and programs to include these 'exceptions to the rule' ". Indeed, same-sex domestic violence, if viewed from the feminist lens, does seem like an exception. This is because sociopolitical theory alone does not fully or adequately explain why the same dynamic of abuse in heterosexual relationships occurs with as much frequency and severity in same-sex relationships.

Psychological Theory

Highly critical of the dominant feminist theory, Island and Letellier break with it altogether. First, they assert that it is heterosexist because it fails to acknowledge or explain the existence of same-sex partner abuse. Second, they make the *controversial* assertion that domestic violence is *not* a gender issue." Island believes that sociopolitical theory has led to ineffective batterer treatment programs and that treatment must be based primarily, if not solely, on the personality and behavioral characteristics of the batterer. Sociopolitical theory, he argues, has over-focused on the experience of battered women and does not focus at all on or explain the source of the problem, that is, the psychology of perpetrators. As a result, Island and Letellier propose a gender-neutral theory of domestic violence which focuses on the psychology of the batterer. They provide batterer diagnostic criteria for the American Psychiatric Association to adopt and support its application to men and women of all sexual orientations. Essentially, Island and Letellier argue that the feminist lens should be replaced by a psychological lens and that batterers should be identified and classified by behavior, not gender.

While their objections are strong and have been controversial in the domestic violence movement, Island and Letellier have more in common with feminists than even they have acknowledged. They agree with the feminist analysis that victims are created by batterers, do not necessarily have pathology that led them to become victims, and are not necessarily in need of treatment (beyond counseling and advocacy to promote safety and to help manage the effects of the abuse). Interestingly, they also devote several pages to the discussion of masculinity as malignant, arguing that male batterers are unclear on the concept of masculinity, having equated it with violence. Finally, Island and Letellier note in the opening of their book that in heterosexual relationships where abuse is occurring, 95% of the perpetrators are male, citing statistics produced by New York's Office for Prevention of Domestic Violence. And yet, if their assertion that domestic violence is not a gender issue were true, one would assume that heterosexual domestic violence would be equally perpetrated by men and women. So, just as feminist theory alone does not fully explain same-sex domestic violence, the strictly psychological theory proposed by Island and Letellier fails to explain the disproportionate number of male perpetrators in heterosexual domestic violence.

Integrating a Social-Psychological Model

What I would like to suggest here is that domestic violence must be understood as both a social *and* a psychological phenomenon and must be examined under both lenses simultaneously in order to be completely understood. Feminist theory and psychological theory are not necessarily mutually exclusive and do not have to negate one another. In fact, if synthesized, they can enhance our vision. Viewing domestic violence through an integrated

framework permits us to see that domestic violence is a gender issue; that heterosexual domestic violence is, in fact, primarily perpetrated by men against women. We also see that gender is only one of several determining social and psychological factors and that the absence of gender inequity, as in same-sex relationships, by no means precludes the possibility that battering will occur.

Zemsky, in conjunction with Gilbert, Poorman, and Simmons, proposes a social-psychological theory of lesbian battering which can be applied to heterosexual and gay male relationships as well. They separate the causation of battering into three categories: learning to abuse; having the opportunity to abuse; and choosing to abuse. The individual who abuses has first learned to abuse through a combination of three psychological processes, usually occurring in the family of origin: one, direct instruction; two, modeling or learning through observation; and three, operant conditioning, or learning by reinforcement that violence is effective and "rewarding." They also suggest that men might be especially prone to learning abuse because of sex-role socialization, but agree with Hart that women in our culture also learn and internalize relationship models that are based upon inequity.

According to Zemsky and Gilbert et al., learning to abuse does not necessarily lead individuals to enact abuse. For that to occur, they must also have the opportunity to abuse without suffering negative consequences. In other words, would-be abusive individuals must perceive that they can "get away with it." Because of the pervasiveness of cultural sexism, homophobia, racism, classism, anti-semitism, ageism, and ableism, some groups are empowered with privileges at the expense of others. For the battered heterosexual woman, the cultural context of sexism and other oppressions which may affect her (such as racism in the instance of a woman of color), as enforced by friends, family members, hospital workers, mental health providers, and the criminal justice system, contribute to an environment in which her abusive partner can batter her without intervention or consequence. Likewise, homophobia, heterosexism, and other oppressions operate in the same way to isolate the battered person in a same-sex relationship, permitting the violence to continue. While the social phenomenon of prejudice does not cause battering, it does create an opportune environment that supports abusive behavior by its refusal to challenge it.

Zemsky uses an apt example to describe the roles of actual and perceived power relations in creating opportunity. She writes that it is unlikely that individuals who had learned to harass the people with whom they work would harass their supervisors because the potential consequence of being immediately fired would decrease the level of opportunity. To extend Zemsky's analysis, if these same people were the supervisors, they would, in fact, be likely to harass their employees, because they would probably believe they could get away with it. To extend this even further, while these same people may not harass their supervisors, they may harass a colleague, someone at their same level of employment. They would be particularly likely to do so if they believed the victim would be unlikely or unable to report it and/or if they believed such a report would not be taken seriously or responded to. Thus, according to this model, abuse against someone with perceived greater power and/or the perceived power to bring effective, negative consequences is unlikely to be expressed, whereas abuse against someone with perceived equal or lesser power and/or a perceived diminished capacity to bring such consequences would be a more ripe opportunity.

Lastly, Zemsky and Gilbert et al. emphasize that although the learning may have occurred and the opportunity might be present, abusive individuals make a conscious choice to abuse. Although many abusive people may not perceive it this way, they have the ability to make alternative choices (or at least to learn alternative choices) and are solely responsible for their violence.

In formulating this theory, the authors successfully integrate sociopolitical concepts and psychological principles and begin to explore their very complex relationship. For instance, the learning process they propose is explicitly psychological since it involves the individual internalizing beliefs and learning behaviors, and yet, Zemsky and Gilbert et al. acknowledge that what is internalized is most definitely shaped by social mores. Their analysis of opportunity is largely informed by feminism and an analysis of power which expands beyond gender, including racism, sexism, heterosexism, and other oppressions. They argue that the social environment, particularly the relation of power and the ability to bring consequences, impacts how the potentially abusive person behaves. And yet they posit that this is not purely sociological either, because as important as the actual power relation is, the abusers' *perception* of the power relation and their *perception* of the partner's capacity to enact consequences (which can be distorted and different from the actual) are also important in explaining battering. Zemsky and Gilbert et al. close their model by promoting a psychological healing model, emphasizing abusers' complete responsibility for their behavior.

This social-psychological theory adequately explains why men predominantly perpetrate heterosexual domestic violence and why women are less likely to perpetrate. Heterosexual men who have learned to batter live in a culture which systematically devalues, discriminates against, and exploits women. In effect, misogyny and sexism increase the opportunity for heterosexual men to batter their female partners without receiving negative consequences. As a result, it is likely that these men would choose to batter. By contrast, heterosexual women who have learned to batter are not as likely to express abuse toward their male partners because their partners generally have more perceived and actual social power and the accompanying access to punish them. Instead, a heterosexual woman who batters might choose to express her abuse toward her children, siblings, elderly parents, or others whom she perceives to have lesser or equal social power and/or a diminished capacity to enact negative consequences against her.

Social-psychological theory also explains the existence of same-sex domestic violence by acknowledging the role of homophobia and by positing that the opportunity for abuse of power can exist not only when recipients have less social power, but also when they have roughly equal social power. This phenomenon of lateral abuse is especially likely to occur in circumstances in which the potential victim is perceived to be unwilling or unlikely to report, and/or in which the abuser believes reporting will have no effect. Like their heterosexual counterparts, same-sex abusers learn to abuse. Homophobia helps to create the opportunity for abuse without consequences by isolating the victims and preventing them access to resources such as their family, appropriate social services, and the criminal justice and legal systems. As a result, battered lesbians and gay men are unlikely to seek assistance, and even if they do, are not likely to be helped. In such a climate of opportunity, it is not surprising that lesbian and gay abusive persons are as likely to express abuse toward their partners as are their heterosexual male counterparts.

The Explanatory Power of a Social-Psychological Model

One challenge to social-psychological theory is its ability to explain exceptions. How does this theory hold up if asked to explain the existence of domestic violence perpetrated against someone who has more power than the perpetrator? Specifically, how does this theory explain the occasional incidence of men who are battered by their female partners? Although most people know that a small minority of men are battered by women, this question and the challenge it poses to theory is rarely addressed. One answer might be that abusive heterosexual women only batter their partners in instances where they have or perceive themselves as having more social power, either economically, racially, or along other dimensions, and/or perceive their partners as being unwilling or unable to enact negative consequences against them.

While this explanation is plausible and remains within the framework of the theory, I believe we also need to add to our analysis a variable that is primarily psychological, the degree of severity of the batterer.[2] Those of us who work with victims and/or batterers know that some batterers will draw the line at pushing or milder forms of abuse while others will stop at nothing, the difference based largely upon their capacity for impulse control. I posit here that the more severe the degree of severity of the batterer, the more likely the batterers are to choose to abuse, regardless of the level of opportunity. For instance, a heterosexual woman who is a "severe" batterer with little impulse control might be likely to abuse her male partner, even though he has more perceived and actual power and can enact negative consequences against her. Because of the cycle of violence in which the abuse escalates over time, the degree of severity might change across time and situations, making it difficult to measure. Other complex variables which influence degree of severity and make it difficult to measure include batterers' own shifting perceptions of being powerless and of not perceiving themselves as having resolution options other than violence.[3] Future work should develop the concept of degree of batterer severity and an appropriate measure, not only because of its explanatory value, but also for its important to treatment considerstions.[4]

I also believe domestic violence theory could benefit from further analysis of power. To date, the analysis of social power, as endowed or denied on the basis of gender, race, sexual orientation, and so on has been extensively explored and is useful. By contrast, the concept of psychological or personal power, referring to a person's ability to access the social and other resources available to him or her has not been adequately explored. Just as some of my clients are physically stronger than their abusive partners and could overpower them if they chose to, some of my clients are also professional gay men who have significantly more social power, and the access it affords them, than their abusers. However, because they have been manipulated emotionally by guilt, shame, fear, attacks upon their self-esteem, a distorted sense of responsibility and other complex psychological tactics frequently employed by batterers, many have been rendered powerless to use resources that are available to them. These cases demonstrate that individuals with greater physical or social power who do not have, or have been robbed of, their sense of personal power can be dominated by an abusive person with less actual power. In other words, the experiences of same-sex domestic violence victims teach us that domestic violence is not always necessarily about the abuser having more physical or social power, but is also about their

willingness to use whatever tools and tactics they may have to subordinate their partner. Further attention to this less evident type of psychological or personal power, which is certainly related to self-esteem, will add a new, psychological dimension, strengthening the theory's ability to account for what otherwise might be considered "exceptions to the rule."

Conclusion

To conclude, this paper argues that in order for domestic violence theory to be comprehensive, it must account for both sociopolitical and psychological dynamics, and their complex, often intertwined relationship. A social-psychological model proposed by Zemsky and Gilbert et al. was discussed as an excellent starting place, and suggestions for future analysis, especially for measuring the degree of severity of the batterer and developing the concept of personal power, were made. As all theories must be tested, researchers are challenged to design tools for assessment and studies which will support or refute a social-psychological model and contribute to our understanding.

For those who strategize to stop domestic violence, the challenge is to devote ourselves to changing the social context so as to reduce the opportunities for abuse, including confronting oppressions, developing culturally-appropriate prevention and early intervention programs, and improving the legal system for all battered individuals, as well as developing a body of knowledge about the psychology of batterers that will aid individual, psychological intervention. If domestic violence is caused by both social and psychological factors, then viable solutions must address both. Finally, researchers are challenged to develop theories based upon behavior rather than upon social identity, theories which explain phenomena for every group that experiences it, not only the majority group. While these theories should not be identity-based, they also should not be blind to the very real impact of identity-based social oppression. These, indeed, are challenges to us all.

Notes

1. A colleague of mine, Cara Page, instructed me in a feminist of color critique of domestic violence theory for which I am sincerely grateful. As Ms. Page brought to my attention, the feminist theory I have summarized here is predominately white feminist theory and does not reflect the valuable contributions of feminist of color. And yet I chose to represent it this way, exclusionary as it may be, because this is the most dominant form of the theory and the one most commonly subscribed. There is much to be gained from advocates for battered women of color and for battered lesbians and gay men of all colors working together to expand the current theoretical lens. To familiarize yourself with relevant feminist of color writings, see *Home girls:*

A black feminist anthology, edited by Barbara Smith; *This bridge called my back,* edited by Cherrie Moraga and Gloria Anzaldua; *Mejor sola que acompanada: Para la mujer golpeada: For the Latina in an abusive relationship* by Myrna Zambrano; *Chain chain change: For black woman dealing with physical and emotional abuse* by Evelyn White and others.

2. The concept *degree of severity of the batterer* assumes that batterers can be placed along a continuum of mild to severe depending upon their capacity for impulse control and the severity of violence used. This concept helps us to distinguish between batterers who have a higher degree of control over their impulses and use "milder" forms of abusive behavior and batterers who have little or no impulse control and regularly use severe, life-threatening forms of violence. I use the words "mild" and "milder" only to provide contrast between degrees of severity, not to suggest that domestic violence in any form, mild or severe, is minor.

3. Thank you to Beth Zemsky for raising this point in her critique of this paper.

4. Further attention to this concept, while crucial, is beyond the scope of this paper and the author's current level of expertise.

References

A list of reference is available in the original source.

Trans and Intersex Survivors of Domestic Violence

Defining Terms, Barriers, and Responsibilities

by Diana Courvant and Loree Cook-Daniels

In the early 1970's, as campaigns to raise awareness of domestic violence were first beginning in the United Kingdom and the United States, domestic violence was seen as a problem of male batterers and female survivors. Although this model still fits the vast majority of cases of domestic violence, it is no longer seen as fully describing the problem. In the 1980's, recognition spread of battering in lesbian relationships, and in the 1990's gay men awakened to battering within their own community. Therefore, over the course of the 25 years of the domestic violence survivors' movement, many communities have evolved programs to assist in meeting the needs of both male and female survivors, and developed intervention programs targeted to male and to female batterers. Within this framework, some few heterosexual men have also received survivor services.

However, even this expanded framework consistently neglects the growing class of survivors who transcend stereotypes of gender expression or physical sex. If these survivors have any interaction at all with supportive agencies, they nearly always confront staff or volunteers who lack even the necessary vocabulary to begin to understand the every day experience of these survivors. So let's begin with that vocabulary.

Defining Terms

Like the water surrounding the proverbial fish oblivious to it, all the various aspects of gender are invisible to most of us. Virtually all of us were given a *gender assignment*—boy or girl—by medical personnel at our birth, based on a visual inspection of our genitals (by using the genitals, doctors hope to match the gender assignment with the child's sex, the genetic or anatomical categories of male and female). Most of us grew into these gender assignments fairly smoothly, adopting them as our own *gender identity:* our personal view of our own gender. *Gender attribution* recognizes that what I think of myself isn't always what counts; this term refers to what someone assumes about my gender when they look at me. On the opposite side of the observer-observed dyad is *gender expression.* This is something I do (a behavior, the choice of clothing, etc.) that influences or is intended to influence another's perception of my gender. A *gender role* is the aggregate of a society's assumptions, expectations and mores for how a person of a particular gender is supposed to act. All of these terms are more likely to be heard in a therapist's office than a shelter, but knowing them can help one understand the complexities facing those who transcend stereotypes of gender expression or physical sex: those who are usually known as intersexual, transsexual, transvestite or cross-dressing, or transgendered persons.

An *intersex* or *intersexual* person has a body with external sexual characteristics typical of both male and female bodies. Nonetheless, in our society, children who are born intersexual are nearly always assigned a male or female gender role, although because of external sexual ambiguities, that assignment may not occur at birth. Intersexual children in the United States typically have their genitals surgically altered before age three to conform to gender assignment.

A *transsexual* is someone who lives full-time in the gender identity "opposite" the gender assignment they were given at birth. Currently in Western European and North American countries, transsexuals usually obtain medical intervention (hormones and surgeries) to alter their bodies to more closely conform physically to their gender identity. Some cultures have roles or institutions that allow what we would call transsexuals to live in their preferred gender identify, often without requiring them to seek medical intervention. Transsexuals may be either female-to-male (FtM) or male-to-female (MtF). They may be "post-operative" or "post-op," meaning they've had one or more surgeries to alter their body's sexual characteristics; "pre-op," meaning they have not yet had any or all such surgeries; or "non-op," a term that acknowledges that some transsexuals feel they can live out their gender identify without altering their bodies surgically.

Unlike transsexuals, *transvestites'* and *cross-dressers'* gender assignment and gender identity match. However, they occasionally wear clothes that social custom says belong to the "opposite" gender role. While crossdressed, an individual might take on a name and/or mannerisms associated with that "opposite" gender role, although this is not always the case.

Transgender is a recently-coined term whose definition is still in some flux. Some people use it to refer to people who don't fit any of the above categories but whose gender identity also won't fit into the society's two given roles of male or female. Others include transsexuals and transvestites under the transgender, or *trans,* umbrella. For the remainder of this paper, this larger definition will be used.

Trans and Intersex Survivors

In preliminary data, the Gender, Violence, and Resource Access Survey of trans and intersex individuals found 50% of respondents had been raped or assaulted by a romantic partner, though only 62% of those raped or assaulted (31% of the total sample) identified themselves as survivors of domestic violence when explicitly asked. Of those who were raped or injured, 23% (12% of the total sample) required medical attention for injuries inflicted by a romantic partner. All of those who received treatment self-identified as survivors of domestic violence when asked.

Clearly, trans and intersex survivors exist. Like other domestic violence survivors, they need the help of service agencies, including shelters, to free themselves from abusive partners and to learn to recognize future abusive relationships before the abuse becomes extreme. Unfortunately, few ever manage to access these services openly. There are many reasons why so few trans and intersex survivors are served by the community that typically aids and advocates for survivors of domestic violence. The next section will discuss these barriers.

Barriers

Despite feminist strides, ours is still not a society that supports and rewards individuals who violate gender norms. Little boys are still kept in line with phrases like, "Don't be a sissy." Little girls and particularly older girls face fierce disapproval if they behave or dress too "boyishly." This early punishment for simply expressing gender identity leaves many scars, but the experiences that lead trans and intersexual domestic violence survivors to believe that it's normal for "people like me" to live with abuse only increase in magnitude as the trans or intersex survivor matures.

Perhaps the most damaging force is the one that teaches transgender and intersexual persons that "helping" institutions are often anything but, and may actually harm them. In Washington D.C., an MtF trans woman named Tyra Hunter, the victim of an accident, was allowed to die by paramedics and emergency room staff who discovered her trans status, then decided to mock her rather than provide aid. In the central United States, an FtM trans man named Brandon Teena was raped by two men who discovered his trans status. Upon reporting the rape to the local sheriff's department, the sheriff asked Brandon, "What are you?" and refused to investigate. Brandon's rapists returned to his house to kill him and two of his friends for reporting the rape. At an annual convention of the Society for the Scientific Study of Sexuality one doctor related the case of a girl child with a large clitoris sexually mutilated by her father, who was angered at the phallic proportions of his infant daughter's clitoris. Amazingly, this doctor completed the child's mutilation by performing a clitoridectomy and was using her story to justify surgery on infants in similar situations, rather than healing the child and calling attention to her abuse. Although these stories' power is anecdotal and not statistical, they and others like them are widely known and retold among trans and intersex individuals. Because of the extreme cruelty and casual indifference of authorities and institutions exemplified in these common stories, a trans or intersex survivor may fear an unknown service institution more than a familiar abuser.

A second level of fear trans and intersex survivors face when seeking help is the possibility that their trans or intersex status, if previously hidden, might become known and expose them to more violence, as in the Brandon Teena case. Exposure might also lead to the loss of a job, as very few jurisdictions provide employment discrimination protection to trans and intersexed persons, and stories of job loss or workplace harassment upon exposure are legion.

Should a trans or intersex survivor decide to brave these risks and seek help despite them, she or he faces other barriers. Some information suggests that trans and intersex survivors have frequently been multiply abused for years or decades. Often a trans or intersex survivor has a unique body and/or a unique vulnerability to the emotional aftermath of sexual violence; either can make difficult or impossible discussing this abuse with an unfamiliar victims' advocate.

Related to this problem is the shame and self-doubt that is endemic in these communities, due to the pressures trans and intersex persons have felt from their earliest years to deny their feelings and conform to others' expectations. Adding to this shame and self-doubt is the widespread perception that trans and intersex individuals are mentally ill. This popular stigma of mental illness is furthered by the existence of Gender Identity Disorder (GID) in the DSM-IV, the guidebook to diagnosis of mental illness and personality disorders, but this perception of mental illness is independent of the DSM-IV and is often strongly felt by those completely unfamiliar with the GID diagnosis. Abusers use this shame and self-doubt against their trans and intersex victims to undermine their victims' perceptions and to convince them that no one else will want them. Combined with stories of dating violence (such as that of Chanelle Picket, an MtF trans woman who was recently murdered by a date enraged at the revelation of her trans status) these "warnings" can convince trans and intersex survivors that they are lucky just to have a partner who doesn't kill them.

Finally, two other barriers that affect some trans and intersex survivors deserve attention. One is the barrier that children present. Although every domestic violence survivor with children worries about the safety and custody of those children, the problem is much greater for trans parents, who know that because of prejudice and ignorance about trans persons, courts are extremely unlikely to grant them custody no matter how abusive the other parent is.

The other barrier is the gender segregation of survivor services. Virtually all trans survivors go through a significant period when they are in legal or medical transition. Some intersex survivors have a unique body that prevents identification with either a male or a female gender. Some trans individuals, including such notable examples as authors Kate Bornstein and Leslie Feinberg, have a gender identity and gender expression that is neither male nor female, but mixes elements of both. For all of these people, turning to a gender-segregated service agency may be inconceivable.

Barriers Specific to MtF Individuals

For those MtF individuals not raised in abusive homes, childhood social education rarely includes any information about domestic violence. An MtF child whose parents are disturbed by the child's femininity may glorify violence or minimize the child's trauma from any peer violence in an attempt to encourage behaviour deemed masculine. As an adult survivor, this may be translated into feelings of guilt for not fighting back in violent situations, reinforcing the common perspective of survivors that they are responsible for their own abuse.

The vast majority of resources for survivors of domestic violence targets women. While this benefits the few MtF individuals who have completed medical, legal and social transitions, it typically excludes the majority. Unfortunately, the few who do have resources nominally available often find themselves feared as invaders if they attempt to access women-based services. In San Francisco, one shelter that had made the decision to welcome openly trans women experienced a case where such a survivor was turned away by a shelter supervisor hired after the initial training. Other MtF survivors may refuse to seek shelter or assistance from women-centered agencies out of a respect for the fears or discomfort of non-trans and non-intersex female survivors. Others may avoid seeking help from those agencies out of low self-esteem or feelings that others will not perceive them as "real" women.

Lastly, MtF survivors battered by women often fear that their stories will not be believed. The existing dominant framework of domestic violence can make this type of violence among the most unexpected. Often it is difficult for survivors' advocates to envision this abuse even though the advocates know that the most important tools for control an abuser possesses are not physical.

Barriers Specific to FtM Individuals

Because their gender identity (and probably also their gender expression) is male, FtM individuals cannot be served by agencies that only serve women. Even if an FtM is lucky enough to be in a place where survivor services are offered to men, he may find himself facing incredulous "helpers." Although many people have heard of Christine Jorgenson or Renee Richards, few realize that FtM's exist. FtM's are so "invisible" that even professionals who are well-versed in trans issues often are surprised at the community's growing contention that there are roughly equal numbers of FtM's and MtF's. An FtM survivor may also hesitate to access services for men out of fear that the other survivors may discover his trans status and ridicule him or worse.

Many FtM's lived within the Lesbian community prior to their transition, and oftentimes their partners still identify as Lesbian and keep ties to that community. Since Lesbian communities are often tightly-interwoven and heavily involved in anti-domestic violence work, an FtM battered by a female partner may well fear that if he seeks help the battery may become public, he will not be believed and/or advocates and community members will side with his partner's version of events. This close interplay between domestic violence workers and an FtM survivor's and/or Lesbian batterer's social network may also heighten an FtM's fears that accessing services will lead to public discussion of his trans status, thus exposing him to the discrimination and violence discussed above.

Barriers Specific to Intersex Individuals

Intersex children are often subjected to multiple genital surgeries in order to ensure that outward shape matches, as closely as possible, a cultural esthetic ideal. Typically, these children are not explained the reasons for these procedures and are made to feel that they have (or, indeed, are) an embarrassing secret. Since doctors still perform these surgeries with a primary goal of preventing psychological stress in the parents, it is not surprising that these children are rarely told the truth: that doctors fear their own parents will hate their bodies enough to mutilate them. It is also not surprising that many of them feel horribly ashamed.

When these children are given reasons for these surgeries and other procedures, they are frequently told that the treatment is necessary if the child wants to be loved as an adult. This message is a brutal double-edged sword: first, it tells the child that people will love or reject them based on their body. Second, it directly states that the child is physically inadequate to be loved. The intermittent affection of honeymoon periods mixed with violent explosions may seem the most loving a relationship for which an intersex adult can hope, if raised with these expectations.

As significant as these other barriers can be, invisibility is by far the most significant barrier. Few even are aware of the existence of intersex individuals in our communities. Large, governmental helping agencies that serve tens of thousands of clients each year may never have heard the word "intersex", much less be aware of a single individual case involving an intersex survivor. This ignorance exists despite the fact that intersexuality and surgical treatment of it in infants is much more common than surgical sex reassignment in adults. When an agency is made aware of intersexuality in a survivor, it may not consider that a factor worthy of special notice or attention. This flies in the face of the motivation for surgical alteration of intersex children: doctors repeatedly state that intersex individuals are at vastly heightened risk of abuse. Even after the May, 1997 breakthrough of this issue to the pages of prominent publications such as *The New York Times* and *Newsweek,* helping agencies have not heard this message, and intersex survivors—both adults and children—are nearly always forced to heal from their abuse alone.

Defining Responsibilities

Because trans and intersex individuals are victims of abuse, and because our society is complicit in creating conditions which perpetuate this abuse, we who have dedicated ourselves to helping survivors of domestic violence must include trans and intersex survivors as a part of that mission. Although the trans and intersex communities, where organized, can provide support to these individuals, we are the ones with domestic violence expertise and should retain primary responsibility for ensuring our services are accessible and responsive to these survivors.

Including trans and intersex survivors within our current mission entails three primary responsibilities. First, we must make certain that every community has a visible place to which survivors may turn, regardless of trans or intersex status. Second, we must not revictimize trans or intersex survivors. Third, we must follow up on our own efforts or referrals in order to ensure that our efforts are positive and effective. Fulfilling these responsibilities (they are never discharged) cannot be a passive resolution. Concrete action is required. An agency can begin by taking these steps:

- At minimum, every staff member and volunteer who works with survivors must be made aware that trans and intersex survivors exist and that the agency is committed to working on their behalf. This is the first step in ensuring that the cardinal rule of domestic violence assistance is implemented for trans and intersex survivors: welcome them, and believe their stories.
- If there are any organized trans or intersex communities in your area, contact them to make sure they know you exist and are prepared to at least counsel any of their members with a domestic violence problem. If possible, establish formal or informal training and consultation procedures with these groups to share expertise and promote referrals. These groups can also help you conduct outreach campaigns to trans and intersex persons.
- If you are the sole service provider in the community, ensure at least one staff member is trained in the unique barriers that trans or intersex survivors face and is empowered to anticipate and remove your agency's barriers to sensitively serving such survivors.
- If your area has multiple providers, use or develop a coalition to determine which agencies in each community will be responsible for providing which services. In larger communities, it may even be possible to define subsections of the trans and intersex communities and assign responsibility for serving each group to a different agency, if care is taken to ensure that no one "between the cracks" is left without options. Agencies in contact with survivors can then be made aware of where survivors should be referred and what questions must be answered before a proper referral can be made.
- This coalition should also publicly identify at least one specific resource that is openly welcoming of trans or intersex survivors. This resource might be an already existing hotline, or a separate number might be created either using regularly checked voice mail or automatic forwarding to an existing hotline or agency. Making a point of advertising the availability of this service tells frightened trans and intersex survivors that what they are experiencing is abuse and that other people feel they deserve better, a concept they may find more novel and life-changing than do many "more typical" domestic violence survivors.
- Once services are prepared to serve trans and intersex survivors, create a strategy of outreach to such survivors, including the addition of information about community resources for these survivors on written outreach materials targeting other communities.
- Finally, create a mechanism to follow up on referrals to other agencies and to make changes to coalition plans as new barriers or problems are identified.

Conclusion

Many of the barriers trans and intersex survivors face when trying to free themselves of domestic abuse are similar to those faced by all survivors: self-doubt, a belief that the known abuse is better than potential future unknown abuse, worry about the children and worry about finances. But because they have had to struggle to find pride in bodies and lives society labels "wrong" and because discrimination against them is so strong, trans and intersex survivors have many more hurdles to leap. One of these hurdles the domestic violence system itself created: a gender-segregated service system. We owe these survivors much more thought and effort to ensure that we do not either force them to stay in the hands of their abusers or revictimize them once they take that first step away.

Resources

For more information about trans or intersex survivors, or for assistance in formulating policies or training staff and volunteers, contact the Survivor Project at:

10 NE Fargo # 2
Portland, OR 97212
(503)288-3191

Women's Use of Force

Complexities and Challenges of Taking the Issue Seriously

by Nancy Worcester

This article discusses the complexities, challenges, and urgency surrounding addressing women's use of force. The author emphasizes that women's and girls' use of force needs to be analyzed using a framework that keeps power and control central to the definition of domestic violence and identifies that violence by men and women takes place within a social, historical, and economic context in which men's and women's roles, opportunities, and social power differ. The article builds on an understanding of women's use of force in heterosexual relationships; however, a similar contextual analysis is also applied to women's use of force in teen dating relationships, lesbian relationships, and against children.

Many people are paying enormous attention to the issues of girls' and women's violence. More women are being arrested for assaulting their partners. Many domestic violence programs are making difficult decisions about whether to run "abuser" groups for arrested women or whether women arrested for fighting back are more appropriately served by being in support groups for battered women.

The antifeminist backlash picks up on "conflict tactics"-type studies or the anti-domestic violence movement's own work to give visibility to lesbian violence in order to promote the idea that women are as violent as men. In most audiences, someone knows one man who has been hurt by an intimate partner and his story must be told. Many well-meaning professionals who have chosen to devote their lives to humanitarian service work pride themselves on publicly demonstrating that their services are equally available to men and women without the information, training, or professional support to develop an analysis of the limitations and dangers of a gender-neutral approach to antiviolence work.

This article examines some of the complexities, challenges, and urgency of reintegrating a gender analysis into violence work and addressing the issue of women using force[1] in ways that build on more than 25 years of work by some of the best thinkers and organizers addressing difficult issues within the battered women's movement. This article particularly draws on my experiences of working with the Education and

Emerging Issues Committee of the Wisconsin Coalition Against Domestic Violence to encourage dialogue on the issue through a series of conference presentations, a 1-day membership meeting, think tanks, a special newsletter on this issue, and hours and hours of discussion. The article also builds on my many years of working within the battered women's movement, collaborating with others to ensure that the movement addresses challenging, cutting edge issues. I welcome the wider readership of this journal and encourage readers to explore how debates around the issue of women and girls using force can help set the agenda for the next decade of antiviolence research and activism.

Core issues of power and control and the context of violence need to be central to discussions and policies regarding domestic violence and battering and women's use of force. Violence by men or women and violence against men or women take place within a social, historical, and economic context in which men and women, in general, still play different roles, have different opportunities, and have different social power. Thus, it is important that violence is not simplistically "counted" separately from the context of societal inequalities and gender roles violence helps to keep in place. In addressing the issue of women using force, counting the violence should never be the goal so much as looking at the meaning and consequences of violence in people's lives. It is urgent that antiviolence thinkers, researchers, workers, and activists take leadership roles in taking women's use of force seriously so that information on female violence is no longer given from just antiwomen, backlash perspectives. The challenge is to take violence by women seriously without losing sight of the fact that the patterns of male and female violence within adult intimate relationships are usually very different, often happen within different contexts, and generally have very different consequences and that both the violence itself and the barriers to ending violence are related to societal inequalities.

Female violence must be taken very seriously. Female perpetrators must be held accountable. I know there are women who are violent. I have been curious about violent women ever since I read MacDonald's book *Shoot the Women First* ("The first book to tell why women are the most feared terrorists in the world," back cover), the cover of which exclaimed,

> "Shoot the women first" is the advice given to German police teams handling terrorist incidents, but is recognized as valid by anti-terrorist groups the world over. Armed men may hesitate before they shoot, women rarely do. They are more ruthless, more determined and consequently more feared than their male comrades, and make the most deadly adversaries.

I am a firm believer that many women are extremely good at whatever they decide to do, so it makes sense that if a woman "decides" violence is necessary, she might be very good at it. It also makes sense to me that when girls and women are rewarded for paying attention to what other people need and for developing good verbal and emotional skills, they could turn those areas of expertise into something that could very much hurt a loved one. Indeed, unless our society starts to give clearer, more consistent messages that will not reward or ignore violence, I think we should expect that more girls will get the message that violence is acceptable or even glamorous. I am obviously writing this article, however, because I want to inspire readers to take female violence seriously without losing sight of the general patterns in intimate partner violence (i.e., male violence keeps women from maximizing their fullest potential) that need to guide antiviolence work. We need to be careful that our curiosity about female violence, our knowledge that some women are violent and thus that some men get hurt in heterosexual relationships, and our commitment to holding abusers accountable do not get in the way of thinking through the complexities of addressing the issues of female violence.

It is time to reframe a number of issues.

Connecting and Disconnecting: Issues of Girls and Women Using Force

The question, "What about girls and women using force?" is so big. There are many answers and many more questions than answers. When the Wisconsin Coalition Against Domestic Violence Education Committee first initiated discussion on this topic, we did not want to leave out any part of the question, so we tried to address all the following questions in our first short workshop:

1. What are the experiences of domestic abuse programs with girls' and women's use of force?
2. What are the political ramifications of asking this question? How do we frame the issue to make sure we are not compromising the integrity of the battered women's movement? What are the dangers of addressing this issue?
3. Do men and women use violence in different ways? Much on the power and control wheel may look the same for male and female violence. But what about the "using male privilege" piece that supports violence against women? A lesbian batterer may use homophobia to hurt her partner, but are there similar privilege or social oppression weapons being used if a heterosexual woman is a perpetrator?
4. What are the similarities and differences of batterers' treatment for men and women? Are there different ways to hold men and women accountable for their violence? Will the same types of intervention work for abusive women and abusive men?
5. What are the similarities and differences between women as perpetrators in lesbian versus heterosexual relationships? (What are the similarities and differences between women as victims or survivors in lesbian versus heterosexual relationships?)
6. If we believe that violence against women is related to gender socialization, are we moving toward boys and men being less violent and/or girls and women being more violent? What are we doing right? What are we doing wrong?
7. Should we make these questions more central to the battered women's movement? If so, how?
8. Are there other forms of girls' and women's use of force we should be addressing? What else should we be discussing?

The fact that more than 100 people attended a workshop, which we expected to be very small (it was scheduled at the same time as many workshops by popular national speakers), demonstrated that people are eager for a chance to talk about the issues. Time ran out much too quickly, and it became obvious that each question needs weeks, not minutes, of discussion time. It was clear that one challenge for the antidomestic violence movement is making the time and creating safe spaces so that we can slowly and carefully develop our thinking about the different ways girls and women may use or are accused of using force at different ages and in different contexts.

Many of us who have worked on a range of violence against women issues have felt connected under the widest violence against women "umbrella" but have found times when we needed to specifically work on lesbian violence, sexual assault, gender harassment, elder abuse, or heterosexual domestic violence; we have done that specific work with the bigger picture of analysis of violence against women in mind. In the same way, it will be important to remember the context of sex-role socialization, societal inequalities, and violence as power and control as the questions about girls and women using force are addressed in relation to teen dating violence, gang violence, lesbian battering, child abuse, elder abuse, heterosexual domestic violence, and other issues. Unique aspects of each of these topics merit much in-depth exploration, and simultaneously, each needs to be contextualized within the broader framework of violence against and by females within a violent, patriarchal society. (Key issues related to several of these topics are introduced at the end of this article.)

Strategy: Acknowledge That Men Get Hurt by Violence

Backlash against a movement is always a sign of how successful a movement has been. No one would be talking about whether women are as violent as men if there had not been more than 25 years of organizing against violence against women; establishing shelters, anti-domestic violence programs, and support groups; working to get the criminal justice system to hold perpetrators accountable; and developing coordinated community responses to domestic violence. Quite rightly, violence against women has received much attention.

Who gets left out of attention focused on violence against women? Men and boys as victims of violence.

Acknowledging that men and boys get terribly hurt by violence may be just as important as exploring the issue of women as perpetrators of violence. It certainly helps shift the discussion in more fruitful directions. Acknowledging that men and boys are killed by violence (mostly by other men and boys) more often than are women and girls in this society may be an effective

strategy for making a gender analysis more central to violence work.

Male violence not only hurts women but also disproportionately kills men, especially men of color. Of homicide victims from 1976 to 1999 in the United States, 76% were men, as were 88% of those who committed homicide. White men between the ages of 15 and 25 are more likely to be killed than White women, and Black men are more likely to be killed than Black women.[2] Male violence particularly devastates Black communities. Black women aged 15 to 24 are killed at nearly the same rate as are White men in the United States, whereas Black men are killed at a rate 8.5 times higher than are Black women or White men.

Both the battered women's movement and many parts of the wider women's (liberation) movement have done an excellent job of making connections among images of women, the socialization of women and their roles in society, and violence against women. An important next stage of working on violence prevention must be to develop a more thorough gender analysis so that the roots of violence are better understood in relation to definitions of masculinity, the socialization of men and their roles in society. Hiding the prevalence of male violence (against both men and women) contributes to the climate in which it becomes acceptable or even fashionable to ask whether women are as violent as men. For example, despite the fact that almost all the so-called school violence that hit the headlines in the 1990s has been perpetrated by (White) male youths, the media have consistently failed to note that, and one could easily get the idea that school violence is a gender-neutral problem. How many people have any idea about the disproportionate amount of violence committed by men?[3] While identifying that both men and women get hurt or killed by living in a violent society, a gender analysis also helps identify that men and women get hurt by violence in very different contexts. Men mostly get hurt by strangers, whereas women mostly get hurt by people they know and care about.[4] Women are more than five times more likely than men to be victimized by a spouse or partner, ex-partner, boyfriend, or girlfriend.

There is not a hierarchy of violence, but the ramifications for intervention, prevention, and long-term consequences are totally different for someone hurt by a stranger and someone hurt by a loved one. These are important issues to identify for anyone questioning the necessity of a gender analysis of violence. Many emergency room and criminal justice system personnel have observed that when someone (usually a man) is hurt by a stranger, they are likely to want to report the crime, to want the other person prosecuted, and to hope they will never see that person again. In contrast, a different pattern is observed when someone (usually a woman) has lived with or loved the person who is hurting them. Reporting the abuse has different ramifications when there are shared children, dreams, identities, finances, and futures and where reporting may cause escalation of the violence. Unlike stranger violence in which men are the main victims of what is usually a one-time occurrence, intimate partner violence, with women as the primary victims, tends to be an on-going pattern of abuse of power and control. Consequently, in general, violence disrupts the lives of men and women in quite different ways.

Gender, Race, and Class

Momentarily focusing on the seriousness of how much male violence hurts men may be an effective way to reassure men that we care about anyone getting hurt by violence, it may help us get on with our presentations and our work, and it may help contextualize the fact that violence against women happens within societies that allow and support the widest range of violence. However, it is also important to recognize the limitations and dangers of this tactic.

First, it is vital to acknowledge that gender differences in homicide rates do not reflect the differences in quality of life for men and women. Many women hurt by violence get hurt every day. The woman who says, "I probably only got hurt once a year for 20 years, but I woke up every one of those other 364 days of the year wondering if that would be the day" (quote from a survivor in the video "Any Day Now," WomanReach, Inc. and the Domestic Violence Advocacy Council of Charlotte/Mecklenburg, 1991) reminds us how violence and the fear of violence affect the quality of women's lives.

Also, it is important to be careful not to leave out an analysis of how other inequalities in society are related to violence. Note that in the previous discussion of homicide victimization of Black and White people aged 15 to 24, gender analysis is meaningless unless the impact of race or racism on homicide is also examined. These figures show that Black women and White men are killed at similar rates and that the homicide rate is 4.2 times higher for Black than for White women. Black men are killed at a rate 35 times higher than are White women.

Both race and class analyses are crucial in addressing violence and understanding that the battered women's movement, the criminal justice system, and other systems have particularly failed to adequately address the needs of many battered women of color, poor women, and other women from marginalized communities. Lack of appropriate services and policies may force some women to resort to using force or other unhealthy coping strategies. In *Compelled to Crime: The Gender Entrapment of Battered Black Women,* Richie wrote,

The extent to which some women experience this predicament [domestic violence] is directly related to the degree of stigma, isolation, and marginalization imposed by their social position. The choices are harder and the consequences are more serious for women with low incomes, women of color, lesbians, women who become pregnant at a young age, and others whose decisions, circumstances, and status violate the dominate culture's expectations or offend hegemonic images of "womanhood."

Studies that have been conducted from the standpoint of battered women have been overwhelmingly concerned with the experiences of White women. . . . The aggregate effect is that while *some* battered women are safer in the 1990s than they were in the 1970s, and while we know more about *general* patterns in the population, we still have very little theoretical or empirical work that speaks to African-American battered women from low-income communities. Consequently, few anti-violence programs, criminal justice policies, or theoretical explanations are sensitive to ethnic differences or address cultural issues that give particular meaning to violence in intimate relationships for African-American or other women of color. Furthermore, those whose lives are complicated by drug use, prostitution, illegal immigrant status, low literacy, and a criminal record continue to be misunderstood, underserved, isolated, and . . . in serious physical and emotional danger. (pp. 2–12)

E. Assata Wright gives examples of well-meaning public policy having an adverse effect for women of color because no one thought through how policies like mandatory arrest might have an impact on these women's lives:

The mandatory arrest policy is particularly problematic for Black women because . . . they are more likely to fight back and protect themselves when being abused. In cases where a woman hits her abuser, she can be arrested along with the attacker.

Many Black women and Latinas may protect the abuser from jail even if it means risking their own safety. In a 1996 report on police brutality in New York City, Amnesty International found that between 1993 and 1994 there was a "substantial" increase in the number of Blacks and Latinos who were shot or killed while in police custody. Advocates point out that while women want protection from their batterers, they don't want him beaten by cops or worse, killed by them. (pp. 550–551)

Economic issues relate to battering a number of ways, such as in both the relationship between poverty and family violence and the potential loss of employment opportunities for self-sufficiency abused women arrested for assaulting their abusive partners may face. Kurz's research found that the poorest divorced women, those on welfare, experienced higher rates of violence than did any other groups of women and that the poorer the woman, the more serious the violence was that she experienced. She questions the relationship between poverty and abuse as follows:

> What is the reason for the higher levels of violence reported by low income women? Are poor women more forthcoming about the amount of violence they experience, or do more of them report the violence to the police because they have less access to other kinds of legal assistance? These are possibilities, but at this point no data answer this question. It is also possible that something about the circumstances of those living in poverty contributes to the higher rates of violence among poorer men. For example, men from lower income groups may have a stronger belief in the legitimacy of violence than other men, since they typically hold more traditional gender ideologies than other men. It is not clear, however, that lower income men actually behave in more gendered ways than do other men. Another explanation for the higher rates of violence reported by poorer women could be that lower-income men have fewer ways of controlling their partners than other men. The higher men's social class, the more ability they have to control their female partners through their greater economic resources. (pp. 136–137)

The National Clearinghouse for the Defense of Battered Women has raised awareness of the economic ramifications of battered women being arrested for and convicted of using force against abusive partners and then having a criminal record, which affects their financial situation.

> We know many women, eager to "get the case over with," accept guilty pleas without being fully appraised of the potential consequences of have a record. Might a conviction bar a woman from certain employment opportunities, public housing situations, welfare benefits, or affect her immigration status or a custody determination? We want to work with defense counsel to help them better understand the consequences of a conviction and the disparate impact on women clients (since so many of the jobs barred by convictions are traditionally "women's work," such as child care and health care jobs, and because so many women, as pri-

mary caretakers for their children, are the ones to apply for public benefits and housing). (p. 8)

It is clear that researchers and practitioners need to more fully understand how gender, race, and class affect battered women's experiences and how and why they may choose to, or need to, use violence.

Domestic Violence = Woman Battering

Domestic violence is certainly not gender exclusive, but the pattern of male perpetrator and female victim reflects and is encouraged by societal power inequalities between women and men and serves to maintain gender inequality. In fact, domestic violence is an extreme example of gender inequality.

The battered women's movement was clearly built on a sophisticated understanding of how violence in intimate relationships relates to and helps perpetuate inequalities between women and men. As the movement grew more visible, as many more players became involved in providing services to victims of intimate violence, and as more funding became available, domestic violence became a hot topic and a very mainstream issue. It was no longer unusual, controversial, or even radical to work to end domestic violence. This was a very exciting phenomenon: Many more people know about and benefited from domestic violence services, and whole communities identified roles different professionals could play in recognizing and responding to domestic violence. This mainstreaming of the battered women's movement coincided with a changing environment where the work of many aspects of the women's movement became less visible and debates about "political correctness" made it much more challenging to figure out how to work on societal inequalities. Although it was no big deal that people involved in this work gradually stopped calling themselves the battered women's movement and became known as people working against domestic violence, symbolically "women" visibly got left out of the name of the movement and out of the analysis of intimate partner violence. (Throughout this article, I use both the terms *battered women's movement* and *domestic violence movement*). Once an issue has a gender-neutral name, it is easy to forget that it is not a gender-neutral issue.

Renzetti illustrated the dangers of a gender-neutral approach to domestic violence in relation to the criminal justice system as follows:

> The police, attorneys, and judges, like the backlash writers, argue that women, like men, must be held accountable for their behavior. To them, prosecuting women who have used violence against an intimate

partner represents a gender-neutral application of the law. However, by decontextualizing women's violence and scrutinizing it in terms of a male normative standard juxtaposed against stereotypes of respectable femininity, the justice system thereby treats unjustly many women who have used violence. The outcome will be—indeed, it already is—"gendered injustice." Women are increasingly being treated like men by the legal system, even though their circumstances typically are quite different. If these differential circumstances are not taken into account, the outcomes can hardly be fair. (p. 49)

With more women getting arrested for domestic violence in heterosexual relationships, it will be increasingly important to have trustworthy assessment tools that help identify when women use force in self-defense or within the context of long-term battering rather than initiate violence as power and control. The complexities of assessing who are the victims and who are the perpetrators have long been issues for discussion in relation to lesbian violence. Burk (C. Burk, personal communications, May 11, 1999, & July 14, 2000) and others have observed that unlike those working on heterosexual domestic violence, people working on lesbian intimate violence have always had to look at how any behavior can be used as power and control, how any behavior can be used as a survival tactic, and the fact that victims may well identify as abusers. There is also an important "reporting artifact" that is recognized in the violence literature: Studies show that women are more likely than men to admit they are abusive. In an article titled "Violent Women: Fact and Fantasy—Social Service Agencies Have the Responsibility to Know the Difference," Edleson stressed that accurate assessment is vital for providing different effective interventions for women who use force in different ways, for different reasons. He summarized how the Domestic Abuse Project's *Women Who Abuse in Intimate Relationships* treatment manual categorizes women who use force into the following three groups:

One group includes women who use violence in self-defense to escape or protect themselves from their partner's violence. Saunders (1986) found that this was the most frequently reported motivation for women's use of violence.

In a second group are women who have a long history of victimization at the hands of previous partners as well as during childhood. These women are described as taking a stance in life that "no one is ever going to hurt me that way again," and their violence is interpreted as an effort to decrease their own chances of victimization.

Violent women in a third group are identified as primary aggressors who use their greater physical power to control their partners. (p. 3)

Obviously, it is of the utmost importance to recognize that many women who use force are battered women who are not safe. Breaking their isolation and helping them be safer may be even more important than it is for women who do not use force because battered women's use of violence may make them even more vulnerable to their partner's aggression.

In general, the context and consequences of male and female violence within intimate relationships is different. Although studies often report that women use violence as a conflict tactic as often as men, women are the recipients of more injurious and life-threatening violence committed by intimate partners than are men. Women are also more likely than men to be killed by intimate partners.[5]

For much of the past decade, anti-domestic violence programs have been conscientiously letting their communities know that they are committed to helping both women and men in violent relationships. Although many anti-domestic violence programs do serve a few men, a committed public effort to reach out to male victims has not resulted in anti-domestic violence programs suddenly discovering they need to rethink their emphasis on serving women. In fact, no man has ever stayed in the first shelter for battered men, established in Britain in 1992 by the group Families Need Fathers. Hanusa (D. Hanusa, personal communication, November 10, 1998) and others who lead abuser groups have observed that the services needed by heterosexual men who identify themselves as abused seem to be different from those needed by abused women because safety is less of an issue and leaving the relationship is not usually associated with increased danger as it is for abused women.

In "Counseling Heterosexual Women Arrested for Domestic Violence," Hamberger and Potente concluded that domestic violence by women and men show distinctly different patterns.

First, although women are domestically violent, often at levels of severity similar to that of men, the impact of their violence is typically less than men's violence. Second, women tend to commit violence less frequently than do men, and for different reasons. Specifically, women tend to initiate physical assault motivated by a need for self-protection or retaliation of a previous assault by their partner. Men, in contrast, tend to identify control or punishment as the primary motivations for assaults on their partners. (p. 59)

Saunders showed that 71% of battered women arrested for domestic violence had used violence in self-defense. Hanusa (D. Hanusa, personal communication,

November 10, 1998) observed that there is a functional difference in how men and women use violence in intimate relationships: Women use it to end oppression geared toward them, whereas men use it to control someone. In 32 in-depth interviews with women court-ordered or referred to counseling because they had used violence, Dasgupta found that "the most pervasive and persistent motivation for women's use of violence is ending abuse in their own lives" (p. 217), and "when viewed in terms of motives, intentions, and consequences, these women's use of violence emerges as instrumental; that is, the incidents are directed toward the resolution of conflicts or control of immediate surroundings" (p. 210), including the fact that "many of the women became physically aggressive with their partners when their children were being abused" (p. 208).

In examining the differences between male and female violence, it may be useful to keep in mind the definition of domestic violence as an on-going pattern in which one person controls the other person and one person thus lives in fear for her or his safety. It is crucial to keep asking who is afraid and who is not safe. We need to explore much more about how men and women use emotional control. We know women can be effective at using emotional control, but whether it takes on the same level of threat to safety and whether the other person lives in constant fear may be a major difference between male and female use of emotional control. In Dasgupta's study of 32 women who had used physical violence, it was clear that even the use of violence did not equalize who was in control and who was afraid in these heterosexual relationships.

> Regardless of the degree of physical force women used, none of the interviewees believed that it made their partners fearful. Neither did it control their behaviors. This perception was not without its base in reality. A group of 10 men whose female partners had been arrested on domestic abuse charges and interviewed as a part of this study also denied that their partner's violence resulted in their experiencing prolonged or significant fear for their safety. This finding is supported by studies that indicate that men in violent relationships, compared to their female counterparts, express little fear of their partners and wives. (pp. 209–210)

In addition to the research quoted throughout this article, most of the ideas and analysis in this article have grown out of on-going discussions with domestic violence service providers, abuser group facilitators, and policy makers. Everyone agrees that much better research is needed on women's use of force. Meanwhile, however, many people agree that they have observed the following different patterns in male and female violence in intimate relationships and the different consequences of male and female violence in intimate relationships:

1. Male violence is more apt to be a pattern to be repeated in subsequent relationships rather than situational in particular relationships. Adult women who are perpetrators in one relationship are less likely to become perpetrators in their next relationship. How many domestic violence programs have served several women hurt by the same man? (Talking about this phenomenon is a good way of reinforcing that most men are not violent. The high percentage of women who get hurt by domestic violence is a reflection of the same men hurting several women rather than a high percentage of men being violent.)

2. Men are more likely to physically injure their partners.

3. Women are more likely than men to be killed by intimate partners and are more likely than men to be punched, hit, burned, thrown out of a window, or strangled by intimate partners (Belluck, 1997).

4. Men have an ability to control women and children by creating an ongoing pattern whereby women and children live in fear. (How much will this situation change when more women have access to guns? In Dasgupta's interviews with women who had used force, she concluded that "only when women picked up weapons, guns, knives, and household objects did their partners become temporarily afraid," p. 210. But the interviewees also said that having used force, including weapons, led to more abusive behaviors in the future by their male partners. What are the dynamics that create an on-going pattern of fear?).

5. A different pattern in ending male and female violence in heterosexual relationships has been observed: If a woman is hurting a man, the violence usually ends when the relationship ends. If a man is hurting a woman, the violence generally escalates and becomes most dangerous when the relationship ends and in subsequent years. Therefore, barriers to ending violence may be fundamentally different for men and women.

In the arena of sexual assault, activists working to end violence against women have been critical of the overemphasis on women learning self-defense when the real issue that needs to be addressed is stopping male violence. Ironically, with domestic violence, the issue of women fighting back is now getting increased negative attention (and more arrests), with too little attention being paid to why women need to resort to violence. Why are other strategies failing to keep women safe within their intimate relationships? Once again, the key issue of how to stop men's abuse of power and control is left out when the discussions focus on whether women should use force to protect themselves.

Violence in Lesbian Relationships

Lesbian battering includes many of the same issues as heterosexual domestic violence (power and control, fear, lack of safety) but is additionally affected by homophobia and a lack of services for victims of lesbian violence. In many communities, neither lesbian organizations nor anti-domestic violence programs have adequately addressed lesbian battering because of the fear that it could rip lesbian communities apart, dilute the issue of male violence against women, draw the "wrong" kind of attention to gay and lesbian issues, or draw the "wrong" kind of attention to a domestic violence program that may need financial support from a conservative community. Unfortunately, it is often the backlash to the violence against women movement that draws attention to lesbian domestic violence in an effort to say that women are as violent as men.

That women tend to be more likely than men to report they are violent must certainly affect studies of lesbian violence. I also wonder whether there is an additional reporting artifact in that women are more likely to identify abuse in a lesbian than in a heterosexual relationship. (Is more equality expected in a lesbian relationship so that an abuse of power and control is more easily identified?). There are extremes related to lesbian violence: It often is ignored or, in contrast, reported at quite high rates (e.g., in surveys at the Michigan Women's Music Festival, although these surveys do not use scientific sampling methods). Why these extremes? Is less known about the prevalence of lesbian violence than about heterosexual violence because of the added complexities of studying it, or are people just more honest about saying that too little is known about the prevalence or consequences of lesbian battering? As someone who teaches women's health topics to 840 university students each year, I have curiously observed that students pay much more attention to the issue of lesbian battering than to other issues, such as legal discrimination against lesbians, lack of partner health insurance for lesbians, lesbian parenting, lesbian alcohol use, or lesbian menopause. Perhaps it is because the battered women's movement has been a major arena for important feminist discussion and debate during the past two decades and the issue rightly belongs here; there have not been similarly effective movements around which to organize other equally urgent lesbian issues. The good news is that because some people have made lesbian battering a visible issue, there are now some very good resources on this topic.[6]

An excellent article, "Ruling, the Exceptions: Same Sex Battering and Domestic Violence Theory" by Merrill, builds on the analysis of power and control in heterosexual domestic violence relationships to look at theoretical frameworks that bring together sociopolitical and psychological theories to include same-sex violence. Merrill identified the following three factors that make someone violent: (a) growing up learning how to be violent (obviously, everyone growing up in the United States learns how to be violent, but many people choose not to act on that); (b) having an opportunity to be violent; and (c) personally choosing to be violent. Merrill said that having the opportunity to be violent can be emphasized as a way to explain same-sex violence because homophobia allows someone to abuse a same-sex partner knowing that homophobia in the outside world will protect abusers from suffering negative consequences for their abusive behavior. Homophobia and heterosexism operate so that battering in same-sex relationships is ignored or not taken seriously; the perpetrators clearly get the message that our society will tolerate it. Potentially violent women in lesbian relationships get the message that they will not be negatively sanctioned for being violent "in that kind of relationship." In contrast, potentially violent women in heterosexual relationships will get strong messages that their violence against male partners would not be socially acceptable or tolerated. Merrill concluded, "While the social phenomenon of prejudice (homophobia) does not cause lesbian or gay battering, it does create an opportune environment that supports this abusive behavior by its refusal to challenge it" (p. 15).

Lesbian battering experts have much to offer the anti-domestic violence field from their years of recognizing the complexities of identifying who are the perpetrators and who may have used force in self-defense. As anti-domestic violence programs work to develop more effective assessment tools for women arrested for using force, this may be an opportunity for activists who have worked on lesbian and heterosexual battering assessment to have more dialogue about what can be learned from each other. Clearly, all communities need to give both men and women consistent messages that violence in any relationship, by either partner, is not tolerated.

Women as Perpetrators of Child Abuse

Of all the areas I work in, child abuse is the area I find the most mother blaming and outright woman hating, and it is the area in which I am most concerned about the increasing levels of woman blaming. Society in general and child protective services in particular assign responsibility for child abuse to mothers, regardless of who assaults the children or the context in which the abuse occurs.

There has now been more than a decade of organizing and education on the effects of domestic violence on children. Ironically, instead of people being better at seeing how child abuse is an extension and predictable component of the ongoing power and control that hurts women in domestic violence, more and more battered women are being charged with child abuse because they "allowed" their children to witness domestic violence or "failed to protect" them from harm, despite the power relations that make it dangerous and impossible for many battered women to keep their children safe.

In their important article "Women and Children at Risk: A Feminist Perspective on Child Abuse," Stark and Flitcraft concluded,

> Representative sample surveys indicate that fathers may be as likely or more likely than mothers to abuse children. . . . More important, there is little doubt that if a man is involved in a relationship, he is many times more likely than a woman to abuse the children. . . . National survey data indicate that men were responsible for two-thirds of the reported incidents of child abuse in which men were present in the relationship. (p. 75)

They are careful to point out that they reach this conclusion despite the obvious fact that women spend many more hours per day, per week with children and that many children are raised by single women.

The issues of child abuse and woman abuse are so clearly interrelated that it feels very intentional that others are not seeing or are choosing to ignore the connection. Years ago, Walker, best know for her important work on battered woman syndrome, noted that if a child is being abused, the most predictable correlation is that the child's mother is also being abused. (That factor—the mother being abused—is more consistent and predictable than is any other variable, including age, income group, and geographic area.) Indeed, if the woman is abusing the child, it is even more predictable that the woman herself is being abused and that her abuse of the child is related to (or a consequence of) the ongoing power, control, and fear in her life. Walker found mothers were eight times more likely to hurt their children when they were battered than when they were safe from violence.

The example of child abuse is a model for how antiviolence activists and researchers can take the issue of women's use of force more seriously, that is, to make sure we take the context of women's violence very seriously. If women are more likely to hurt their children when they themselves are being hurt, it of course rein-forces the need for ending violence against women, but it also reinforces our need to find more effective ways to communicate and collaborate with agencies and institutions that have not always seen violence against women as their issue. The Advocacy for Women and Kids in Emergencies Program at Boston Children's Hospital (Schechter & Gary) is a model that takes both child abuse and woman abuse seriously and does not leave anyone pulled between two systems or two victims. Schecter's work at the Advocacy for Women and Kids in Emergencies Program inspired others to work on the premise that if a child is being hurt, the mother may also be getting hurt and that child abuse intervention needs to be consistently done in a way that ensures the violence in a mother's life will be addressed. Different sets of advocates are available to help the child through the child protective service system, and another set of advocates helps the mother end the violence in her life. Instead of seeing a conflict between the interests of abused children and their mothers, a reframing of the issue helped this agency identify that in many cases, helping women to be safe is a very effective way to help children be safe.

Teen Dating Violence

This issue of women getting mixed messages about whether it is acceptable to initiate violence or to fight back for self-protection is particularly crucial in relation to work on girls' use of force in teen dating relationships.

An example of what is happening in teen dating violence is apparent in Molidor and Tolman's article, "Gender and Contextual Factors in Adolescent Dating Violence," which reported a study of 635 students surveyed about dating violence. The study found that male and female adolescents did not differ in overall frequency of violence in dating relationships. However, when researchers went beyond simply counting experiences of violence to looking for the context and consequences of teen intimate violence, they found that adolescent girls experienced significantly higher levels of severe violence and emotional reactions to the violence than did boys.

This is an important example of an article that clarifies the difference between the amount of violence and the consequences of violence for male and female teens. But most observations of teen violence do not make that important distinction. All too often, it is simply stated that girls are pushing and shoving just as much as boys these days. How many of us have been a part of meetings where researchers indicate they know there are limitations to the usefulness of conflict tactics scales but then quickly move on to simply report the interesting data they have that girls say they are using considerable amounts of violence? Once a girl has identified herself as "using violence," how much more difficult will it be for her to identify herself as needing support and safety planning if she is in a pattern of ongoing power and control?

The American Association of University Women Educational Foundation study on sexual harassment at school reported that sexual harassment was an issue for both girls and boys but stressed that the consequences were distinctly different. Boys reported knowing they had been harassed, but they could not remember when it started. In contrast, girls could remember exactly when they were harassed and the serious consequences (i.e., hating school, skipping school, not speaking up in class) that resulted from the harassment.

There is a dangerous trend in the resources designed for teens. Concern has been expressed about the lack of antiviolence resources appropriate for young men. There is a need for resources that are male positive but clearly antiviolence, in contrast to some of the present dating violence materials that some young men feel are antimale. Unfortunately, in aiming for this newly defined "market," there is a trend toward dating violence resources showing equal levels and consequences of male and female violence. It is crucial that resources and messages are developed and disseminated that appeal to young men but do not hide the different patterns and consequences of male and female violence.

The arena of the middle school is a most urgent one in which to address the question, "What about women or girls as perpetrators?" In many ways, middle school is "no person's land: Everyone is powerless" (D. Hanusa, personal communication, November 10, 1998), but it is also the key opportunity for helping young people learn healthy ways of reclaiming their personal power and setting very high standards for themselves as to how they will perform and what they will expect from future relationships. As more and more dating violence prevention resources and messages are rightly being aimed at this age group, it is important that educators and policy makers find effective messages that do not downplay the seriousness or prevalence of male violence or present violence in intimate relationships as a gender-neutral topic.

Whenever violence in a group is first noticed, attention is wrongly paid to the fact that much of the violence is probably "mutual violence." This is what happened with the initial observations of both adult heterosexual domestic violence and lesbian violence. Then, as people were more careful about understanding the dynamics and consequences, it became apparent that most domestic violence and lesbian battering was the ongoing pattern of one person abusing power and control in all or most aspects of the relationship. Now, middle school violence is increasingly labeled *mutual abuse*. Many well-meaning educa-

tors and youth leaders describe middle schools girls as being as violent as middle school boys. What is happening here? Is there a short time in that "no person's land" when girls and boys have not yet learned their "appropriate" social roles regarding who should and should not be violent? Do they grow out of this a couple of years later when gender roles become exaggeratedly defined in high school? Is this another case in which it is dangerous not to be identifying the perpetrators (who are otherwise not held responsible or are sent to mediation)? Substantial resources need to be devoted to studying and preventing the dynamics and consequences of middle school violence.

On the other hand, if there is a real trend toward girls becoming more violent (either as perpetrators or learning that violence is the most effective way to not be controlled by someone else), it is urgent that this trend be recognized and addressed. If girls are learning that it pays to be violent, this raises important issues for the antiviolence movement. After more than 25 years of activism against violence against women, we should be reaching a point where we are starting to notice a decline in male violence. Is it possible that wider societal influences are so strong that instead of decreasing violence against women, we are seeing more young women get the message that their own violence is acceptable?

Conclusion

It is time for antiviolence researchers and activists to take the question "What about girls and women using force?" seriously. The question is useful for reframing the analysis of violence to examine more carefully how male violence hurts both women and men, although in different ways and in different contexts. We also need to find ways to take female violence seriously without taking a gender-neutral approach to violence. It is possible to simultaneously acknowledge individual female violence and show how the pattern of male violence against women reflects and perpetuates societal inequalities between men and women. We also must more carefully examine the intersection of race, class, sexuality, and gender in our antiviolence work.

The battered women's movement has been good at listening to each victim's story. Sometimes people's stories help us see general patterns that help us predict, understand, and interrupt ongoing power and control in relationships; sometimes a person's situation needs to be understood and addressed uniquely. We are fully capable of taking female violence against men seriously and serving individual men hurt by intimate partner violence without losing sight of the societal patterns of male violence hurting both men (usually as strangers) and women (usually within intimate relationships).

We can also use the question "What about female violence?" to explore other difficult issues. The gun industry, video games, and the media have been giving girls and women powerful messages about using violence. After more than 25 years of violence against women activism, is it possible that instead of diminishing or ending violence against women, we are seeing an increase in the number of girls and women who are learning that violence is an effective way to have power in a society that often limits their opportunity for healthy control in their own lives? What are we going to do about this?

Violence is a social issue. There is nothing "natural" about men being violent and women being less violent or passive. Male violence is rooted in the socialization processes our society has consistently imposed on boys and men. If there is an increase in girls and young women (and maybe even women of all ages) using force, it is a reminder that we need to start now to address socialization toward violence in new ways. The anti-violence against women movement, as with women's movements more generally, was never about making girls and women more like men. It was about building a fundamentally different, violence-free society. Asking hard questions about women's possible use of force may be an important way of remembering the social change work that still needs to be accomplished. Much work needs to be done to create a world in which girls and boys learn they can have a healthy amount of control in their own lives without controlling someone else. All communities need to give clearer, more consistent messages that neither male nor female violence is ignored or rewarded. In our work for a violence-free society, what are we doing right and what do we need to do differently? How can we use the question "What about women and girls using force?" to help set the agenda for the next decades of violence research and activism?

Notes

1. Erin House (n.d.) has encouraged the use of the term *force* rather than *violence,* noting that

   > according to Webster's Dictionary, violence is defined as "rough or injurious physical force," "an unjust or unwarranted exertion of force and power." Thus, violence can be defined as a type of force, used unjustly, with the intention of causing injury. Force itself is descriptive of the use of physical strength to accomplish a task—but does not imply the same degree of wrong-doing or harmful intent. (p. 2)

2. In 1997, White men aged 15 to 24 were killed at the rate of 13.2 per 100,000 compared with White women aged 15 to 24, who were killed at the rate of 3.2 per 100,000 (Kumanyika, Morssink, & Nestle, 2001). Thus, White men are 4.2 times more likely to be killed than White women. Black women aged 15 to 24 are killed at nearly the same rate (13.3) as are White men in the United States. With a homicide rate of 113.3 per 100,000, Black men are killed at a rate 8.5 times higher than Black women (Kumanyika et al., 2001).

3. For example, men committed 88% of homicides in the United States between 1976 and 1999 (Fox & Zawitz, 2001b).

4. According to the National Crime Victimization Survey, in 2000, 54% of nonfatal violent crime (rape or sexual assault, robbery, and aggravated or simple assault) against men was committed by strangers and 44% was committed by intimates, other relatives, or friends or acquaintances. In contrast, 33% of nonfatal violent crime against women was committed by strangers and 66% was committed by intimates, other relatives, or friends or acquaintances (Rennison, 2001).

5. In 1999, 32.1% of female homicide victims were killed by intimates (in the cases in which the victim-offender relationship was known) compared with 3.6% of male homicide victims (Fox & Zawitz, 2001a).

6. Lesbian resource lists are available from both the Wisconsin Coalition Against Domestic Violence (phone: 608-255-0539) and the Wisconsin Domestic Violence Training Project (phone: 608-262-3635).

References

A list of references is available in the original source.

WORKSHEET — CHAPTER 6
Intimate Partner Violence and Health

1. Societal Responsibility for Violence Against Women

   a. How do boys and men get the message that "it's ok," "it's socially acceptable" for men to be violent towards women? Give examples of ways in which boys and men are given this message. (Use examples from advertising, t.v., literature, movies, etc.)

   b. For one day in your own life, keep track of all the situations (t.v. shows, video games, cartoons, jokes, lectures, friends, language, etc.) in which violence is allowed or even encouraged.

   c. Identify ways that gender-role socialization may play a part in violence against women.

   d. Building on the articles "Battered Women of Color in Public Health Care Systems: Racism, Sexism, and Violence" and "Ruling the Exceptions: Same Sex Battering and Domestic Violence Theory," identify how sexism intersects with another form of oppression to explain "who has the opportunity to abuse" in this society.

2. **Many forms of violence against women:** Sexual harassment at school or work, pornography, child sexual abuse, date rape, sexual assault, battering, and elder abuse are all ways in which violence against women gets expressed. Choose any two of these forms of violence. Show ways in which those two forms of violence are similar, what they reflect about attitudes towards women, how they limit women's roles in society, and why they are mental and physical health issues.

3. **Continuum of family violence:** The continuum of family violence (p. 258) would look different for different women because what most hurts us is different for each of us and many hurtful actions are not listed on the continuum. Work with friends, especially survivors, to design continuums that better reflect your feelings and experiences. Be sure to add other ways abusers can control their partners, such as stalking, spreading rumors, using friends, threatening to "out" a same-sex partner, hurting a pet, hurting a child or parent, or threatening to be unfaithful.

4. Identify ways dating violence for college women is the same as and different from domestic violence for adult women. What resources are there for young women in abusive dating relationships on your campus and in your community? Who would you ask for help if a partner was controlling you?

5. Identify ways in which domestic violence in lesbian relationships is the same as and different from heterosexual domestic violence. (Think about what would be the same and different in a lesbian power and control wheel compared to the power and control wheel on page 259.)

6. Identify some of the barriers the following women might face in trying to safely end violence in their lives:

a poor woman _____

an undocumented woman from another country _____

a woman who is very ill _____

a woman whose abuser is ill _____

a very rich woman _____

a doctor's wife _____

a minister's wife _____

a woman who is a minister _____

a Latina woman _____

a woman with serious disabilitites _____

an alcoholic _____

a 40 year old trying to get pregnant _____

7. **Health workers response to violence:** This chapter addresses the importance of health workers' response to domestic violence. Health practitioners *should* now routinely screen for domestic violence. Describe whether or not you have been screened by a health practitioner for intimate partner violence. Describe what actually happened and whether it felt appropriate to you. If you have not been screened, describe how it should have been done.

8. **Institutional response to domestic violence:** The Medical Power and Control and Medical Advocacy/ Empowerment Wheels (p. 268) were designed to help health workers identify whether their responses were hurtful/controlling or helpful. Create similar "unhelpful" vs. "helpful" wheels for another system's response to domestic violence. For example, what would the "wheels" look like for dentists, house fellows, social workers, landlords, teachers, clergy, or police?

9. **Institutional power and control:** The power and control wheel (p. 259) was designed by battered women to describe the many ways their individual abusers controlled them. Create an institutional power and control wheel to describe how institutional oppressions work to control people. Sexism as power and control would include men getting paid more than women, men using male privilege, women having major responsibilities for contraception and children, women's issues not being taken seriously. What would racism as power and control, homophobia as power and control, or ageism as power and control, include?

CHAPTER 7
Alcohol and Tobacco Issues

Both women and men smoke cigarettes and use alcohol, so it might be easy for someone to think that alcohol and cigarettes are gender-neutral issues. Nothing could be further from the truth. In fact, issues related to cigarettes and alcohol consumption or addiction are sufficiently different for women and men that these topics serve as good "teaching tools" to help students learn why a gender analysis is essential for almost all health issues and how to develop a gender analysis.

To develop a gender analysis of tobacco and alcohol issues, we would want to ask questions about the widest range of ways that physiological sex differences, acceptable social roles for women and men, and institutional responses to women and men might influence cigarette and alcohol use, misuse, and consequences. Here are some of the questions we might want to explore: How do sex-role stereotypes impact on women's and men's use or non-use of cigarettes and alcohol? How does the physiology of women's and men's bodies affect how tobacco and alcohol are used and metabolized and what are the consequences? How do hormonal changes associated with contraception, pregnancy, lactation, and menopause affect tobacco and alcohol metabolism and consequences? How do social/cultural roles make cigarette and alcohol use or addiction different issues for women and men? How do issues of pregnancy, breast-feeding and women-as-caregivers affect the issues of substance use, dangers of use, and stigma of use? What are health practitioners' attitudes towards women's and men's use and abuse of tobacco and alcohol? Is the health system equally effective at diagnosing and helping women and men addicted to tobacco or alcohol?

Articles in this chapter provide some answers to these questions and address some unique issues for college students. Readers are also referred to the excellent chapters on tobacco and alcohol in the Boston Women's Health Book Collective's *Our Bodies, Ourselves for the New Century* (Simon and Schuster, 1998) and Jean Kilbourne's *Can't Buy My Love: How Advertising Changes the Way We Think and Feel* (Simon and Schuster, 1999).

Lorraine Greave's thought-provoking work on theories of women's smoking demonstrates how societies benefit from women's smoking:

> When smoking reduces or erases women's demands, emotions, or challenges, women can be seen as compliant and less troublesome. The true scope of women's feelings, particularly anger, remains invisible. Women smokers describe "sucking back anger" with each drag on a cigarette. If women smokers continue to internalize the tensions of interpersonal and societal relations, the responsibility of others in their lives to deal with legitimate emotions is lifted . . . Women smokers are using a socially acceptable (among some cultures) form of self-medication. Unlike alcohol and most other drugs, tobacco does not render a woman incapable of carrying out her more traditional nurturing and caretaking social roles. In fact, as we have seen, it often helps women carry out numerous social roles that are unequal and unsatisfying.

After summarizing that "worldwide cross-cultural studies reveal that depression and anxiety disorders are two to three times more common in women than in men," Jean Kilbourne goes on to connect cigarette use and addiction to women's negative emotions:

> Women are also more likely than men to use cigarettes, food, alcohol, and other drugs to deal with stress and depression and negative feelings, such as anxiety, nervousness, and especially anger. Depressed women are also more likely than depressed men to eat, smoke, and blame themselves, whereas men are more likely to become aggressive, to isolate, or to engage in sexual behavior . . . Some studies indicate that women experience greater anxiety than men when they attempt to quit and seem to have a higher rate of relapse. Although this could be at least partially due to weight gain or premenstrual stress, several researchers, including myself, believe that it is women's use of cigarettes to cope with negative feelings, especially anger, that makes it easier for women both to start smoking and to relapse in situations involving negative emotions, such as anger and stress, whereas men relapse more in positive situations such as social events. (*Can't Buy My Love*, p. 190.)

Robert Weissman's "Women and Tobacco" article describes why the phenomenon of cigarettes being "the single most important preventable cause of death and disease in society" has particular dire consequences for women as "lung cancer kills 50% more women than does breast cancer" and cigarettes are linked to everything from cervical cancer, infertility, osteoporosis, and heart disease to wrinkles and premature graying. Greaves argues that women's alcohol use is much less socially acceptable than smoking because it interferes with women's roles as mothers. However, it is tragic to read how little alcohol treatment programs have catered to the unique needs of women, especially their roles as mothers and people socialized to take care of others' needs before their own. "Alcoholics Invisible: The Ordeal of the Female Alcoholic" is Marian Sandmaier's classic 1980 article that first identified the many ways the health system had failed to deal appropriately with women's problems with alcohol. Over the years, with different editions of this book, we have tried to contrast the 1980 Sandmaier article with a newer article showcasing a model alcohol treatment program designed to empower women and recognize their unique needs. It becomes obvious that good alcohol treatment programs for women come and go, funding for such programs is too rarely stable, and it is very hit and miss whether such a program will be available to a woman if she needs it, especially if she is poor or has children. Nearly 25 years after Sandmaier's article, women-centered programs remain the exception to the male "norm" of alcohol treatment. The authors of an article, "Special Needs of Pregnant and Parenting Women in Recovery: A Move Toward a More Women-Centered Approach" conclude: "Changing the mindset from one that colludes with the larger culture's sometimes subtle critique of women's relational orientation to one that recognizes these tendencies as strengths to be built upon in treatment was (and is) not an easy task." (Sue Creamer and Claire McMurtrie, *Women's Health Issues,* Volume 8, number 4, 1998, pp. 239–245.)

Alcohol consumption has different consequences for women and men and this may be especially serious for young women:

Adolescent females are significantly more at risk for becoming dependent on alcohol than are women in any other age group . . . Young women are drinking more heavily than ever before and are suffering terrible consequences. Females have less gastric alcohol dehydrogenase, an enzyme that digests alcohol in the stomach, than males do, so alcohol passes more quickly into the bloodstream. Thus females tend to get drunk faster, become addicted more quickly, and develop diseases related to alcohol abuse sooner than males. In addition to sharing the risks of early death with men, young women who drink heavily are more likely than their non-drinking counterparts to be the victims of rape and sexual assault and to have unwanted pregnancies. Those who become alcoholic are far more stigmatized than their male counterparts. (Kilbourne, *Can't Buy My Love,* pp. 167–168.)

Aaron Brower's inspiring article, "Are College Students Alcoholics?" stimulates us to think about responding to alcohol consumption in new ways. The article addresses unique challenges of binge drinking on college campuses, stressing that, "Instead of focusing on the drinking behaviors of individual students, we have focused on the problems for the campus and community . . . Alcoholism is best addressed through individualized treatments that emphasize abstinence. College binge drinking is best addressed through several types of initiatives that stress shifting the role that alcohol plays in the college environment." Ironically, while the "special issues" for college students and a unique problem in how women often use alcohol—i.e., pressure to drink with a group of friends vs. drinking alone to drown one's sorrow about personal/relationship issues—appear to be worlds apart, looking for a *collective* answer instead of individualistic approaches certainly seems worth trying. What would be a collective, social-change approach to help women find healthier, safer coping mechanisms for stress-reduction and to address alcohol abuse in more women-centered ways?

Charlotte Davis Kasl, a psychologist and former member of 12-step programs, contributes to this discussion by examining programs modeled after Alcoholics Anonymous, which was originally designed for and by men. In her 1990 article, "The Twelve Step Controversy," Kasl proposed a 12-step model built on the reality of women's lives, which would be more useful to women trying to heal and move from "recovery to discovery." The good news is that this article and others like it have influenced 12-step programs in some communities to be much more appropriate to women's needs.

Despite the fact that tobacco and alcohol consumption harms women and cuts their lives short at speeds which exceed the harm done to men using an equivalent amount of these products, women are most likely to receive information on the dangers when they are pregnant. In fact, Lorraine Greaves says that pregnancy is really the only time when society worries very much about women's smoking: "Indeed, as long as it (smoking) does not interfere with childbearing, childrearing and the maintenance of heterosexuality, women's smoking can be regarded as useful by advocates of the status quo to both the woman and her society." Much information given to pregnant women is very victim-blaming and the protection of the fetus is often presented as more important than the health of the woman herself. Compare the messages women receive about smoking or drinking during pregnancy to *any* information you can find for men about their social roles in creating a healthy safe environment for their pregnant partner or how their reproductive physiology might be impacted by substance use.

Some of the most blatant victim blaming happens in relation to fetal alcohol syndrome, yet the social, economic, and political causes and consequences are practically never addressed. The devastation of fetal alcohol syndrome (FAS) in Native American communities is analyzed by Charon Asetoyer, a Native American health activist and educator, in "Fetal Alcohol Syndrome: A Nation in Distress." She emphasizes the need to end victim blaming approaches and repressive measures (such as forced sterilization) and calls for leadership to examine and correct the underlying societal and economic factors that lead to alcohol abuse among Native Americans. A follow-up letter to Asetoyer's article by Ruth Hubbard, "Fetal Alcohol Syndrome Class Related," adds research data to support the importance of the role of economic and social factors in FAS.

What Is a Theory of Women's Smoking? and How Do Societies Benefit?

by Lorraine Greaves

The analysis expressed in the first part of this chapter forms a useful starting point from which to develop a more thorough explanation of women's smoking:

> Smoking may be an important means through which women control and adapt to both internal and external realities. It mediates between the world of emotions and outside circumstances. It is both a means of reacting to and/or acting upon social reality, and a significant route to self-definition.

This view reflects the words of the women in this book. A consciousness and self-analysis is revealed by the women smokers, showing awareness of the discrepancies between emotional states and cultural and social expectations. Smoking mediates between these two fields. Women smokers use cigarettes to assist with their taking responsibility for social relationships and the maintenance of emotional equilibrium in their social groups.

Each cigarette serves as a temporary answer to these women's search for meaning. But as each one is stubbed out, the limitations of the answer it provided likely becomes clear. Not only do unpleasant aspects of life reenter consciousness, but the guilt. contradiction and tension associated with smoking also re-emerge.

Smoking a pack of cigarettes per day may offer repeated "meditations." It protects against full engagement with reality, allowing those realities to continue unabated. This is how smoking benefits the social order surrounding women. Not simply a lucrative and desirable aspect of commerce, fashion or femininity, smoking is also a way of perpetuating unsatisfying and unequal social relations.

The question remains whether women's smoking is a passive or active response to the world. Women can be either "passive victims" of or "active resisters" to patriarchal domination or possibly both, depending on their cultural or subcultural milieu. In some instances, women are victims and are limited to reacting. Other times, we have the energy and opportunity to be proactive in defining the self and negotiating social life. Depending on time, place and personal circumstance, women can use smoking to absorb inequality or resist it.

It is facile to assume that all women are victims. Seen this way, women smokers would be understood to be either completely duped by the culture or driven to smoke as a direct result of their treatment in the world. Neither of these is true. But it is equally facile to assume that a clear sense of self can be forged in a world that largely excludes the female experience in defining female identity. Smoking seems to assist in the assertion of the self in such circumstances.

Women across the social spectrum experience the failure of the ideal, but specific experiences such as abuse help expose the range of ways in which smoking can serve women. These interviews suggest that cigarettes are shock absorbers for abused women; smoking mediates between reality and ideal and eases the rawness of women's pain and life. Not surprisingly, suppressing negative emotions and using cigarettes as comfort were both more common in the testimony of abused women smokers. Many abused women know that directly expressing emotions could be perceived as aggressive and, as such, could potentially further endanger them.

The feminist smokers interviewed consciously analyze their reality. Their conflict centres on the discrepancy between their experience (as feminists and smokers) and their own and others' definitions of feminists and smokers. Is smoking liberating or did they just buy the advertising line? Is their continuing to smoke evidence of disempowerment? Is there a way to analyze this that fits with a feminist critique of the world? Tensions surround the personal and the political are the source of self-punishment and guilt. The politics of empowerment clash with the fact that these women are being controlled to varying degrees by their need to smoke. But throughout, smoking is useful in negotiating life circumstances.

How *Do* Societies Benefit?

In industrial countries when women use smoking to mediate existence, whether taking the edge off their emotional reactions, giving themselves space and time away from pressures or even staying thin and looking sophisticated, there is often a tangible benefit to others in their society.

Culturally and economically, women's smoking is approved of (in some cultures) in advertising, movies and fashion and as a weight control method. Women's image, size and superficial beauty is treated as a commodity. Generally, when a fashion magazine shows a thin model with a cigarette or a film shows an independent woman defiantly smoking, smoking is seen as positive in the industrial world. Several industries, including the tobacco industry, will benefit directly. Naomi Wolf describes the Western patriarchal definitions of women's beauty and the lucrative industries and practices that support these definitions. She argues that women who smoke to control their weight are actually reflecting the logic of the (North American) culture where women's external body image is valued far more than their internal health. She says women should not be blamed for making the decision to smoke as there is no real social or economic reward for choosing otherwise, nor is there any particular reward for women who live longer (1990, 229–30).

When smoking reduces or erases women's demands, emotions or challenges, women can be seen as compliant and less troublesome. The true scope of women's feelings, particularly anger, remains invisible. Women smokers describe "sucking back anger" with each drag on a cigarette. If women smokers continue to internalize the tensions of interpersonal and social relations, the responsibility of others in their lives to deal with legitimate emotions is lifted.

Some women describe quit attempts that appear to be sabotaged by partners or family members. Sometimes cigarettes will be presented to a woman struggling to quit simply because she is being too irritable or difficult. In fact, this pattern indicates the strength and impact of emotions concealed by smoking.

When women depend on cigarettes instead of a partner or friend in cultures which approve of women's smoking, the pressure and collective responsibility to offer comfort and care is often relieved. The intensity of feelings toward cigarettes as friends and the grief connected to giving them up is a key indicator of some women's security needs that go unfulfilled by others.

Both individual and collective responsibility for providing comfort and consistency to women may be abrogated. Recognizing and countering this situation is critical to effective and ethical cessation programming for women. If women are being asked to give up smoking, what can be offered to replace it?

Women smokers are using a socially acceptable (among some cultures) form of self-medication. Unlike alcohol and most other drugs, tobacco does not render a woman incapable of carrying out her more traditional nurturing and caretaking social roles. In fact, as we have seen, it often helps women carry out numerous social roles that are unequal and unsatisfying.

The women in this study generally have few legitimate avenues for expression of negative emotion and angst. While smoking is profoundly self-destructive for a woman, it does not undermine the patriarchal family. Indeed, as long as it does not interfere with child bearing, childrearing and the maintenance of heterosexuality, women's smoking can be regarded as useful by advocates of the status quo to both the woman and her society.

On the other hand, women who get drunk or stoned are unable to care for children or continue working. This is one explanation why women's use of alcohol and drugs is much less acceptable from a Western societal point of view, despite the fact that alcohol consumption and drug use cause much less death and disease than does smoking. Several of the women interviewed, especially the First Nations women, were particularly clear about this. Smoking is most similar to the use of legal drugs—the traditionally overprescribed tranquilizers and sedatives—which have also been used in the service of pacifying women. In this sense, tobacco is a preferred drug, a socially acceptable form of medication.

There are rare exceptions to this. Pregnant women who smoke are the subject of a great deal of attention regarding women and smoking. Indeed, for many years in industrial countries the only form of attention paid to women smokers focused on smoking in pregnancy. Even now, there is an overemphasis on pregnant smokers. Not discounting the serious health problems created by smoking during pregnancy, the best intervention would be respectfully focused on women, not the fetus, long before and long after pregnancy.

A related, more recent concern among anti-smoking activists is the effect of women's smoking on children they are looking after. The issue of children being exposed to smoke, while very important, arouses passions in anti-smoking activists far in excess of the concern invested in women's health. In many instances involving children, societal reaction and attention from the international tobacco control movement has been, and continues to be, swift, sexist and woman-blaming (see Jacobson 1986, 124–26). There is a widespread and strong motivation to intervene in these circumstances.

How can we specify the benefits of women's smoking to a society? The cultural meaning of women's smoking changes rapidly over time and from place to place. These shifts often affect the development of women's identity and pressure it to fit with new prevailing values and political realities. Over time, this has led to many social meanings being applied to women's smoking. Cultural meanings have demarcated occupations and class groups and evoked images, qualities and aspirations. In contemporary industrialized societies, smoking serves as a socially useful and legal method of self-medication for some women. In Third World countries, or countries where women's smoking rates are low

it may still be a mark of resistance, the emblem of the "bad girl." In either case, smoking is a form of social control.

What would industrial societies do if women did not suppress emotions through smoking? What would happen if women refused to overwork instead of coping through smoking? What would happen if women took control and stopped adapting? Even anti-tobacco activists in the West fail to consider these questions! Could it be that women's health is so undervalued that the benefits to industrial societies of women's smoking will likely be perpetuated and the negative effects of smoking on women will not arouse a great deal of effective concern?

For references, see original.

Women and Tobacco

by Robert Weissman

Phillip Morris is now conducting a $100 million advertising campaign to refurbish its image. Central to its television advertising strategy are spots that highlight the company's contributions to battered women's shelters.

Is Phillip Morris a friend of women?

Consider this fact: Between 1960 and 1990, the death rate from lung cancer among American women increased by more than 400 percent, and the rate is continuing to increase, according to the Centers for Disease Control (CDC). Eighty percent of lung cancer deaths are due to smoking.

Lung cancer kills 50 percent more women than does breast cancer. The American Cancer Society estimates 67,000 women died from lung cancer in 1998, while 43,500 women died from breast cancer. Lung cancer surpassed breast cancer as the number one cause of cancer deaths among women in 1987.

All told, more than 152,000 American women died from smoking-related disease in 1994.

Overall, reports the Centers for Disease Control, "tobacco use is responsible for approximately one of every five deaths in the United States and is the single most important preventable cause of death and disease in our society."

Although smoking rates among American women historically fell far below those for men, the gap has dramatically narrowed. Increased smoking prevalence among women and girls tracks closely with tobacco industry advertising and marketing campaigns.

Well-produced ads to the contrary notwithstanding, Philip Morris, R. J. Reynolds, Brown & Williamson and friends should be labeled among women's worst public health enemies.

Women, Tobacco and Health

Smoking is linked not just to lung cancer, but a stunningly long list of diseases. It contributes to: bladder, cervical, esophageal, kidney, laryngeal, oral and pancreatic cancers, arteriosclerosis, cardiomyopathy, circulatory problems, emphysema, hearing loss, heart attacks, hypertension, osteoporosis, stroke and ulcers, among other health problems. It also contributes to wrinkles, premature graying, and halitosis.

Cigarette smoking doubles the risk of coronary heart disease among women. Smoking is associated with reduced fertility—with one study showing women smokers 3.4 times more likely to take longer than a year to conceive than nonsmokers—and early menopause.

Smoking during pregnancy poses serious risks to mothers, developing fetuses and newborn. These risks include pregnancy complications, premature birth, low-birthweight infants, stillbirth and infant mortality. Cigarette smoking during pregnancy accounts for 17–26 percent of low-birthweight babies.

Second-hand smoke is also a major cause of death and disease, estimated by University of California San Francisco Professor Stan Glantz to cause more than 50,000 deaths a year, placing it only behind active smoking and alcohol use as the third leading cause of preventable death in the United States.

Women bear a special risk for exposure to second-hand smoke: exposures to second-hand smoke can be as much as five times worse in restaurants and bars as other workplaces, reports Boston University Professor Michael Siegel. And, as the Center for Tobacco-Free Kids points out, women make up 80 percent of wait staff.

Mothers who smoke, along with fathers, expose their children, from birth throughout childhood, to serious health risks.

The Surgeon General reports that intrauterine exposure and exposure to second-hand smoke after pregnancy increases the risk of Sudden Infant Death Syndrome (SIDS) in infants. One study found that 6,200 children in the United States die each year from lung infections, low-birth weight, SIDS and burns caused by parents' smoking.

The odds of developing asthma are twice as high among children whose mothers smoke at least 10 cigarettes a day. Between 400,000 and 1 million children in the United States have asthmatic conditions worsened by exposure to second-hand smoke. Parental smoking, especially by mothers, who tend to spend more time with children, each year contributes to 150,000 to 300,000 cases of lower respiratory tract infections (such as pneumonia and bronchitis) in infants and children under 18 months.

Finally, parents who smoke greatly increase the chance that their children, especially their daughters, will smoke. One study found that white girls whose families smoked were more than three times as likely to try cigarettes than white girls from non-smoking families.

Women's Smoking: Still Too Prevalent

Approximately 22 percent of all American women—22 million women in total—smoke. Smoking rates are highest among young women, according to the CDC. Approximately one in four women aged 18–24 (24.5 percent) and 24–44 (25.6 percent) smoke. Smoking rates decline as women get older—22.5 percent of women aged 45–64 smoke, and only 11.2 percent of those 65 or older.

Smoking rates among teenage girls have jumped significantly in the 1990s. Smoking rates among high school girls—measured as having smoked in the last 30 days—zoomed from 27 percent to 34.7 percent from 1991 to 1997.

Smoking rates among American women vary significantly by race, to a considerable extent reflecting differing cultural attitudes toward smoking and women smoking. The smoking rate among non-Hispanic white women was 23.6 percent in 1998, 21.3 percent among non-Hispanic African-American women, 13.3 percent among Hispanic women, 38.1 percent among American Indian/Alaska Native women, and 9.9 percent among Asian/Pacific Islander women.

With rising health consciousness among higher income and better educated people, smoking rates are now significantly correlated with income and education. Among women living below the poverty level, 29.3 percent smoke—only 21.3 percent of those above the poverty line are smokers. Among women with 9–11 years of education, 34.3 percent smoke—more than three times the rate (11.2 percent) for those with 16 or more years of education.

Targeting Women

When he sought to regulate tobacco in 1995, Food and Drug Administration Commissioner David Kessler declared nicotine addiction a "pediatric disease." It is that, but it is much more.

Would Health Organization Director General Gro Harlem Brundtland may have gone more to the core of the issue in labeling tobacco consumption a "communicable disease." The vector of transmission is not mosquitoes or bacteria, but the multinational tobacco companies.

Big Tobacco's marketing, advertising and promotional efforts are perhaps the most sophisticated of any industry. And a considerable portion of the industry's investment in promotion—tabulated by the Federal Trade Commission as totaling $6.73 billion in the United States in 1998—is targeted at women. This includes heavy investments in magazine advertising, especially women's magazines, direct marketing and promotion, new innovations like Camel Nights at nightclubs and bars, and internet advertising.

The industry practice of luring women into smoking goes back to early in the twentieth century. Edward Bernays, one of the pioneers of the advertising industry, persuaded women's rights marchers in New York City to hold up Lucky Strikes as "torches of freedom."

The association of smoking with women's liberation—an ironic linkage, since the means of "liberation" is enslavement to a fatally addictive product—helped spur smoking among women, especially urban and better-educated women. The industry has never abandoned this theme.

In the late 1960s, Philip Morris began its Virginia Slims "You've Come a Long Way, Baby" advertising blitz. Smoking rates for teenage girls rose from 8.4 percent in 1968 to 15.3 percent in 1974, by which time other companies had begun hawking cigarettes to girls (with products like Silva Thins and Eve). The marketing campaigns were particularly effective with girls. Between 1967 and 1973, smoking initiation rates for 12-year-old girls increased by approximately 110 percent, by 55 percent for 13-year-olds, 70 percent for 14-year-olds, 75 percent for 15-year-olds, 55 percent for 16-year-olds and 35 percent for 17-year-olds.

Liberation, freedom, sophistication and slimness remain the top themes of the tobacco merchants. Women in tobacco ads are uniformly thin, and the industry plays on and exacerbates prevailing cultural obsessions with women's weight. This is an especially effective strategy with girls and young women.

Virginia Slims remains the trendsetter for cigarette brands targeting women. "You've Come a Long Way, Baby" was followed by "It's a Woman Thing," and recently by the "Find Your Voice" campaign. Philip Morris abandoned the "Find Your Voice" campaign, which featured attractive women from around the world, after Philip Morris' CEO was questioned about it in the Engle litigation—the Florida case which led to a $154 billion punitive damages verdict against the tobacco industry.

But Philip Morris hasn't given up. Virginia Slims recently launched a "See Yourself as a King" campaign, which women's health and tobacco control groups have roundly denounced.

"Philip Morris, the world's largest tobacco company, insults and degrades women with its new magazine ad for Virginia Slims cigarettes," says a statement issued by more than a dozen organizations including the Boston Women's Health Book Collective, the American Medical Women's Association, the American Lung Association and the Campaign for Tobacco-Free Kids.

"The company, in an expensive and lavish presentation, uses the metaphor of an ancient Egyptian female pharaoh to encourage women to 'See Yourself as a King' by smoking Virginia Slims," the statement explains. "By once again suggesting that women are empowered by smoking, Philip Morris shows contempt for women's health issues. The Virginia Slims ads are the most recent evidence that Philip Morris' attempts to portray itself as a socially responsible company are a sham."

Internationally, the scale of the problem is mind boggling. Tobacco-related disease kills 4 million a year worldwide, a number projected by the World Health Organization to rise to 10 million by 2030, with 70 percent of those deaths occurring in developing countries. In most developing countries, smoking rates among men are much higher than women. The unique contribution of the tobacco multinationals—led by Philip Morris, British American Tobacco and Japan Tobacco (which now owns R. J. Reynolds' international operations)—is to hook women on smoking through slick advertisements and promotions. In the year after South Korea opened its market to foreign cigarettes, for example, smoking rates among girls nearly quintupled, rising from under 2 percent to nearly 9 percent.

Addiction, Dependence, Kicking the Habit

There is overwhelming evidence that tobacco advertising and marketing has a major effect on smoking initiation rates. The industry strategy is focused on finding new smokers, because it is so hard to quit once a person begins smoking. (The tobacco companies also need new smokers to replace those they kill and the not insubstantial number who manage to overcome nicotine dependence and kick the habit.)

Unfortunately, quitting smoking is even harder for women than men, though it is hard for everyone. Although many young people start smoking with the expectation they can and will quit, nearly three quarters of adolescent smokers who intend not to be smoking 5–6 years after starting are in fact still smoking five years after starting, according to the CDC. Girls and women aged 12–24 are even more likely to report being unable to cut down on smoking than boys and men of the same age.

In CDC surveys, 73 percent of women smokers say they want to quit smoking, nearly 80 percent report symptoms of addiction and three quarters say they are dependent on cigarettes. Only 2.5 percent of all smokers quit each year.

The good news in this story is that, although smoking is very hard to stop, cessation programs for those who want to quit significantly improve quit rates.

Even more important, large-scale social interventions can have a dramatic effect on both smoking rates and on the number of cigarettes smokers consume. In recent years, states such as California, Massachusetts and Florida have shown dramatic results from comprehensive tobacco control plans featuring a mix of community-based programs, smoke free ordinances, cigarette price increases and television counteradvertising—with an emphasis on ads that demonize Big Tobacco and portray industry executives as deceitful and manipulative.

Alcoholics Invisible
The Ordeal of the Female Alcoholic
by Marian Sandmaier

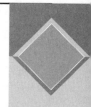

Even under the best of circumstances, the ability to turn away from a drug to which one is physically and psychologically addicted requires uncommon courage and determination. But most of the women whom I interviewed recovered from alcoholism in the face of an appalling lack of support from the doctors, therapists, alcoholism personnel, and others charged with diagnosing and treating their illness. With a few notable exceptions, these women were discouraged by the health system from embarking on alcoholism treatment to begin with, and once involved in treatment, were denied supports and services important to their recovery. They discovered what most alcoholic women who seek help are forced to recognize: that contemptuous attitudes and sheer ignorance about women with alcohol problems pervade the health system as thoroughly and destructively as any other segment of society. There, as anywhere, the real needs and the very humanity of alcoholic women remain invisible.

Within the health system, the first person an alcoholic woman is likely to encounter is her own doctor. And at first glance, he* would seem to be in an excellent position to identify her alcohol problem and steer her toward appropriate treatment.

Diagnosis

Yet physicians appear highly unlikely to diagnose alcoholism in their female patients. In a 1975 survey of 89 women in Alcoholics Anonymous, fully half of the women surveyed said they had tried to discuss their drinking problem with someone who told them they couldn't possibly be alcoholic; twelve received such advice from physicians, five of these psychiatrists.[1] Of the 50 women I interviewed, 45 had been seen by doctors while they were drinking alcoholically, but only seven were ever confronted by their physicians about their alcohol abuse. A 54-year-old Boston woman recalled: "In all of the times I landed in the hospital during my drinking years, no doctor ever said anything to me about alcoholism. I always either had colitis or a kidney problem or pneumonia, and when they couldn't think of anything else, I would have nerves. Twice I attempted suicide and once wound up in a hospital afterward for three months. And in those three months, I saw a psychiatrist every day and not once did he say a word to me about being alcoholic. And at that point I had been drinking almost around the clock."

Some physicians fail to respond to even clear-cut evidence of alcohol problems in their women patients. "I used to carry a big purse full of beer into my psychiatrist's office and drink right through the sessions," recalled a young social scientist from Virginia. "He never said a word to me about it. As I look back, I think I was probably challenging him to say something, to do something, to help me. But he never dealt with it." A Detroit homemaker who had a drinking problem while still in college encountered the same kind of reaction from her therapist at a university health service. "There were times when my husband called my psychiatrist in the middle of the night because I'd be so out of control and drunk and hysterical. . . . But when I would come in for my next session . . . the drinking would never get mentioned as a problem in itself."

Probably the primary reason for many doctors' failure to confront alcohol problems in their patients is, perhaps surprisingly, sheer ignorance of alcoholism itself. Although alcohol abuse affects at least 10 million persons in the United States and is considered the third largest health problem in the country, it is one of the most neglected areas of study in medical schools. Although this situation is slowly being corrected, few medical schools even today offer more than one course on

From *Social Policy.* Jan/Feb 1980, pp. 25–30. Reprinted with permission of the author from *The Invisible Alcoholics,* McGraw Hill, New York.

*I use the pronoun "he" deliberately because the medical profession is still overwhelmingly masculine; at present only 12 percent of physicians are women.

the subject, and many limit their coverage to a single lecture. This gap in education is largely due to alcoholism's heritage as a moral problem rather than a medical one, despite its obvious physical and emotional consequences. In a 1972 nationwide survey of 13,000 physicians who treat alcoholism, 70 percent declared alcoholics to be difficult and uncooperative patients, while a sizable minority believed alcoholism indicated a "lack of will or morality."[2]

Further, as the research of Phyllis Chesler and others has demonstrated, doctors as a group hold notably stereotypical attitudes about appropriate behavior for women.[3] Consequently, many physicians who believe that alcoholism is a sign of moral laxity may well also subscribe to the double standard rendering alcoholism—i.e., immorality—more shameful in a woman than a man, and thus more discomfiting to discuss with a female patient. Indeed, a study of the attitudes of 161 physicians toward their alcoholic clients revealed that a substantial number of doctors believed that, compared to the alcoholic man, the alcoholic woman "had loose sexual morals, had more psychosexual conflict such as homosexuality, and was more likely to get into social difficulties."[4]

But if a doctor is unable or unwilling to diagnose a woman as alcoholic, he may give her condition another label instead. All too often, a physician notes the distraught state of his alcoholic female client, makes a primary diagnosis of "depression" or "anxiety," and proceeds to prescribe a pill to alter her mood, most commonly a tranquilizer, sedative, or antidepressant. Consequently, many alcoholic women walk out of their doctors' offices not only with their alcoholism undiagnosed but with a second powerful potentially addictive psychoactive drug in hand. A 50-year-old Maryland woman who abused both alcohol and a variety of pills described her introduction to mood-altering drugs: "I was incredibly jumpy from all the booze I was drinking, so my doctor put me on both Librium and Nembutal—one to calm me during the day and the other to get me to sleep at night. Then about a year later, he put me on Dexedrine to get me going in the morning, to counteract the effects of the pills—and the alcohol. He actually knew I was drinking, but he never seemed to see it as a major problem." A young Black woman from Washington, D.C. recalled her first visit with a psychiatrist during one of her worst periods of drinking. "I told this man I was depressed and exhausted all the time, but I also told him I thought my drinking might be getting a little out of hand. He told me to be cool about it and handed me a prescription for an antidepressant. In three months, I was going through a month's worth of that prescription every ten days."

Both their professional training and prevailing societal attitudes influence doctors and therapists to view women as inherently less stable emotionally than men by virtue of their female biology, and therefore more prone to psychological disturbances. Consequently, many doctors may be likely to misread a number of serious medical problems in women—including alcoholism—as merely "nerves," depression, or another emotional ailment. This image of women as "naturally" given to mental disorders is the content of much of the advertising by which the powerful American drug industry, at a cost of 1 billion dollars per year—approximately $5,000 per physician—tries to persuade doctors to prescribe mood-altering drugs to their patients.

Psychoactive drug use is not risk free for anyone, but it is especially dangerous for problem drinkers for several reasons. Perhaps the most obvious danger is that of mixing a mood-altering drug with alcohol. The combination of alcohol and certain psychoactive drugs produces a supra-addictive effect substantially more powerful than the effects of any of the drugs taken alone, and consequently increases the possibility of accidental death by an overdose. Access to both alcohol and psychoactive drugs also makes suicide attempts a relatively easy matter, a serious concern in view of the high rate of such attempts—many of them successful—among alcoholic women.

The other major danger of prescribing mood-altering drugs to an alcoholic is the possibility of cross-addiction, that is, dependence on both alcohol and one or more other drugs. Anyone who habitually uses psychoactive drugs may become addicted to them, but the alcoholic is a particularly high risk as she has already established an addictive drug use pattern with alcohol. Cross addiction sometimes keeps a woman drinking for a longer period of time, because she may be able to switch to Valium or another pill temporarily when the effects of alcohol become too staggering for her body to bear. And a woman addicted to both alcohol and pills is likely to face more difficulties in treatment, because she must withdraw and recover from the effects of two or more powerful drugs instead of alcohol alone.

Yet despite these multiple dangers, many physicians distribute these drugs to alcoholic women with an alarmingly free hand. According to Dr. LeClair Bissell, chief of the Smithers Alcoholism Center of New York City's Roosevelt Hospital, it is so easy for alcoholic women to get prescriptions for these drugs that, once addicted, many obtain their maintenance supply from several physicians simultaneously. "If a doctor is giving an alcoholic woman pills, don't imagine he is her only source. He is probably part of a long succession of people who are prescribing for her. For instance, the gynecologist is quite capable of writing prescriptions for Librium and Valium. The general practitioner, if there is one, will hear some of her problems and prescribe pills too. If there's been an emergency room visit afterward, that may result in yet another prescription for tranquilizers. Even the ophthalmologist taking care of the glasses can prescribe pills. The possibilities are endless."

Since physicians prescribe psychoactive drugs for women in the general population at almost twice the rate they prescribe them for men,[5] it is perhaps not surprising that alcoholic women are far more likely to be cross-addicted than alcoholic men. A 1977 nationwide survey of more than 15,000 Alcoholics Anonymous members showed that 29 percent of the women but only 15 percent of the men were addicted to other drugs besides alcohol. Of new AA members 30 years old or younger, a startling 55 percent of women were cross-addicted, compared to 36 percent of men.[6] Smaller surveys report similar findings: a study of residents in 36 alcoholism halfway houses in Minnesota, for example, found that nearly twice as many women as men were addicted to both alcohol and drugs.[7] Studies of individual treatment programs report similar female-male ratios for cross-addiction.[8]

Treatment

Not every physician, of course, acts as an obstacle to treatment. Some doctors are not only impressively knowledgeable about alcoholism, but will forthrightly confront any patient, regardless of sex, who shows symptoms of the illness. But even if an alcoholic woman is fortunate enough to come into contact with such a physician—and the odds are not good—he can provide no guarantee that she will ultimately receive caring and effective treatment. For once a woman acknowledges her alcohol problem and is ready to seek help, she is then faced with an alcoholism treatment system that, by and large, neither welcomes nor understands her.

The first challenge a woman may confront is simply finding an alcoholism program that has room for her. A 1976 study conducted by the Association of Halfway House Alcoholism Programs of North America reported that of a representative nationwide sample of 161 alcoholism halfway houses, 56 percent served men only, 35 percent were coed, and only nine percent were open only to women. Further, and perhaps more important, women occupied only 19 percent of all available beds in the 161 houses, because the "coed" units reserved only ten to 30 percent of their beds for women.[9] Another survey, conducted by the New York State Commission on Women and Alcoholism, found that in 45 inpatient alco-

holism facilities in the state, only 17 percent of all beds were allocated for women. Some surveyed centers refused to treat women at all, citing inadequate budgets and, in one case, the lack of space for a second bathroom.[10]

The scarcity of treatment space for women stems largely from the long-standing assumption by the health system that alcoholism is essentially a male illness. Prior to 1970, the year Congress passed legislation requiring alcoholism programs to offer services to women as a criterion for receiving federal funding, relatively few alcoholism programs admitted women on any basis. And even after the legislation was enacted, many programs added only a few token beds for women rather than providing space on a par with the actual numbers of alcoholic women in the population. It is not uncommon, even today, for a 30-bed treatment center to reserve only four or five beds for women clients.

Consequently, some women seeking help for alcoholism become names on waiting lists, or are forced to travel far out of their communities to find programs with room for them. Others, like the many women in our society who are considered troublesome and who lack other options, end up in mental institutions. Although they are resorted to less often now than in the past, psychiatric hospitals are still used as dumping grounds for some women with drinking problems. Dr. LeClair Bissell described the typical experience of an alcoholic woman consigned to a psychiatric ward: "First of all, it's usually not hard to get her in there because women have always been willing to self-define as mentally ill more readily than men, especially if the alternative is to be called an alcoholic. And as for her drinking, it plays right into the psychiatric approach that says, 'Find the underlying cause, get a lot of insight, pull up your socks, honey, and guess what? You won't be drinking like that anymore and you'll be having two drinks before dinner just like everybody else.' Never mind that she is physically addicted to alcohol."

The "treatment" of alcoholic women in mental wards is sometimes marked not only by ignorance but outright brutality. A Washington, D.C. businesswoman remembered: "My husband told me he was taking me to a hospital and I went willingly, no questions asked. I was diagnosed as alcoholic. My husband left and I was told to follow the man who was carrying my bags. And as we walked along I noticed that he was locking doors behind him and I said: 'What are you doing that for?' And he said, 'Don't you know where you are?' And I said, 'No' and he said, 'You're at a federal facility for the insane.'

"It turned out that the hospital had an alcoholism program for men but none for women, so if you were unfortunate enough to be taken there as an alcoholic woman, you got thrown in with the violently insane. I will never forget it. I was put in a ward where people were defecating in the corner and ladies were walking around nude. And the people working there were just brutal. Really brutal. Full of contempt. I was treated like an animal just like everyone else there. There were no doors on the johns. You had to take a shower with somebody watching you. The blanket on my bed smelled like urine. For the first three days I just shook— I was having junior grade DTs. I was withdrawing from alcohol for the first time in my life and they didn't give me any drugs or any other kind of help. I just lay on my cot and shook."

But even if a woman is able to avoid the route of the psychiatric ward and finds an alcoholism program that has room for her, adequate treatment is by no means guaranteed. For by and large, the alcoholism treatment system is still very much a man's world, with most recovery programs primarily used, staffed, and directed by men and designed to meet male needs. As Rita Zimmer, director of a New York Bowery area alcoholism program, summarized the situation: "Just because most facilities now admit some women doesn't mean that most of them make any attempt to develop programs that relate to women. It doesn't mean they really try to reach out to find alcoholic women in the community. It doesn't even mean they hire staff who have an interest in working with women or who have any knowledge of how to work with women." Consequently, many women find themselves in treatment programs which are neither prepared nor committed to meeting many of their fundamental psychological and practical needs.

Perhaps more than anything else, a woman beginning treatment for alcoholism needs to feel cared about and believed in. In most cases, she has weathered years—sometimes decades—of a brutalizing addiction that has left her overwhelmed with feelings of failure and hopelessness about the possibility of acceptance by others. Dr. Edith Gomberg, professor of psychology at the University of Michigan and a pioneering researcher on women and alcoholism, noted from her experience: ". . . in a deviance disorder like alcoholism, the attitude (conscious and unconscious) of the therapist toward women and toward alcoholism and the enthusiasm and interest of the therapist seem far more related to outcome than the technique used."[11] Given the importance of these factors, the attitudes of many treatment professionals toward alcoholic women are deeply disturbing. A survey of 161 physicians involved in alcoholism treatment revealed that they generally believed that "women have more basic personality disorders: they are more hostile, angry, unhappy, self-centered, withdrawn, depressed and more subject to mood swings; they are more

emotional, lonely, nervous; they have less insight, and are not as likable as men alcoholics."[12] Other surveys note similar negative views of women among treatment personnel, in particular the notions that alcoholic women are more emotionally unbalanced than alcoholic men, and by implication, more difficult to treat. Such attitudes are deeply destructive to recovering women because they are likely to become self-fulfilling prophecies.

As the theory that women are more psychologically maladjusted than men appears to be widespread among alcoholism-treatment personnel and can seriously undermine a woman's successful recovery, its origins need to be examined more closely. It is possible that on the average, an alcoholic woman may actually enter rehabilitation more emotionally impaired than an alcoholic man, due to the psychic strain of the particularly harsh stigma attached to female alcoholism. But it is also likely that the "sicker" label springs from deeply sexist notions about the psychology of women held by mental health professionals. In the study most clearly illustrating these attitudes, conducted in 1970 by Dr. Inge Broverman and Dr. Donald Broverman, a group of psychotherapists was asked to define, respectively, a mature healthy man, a mature healthy woman, and a mature healthy adult. The clinicians, who displayed a high level of consensus in their conclusions, described a healthy male and a healthy female in very different terms. Specifically, they characterized a healthy, mature woman as more submissive, less independent, less adventurous, less competitive, more excitable in minor crises, more easily hurt and more emotional than a mature, healthy man. Equally significant, their description of a healthy adult closely paralleled their characterization of a healthy man, and thereby differed radically from their assessment of a healthy woman.[13] This landmark study, along with others which have replicated its findings, indicates that the standard of mental health in our culture is a clearly masculine one, and conversely, that feminine behavior is basically inconsistent with society's concept of adult mental health.

Stereotypical views of women among alcoholism professionals not only earn many women the damaging labels of "sick" and "hard to treat" but almost inevitably shape the criteria used for women's recovery. If a "healthy" woman is considered relatively submissive, dependent, and noncompetitive, such behaviors are likely to be urged on alcoholic women as evidence of emotional maturity, while behaviors that fail to conform to conventional feminine norms are apt to be punished. When Ardelle Schultz first joined the staff of a drug-alcohol program near Philadelphia in the early 1970s, she found that the staff—until her arrival entirely male—was bent on such a "reeducation" program for women clients:

Women were being taught a new set of behaviors to please males. They were told to give up their sleazy bitch ways. . . . If a woman happened to be naturally sexy and sensuous, she was accused of seducing the men and chastised. If she was unfemininely aggressive and angry, she was told she was treacherous and that she was losing her sensitivity and humanity. If she was lesbian, she was accused of being a man-hater and "sick." In other words, she was learning, again, to repress a part of herself that belonged to her and to become an "honest paper doll" cut out in man's image.[14]

Pressure to conform to such narrowly sexist standards of behavior is seriously damaging to any woman, but it is apt to be particularly destructive to a woman who is alcoholic. The heavy load of guilt, self-hatred, and worthlessness that an alcoholic woman drags with her into treatment is inextricably linked to her failure to live up to a self-denying and impossible ideal of womanhood—the sexual innocent, the nurturing mother, the dutiful wife, the consummate "lady." To be assaulted in treatment with further accusations of her sins against femininity—whether blatantly or subtly conveyed—can only reinforce her already profound conviction of failure as a woman.

Indeed, therapy that imposes a stereotyped vision of femininity on recovering women may also intensify the very kinds of conflicts that triggered their abusive drinking in the first place. Recent research by Dr. Sharon Wilsnack and others indicates that many women who become alcoholic suffer painful sex-role conflicts, usually between a consciously desired "feminine" self-image and unconscious "masculine" strivings which they experience as unacceptable and acutely threatening to their identities. This research shows that drinking may stifle this conflict, allowing a woman to temporarily integrate the masculine and feminine sides of her personality, and that uncontrolled drinking may be activated by a crisis that forces her forbidden "unfeminine" feelings to the fore.

The Social Context

Insensitivity to the psychological needs of alcoholic women is often coupled with apparent indifference to some of their most urgent practical concerns. For example, the typical woman entering an alcoholism treatment program is in serious financial difficulty and badly needs job training. More often than not, she is divorced, has custody of her children, and is receiving little or no support money from her ex-husband. Her job skills are likely to be minimal and she probably has been unable

to work steadily for some time. A 1977 survey by the National Institute on Alcohol Abuse and Alcoholism revealed that of the some 60,000 women in federally funded treatment programs, approximately 30 percent were unemployed at the time of entering treatment, and only about seven percent held professional-level jobs. The mean household income of all the women surveyed was about $7,000.[15]

Yet, regardless of these stark financial realities, few alcoholism programs offer serious job training to recovering alcoholic women, either within the facilities themselves or through arrangements with outside agencies. The myth appears to linger among program staff that women don't really need jobs, that their own and their children's survival are never wholly or even primarily dependent on their own wage-earning abilities. This obliviousness to the economic realities of women's lives was underscored in a recent study of staff attitudes toward clients at a Newark, New Jersey, drug-alcohol program, in which researchers asked the 25 male and nine female staff members their perceptions of the major problems faced by their clients. Less than a quarter of the staff believed that lack of job training was a significant problem for women, although it was seen as a major need for male clients. But when the clients themselves were asked what they perceived as their most serious problems, an overwhelming 96 percent of the women named lack of job training. No other single problem was named by as many women.[16]

When job training is offered to women at all, it is usually for low-paying "women's work" such as typing and other clerical functions, while men in the same program are often trained for more lucrative, highly skilled occupations. Many alcoholism programs provide no job training opportunities whatever for women, instead assigning them the "occupational therapy" of household chores within the program residence, or brush-up courses on cooking, sewing, and home management. Although these skills may be useful and even necessary to some women, to offer them in lieu of hard-nosed job training almost ensures continuing financial hardship for many women once they leave a treatment program. Unable to find a job that pays enough to support themselves and possibly children as well, many find themselves on welfare shortly after completing treatment, or are forced to work two jobs simply in order to pay the bills. Clearly, it is not a way of life conducive to staying sober.

Child care is another service crucially needed by recovering women and almost never provided by alcoholism programs. As most recovery facilities are designed for and by men, this gap is not altogether surprising, since men who enter rehabilitation programs ordinarily leave their children in the care of their wives.

But women who begin alcoholism treatment have no such convenient caretakers. Even if a woman's husband is still living with her, which is unlikely, he is rarely able or willing to undertake primary care of the children while she gets help for her alcoholism. Foster care is generally a risky choice, since poor women in particular may be declared "unfit mothers" on the basis of their alcoholism and lose custody of their children, sometimes permanently. As for private day care and other kinds of child care services, New York City family alcoholism counselor Sheila Salcedo observed: "Day care centers are prohibitively expensive and have incredible waiting lists, and the homemaker services charge so much money that your average woman could never afford it. So if you have a lady in need of immediate detoxification and other treatment and she happens to have children, you're really in trouble."

Despite this clear and pressing need for child care services, to date only two alcoholism programs in the entire country offer in-house child care, and few others offer even minimal outside arrangements. Consequently, many women are literally prevented from getting any kind of alcoholism treatment because they can't find anyone to take care of their children. And if a woman tries to begin treatment without having made workable child care arrangements, her recovery is undermined from the start. Salcedo noted: "It is very difficult for most women to get the rest they need in treatment if the kids aren't in good hands. It's easy enough to say, 'OK, let's send the woman into rehab', but if she's got five kids at home, one of whom is on drugs and another who is failing school, and a husband who never really wanted her to go into treatment in the first place, nothing that happens in that treatment program is going to make any kind of impression on her. She gets phone calls from home, she worries, she feels guilty. What kind of treatment does that amount to?"

The realities of women's lives are such that they also may need more intensive follow-up than men after completing a formal program of treatment. In general, women are likely to both face greater pressures than men and receive less support from others once they return from a rehabilitation program to the "real world." Dr. LeClair Bissell observed: "There is much less support from the family of the alcoholic woman than the man. As soon as she returns from treatment she is expected to begin taking care of the children and cooking dinner for the husband and whatnot. And AA (Alcoholics Anonymous) sometimes rather blandly advocates '90 meetings in 90 days' at the beginning, which is fine in theory, but what about the woman who has a job and whose babysitter leaves every day at five o'clock? Or whose husband refuses to take care of the kids every night? How is she going to work the mechanics of that?"

The acute stress and isolation faced by many women following treatment can seriously threaten their sobriety. "You can't just treat a woman, show her how to stop drinking and then tell her to go out and do her own thing," said Clara Synical, founder and director of Interim House, a halfway house for alcoholic women in Philadelphia. "You have to go step by step, follow through, and keep in touch with her so she knows she has a home where she can get support at all times." Yet few alcoholism facilities provide any sustained follow-up services to clients once they complete treatment, in terms of either counseling or practical help in rebuilding their lives. Without such support, many women become quickly overwhelmed by the multiple pressures of their new situations and, sometimes within a few months or even weeks of completing treatment, turn back to the bottle for relief.

The disregard for women's concerns which marks many rehabilitation programs has sparked a small but vigorous movement within the alcoholism field to develop treatment programs specifically designed for women. These programs, which are often staffed and used entirely by women, are committed to providing alcoholic women with a strongly supportive, caring environment and to approaching their recovery needs in the context of women's total experience in society.

Yet, within the alcoholism field, support for women's programs has been grudging at best. Organizers of such programs have found funding hard to come by in a field that has yet to fully recognize the extent of female alcoholism, much less the inability of many traditional programs to meet women's needs. The National Institute on Alcohol Abuse and Alcoholism has funded only 29 women's programs in a total of some 500 treatment facilities, and although some of these federally supported programs are excellent, they clearly do not begin to meet the extent of women's needs. At present, many major metropolitan areas and even entire states are without a single women's program or even a coed program that has instituted special services for female clients.

Since alcoholism programs sensitive to women's concerns still comprise only a tiny percentage of existing programs, the vast majority of women continue to be treated in facilities that fail to meet many of their most pressing needs. Many women drop out of these programs before completing treatment. The reasons they cite are varied: lack of emotional support from staff, an inability to make suitable child care arrangements, diffuse feelings of alienation and isolation, sometimes simply an overwhelming sense that "it's not helping." Occasionally, women leave because of sexual harassment or abuse from male staff or residents. Of those who complete treatment, most studies show a significantly lower rate of recovery by alcoholic women than men, in some cases less than half the rate for men.[17] A good number of women who resume abusive drinking after leaving treatment become part of the "revolving door" syndrome, making their way in and out of treatment programs over and over again for years, endlessly searching for a way out of their addiction, and endlessly failing to find it.

Notes

1. Jane E. James, "Symptoms of Alcoholism in Women: A Preliminary Survey of A. A. Members," *Journal of Studies on Alcohol,* 36 (1975), p. 1567.

2. Robert W. Jones and Alice R Heinch, "Treatment of Alcoholism by Physicians in Private Practice: A National Survey," *Quarterly Journal of Studies on Alcoholism,* 33 (1972), pp. 117–131.

3. Phyllis Chesler, *Women and Madness* (New York: Avon Books, 1972).

4. Marilyn W. Johnson, "Physicians' Views on Alcoholism with Special Reference to Alcoholism in Women." *Nebraska State Medical Journal,* 50 (1965), p. 380.

5. Herbert I. Abelson et al., *National Survey on Drug Abuse: 1977,* vol. 1 (Rockville, Md.: National Institute on Drug Abuse. U.S. Department of Health, Education and Welfare, 1977). p. 102.

6. John L. Norris, "Analysis of the 1977 Survey of the Membership of Alcoholics Anonymous" (Paper presented at the Thirty-second International Congress on Alcoholism and Drug Dependence. Warsaw, Poland Sept. 3–8, 1978), p. 20.

7. Luise K. Forseth, "A Survey of Minnesota's Halfway Houses for the Chemically Dependent" (Unpublished paper, 1976), p. 9.

8. Ingrid Waldron, "Increased Prescribing of Valium, Librium and Other Drugs: An Example of the Influence of Economic and Social Factors on the Practice of Medicine," *International Journal of Health Sciences,* 7 (1977), p. 55.

9. Association of Halfway House Alcoholism Programs of North America, "Statistical Survey of Full Member Halfway House Alcoholism Programs" (St. Paul, Minn.: 1976), pp. 6–7.

10. Cheryl Gillen et al., "Report on Survey of Eighty-Eight New York State Outpatient Detoxification Halfway House and Rehabilitation Facilities" (New York: Committee on Women and Alcoholism in New York State, 1977), p. 1.

11. Edith S. Gomberg, "Women and Alcoholism," in V. Franks and V. Burtle (ed.), *Women in Therapy* (New York: Brunner/Mazel, 1974), p. 183.

12. Johnson, "Physicians' Views on Alcoholism," p. 380.

13. Inge Broverman et al., "Sex Role Stereotypes and Clinical Judgments of Mental Health," *Journal of Consulting and Clinical Psychology,* 34 (1970), pp. 1–7.

14. Ardelle M. Schulz, "Women and Addiction" (Paper presented to Ohio Bureau of Drug Abuse, Cleveland, Oh., June 17, 1974), pp. 23–24.

15. National Institute on Alcohol Abuse and Alcoholism, U.S. Dept. of Health, Education and Welfare, *Women in Treatment for Alcoholism in NIAAA Funded Facilities,* 1977 (Rockville, Md.: 1978), p. 8.

16. Stephen J. Levy and Kathleen M. Doyle, "Attitudes Toward Women in a Drug Treatment Program," p. 431.

17. David A. Pemberton, "A Comparison of the Outcome of Treatment in Female and Male Alcoholics," *British Journal of Psychiatry,* 133 (1967), pp. 367–373.

Are College Students Alcoholics?

by Aaron M. Brower, PhD

Are college students alcoholics? We get this question a lot. It is a different question from "Is student drinking worse than ever before?" or "Is student drinking out of control?" This question is specifically about whether college students are alcoholics—whether their drinking is making them alcohol dependent or whether they are headed down a road to long-term alcohol abuse.

We get this question from people with different agendas: from those who are sincerely interested in whether college students are alcoholics and from those who want to discuss why students drink, what harm drinking causes in a campus community, and how universities should best handle it. But we also get this question from those whom we call the *Carrie Nations.* Their question often leads to a one-sided lecture about the evils of alcohol (and society) and their contention that prohibition is the only real stance to take and that universities should promote abstinence.

We also get the question from people who simply want the issue of college drinking to go away. Very often these questioners are bar owners or others with ties to the alcohol industry, although equally often they are alumni who are remembering their college days and are asking us what all the fuss is about. From these people, the real statement they are making is, "I know students aren't alcoholics, so what's the big deal?" College students, they say, have been drinking excessively since colleges began, so the best thing a university can do is just get out of the way. Students, they say, need to experiment and learn through trial and error—just as they did when they were in college.

From *Journal of American College Health,* Vol. 50, March 2002. Reprinted with permission of the Helen Dwight Reid Educational Foundation. Published by Heldref Publications, 1319 Eighteenth St., NW, Washington, DC 20036-1802. Copyright © 2002.

My associates and I do *not* believe that college students are alcoholics or are alcohol abusers as diagnosed from a psychiatric point of view. At the same time, it is clear to us that college students do abuse alcohol, according to the most common-sense definition, and that this abuse inflicts real consequences on themselves and others. We also believe that a university should do certain things to monitor and manage this behavior for its students. Those things, however, are unique to a college community and would not work in a community at large or even with these same people if they were not in college. By confusing college drinking with alcoholism or traditional alcohol abuse, we muddy the view of college drinking and create roadblocks for intervention.

But I've jumped ahead. Alcohol and drinking have a long tradition at the University of Wisconsin–Madison, so mush so, in fact, that our recent drop in the "party schools" rankings was met with chagrin in some circles. As a university, we approached this problem in all the typical, piecemeal ways: with alcohol awareness campaigns, with alcohol-free programs, and with offers of help to those we identified as having serious drinking problems. We were about as successful with these efforts as was everyone across the country, which is to say that we weren't making much of a dent in the problem.

We needed a new approach. The realization that our efforts had been wrongly based on the view that college drinking was a subset of the types of problem drinking that show up in society at large helped us search for that new approach. Seeing problematic college drinking as a type of traditional alcoholism or alcohol abuse was getting us nowhere; we needed to view the problem from a completely new vantage point. We began to look at public health approaches and community action programs that see problems as supported by forces in the immediate and distant environment and recognize that the solutions need to come from broad-based community partnerships. We began to focus on campus and community norms and expectancies and the policies, regulations, and enforcement of laws to control the alcohol supply and demand. In addition, we examined who benefits economically from student alcohol use. And we considered weekend and evening options that were truly viable from the students' points of view.

Our efforts received a huge boost when we received a grant from the Robert Wood Johnson Foundation 5 years ago. Similar grants were awarded to 10 campuses across the country and were provided specifically to direct campus and community leaders to the problem of college drinking as a phenomenon unique to colleges and universities. The grants have been a godsend that is all too rare, particularly given the enormous amount of money and attention that the alcohol industry devotes to developing college drinkers. The grants have created an opportunity for people on campus and in the surrounding community to focus significant amounts of time and attention on a specific and serious problem in a way that has allowed real change to take place.

With this grant, we have extensively studied why students drink, how they drink, when they drink and what they drink. We have evaluated approaches that have worked and strategies that have not worked on our campus. Several themes arose.

First, our definition of the problem of student drinking for a campus has been an important guidepost to reorient our efforts. Instead of focusing on the drinking behaviors of individual students, we have focused on the problems for the campus and community. That is, if a student goes out, gets drunk, comes home, falls asleep, and gets up the next morning without any problems, even if he or she does it every single night, we do not consider this a problem that requires university action. Of course, this type of behavior is not what we want to encourage in our students, but we have taken the explicit position that college students are adults who can make their own decisions about how they use their time. Instead, we have defined student drinking as a problem for the campus and the community when students physically and sexually hurt themselves and other students, when they destroy property, and when their behavior disrupts others and prevents them from doing well in school. We have defined student drinking as a problem that is based on its community consequences rather than on an individual's drinking behaviors.

Second, we have found it important to help others understand that college problem drinking is a product of the college environment. The commonly used definition of *college binge drinkers*—male students who consume 5 drinks in one sitting and female students who consume 4 drinks in one sitting—has been useful for us. We know that this definition remains somewhat controversial, but for us it creates a reasonable threshold when student drinking becomes associated with serious consequences (eg, violence, sexual assaults, vandalism, and school failures).

The more descriptive term that we sometimes use is *episodic high-risk drinking,* which conveys a more accurate picture of how students drink: ingesting a large quantity of alcohol in a relatively short period of time and doing so relatively infrequently (ie, not every night or even regularly). But note that this definition and that used for college binge drinking are wholly different from the way the American Psychiatric Association defines alcoholism and alcohol abuse. In the association's *Diagnostic and Statistical Manual of Mental Disorders,* 4th edition (*DSM-IV*),[1] the definitions of alcohol dependence and alcoholism focus on the individual's need to drink more and more for the same effects and his or her inability to stop drinking. Continuing to drink in the face of repeated interpersonal, legal, and work-related problems is termed *alcohol abuse*. Again, the problems with college drinking are entirely different from problem drinking in society as a whole.

Third, the binge-drinking pattern for students on our campus is typical for a heavy-drinking campus according to several national studies—going out and getting drunk one night on the weekend. A lot of students drink this way occasionally (from once a week to once a month or less), although a small portion drink this way much more frequently. Overall, we find that about 60% of our students occasionally binge this way, whereas about 6% to 8% of those who drink are considered frequent binge drinkers—they binge either 2 or 3 times a week or on several weekends in a row. Even on our campus, about 10% of the students do not drink at all.

We find that students go through cycles of this type of drinking. It is worse at the beginning of the school year and subsides as the semester wears on and as school demands increase. Binge drinking also peaks following exam times, during home football weekends, and during spring break. Some "developmental" progressions can be seen in these patterns, with many new students engaging in this type of binge drinking for the first time very soon after they arrive on campus and then moving away from it in their subsequent years at school.

Finally, we find that college binge drinking, as a consistent pattern, ends for almost all students when they graduate from college and move on. Thus, this is a pattern that is strongly determined by living in a college environment and by the developmental life stage of being a college student. The vast majority of students never drink in this way again or engage in this same type of drinking only when they return to campus for alumni weekends or for football games. "Real life" is a strong disincentive to this type of drinking.

That college binge drinking is largely determined by and is a product of the college environment has been an extremely important point to get across as we have talked to people on our campus and in our community. Unlike alcoholics per se, students in college seem to be able to turn their willingness to binge drink on and off, depending on their environments (eg, whether they have exams to study for or whom they are with). And although a small segment of our students become alcoholics, this percentage is roughly the same as the percentage of alcoholics in the general population. We have found no studies whatsoever that show that drinking in college leads to later-life alcoholism or long-term alcohol abuse. On the other hand, we have found many studies that show that the drinking habits of 18- to 22-year-olds attending college are different from the drinking habits of 18- to 22-year olds who do not attend college.[2] (The focused "drinking to get drunk" of college students who put the drinking itself as the centerpiece of that night's activity does not characterize 18- to 22-year-olds not in college.) Again, real life is a strong disincentive for the kind of binge drinking that college students do.

The facts that the campus and community problems result from college drinking patterns and that college binge drinking is a college-environment phenomenon distinguish college binge drinking from alcoholism. With this distinction clear, we can continue to direct campus and community efforts toward interventions that work, Alcoholism is best addressed through individualized treatments that emphasize abstinence. College binge drinking is best addressed through several types of initiatives that stress shifting the role that alcohol plays in the college environment. From our reviews of the literature and from our own efforts, we have concluded that college binge drinking is best addressed by decreasing student anonymity, by providing consistent and coherent expectations about what it means to be a college student on campus, and by consistently enforcing policies that maintain these expectations. In contrast, we have found that the approaches that are *most* effective against alcoholism are the *least* effective for combating drinking as a campus and community issue.

Individual, one-on-one approaches, by definition, focus people's attention on how they must change their own behaviors. Environmental approaches, on the other hand, focus attention on the central role that campus and community departments, units, divisions, and other groupings, as well as economic, political, and social factors play in the solution to this serious problem.

Equating college binge drinking with alcoholism has only served as a distraction for our campus—it obscures both a clear view of the phenomenon itself and the intervention strategies that work. Ironically, we have found that the group most invested in maintaining this confusion has been the alcohol industry. Although viewing college binge drinking as alcoholism can create more public "buzz" on the issue (which one might think the alcohol industry would downplay), we have found that this confusion ultimately leads people to absolve the alcohol industry of its responsibility in effective solutions. If college binge drinking is an individual problem determined by individual choices and responsibilities, then the solutions rest with individuals who seek help and who stick with their resolutions to change. If, instead, college binge drinking is an environmental problem determined by a set of campus, community, and individual/developmental factors, then the responsibility for the solutions rests with all of us who can ensure that our campuses and communities do not encourage and support these behaviors.

Note

For further information, please address communications to Aaron M. Brower, PhD, Principle Investigator, Coalition for Campus and Community Change, School of Social Work and Integrated Liberal Studies, University of Wisconsin–Madison, 1350 University Avenue, Madison, WI 53706 (e-mail: ambrower@facstaff.wisc.edu).

References

1. *Diagnostic and Statistical Manual of Mental Disorders.* 4th ed. Washington, DC: American Psychiatric Association; 1994.
2. Schulenberg J, Bachman JG, O'Malley PM, Johnston LD. High school educational success and subsequent substance use: A panel analysis following adolescents into young adulthood. *J. Health Soc Behav.* 1994;35:45–62.

Fetal Alcohol Syndrome
A Nation in Distress
by Charon Asetoyer

And indeed, if it be the design of Providence to extirpate these Savages in order to make room for cultivators of the earth, it seems not improbable that Rum may be the appointed means. It has already annihilated all the tribes who formerly inhabited the sea coast.

—from the diary of Ben Franklin (1700s)

Let us put our minds together and see what kind of life we can make for our children.

—Sitting Bull (1800s)

It becomes clear who was the savage and who was the civilized man.

Historical Overview

In 1973, two doctors from Seattle, Washington, David Smith and Kenneth Jones, identified an irreversible birth defect that occurs when alcohol is consumed during pregnancy. They called it fetal alcohol syndrome (FAS) and noted its effects: mental retardation, deformed facial features, and stiff joints in the hands, arms, hips, and legs.

This naming of FAS by "modern man," however, was not our first knowledge of the connection between alcohol and the birth of unhealthy children. As early as 428–347 B.C., in the Laws of Plato, we find warnings about alcohol consumption during pregnancy: "Any man or woman who is intending to create children should be barred from drinking alcohol." Plato believed that all citizens of the state should be prohibited from drinking alcohol during the daytime and that children should not be made in bodies saturated with drunkenness. He went on to say: "What is growing in the mother should be compact, well attached, and calm."

In 322 B.C., Aristotle was quoted as saying: "Foolish, drunken, hair-brained women most often bring forth children like themselves, morose and languid." In ancient Sparta and Carthage, the laws prohibited bridal couples from drinking on their wedding night for fear of producing defective children. Even in the Bible (Book of Judges 13:7), an angel warns the wife of Manoah: "Behold, thou shalt conceive and bear a son, and now drink no wine or strong drink."

If the great philosophers were aware of the relationship between alcohol and birth defects, why has it

Charon Asetoyer is the founder and director of the Native American Women's Health Education Resource Center in Lake Andes, South Dakota.

taken so long for modern medicine to reach the same conclusion?

Ben Franklin's diary serves as a reminder that the colonial governments of what are now referred to as the United States, Africa, and Australia all used alcohol, in one form or another, to manipulate and control the local inhabitants of the continents they invaded. Alcohol was often used as a form of money with which to barter with local inhabitants for land, food, and animal hides. Colonial governments knew that indigenous people had no experience with alcohol and, therefore, were vulnerable to its effects. As Franklin makes clear, annihilation of indigenous people through alcohol became the unofficial policy of the colonial (U.S.) government.

Throughout U.S. history, the government has continued to use alcohol to control, manipulate, and murder Native Americans. Alcohol has been legal, illegal, and legal again at the whim of various presidents. The most recent change in the law pertaining to alcohol use among Native Americans was in 1953, when the Eisenhower administration once again legalized the sale of alcohol to Native Americans. Knowing this history, we should not be surprised that alcoholism remains a major health problem among Native Americans, nor that alcoholism results in the birth of significant numbers of children with FAS.

The Women and Children in Alcohol Program

Of all women who drink alcohol during pregnancy, 40 percent will give birth to children suffering from either FAS or a lesser condition known as fetal alcohol effects (FAE). FAE occurs four to six times more often than FAS, and though a less serious birth defect, we must not underestimate it. The effects are: below average intelligence; learning disabilities; visual, speech, and hearing problems; hyperactive behavior; and a short attention span. FAE may also be accompanied by some of the same physical disabilities as FAS. FAE children usually are not detected until they enter school, where they are often seen as children with discipline problems. On Native American reservations, it is estimated that anywhere from one in nine to one in four children are born with FAS or FAE.

To address the problems of alcohol consumption among Native American women and its impact on their children, the Native American Community Board (NACB), a nonprofit project based on the Yankton Sioux Reservation in Lake Andes, South Dakota, developed the Women and Children in Alcohol program. NACB was founded in 1985 to improve the quality of life for indigenous people and to ensure the survival of our culture through increasing awareness of health issues pertinent to our communities and encouraging community involvement in economic development efforts.

Women and Children in Alcohol was the first program of the NACB, and this focus resulted in NACB opening the first Native American Women's Health Education Resource Center in 1988. Located on the Yankton Sioux Reservation, the center addresses many of the unmet needs of women and children identified during the initial program, including child development; nutrition; adult learning; women's health issues, especially reproduction, AIDS and other sexually transmitted diseases, and cancer prevention; and environmental issues. It is not enough to go out into the community and spread the word about FAS/FAE. Information is important; however, there is more to it than that.

Blaming the Women

Early on, we discovered that when people learned of FAS/FAE, they were quick to blame mothers and their children. No one wanted to examine the larger picture, to ask questions about why women drink when pregnant. What about men's involvement in this, the peer pressure to drink in a community where alcohol use has become the accepted norm? What about the idle time in communities where the unemployment rate is often as high as 85 percent and the high school drop-out rate is over 60 percent? What about the high rates of domestic violence and sexual assault in our communities and the lack of community agencies to address these issues? It is easy to say that a mother's drinking causes an FAS/FAE child to be born, but it is far from the whole truth.

Women who are chemically dependent don't plan to get pregnant and give birth to unhealthy children. They are often the products of abusive childhoods or of homes where their parents drank. They were introduced to alcohol at an early age—I've known children on reservations addicted by the time they were ten or eleven years old. As adults, these women have many health problems of their own—liver damage, diabetes, and other conditions related to alcohol abuse. But these are not uncaring mothers. Chemically dependent mothers love their children as much as other mothers—no matter how unlikely this may seem to outsiders. They must also live with the guilt that society imposes upon them for having given birth to imperfect children. Every day they are reminded that had they not consumed alcohol during pregnancy, their children would probably have been normal and healthy. Chemically dependent women who seek treatment find one barrier after another blocking their paths. Only a small number of alcohol and drug treatment centers take pregnant women. In our four-state area, there is only one such center designed for Native American women. The Kateri program, in St. Paul, Minnesota, will take women through their sixth month of pregnancy (due to complications with Title 19, women cannot receive medical coverage if they stay beyond this point). This program, however, is in the process of being closed down because of problems with state and county funding.

Even if a woman is able to find a treatment center, in most cases, she will be unable to have her children there with her. If she is lucky enough to have supportive and available family members, she can leave her children with them; otherwise, she must turn them over to foster care, where she may fear that they will be abused and neglected. Most Native American women will not turn their children over to foster care unless ordered to do so by the courts.

Of course, someone must pay for women to enter treatment centers. Often, for poor women, the only means of gaining access to treatment is through a court order. But more often than not, when a woman is prosecuted for crimes related to chemical dependency, the courts find it easier and cheaper to terminate parental rights or to sentence a woman to jail than to provide treatment.

In recent years, it has become more and more common for prosecutors to charge women with child abuse or with giving a controlled substance to a minor in cases where a woman has continued to drink or take drugs during pregnancy. Judges want to punish women for engaging in what they consider self-indulgent behavior. They see these mothers as abusive rather than ill. The court may not even consider the fact that the woman being prosecuted may have tried to gain access to unavailable services.

Women of color are reported to authorities eight times more often than white women for giving birth to babies who are drunk or who have controlled substances in their blood. These women are often brought to the attention of authorities by social workers or doctors who deliver their children. But what have these service providers done to help these women deal with their addictions? In our communities, it is a sad fact that social-service and child-protection workers are often aware of alcohol problems among children and adults but are unwilling to intervene because those in need of assistance are part of their own extended family or the family of a tribal council member. Because of the politics involved, a social worker may lose his or her job for trying to assist a child in need of services.

Several years ago, a doctor at the Indian Health Services Hospital on our reservation diagnosed a child with FAS. It turned out to be the tribal chairman's child. The doctor was transferred out of our hospital. It is easier for the problems of families and children to be ignored, for the entire system to become dysfunctional, and for all of the blame to fall on alcoholic mothers, who are given little or no support in the first place.

Sterilization Abuse

Since the courts are rarely interested in helping women to overcome their addictions, they have instead focused on how to prevent alcoholic and drug-addicted women from having children. Although judges have shied away from permanent surgical sterilization of women because of fear of violating women's civil rights, new contraceptive technologies have allowed judges to order women to be temporarily sterilized. This, too, is a violation of civil rights.

Norplant, a surgically implanted contraceptive that prevents pregnancy for up to five years, has become the sterilization method of choice among judges. Norplant must be implanted, and removed, by a physician; thus, the woman who is subjected to Norplant has no control over her fertility. She is sterilized. The same is true with the contraceptive Depo-Provera (an injected contraceptive that lasts for approximately three months), which was used to sterilize mentally ill Native American women in the 1980s. Not only were these Indian women injected with Depo-Provera without their approval, but they were given the contraceptive before the FDA had even approved it for use in this country.

The first case in which a judge, as part of a plea bargain, ordered a woman to use Norplant, was in California in 1991. The woman, Darlene Johnson, was African American. The judge had little, if any, understanding of the potential harm that Norplant might do to this woman. He did not know that Johnson had health conditions that could become life-threatening if she were to be given Norplant. Should court officials who have no medical background be prescribing powerful medications? Will the courts assume legal responsibility if they endanger a woman's life in prescribing a potentially harmful drug?

Poor women, many of them women of color, have been targeted for sterilization not only through the courts but through bills in a number of states that require the use of Norplant as a condition for receiving welfare. Clearly, society takes the attitude that you reduce the risk of FAS/FAE babies by sterilizing women at high risk for giving birth to these babies. Reducing the risk of alcoholism and drug addiction among women of color and providing treatment for those in need is not a priority. This means that FAS/FAE and chemically dependent children often end up as orphans, dependent on the state for medical treatment as well as other social services.

Addicted mothers end up absent from home because they are still "using" and are out in the streets, in jail, or are dead after many years of substance abuse. Others must care for the children who may end up in foster homes or state facilities for the remainder of their lives. I have a close family member who has FAE. He lost his mother when he was seven years old due to an alcohol-related car accident. By the time he was fourteen, he had been in ten foster homes. Some were so bad that he experienced sexual abuse, drug abuse, and neglect. He is now 25 and has many problems with chemical dependency as well as with the law.

Society must take some responsibility for allowing a system to continue to function in this manner. It seems that it is easier to allow a system to be ill than to assist it in trying to get healthy. Both tribal and state courts have overstepped their authority in recommending or sentencing women to use Norplant or Depo-Provera. The bottom line is that this is sterilization, whether short-term or permanent, and such a policy carries with it strong connotations of racism and genocide when women of color are the intended targets. We cannot forget that in the mid '70s, the surgical sterilization of Native American women was common practice, with estimates running as high as 25 percent of all child-bearing age women having been permanently sterilized against their will.

Conclusion

It is easier to blame women for being alcohol- or drug-addicted than to admit that society has failed to provide services that will help these women to work toward a healthy lifestyle. Though not entirely surprised by the response of the courts, I have been shocked by hearing health care professionals support sterilization policies. In a recent interview with an Indian Health Service doctor concerning Norplant and Native American women, he said that he "would support court ordering of Norplant for the prevention of FAS/FAE." Never during the entire interview did he mention or suggest that the system had failed in trying to assist women who are alcohol or drug addicted.

Fetal alcohol births are an indicator of a Nation in distress. What does this mean for the future of a Nation? For the existence of a culture? The quality of a Nation's leadership is derived from its people and the vulnerability of a Nation lies in its leadership. Health care professionals, social service workers, tribal leaders, lawyers, and judges—people in a position to create a positive response to this issue—have chosen not to do so. Thus, they must share the burden of guilt each time an FAS/FAE or chemically dependent baby is born.

Fetal Alcohol Syndrome Class Related

by Ruth Hubbard

Readers of Charon Asetoyer's article about fetal alcohol syndrome in the March health supplement might like to know about a paper published in the journal *Advances in Alcohol and Substance Abuse* in summer 1987. The article, written by Nesrin Bingol and six others and entitled "The Influence of Socioeconomic Factors on the Occurrence of Fetal Alcohol Syndrome," reports the results from a study comparing the children of 36 upper-middle or upper-class chronic alcoholic women and the children of 48 chronic alcoholic women receiving public assistance in New York City. The authors found that whereas 4.6 percent of the children of the affluent mothers exhibited Fetal Alcohol Syndrome and other alcohol-related effects, 71 percent (or 15 times as many) of the children of the poor mothers did. Both groups of women were heavy drinkers, but their lives differed in many ways. For example, the poor women were more likely to have had alcoholic parents and grandparents and less likely to eat regular and balanced meals than the affluent women. The results of this study show clearly that Fetal Alcohol Syndrome is not just the result of pregnant women drinking too much alcohol, but of the economic, social, and physical neglect entire segments of our population experience all their lives.

The Twelve-Step Controversy

by Charlotte Davis Kasl

Drug addiction, codependency, incest, compulsive eating, sex, gambling, and shopping—multitudes of people are using 12-step programs modeled after Alcoholics Anonymous (AA) to recover from these problems. But beneath the surface of this massive movement, women are asking, is this really good for women? While female dissatisfaction with AA is not new (Jean Kirkpatrick founded Women for Sobriety in 1976), widespread questioning of these programs has only begun recently.

In workshops and group interviews, women repeatedly expressed fear about opening up the sacrosanct 12-step institution to scrutiny: "I'm afraid if we talk about this I'll lose something that helped me," or "I questioned the steps in my training program and they said I'd have to leave if I kept that up."

Women who question "the program," as it's often called, have been shamed, called resistant, and threatened with abandonment. They have been trained to believe that male models of nearly anything are better than whatever they might create for themselves.

Some women are grateful for what 12-step programs have given them: a generally available peer model providing support and understanding at no cost. Yet no one way works for everyone. The steps were formulated by a white, middle-class male in the 1930s; not surprisingly, they work to break down an overinflated ego, and put reliance on an all-powerful male God. But most women suffer from the *lack* of a healthy, aware ego, and need to strengthen their sense of self by affirming their own inner wisdom.

Research strongly indicates that alcohol addiction has links to genetic predisposition. A vital point that seems overlooked in AA is that in the case of nearly all substance abuse, the brain chemistry and the body ecology need extensive healing in order to prevent the protracted withdrawal syndrome of depression, anxiety, volatile emotions, and obsessive thinking that can last for years. Too often women endlessly attend groups, have psy-chotherapy, or take antidepressants when their emotions are actually being influenced by a chemical imbalance that could be helped by proper nutrition and exercise.

Other addictions, and codependency (as well as the will to recover), are influenced by cultural *oppression,* which includes poverty, battering, racism, sexism, and homophobia. Treatment programs need to incorporate understanding—and advocacy—regarding these concerns.

As a psychologist and a former member of 12-step programs, I have encouraged women to write steps that resonate with their own inner selves, putting the focus on self-empowerment.

Here are the 12 steps (as published by AA World Services) followed by a critique and by some possible empowerment steps:

1. "We admitted we were powerless over [our addiction]—that our lives had become unmanageable." The purpose of this step is to crack through denial or an inflated ego and acknowledge a destructive problem. It can be helpful to say "I am powerless to change my partner," but many women abuse chemicals or stay in harmful relationships *because* they feel powerless in their lives. Thus, many women prefer to affirm that they have the power to *choose* not to use chemicals or have dependent relationships. So, alternatively: *We acknowledge we were out of control with _____ but have the power to take charge of our lives and stop being dependent on others for our self esteem and security.*

2. "Came to believe that a Power greater than ourselves could restore us to sanity." I believe that spiritual power is neither higher nor lower but all pervasive. I would replace the passivity implied in this step—that something external will magically restore us to sanity—with "affirmative action": *I came to believe that the Universe/Goddess/Great Spirit would awaken the healing wisdom within me if I opened myself to that power.*

3. "Made a decision to turn our will and our lives over to the care of God *as we understood Him.*" This conjures up images of women passively submitting their lives to male doctors, teachers, ministers, often with devastating consequences. Instead: *I declared myself willing to tune into my inner wisdom, to listen and act based upon these truths.*

The following steps are grouped together here because they all ask women to focus on negative aspects themselves:

4. "Made a searching and fearless *moral inventory* of ourselves."
5. "Admitted to God, to ourselves, and to another human being the exact nature of our *wrongs.*"
6. "Were entirely ready to have God remove all these *defects of character.*"
7. *"Humbly* asked Him to remove our *shortcomings.*"
8. "Made a list of all *persons we had harmed,* and became willing to *make amends* to them all."
9. *"Made direct amends* to such people wherever possible, except when to do so would injure them or others." (All emphases mine.)

We women need to make a searching and fearless inventory of how the culture has mired *us* down with guilt and shame, recognizing how hierarchy has harmed *us* and how *we* have been complicit in harming ourselves and only then look at how we have harmed others. So, instead:

We examined our behavior and beliefs in the context of living in a hierarchal, male-dominated culture.

We shared with others the ways we have been harmed, harmed ourselves and others, striving to forgive ourselves and to change our behavior.

We admitted to our talents, strengths, and accomplishments, agreeing not to hide these qualities to protect others' egos.

We became willing to let go of our shame, guilt, and other behavior that prevents us from taking control of our lives and loving ourselves.

We took steps to clear out all negative feelings between us and other people by sharing grievances in a respectful way and making amends when appropriate.

10. "Continued to take personal inventory and when we were wrong promptly admitted it." As one woman said in a group, "Admit that I'm wrong? I say I'm wrong for breathing air. I need to say I'm *right* for a change." *Continued to trust my reality, and when I was right promptly admitted it and refused to back down. We do not take responsibility for, analyze, or cover up the shortcomings of others.*
11. "Sought through prayer and meditation to improve our conscious contact with God *as we understood Him,* praying only for knowledge of His will for us and the power to carry that out." Instead of looking to an external power, women need to reach inside and ask, What do I believe, what feels right to me? For example:

Sought through meditation and inner awareness the ability to listen to our inward calling and gain the will and wisdom to follow it.

12. "Having had a spiritual awakening as the result of these steps, we tried to carry this message to [others], and to practice these principles in all our affairs." The desire to reach out to others is a natural step that comes with healing, but women need to remember to first care for and love themselves and then to give from choice, not from guilt, emptiness, or to prevent abandonment.

Most important is that we not identify ourselves with such labels as codependent or addict, or get stuck in chronic recovery as if we were constantly in need of fixing.

The goal is to heal and move on, embrace life's ups and downs, and move from *re*covery to *dis*covery. Then we can break through the limitations imposed by hierarchy, work together for a just society, and free our capacity for courage, joy, power, and love.

WORSHEET — CHAPTER 7
Alcohol and Tobacco Issues

1. The article by Lorraine Greaves describes how cigarette smoking helps women cope with rather than change their lives and that this helps maintain the status quo. Interview two women who smoke now or have smoked to see if their experiences support or contradict Greaves' ideas.

2. **The marketing of alcohol and tobacco products:** Collect or photocopy a number of ads, from a range of magazines, selling alcohol and cigarettes. For this project, deliberately look for magazines aimed at both women and men, aimed at both teenagers and adults, and aimed for both white audiences and women of color.

   a. Compare ads for alcohol and cigarettes. What themes emerge in how these products are marketed?

   b. Compare the strategies in the ads that seem to be directed at women and those aimed at men. Are there re-curring themes?

   c. Compare the messages to white people and the messages to people of color.

   d. Describe the ads which seem to be aimed at young people. Are there educational strategies you can think of to counter the ads aimed at young people?

3. You have been asked to consult on a new alcohol treatment center for your community. All the other "experts" on the committee have years of experience in setting up treatment centers for men. Drawing on articles in this chapter and other information and experience, identify a number of issues which you may need to address to ensure that this new facility will be appropriate for women. Can you identify an example of an alcohol treatment program in your community which has worked to make sure it is appropriate for women?

4. The article, "Are College Students Alcoholics?" talks about focusing on drinking problems for the campus and community and shifting the role that alcohol plays in the college environment instead of focusing on drinking behaviors of individual students. Give several specific suggestions of how this could be done.

5. Much anti-smoking and anti-drinking information aimed at pregnant women is very victim-blaming and implies the health of the fetus is more important than the health of the woman. Suggest a different kind of anti-smoking and anti-alcohol health education "information piece" which could be aimed at pregnant women or their partners.

CHAPTER 8
Food, Body Shaping, and Body Projects

Body images, keeping our bodies healthy, and how we feel about our bodies are core women's health issues. This chapter should be several volumes covering every inch of women's bodies from heads to toes! Think about the messages women are given about every part of the body. What unhealthy things are women encouraged to do in order to "fit" society's ever changing definition of "attractive"?

The first articles in this chapter address body image issues from the perspectives of women, food, and fat. "Nourishing Ourselves" pulls together many of the interrelationships between women's roles as food producers, and how women's inferior status and internalized sexism may affect women's access to the very food they have produced. The similarities are drawn between malnutrition in poor countries/poor communities and in richer communities where, whether due to a lack of food, unequal distribution of food, or pressure to be thin, girls and women are too often deprived of the quality of diet they need for maximum mental and physical health.

The next articles concentrate on the ramifications of learning to hate fatness in others and especially in ourselves. "Fatphobia" looks at one of the most prevalent, yet uncriticized, forms of prejudice in our society, and "Mental Health Issues Related to Dieting" discusses mental health consequences of this cultural obsession with trying to be thin. Healthier attitudes towards one's non-skinny body are expressed in "We'll Always be Fat but Fat Can Be Fit." This approach, which uncouples health promotion activities (regular exercise, consumption of fruits, vegetables, and fibers, increasing social support) from weight loss, is the approach that McAfee and Lyons are asking for in "Weight and Health," their critique of the Surgeon General's recent "Call to Action to Prevent and Decrease Overweight and Obesity." They express grave concern that this much publicized national call to action promotes attitudes which increase the social stigma of being overweight and totally "ignores research over the past 40 years that has found sustaining weight loss to be nearly impossible."

Until quite recently, much of the research and writing on women, dieting, and "eating disorders" has been focused primarily on white, middle-class women. Women of color have often expressed frustration that such information did not reflect their experiences. Haubegger's "I'm Not Fat, I'm a Latina" is a reflection on what it feels like not to fit the too narrow societal definition of what women should look like. Becky Thompson has done cutting-edge work examining how race, class, and heterosexism intersect with sexism and other psychic and physical invasions to impact body image and "eating disorders" issues. Thompson's chapter pushes us to think about "eating problems" in new, complex ways.

As reminders that body modification and manipulation are about much more than just what we do or do not eat, this chapter ends with articles about breast implants, tattooing, and piercing. Diana Zuckerman, a longtime leader on breast implant issues, draws attention to the scientific, medical, and political factors which *should* come together for good decisions about which products and procedures are and are not safe enough to be allowed on the market.

The two extremely different, both fascinating and informative, articles on women's tattooing are meant to stimulate conversations on the politics of women's health *information* as well as the topic of tattooing itself. The very sophisticated, highly academic "Pretty in Ink: Conformity, Resistance, and Negotiation in Women's Tattooing" published in the very respected academic journal *Sex Roles* is an example of a research paper which brings together a qualitative study of women's experiences and attitudes, feminist theories about bodies, and a vast literature on the widest range of related issues. "Women's tattooing activities and their subsequent tattoo narratives are critically inspected as deeply gendered practices and discourses" by the researcher who emphasizes "how women employ tattooing as a communications signifier of 'established' and 'outsider' constructions of femininity." In contrast, an article on tattooing and piercing, "Ouch—You Call That Body Art?" is from *Teen Voices,* an alternative feminist magazine *for* teens, *by* teens, designed to give teenage girls different non-commercial kinds of pro-girl messages than they get from mainstream, product-orientated teen magazines. Both *Sex Roles* and *Teen Voices* represent achievements of the women's movement in making certain that sex and gender roles in society are seriously studied and critiqued and that a much wider range of girls' and women's voices and perspectives are heard.

Nourishing Ourselves

by Nancy Worcester

What could be more ironic? Nourishing others is a fundamental part of women's lives but that very role itself limits the ability of women to take care of their own nutritional needs.

Women are the world's food producers and throughout the world, within a wide range of family units, women have responsibility for purchasing and/or preparing the daily food. Yet, both globally and within families, women are much more likely than men to be malnourished. Nearly universally, wherever there is a shortage of food or a limited supply of quality food, women's diets are inferior to men's quantitatively and qualitatively. Even when food supply is adequate or abundant, women's diets may be nutritionally inferior to men's.

It matters! At some level we all have a feel for how important a good diet is: "We are what we eat." If we feed our bodies the basic nutrients, the healthy body is amazingly clever at being able to take care of itself. An adequate diet is obviously important for *every* man, woman and child. However, both societally and individually, a terrible mistake is being made when women's diets are inferior to men's.

A woman's diet must be more "nutrient-concentrated" than a man's in order to be nutritionally adequate. Most women require considerably less energy than most men. For example, the US Food and Nutrition Board recommends an intake of 1600–2400 Calories per day for women age 23–50, compared to 2300–2700 Calories per day for the same age men. A US Food Consumption Survey showed that the average 23 year old woman consumes only two-thirds as many Calories as the average 23 year old man, 1600 compared to 2400.[1] However, women's requirements for many specific nutrients are identical or greater than men's. The ramifications for this are most serious for calcium and iron. US Food and Nutrition Board Recommended Daily Allowance (RDA)[2] for calcium is the same for men and women. The RDA of 15 mg. of iron per day for reproductive aged women is 50% higher than the 10 mg. RDA for men.

Picture a woman and a man sitting down to consume their daily nutritional needs. The man's pile of food will be 50% bigger than the woman's but in the woman's smaller pile she will need to have the same amount of calcium and 50% more iron. Each bite the woman takes must contain 50% more calcium and twice as much iron! Put another way, even if a man does not have a particularly nutrient-rich diet, he will probably be able to meet his body's needs and he will even get away with consuming quite a few empty-calorie or low-quality foods whereas a woman's diet must be of a relatively higher quality. A man's diet can be nutritionally inferior to a woman's and still be adequate for his needs. The world and millions of individuals are paying a high price for the fact that women's diets are often inferior to men's.

Sex Differential in Food Distribution and Consumption

The trend to feed boys better than girls gets established early in life. In Kashmir, girls are breastfed for only 8–10 months but boys are allowed to suckle for three years or longer.[3] In Arabic Islam, girls are breastfed for only 1–1-1/2 years while it is common for a boy to be nursed until the age of 2–2-1/2.[4]

A recent Italian study also showed differences in the patterns of feeding baby boys and girls—girls are breastfed less often and for shorter periods; girls are weaned an average of three months earlier than boys. Additionally, it was observed that boys were more irritable and upset before feeding but went to sleep immediately after feeding. In contrast, the girls were less aggressive in asking for food but settled down less easily after feeding.[5]

Throughout the world, men and boys get feeding priority. In many cases, men literally eat first and women and children get what food is left-over, such as in Bangladesh where the tradition of sequential feeding means adult men are served first, followed by male children, then adult women and female children. Ethiopian women and girls of all classes must prepare two meals, one for the males and a second, often containing no meat or other substantial protein, for the females.[6] Boys' better access to food based on a gender defined division of labour can get started early in life. For example, in Alor, Indonesia, very young boys are encouraged to do "masculine" work and food serves as an important incentive and reward for that work. Boys receive "masculine" meals as guests of adult men for whom they have performed some service. In contrast, young girls do less valued work like weeding and get a lower quality vegetable lunch.[7]

In whatever way a particular society works it out, there is a nearly universal pattern of men getting fed more and better. Most women recognize this pattern and can identify ways in which they feed their children and their partners better than themselves. Although this may mean nothing more serious than taking the burnt slice of toast or the least attractive piece of dessert for oneself, in times of shortage this pattern means that women are the most likely to be malnourished.

Family members may not even be aware of the sacrifices the woman is making. A British woman who fed her husband and her children even when she could not feed herself during the 1930s remembered, "Many a time I have had bread dripping [animal fat on bread] for my dinner before my husband came home and I said I had my dinner as I would not wait."[8] That pattern is becoming prevalent again as many families do not have enough food. How many women say they are on a diet when in fact they would love some of what they are serving up to their family?

Hilary Land's study of large families in Britain concluded, "It was very evident that the mother was the most likely to go without food for she was the most dependent on meals provided at home. . . It was clear that the father's needs were put first, then the children's and finally the mother's." Over half of the women had no cooked meal in the middle of the day. A quarter had no breakfast and nothing more than a sandwich for lunch. One in twelve women *never* had a cooked meal.[9]

Studies in both Britain and the US have shown that poor parents go without food in order to leave enough food for their children. A British survey found that children were generally better and more regularly fed than their parents. "Only" 15% of the children had fewer than three meals during the previous twenty-four hours in contrast to 75% of the parents having had fewer than three meals, 50% having had two meals and 25% having had only one meal in the twenty-four hour period.[10] A 1983 New York study interviewed people at various sites including emergency feeding centers, food stamp offices, health centers and community centers. When asked, "Do your children eat and sometimes you're unable to?", over one-third of all respondents answered yes and 70% of the parents interviewed at the emergency feeding sites said yes.[11] (These studies did not look for different impacts on mothers and fathers.)

The feminization of poverty means that women in singleheaded households are often the worst affected. A Northern Ireland survey of 700 lone parents found that food was the item on which economies were most likely to be made and inevitably the savings were made by the mother herself going without food.[12] An English woman living on Supplementary Benefits describes the stark "choice" between her needs and the children's:

> It has to be me cutting down on what I eat. It's the only way to find the extra money you need. The rest of it, they take it before you can get your hands on it really. So it's the food. It's the only thing I can cut because I use as little heating as I can and I don't smoke.[13]

Providing food for the children is such a worry for women who are the only parent that they may actually deprive themselves more than is necessary. Marsden's study of 116 lone mothers found that they hoarded food to be able to feed the children. He observed a stress reaction to living on low income in which the caregivers economized on their own food more than the size of their income required.[14]

Efforts specifically designed to improve women's diets are not successful if programmes are not planned around the recognition that women feed their families before they feed themselves and that men tend to get the high status foods. For example, a very ambitious 86 million dollar (US dollars) World Food Programme (WFP) project set up to improve the nutrition of pregnant and nursing mothers and their young children in Pakistan has had practically no nutritional impact. The major problem with the programme was that food was rationed so that each woman would receive an individual dietary supplement of 850 Calories per day, but, of course, the women shared the extra food with their families. The average family had six people so one-sixth of the supplement, less than 150 Calories a day, did not make a significant improvement in women's diets.

The acknowledgement that women do not give themselves priority in food allocation posed new problems for evaluators of the Pakistan WFP project:

> Another possibility that has been mentioned is to simply accept the realities of family structure and food habits in Pakistan and expand the rations given to the women so that they are enough to provide supplements to the entire family. Obviously, a major drawback to this approach is that the same amount of food would then supply fewer women because of the increased ration size and not nearly as many women would be drawn to the centers.[15]

Judit Katona-Apte, consultant to the World Food Programme (but apparently not terribly influential!), suggests that one way to make certain that women benefit from food aid is to provide foods which are nutritionally-rich but less desirable than traditional foods. In such situations, the high status traditional foods will be given to the men and the newer, less desirable but nutritional foods will be relegated to the members of low status in the household—the women and children![16]

The differential access to food is often exaggerated by food taboos, which have more impact on women that men. Food habits, including rituals and taboos are an integral part of defining cultures ("we" versus "others"). Food taboos serve the function of reinforcing social status differences between individuals and social groups and symbolize the place one has in society. Taboos characteristically involve the prohibition of the highest quality protein foods. Jelliffe and Jelliffe suggest that, "The reservation of the best foods for the males reflects the ancient situation where it was imperative that hunters be well fed." However, Trant's explanation seems more to the point, "Widespread prohibitions applied to women against the eating of flesh foods may have partly derived from the male wish to keep the foods for themselves."[17] Those Italian baby boys aggressively demanding their food are just perpetuating a very ancient pattern!

Overall, it seems that most permanent taboos and avoidances have little effect on the nutrition of individuals practicing them because the group's diet will have evolved so that other foods supply the nutrients found in prohibited foods. However, temporary avoidance, particularly at crucial periods of the life cycle can have grave consequences.

Such limited duration taboos particularly affect women because they occur at the most nutritionally sensitive periods. For example, hot and cold or yin and yang classifications of food are common throughout the world and are especially important in Latin America and parts of Asia. Although hot and cold and yin and yang are defined differently in diverse cultures, in all cultures practicing these classifications, the balancing concept is closely tied to women's reproductive cycles. So, however menstruation, pregnancy and lactation get defined, it will be particularly important that women avoid certain "unbalancing" foods during those times. The foods which must be avoided are often foods of high nutritional value. Some Puerto Rican women consider pregnancy to be a hot state so avoid hot foods and medications, including vitamin and iron supplements, to prevent babies from being born with a rash or red skin. Bangladeshi women must not eat meat, eggs, fish or hot curries for several days after childbirth because those foods are believed to cause indigestion. Women are expected to eat only rice, bread, tea and cumin seed for those nutritionally-demanding post-partum days.[18]

There are two more points to consider in looking at the impact of food taboos and avoidance on women's nutrition. First, food taboos, as a cultural construct, are a part of the values of the society which are taught to people as they grow up. People learn those taboos as patterns of behavior which are right, normal, best. Other ways of doing things are viewed as wrong, misguided, or irrational. Understanding and appreciating another culture will require getting to know the food habits and vice versa. Second, sound nutritional practices can, with thought and planning, be developed and reinforced within the context of most existing food patterns.

This relates to an important theme I am introducing here which I will then weave throughout this chapter. I am suggesting that our society's fear of fat and obsession with dieting play a role in limiting women's access to optimum nutrition similarly to the way food taboos can affect women's nutrient intake in more traditional cultures. Dieting certainly has more impact on women than men, reinforces social status differences, and leaves more food for others. As a cultural phenomenon, there can be no denying that women from many parts of the world would find the notion of purposefully restricting food intake to lose weight to be "wrong" or "misguided". Imagine trying to explain the pattern of American college women who intentionally skip meals to save calories for snacking and beer drinking at parties to Western Samoan women who exaggerate the amount they eat on diet surveys because, "The more they could say they had eaten . . . the more powerful that meant the village was in being able to amass lots of food."[20,21] When we hear that many nine year old girls are already on slimming diets, we must recognize dieting to be a part of the values which our society now teaches to young women. Because much dieting is erratic behavior, "a temporary drastic measure just to take off a few pounds" (repeatedly performed!), it is more similar to temporary taboos with the potential for grave consequences than to permanent taboos for which people have learned to compensate. Just as one can eat a nutritionally adequate or even nutritionally superior vegetarian or vegan diet if one knows animal products are going to be consciously avoided or unavailable, it is certainly possible to consume nutrient-rich low calorie or weight-maintenance diets. But, that is not how the dieting taboo is usually practiced in this society.

Nutritional Consequences of Sex Differentiation

Clearly there is no way to summarize the effects of sex differentiated nutrition. Nutritional vulnerabilities vary enormously from one part of the world to another, from one region to another, and between classes in the same small community. Malnutrition, of course, is not inevitable and is totally preventable. There is enough food and land available to feed the world's population if our governments considered that to be an important priority.[22] Factors such as cultural food preferences, storage and transport facilities, the soil the food is grown in and the value placed on equal food distribution within a community will have more influence on one's chances of being malnourished than whether one is a woman or a man. But, a pattern emerges which shows that universally malnutrition is far too common and that it affects girls and women more than boys and men.

> Hunger affects whole regions and classes of people and sweeps men as well as women into its nets. It seldom happens that the male members of a family are well-fed or overfed while the females starve. The differentials are narrow, and the question is that of which sex first crosses the line between health and sickness. In general, those who skate closest to the margin of deprivation are the most powerless—the very young, the old, and, everywhere, the women.[23]

Nutritional studies do not always look for or find sex differences in nutritional deficiencies. However, when nutritional sex differences are found it is almost always in the direction of the higher occurrence being in females. *Women and Nutrition in Third World Countries*[24] summarizes hundreds of nutritional studies in poor countries and concludes:

> Calorie intake is often low among women, although a few populations show adequate intake (Mexico, Tarahumaras, Korea) or excessive (Micronesia) ones. Deficiencies in caloric intake are common, regardless of physiological status . . . where intakes are reported by income, low-income women appear to consume less than their middle and high income counterparts. Not only do women consistently eat less than men, in a number of studies, they consume, on average a smaller percentage of their recommended daily intake . . . Women often consume lower quality, vegetable protein while men receive the larger share of whatever animal protein is available . . . On the basis of quantity alone, women of-ten consumed a smaller percentage of their protein requirements than did men.

> The adequacy of vitamin intake varies greatly by culture. Riboflavin intakes are adequate in almost every country reviewed. The adequacy of vitamin A varies considerably, while most women (except those in Singapore, Iran, and the Tarahumara Indians) are deficient in their vitamin C intakes.

> Calcium and iron are the two minerals most commonly studied and in a majority of the countries reviewed, women are seriously deficient in their intakes of both.

The particular ramifications of women's iron and calcium deficiencies will be recurring themes in this book.

Iron is vital to the oxygen-carrying capacity of the blood and muscles but iron deficiency anaemia is the most common nutrition problem in rich and poor countries and in rich and poor people. Iron is available in many foods including meats, eggs, vegetables (especially greens), cocoa powder, apricots, breads and cereals, but in light of the prevalence of iron deficiency, the United Nations Committee on Nutrition recommends that more priority be given to iron fortification and supplementation.[25]

Reproductive age women are particularly vulnerable to iron deficiency because iron lost through menstruation must be replaced and highly increased circulatory requirements of pregnancy must be supplied in addition to the body's other needs for iron. Iron deficiency anaemia's incapacitating physiological and psychological effects influence the lives of women three or four times as much as men in many parts of the world. In low income countries, about half of non-pregnant women and nearly two-thirds of pregnant women show signs of iron deficiency anaemia.[27] Bangladesh is the most extreme example where a national survey discovered abnormally low iron (measured as blood haemoglobin) levels in 95% of rural women.[28]

Serious anaemia increases the risks of difficulty and death in childbirth of these women. While the consequences of iron deficiency anaemia are usually less severe in richer countries, the debilitating condition is far too common. Anaemia was identified in 40% of pregnant women in New Mexico's Women, Infant, and Children (WIC) Program and in 33% of poor pregnant women in Minneapolis, Minnesota. Black children show consistently higher rates (often more that twice as high) of anaemia than white children, so the effects of anaemia are probably even more exaggerated for Black than white US women.[29]

The consequences of sex differentiated nutrition become most obvious at the vulnerable times just after weaning and during the childbearing years. These are the two stages of life at which the female to male sex ratios take a dive.[30]

Biologically, it seems females are stronger than males. In general, life expectancy in females is greater than that in males. More males than females are conceived (120–150 males: 100 females), seemingly to "prepare" for the male biological vulnerability. More male fetuses are spontaneously aborted or stillborn, so the male to female ratio is down to 103–105:100 at birth.[31] Fifty-four percent more males die of birth injuries, 18% more males die of congenital malformations, and males account for 54% of all infant deaths in the first year of life.

Given the apparent biological advantage of females, a fascinating exercise is to try to identify the biological versus social and political causes of sex differences in death rates. Obviously, the fact that 68% of the US deaths at age 21 are male is more related to societal messages about who should play with guns and drive fast cars than a biological difference. Whether the supposedly higher rate of coronary heart disease in middle aged men than in women is more related to different roles in society, women's higher oestrogen levels, or a difference of who gets diagnosed, is a much more complex debate. Wherever there is a higher death rate for males, there may be a combination of biological and social factors working. Higher death rates for females clearly indicate that there are social, political or economic conditions overriding the female biological advantage.

The most marked sex discrimination in nutrition occurs after disasters in which there is a food shortage. Although physiological differences between males and females suggest that figures would show an excess mortality among males, statistics which exist consistently show that it is females and especially girl children who are at highest risk.[32] In the economic disasters after flooding in West Bengal, girls under five had a 60 percent higher incidence of third-degree malnutrition than the same age boys.[33]

A number of studies in South Asia have shown dramatic differences in the food and health care available to girls and boys. Preferential treatment of boys begins at birth when the birth of a boy is almost always viewed as a splendid occasion. Attitudes to the birth of a baby girl are at best ambivalent. While explicit female infanticide is no longer commonly practiced, the withholding of food and health care resources from girls can be viewed as a modern day version of female infanticide. The end result is the same: female mortality exceeds male mortality by as much as 50 percent in the 1–4 year age groups in rural Bangladesh.

A detailed study of six rural Bangladeshi villages pinpoints how this happens.[34] Intrafamily food distribution surveys carried out by 130 families showed that energy and protein intakes were consistently higher for males than females in all age groups.

Protein consumption in males compared to females was 14% higher in 0–4 year olds, 22% higher in 5–14 year olds, 25% higher in 15–44 year olds, and 53% higher in males over 45. Malnutrition rates reflected the intrafamily distribution pattern. Of 882 children surveyed, 14.4 percent of girls were classified as severely malnourished compared to 5.1 percent of boys.

There is usually a distinct, almost synergistic relationship between malnutrition and infection. Malnutrition severely compromises the body's ability to resist infection, and resisting or succumbing to infection increases the body's nutritional needs, thus enhancing the degree of malnutrition. The effects of malnutrition will usually be exaggerated by this malnutrition—infection—increased malnutrition cycle and malnourished children can die from normally non-lethal diseases like measles.

Surprisingly, the six village rural Bangladesh study found rates of infection among female children were consistently lower than among males, although the differences were small and statistically insignificant. (More proof of the biological strength of little girls!) The tragedy was that girls were valued so much less than boys that health resources were made available to ill boys but not to ill girls *even when transport and health care was provided for free.* Despite nearly comparable incidence levels of diarrhea, boys exceeded girls at the treatment center by 66 percent: diarrhea treatment rates averaged 135.6 per 1000 for male children in comparison to 81.9 for female children.

Studies from India show even more starkly the consistent and systematic discrimination against females in the allocation of food and health care resources. Kwashiorkor (protein-calorie malnutrition) is four to five times more common among girls than boys. Though girls were more likely to be suffering from this life-threatening form of malnutrition, boys outnumbered girls at the hospital for treatment by a ratio of 50:1. When treated, children of both sexes responded equally well, but the mortality rate was considerably higher in girls due to both a lack of food and a lack of health care.[35,36]

Male-preferential distribution of food and other resources is certainly not a phenomenon only in poor households. Excess female to male mortality in 1–4 year olds is observed even among wealthy landowning families in Bangladesh, demonstrating that competition for scarce, insufficient resources does not explain all the disparity. It is not known whether this pattern is more marked in poor families when there is simply not enough for everyone so less valued members must be "sacrificed" for the sake of others or whether it is exaggerated in wealthier families where the social role of rich women is even more inferior in comparison to the status of rich men. In Bangladesh, excess female mortality is higher in rich households some years but other years excess mortality is higher in poor families.[37]

Intergenerational Consequences of Female Malnutrition

Malnutrition in girls and women can have long term and intergenerational repercussions, because of women's reproductive role. Any nutritional deficiency, such as rickets, which interferes with the physical development of little girls can cause problems, including maternal and infant death, decades later in pregnancy and childbirth.

The most profound and long term effect of women's malnutrition is demonstrated by the link between poor maternal height and weight and low birth weight babies. Low birth weight babies, defined as weighing less than 2500 grams (five and one-half pounds) at full gestation, have a much higher mortality rate and are more susceptible to illness throughout childhood than normal weight babies. A Sri Lankan study found an average maternal height of 150 cm (4'9") for low birth weight babies and a modal maternal height of 155 cm (5'1") for well-grown babies.[38] Poor maternal height and weight can be a reflection of the mother's own intrauterine growth retardation and inadequate childhood nutrition. Healthy diets for all potential mothers from pre-conception through pregnancy can be seen as a high societal priority when one realizes that *it takes at least two generations to eliminate the effect of stunted maternal growth on future generations of women and men.*

Reversing the effect of malnutrition brings new challenges. When a basic nutritionally-adequate diet for everyone becomes a national priority, young women with a family history of malnutrition will have access to a healthy diet after their own development has been stunted. In revolutionary China, as a consequence of major improvements in food production and distribution, birth weights rose dramatically within one generation. In order to maximize on its nutritional achievements, China's health services had to be able to cope with an increased rate of complicated deliveries as there was a generation of small mothers producing relatively large babies.[39]

While the relationship of women's malnutrition to generations of limited development may be most exaggerated in the poorest countries, it is certainly also an issue for wealthier countries. Some figures will help us follow through the impact of restricted nutrition on poor women in Britain and the US but one has to be critical of categories of analysis. Not by accident, measures of social class such as wealth, income, education and job classification are seldom recorded on US records such as death certificates.[40] Britain is much better at recognizing/not hiding the importance of social class information but the information is more appropriate to men than to women. Women's social class is based on husband's occupation. Even when categorization is based on the woman's own job, as with unmarried heterosexual or lesbian women, women's jobs certainly do not sum up women's lives.[41]

In Britain, 41 percent of wives of professional men have a height of at least 165 cm (5'5") compared to only 26 percent of wives of manual workers. Similarly, in the US, women in low income families have an average height of 160.4 cm (5'3") compared to 163.4 cm (5'4") for women in higher income families.[42] Heights for US children have, on average, been increasing throughout the last century, but the average height for poor children lags behind that for nonpoor children by more than a generation. The average height of ten year olds from families above poverty level is now significantly higher than the average height of ten year olds living below poverty. (This is not a race difference, for the average height of Black children is slightly higher than that of white children of the same income.) Sweden has recently managed to eliminate growth differences between social classes and is probably the only country with this achievement.[43]

In Britain, low birth weight babies and stillbirths are nearly twice as common in poor families (social classes IV and V) as in wealthier families (classes I and II). In the US, infant mortality rate is thirty times higher in low birth weight babies than normal weight babies.[44] Infant mortality rate (IMR = the number of babies per thousand live births who die in the first year of life) is an invaluable tool for comparing the health status of groups because it is a figure which is calculated similarly all over the world and is an excellent reflection of maternal and infant nutrition, as well as general standard of living and access to preventative and curative health care. IMR is 50 percent higher for US whites living in poverty areas than for US whites living in nonpoverty areas and IMR is at least 2.5 times higher in poor than in wealthy families in the UK. The intersection of poverty and racism is obvious from national (US) figures showing IMR more than twice as high for Black babies as white babies. Blacks in poor areas have a far higher IMR than Blacks in nonpoor areas although Black IMR is higher than white IMR in both income areas.[45,46]

The potential for change with an improved standard of living, including an emphasis on nutrition and access to health care, is most striking when IMRs are compared for small geographical areas. The Physician Task Force on Hunger in America contrasts the New York City

IMRs of 5.8 in the Sunset Park section of Brooklyn with the 25.6 rate for Central Harlem and the Houston, Texas IMRs of 10.0 in the Sunnyside areas versus 23.5 in the Riverside Health Center community.[47] When we see that two or four times as many babies are dying in one part of town than in another, little guessing is needed to figure out where the poor, malnourished people live in New York City or Houston.

Malnutrition: Cause and Effect on Women's Role in Society

It is women not men who are unequally distributing food within the family, giving men and boys more than their share of what is available for the household. Women depriving themselves and their daughters of life-sustaining nourishment is the ultimate example of internalized sexism. Men do not need to discriminate against women or carry out nasty plans to "keep women in their place" if women are sufficiently well socialized to their inferior role that they themselves perpetuate keeping women in inferior roles.

A profoundly intermeshing relationship exits between women's status in society and the responsibility for food production and distribution. Women's responsibility for domestic work, especially food production, is so undervalued that women internalize that low value and starve themselves literally or figuratively. Although millions of women and girls die each year as a result of malnutrition, that number is a mere fraction of the number of women and girls who cannot maximize on their full potential because of undernutrition and because their responsibilities for feeding others do not leave them food, time or energy to nourish and nurture themselves.

Women's role as food producer can actually restrict a woman's ability to feed herself and others. How often have we observed a woman who eats practically nothing herself after spending hours preparing a meal for others? How often have we seen a woman so busy serving others that she barely sits down herself? A woman's standards for feeding herself may be totally different than those she holds to for her family. For example, a (London) *Daily Mirror* survey showed that even though mothers of school-age children make sure their children have breakfast, a fifth of mothers do not take time to eat breakfast themselves.[48]

Charmian Kenner's interviews with English women who have survived times of economic hardship show how the family's dependence on mum's food can make mum so ill that she cannot feed them:

> There was a vicious circle in which sickness bred further sickness. Lacking food, women had less resistance to infections. And when a woman fell ill

and especially needed better food nobody else could take over and stretch the budget. Some women did not even feel able to set aside valuable time to teach their children to help them.[49]

It is exactly the women who face the most demanding food preparation tasks who have the least time and energy for this work. The woman who can afford the latest food processor and microwave may also be able to afford to buy easy-to-cook or partially prepared nutritious foods when she is too busy to cook. The woman who has to work overtime to have money to buy beans may not be able to buy a pressure cooker to reduce cooking time. Before or after a long day, she may have to decide between spending several hours on food preparation and eating less nutritional foods.

In many agricultural communities, it is *because* women have put all their time and energy into growing and harvesting the food that they may not be able to take the final steps, often extremely time and energy consuming, of turning the raw products into an edible form so that they can feed themselves and others.

> One report speaks of African women "sitting about hungry with millet in their granaries and relish in the bush" because they were too exhausted to tackle the heavy, three-hour work of preparing the food for eating.[50]

The seasonal nature of agriculture exacerbates this. Peak periods for women's work in the fields are normally at planting, harvesting and post-harvesting processing times when the working day can average fifteen hours. This coincides with the food supply being scarcest, most expensive, least varied and least well prepared. As a consequence, it has been noted that in Gambia, pregnant women actually lose weight during the peak agricultural time and, in Thailand, there is a marked increase in miscarriages and an early termination of breastfeeding during the rice planting and harvesting seasons.[51,52]

The relationship between productivity and nutrition works in several ways. Not only does extreme work keep women from feeding themselves, but also undernutrition is clearly a factor limiting women's productivity. Intensity of work, the productive value of work activities selected, and labour time are all dimensions of productivity which have been shown to be affected by nutrition. If women are not able to maximize on their productivity, food production is limited; several studies have identified women's labour input as the critical constraint on crop production. Although the value of women's productivity is universally and consistently *not* recognized, any signs of poor performance are definitely used to prolong women's low status.

The case of Sri Lankan women tea workers illustrates the cycle whereby low status affects diet, then malnutrition perpetuates low status. Tea workers' poor social and economic position is reflected by high morbidity and maternal mortality rates. Due to poor diets and hook worm manifestation, the women also have high rates of iron deficiency anaemia (measured as low haemoglobin levels). Studies found that this iron deficiency restricted work performance; a significant relationship was found between haemoglobin levels and various treadmill tests of physiological capacity. (Iron deficiency anaemia affects work intensity by decreasing the blood's oxygen transporting capacity.) After the women were given iron supplements for one month, significantly more tea got picked! These studies were of particular interest to the Sri Lankan government because tea has been the main asset for foreign exchange and the poor nutritional status of the female labour force was seen as having far reaching socio-economic consequence. Assuming women's increasing productivity was appropriately financially rewarded, one can see where something as seemingly simple as iron supplements can be an important step to improved economic status for some women.[53,54]

This specific example suggests an even bigger question: How much does the image and reality of the malnourished woman as weak, lethargic and not maximizing on her potential become the generalized description for "women" which then justifies and perpetuates women's inferior status?

Worldwide the high incidence of iron deficiency anemia has to be seen as a major, often unrecognized, component of women's low status. We know that this one nutrition issue affects as many as 95 percent of women in some communities and has profound physiological and psychological repercussions, including impaired work capacity, lassitude, lowered resistance to infection, and increased complications of pregnancy and childbirth. The Sri Lankan tea workers' example is worth remembering as a positive example of both how easily some consequences of iron deficiency can be reversed and the need to make sure our governments become better educated about what they have to gain from a well nourished female labour force.

A wide range of other nutrition problems also have an impact on women's status. As an illustration which has nearly universal ramifications, low Calorie diets serve as an important example of undernutrition which, for very different reasons, can interfere with women maximizing on their potential and limiting their role in society in both rich and poor countries and for both rich and poor women. It is well known that low energy intakes restrict work potential and conversely that Calorie supplementation significantly increases work intensity and capacity.[55] The body, of course, has to work equally hard at coping with the limitations of a low Calorie diet whether that restriction is imposed because of a natural disaster food shortage or the fact that someone "chooses" to diet down to a smaller size. Research from poor countries indicates that the body does have adaptation mechanisms for adjusting to *permanently* restricted food intake but the body has a particularly chaotic job adjusting to great dietary fluctuations such as erratic food supply or yo-yo dieting.

What price do individuals and society pay for women's undernutrition caused by lifelong dieting? Hilde Bruch, psychiatrist respected for her groundbreaking work on eating disorders, describes "thin fat people" as people (usually women) who routinely eat less than their bodies require in order to stay at a weight which is artificially low for themselves. Very often these women are tense, irritable and unable to pursue educational and professional goals as a direct result of their chronic undernutrition. But, if they never allowed themselves to eat properly they do not recognize the signs that these limitations are due to undereating rather than personal weaknesses. Characteristic signs of malnutrition—fatigue, listlessness, irritability, difficulties in concentration and chronic depression—often escape correct professional diagnosis because the starved appearance (and especially average weight appearance in someone meant to be heavy) is a matter for praise rather than concern by our fatphobic society. "It has become customary to prescribe tranquilizers for such people; three square meals a day would be more logical treatment, but one that is equally unacceptable to physicians and patients because they share the conviction that being slim is good and healthy in itself."[56]

Is it possible that the relationship to food is sufficiently different between women and men that it helps determine gender differences in how women and men operate in the world? What if our scientific studies which "prove" that men are superior at performing certain tasks are actually measuring men's superior ability to fulfill their nutritional requirements rather than measuring task performing abilities? How would we even begin to start to think about or "measure" such things?

Claire Etaugh and Patricia Hill have started on some fascinating research to test their theory that gender differences in eating restraint (dieting) influence previously reported gender differences in cognitive restructuring tasks. Their initial study found that gender differences were in fact eliminated on one of two tasks when men and women were matched for eating restraint. On the other task, eating-restricted females performed the task more poorly than unrestricted females, thus exaggerating the male-female difference.[57] This work certainly confirms the need for eating restraint to be a factor which must be controlled in any study which attempts to measure gender differences. This research builds on previous work which showed that many differences found between fat and thin people are actually differences between restrained eaters (dieters) and non-restrained eaters (non-dieters). Even without further research, we know that some cognitive restructuring task gender differences disappear when dieting is controlled for and we know that dieting can result in poorer performance on a range of tests. What more proof do we need that dieting can prevent women from maximizing on their potential?

Although we have started to explore how the nearly universal pattern of men and boys getting fed more and better than women and girls can play a part in perpetuating women's inferior social and economic roles, it is hard to imagine all the many subtle and unnoticed ways in which this may manifest itself.

Hamilton, Popkin and Spicer suggest that nutritional status affects one's selection of work activities. Only well-nourished workers would be expected to qualify for the higher paying jobs if they are more physically or mentally demanding. Conversely, they suggest, individuals adapt to low energy intakes by being involved in less demanding occupations.[58]

Not surprisingly, most studies concentrate on nutrition-productivity relationships in men. Much less is known about the interaction of nutrition and productivity in women and, of course, even less is known about how nutrition affects women's roles outside the paid labour force. One study reported that supplementation of women's diets improves the mother-child interactions and enhances child development by providing women with greater energy and increasing their potential capacity for physical effort and active time for interaction with the children.[59] A study of Guatemalan peasants found that women who receive dietary supplements spent more leisure and market time in physically active tasks than women who did not receive supplements. Sixty-seven percent of the supplemented group were considered "fully active" compared to only five percent of the unsupplemented group.[60]

The long term and intergenerational costs of the malnutrition-low status relationship in girls is just starting to be recognized. It is now known that cognitive development is dependent on both adequate nutrition and intellectual stimulation. Ten year follow-up studies of children who were treated for severe protein-calorie malnutrition showed no significant difference in mental performance when compared to their siblings or controls. But, there was a strong correlation between their intellectual achievement and years of schooling. It was noted that malnourished children sometimes took a few years to recover from any mental consequences of early childhood malnutrition and that the normal curriculum might not be appropriate during that time. This finding has particular significance for girls since in many communities girls will have already been withdrawn from school before the recovery time and thus girls will be deprived of the educational opportunity even if they were lucky enough to be treated for malnutrition.[61]

Several studies have now demonstrated the crucial importance of female education as a factor contributing to lower child mortality even when family income is controlled.[62] These studies do not try to explain the complex mechanisms through which improved female education operates to reduce child mortality, but they help emphasize that women, their children, and society are deprived when women do not get to explore their educational potential.

The relationship of girls' undernutrition and girls' not being able to maximize on their mental development and educational capabilities obviously has enormous ramifications for what women can contribute to society, what women are expected or encouraged to do, and the recognition they are given for their achievements. We saw how a child's birth weight, and thus "good start in life", was influenced by the mother's height and weight which was affected by the grandmother's nutrition. We now see the vital link among childhood nutrition, female educational opportunities and child mortality. Although this may be two different ways of looking at similar information, it is also a reminder of how these social and economic factors work together and exaggerate each other.

Consequently, the low value of females can cause the mothers to feed boys better than girls so that boys are less apt to be malnourished and more likely to be capable of benefitting from, and having access to, educational opportunities. Boys will then be far more likely to be the "well-nourished workers to qualify for the higher paying, higher status, physically or mentally demanding jobs" than their undernourished sisters. In one generation, in one community, the pattern could be clear cut— the boys worked to their potential more than the girls and the boys have more status than their sisters. When the sisters have their own children, how equally will they distribute the food and will they be aware of the unequal distribution if they give more to their sons than their daughters? In the extreme Bangladesh example, women tended to deny unequal distribution except when male child preference was expressed in relation to marked food shortages or in reference to sex differentials with regard to food quality.[63]

Does this extreme but not exaggerated example give us clues to how this process may operate more subtly? Having seen that cognitive development is dependent on both adequate nutrition and intellectual stimulation and having seen gender differences disappear (in one test) when men and women were matched for eating restraint, what significance is there in the fact that many nine year old girls are now dieting? We know the physical abilities of girls and boys are pretty evenly matched until age 10–12 when social pressure discourages young women from developing their physical potential. We know that many girls excel in maths at an early age but then internalize the "girls aren't good at maths" idea by adolescence. In what ways do these messages which limit young women from maximizing on their potential now get exaggerated by the pressure on them (and their mothers) not to let themselves get fat?

A young woman's nutritional needs are among the highest of her life when she is 11–14 years: an average 100 pound girl uses up 2400 Calories a day and needs a very vitamin and mineral concentrated diet. This is also one of life's most crucial times for making educational decisions which will influence future choices. If individuals or society wish to improve the role of women in society, this is the worst possible stage for young women to start practicing their lives as "thin fat people"!

References

1. Judith Willis, "The Gender Gap at the Dinner Table", *FDA Consumer,* June, 1984, pp. 13–17.
2. 1989 RDA
3. Mary Roodkowsky, "Underdevelopment Means Double Jeopardy for Women", *Food Monitor,* September/October 1979, pp. 8–10.
4. Lisa Leghorn and Mary Roodkowsky, *Who Really Starve? Women and World Hunger,* New York: Friendship Press 1977, p. 20.
5. Colin Spencer, "Sex, Lies and Fed by Men", *Guardian,* November 4–5, 1989, p. 11.
6. Leghorn and Roodkowsky, *op. cit.*
7. E. M. Roenberg, "Demographic Effects of Sex Differential Nutrition" in N.W. Jerome, R.F. Kandel and G.H. Pelto (ed.) *Nutritional Anthropology—Contemporary Approaches to Diet and Culture,* Redgrave Publishing Co. 1980, pp. 181–203.
8. Charmian Kenner, *No Time for Women—Exploring Women's Health in the 1930s and Today,* London: Pandora 1985, p. 8.
9. Hilary Land, "Inequalities in Large Families: More of the Same or Different?" in Robert Chester and John Peel (ed.) *Equalities and Inequalities in Family Life,* New York: Academic Press 1977, pp. 163–175.
10. Hilary Graham, *Women, Health and the Family,* Brighton, Sussex: Wheatsheaf Books 1984, pp. 120–135.
11. Ruth Sidel, *Women and Children Last—The Plight of Poor Women in Affluent America,* New York: Viking 1986, p. 149.
12. E. Evason, *Just Me and the Kids: A Study of Single Parent Families in Northern Ireland,* Belfast: EOC 1980, p. 25, quoted in Graham, *op. cit.*
13. "Food for All?" *London Food News,* no.4-Autumn 1986, p. l.
14. D. Marsden, *Mothers Alone: Poverty and the Fatherless Family,* Harmondsworth, Middlesex: Penguin 1973, p. 43, quoted in Graham, *op.cit.*
15. Neil Gallagher, "Obstacles Curb Efforts to Improve Nutrition", *World Food Programme Journal,* no.3, July–September, 1987, pp. 19–22.
16. Judit Katona-Apte, "Women and Food Aid—A Developmental Perspective", *Food Policy,* August, 1986, pp. 216–222.
17. Paul Fieldhouse, *Food and Nutrition: Customs and Culture,* London: Croom Helm 1986, pp. 168–169.
18. *Ibid.,* pp. 41–54.
19. *Ibid.*
20. Betsy A. Lehman, "Fighting the Battle of Freshman Fat", *The Boston Globe,* September 25, 1989, pp. 23,25.
21. Joan Price, "Food Fixations and Body Biases—An Anthropologist Analyzes American Attitudes", *Radiance,* Summer 1989, pp. 46–47.
22. See for example the excellent resources of the Institute for Food and Development Policy, 1885 Mission Street, San Francisco, CA. 94103 (USA) or Oxfam, 274 Banbury Rd., Oxford OX2-7DZ (England).
23. Kathleen Newland, *The Sisterhood of Man,* London: W.W. Norton 1979, pp. 47–52.
24. Sahni Hamilton, Barry Popkin and Deborah Spicer, *Women and Nutrition in Third World Countries,* South Hadley, Massachusetts: Bergin and Garvey Publishers 1984, pp. 22–26.
25. United Nations Administrative Committee on Coordination—Subcommittee on Nutrition, *First Report on the World Nutrition Situation,* Rome, Italy: FAO Food Policy and Nutrition Division 1987, pp. 36–39.
26. UNICEF News Fact Sheet printed in Leghorn and Roodkowsky, *op. cit.*
27. Hamilton, Popkin and Spicer, *op. cit.* p. 55.
28. Shushum Bhatia, "Status and Survival", *World Health,* April, 1985, pp. 12–14.
29. Physician Task Force on Hunger in America, *Hunger in America—The Growing Epidemic,* Middletown, Connecticut: Wesleyan University Press 1985, pp. 119–120.
30. Newland, *op.cit.*
31. Ethel Sloane, *Biology of Women,* 2nd Edition, New York: John Wiley 1985, pp. 122–123.
32. J. P. W. Rivers, "Women and Children Last: An Essay on Sex Discrimination in Disasters", *Disasters,* 6(4), 1982, pp. 256–267.
33. Amartya Sen, "The Battle to Get Food", *New Society,* 13 October, 1983, pp. 54–57.
34. Lincoln C. Chen, Emdadul Huq and Stan D'Souza, "Sex Bias in the Family Allocation of Food and Health Care in Rural Bangladesh", *Population and Development Review,* vol. 7, no. l, March, 1981, pp. 55–70.
35. Newland, *op. cit.*
36. Bhatia, *op. cit.*
37. Chen, Huq and D'Souza, *op. cit.*
38. Priyani Soysa, "Women and Nutrition", *World Review of Nutrition and Dietetics,* vol.52, 1987, pp. 11–12.
39. Discussions with Chinese health workers and the All China Women's Federation, March 1978 and March 1983.

40. Victor W. Sidel and Ruth Sidel, *A Healthy State—An International Perspective on the Crisis in United States Medical Care,* New York: Pantheon 1977, p. 15.
41. Jeannette Mitchell, *What Is To Be Done About Illness and Health?* Harmondsworth, Middlesex: Penguin 1984, p. 22.
42. Soysa, *op. cit.*
43. Sidel and Sidel, *op. cit.,* p. 26,
44. Physician Task Force on Hunger in America, *op. cit.,* p. 99.
45. Melanie Tervalon, "Black Women's Reproductive Rights" in Nancy Worcester and Mariamne H. Whatley (ed.) *Women's Health: Readings on Social, Economic and Political Issues,* Dubuque, Iowa: Kendall/Hunt 1988, pp. 136–137.
46. Sidel and Sidel, *op. cit.,* p.17.
47. Physician Task Force on Hunger in America, *op. cit.,* p. 109.
48. Kenner, *op. cit.,* p. 10.
49. *Ibid.,* p. 8.
50. Ester, Boserup, *Women's Role in Economic Development,* London: George Allen and Unwin 1970, p. 165 quoted in Barbara Rogers, *The Domestication of Women—Discrimination in Developing Societies,* London: Tavistock 1981, p. 155.

51. Hamilton, Popkin and Spicer, *op. cit.* p.45.
52. Ellen McLean, "World Agricultural Policy and Its Effect on Women's Health", *Health Care for Women International,* vol.8, 1987, pp. 231–237.
53. Hamilton, Popkin and Spicer, *op. cit.,* pp. 20– 21.
54. Soysa, *op. cit.,* pp. 35–37.
55. Hamilton, Popkin and Spicer, *op. cit.*
56. Hilde Bruch, "Thin Fat People" in Jane Rachel Kaplan (ed.) *A Woman's Conflict—The Special Relationship Between Women and Food,* Englewood Cliffs, New Jersey: Prentice-Hall 1980, pp. 17–28.
57. Claire Etaugh and Patricia Hall, "Restrained Eating: Mediator of Gender Differences on Cognitive Restructuring Tasks?", *Sex Roles,* vol.20, nos.7/8, 1989, pp. 465–471.
58. Hamilton, Popkin and Spicer, *op. cit.*
59. *Ibid.*
60. *Ibid.*
61. Soysa, *op. cit.,* pp. 13–14.
62. Chen, Huq and D'Souza, *op. cit.*
63. *Ibid.*

Fatphobia

by Nancy Worcester

We learn not to like fat people, then we internalize that as anxiety of gaining weight ourselves or self-hatred if we are already overweight. Both English and American studies consistently show that excess body fat is the most stigmatized physical feature except skin color.[1,2] Fatphobia differs from racism in that being overweight is thought to be under voluntary control. Anti-fat attitudes are well established before a child reaches kindergarten. "Even at that young age, children attribute negative characteristics to the heavy physique, do not want to be like that themselves, and choose a greater 'personal space distance' between themselves and a heavy child than from other children."[3]

The animosity towards fat people is such a fundamental part of our society, that people who have consciously worked on their other prejudices have not questioned their attitudes towards body weight. People who would not think of laughing at a sexist or racist joke, ridicule and make comments about fat people without recognizing that they are simply perpetuating another set of attitudes which negatively affect a whole group of people.

The pressure to look like the "ideal" is so strong that we do not question the implications behind teaching that routinely instructs young women on how to make their bodies look "as perfect as possible". Home economics classes teach young women that horizontal stripes make one look wider, vertical stripes make one look thinner. I was so well socialized by such instruction that I still find it hard to be comfortable in horizontal stripes, unless, of course, they are strategically placed so as to make the chest look larger! Even after years of criticizing the pressure on women to look thin, instead of admiring a large woman who has the courage to wear the "wrong" stripes, I still find myself wondering, "But, doesn't she know . . . ?"

Although the prejudice against fat people affects both men and women, its impact is most exaggerated on women and their lives. Women put on body fat more easily than men for a number of social and physiological reasons. Of course, every topic in this book is a part of the explanation. The physical abilities of females and males are identical until puberty, but by that time socialization in most western cultures discourages physical fitness in young women thus encouraging weight to be put on as fat rather than as muscle. (At the age of 25, body fat content averages 14% for men and 23% for women.[4]) Although both females and males have a mixture of the sex hormones estrogens and androgens, the average female tends to have higher levels of estrogens than androgens and this influences the deposition of fat. Times of hormonal changes, adolescence, going on oral contraceptive pills, pregnancy, and menopause, are all times when some women notice that they put on fat easily.

Women are judged by appearance far more than men and a much wider range of sizes and shapes is considered attractive in men. For example, a 1982 study of the most popular North American television programs, found that of male characters, less than one-fifth were slim and more than one-quarter were plump, whereas of the female characters, over two-thirds were slim and only one-tenth were plump.[5] Women, not men, are bombarded with information that the size and shape of their bodies is central to who they are and if it is less than perfect they should be working to try to change it. Comparing the most popular of men's and women's magazines, we see that articles and advertising relating to body weight and dieting appear 17 times more often in women's magazines.[6]

At any moment in history, the ideal female figure is quite precisely defined. Studies have shown that both men and women judge women's bodies by how closely they measure up to that supposed ideal. The more a woman deviates from that 'norm', the more her appearance will adversely affect her social life, her acceptance at college, her employment, and her status.

In both England and North America, obesity is more common in working class women than in women of higher socio-economic groups. With men, the relationship of class and body weight is not so well defined.[7,8]

It seems relevant to suggest that the relationship between social class and obesity is not as simple as just the fact that poor people have less access to healthy, non-fattening foods. It is *both* poor women and men who have less access to these foods so we would expect that the relationship of class to obesity to be more consistent for both women and men. I am not convinced that differences in manual labor provide an explanation. (It has been suggested that working class men offset a tendency to obesity by doing more physical labor than middle class men. This explanation does not take into account that middle class men have more access to leisure exercise opportunities and facilities than do working class men and that working class women are also more likely to be involved in physically active jobs than middle class women.)

Is it possible that in our society a woman's body build is a factor in *determining* her socio-economic status? Nearly twenty years ago, a paper on the stigma of obesity concluded that, "Obesity, especially as far as girls is concerned, is not so much a mark of low social economic status as a condemnation to it."[9] A study of 1660 adults in Manhattan observed that overweight women compared to non-obese women are far less likely to achieve a higher socio-economic status and are much more likely to have a lower socio-economic status than their parents.[10] This relationship was not found in men. A now classical study of the late 1960's found that non-obese women were more likely to be accepted for college than obese women even though the obese and non-obese women did not differ on intellectual ability or percentage who applied for college admission.

> If obese adolescents have difficulty in attending college, a substantial proportion may experience a drop in social class, or fail to advance beyond present levels. Education, occupation, and income are social-class variables that are strongly interrelated. A vicious circle, therefore, may begin as a result of college admission discrimination, preventing the obese from rising in the social-class system.[11]

As long as women are valued and rewarded for their roles as sex objects, and the non-skinny woman is not seen as fitting this image, it is easy to see how the stigma of excess weight limits a woman's status through job discrimination, apparently less marriage to high-status men (sic!) and fewer social and economic opportunities. The discrimination against fat women should serve as a reminder to all of us that we need to change the basis upon which the worth of all women is determined by society. Tragically, instead of viewing fatphobia as *society's* problem, many women internalize the fear and intolerance of fat as their *individual* problem. Instead of trying to change the world, women end up trying to change themselves.

> In this era, when inflation has assumed alarming proportions and the threat of nuclear war has become a serious danger, when violent crime is on the increase and unemployment a persistent social fact, 500 people are asked by pollsters what they fear the most in the world and 190 of them answer that their greatest fear is 'getting fat'.[12]

References

1. S. J. Chetwynd, R. A. Stewart, and G. E. Powell, "Social Attitudes Towards the Obese Physique" in Alan Howard (ed.) *Recent Advances in Obesity Research: 1,* London: Newman Publishing 1975, pp. 223–225.

2. Susan C. Wooley and Orland W. Wooley, "Obesity and Women—I. A Closer Look at the Facts", *Women's Studies International Quarterly,* vol. 2, 1979a, pp. 69–79.

3. Orland W. Wooley, Susan C. Wooley, and Sue R. Dyrenforth, "Obesity and Women—II. A Neglected Feminist Topic", *Women's Studies International Quarterly,* vol. 2, 1979b, pp. 81–92.

4. Marion Nestle, *Nutrition in Clinical Practice,* Greenbrae, California: Jones Medical Publications 1985, p. 222.

5. Brett Silverstein, *Fed Up—The Food Forces That Make You Fat, Sick and Poor,* Boston: South End Press 1984, p. 107.

6. Silverstein, *op. cit.*

7. Wooley, 1979b, *op. cit.*

8. J. Yudkin, "Obesity and Society", *Biblthca Nutri Dieta,* vol. 26, 1978, p. 146.

9. W. J. Cahnman, "The Stigma of Obesity", *Sociological Quarterly,* vol. 9, 1968, pp. 283–299, quoted in Wooley, 1979b, *op. cit.*

10. P. B. Goldblatt, M.E. Moore, and A. J. Stunkard, "Social Factors in Obesity", *Journal of the American Medical Association,* vol. 192, 1965, pp. 1039–1044.

11. H. Canning and J. Mayer, "Obesity—Its Possible Effect on College Acceptance", *New England Journal of Medicine,* vol. 275, 1966, pp. 1172–1174.

12. *San Francisco Chronicle,* January 17, 1981, quoted in Kim Chernin, *Womansize—The Tyranny of Slenderness,* London: The Women's Press 1983, p. 23.

Mental Health Issues Related to Dieting

by Nancy Worcester

The assumption is that if anyone is overweight they must be trying to lose weight and if they are not trying to lose weight, they certainly should be. The slimming industry has sold us this assumption and it is time that we stop swallowing it. The dieting experience is pretty disastrous for many women. We need to be more aware of the mental hazards of slimming and figure out ways to be more supportive of women who choose not to lose weight.[1] The more that women discover that they can live in large bodies without having to torture themselves with endless slimming diets, the less pressure there will be on all women to carve themselves down to smaller sizes.

1. Women Feel Guilty if They Are Not Slimming

The most liberating gift many women can give themselves is the decision that they are not going to try to lose weight. Until that decision is made, it is tempting to put off everything else and meanwhile dislike oneself both because of the fat itself and because the fat becomes symbolic of an unfulfilled goal.

As long as someone is thinking about changing her body, she is not going to be putting energy into learning to like her body the way it is.

As long as someone is postponing accepting and liking her body, there is a tendency not to work at making that body healthy and fit. This is a part of a self-perpetuating cycle. The more 'out-of-shape' one is, the more dissatisfying (and hard!) it is to undertake even ordinary exercise, the less exercise the body has the worse it feels and fewer calories will be burned up. This, of course, contributes to the tendency to gain weight and feelings of sluggishness.

See "We'll Always Be Fat But Fat Can Be Fit"[2] which takes a positive approach to accepting one's body weight and improving both mental and physical health (p. 341).

2. Dieting Makes a Person More Aware of Food

We have all heard of someone who works through lunchtime without realizing they have not eaten or the person who loses weight because they are too busy to eat regularly.

One of the primary purposes of food advertising is simply to keep food on the mind so that the consumer is aware of her appetite. Secondly, of course, advertising aims to influence which particular product is on the mind.

In much the same way, the very act of dieting works to keep food on the mind. The constant preoccupation with not overeating (or more often, not eating normally) makes food take on a new significance. Thus, paradoxically, the most unmanageable time to restrict food consumption is when one is consciously attempting to limit food intake. Can you imagine committed dieters working through a lunchtime without realizing it or being so busy that they did not eat regularly?

Old studies claimed that a difference between fat people and thin people was that fat people ate according to external cues—set meal times, attractive foods, social situation—whereas thin people ate in response to internal cues such as hunger signals. Thus, this explanation implied, thin people were less likely to eat more than their bodies needed. This work is now being reinterpreted.[3] It seems that dieting is a major factor in determining whether one responds to external or internal signals. A dieter cannot respond to internal cues saying she is hungry because dieting creates a state of almost constant hunger. The old studies simply overlooked the fact that fat people are far more likely to be dieting than thin people. Instead of looking at the differences between fat and thin people, researchers were looking at the differences between dieters (restrained eaters) and non-dieters (non-restrained eaters). Dieting makes people unable to listen to their own body signals.

Dieting may be responsible for setting up a vicious cycle which increases the need for further dieting. Once a dieter's restraint is broken, the dieter can easily move in the opposite direction and 'overeat'. Depression and anxiety are emotions likely to break a dieter's restraint. Yet, dieting itself can cause anxiety, depression, and apathy.[4]

In attempting to change food habits, we are embarking upon changing one of our most conservative behaviors, something often intricately related to our inner sense of security. Food habits are the last patterns to change even when a person is living in a new environment and living a new lifestyle, e.g., immigrant food habits often more nearly resemble the diet of the homeland than of the new country even years after settling.

Additionally, changing one's pattern of food consumption presents a uniquely arduous challenge in that one has to deal with it daily, at regular intervals throughout the day. Difficult though it is, someone who is concerned about their smoking or drinking habits may choose to give up cigarettes or alcohol. Someone concerned about their eating habits does not have the option of giving up food.

These problems are all distinctly exaggerated for a woman responsible for others. She does not have the luxury of escaping from thoughts of food. While trying to ignore her own preoccupations with food/hunger, she will need to be making grocery lists, shopping in environments filled with visions and aromas of food, preparing food, serving food to others, and then cleaning up after the meals.

Such a seemingly unappetizing task as clearing up after a meal can be an immense challenge for the dieter. Keeping food intake records for nutrition classes, my students with young children have often discovered that a high percentage of their calorie intake comes from cleaning up the children's plates. They find themselves constantly torn between their lines not to waste food and their waistlines.

A major reason why women are somewhat less successful at losing weight than men is because their domestic responsibilities are so directly contradictory to the optimum conditions for dieting. Responsibility for food preparation is the worst imaginable antidote for the diet-induced obsession with food.

3. Dieting Often Fails

Few people would encourage a loved one, a friend, or a professional client to embark upon an activity which they knew was destined for failure. Yet, knowing that most dieting fails (probably 90%–98% in the long term), people in all types of capacities are constantly advising and cajoling each other to "try to lose some weight", to check out the newest slimming gimmick, or to try the most recent best selling diet.

While it may be an overstatement to say that it is sadistic to encourage someone else to diet, it is time to acknowledge that it is often irresponsible to influence someone else to diet. The act of encouraging dieting needs to carry with it the obligation to support the dieter practically and emotionally through the challenges of the dieting process and to nurture the dieter if the attempt to lose weight is not successful. How many people would be willing to commit themselves to something so risky and potentially demanding? There would be far less pressure on people to diet if such pressure had to be accompanied by appropriate supportive commitments.

No one likes failure in any aspect of their life. Too often failure at dieting can take on a significance unexpected and unrecognized by the dieter and her friends. Media bombardment of fictitious slimming success stories completely nullifies the fact that only one to ten percent of dieting is "successful". Therefore dieting gets experienced as "something anyone should be able to do" and is not seen as a particularly ambitious goal. Failing at such a seemingly simplistic task can be especially disheartening.

Because of all the factors which influence body weight and the unpredictable ease with which one can or cannot lose weight, body weight is one of the most difficult areas of one's life to control. But, because body image is so central to a woman's self-image and confidence and is so related to her actual experiences in the world, a woman's inability to lose weight too often becomes symbolic for her of her failure to be in control of her own life.

4. Dieting May Be 'Successful'

If a woman is successful at losing weight, she will lose the advantages of being fat.

Advantages of being fat are imperceptible to most dieters. Yet having managed to lose weight, many women are shocked to discover that the expectations of a slim woman are different than those of a fat woman in this society. I have stopped being surprised by how regularly I meet women who have purposefully gained back weight because they found that "sexual attractiveness" and not being taken seriously as thin women were so problematic. *Fat Is a Feminist Issue* has been immensely popular because it explores the meaning of being fat or thin in our society and enables women to discover why they may be subconsciously choosing to stay fat.

> My fat says 'screw you' to all who want me to be the perfect mom, sweetheart, maid, and whore. Take me for who I am, not for who I'm supposed to be. If you are really interested in me, you can wade through the layers and find out who *I* am.[5]

Food can be an invaluable tool for relieving tension, coping with stress, or rewarding oneself. Successful dieting inevitably means changing those food habits that one has developed over a number of years. Additionally, the stress of dieting itself may undermine even the most well established coping mechanisms. Ingenuity is necessary in providing oneself with healthy alternatives to the role that food has played in keeping life in balance.

Education against child abuse is increasingly suggesting that adults hit a pillow or eat something to relieve tension involved in some adult-child interactions. This is a questionable and simplistic approach to decreasing child abuse, but it is a reminder of the role that food can play in defusing tension which could lead to physical violence or verbal confrontation with a child or an adult. Eating, even if that means overeating, will often be the healthiest way of dealing with immediate distress. We need to be alert to the dangers of dieting blocking that outlet.

There is also an obvious problem with the inverse relationship between cigarette smoking and weight. Women have been encouraged to use cigarettes as a means of weight control since the American Tobacco Company introduced the slogan "Reach for a Lucky instead of a sweet" in 1928.[6] Probably because of the way cigarette smoking affects metabolic rate, most people gain some weight when they stop smoking. Fear of weight gain is a major reason why women are less successful than men at quitting smoking.[7] Thus, lung cancer has now surpassed breast cancer as the leading cause of death in middle-aged women (in the US).[8] Women are paying with their lives for their success in keeping off a few pounds.

5. Suicide Is Less Common in Obese

A most intriguing figure never gets explained. Hidden near the bottom of all the charts showing the differences in mortality for obese and non-obese are the figures for suicide. Suicide rates are noticeably lower in both obese men and women. If obese and non-obese committed suicide at the same rate, suicide rates for obese would be recorded as 100% of actual expected deaths. Instead, the figure is only 73% for obese women and 78% for obese men.[9]

There seems to be at least one mental health advantage of obesity that is overlooked and not understood.

References

1. Many of the ideas in this section have grown out of discussions of *Fat Is a Feminist Issue* with students and women's groups. (Susie Orbach, *Fat Is a Feminist Issue,* London: Paddington Press, 1978.)
2. Carol Sternhell, "We'll Always Be Fat But Fat Can Be Fit", *Ms,* May, 1985, pp. 66–68 and 142–154.
3. William Bennett and Joel Gurin, *The Dieter's Dilemma,* New York: Basic Books, 1982, pp. 34–45.
4. Valerie S. Smead, "Anorexia Nervosa, Bulimarexia, and Bulimia: Labeled Pathology and the Western Female", *Women and Therapy,* vol. 2, no. 1, 1983, pp. 19–35.
5. Susie Orbach, *Fat Is a Feminist Issue,* London: Paddington Books, 1978, p. 21.
6. Bennett and Gurin, *op. cit.,* pp. 92–93.
7. Bobbie Jacobson, *The Ladykillers—Why Smoking Is a Feminist Issue,* London: Pluto Press, 1981, pp. 14–15.
8. *1986 Cancer Facts and Figures,* American Cancer Society, 90 Park Avenue, New York, N.Y. 10016.
9. Jean Mayer, "Obesity" in Robert S. Goodhart and Maurice E. Shils (ed.) Febiger Press, 1980, pp. 721–740.

We'll Always Be Fat But Fat Can Be Fit

by Carol Sternhell

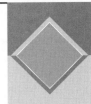

Sometimes I think we've all gone crazy. Sometimes I feel like a feminist at a Right-to-Life conference, an atheist in Puritan New England, a socialist in the Reagan White House. Sometimes I fear that fat women have become our culture's last undefeated heretics, our greatest collective nightmare made all too-solid flesh. I worry—despite our new ethos of sexual freedom—that female bodies are as terrifying and repulsive as ever, as greatly in need of purification and mortification. Certainly these days, when I hear people talking about temptation and sin, guilt and shame, I know they're referring to food rather than sex. When my friend Janet calls me up and confesses "I was bad today," I don't wonder whether she committed adultery (how archaic that sounds!); I know she merely means she ate dessert. When posters quoting Mae West appeared recently on Manhattan buses ("When choosing between two evils, I always like to take the one I've never tried before"), I wasn't surprised to find her remark illustrated with a picture of two different ice cream sundaes. (As I recall, however, when Mae West talked about evil, she generally wasn't thinking of hot fudge.) Kim Chernin, in *The Obsession: Reflections on the Tyranny of Slenderness* (Harper & Row), compares the language of diet books to "The old fire-and-brimstone sermons, intended to frighten men and women away from the delights and pleasures of sexual experience of their bodies." The sins of the flesh have been redefined, but the message is the same; a tremendous fear that women's natural appetites, uncontrolled, will bring about destruction.

Everything in this world, for women, boils down to body size.

We all know the story—the ugly duckling transformed into swan after years of liquid protein, the virtuous but oppressed stepdaughter whose fairy godmother appears with a pumpkin and a lifetime membership in Weight Watchers. Our fantasies of transformation are desperate, thrilling; when women imagine changing our lives, we frequently begin with our weight. "I always feel as if real life will begin tomorrow, next week, some-

time after the next diet," said one friend, a talented writer who has been cheerfully married for 12 years and a mother for five. "I know it's crazy, but I won't be happy until I lose these fifteen pounds." So far her efforts—like 98 percent of all diets—have been unsuccessful. A few years ago, when public opinion pollsters asked respondents to name their greatest fear, 38 percent said "getting fat." Even very slender women believe that their lives would be better if only they could take off five pounds, or three, or two. In a recent survey conducted for *Glamour* by Susan Wooley, an associate professor in the psychiatry department of the University of Cincinnati College of Medicine, 75 percent of the 33,000 women who replied said that they were "too fat," including, according to Wooley, "45 percent who in fact were underweight," by the conservative 1959 Metropolitan Life Insurance Company Height and Weight Table. (By the revised 1983 table, which set generally higher levels of up to 13 pounds for desirable weights, these women would be even more underweight.) Wooley, who is also codirector of the university's Eating Disorders Clinic, sees our contemporary obsession with weight in part as a perversion of feminism. "This striving for thinness is striving to have a more masculine-type body," she points out. "As we join men's worlds, we shouldn't be cashing in women's bodies. We have to reclaim the right to have female bodies and still be respected. Thinness has become the cultural symbol of competency—if we buy that symbol and foster it ourselves, that's a very self-mutilating stand to take."

Everything in this world, for women, boils down to body size.

Cinderella's unfortunate stepsisters cut off chunks of their feet in order to fit into the prince's slipper. He knew they were impostors when he saw their blood oozing insistently over the delicate glass. These days women merely wire their jaws, staple their stomachs, and cut off chunks of their intestines in their effort to win the prince. "Stomach stapling" operations—50,000 are reportedly performed each year, 80 to 95 percent of

---

Reprinted with permission from *Ms.* Magazine, May, 1985, pp. 66–68; 141–154.

them on women—can have side effects, such as abdominal pain, severe malnutrition, nausea and vomiting, osteoporosis, brain damage, and possibly even cancer. "Weight-loss surgery, including intestinal bypass operations, has probably already killed well over a hundred times as many people as the toxic shock syndrome, and has caused more than ten times as many deaths as AIDS," notes Paul Ernsberger, a postdoctoral research fellow at Cornell University Medical College. "More Americans have died in the surgeons' War on Fat than died in the Vietnam War." Yet desperate fat women—veterans of Stillman and Atkins, Scarsdale and Beverly Hills, diet camps and amphetamines—gratefully welcome the surgeon's knife, perhaps dreaming of old fairy tales. "I sometimes wish I had cancer," said a large, pretty woman in her early twenties at a diet workshop I once attended in San Francisco. "I sometimes think I wouldn't mind dying, if only I could die thin."

Everything in this world, for women, boils down to body size.

I still remember those little girls drinking diet soda and waiting for the miracle. I was 14 years old and 145 pounds that summer, at Camp Stanley for overweight girls, but many of the campers were younger, chubby little kids who already knew their bodies were their shame. When some of us failed to lose weight even on the camp's low-calorie regime, we were put on a special plan: three scoops of cottage cheese a day and all the diet soda we could drink. I remember the hunger (I would roll my pillow up under my stomach at night, trying to fill the hollow so I could sleep), the dizziness, but also the exhilaration; I felt like a secular saint, virtuous, disembodied, utterly pure. We sat around, starving, and talked about food, food we recalled from our profligate pasts. We talked about the new lives we would inhabit in the fall, transmuted all into magical swans.

I lost 15 pounds that summer and felt quite swanlike for a while, particularly among my relatives, who often seemed to admire weight loss the way other families might esteem an Olympic medal. By Christmas, however, when a group of campers gathered for a mini-reunion, every one of us had recouped our loses, and then some. We talked about the new lives we would inhabit in the spring, after the next diet had made us swans.

After the next diet, of course, most of us were fatter than before. Not only do almost all diets fail; according to Kim Chernin, "ninety percent of those who have dieted 'successfully' gain back more than they ever lost." This is not because "overweight" people are weak-willed compulsives, unable to pull our faces out of the Haagen-Dazs. (The medical profession may still disagree, but the medical profession, remember, once advised women that our reproductive organs would shrivel if we made the mistake of obtaining a higher education.) In fact, observes Wooley, "On the whole fat people eat no more than thin people—often women who believe they're compulsive eaters are trying to deny the need to eat at all." The one thing fat women do more than other people is diet—and continual dieting, we now know, actually causes weight gain. "Repeated starvation can encourage fatness at the same time it destroys somebody's health," explains Ernsberger. "Cutting calories turns out to be the great fattener. The body—threatened with famine—overcompensates and creates new fat cells when normal eating is resumed. The cells may even double in number, and these new fat cells are forever. The body can now store more fat—the next diet will be harder."

A decade or so after my summer at Camp Stanley, I failed at a much more ambitious diet. This time I felt like a swan humiliatingly transformed into an ugly duckling. Even worse, I felt like a criminal; I was wearing my scarlet letter for all to see. My shame was intense—but as Wooley has remarked, "If shame could cure obesity, there wouldn't be a fat woman in the world."

During this period while attending graduate school in California, I sampled a variety of weight-loss groups. Two in particular were so disturbing that they made me question for the first time my own obsession with slimness. At the first, an Overeaters Anonymous meeting in Palo Alto, a depressed group of middle-aged people—mostly large and mostly women—sat on uncomfortable chairs in a chilly church basement and acknowledged that they were helplessly controlled by food. Only the aid of their "Higher Power" could save them, they agreed. At the height of the meeting one sad, gray-haired woman got up to tell us that she "really was shit." She didn't understand why, now that she'd lost weight, her husband had left her, but she said she was sure it must be for the best because everything—of course—was part of her Higher Power's plan. She said again and again that without the guidance of her HP she was "a piece of shit," and many group members murmured that they were too.

Then, in a San Francisco workshop ironically titled "Fat Liberation"—a supposedly progressive approach to weight loss in which participants "got in touch" with their feelings about fat and food—a group of women, almost all slender (but feeling fat), sat in a circle and imagined meeting a fat person in the street. "You were huge, gigantic, obese," one women wrote, "a man or a woman, androgynous in fat. I feel uncomfortable around you, and guilty. I avoid looking at your body, I feel sorry for you, threatened—you don't have to look like that. Under the surface you have nothing. I follow you to a dark room; you go in alone and sit. I leave you sitting there in the dark. When I leave, I am happy, whistling." We then sat on the floor and told a pile of food that it couldn't scare us any more.

After this workshop I bought a new political button: "How Dare You Presume I'd Rather Be Thin?" I've never had the nerve to wear it.

Fat women are continually told to lose weight in order to improve our health—but, in fact, we are likely to damage our health while trying to lose weight. Women don't drink liquid protein, pour saccharin in our coffee, and staple our stomachs in order to be healthy; instead, women risk death in order to be thin. According to Dr. Faith Fitzgerald of the University of California at Davis, "Obesity, as we commonly use the term, may be more of an aesthetic and moral problem than one of physical health." Certainly our horrified revulsion at the sight of a fat body springs from deeper sources than a disinterested concern for that body's well-being. If it did, the billions of dollars poured into the diet industry each year would be transferred to an anti-smoking campaign.

"In general, the healthiest eaters we see are fat women," adds Susan Wooley. "Most would have to be on a starvation diet their whole lives to get them down to a weight the culture considers normal, and the physical and emotional effects of starvation are much worse than the effects of overweight."

Nevertheless, most Americans—including most medical professionals—believe that fatness and good health are antithetical. A panel convened by the National Institutes of Health recently proclaimed obesity a "killer" disease. The 14-member panel set the danger point at a level of 20 percent or more above "desirable" body weight, but said that even five to 10 pounds above recommended weights could pose increased health risks to those people susceptible to or suffering from diseases like high blood pressure, adult onset of diabetes, and some cancers. A woman of my height, five feet four, would be 20 percent overweight at about 160, 40 pounds less than I weigh. The health charge is disturbing. No one—however terrific, energetic, and attractive she may feel—wants to walk around with a "killer" disease.

According to Ernsberger, the NIH report is simply wrong. "Fatness is *not* associated with a higher death rate," he says. "In fact, in every given population examined, the thinnest people have the highest death rate." The new NIH panel "flatly contradicts" previous reports of the same data, the well-known Framingham Heart Study, he adds. "The fact is the very fattest women in Framingham had a lower death rate than women who were at their 'correct' insurance table weights." The heaviest Framingham women, ranging from 40 percent to 172 percent over the 1959 tables, had lower mortality than both underweight women and women within a few

pounds of their "desirable" weight. The *lowest* death rates, Ernsberger points out, occurred in women who were between 10 percent and 30 percent over the insurance tables. About 30 controlled studies correlating mortality and weight have reported similar findings. Dr. Ancel Keys of the University of Minnesota, a cardiovascular researcher, coordinated such studies in 16 different geographical areas with an emphasis on risk factors leading to heart attacks. He concluded that "in none of the areas of this study was overweight or obesity a major risk factor for death or the incidence of coronary heart disease."

"Cancer deaths actually decrease with increasing fatness," says Ernsberger. "Only one study, the study cited in the NIH report, showed an increase in cancer rates," he adds, "while five or six that I know of show a decrease with increasing fatness." The NIH panel chose to ignore the decreased overall cancer rate in obesity, mentioning only that a single type of cancer, uterine cancer, is more common in obese women.

Wooley concurs. "A person can definitely be fat and healthy," she says. "My reading of the literature tells me that for women there's a very sizable weight range in which extra weight does *not* constitute a risk in mortality." Wooley notes that some studies have shown that women can weigh up to 200 pounds, without increased mortality risks, and even after that point, she says, being overweight may be healthier than dieting.

Many of the health problems commonly associated with fatness are probably caused by fat people's incessant pursuit of thinness, Ernsberger points out. Thus the "yo-yo syndrome"—that deadly cycle of weight loss and weight regain—may cause hypertension; diet pills can also cause high blood pressure and amphetamine psychosis; low carbohydrate diets can raise cholesterol; and liquid protein diets have led to heart disease and sudden death. "We don't know how unhealthy overweight is in and of itself because most overweight people have been doing these things," Ernsberger comments.

Furthermore, fat people receive terrible health care, partly because doctors see them as "bad patients" and partly because the overweight person herself tends to give up in despair. "We've had it drummed into our heads that the *only* route to fitness is through weight loss," explains Nancy Summer, member of the board of directors of the National Association To Aid Fat Americans (NAAFA), a nationwide fat rights organization based in New York. Summer, a dynamic blond who weighs more than 300 pounds, swims twice a week on Long Island with a group of large women. "Many of us have developed an all-or-nothing attitude. If we can't be thin, we may as well not worry about nutrition or exercise—we are going to die young anyway. I think it's time we reject that concept."

The medical evidence may be contradictory—obesity "experts" may disagree—but the message to me as a self-accepting fat woman is fairly simple. People come in lots of different sizes, and our frantic struggle to squeeze—all of us—into the thinnest 10 percent of a once-normal bell-shaped curve is driving us all crazy (and at the same time making us fatter). Self-hatred and cultural stigmatization doesn't do anyone any good; indeed, many of the diseases frequently associated with overweight are stress-related illnesses. Even, if all the other things being equal, it is "healthier" to be thin, weight-reduction programs fail 98 percent of the time, according to Chernin. Therefore I have two choices: I can be fat and unhealthy or I can be fat and healthy. I can find a new miracle diet, or I can eat sensible food (fruit and veggies, fiber, not too much fat, sugar, or salt), avoid cigarettes, and get plenty of exercise.

I'll still be fat, but fat can be fit.

The six women flash brightly colored tights and leotards, shake to a driving rock beat, smile at their reflections in shiny mirrors, bend and stretch, tap some feet. It's just another Manhattan exercise class, but here all the women look like Rubens' models, ranging in size from perhaps 150 pounds to well over 200. At the Greater Woman, "New York's first exercise studio for the large woman," clients are expected to be at least 30 pounds over their "ideal" weight—some weigh nearly 300 pounds—but the program emphasizes fitness and self-esteem rather than weight loss.

"There's a great difference between fitness and skinniness," says Mary Sams, a family psychotherapist who heads the studio. "Women are told that fat is immoral, that everyone who is overweight is out of control, consuming massive amounts of food. That's garbage."

According to Sams, the purpose of Greater Woman "is not to get people to lose weight, but to help people become fit and healthy and change their feelings about themselves. A lot of women come here wanting to get thinner," she adds, "but three weeks into the program they're thinking entirely differently." Clients are likely to lose inches rather than pounds. "Over several months, their dress sizes may go down," says Greater Woman's nutritionist, Jeannette Harris, "but they don't see a decrease on the scale." "Fitness isn't a scale measurement," agrees Sams. "Our goal is to increase lean body mass and raise the metabolic rate." In order to accomplish this, the studio has developed exercise classes specifically tailored to the needs of larger women. "The only exercise that really increases metabolic rate is aerobics," explains Sams. "We have learned to choreograph aerobic dances that are very lively but don't involve pounding exercises, which put too much stress on the knees and back."

The class members I speak with seem genuinely enthusiastic, and sometimes amazed to find themselves moving about so vigorously. One, a psychiatric social worker who has lost 30 pounds in the last year, explains earnestly, "People don't come here to lose weight, just to feel human about their bodies."

Remember the old fairy tales, the ugly ducklings and crippled stepsisters and hungry little girls all waiting for their miracle? Well, it's not exactly the story I'd imagined, but my transformation finally took place. My chronicle has a happy ending, but it's an ending with a twist, for as Susan Wooley once remarked, "When it comes to weight, people can't accept a happy ending that leaves us different shapes and sizes. To me, a happy ending is when someone can accept her body as it is."

My fairy godmother showed up after all, but she didn't change my body: she changed my mind.

Resources

Shadow on a Tightrope: Writings by Women on Fat Oppression, edited by Lisa Schoenfielder and Barb Wieser, foreword by Vivian Mayer *(Aunt Lute Book Company. Iowa City).* The best feminist collection I know of on the subject of fat. Includes much material from the original Fat Underground, a feminist fat liberation group that formed in Los Angeles in 1973.

The Obsession: Reflections on the Tyranny of Slenderness, by Kim Chernin *(Harper Colophon Book).* A subtle, well-written, and sometimes brilliant dissection of our cultures' frenzied pursuit of thinness, and its terror of female flesh.

The Dieter's Dilemma, by William Bennett, M.D., and Joel Gurin *(Basic Books).* A thoughtfully presented and scientific case against dieting as a means of weight control.

Such a Pretty Face: Being Fat in America, by Marcia Millman, with photographs by Naomi Bushman *(Norton).* A sociologist's investigation of what it is like "to live as a fat person in our society." Much of the material is drawn from interviews with fat people and from observations of organizations like NAAFA and Overeaters Anonymous.

Fat Is a Feminist Issue: a Self-Help Guide for Compulsive Eaters, by Susie Orbach *(Berkley).* Some feminists have found Orbach's discussion helpful, but it disturbs me because its emphasis is still on achieving thinness. Here fatness is seen not as a sin, but as a means of adapting to a sexist society. When women learn better ways of coping with sexism, Orbach believes, they will become slim. She also makes the mistake of confusing fatness with compulsive eating. They are two distinctly different conditions.

Big & Beautiful: How To Be Gorgeous on Your Own Grand Scale, by Ruthanne Olds *(Acropolis Books).* A fashion guide for women size 14 and up.

BBW: The World's First Fashion Magazine for the Large-Size Woman. Six-issue subscription is $13 from BBW *(Suite 214. 5535 Balboa Blvd. Encino. Calif. 91316).* A fashion magazine published six times a year. BBW stands for Big Beautiful Woman.

NAAFA—The National Association To Aid Fat Americans (P.O. Box 43. Bellerose. N.Y. 11426). The country's premier fat rights organization, active since 1969. Call 516–352–3120 or write for information. Sponsors both political action and social events.

The Greater Woman (111 East 65 St., N.Y., N.Y. 10128; telephone: 212–737–4889). Exercise classes for the larger woman.

Weight and Health

Analyzing the Surgeon General's "Call to Action"

by Lynn McAfee and Pat Lyons

We'll begin with the good news about the Surgeon General's December 2001 "Call to Action to Prevent and Decrease Overweight and Obesity": This is the first government report on weight and health to conclude with a desire to create a future where the "social stigmatism (sic) associated with overweight and obesity is eradicated."[1] The bad news is that many of the report's recommendations work against such a future, and could instead dramatically increase the prejudice and discrimination fat people already experience. Furthermore, it relies on weight loss strategies with a consistent failure rate in excess of 90 percent. Women's health advocates need to read this report with a critical eye directed both to what it says and what it ignores.

What Is the Problem?

Much of the report focuses on fostering cultural changes that we agree are very positive: putting physical education back in the schools and making it accessible to all children; promoting healthier meals and snacks in schools; creating more opportunities for physical activities for adults in their communities and workplaces; and promoting healthy eating habits and food choices. Women's health advocates can play a leading role in implementing these strategies, which could certainly improve community health. But strong collaborative relationships and long-term public health funding commitments are also necessary, as the suggested strategies require challenging vested corporate interests of the food, soft drink, media, advertising and weight-loss industries, to name a few.

The underlying problem with the report is apparent in the title. While the strategies suggested might prevent the development of overweight and obesity in some people, they are unlikely to bring Americans' weight in line with the stringent standards of leanness identified as "healthy" by the National Institutes of Health. (See "The Great Weight Debate," The Network News, September/October 1998.) By defining weight as the problem and "preventing and reducing overweight and obesity" as the solution, the report ignores research over the past 40 years that has found sustaining weight loss to be nearly impossible.

Although the Surgeon General recommends that the 60 percent of the population now considered "overweight" try to attain weight loss of "only" 5-10 percent, what it doesn't mention is that, even at the best academic weight-loss centers, only about 10 percent of participants experience long-term success.[2] The report also ignores the health risks associated with repeated failed weight-loss attempts, including the risks to life and health exemplified by the Phen-Fen/Redux diet pill debacle.[3] Just because theoretically more people might benefit from weight loss doesn't make the treatments we have more successful.

A major concern about the increasing weight of the population is due to the rising rates of Type 2 diabetes. The report discusses the recent Diabetes Prevention Program (DPP), which showed that weight loss, a healthy diet and exercise helps prevent the development of Type 2 diabetes. However, the report fails to mention that the DPP research group attained only a 7 percent weight loss in a very intensive lifestyle intervention carried out by a top behavior-modification expert. Each person had regular meetings with her or his own case manager for several years, and was given gadgets such as pedometers along with nutrition classes and exercise opportunities. Motivated to be part of a highly structured clinical trial, these folks clearly were not the typical mom with two kids told by her doctor to lose weight and sent on her way. Unfortunately, the DPP trial did not separate the effects of exercise, diet composition and weight loss, so we really don't know to what extent any or all of these variables were responsible for preventing diabetes.

What about the person who tries to follow her doctor's advice and goes to a commercial weight-loss program? During several years of negotiations in a group put together by the Federal Trade Commission, the top diet industry programs refused to track their long-term results. Their lawyers sat across the table from consumer advocates and said: "We've all decided it would be too depressing for our customers to know failure rates are extremely high, so we're not going to track results." Outside groups that tracked results saw failure rates well in excess of 90 percent.

For that reason, we oppose the Surgeon General's repeated calls in this document to "create mechanisms for appropriate reimbursement for the prevention and treatment of overweight and obesity." The diet industry should not be reimbursed for anything until it commits to long-term follow-up studies of its programs and demonstrates greater success.

Reduce Weight Prejudice and Promote Health at Every Size

The "Call to Action" was released one year after the Surgeon General held a federal "listening session" that we both attended. At that session we raised concerns that this document would, like previous governmental health pronouncements, add to weight discrimination rather than ameliorate it. We were assured that would not happen. But the report recommends: "Inform employers of the direct and indirect costs of obesity." And "Create incentives for workers to achieve and maintain a healthy body weight." Weight discrimination in all areas of life is very well documented, none more so than in job discrimination. In a review of 28 studies on workplace bias, employers consistently stereotyped fat people as "lazy, lacking in self-discipline, less conscientious, less competent. . . ." One study showed that participants "displayed more negative attitudes toward overweight employees than ex-felons or ex-mental patients."[4] Into this negatively charged environment, the Surgeon General proposes telling employers how expensive it is to hire people they already view as inferior. It is difficult to fathom how this could possibly improve worker health.

We believe the best approach to improving the health of Americans of all sizes is to uncouple healthy lifestyle behaviors from weight loss. Studies show considerable health benefit in increasing an individual's social support, regular exercise and consumption of fruits, vegetables and fiber independent of weight loss. These health benefits are what should be stressed. Yes, these

activities could contribute to some weight loss or prevent weight gain in some people. But this can be seen as a byproduct, not the goal. When weight loss is the focus of success, and people adopt healthy behaviors but find that their weight loss stops at 5 percent, the healthy behaviors often stop when the weight loss stops. And even if a 300-pound person successfully loses the recommended 10 percent of her weight, the world will not treat her much differently.

And what about those people who say, "I'm thin; why do I need to eat broccoli or go for a walk?" Assuming that people are thin because they eat well and exercise is just as misguided as assuming that fat people eat too much and don't exercise. But the consequences are greater for fat people; thin people will not be denied jobs or health insurance. Assuming that we can assess a person's overall health just by looking at her or comparing her weight to a number on a chart is simply untrue and reinforces persistent weight prejudice.

As long-time advocates for the Health @ Every Size approach, we asked to be involved in the process of defining the Surgeon General's plan. But no one from an anti-weight discrimination advocacy group not funded by the diet industry was involved. We asked to see the document before it was released and were denied. Would any federal policy-making group addressing women's health issues refuse to include women advocates without an outcry? We think not.

Many of the recommendations in the "Call to Action" are healthy choices for everyone, fat or thin. If the Surgeon General really wants to see improved health in a world free of weight-related social stigma, we urge going back to the drawing board to rethink the problem and include anti-weight discrimination advocates in developing intervention approaches and public health policies. That is a future we could all applaud.

References

1. The Surgeon General's report can be obtained from *www.surgeongeneral.gov/topics/obesity*.
2. NIH Technology Assessment Conference Panel. "Methods for Voluntary Weight Loss and Control." *Annals of Internal Medicine* 1993; 119:764–760.
3. Mundy A. *Dispensing With the Truth: Behind the Battle Over Fen-Phen*, 2001. St. Martin's Press.
4. Roehling MV. "Weight-Based Discrimination in Employment: Psychological and Legal Aspects." Personnel Psychology 1999; 52, 969–107.

I'm Not Fat, I'm Latina

by Christy Haubegger

I recently read a newspaper article that reported that nearly 40 percent of Hispanic and African-American women are overweight. At least I'm in good company. Because according to even the most generous height and weight charts at the doctor's office, I'm a good 25 pounds overweight. And I'm still looking for the pantyhose chart that has me on it (according to Hanes, I don't exist). But I'm happy to report that in the Latino community, my community, I fit right in.

Latinas in this country live in two worlds. People who don't know us may think we're fat. At home, we're called *bien cuidadas* (well cared for).

I love to go dancing at Cesar's Latin Palace here in the Mission District of San Francisco. At this hot all-night salsa club, it's the curvier bodies like mine that turn heads. I'm the one on the dance floor all night while some of my thinner friends spend more time waiting along the walls. Come to think of it, I wouldn't trade my body for any of theirs.

But I didn't always feel this way. I remember being in high school and noticing that none of the magazines showed models in bathing suits with bodies like mine. Handsome movie heroes were never hoping to find a chubby damsel in distress. The fact that I had plenty of attention from Latino boys wasn't enough. Real self-esteem cannot come from male attention alone.

My turning point came a few years later. When I was in college, I made a trip to Mexico, and I brought back much more than sterling-silver bargains and colorful blankets.

I remember hiking through the awesome ruins of the Maya and the Aztecs, civilizations that created pyramids as large as the ones in Egypt. I loved walking through temple doorways whose clearance was only two inches above my head, and I realized that I must be a direct descendant of those ancient priestesses for whom those doorways had originally been built.

For the first time in my life, I was in a place where people like me were the beautiful ones. And I began to accept, and even like, the body that I have.

I know that medical experts say that Latinas are twice as likely as the rest of the population to be overweight. And yes, I know about the health problems that often accompany severe weight problems. But most of us are not in the danger zone; we're just *bien cuidadas*. Even the researchers who found that nearly 40 percent of us are overweight noted that there is a greater "cultural acceptance" of being overweight within Hispanic communities. But the article also commented on the cultural-acceptance factor as if it were something unfortunate, because it keeps Hispanic women from becoming healthier. I'm not so convinced that we're the ones with the problem.

If the medical experts were to try and get to the root of this so-called problem, they would probably find that it's part genetics, part enchiladas. Whether we're Cuban-American, Mexican-American, Puerto Rican or Dominican, food is a central part of Hispanic culture. While our food varies from fried plaintains to tamales, what doesn't change is its role in our lives. You feed people you care for, and so if you're well cared for, *bien cuidada,* you have been fed well.

I remember when I used to be envious of a Latina friend of mine who had always been on the skinny side. When I confided this to her a while ago, she laughed. It turns out that when she was growing up, she had always wanted to look more like me. She had trouble getting dates with Latinos in high school, the same boys that I dated. When she was little, the other kids in the neighborhood had even given her a cruel nickname: *la seca,* "the dry one." I'm glad I never had any of those problems.

Our community has always been accepting of us well-cared-for women. So why don't we feel beautiful? You only have to flip through a magazine or watch a movie to realize that beautiful for most of this country still means tall, blond and underfed. But now we know it's the magazines that are wrong. I, for one, am going to do what I can to make sure that *mis hijas,* my daughters, won't feel the way I did.

Making "a Way Outa No Way"

by Becky W. Thompson

Compulsive eating, bulimia, and anorexia have taken on complicated symbolic significance in late twentieth-century culture in the United States. Those suffering from eating problems invariably are thought to be young, middle- to upper-class, heterosexual white women desperately trying to mold their figures to standards created by advertisers and clothing designers. The most popular terminology used to describe these problems is "eating disorder," which suggests that some psychological frailty or inadequacy is the agent of the illness. In short, those suffering from eating problems are thought to be decadent, self-absorbed, and heavily implicated in their own troubles. Such conceptions are misguided, short-sighted, and harmful. They are built on skewed assumptions about race, class, and sexuality that belittle the putative victims—white, middle-class, heterosexual women—while they ignore women of color, working-class women, and lesbians.

Talking with Latina, African-American, and white women—including both heterosexual and lesbian women—reveals that the origins of eating problems have little or nothing to do with vanity or obsession with appearance. In fact, eating problems begin as survival strategies—as sensible acts of self-preservation—in response to myriad injustices including racism, sexism, homophobia, classism, the stress of acculturation, and emotional, physical, and sexual abuse. The women I interviewed for this book told me stories that starkly expose how eating problems often begin as an orderly and sane response to insane circumstance.

Their candid stories about how and why they turned to food to cope requires that the reader grapple with the idea of both subtle and overt injustices regularly visited upon women. Some of the experiences the women described are of outrageous, deliberate, and sometimes brutal acts that compromised their ability to feel safe—to be comfortable and sure—in their bodies and in the world. Their experiences reveal both how they developed eating problems and how their ingenious methods of healing are nothing less than testimonies of endurance and empowerment. Their creative strategies for carrying on with their lives—often against great odds—along with their dedication to healing their minds, bodies, and spirits, give yet another face to Minnie Ransom's wise words in Toni Cade Bambara's novel *The Salt Eaters:* "Wholeness is no trifling matter."

On a concrete level, then, the book explains why eating problems are logical, creative responses to trauma, and it identifies effective methods of healing. On a political level, the book posits that bingeing, purging, and starving will continue until women's access to racial, social, sexual, and political justice is ensured. On a more philosophical level, it suggests that women who face injustice have much to teach about faith and resistance, trauma and coping, creativity and despair. My hope is that the book does justice to the experiences of the women I interviewed, reinforcing their ability to—in the words of Richard Wright—"create a sense of the hunger for life that gnaws in us all, to keep alive in our hearts a sense of the inexpressibly human."

Origins of This Book

Embedded in public and medical perceptions of health and disease are metaphors created to explain, engage with, and sometimes dismiss illness. In her creative and expansive approach to scholarship, Susan Sontag has unpacked metaphors surrounding cancer, documenting how cancer has been regarded as a disease of the psychically defeated, the inexpressive, and the repressed. As a cancer patient herself, Sontag was enraged by how much "the very reputations of this illness added to the suffering of those who have it." In her later work, Sontag expanded this framework with her illuminating insights about AIDS, detailing how metaphors about illness reveal much about current states of social disease. She is particularly interested in illness metaphors that, she believes, are used to justify authoritarian rule and militarism. She traces the origins of these militaristic metaphors back to World War I in explanations about syphilis and tuberculosis. These afflictions were described as invasions of alien organisms to which the body responds with its own militaristic operation. While militaristic metaphors still predominate in descriptions about disease, particularly with regard to AIDS, the identity of the enemy has changed. In this shifting use of metaphors, the threat to supremacy is no longer Russia or communism; rather, it is domestic, a result of changing relations in an increasingly multicultural world. In a quintessential social constructionist analysis, Sontag roots conceptions of disease within their historical contexts, capturing public anxiety and political conflicts as they are projected onto human illness.

Like many illnesses represented in the public imagination—such as cancer and AIDS—eating problems are imbued with their own images. Among them is the image of anorexia and bulimia as transitory, self-inflicted obsessions developed by young women lost in their own worlds of fashion, scales, and calorie counting. The cost of the dedication to this idea is paid by those with eating problems, sometimes with their lives. While many know that Karen Carpenter's death was caused by anorexia, few are aware that she was only one of about 150,000 women who die of anorexia each year. More people die of anorexia in a year than died of AIDS in the Untied States from the beginning of the epidemic until the end of 1988. This comparison is not meant to minimize the tragedy of AIDS, but to uncover one of the most powerful popular assumptions about eating problems: that, although they are prevalent, they are decadent acts of self-obsession that are only in rare situations life threatening.

In 1984 I began to conduct workshops on eating problems among women and men, and, over time, I started to question this vexing portrayal along with the standard profile that has been attached to it. I soon saw that while many women fit the usual profile—white, middle and upper class, heterosexual—many did not. I began to look, largely in vain, for research about women of color and lesbians, and I resorted to incorporating any anecdotal evidence I could find. I cited, for example, Dinah Washington, the jazz singer whose untimely death resulted from a lethal combination of alcohol and diet pills; Oprah Winfrey, whose struggles with her weight have been followed by millions of television viewers; the multigenerational eating problems among African-American women in Gloria Naylor's *Linden Hills;* and poetry about anorexia by the prominent Puerto Rican writer Luz Maria Umpierre-Herrera. My friend Mary Gilfus, a social worker and sociologist who has worked in a women's prison, told me that many incarcerated women are bulimic. Other prison activists have also noted the widespread use of laxatives among women in prison. Prison policy supports the development of eating problems. Healthy food is rarely avail-

able; the meals are high in fat and starch, which makes it difficult not to gain weight. Because of severe restrictions on freedom of movement, the act of eating takes on an importance that makes incarcerated women vulnerable to bingeing. The fact that they are disproportionately African-American, Latina, poor, and working-class women raises further questions about the standard profile of women with eating problems.

My interest in women's health in general and my increasing frustration with the dearth of information on eating problems among women of color and lesbians led me to write this book. I conducted eighteen in-depth interviews with African-American, Latina, and white women with eating problems, which allowed me to scrutinize the standard profile and to develop a framework in many ways different from the one offered by the popular media and held by many researchers. Of the women I interviewed, two-thirds have had eating problems for more than half their lives—which counters the popular conception of anorexia and bulimia as transitional and temporary. The fact that the average age among the women I interviewed was thirty-three does not support the common belief that eating problems are primarily teenage problems. Several women were taught to diet, binge, and purge by older relatives—who had done so for years themselves—which suggests that eating problems may not be as historically specific as is typically thought. When eating troubles are seen as survival strategies rather than as responses to strictures about size and shape, they can be identified long before Twiggy's arrival on the fashion scene and Jane Fonda's exercise regimes.

A multiracial focus also raises questions about the adequacy of the theoretical models used to explain eating problems. The biomedical model offers important scientific research about possible physiological causes of eating problems and the physiological dangers of purging and starvation. However, this model adopts medical treatment strategies that may disempower and traumatize women, and it ignores many historical and cultural factors that influence women's eating patterns. The psychological model identifies eating problems as "multidimensional disorders" that are influenced by biological, psychological, and cultural factors. While it is useful in its exploration of effective therapeutic treatments, this model, like the biomedical one, tends to neglect women of color, lesbians, and working-class women.

A third model, offered by feminists, opened up the field of inquiry in crucial ways. With the emergence of feminist work, eating problems were rescued from the realm of individual pathology. When Susie Orbach's *Fat is a Feminist Issue* was published in 1978, its critique of dieting and self-denial and its convincing plea for understanding bingeing as a way women cope with living in a society that relegates them to second-class citizenship made it a handbook for thousands of women. This was one of many important books by therapists, sociologists, physicians, and researchers that focused on gender. The fact that most people with eating problems are women was no longer considered simply a factor in but rather integral to understanding anorexia and bulimia.

Feminist argue that patriarchy—which limits women's access to power both within and outside the family—is at the root of women's eating problems. Most women are relegated to sex-segregated jobs that pay them less well than men are paid for comparable work. What is typically referred to as the "glass ceiling" in employment is actually a euphemism for real men's bodies blocking most women's advancement. These barriers, coupled with educational systems that still steer girls away from mathematics, science, and competitive sports, help explain why adolescent girls' self-esteem declines as boys' self-esteem increases. In this context, eating problems signal women's many hungers—for recognition, achievement, and encouragement. It is no surprise that appetites and food take on metaphorical significance in a society in which women typically are responsible for food preparation and yet are taught to deny themselves ample appetites; girls are taught that the barriers they face are their own fault and therefore require individual solutions; and female socialization means caring for others, often at one's own expense.

Rightfully, feminists have raised questions about why the emphasis on dieting and thinness has become so severe. In her groundbreaking book *The Obsession: Reflections on the Tyranny of Slenderness,* Kim Chernin argues that in this historical period of women's increased struggle for economic, legal, and sexual power, one form of patriarchal backlash is defining female beauty as childlike and thin. Chernin writes, "In this age of feminist assertion men are drawn to women of childish body and mind because there is something less disturbing about the vulnerability and helplessness of a small child and something truly disturbing about the body and mind of a mature woman."

In the United States, this image is upheld by interlocking institutional powers: a multi-million-dollar weight-reducing industry in which most of the consumers are women; medical professionals who maintain the dubious assumption that fat is by definition unhealthy and ought to be eliminated; a multi-million-dollar advertising industry that promotes demeaning images of women; a job market in which women who do not fit this model of beauty face discrimination; and an insurance industry that upholds medically prescribed standards of what constitutes a healthy body size. A 1984 national poll of 33,000 women conducted by *Glamour* magazine found that the majority of women surveyed were ashamed of their stomachs, hips, and thighs—parts of the body that contribute to female shapes. The pressure to diet that many girls face from a very young age is an example of an assault aimed directly at the very parts of bodies that are decidedly female—as women throw up and out, excise or diet away breasts, hips, and buttocks. Feminists rightfully ask how different the quality of women's lives might be if the enormous energy they are taught to invest in denying themselves food were redirected toward dismantling sexism in all its many manifestations.

Feminists have also spearheaded research on the connections between eating problems and sexual abuse. In so doing, they have laid the foundation for understanding other traumatic origins of many eating problems. Identifying the functional basis of bingeing and purging helps take eating problems out of the realm of "disorder" and into the realm of coping mechanisms. As is true of feminist frameworks on the field of health in general, feminist research on eating problems has refused to diagnose them as individual psychic conflicts. Portraying them as individual "disorders" rather than as responses to physical and psychological distress is part of a historical tendency to mislabel the results of social injustices as individual pathologies. It is for this reason that some feminist theorists, including me, avoid using the term "disorder" altogether in relation to women's eating patterns, particularly since, for many women, bingeing, purging, and dieting begin as creative coping mechanisms in highly "disordered" circumstances.

Despite significant feminist contributions, scholarship typically has focused on gender to the exclusion of other analytical categories—specifically, race, sexuality, and class. This imbalance in the literature on eating problems mirrors similar exclusionary practices in much white feminist scholarship that bases its theoretical framework on a false universalism. In this way, scholarship on eating problems is not particularly behind in its lack of attention to race, sexuality, and class. Unfortunately, it mirrors health scholarship in general.

This research historically has failed to consider race a significant focus, often treating race or gender or both as "afterthoughts in analyses rather than main points of research studies." Until recently, research on cancer and alcoholism, for example, has paid little attention to African-American women, despite the fact that black women die of cancer far more frequently than white women do. The initial nomenclature for AIDS—gay-related immunodeficiency—identified an "at risk" population that erroneously excluded women and heterosexual men. Although women of color in the

United States are now the fastest-growing group infected with the HIV virus, government programs and most private agencies are still poorly equipped to respond to their health care needs.

Rethinking biased assumptions in the literature on eating problems begins with scrutinizing ideas about femininity and gender socialization. For example, the belief that women's bodily insecurities are fueled by lessons about femininity that teach women to be passive and complaint may accurately describe socialization patterns among middle- and upper-class Protestant white women, but this does not apply to many African-American and Jewish women, who are often encouraged to be assertive, self-directed, and active both within their families and publicly. Nor do passivity and dependence accurately describe lesbians and single, divorced, and widowed women who do not rely upon men for economic support and who tend to work in the paid labor market all of their lives. The notion that an institutional imperative toward thinness is a backlash against women's economic gains does speak to the advances of white middle-and upper-class women. But, as these women have been struggling to move up the occupational ladder, working-class women of all races have been striving simply to stay on the ladder—a ladder that, for them, has been horizontally rather than vertically positioned. While women of all classes and races are affected by a backlash Susan Faludi rightfully termed "the undeclared war against American women," the link some theorists draw between this backlash and augmented economic power is a race- and class-specific supposition that reinforces the association of eating problems with "achievement-oriented" business and professional women. Once again, anorexia and bulimia are rendered invisible among working-class women.

Similarly, the connection drawn between an increase in eating problems and "superwoman" expectations—as more women juggle careers and family responsibilities—accurately identifies changes in the participation of white middle-class women in the paid labor market. More middle-class white women are balancing two full-time jobs, but this double duty is not new for working- and middle-class women of color, lesbians, and single mothers. As white middle-class women have been fighting for the right to work outside the home, many black and Latina women have been fighting for the opposite: a chance to stay home with their children.

Race and class stratification breaks apart a singular reliance upon sexism as the underlying cause of eating problems. The women I interviewed linked the origins of their eating problems to many different types of trauma, many of which have received scant attention from researchers or the media. More than half of them—across race and class—were survivors of sexual abuse, which was often peppered with racism or anti-Semitism. Some women tied eating problems to a range of class factors, including poverty and stress caused by upward class mobility. Among the lesbians, some developed eating problems to cope with homophobia. Other traumas women linked to eating problems were emotional and physical abuse, often laced with racism, and witnessing abuse of siblings or parents.

The multiple traumas women link to their eating problems do not discount the important feminist analyses of the impact of sexist assaults against women's bodies and appetites. A multiracial focus, however, complicates the picture considerably. While feminists have shown how emotional, physical, and sexual abuse may lead women to binge or purge, little attention has been given to how inequalities besides sexist ones change women's eating patterns. Such a focus requires an expanded understanding of trauma that includes not only physical but also psychic injuries. In this way, trauma may include what Harriette McAdoo has termed the "mundane extreme environmental stress" of racism, injuries from poverty, incest and other sexual abuse, physical and emotional abuse, immigration, battery, heterosexism, and a variety of other socially induced injuries.

It is frightening to consider that the many extraordinary and harrowing accounts of trauma the women I interviewed identified may not, in fact, be uncommon. One African-American woman began bingeing when she was four years old because it gave her reliable comfort from the pain of sexual abuse, racism, and witnessing the battering of her mother. A white upper middle class Jewish woman attributed fasting for days on end to sexual and emotional abuse by her boyfriend. Pressed into isolation with the threat of further abuse, this woman began to think she deserved no pleasures—eating, seeing people, or even going out in the sunlight. She locked herself up in her dormitory room, sometimes even in her closet, and starved herself. A Latina woman described her body as a "shock absorber" that attracted the "world's pain," going back as far as she could remember. She ate to buffer herself from this pain. She remembered wondering at the age of five if an entire picnic table of hot dogs, hamburgers, chips, potato salad, and buns would be enough to fill her. Beset by emotional abuse and her relatives' constant criticism of her weight, she had little chance to understand either her body or her appetite as trustworthy or safe.

Identifying the traumatic bases of many eating problems reveals the dangers of labeling a common way women cope with pain as an appearance-based disorder. One blatant example of sexism is the notion that women's foremost worries are about their appearance— a belittling stereotype that masks women's worries about paying the bills, keeping their children off the streets and in school, and building loving and egalitarian relationships. By highlighting the emphasis on slenderness, the dominant imagery about eating problems falls into the same trap of assuming that difficulties with eating reflect women's "obsession" with appearance. This misnaming fails to account for the often creative and ingenious ways that girls and women cope with multiple hardships, quite frequently with no one's help but their own.

The culture-of-thinness model has also been used, erroneously, to dismiss eating problems among women of color based on the notion that they are not interested in or affected by a culture that demands thinness. This ideology lumps into one category a stunning array of racial and ethnic groups—Japanese-Americans, Chicanas, Hopi, Puerto Ricans, Amerasians, and African-Americans, to name just a few. The tremendous cultural, religious, and historical diversity among these groups of people makes the notion that they are—as a whole— invulnerable to eating problems dubious at best.

Emphasis on thinness is certainly not universal or equally tenacious across race and ethnicity. There are aspects of African-American culture, for example, that historically have protected against a demand for very thin bodies. In addition, festivities that take place when food is being prepared and eaten are key aspects of maintaining racial identity. Many black women writers, for example, include positive images of physically large women who enjoy food, and celebrate women of varying shapes and sizes. In fact, Alice Walker's definition of "womanist" includes a woman who "loves love and food and roundness." In her poem "Song for a Thin Sister," Audre Lorde also celebrates size and rejects the notion of thinness as an ideal:

Either heard or taught
as girls   we thought
that skinny was funny
or a little bit   silly
and feeling a pull
toward the large and the colorful
I would joke you   when
you grew too thin.

But your new kind of hunger
makes me chilly   like danger
I see you forever retreating
shrinking   into a stranger
in flight
and growing up
Black   and fat

I was so sure that   skinny
was funny   or silly
but always
white.

In her poetic voice, Lorde associates "skinny" with whiteness and a culture outside her own. One African-American woman I interviewed was raised in a rural community in Arkansas that valued women of ample proportions. One Puerto Rican woman was given appetite stimulants as a child because her mother thought that skinny children looked sickly.

This ethic did not, however, stop either of them from developing eating problems. In her chronicle about eating problems, Georgiana Arnold, an African-American health educator, identifies dual and conflicting patterns about food. While eating was a joyful part of family life, fat was a topic that the family avoided:

> In our home, food was a source of nourishment, a sign of love, a reward and the heart of family celebrations. It was also a source of ambivalence, guilt, shame, and conflict. Our "family fat" issues descended into the same cavern of silence that housed my father's alcoholism, gambling and willful disappearance from our lives. There was no talking about it and there were no tears.

Ironically, an ethic that celebrates food and protects against internalizing a value of thinness can work against identifying and getting help for eating problems. Furthermore, since there is no such thing as a monolithic "black community," any attempt to identify a single idea about weight, size, and food quickly breaks down.

A multiracial focus does not make the culture of thinness insignificant, but shows that its power needs to be understood in the context of other factors. For some girls, an imperative toward thinness initially has little or nothing to do with their eating problems. They link other social injustices to their eating difficulties. Furthermore, those who do internalize an emphasis on thinness also attribute other injustices to anorexia or bulimia.

By questioning the prominence of the culture-of-thinness model, I do not want to suggest that women avoid talking about their desires to be thin. Issues of appearance are essential currency for women's access to power in this country, and thinness is a critical component. While fat men are vulnerable to ridicule and discrimination, the standards are clearly gendered: being a fat woman is a far graver "mistake" than being a fat man. For white young women, thinness may, in fact, be the most powerful marker used to judge their physical attractiveness. But for women of color, body size is only one of many factors used to judge attractiveness. For older women of any race, the approval of thinness is countered by disdain for wrinkles and an aging body. For lesbians, cashing in on the power of thinness depends upon taking care not to look too "butch." Stereotypes aimed at lesbians of color who are not thin are a stark example of what Barbara Smith termed the "simultaneity of oppression." Nedhera Landers, a black lesbian who is fat, explains:

> My mere existence shows up society's lies in great relief. Being Black (and a chick) would eliminate my being fat. But since I am fat, young and childless, that must mean I'm a whore out of desperation for a man. But, since I am a lesbian and men aren't central to my life, that would eliminate my whore status. So, according to the current myths, I don't exist. When I assert my presence and insist that I am indeed fully present, I become an object of ridicule.

Ultimately, more troubling than what the reliance on the ideal of thinness reveals about health research is what it may signal about U.S. society in general: it speaks to a social inability to openly confront and deal with the results of injustice. In a country brimming with glorified images of youth, whiteness, thinness, and wealth, it makes painful sense that dissatisfaction with appearance often serves as a stand-in for topics that are still invisible.

In fact, it is hard to imagine what the world might be like if people were able to talk about trauma and the ways they cope with it with the same ease as they talk about dissatisfaction with their weight and appearance. The fact that Anita Hill was herself put on trial for testifying about sexual and racial harassment is a glaring indicator that much that we need to know about injustice and people's responses to it is still "unspeakable." The fact that more energy has been spent taking the hateful images of Public Enemy off the music racks—on the premise that the lyrics incite violence—than regulating the guns responsible for the death of thousands of young people is a glaring example of the politics of distraction. The Bush and Reagan administrations' use of the military term "vertical insertion"—a euphemism for the bombing and death of human beings—is a searing example of how language is used to hide violence and violation. In the words of Judith Herman, the "ordinary response to atrocities is to banish them from consciousness. Certain violations of the social contract are too terrible to utter aloud: this is the meaning of the word unspeakable." For a staggering number of women, atrocities done to them have been rendered unspeakable. In the place of this unuttered language are symbolic representations of their traumas— often manifested in unwanted eating patterns and supreme dissatisfaction with appetites and bodies.

Of course, not all women with eating problems have developed them to cope with trauma. The fact that 80 percent of fourth grade girls in one large study said they were on diets and that dissatisfaction with weight and size is in fact normative for women in the United States indicates the danger of such a sweeping generalization. A key distinction between periodic dieting and body disapproval and potentially life-threatening and long-term eating problems may be the history of abuse underlying them. Different exposure to trauma may distinguish a young girl who constantly worries about her weight from a woman for whom bulimia is the centerpiece of her day, a woman who occasionally uses liquid diets from a woman who, at eighty pounds, remains afraid to eat. Explicating possible distinctions like these would require examining trauma in different categories of women. This is a study yet to be done. But the experiences of the women whose lives form the basis of this book reveal that discomfort with weight, bodies, and appetite are often the metaphors girls and women use to speak about atrocities. To hear only concerns about appearance or gender inequality is to miss the complex origins of eating problems

The Politics of Invisibility

How were women of color and lesbians left out of media attention and research on eating problems in the first place, given that the stereotype of eating problems as a golden girl's disease is probably more indicative of which women have been studied than of actual prevalence? Certainly, the common reliance on studies conducted in hospitals, clinical settings, private high schools, and colleges skewed public perceptions of those most vulnerable to developing anorexia or bulimia. Basing theory on studies restricted to these locations has limited knowledge of women who are not in college, of women of color, of older women and poor women.

This skewed focus has long-term and potentially debilitating consequences. The stereotype that eating problems are "white girl" phenomena has led many highly trained professionals to either misdiagnose or ignore women of color. Maria Root explains that "social stereotypes of plump or obese Black, Latina or American Indian women may avert the therapist from examining any issues around food and body image. Similarly a thin, Japanese American woman may not be assessed for an eating disorder." When women of color are treated, their eating problems tend to be more severe as a result of delays in diagnosis. Among the women I interviewed, only two had been diagnosed bulimic or anorexic by physicians, yet all who said they were anorexic or bulimic fit the diagnostic criteria (DSM-111) for these diagnoses.

Given these realities, a more important question than *how* these groups of women have been made invisible may be *why* theorists and the media have been dedicated to stereotyped images of eating problems. The answer to this question lies in the way that ideology about black women's bodies has been invisibly inscribed onto what is professed about white women's bodies. In her work on biases in higher education curricula, Patricia Hill Collins explains, "While it may appear that the curriculum is 'Black womanless' and that African-American women have been 'excluded,' in actuality subordinated groups have been included in traditional disciplines through the groups' invisibility." Toni Morrison also offers essential tools for uncovering ideology about race and racism in literature, tools that apply well to developing race-conscious health research. In her groundbreaking essay "Unspeakable Things Unspoken: The Afro-American Presence in American Literature"—which she later expanded into the book *Playing in the Dark*—Morrison unravels the illusion that traditional literature in the United States has been "race free" or "universal," recognizing the presence of Afro-Americans, whether spoken or not, in the work of such well-known white writers as Melville, Poe, Hawthorne, Twain, Faulkner, Cather, and Hemingway, to name a few. Using Melville as a case in point, Morrison recognizes the presence of Afro-Americans and slavery in *Moby Dick,* pointing out that traditional American literature is both informed and determined by this presence. For Morrison, this analysis doubles the fascination and power of the great American writers. She warns us that "defending the Eurocentric Western posture in literature as not only 'universal' but also 'race-free' may have resulted in lobotomizing that literature, and in diminishing both the art and the artist." Avoiding future lobotomies, she writes, depends on excavating the "ghost in the machine"—the ways in which the "presence of Afro-Americans has shaped the choices, the language, the structure and the meaning of so much American literature."

Morrison's method of searching for the ghost in the machine of American literature can reveal substantial biases in research on women's mental health. This tool for theoretical excavation dredges up stereotypes of women of color, lesbians, and working-class women that not only are debilitating for these women but also ultimately backfire on white heterosexual women as well.

The portrayal of bulimia and anorexia as appearance-based disorders is rooted in a notion of femininity in which white middle- and upper-class women are presented as frivolous, obsessed with their bodies, and accepting of narrow gender roles. This representation, like the reputation of AIDS and some cancers, fuels people's tremendous shame and guilt about them. The depiction of middle-class women as vain and obsessive is intimately linked to the assumption that working-class women are the opposite: one step away from being hungry, ugly, and therefore not susceptible to eating problems. The dichotomy drawn between working-class and middle-class women reflects the biased notion that middle-class people create symbolic, abstract relations through their actions and thought while working-class people relate to the world in literal, concrete ways. Within this framework, middle- and upper-class women's eating patterns are imbued with all kinds of symbolic significance—as a way of rebelling against parents, striving for perfection, and responding to conflicting gender expectations. The logic that working-class women are exempt from eating problems, by contrast, strips away any possible symbolic significance or emotional sustenance that food may have or give in their lives. Recognizing that women may develop eating problems to cope with poverty challenges the notion that eating problems are class bound and confirms that both middle- and working-class women are quite capable of creating sophisticated and symbolic relations with food that go far beyond a biological need for calories.

Like biased notions about class, the belief that African-American women are somehow untouched by the cult of thinness is built on long-standing dichotomies—good/bad, pretty/ugly, sexually uptight/sexually loose—about white and black women. These divisions feed into an erroneous notion of black women as somehow separate from a society in which beauty standards are an integral part of the socialization of all women. The portrayal of white women as frivolous and obsessed with their appearance is linked to the presentation of black women as the opposite: as unattractive "mammies" who are incapable of being thin or who are not affected by pressures to be thin. With these multiple distortions, the fact that the dress and "look" of black youth have frequently set the standard for what constitutes style in the fashion industry is entirely unaccounted for.

In an autobiographical account, Retha Powers, an African-American woman, describes being told not to worry about her eating problems because "fat is more acceptable in the Black community." Stereotypical perceptions held by her peers and teachers of the "maternal Black woman" and the "persistent mammy-brickhouse Black Woman image" added to Powers's difficulty in finding people willing to take her problems with food seriously. The association of eating problems with "whiteness" has made some women of color unwilling to seek help. Getting help may feel like "selling out" or being treated as an oddity by friends or medical professionals. The racist underpinnings of some health care policies historically have also led some women of color to avoid seeking help out of fear of being treated in a prejudicial way. Furthermore, the historical view of black women as bodies without minds underlies their invisibility in the frame of reference; they are dismissed as incapable of developing problems that are both psychological and physical. With the dichotomy drawn between black and white women, Latinas drop out of the frame of reference altogether.

Failing to consider eating problems among lesbians reflects the unwritten but powerful belief that lesbians are not interested in or capable of being "attractive" in the dominant sense of the word. This reflects stereotypical notions of "butches" who are too ugly to care about their weight; women who have "become" lesbians because of fear of men and who have subsequently lost touch with "mainstream" society; and women who settle for women after being rejected by men. As biased notions about race reflect racial fears, so distorted ideas about sexuality reflect fears about sexuality in general, and these fears historically have been projected onto lesbians' bodies. These distortions have not only pushed attention to lesbians with eating problems out of the frame of reference, they have also rendered invisible the many ways lesbian communities have refashioned what constitutes beauty in ways that nurture multiple versions of style, glamour, and grace. It is no coincidence that much of the activism and scholarship opposing "fat oppression" has been spearheaded by lesbian feminists who astutely analyze how discrimination against fat women reflects a society hostile to women who take up space and refuse to put boundaries around their hunger for food, resources, and love.

The notion that eating problems are limited to heterosexual women has also contributed to some lesbians' secrecy. The historical association of lesbian sexuality with mental illness and deviance undercuts many lesbians' willingness to identify themselves with any stigmatizing illness. This institutional bias has been coupled with secrecy among lesbians based on the fear of being misunderstood or rejected by other lesbians. The connotation of anorexia and bulimia as problems developed by those who accept male models of beauty means that a lesbian with an eating problem is admitting to being male-centered and therefore not appropriately lesbian. In this way, linking eating problems with appearance rather than trauma has impeded lesbians' self-diagnosis.

Pioneering research on lesbians has confronted the problematic assumptions underlying their invisibility. Like the emerging research on race, this scholarship links unwanted eating patterns and internalized oppression—the process by which people from subordinated communities accept negative attitudes about themselves

that are created by the dominant culture. In addition, although lesbian communities may offer women more generous versions of what constitutes health and beauty, this ethic may not be able to compete with dominant cultural beliefs about body size and weight. The scholarship on lesbians, like that on African-American women, reveals cultural methods of protection against harmful social standards previously missing in research that treated white heterosexual women as the standard.

The intricacies of race, class, and sexuality encourage us to rethink demeaning assumptions about white middle-class femininity and racist assumptions about women of color and to consider bulimia and anorexia serious responses to injustices. At their core, bulimia and anorexia are not signs of self-centered vanity and obsession with appearance but rather, at least in their initial stages, are sensible ways women cope with the difficulties in their lives. Reexamining split and oppositional images about race, class, and sexuality with a wide-angle lens reveals a single complicated frame. A multiracial focus shows that distorted notions about black, Latina, and lesbian women are embedded—both explicitly and implicitly—in notions about white heterosexual women, and that it is impossible to understand any of them without the others.

Body Consciousness

The traumatic basis of many women's eating problems can teach us much about bodies and embodiment, for trauma often disrupts an intact sense of one's body. Women's ways of using food are emblematic of a rupturing of women's embodiment, of their ability to see themselves as grounded in and connected to their bodies.

When I first began to ask women about their relationships to their bodies, I asked them to tell me about their body images, but I soon realized a basic conceptual problem in my question. By inquiring about their body "image" I was taking for granted that they imagined themselves as having bodies, an assumption that many women quickly dispelled. The notion that someone can imagine her body assumes that she considers herself to have a body. Some women do not see themselves as having bodies at all.

This painful reality is partly a consequence of oppression that has both historical and contemporary manifestations. The more than three hundred years of slavery in this country robbed African-American men and women of the right to own their own bodies. African-American women were forced into this country as pieces of property "whose purpose was to provide free labor. . . . Their roles in U.S. society were synonymous with work, labor outside of the home, and legitimized sexual victimization from the very outset." In the existential nightmare of slavery, no self was legally recognized, and therefore the body could not exist for the self either. Once slavery was abolished, all that black people had were their bodies. The legal right to own one's body, however, does not in itself ensure that one can claim this right. The legacy of slavery still informs black women's experiences of their bodies in profound ways. The portrayal of black women as mammies (women incapable of being sexual), as Sapphires (women who dominate in the family and in the bedroom), and as Jezebels (sexually promiscuous women who willingly participate in sexual exploitation) reflects the projection of white fantasies and sexuality onto black women's bodies. The idea that white women needed protection was build on seeing black women as their opposite—neither worthy of protection nor wanting to be free of sexual violation.

Debilitating and contradictory stereotypes of Latina women are among the complex and limiting messages against which Latinas have struggled. They have been viewed both as highly sexual, irrationally flamboyant temptresses and as obedient, subservient, fat, and passive—good Catholic mothers. In both their historic and contemporary versions, these stereotypes have long-lasting effects on embodiment and physical presence for Latinas. The existence of these stereotypes does not mean they are inevitably internalized. But what embodiment means for black and Latina women cannot be understood without awareness of the struggle and impact of these stereotypes on self-consciousness.

For many women, responding to social injustices directed at their bodies includes trying to escape what seems like the very location of that pain—their bodies. Pecola, a character in Toni Morrison's *The Bluest Eye,* tries to make her body disappear in response to incest, racism, and poverty:

> Letting herself breathe easy now, Pecola covered her head with the quilt. The sick feeling, which she had tried to prevent by holding in her stomach, came quickly in spite of her precaution. There surged in her the desire to heave, but as always, she knew she would not.
>
> "Please, God," she whispered into the palm of her hand. "Please make me disappear." She squeezed her eyes shut. Little parts of her body faded away. Now slowly, now with a rush. Slowly again. Her fingers went, one by one; then her arms disappeared all the way to the elbow. Her feet now. Yes, that was good. The legs all at once. It was hardest above the thighs. She had to be real still and pull. Her stomach would not go. But finally it, too, went away. Then

her chest, her neck. The face was hard, too. Almost done, almost. Only her tight, tight eyes were left. They were always left.

Pecola's wish to make her body disappear dramatizes the destructive intersection of sexual abuse, racism, and poverty as no statistic can. Trying to disappear is an immediate and logical strategy to escape what Pecola came to believe caused her pain—her brown eyes and brown body. Her attempt to slip out and away from the reality of a world bent on destroying her is a vivid example of how women's embodiment is compromised. People facing these injustices cannot take for granted such a basic and elemental capacity as being able to reside comfortably in their bodies. And yet the costs of leaving one's body are monumental.

Ultimately, I put aside the concept of body image and instead thought about women's relationship to their bodies as forms of consciousness. Body consciousness is shaped by biological changes common to all women—growth spurts during childhood, puberty, menstruation, menopause, and the aging process—and by the changes of pregnancy and birthing. People are born with a self-consciousness of mind and body, with an internal body image, and a "sixth sense"—a body self-awareness and a sense of mind-body integration. It is through body consciousness that people can often sense danger, intuitively know what to do, and identify how they feel. These elemental and substantial capacities depend on residing within one's body. Embodiment that allows a person to know where his or her body stops and another's physical body begins may be at the root of a person's capacity to know him/herself as simultaneously unique and connected to the world.

Although everyone is born with a sense of embodiment, experience of it is not universal. The meanings people ascribe to their bodies and the social injustices that violate embodiment vary across gender, race, sexuality, class, religion, and nationality. Unlike the term "image," which has a psychological, individual connotation, the etymology of "consciousness" links an awareness of one's social standing directly to social conditions. Consciousness, as Karl Marx used the term, links individual people's social realities, opportunities, and perspectives to class. In a similar way, one's body consciousness is linked to one's race, gender, and sexuality. This connection more accurately captures women's complicated relationship to their bodies than is conveyed in the term "image." Representations of black and Latina women's bodies and their body consciousness are profoundly different from those of white women. Class stratification also shapes body consciousness. Poverty, for example, can significantly alter a woman's relationship to her body. Being denied the chance to own a car, a house, or even furniture can make a poor woman feel as if her body is all she has left.

Women with eating problems certainly do not have a corner on the market in terms of having difficulty residing comfortably within their bodies. As Emily Martin chronicles in her research on women's reproduction, medical and social processes of birthing, menopause, and puberty in the United States fragment women's embodiment. Feminist theorists on disability offer rich analyses of how disability changes women's embodiment. Discriminatory practices against people with disabilities—including limited access to education, employment, independent living, and sexual freedoms—are typically more restricting than actual physical conditions.

The essential issue may not be *if* women struggle to claim their bodies as their own, but rather the differing ways that embodiment is disrupted. Adrienne Rich writes:

> I know no woman—virgin, mother, lesbian, married, celibate—whether she earns her keep as a housewife, a cocktail waitress, or a scanner of brain waves—for whom her body is not a fundamental problem: its clouded meaning, its fertility, its desire, its so-called frigidity, its bloody speech, its silences, its changes and mutilations, its rapes and ripenings.

In her poetic way, Rich captures the contradictions and complexities of living in one's body.

To complicate this further, women employ a variety of survival strategies in response to violations of their bodies. The poet Wanda Coleman writes:

> The price Black girls pay for not conforming to white standards of beauty is extracted in monumental amounts, breath to death. We bend our personalities, and sometimes mutilate our bodies in defense. Sometimes that bent is "bad attitude," perhaps accompanied by a hair-trigger temper, ready to go off at the mildest slight: neck-wobbling, hands to hips, boisterous, hostile, niggerish behavior.

Women may also respond to psychic and physical assaults with silent refusals to engage or show rage. They may run away from home or never leave their apartments. They may flunk out of school or hide behind books. The reasons for these coping strategies are complicated and not easily predicted—just as it is not easy to explain why some women develop eating problems and others do not.

Women with eating problems, however, offer special insights about body consciousness because they respond to trauma in particularly bodily ways. Their stories reveal how bingeing, purging, and dieting can change a woman's embodiment, and they provide vivid examples of what it means for a woman to "leave her body."

Leaving the body is a survival strategy many women use when they see no other alternatives. The sophisticated ways in which the women I talked with describe their experiences of their bodies originate in part in their having had to grapple—seriously and over the long term—with the discomfort of being in their bodies. Their stories reveal the social inequalities that whittle away at a woman's ability to identify her body as her own. They explain what it means to be in exile from one's own body, and why this is common. Their testimonies reveal why sexual abuse and racism can lead a teenager who weighs 110 pounds to see herself as fat and to consider her body the cause of her pain. Their stories also highlight the consequences of drastic weight loss and gain on a woman's sense of her body's shape and size. The average weight fluctuation among the women I talked to was seventy-four pounds. Many of the women's weight changed several times in their lives. Substantial and recurrent weight fluctuation raises complicated and painful questions about what it means to be "embodied" since a woman's possession of a significant portion of her body may be in constant flux.

The women's stories reveal that body consciousness is a highly imaginative and simultaneously concrete ability to see one's self as part of one's body and to draw upon the power generated from this embodiment. It is a concrete reality in that, regardless of one's relation to one's body, breathing, eating, sleeping, and simply being require some consciousness of one's body. But body consciousness occurs at the imaginative and symbolic level as well. In the face of debilitating stereotypes and injustices, women do struggle to claim their bodies as their own. The struggle requires being able to see one's own image of one's body rather than the images projected onto it. Consciousness both takes into account oppressive perceptions of the body and rejects what is debilitating about them.

The women's stories also reveal the often ingenious and creative strategies they develop to counter various assaults, strategies that are at the core of their journey toward self-love and empowerment. Self-love and empowerment are profoundly related to the body. Cornel West writes:

> The issue of self-regard, self-esteem, and self-respect is reflected in bodily form. . . . Toni Morrison would say, "Look you've got to love yourself not only in the abstract; you've got to love your big lips; you've got to love your flat nose; you've got to love your skin, hands, all the way down."

The women whose experiences form the basis of this book identify their injuries and their resistance with honesty and insight. In so doing, they chronicle their despair and resilience, their depression and fortitude, their ingenuity in taking care of themselves.

Methods and Ethics

Conducting life-history interviews enabled me to hear in women's own words how they interpreted the meaning of and reasons behind their eating patterns: what it feels like to turn to food for comfort, how they come to see their bodies as liabilities, and what resources have most helped them develop sane relationships with food and their bodies. They also explain why food begins as, and often remains, the drug of choice for many girls and women.

I interviewed eighteen women ranging in age from nineteen to forty-six, five of them African-American, five Latina, and eight white. All of the white women and four of the women of color are lesbian. I wanted women of color and lesbians to be at the center of my analysis since we know so little about their eating problems. A third of the women are mothers. Five are Jewish, eight are Catholic, and five are Protestant. Three of them grew up outside the United States. They represent various class backgrounds, in terms of both their families of origin and their own current situations.

The majority of the women had a combination of eating problems (at least two of the following: bulimia, compulsive eating, anorexia, extensive dieting), and the particular types often changed during their lives. The most common problems were bingeing and extensive dieting, although half of the women were also anorexic, bulimic, or both. All had problems that were long-term and serious—for some, even life-threatening. The specific types of eating problems did not correlate with race, class, sexuality, or nationality, although the types of trauma the women associate with their unwanted eating patterns did vary with social position. (There are brief biographical sketches of the women at the end of the book.)

I found women willing to be interviewed by letting people know—where I work, in my neighborhood, in political and community groups—about my study. Some of the women approached me, others I asked. I typically had many conversations with them before the interviews, an important step given the secrecy, vulnerability, and fear that many people feel when they talk about eating problems and the pain underlying them.

The women and I also often discussed the origins and purpose of the study, including my personal and intellectual interest in eating problems. Like many feminist scholars, I believe that a researcher's self-disclosure counters power imbalances; people who consent to talk openly about their lives deserve the right to ask the researcher potentially personal questions as well. Self-disclosure does not eliminate power differences based on race, generation, sexual identity, or class, but our common experiences—as lesbians, as women with eating problems, as neighbors, as antiracist activists, our work-related affiliations—did serve as an initial bridge that made it easier to talk about our differences. One Latina woman asked me why a white and perhaps heterosexual woman was doing research about African-American women, Latinas, and lesbians. I explained that my research emerged from antiracist work and my frustration about the dearth of information on mental and physical health concerns of African-American and Latina women. I also talked about how relying upon friendship networks and alliances at work to find women to interview was partially based on my knowledge that women of color might understandably be skeptical of my background and motivations. Her questions about me and the study also gave us a chance to talk about the complexity of sexual identity—how lesbian identity is not necessarily apparent. This ambiguity parallels the complexity of identification for many light-skinned Latinas (such as herself).

A white woman who is a survivor of sexual abuse was quite hesitant and wanted to be sure that she could stop the interview at any time. Learning that her right as the speaker superseded my rights as the researcher influenced her eventual decision to participate. I also spoke about my own worry, as a survivor of sexual abuse and someone who had a long-term eating problem earlier in my life, about talking about this subject with people I did not know well. In both of these situations, the women's candid questions and our discussion about methods and ethics influenced the tenor of the interview process. These conversations allowed women to talk about their fears and worries about not being understood or having to "start from the beginning all the time" in order for their story to make sense.

Tapping into friendship, work, and community networks was an effective way to find women willing to be interviewed since it allowed them to scrutinize me and the project. Many people of color have had to reckon with false generalizations and distortions put forward by white social workers who have not examined their own understanding of race. People who are willing to talk about private, painful, and power-laden issues deserve to know something about both the research and the researcher.

Clearly, the study was in no way random. I was very specific in terms of race and sexuality about who I was hoping to interview. In addition, I sought women who considered themselves to be in the process of healing, surmising that their understanding of the roots of their eating problems would be greater than that of women whose eating difficulties were at their height. I did not approach the research process as an objective observer, in part because I do not think that, for a study of this kind, "objectivity" is possible or ethical. I came to the interviews with biases: believing that the women were courageous to talk on this subject and already skeptical of the dominant imagery associated with eating problems.

During the interviews I used what Patricia Hill Collins calls "an ethic of care," which she defines as understanding that "personal expressiveness, emotions and empathy are central to the knowledge validation process." I had been conducting workshops on eating problems for several years prior to beginning the book and had been personally immersed in the topic for many years before that. From that experience, I responded to the women's stories in a way that I believe heightened their trust and therefore the integrity of the interviews. Had I approached the interviews as an objective observer, I would have been betraying myself and the women who shared their life stories with me.

Because I interviewed only a few women—who were not randomly selected—generalizations based on their experiences need to be made with caution. My point is not to confirm prevalence or even incidence but rather to examine the meaning of eating problems in these women's lives and what they have to teach us about coping, embodiment, and recovery. At the same time, I do not want to overlook the possibility that their experiences reflect a larger reality. The stakes involved in speaking openly about the traumas underlying many eating problems are high, and much injustice remains underground (only one out of ten incidences of sexual abuse is reported, for example). Perhaps the balance lies in both recognizing what makes each of the women's stories unique and understanding how their experiences reflect common injustices and methods of resistance.

Like many feminist and qualitative researchers, I approached the interviews believing that the people being interviewed, not the researcher, are the experts on their lives, that they know the best chronology, emphasis, and methods of telling about their lives. My task was to remind myself of that when I began to proceed otherwise. In some of the interviews I spoke very little, only infrequently asking for clarification. Other interviews were more like conversations, in which I followed along with questions and comments as the women talked about their lives. The ways the women told their stories mirrored the complex detours, the starts and stops, of their lives.

The multiple and textured meanings of their stories often reflected the ways they lived their lives. People often don't remember or describe their lives in a linear sequence, particularly when they're relating experiences of injustice. Judith Herman explains that people who have survived trauma often tell their stories in a "highly emotional, contradictory, and fragmented manner." In open-ended interviews the women explored subjects from more than one angle, which helped me piece together events and emotions that otherwise were too complicated or confusing for me to follow. Their stories revealed why hesitations, silences, and omissions were understandable and inevitable. Like many qualitative anthropologists and sociologists, I am not sure there is such a thing as a complete story: future experience keeps adding to and revising what the present offers. Partial truths and circuitous narratives of lived experience are often the closest approximation of the whole story available.

Body language—particularly the women's eyes—often helped me know when to move on. Typically, I waited for the woman to talk about a topic so I could use her terms rather than impose my own, so she could decide when it was all right to broach a particular subject. I deliberately did not assume a definition of eating problem or recovery, and I tried to avoid specific terms until the women used them. Humor often played a key role in their stories; laughter frequently mingled with tears.

Almost all of the interviews took place in the women's homes, which gave me vivid insights into their lives, struggles, and dreams. An African-American woman explained that a key component of her healing was to travel to Egypt "to see the birthplace of black people prior to slavery." Her living room was a shrine: statues of Egyptian gods, portraits of Jesus with brown face and curly hair, candles, stones, and other religious instruments she had collected. Seeing her home gave me an understanding I would otherwise have been unable to grasp. A woman who linked her eating problems to poverty let me into her apartment and then bolted her door with four locks and a long metal police bar that she jammed between the door and a wall as she explained that her home had been broken into three times. She served me tea with powdered milk crystals, having run out of milk—and money—much earlier in the week. A woman who detailed the psychological abuse she suffered at the hands of her husband was forced to stop talking perhaps a dozen times as her husband came crashing into the house, screaming and yelling, interrupting her despite her pleas for privacy.

One woman explicitly requested that the interview occur outside of her home—a request that taught me a lot about language, culture, and acculturation. This young Dominican woman insisted upon meeting me in my office for the interview, which initially worried me because I associated the office with business, distance, and formality. It turned out that this was her way of seeking rather than avoiding intimacy. She lives with her parents and brothers and has never told any of her relatives about her eating problem. She has no privacy at her house, so it would have been impossible for her to talk there. Also, when she thinks about her eating problem, she thinks about it in English (even though she did not learn English until she was sixteen years old). Because she speaks Spanish at home and English at the university, the university seemed like the natural place to talk about this subject.

I transcribed my tapes of the interviews and gave copies to the women who wanted them. I had further conversations with some of the women in which they clarified ideas and made additions to the transcript. Some women said they were glad to have the transcripts but found it too hard to read them. Many said they felt exhilarated, relieved, satisfied, and glad to have told their life stories, although the costs for some were intense. One woman had a number of painful flashbacks during the interview and later told me she had left her body at some point during the interview; she had to have emergency sessions with her therapist and increase her medication for several days after the interview. Another woman had a hard time emotionally after the interview because she had remembered instances of abuse she had not previously recalled. While these two women's experiences were in the minority, they highlight the courage it takes to speak about eating problems and the traumas that often underlie them. I often felt dazed and exhausted after an interview. Sometimes I had difficulty staying fully "present," which I attributed to the pain in some of the women's stories. My reaction is yet another example of why silence about trauma—and the ways people cope with it—remains and why telling life stories is a risky endeavor.

The women's experiences that are the centerpiece of this book play a central role in each chapter. Chapter 2 examines conditions that may make girls vulnerable to developing eating problems. The women's stories offer essential clues about why many girls grow up distrusting their bodies and their appetites. Lessons they are taught about race, religion, sexuality, and ethnicity are the filters through which they learn about food and eating. Chapters 3 and 4 identify connections between eating problems and several forms of trauma—sexual abuse, racism, heterosexism, poverty, acculturation, and emotional and physical abuse. These chapters show how bingeing, purging, and dieting begin as ways women numb pain and cope with violations of their bodies and how survivors of trauma use food as a logical response to injustices, given the limited alternatives available to them. The lives of the women I interviewed show why we need an expansive understanding of how trauma can be inflicted. Many of the women linked eating problems to physical violations, and others associated them with the psychic invasions of heterosexism, poverty, acculturation, racism, and emotional abuse. Recognizing both psychic and physical invasions avoids the historical tendency to identify the body and mind as somehow disconnected entities.

The concluding chapters examine why food is women's drug of choice, how embodiment is shaped by social inequalities, and the women's healing methods. The women's stories reveal that although eating problems begin as sensible responses to various injustices, they may eventually become liabilities. Healing depends upon making the connection between trauma and eating and understanding how violations distort "body consciousness" and appetites. The healing strategies often entail recovering memories through self-help, community, religious, political, and therapy groups. Finding resources that support women financially, emotionally, and spiritually are also keys to recovery.

Regarding the FDA's Approval of Saline Breast Implants

by Diana Zuckerman, PhD

The decision to approve saline breast implants brings FDA's standard of safety to a new low. The FDA's decision is baffling on many levels. On the scientific level, it is baffling because the manufacturers' own studies, analyzed by FDA scientists, showed that between 73–82% of the breast cancer patients who tried saline implants had complications within three or four years. Those complications included additional surgery, implant deflation, excruciating pain, and serious infections—not the kinds of outcome a reasonable person would call "safe."

On the medical level, it is baffling because breast implants are known to interfere with mammograms, sometimes obscuring cancer in its early stages. Of the two million women who already have breast implants, 20,000–40,000 will be diagnosed with cancer at a later stage as a result.

On the political level, the decision was baffling because the FDA seems to have turned a deaf ear to the Clinton Administration's efforts to improve health care in America. Improving access to care has been a major focus of this Administration, but providing a strong watchdog when medical products are reviewed is also an essential component of health care in America. The approval of saline implants is just the latest FDA misstep, which has included the approval of numerous medical products that were recently removed from the market after killing and seriously injuring patients.

Women are smart enough to make their own choices, but they need accurate information to do so.

Why would any woman put a questionable product in her body, knowing that it will break after a few years, knowing that it can grow bacteria or fungus inside, knowing that her breast may get hard and painful, and knowing that each additional surgery will result in the removal of her healthy breast tissue and new scars where the implants are inserted and removed? Unfortunately, the answer seems to be that women don't know the facts. The FDA hopes to improve that situation by providing an *informative brochure* and disturbing *photographs* of breast implant complications to warn women about the risks. They will try to require that plastic surgeons distribute this brochure, but the FDA is unlikely to enforce that.

Since virtually everyone—at FDA and elsewhere—agrees that better, longer-term research is needed, it would have made sense to require additional research before approving these products. Consumers have not been protected by the FDA's decision: let the buyer beware.

The *National Center for Policy Research for Women and Families* is a nonprofit, nonpartisan organization that is dedicated to improving the lives of women and families by using objective, research-based information to encourage new, more effective programs and policies. CPR for Women and Families has fact sheets, research analyses, information about FDA's regulation of implants, and information about other experts and implant patients' experiences that are available upon request.

Pretty in Ink

Conformity, Resistance, and Negotiation in Women's Tattooing

by Michael Atkinson[1]

Since the early 1990s, Canadian women have participated in tattooing in unprecedented numbers. These women are utilizing tattoo "body projects" to communicate a wide range of personal and cultural messages, and challenging the long-standing association between tattooing and masculinity. However, and perhaps more consequentially, women's tattoo projects express diverse sensibilities about femininity and the feminine body. For some Canadian women, contesting culturally "established" constructions of the female body is central in their tattoo body projects, whereas others participate in tattooing as an explicit form of consent to such constructions. In this paper, women's tattooing activities and their subsequent tattoo narratives are critically inspected as deeply gendered practices and discourses. I present participant observation and interview data on tattoo enthusiasm in Canada. The focus is directed toward the ways in which conformity to, resistance against, and the negotiation of established cultural ideas about femininity are equally embedded in women's tattooing. Drawing upon feminist theories about bodies and central tenets of process-sociology, emphasis is given to how women employ tattooing as a communicative signifier of "established" and "outsider" constructions of femininity.

Introduction

Shilling described the deliberate modification of one's physical size, shape, appearance, or ability for movement as purposive "body projects," and contended that such projects are integral in constructing and representing identity over the life course. Shilling noted that individuals are socially encouraged and expected to engage in body projects that range from the routine (e.g., a hair cut) to the physically invasive and traumatic (e.g., breast augmentation). In response to the increased exploration of bodies as floating symbols of cultural identification, sociologists have critically inspected a wide range of body projects. Research efforts are usually directed toward the myriad ways cultural ideologies are inscribed upon/into bodies, and how the preponderance of North Americans' body projects are dialogical with normative standards about bodies and their representation. In particular, most of the research has focused on North American women's experiences with corporeal modification and how women's body projects are typically congruous with "hegemonic masculine" constructions of femininity. Forms of cosmetic surgery, excessive dieting, and aerobic exercise have been interrogated as highly ritualized, commonplace, and deeply gendered projects that embody patriarchal ideas about femininity.

One of the more popular body projects among North American women since the late 1980s has been tattooing—despite the fact that North American women have been dissuaded traditionally from involvement in tattooing as a result of cultural prohibitions that emanate from both inside and outside of the larger collective of "tattoo enthusiasts."[2] In general, sanctions against the widespread participation of women have come from (sub)cultural associations between tattoos and masculinity, as tattooing has been historically relished within male-dominated subcultures (e.g., military groups, prisoners, street gangs, motorcycle clubs) as a mechanism for creating and confirming aggressively strong, or "dangerous," masculinities.[3]

Some authors, however, have suggested that non-normative body projects such as tattooing are increasingly adopted by North American women *precisely* because radically marked bodies tend to subvert hegemonic ideologies about femininity—especially images of the weak, sexually objectified, or otherwise submissive woman. The overriding meta-narrative in the emerging literature on the practice is that tattooing is intentionally structured by North American women as political resistance against misogynist ideologies and social structures of oppression. Almost without exception, contemporary discourses point to the socially rebellious and personally emancipating nature of tattooing for women.

I argue, however, that such homogenizing accounts of women's tattooing are somewhat misleading—in that only a portion of women's experiences are represented by this line of inquiry. Clearly, although more women include tattoos in their respective repertoires of self-expression, and choose to articulate their body modification practices as political protests against culturally preferred, masculinist constructions of the female body in North America, researchers have not sufficiently examined the largely hidden, private, or *negotiated* nature of these protests. Furthermore, investigators have overlooked the extent to which many North American women's tattooing projects express a degree of consent to "hegemonic masculine" constructions of femininity.

In this article, tattoos are analyzed as embodied signifiers of gender. More specifically, I tap into critical feminist and profeminist research on the body, and Elias and Scotson's theory of established/outsider social relationships, *to argue that women's tattoos are layered with culturally established, resistant, and negotiated images of femininity.* Through the examination of 40 Canadian women's tattoo narratives, a critical investigation of how bodies are encoded with cultural messages about femininity is offered. Emphasis is given to both the intended (encoded) messages about gender embedded in tattoos by female wearers and the established cultural codes about "appropriate" gender display that influence how tattoos are decoded by audiences.

Theoretical Underpinnings

Curiously absent from the burgeoning literature on contemporary body projects are many in-depth, *empirical* analyses of tattooing. Given the booming popularity of tattooing in North America (especially among the 18-35-year-old age group), this stands out as a rather peculiar gap in the literature. Even though extant sociological, cultural anthropological, and psychological analyses of tattooing are unquestionably groundbreaking along a number of theoretical and substantive lines, the bulk of the research is relatively unreflective of the array of sensibilities toward the practice held by the newest genera-

tion of tattoo enthusiasts. This is compounded by the fact that sociologists who have addressed the subject have almost uniformly failed to explore sociological theories about bodies and body modification in their respective works.

One of the most neglected areas within research on tattooing is women's involvement in the practices. As tattooing has long been associated with masculinity, only a handful of researchers have attended to issues in the cultural construction and expression of femininity through tattooing. When issues related to femininity have figured into analyses of tattooing, emphasis is principally directed toward how acquiring tattoos can significantly jeopardise a woman's femininity. For example, Steward classified North American women who have participated in tattooing as "tramps," "dykes," and "farm wives." Adopting the position that women who choose to mark their bodies with tattoos wilfully violate existing norms about gender, links have been made between tattooing and the "fallen" or overtly masculine woman. In a similar way, recent research has focussed on (and perhaps overemphasized) the liberating nature of tattoos for women, as marking the body with tattoos immediately connotes a significant violation of feminine body practice.

Although information gleaned from existing research illuminates a series of relevant questions pertinent to women's tattooing, we ultimately know very little about how tattoos are actively constructed and experienced by women—especially in the Canadian context, as no empirical research has been conducted on Canadian women's experiences with tattoos save for the partial analyses provided by Atkinson, and Atkinson and Young. In order to pursue a more theoretically stimulating and empirically informed account of Canadian women's tattooing experiences (as theoretical understandings of tattooing have been largely constructed around men's experiences with the body project), several concepts central in feminist and profeminist research on the body are worth (re)consideration.

Feminisms, Bodies, and Tattooing

Building largely upon the works of Foucault and other poststructuralists, feminist researchers have illustrated how hegemonic masculine authority in Western cultures is partly maintained through the active biological (i.e., medical) and social (i.e., norms, values, beliefs) control of women's bodies. In these processes, women's bodies become socially constructed, monitored, and regulated in accordance with a dominant image of the "feminine body" as thin yet curvy, placid yet playful, sexy yet wholesome. In describing the female body as a "text of culture," Bordo wrote:

> Through the pursuit of an ever-changing, homogenising, elusive idea of femininity—a pursuit without a terminus, a resting point, requiring that women constantly attend to minute and often whimsical changes in fashion—bodies become what Foucault calls "docile bodies"—bodies whose forces and energies are habituated to external regulation, subjection, transformation, and improvement.

Bordo maintained that socially accepted women's body projects such as breast augmentation or excessive dieting are best viewed as caricatured expressions of dominant ideals of the female body, because these body projects express traditional images of the female body (and women's marginalized positions within social structures that produce them) in excess. Central in the feminist literature is, then, the relationship between body modification and social structures of power/authority:

> It is no coincidence that this sexual ideal (of the slim, soft, innocent body) is an image which connotes powerlessness. Admittedly, the actual ideal is not of a demure, classically "feminine" girl per se, but a vigorous and immature adolescent . . . it is not a shape which suggests power.

In order to conceptually synthesise the pioneering work of feminist scholars in this area, we may draw upon Elias and Scotson's process-sociological understanding of "established" and "outsider" figurational relationships. Elias and Scotson principally argued that community life is moulded around the relationship between established and outsider social groups. Elias and Scotson inferred a model of figurational dynamics that takes into account the distribution of power chances between and within a series of mutually identified social groups. Established social groups are those that are more deeply embedded in both the base and superstructural segments of a figuration—typically because they have a longer history there, and/or greater access to resources (e.g., material, cultural, political, and educational) in the figuration—and consequently control key ideological state apparatuses. Established groups have considerable ability to influence the construction of social laws, promulgate cultural norms, and promote collective ways of interpreting social rituals, such as body modification practices.

Conversely, outsider groups are more marginal members of a figuration, less embedded in power positions, and socially/culturally dominated (in varying degrees) on the basis of their marginalized statuses and associated roles. Outsiders are generally excluded from participation in socially influential power structures within a figuration, and as a result, their social opportunities and cultural experiences are often "given" to them (or interpretively configured) by members of established groups. Thus, what is deemed to be acceptable for an outsider to participate in as a form of social interchange or cultural expression is restricted in accordance with established conventions and practices (including, e.g., how to modify one's body). To break established rank and violate cultural idiom within a figuration by transgressing established norms can be risky social practice for an outsider, as it may warrant social contempt or some other control response. Jibing, then, with the more central principles of Elias' work on civilizing processes in Western cultures—and feminist research on body projects more generally—Elias and Scotson revealed how social standards (including norms of acceptable bodily display) protect the vested interests of established groups, such as figurational patriarchy.

Feminist and process-sociological researchers have argued that body projects can accomplish more than the simple reproduction of established gender codes. That is, although many have inspected body projects that reaffirm and reproduce established images of the beautiful female body, the study of how body projects can be used by outsiders to resist established cultural ideology is equally germane. For example, Maguire and Mansfield suggested that the "unnatural" strength cultivated by women who participate in aerobic exercise breeds both a physical and a social power that challenges the established masculine hegemony. By poaching an established male body practice (i.e., athletic exercise) women challenge the gender order. Through the study of radical forms of cosmetic manipulation, Davis illustrated how women contest established cultural codes by engaging in certain types of "gender appropriate" plastic surgery to the extreme, and in the process, excessively embrace the images and practices of the socially marginalized. These theatrical body modifications are vulgar or "grotesque" in comparison to established images of the beautiful woman.

Without question, research on women's body projects has greatly advanced our theoretical understanding of how bodies are socially constructed and monitored. Feminist, profeminist, and process-sociological research underscores how bodies are texts upon which established and outsider relationships are reproduced and contested—as body projects can involve the ongoing maintenance of established ideology and/or the conscious attempt to subvert established ideologies by employing the body as a site of outsider resistance. Unfortunately, few who have conducted empirical research on tattooing body projects have explored the wealth of theoretical insight offered about bodies by feminist or process-sociological research. Even fewer have considered the ways in which tattoo body projects are used by women in the process of *negotiating* established gender ideologies and codes of physical display.

Method

Data were collected during a 3-year participant observation-based study of tattoo enthusiasm in Canada. During the research, I spent over 400 hr "hanging out" with tattoo artists and their clients in various tattoo studios—mainly, in the cities of Calgary (AB) and Toronto (ON). Through the research process I interacted with hundreds of tattoo enthusiasts, and eventually approached 92 of them to ask if they would be willing to be interviewed. Although both men and women were interviewed in the study, data discussed here pertain to the women I interviewed about their tattoo body projects.

I met the women involved in this research in several different locations, but first encountered a majority of them at tattoo studios in either Calgary or Toronto. Some of them were regulars within the studios; others were entirely new to the tattooing process. Almost all of the women with whom I spoke were overtly receptive toward the prospect of being interviewed—even though most had no prior experience with interviewing for any purposes other than employment. Interviewees were also met through the friendship networks I cultivated in the participant-observation phase of the research (i.e., friends of individuals I became acquainted with in the tattoo studios). A smaller number of interviewees were students or friends of mine at a university in western Canada.

In total, 40 women were interviewed. Although the group of interviewees initially developed as a convenience sample, I eventually targeted several categories of tattoo enthusiasts for interview purposes including women with different socioeconomic backgrounds, ethnic affiliations, religious beliefs, and sexual or lifestyle preferences. Furthermore, I sought out women with assorted levels of involvement in the practice—in reference to how long they had been tattooed (in years); how many tattoos they had acquired (total number); how many times they had been tattooed (number of sittings or total number of hours); and, how extensively they had been tattooed (amount of skin covered by tattoos and locations of tattoos on the body).

The mean age of the women I interviewed was 24, with an overall age range from 18 to 50. Despite the long-standing association between tattooing and the working-class, only 6 (15%) of the women interviewed had working-class backgrounds. Of the women interviewed, 21 (52.5%) were employed at the time of the study, with an average annual income of approximately Cdn$24, 000. Considering that the majority of the unemployed women were students at the time of the study—

most of whom had a modest income—this figure appears to be a rather conservative estimation. The women I interviewed in this study were also rather well educated. Thirty-one (77.5%) had a university degree or at least 1 year of university education. Of the group, 24 (60%) were single at the time of the study, and 12 (30%) of the women had children. Also, 35 (87.5%) of the women interviewed were White, and 5 (12.5%) were Asian-Canadian.

A majority of the women interviewed, 27 (67.5%), had one tattoo at the time of the interview. Seven (17.5%) of the women had two tattoos, 2 (5%) had three tattoos, and 4 (10%) had three or more tattoos. Experience in tattooing also varied; the age of entry into the practice ranged from 14 to 48 (with a mean of 22). Twenty-nine (72.5%) of the women were tattooed in either Calgary or Toronto (including seven different studios in Calgary and four different studios in Toronto). Other Canadian cities in which individuals were tattooed included Vancouver (BC), Edmonton (AB), Lethbridge (AB), Regina (SK), Winnipeg (MB), Kitchener-Waterloo (ON), Montreal (PQ), Halifax (NS), and St. John's (NF).

The interview strategy adopted in this research closely followed the prescriptions for open-ended interviewing as outlined by Glaser, Glaser and Strauss, Lofland and Lofland, and Prus, and simultaneously incorporated Gubrium and Holstein's suggestions for exploring and dissecting narratives via the "active interviewing" process. As little is known about the actual forms and meanings of women's tattooing in Canada, I required an interview strategy that would elicit free-ranging and highly descriptive responses from women about their experiences with the body project. Therefore, the interview sessions were designed to "open up" narratives about tattooing experiences in the quest of developing an understanding of how and why women select tattooing as a body project. Simply put, I needed an open-ended interview approach that would allow for a considerable amount of empirical exploration into how women decide to become tattooed, experience tattooing, and draw upon a series of "interpretive resources" when creating narratives about their tattooing body projects.

Interviews were conducted in a variety of settings such as my office at the university, coffee shops, local restaurants, or tattoo studios (typically, the interviewee would choose the location). In all but a few instances, I avoided using a tape-recorder or other technological device in the sessions; instead, notes were taken both during and after the interviews. Notes were (within several hours, or at maximum within 1 day) transcribed onto computer files and filled in considerably as I analyzed the texts. Interviewees were given an explanation of informed consent prior to and after each interview. Interviews ranged in length from 45 min to (in some rare cases) 4 hr. All of the participants involved were interviewed one time, and each of them (with the exception of 6) were shown transcripts of the interview sessions at a later date so that they might review their own narratives (i.e., to freely amend or delete any portions of text). In all cases here, pseudonyms have been used to protect the identities of the participants.

It is interesting that my being a male researcher seemed to stimulate a heightened degree of exchange about the subject of gender and tattooing. I found that in sharing stories about our social experiences with tattoos, the interviews became lively discussions geared toward dissecting how gender is central in framing one's interpretations of tattoos. Being able to relate to the women as fellow tattoo enthusiasts, but discussing our lived experiences with tattooed skin from different gender standpoints, became central in developing a grounded understanding of how tattoos are constructed along gender lines. Stories about, and theoretical interpretations of, women's tattooing presented in this article have been assembled as a result of these "active" conversations. Although a degree of theoretical and conceptual abstraction is undertaken in order to cull the women's tattoo narratives around the theme of gender, my overarching goal is to present their gendered understanding of tattooing by using their own terms and categories.

Results

In the sociological literature on body modification, cultural conformity and resistance via physical representation are recurrent themes, yet they are typically separated as dissonant forms of social expression. Conformity and resistance through body modification are often analyzed as the polar extremes of cultural identification. As I contend here, this is a conceptually misleading approach to the study of cultural expression, as acts of conformity or ⋅ resistance to social edict (which form the basis of most body projects) are inexorably intertwined. In the case example of tattooing, women's involvement in the body project illustrates the ways in which forms of body modification are simultaneously replete with cultural messages about conformity and resistance.

Established Conformity and Women's Tattooing

As critical feminists have suggested, established North American standards of feminine beauty tend to produce passive female bodies. The established female form is not a physical shape (i.e., we may think of the quintessential runway model or beauty pageant contestant as

the ideal-type) that demands social attention for its foreboding, powerful, or authoritarian stature. Whereas masculinity is partially achieved through the corporeal display of strength, aggression, risk-taking, and the ability to withstand pain and injury, preferred understandings of femininity consider such display among women as repugnant. As a result, established feminine body projects (which, ironically, are often rife with pain) highlight the docility of women's bodies.

For many of the women I interviewed, attending to the body as a communicative symbol of established femininity is everyday ritual. Common body projects such as applying make-up; blow-drying, colouring, or fixing one's hair; wearing dresses or skirts; exercising at the gym; dieting; and of course, shopping for body modification projects, are clearly ingrained in the gendered habitus. In the process of linking body ritual to one's social status as a feminine woman, many women's tattooing projects are performances of established femininity. *In this study, almost two-thirds (25, 62%) of the women I interviewed conformed to established constructions of femininity through their tattooing projects.* This was initially evident in portions of their tattoo narratives that detailed the "pre-tattoo enthusiast stage," in which the women were debating whether or not to partake in the body project:

> I couldn't decide whether or not I was going to get tattooed. One of the main reasons was that, I dunno, I guess I never thought it looked lady-like. And all the guys I knew, were like, "you want to do what?" They looked at me like I was crazy . . . But then I started talking about getting a string of roses tattooed across my lower back, right at the top of my butt. I think it looks sexy, and so do all my male friends. Like, when you go out with a high cut t-shirt on, and low-rise jeans, you can see it really well, and it looks great. I've got a pretty flat stomach too, and when I'm dressed up in the right clothes it makes my body look killer. (Janine, age 22)

As confirmed by Janine and 16 (40%) of the other women I interviewed, by taking into account how men would decode the tattooing project as a signifier of femininity, some women enter into the process only if it will homologically complement their established feminine body projects.

On these grounds and others, established female body projects are not simply the embodiment of diffuse cultural constructions of femininity, they are acts of consent to the underlying structures of figurational power distribution that help create such established images of femininity. The ongoing self-monitoring of one's daily physical regimen and preferences for body modification, as part of "doing gender," help reproduce relational structures of authority and power between established and outsider gender groups. As a vital part of social organization within a figuration, these seemingly banal cultural rituals translate into justifications for and confirmations of the ways in which social statuses and roles are hierarchically divided along gender lines. This was clearly evidenced in Celeste's (age 24) narrative about her decision to be tattooed:

> My boyfriend always said that he didn't want me to get tattooed . . . but I harped at him for about a year and then he finally agreed that it was okay. He wanted to help me decide what to get exactly and where. He seemed really happy when I said that I wanted a tattoo on the front of my stomach, right under my bikini-line. He thought it would be special if only he and I could share it, well, you know when, right? I want him to be attracted to me, and appreciate how I look, and I don't want a tattoo to ruin that . . . He threatened to leave me a couple of times when I said I wanted to cut all my hair off and go real short. He hates short hair, and said "no way." I thought if he liked the tattoo, and so did I, then everybody would be happy.

In Celeste's case, and that of 9 (23%) other women I interviewed, her desire was to enhance her body aesthetically through tattooing. As with many other mainstay forms of female body modification such as liposuction or excessive dieting, the underlying act is not simply a process of beautifying the female form, it is also an act of self-imposed gender stratification. Celeste's tattoo project is an embodied reproduction of the established cultural standard that women conform to men's desires and sexual interests—to the extent that a woman will radically modify her body in the process of such conformity. Akin to the process of breast augmentation, then, tattooing the body for these reasons symbolically justifies women's (and femininity's) cultural position as the outsider, as the Other.

As suggested in Celeste's and others' tattoo narratives, although women have historically shunned widespread participation in tattooing, newly established sensibilities about female sexuality have incorporated this body practice into the mix. Reminiscent of the "carnival era" of tattooing in North America (ca. 1920-50) in which scantily clad tattooed women were paraded through side-shows to titillate male audiences, women's current tattoo practices are often constructed as a sexual curiosity by men. Women's participation in this traditionally masculine body practice is often mediated by the ways in which it can be sexualized. Once more, the body project becomes an act of corporeal beautification

if undertaken with reverence to established constructions of femininity. For example, Ashlyn (age 28) stated:

> Some girls get big boobs [implants] and others get their lips or hips done. I chose tattooing because it makes me look great, and it draws attention to my body. When I'm out at a club, I know guys will see my tattoo [on her upper right breast] and come over and talk to me. Not a lot of women have them, and I know it sets me apart from the crowd . . . guys are really cool about my tattoo, and no one has ever said that I look like less of a woman for having it. I mean, as long as I don't go out and tattoo a snake across my neck.

We must be careful not to reduce the manners by which women conform to gender codes through tattooing into such a neatly packaged process. Although the narratives above strongly suggest that pursuing established standards of femininity through body work may motivate one's involvement in the practice, it does not capture the myriad ways in which established constructions of femininity are (re)produced through tattooing.

As I have argued elsewhere, for example, another *learned* motivation that underscores how tattooing is undertaken in the process of conforming to established femininity centres on the manners by which a tattoo body project can be generically cast as a tool for "exploring femininity" in a culturally fragmented, postmodern world. Given that emotionality and introspection conform well with established interpretations of femininity, it make sense that tattooing (if done as an expression of emotionality or self-exploration) can be reconciled in some cases as a feminine practice. Wrapped in discourses of empowerment, identity-exploration, and personal meaning, some women offer elaborate justifications for their involvement in tattooing as a "woman's" form of expression. For at least 7 (18%) of the women I interviewed, these quests for individuality, as personally emancipating as they may be conceived, concern established ideas about femininity:

> Women are a lot freer to be who we want to be nowadays. I'm not like my mom, right, who looks and dresses exactly like the men in her life always expected her to. I love my mom, but she has an outdated way of thinking about how women should look. All prim and proper like a little schoolgirl. If you want to get a tattoo, get a tattoo. That's what I say . . . be careful, though, and don't go attracting all kinds of unwanted criticism you don't need . . . I decided to have my lower back tattooed [a sun and moon] about 10 months ago, and my friends all love it; especially my close girl friends. But I didn't do it for anybody else other than me. It's my own way of personalising my body. (Heather, age 21)

Even though these projects tend to be whitewashed with nouveau-hip sentimentalities about "girl power" and the freedom of choice (vis-à-vis the dismantling of established gender codes), they almost invariably *reproduce* established ideas about femininity and the feminine body. This is plainly evidenced by the specific images chosen by the women, the location/placement on their bodies, and the actual sizes of the tattoos selected.

First, among women who are exceedingly sensitive about jeopardizing their established femininity through the tattooing process, the design of the tattoo is normally the principal concern. As tattooing is precarious social practice if undertaken with reckless abandon (re: one's gender status), the image selected must resound with established images of femininity:

> I love the butterflies that I have done around my ankle. I know it's not cool to say it these days, but it looks cute and girly. Sometimes women like to look pretty, and I think that tattoo makes my leg look really pretty. That's why I asked Phil [tattoo artist] to colour them pink and yellow, because I want my butterflies to look beautiful. (Selena, age 29)

Floral imagery (e.g., roses, orchids, lilies, or abstract vine work), animals or insects (e.g., birds, dolphins, turtles, cats, butterflies, beetles, or ladybugs), celestial motifs (e.g., suns, moons, or stars), and cartoon characters (e.g., Minnie Mouse, Hello Kitty, Snoopy) are commonly chosen as they immediately connote established feminine qualities and attributes such as being gentle, nurturing, playful, and delicate. They are deemed less gruesome or violent than "typical" men's tattoos, and thus they become feminized. As Lenskyj described in her research efforts on female athletes, women who encroach onto a traditionally male terrain like sport must engage in a certain degree of "apologizing" for their conduct. In the case of tattooing, the only way the practice is acceptable for women in some social circles is to feminize the project overtly in accordance with established gender codes.

Second, the strategic placement of some women's tattoos brims with conformity to established constructions of femininity. For instance, the overarching "rule of placement" for more conforming women is concealability. Fearing reprimand or scorn from others, these women do not publicly flaunt their dalliances into tattooing, and thus the lower back, the hips, and the upper back are the most common locations for their tattoo projects:

> The only thing that kept going through my mind was, "what about my wedding dress." There was no way in hell that I could see myself standing at the altar, right beside my future husband, right in front of the whole congregation, with a fat tattoo of a heart stuck up there on my bare arm. That would look so tacky, and it would ruin the whole experience of being a bride. Brides in their lace gowns with huge tattoos showing don't paint a very attractive picture . . . My tattoo is on my lower back, where no one has to ever see it except me. (Devon, age 26)

However, regularly concealed parts of the female body are also those that tend to be highly sexualized. As a fringe benefit of concealing her tattoos, Trina (age 30) explained that by having them on her lower back (traced around the contours of her upper buttocks, and around the front of her pelvis), she had received "positive feedback" from her sexual partners:

> There's quite an aesthetic pleasure that comes from seeing a naked body with elegant markings around its sensuous parts. We've all seen dozens of naked bodies in our lives, and when you are having sex with a partner, it's always exciting to experience difference . . . I remember one man I dated became immediately aroused when I told him about the tattoo across the top of my ass. When we eventually had sex, he couldn't wait to find out what it looked like. It's funny because he only wanted to have sex from behind so he could see it the whole time. He's not the only guy that I've slept with who has said that I have the most beautiful ass ever, and that they would have never guessed that I would be someone who was into tattooing.

In a conceptually related way, if the tattoo is placed "out in the open" (e.g., the ankle or lower leg), it can be discursively configured as a form of feminine/sexual ornamentation akin to a piece of jewellery. If viewed by the tattoo enthusiasts and their social networks as an act of compliance to established femininity, then, tattooing and femininity may become closely related.

Third, concerns about jeopardizing one's femininity will bear on the size of the tattooing project. Describing extensively, or "heavily" in the common parlance, tattooed bodies as "disgustingly unfeminine," Cora (age 28) articulated her thoughts about the size of her tattoo in the following way:

> There's a fine line between something that is dignified and understated, and something that is boorish and ugly. When I see a woman with a lot of really large tattoos, I think, that doesn't become her at all. I can't see a heavily tattooed woman and say to myself, wow, that's really feminine. Aesthetically, it doesn't work.

Heavily influenced by the locations on the body preferred by these women for their tattoo projects, the size of their tattoos are relatively dictated by dominant understandings of how femininity and tattooing are related. On the basis of the narratives of 32 (80%) of the enthusiasts I interviewed, there is little to suggest that a "large" tattoo is consistent with established constructions of femininity.

In sum, the desire to maintain a culturally established feminine status is either explicit or implicit in many Canadian women's tattooing body projects. In some cases, the women readily acknowledged the nature of their compliance; others were more reluctant to acknowledge any conformity. In either case, it became evident through the exploration of their tattoo narratives that the interpretive resource provided by one's gender mediates most aspects of the tattoo body project—from the selection of a tattoo, to the way it is displayed, to the way tattooed skin is socially experienced. It is this mediation that is key for understanding the processes of cultural conformity in women's tattooing. As suggested below, however, it is similarly crucial for interpreting processes of cultural resistance and negotiation in women's tattooing.

Cultural Resistance and Women's Tattooing

Even a cursory review of the sociological literature reveals a meta-narrative that suggests that tattooing is undertaken by North American women as acts of cultural rebellion. It is argued that North American women pursue alternative cultural constructions of femininity and the feminine form by wilfully violating established body idiom through tattooing. Rejecting the idea that women's bodies are passive and best unscathed, women tattoo enthusiasts express different standards for what they consider to be feminine through their tattoo projects. This version of femininity starkly contrasts established gender ideologies and traditionally feminine forms. As Caroline (age 31) described,

> I've never heard anybody say, I think women are all about bows, daisies, sunny days, and tattoos. When you say the word "tattoo," I mean, you think of a guy right away . . . Women nowadays believe that whatever men can do women can do better, and that includes tattooing. We're taking over the whole business [laughs].

For Caroline and likeminded women tattoo enthusiasts, indelibly marking the skin with tattoos is a social

crusade into historically masculine body practice. *Among the women I interviewed, 15 (38%) stated that one of their main interests in tattooing projects is derivative of the extent to which a woman's tattooed flesh is a breach of established body convention.* Inferring the body as a communicative text of culture, emphasis is given to the ways in which the marked body resists established constructions of the "body beautiful," a body that is recognizable in its docility and attractive for its fleshy curves, shapes, and contours. By cleverly using a profane body modification project to disrupt entrenched cultural images of the beautiful female body, some Canadian women are drawing alternative images of femininity through their body work.

As body projects are typically expressions of conformity to established gender ideologies, modifying the skin to wage cultural resistance is an act of cultural subversion. The bricolage involved in the tattooing process bespeaks of a conscious attempt to expand the cultural boundaries of women's body projects. Rather than passively partaking in ritualized, mass-marketed, and painful body projects in the pursuit of ideal-type feminine forms, some Canadian women promote individuality and alternate constructions of femininity through body play:

> Squeezing your breasts into a tight bra doesn't feel comfortable. Neither does pasting fake eyelashes to your eyelids, or going hungry all day just to stay a size 4. Pushing, pulling, stretching, or binding your body to look good for a man isn't my idea of fun . . . So when people tell me that I'm nuts for getting tattooed [because it's painful], I respond by telling them that I'm not the one who mutilates my body everyday to look like the fashion models in magazines. Punishing your body to appease somebody else is psychotic, and most of the women I know don't get that. But they still have the nerve to stare at me and think I'm less of a "woman" for choosing this [tattooing]. (Laura, age 24)

Just as some women have learned to inscribe cultural conformity upon their bodies through ritual projects of identity construction, other women have equally learned to confront the established gender order through body modification. A "flesh journey" such as tattooing can, then, disturb the established order as it creates a certain amount of cultural "noise" as a non-standard body project.

But why stir such cultural noise through tattooing body projects? Given the litany of non-invasive methods of contesting oppressive gender ideologies through physical style, why would someone choose to mark the body permanently with tattoos? Eight (20%) of the women I interviewed suggested that a tattoo's permanence is actually one of the primary allures behind the body project. This was symbolized by Zeta's (age 25) words:

> I'm going to the grave and beyond with my tattoos. If you are really committed to a cause, then you're prepared to give over your body and mind forever. I could talk, and talk, and talk about wearing grungy clothes or not dyeing my hair to look like a Barbie doll, and no one would care since all of that is superficial. A body is a temple, and how I decorate mine is a forever thing. I am not a Barbie doll, and will never be one. That's a played out image of women, and my temple is marked with symbols that read, "a strong and independent woman lives here . . . forever."

The personal significance of the body project is accented because tattoo enthusiasts are able to "customize" the images with which they choose to contest established social convention over the life-course.

Tattooing can also be a rather flamboyant way to violate diffuse cultural rules about the gendered body. Although colouring one's hair with bright green or purple hues, wearing men's suits, or exercising the body to the point of hypermuscularity can be designed by women as spectacular forms of resistance to gender codes, some Canadian women believe the message is most dramatically conveyed through radical forms of body modification. Given the enduring cultural association between tattooing and the masculine social underbelly in Canada (i.e., gangs, prisoners, carnival workers, or deviant youth subcultures), the body project *itself* conjures images of the outsider, and is socially prepackaged as the practice of the rebel. Furthermore, because women have traditionally participated in tattooing in more limited ways than men, the social practice is, as Hebdige might describe, "pregnant" with social significance for women with vested interests in challenging the established gender order.

In the process of engaging in cultural resistance through tattooing, the idea that women are symbolically liberated via this "liminal rite of passage" is often promoted through situated narratives. Associating one's tattooing projects with gender discrimination and social stratification (i.e., as a method of struggling against such marginalization), the body project is inserted into collective identity politics. Exploring the ways tattooing can serve a mimetic function for social outsiders in patriarchal figurations, Canadian women reveal their tattoos as a means of exhibiting their gender wounds:

> I participate in a women's group that meets once a month. About a year and a half ago one of the women mentioned she received a tattoo a couple of days prior to our meeting. All of the women in the group are very middle-class and we were pretty startled by this. We all clamoured around her, poking and prodding to see if we could guess where it was placed. After about 5 minutes of persistent badgering she lifted up the back of her shirt and showed us a tattoo of an angel with broken wings. I couldn't get over how beautiful it looked, and it made me gasp when she told us how it helped her manage her feelings about being raped when she was a teenager . . . We talked about her tattoo for hours and how she felt as a woman about being sexually abused. By the end of the session, 5 of us decided we were going to have tattoos done as well. I mean, the way it helped Sandy deal with her victimization was incredible. I think most women have been abused like that at some point in our lives . . . Ten of the women in the group now have tattoos, and each one of us has taken a turn writing a story about our tattoo and what it means. We present them at group meetings and go over how tattooing helps women feel in control of our bodies. It's absolutely exhilarating to hear the stories, and to be friends with such strong women. (Marion, age 29)

The resulting narratives become widely circulated scripts for decoding the significance of tattooing as acts of personal reclamation, self-definition, and gender empowerment. In this way, gender resistance through tattooing becomes discursively configured as an interdependent and intersubjective enterprise among Canadian women.

Not only are discourses shared among some Canadian women in the process of "doing" resistance to established gender ideologies, certain tattoo designs are also commonly worn. Rather than inscribing roses, butterflies, or moons onto the body, traditionally masculine tattoo designs are strategically chosen by some women. For instance, skulls and crossbones, hearts and daggers, eagles, or tribal (e.g., Polynesian, Melanesian, or African) motifs are often utilized to disassemble established cultural associations between femininity and weakness:

> Why should men get to wear all the really cool "traditional" tattoos? All of the really boss designs that I like are from the old school days, like all the sailor tattoos . . . I'm not stupid, and I know tattooing is this macho thing, and that's why girlies have worn little rainbows or baby pandas or whatever, and dance around saying "ooh, look at my cute little tattooed ass." More of the girls I hang out with don't care about that crap, and don't buy into a tattoo because it's what looks right on a woman. I have these

tattoos [heart and banner, navy ship] to show I'm strong-willed, just like the tradition of tattooing in our culture. (Jenna, age 19)

Similarly, by tattooing "pin-up girls" on her body, Clarice (age 26) sought to reclaim and redefine the naked/partially nude body as a symbol of femininity. As an avid tattoo "collector," she described her pin-up girl tattoos in the following way:

Every time I go into Chapters or some other bookstore and pick up magazines, all I see are half-naked women. Turn on the T.V., and it's exactly the same. All men know about women are their naked bodies, and usually it's men who get to control how many naked women are in a film or whatever . . . Guys flip out when they see the two pin-up girls I have tattooed on my arm. Some of them, right, the first question they ask me, or want to ask me, is, "are you a dyke?" Guys are so predictable. But that is the reaction I want from men. I want a guy to look at me, look at my tattoos, and have everything he thinks about women screwed up.

In these cases, the tattooed body is literally designed to fracture established gender ideologies by inverting typical masculine or feminine icons and attributing alternative cultural meanings to them through a process of bricolage.

The strategic placement of the symbol on the body is also central in women's tattoo projects that are motivated by cultural resistance. Choosing parts of the body that tend to be exposed or exposable in everyday life situations, some Canadian women offer their bodies to be decoded as confrontational or different. By tattooing arms/forearms, hands, lower legs/calves, upper chests, and necks, women consciously breach established body idiom as part of their rejection of established cultural understandings of femininity. The designs tend to be larger than those selected by more conforming tattoo enthusiasts and encompass greater portions of body space. Even though the tattoos are concealable in most cases, enthusiasts often believe that tattoo body projects intended for social resistance must be visible to be effective. As a segment of Karen's (age 25) tattoo narrative described,

When it comes to tattooing, bold is beautiful. I hate women who talk tough about their tattoos, pretending like they've done something rebellious with their bodies just because they have an ant dot [tattoo] on their hip. What's the point in even getting tattooed if people aren't going to see it? For young women it's important that we aren't embarrassed about having tattoos, and we can't let what's expected of us "girls" restrict our involvement . . . People don't respect half-stepping. If we're going to bother saying something through our tattoos, make everybody listen or the message gets lost.

According to Karen and her peers, without actually confronting others in the process of "being confrontational," no discernable challenge to established understandings of the body can be initiated.

To imply, however, that all forms of resistance to established constructions of the female body through tattooing are similar to those described above would be patently false. Although the strategies outlined above seem to be the standards for interpreting when and how resistance through women's tattooing and other radical forms of body modification is undertaken, they simply do not capture the full range of resistance expressed by women through this type of body work.

In this study, 6 (15%) of the women I interviewed stated that their resistance to established gender codes is more subtle and private than the wildly spectacular variation displayed by, what they perceive to be, more "radical" feminists. These women are astutely aware of the ways in which tattooing a "feminine" body undermines established body codes, and have become drawn into the recent popularity of women's tattooing in Canada for this reason. Many of these women have also become privy, in one context or another, to tattooing narratives that detail the liberating nature of the body project for women. Hence, some Canadian women are fascinated by the possibilities of using the body in a popularly rebellious way. At the same time, they are not eager to be labelled a "deviant female" through their participation in tattooing.

The pragmatic position that some Canadian women adopt toward tattooing is, then, founded upon a desire to engage in resistance to established gender codes while maintaining a semblance of conformity to such edicts. The contestation of established cultural body images and practices (and relationships of social inequality that produce them) is crucial here, but is not undertaken with social/cultural recklessness. The *negotiated* centre-point between outright conformity and unapologetic resistance allows a tattoo enthusiast to be compliant or rebellious in situated contexts of interaction. Assessing when the marks might be stigmatizing (i.e., involving an unbearable loss to identity, status, or role-set), or socially rewarding (i.e., having one's resistance to gender codes respected and appreciated, or receiving kudos from others about one's tattoos), is central in the negotiation process and can shape a woman's involvement in tattooing.

The main rationale for negotiating one's involvement in resistant forms of tattooing articulated by the women I interviewed hinged upon the idea that tattooing should be a private customization of the female body. For these women, resistance to gendered ways of thinking and acting is accomplished through subtle acts of protest rather than overt and easily targeted forms of gender "bending." The tattooed body does not necessarily have to be publicly displayed to others in this process, as a tattoo body project reflects a deeper and more symbolic dialogue with the self. The tattooed body is an illustrative diary of one's innermost thoughts and feelings about established constructions of femininity and established gender ideologies:

> To change Descartes' terms slightly, "I tattoo, therefore I am." Personally, I didn't do any of this [points to tattoos on her arms] for anyone other than myself. When it comes to my body, I make the decisions. If I want to look different than I'm supposed to [as a woman], because that's how I feel, then I can deal with that through my tattoos. I don't have to stand on the top of buildings and scream out that I lived as an anorexic, or that I have been taught to hate the way my body looks—or, I should say, how it used to look . . . It wasn't until I started to express myself though tattooing, and figured out how I wanted to look as a woman, that I had a grip on my identity and a strong sense of who I am. I don't see any reason why I should include anyone else in that either. A tattoo is something that is supposed to be personally satisfying and meaningful . . . for me, it's not about the public consumption of my identity anymore. (Chasey, age 22)

As McRobbie and Muggleton have pointed out, negotiated forms of social resistance can be injected into a gamut of private, personal practices that are never given to audiences for consumption. In the case of tattooing, there is an inner satisfaction derived from simply expressing anger, frustration, or depression about established constructions of femininity through a tattoo body project.

Still, from the moment that a woman begins to think about a tattooing body project as a private form of resistance, other people enter into the equation. On the basis of previous interaction with others (e.g., sisters, fathers, daughters, school mates, or employers), including the exchange of physical cues and body language, women develop "stocks of knowledge" concerning others' attitudes toward tattooing and the female body. From the onset, it seems that social reactions figure prominently in deciding how and when to participate in tattooing as negotiated gender resistance, including what image will be tattooed, the location of the tattoo, and the size of the design:

> I knew that if I went overboard and had the tattoo take up most of my arm or something, then people would go bonkers. It's quite a jump to make from having no tattoos to having this massive one. You have to ease people into it, right, let them get used to the idea that your body is going to be "different" looking woman forever. I didn't want everybody to think I was basically saying, I'm not myself any-

more . . . so I figured I would start small and if I liked it, and people didn't get too huffed, I could always go back and get something bigger [on another part of my body] if I decided. If you let your friends know that you've haven't really changed that much, you can get into it as much as you like. (Rosalyn, age 22)

Rena (age 23) stated that her inclinations to be tattooed were tempered by the fear that her modified flesh would meet with significant disapproval from her family:

> I wanted to get tattooed so badly. But my dad always said that he thought women with tattoos look like whores. And, he said that if people look at you like a whore, they will treat you like one. But that was the point for me, right . . . not looking like a good little girl, or always doing what I was told. My mom always agreed with him, and even my brother asked me why I wanted to do it. I have this friend named Marcy, and she has a devil girl tattooed on her shoulder. My dad won't even talk to her anymore when she comes by the house, and has basically told me he doesn't want me to hang around with her . . . So, I finally screwed up enough courage to be tattooed with the Chinese symbol of eternity and took the plunge. I thought my butt would be the best place because even when I am in a bikini, my dad would never see it. He's never seen it to this day, and I don't think I could ever bring myself to even tell him.

In Rena's case, she interpreted her family members' negative sentiments about tattooing as a form of social protection. By condemning the body project as outside the established gender norm, family members impress upon the budding enthusiast the importance of following established cultural practices. By selecting locations on the body for the project that are regularly covered by clothing, however, these tattoo enthusiasts are able to negotiate their involvement and "pass" as norm abiding.

The reactions to tattooing body projects (experienced or anticipated) expressed by employers and coworkers can be even more tenuous than those provided by family members or friends. A primary concern for women tattoo enthusiasts, especially in neo-conservative business environments, is that negative reactions from coworkers will interfere with their achieved statuses at work. For the most part, they come to view their tattoo projects as a form of "intolerable deviance" in the workplace—a profane form of representation that carries immediate career ramifications:

> When I go to work I'm not there completely on my own terms. I feel like the company pays my salary,

and gets to tell me how to behave. That's the price you pay to get paid . . . I work in an office as a personal assistant and if you come in looking bizarre in front of all the stuffed shirts who hit on you all day, you catch hell. You have to maintain a business persona at work, and apparently you can't have a tattoo and be professional . . . especially if you are a woman. At work, I can't bring my [gender] politics there everyday, and I have to cover it up. I've had nightmares about going to work naked—not because everyone can see my breasts, but because everyone could see the tattoos on my breasts. [The company] gives off this image like they're hip and young and urban, but we'd see how hip they are if I came in with a low-cut top on. I'd be the hippest girl on the unemployment line. (Laura, age 24)

In recognizing that one's attitudes about gender resistance through tattooing may not be intersubjectively appreciated in the workplace, enthusiasts may negotiate their involvement in tattooing as personal necessity; that is, women enthusiasts are not oblivious to their economic interdependencies and curtail their body modification projects accordingly.

The impetus to negotiate one's involvement in this form of self-expression can, however, create internal tensions for women who perceive their conformity to established body politics as a character deficiency. Five (13%) of the women I interviewed used the term, "selling out" to describe their sense of public inauthenticity:

> I made the conscious choice to tattoo my body, and I'll never regret it. It was probably the defining moment in my life so far . . . it was the only time I did anything solely for myself, to display who I am as an individual. Still, I'm not indifferent to ridicule from other people about my tattoos, so I keep them under wraps most of the time. I go home at night and cry sometimes because I don't have the brass to stand up and ask people to accept me for how I look. I had this vision of how tattooing was going to change my life for the better, and make me more socially confident. And when I sell out by hiding my body under the clothes I wear, I feel like a shy little girl again, peeking around my mother's skirt to see who's talking to me. (Adele, age 23)

Complying with pressures created by established gender codes and supported in institutional contexts such as the family, school, or workplace, some women enthusiasts believe that they compromise a part of their resistant philosophies by putting on a conforming front. In socially presenting a disingenuous persona in the front regions of everyday settings, these women experience an unsettling bifurcation of identity. By undertaking a series of body management techniques in order to hide their tattooed flesh when in the presence of others, some Canadian women come to view their negotiation as an act of cowardice.

In brief, the decision to engage in cultural dissent through body projects such as tattooing appears to be mediated by one's purpose or motivation for the project and the degree to which the resulting body modification jeopardizes one's achieved/ascribed cultural statuses. Although the central purpose of the body project may be to challenge the very basis of such statuses and associated roles (i.e., as they support established constructions of femininity), Canadian women are not impervious to established cultural norms about gender and its representation. Resistance, therefore, to established social constructions of gender through tattooing exists on a sliding scale. Although some women's tattoo body projects are flagrant violations of established body play and dominant images of masculinity/femininity, others are privately negotiated acts of dissent.

Discussion

Canadian women's involvement in tattooing has risen dramatically over the past 10 years. Despite this noticeable shift in the demographics of tattoo enthusiasts in Canada, sociologists have failed to address adequately how and why women are now active in the practice. Contemporary analyses of tattooing in North America reveal a keen awareness that women's interest in the body project is burgeoning, but do not offer many theoretical interpretations of this boom in popularity, or its consequences on established constructions of femininity. Furthermore, authors have misguidedly conjoined the entirety of men's and women's uses for, and interpretations of, tattoos around a core set of principles that were originally intended to explicate men's tattooing practices only. The preoccupation with men's tattoo experiences, and the subsequent creation of academic understandings/discourses about tattoos from this gaze, has conceptually homogenized the body project between the genders and systematically persuaded individuals to overlook ways of knowing/seeing the tattooed body as a gendered entity.

Feminist theories and related theories about the body richly enhance researchers' understanding of how and why women participate in the body project. By attending to a full range of body projects commonly undertaken by women, feminist and profeminist researchers have struggled to expose the gendered ways through which corporeality is physically and socially constructed. In underscoring that one's preferences for body modification are partially reflective of one's socially achieved gender status, we are able to appreciate the ways in which tattooed bodies are defined via this key interpretive resource. Although a conceptualization of the gender-body link described in this paper is not a revelation within the larger literature on body projects, it is a major revelation in the study of tattooing as sociologists, psychologists, and cultural anthropologists have discussed gender and tattooing without theoretically interrogating the relationships between tattooing, gender, and gendered bodies.

To recognize the gendered parameters within which women participate in the body project is critical at this juncture. Recent estimates suggest that more women than men comprise the newest generation of tattoo enthusiasts in Canada, and a vast array of meanings have been attributed to women's tattooed bodies. By going beyond the popular idea that women's tattoo body projects are simply crass refutations of established gender codes (perhaps a lingering product of mainstay decodings of women's tattooing projects as the antithesis of men's), we open up a possibility for understanding why women tattoo their bodies in the conscious effort of reproducing or negotiating established constructions of femininity.

As the women I interviewed articulated through their narratives, feelings about one's gender status dictate one's tattoo body projects and subsequent interpretations of them. The women structured much of their tattooing narratives around the ways in which they decode their tattoos *as women,* or were tattooed as an expression of some "femininity." Almost without exception, the women's underlying reasons for being tattooed; the shapes, sizes, and placements of their tattoos; the social presentation of their tattoos; and the active construction of their tattoos reflected desire to communicate specific messages about gender to particular audiences.

These contextual communiqués are evidently dialogical with established constructions of femininity and the feminine body in Canada. For the most part, the women I interviewed voiced an awareness of the outsider social status women continue to hold in Canada and how women are expected to modify their bodies for the pleasure of men (i.e., men prefer soft, supple, thin, sexy, and unblemished feminine bodies). Recognizing the extent to which they regulate their bodies in accordance with prevailing established images of femininity, almost all of the women I interviewed recounted how their forays into tattooing were mediated (in some basic way) by this cultural understanding. In the majority of cases, traditional or established cultural constructions of femininity in Canada formed the mortar of the women's tattoo projects.

Canadian women who actively comply with established constructions of femininity through their body work deftly mould their tattooing projects into acts of gender conformity. Caught up in the current popularity of tattooing among the younger generations, and the ways in which it has been fashionably inserted into the mainstream, these women narratively and physically construct the projects with deference to established gender expectations. By drawing attention to the beautiful/sexual feminine body and highlighting the docility of the female form, these women's tattoo projects are conceptually equivalent to other body projects such as liposuction, breast enlargement, excessive dieting and corseting in that each reinforce the established feminine form as the cultural norm. Furthermore, such tattoo projects garner favourable attention from others (e.g., parents, peers, boyfriends, husbands) as they are explicitly assembled as acts of consent to established constructions of femininity. As a result, these body projects symbolically reproduce women's outsider social status in Canada, and physically illustrate the ways women's bodies are sexualized, objectified, regulated, and monitored in accordance with established cultural constructions.

However, other women tattoo enthusiasts reject the oppressive outsider social standing that established femininity carries in Canada, and they challenge such depictions of femininity through their body projects. Subverting established reasons for engaging in body projects (i.e., the pursuit of an ideal-type femininity), these women utilize the tattooed body as a billboard for political protest. Instead of consenting to masculinist preferences for the female body through painful processes of body manipulation, these women seek to dismantle established ideologies and the structures of gender stratification they buttress. In de Certeau's terms, they use "what they have" in order to wage resistance. As the body is one of the most socially recognized signifiers of one's gender, immediate confrontations to the established patriarchal hegemony in Canada can be initiated through bold and highly visible tattoo projects.

We must question, however, whether or not these acts of cultural defiance are merely "magical solutions" to common problems of status adjustment among women in Canada. Because the flamboyantly tattooed woman's body tends to elicit negative responses from established others (i.e., as a "freakish," "unattractive," or "deviant" body), does the campaign of resistance through tattooing further entrench these women into the status of the outsider? Just as Punk Rockers solidified their marginalized social class positions by adopting radical physical styles to express their collective sense of alienation and disenfranchisement, these women may very well be *reinforcing* the sanctity of established images of femininity (and related established body practices) as the cultural norm.

It is not surprising, then, that many of the women I interviewed preferred to negotiate their involvement in tattooing. Neither accepting nor consenting to established constructions of femininity in Canada (yet not ignoring their cultural saliency), some women tactically engage in tattooing as a form of *negotiated* resistance to dominant gender codes. Established and outsider social relationships (vis-à-vis gender) are partially maintained in this process of negotiation, but the women nonetheless derive an inner satisfaction from their negotiated cultural transgressions. The negotiation is justified by women as social necessity in most cases—as an overt tattooing body project may jeopardize key interdependencies one shares with conforming others. It is further justified as a deeply personal form of self-expression, and the tattoo designs or symbols represent an individual's unique biography. In all cases, the negotiation permits women to explore tattooing as a self-directed "flesh journey" of self-discovery without raising the ire of, or stirring unwanted critique from, "unenlightened" audiences.

In conclusion, the discussion presented in this article is not a totalizing, static, or definitive account of women's experiences with tattooing in Canada or elsewhere. We must recognize that women's tattooing experiences are highly varied, culturally contextual, and temporally bound. In this respect, there is a pressing need for extended and concatenated research on women's tattooing—both within Canada and elsewhere. Within this lacuna, we would immediately benefit from in-depth empirical analyses of the ongoing social construction of tattooing as an intersubjectively meaningful body project among women, the long-term and unintended impacts of women's participation in the body project on men's involvement in tattooing, and of course, the stylistic changes in North American tattooing as a result of the increasing "feminization" of the tattoo business. Future researchers should strive to enrich our knowledge about women's involvement in tattooing through theoretical innovation, methodological experimentation, and substantive exploration. As women's participation in the body project continues to expand and diversify, so must our sociological understanding of women's tattooing.

Acknowledgments

I thank Kevin Young, Joan Chrisler, and the anonymous reviewers for their helpful comments on earlier drafts of this article. This study was funded in part by the Social Sciences and Humanities Research Council of Canada.

Notes

1. To whom correspondence should be addressed at Department of Sociology, Memorial University of Newfoundland, St. John's, Newfoundland, Canada A1C5S7; e-mail: atkinson@mun.ca.
2. The term "enthusiast" refers to all individuals who have voluntarily chosen to tattoo their bodies at some point. Although there are qualitative distinctions to be made between various types or categories of tattoo enthusiasts, the term is employed here simply as a tool for discussing the conceptual similarities between people's experiences with tattooing.
3 One should be careful to note that women have a long history of participation within the larger tattoo figuration in North America—particularly among circus or carnival groups, as part of elite fashion and haute couture trends, as part of women's liberation movements, and in some nefarious subcultures or lifestyle enclaves. In comparison to men, however, women have played a marginal role in tattooing practices until recently.

References

A list of references is available in the original source.

Ouch!

You Call That Body Art?

by Teen Voices

Recently, even within the last five to 10 years, what was once popular only among sailors and bikers has now become a new trend among teenagers: body art. Suddenly teens everywhere are getting their bodies pierced and tattooed. Before, tattoos and piercings were associated either with criminals and street punks, using these markings as their battle flag, or with people who belonged to certain cultures such as the Maori of New Zealand, the Samoan of Polynesia, the Hindi of the Fiji Islands, and the Mehinaku and Kayapo of the Amazon. During the 1990s, young women of all socioeconomic classes have started taking part in this fad. These piercings and tattoos are used as a tool, allowing individuality to be expressed. However, this rebellion against conventional standards of beauty has now made its way into mainstream culture; instead of being the exception, it is commonplace.

Another reason for this popularity is that many familiar faces in the media have jumped on the bandwagon. Musicians including Madonna, Ani DiFranco, the Spice Girls, and Janet Jackson flaunt their body art. In a music video featuring Aerosmith, Alicia Silverstone is shown getting her navel pierced. Supermodels Christy Turlington and Naomi Campbell show off their navel piercings on the runway, while Eve's shaved head reveals a tattoo below. Actresses like Alyssa Milano, Tiffani Amber Thiesen, Pamela Lee, and Drew Barrymore are not shy about showing their tattoos.

In fact, this trend has skyrocketed to the point where some of us are going to extremes to fit in with our peers. Some are piercing themselves with sewing needles or safety pins. Others are sporting homemade tattoos made using a needle and thread dipped in ink. However, there is danger involved in what some of us are doing, even if the work is done professionally.

Body Piercing

Body piercings are more common than tattoos for several reasons. For one, they are definitely easier for underage teens to get. Piercers are more likely to work on those who are underage than tattoo artists are. Another reason that piercings are more popular is that, unless stretched, the hole is not "permanent." If piercing ever goes out of style or the teen simply decides she does not want the piercing anymore, the jewelry can be removed and the hole will close. The most popular places for these piercings seem to be the eyebrow, navel, nose, tongue, lip, nipple, and genital area.

Getting My Tongue Pierced

Stephanie Kutzer, 16

Pensacola, Florida

I got my tongue pierced on January 20, 1998, when I was fifteen. I didn't go to a professional piercer. My friend did it for me. Don't get me wrong, though, because she knows what she's doing. She used to be a piercer in New Orleans. She even ordered sterilized needles and everything. [When] I went over to her house . . . we talked for a while and hung out. Then I washed out my mouth and she looked at my tongue to find the spot where I wanted it. She had to pierce it kind of off-center to miss the web and the vein. I watched everything in the mirror that was behind her. Her friend, Randy, and her sister's boyfriend watched the whole time. She pierced it from the bottom to the top. The only time it hurt was when she went to push the needle through the top of my tongue. This is the only time I even said anything, which was, "Ugh!"

Randy was really surprised that I didn't bleed. After the needle was all they way through, my friend put the barbell in. It was a 14 gauge, one inch barbell. The reason it was one inch was to allow for swelling. She put the barbell through. Then it was over. I washed out my mouth again.

I went home later that night, but I didn't eat anything. My tongue was kind of sore, but not as bad as I thought it would be. Sunday morning I woke up and washed my mouth out with Listerine.* At this point, my parents . . . didn't know. Sunday night I went out with the guy I was seeing at the time. He said I was talking kind of funny, but it wasn't that bad.

When I woke up on Monday, my tongue still wasn't really that swollen. Actually, it never swelled up that bad. At first when you are getting used to having a barbell in your tongue, you slobber when you talk. That night, I was on the phone when my mom saw my Listerine. Don't ask me what made her do it. My mom came into my room and made me open my mouth. Then she told my dad. He told me to make sure I kept it clean in order avoid infection. My mom didn't talk to me for a week after that.

The whole experience was great. I would do it again in a second. It doesn't hurt as much as you think it will because your body knows what is happening. It's June now and I've stretched out my piercing to a 12 gauge barbell. My mom still doesn't like it, and my dad still doesn't care. If you want to pierce a body part, make sure the person knows what they are doing. It's your body, and you should take a stand for the right to do what you want with it.

Eyebrow Piercing Procedure

Jen, 15

Allentown, New Jersey

First of all, I have my right eyebrow pierced and I think it kicks some major butt . . . Anywayz . . . about the procedure . . . First, the dude will ask which side ya want it on. Then he'll put a 'lil black dot on the spot where he/she thinks it will look best. You can look in the mirror to see if ya like it. They clean the area really well with some stuff that I don't know the name of. Then they put a clamp where the dot is and stick a pin through it. There ya go, you're pierced. Then they put the ring in, and you're set to go.

Before you leave, they tell you how to clean it. You use the same stuff as when you get your ears pierced.

You just have to put it on the ring and keep turning it. I love my piercing, but you have to be careful with it. Clean it at least two or three times a day and turn it so the ring doesn't get stuck. Yucky. Oh, and if it gets infected, it gets mad raunchy, all pussy and crusty. Ewww. So if you plan on getting a piercing, make sure you take good care of it. You have to keep the ring in for about a month before you can take it out.

A big disadvantage to getting your eyebrow pierced is that the skin gradually grows over it. It can take a year or longer before it grows out. Oh, and try not to get it caught on anything because it can rip the skin and make the hole bigger. Lots of people comment on how cool it is or how cool it isn't. I get attention wherever I go. It's awesome.

My Eyebrow Mishap

Jaisa Olasky, 17

Framingham, Massachusetts

I thought that getting an eyebrow ring was going to be simple. You see, I already had, and still have, my navel pierced. I have had it for two years, and it has only become infected once and did not cause me much pain at all. As I expected, the procedure of getting my eyebrow pierced was quick and virtually painless. As early as the night I received the piercing, I started having problems. Every time I tried to hug anyone or lie down, it seemed as if it was in the way, always getting knocked around. I remember the immense pain every time I casually brushed my hair out of my eyes and accidentally hit the ring. It was also every complicated to try and put on sweaters, turtle necks, or shirts with collars. After a while I got used to having it and really started to like it.

By January, I had grown quite attached to it since it had finally stopped sticking straight out. Unfortunately, I was still having painful incidents. On two separate occasions, friends of mine hugged me and knocked the ring really hard. That was around the time that I started to notice that it was really hanging kind of low. The hole started to feel a little loose as well. I talked with a couple of people who also had eyebrow rings. Incidentally, they have both taken them out since. They agreed with me that it was growing out.

I went back to the same place I got it pierced to get the ring taken out. The piercer there said it was common for eyebrow piercings to "grow out" and was often "unavoidable." Since then I have found out from other piercers that if the procedure is done with a large gauge and is very deep, it won't grow out.

---

*Listerine is not a good mouthwash to use because it contains alcohol. If you want to use a mouthwash with alcohol, it must be diluted by half with water.

I've had a lot of people ask me if I'm going to get it pierced again. Since it healed well and did not scar, I would like to, but I don't think I will. It just seems like there's too big a chance that it will grow out again. It also costs a lot, and it's a pain have it in the way all the time.

Tattooing

While tattooing has not become as trendy as body piercing because it costs more, is permanent, and hurts more, many teens are still getting this type of work done.

My Itsy Bitsy Spider

Jessica Laura Lila, 17

Los Angeles, California

When I turned fifteen, I wanted a tattoo. My dad already had one of a hummingbird on his arm and his girlfriend had a Pegasus on her back. My dad's a pretty fair guy. I guess he figured if this was something I really wanted, and he would be able to check out the tattoo studio beforehand, it would be okay.

I took him down to the place where I wanted to get the work done and we met with the artist who would do the work. We chatted with him about cost, size, and placement concerns. Then we made my appointment.

I had planning in getting a design, a spiral, for at least a year. However, a day or two before the appointment, I had a sudden idea. I drew up a little black spider and decided I wanted that instead. I also changed my mind about where I wanted the tattoo. Originally, I had planned to get it put in the center of my chest. That same sudden idea made me decide to get it placed off-center, though, between my breast and shoulder. If you've seen the movie Foxfire, it's the same spot where all those girls got their tattoos. I didn't know this at the time, though.

On my birthday, after a nice breakfast, my dad, my boyfriend, and I went to get the work done. I was having some serious butterflies in my stomach, but I bit my tongue and sat down in the chair anyway. After some time, the spider was done, and I was bouncing around showing it to anyone who would stay still. I had to go back a year later to have white highlights put in and to darken his legs a bit.

For me, getting a tattoo was great. It did hurt, though. I would rank mine at just a bit more painful than waxing your bikini line. Some people say it's much worse. Others say they hardly even felt it. It takes a while to heal and the skin on top of the tattoo will scab over. You have to make sure you don't pick at it. After the scab flakes and peels off, the design you have left is what you'll have for the rest of your life.

Dear Teen Voices,

Your magazine is wonderful. I only wish that there was a magazine like yours when I was growing up. I applaud you on covering the topics that you do. However, I do have a health concern about the young lady with a pierced nose on one of your past covers.

As a health care professional, [I know] most states do not have guidelines for body piercing. The potential for HIV, Hepatitis B and C, etc. are substantial. Oral piercing is extremely dangerous with those complications as well as Ludwig's angina, hemorrhage, aspiration of parts of jewelry, traumatic injury to teeth, etc.

Thank you for your attention. Keep up the good work!

Sincerely,
June Caine
Spring Hill, Tennessee

Here are some words of advice I want to offer any teenager who's thinking of getting a tattoo:

1. I recommend you wait. I know you want to get it done now, but you'll probably regret it later if you do it now. Also, most respectable tattoo studios won't work on someone who is underage because they will lose their licenses. That's why I'm not giving the name of the place where I got mine done.

2. Know your design very well. Think about it for at least a year beforehand to make absolutely sure it's what you want. It's not a good idea to walk into the studio and get something just "because it looks cute." Those are the tattoos that people regret the most. Try getting the design you want done in ink or henna first. That way you can get used to having it and, if you change your mind, the henna will wash off, but a tattoo won't.

The Truth About AIDS and Tattooing

Randie Farmelant, 18
Framingham, Massachusetts

In the age of AIDS (Acquired Immunodeficiency Syndrome), many people have become paranoid and have

(Adapted from *Safe Tattooing* by Steve Gilbert and *Can I Get Infectious Diseases From Tattoo Needles?*, by Nick Baban)

Is This Artist's Studio a Safe Place For Me?

Here's a list of things to look for in an artist's (referring to tattoo artist or piercer) studio. If you cannot answer yes to the following questions, the studio is not a safe, sterile environment.

- Is the area well lit, allowing the artist to see what s/he is doing?
- Is there a sink besides the one in the bathroom?
- Are the counter and floor light colored, allowing dirt to show up easily?
- Is the artist wearing gloves? If yes, s/he should not touch anything besides your skin, the needle, and the jewelry.
- Did you see some of the artist's previous work? Pictures are good, but seeing the real thing is even better. This applies to piercings, as well as tattoos. You should also talk with people who have had work done by the artist to see how they felt about the person and their work.
- Does the artist clean your skin and disinfect it before the procedure?
- Are all the needles either discarded or autoclaved after each use?
- If your skin has to be shaved, is the artist using a disposable razor?
- If you are getting a tattoo, is the ink being poured from the large container into separate, smaller cups?
- Do you feel comfortable to ask the artist any questions you may have so that you fully understand everything that is happening?
- Are the needles being used as soon as they are unwrapped? They should not be set down anywhere.

exaggerated the risk that certain activities present. One of these is tattooing. So here's the real scoop on the risk factor.

First of all, the needles used in tattooing and those employed by drug users are very different. When drug users inject drugs, they use hollow needles to get the drugs directly into their bloodstream. Since some blood usually remains in the syringe, AIDS is transmitted when the next person uses the needle. The needles used in tattooing are not hollow, however. What happens when you get a tattoo is that the needle travels back and forth through a tube, which holds the ink. As the needle goes into the tube, it becomes coated with ink. As it moves forward, it pierces your skin and deposits the ink. When the needle makes a hole in your skin, you bleed a little. If the needles are sterile, which they should be, the needle only touches your skin and your blood. Thus, the only person who is really at a risk for (HIV), the virus that causes AIDS, is the artist because s/he is the only one coming in contact with another person's skin and blood.

In fact, Hepatitis B is one of the most serious complications that can arise from getting a tattoo. The reason for this is that it is more prevalent than HIV and a lot easier to catch. The HIV virus is also much easier to kill than Hepatitis B. Boiling water or immersion in alcohol, bleach or other disinfectant will be as effective in killing the HIV virus as autoclaving. The HIV virus can only survive outside the human body for a few days, in comparison to Hepatitis B which can survive indefinitely.

HIV is also less contagious than Hepatitis B. Infection with the Hepatitis B virus can occur if as little as .00004 ml of blood is transferred. The HIV virus can only be transmitted if .1 ml or more of blood is transferred. In fact, the reason that tattooing was outlawed in New York in 1960 is because health officials blamed tattooing for thirty cases of Hepatitis B.

If all the needles and equipment have been properly sterilized in an autoclave and the tattoo artist wears rubber gloves, there is almost no risk of infection with the HIV virus. If you are planning on getting multiple piercings or tattoos done, it is in your best interest to become immunized against the Hepatitis B virus, however.

But Is Body Art the Right Choice for You?

As you have seen, body art may be an outlet through which to express yourself. If you do choose to get a piercing or tattoo, make sure you are safe. Think about the decision very carefully. Will you still want a hole in your nose ten years down the line? Is the heart tattoo on your arm going to look nearly as cute when you are eighty? Remember, these are permanent body modifications. Yes, piercings too. Even if you take the jewelry out, there will still be a scar and maybe even a hole if you have stretched the piercing at all.

If you still think that you want to get the body art, do it safely and carefully. Make sure you have your parents' permission. It is illegal in most states to get tattoo or piercing without parental permission if you are under eighteen. Always go to a licensed professional. Never have a friend do it for you. No matter how clean it seems and no matter how much you trust the person, this is never a good idea. Make sure the conditions of the studio where you get your work done are comparable to those of your dentist or doctor's office. Remember, as shown in Jaisa's situation, just because someone is licensed does not necessarily mean s/he knows what s/he is doing. Before you have the artist do anything to you, ask some questions and ask to see samples of the artist's previous work. This way, you will at least get a feel for how much experience the artist has. After you get the work done, make sure you follow all the after-care directions given to you by the artist.

Also, remember you are a strong female. If you want to get this work done because you want it, fine. But if you are getting your body permanently altered because you think someone else will think it looks good, you may want to think twice. There are also many other considerations to keep in mind. For example, everyone has her own tolerance for pain. Just because one person does not think it hurt to get her navel pierced does not mean that it will be the same painless experience for you.

Before You Decide to Get a Piercing or Tattoo, Read These Books

- *Coping with the Dangers of Tattooing, Body Piercing, and Branding,* By Beth Wilkinson
  This book is aimed especially at older teens. It has lots of good stuff, including: personal stories, historical information, dangers, after-care, and basic facts.
- *Everything You Need to Know About the Dangers of Tattooing and Body Piercing,* by Laury Reybold
  Written specifically for teenagers, this book contains a lot of cautions and warnings about body art. It also suggests some non-permanent alternatives.

WORKSHEET—CHAPTER 8
Food, Body Shaping, and Body Projects

PART 1: The Continuum of women and food relationships

This study guide is designed to help us see the similarities among a wide range of behaviors which get labeled as "eating disorders" and very related patterns which do not get labeled as "eating disorders."

The so-called "eating disorders" feel less threatening to us if we can view them as extreme cases which have nothing to do with us. However, even if we look at how common the extremes are, we must already face the fact that "eating disorders" are very much a part of our lives.

It may be more helpful to understanding the ambivalent relationship many women (in most western countries) have to their bodies and their food if we look at a wide range of eating patterns as a part of a continuum. If anorexia, bulimia, and compulsive eating are seen as exaggerated manifestations of dieting, we may be better able to understand both how our society encourages "eating disorders" and the unnaturalness and unhealthiness of most dieting.

    a. Make a list (collect examples from magazines, t.v., conversations, jokes) of messages women get about what they should look like. Make a list (collect examples from magazines, t.v., conversations, on-street advertising) of messages women get about delicious food available to them to eat or prepare. What is contradictory about these messages? How do women internalize these confused messages?

    b. Read the definitions for all the "eating problems" (pp 383-384) Look for similarities between the different patterns. Be creative! Think of a way to show the similarities between different patterns by connecting them with overlapping circles or lines. You may want to photocopy the words for eating problems and do a "cut and paste" job. You may want to use several different colors to identify themes which keep occurring.

    c. Reread definition #9 for "unnatural relationship to food and eating." Do you think this description of women for a body image study reflects *all* women or is it peculiar only to women concerned with body image? Can you think of ten women you know who are not concerned about body image? Can you think of ten women you know who are not very conscious of food/weight/exercise issues?

d. Based on your own experiences and the two articles by Christy Haubegger and Becky Thompson, describe whether you think body image issues are the same or different for white women and women of color.

e. Describe how you think race, class, and heterosexism impact on body image issues.

f. Many girls and women are pressured to be thinner than they are genetically meant to be. Based on the articles in this chapter and your own observations, identify some of the consequences of this for individual women and society.

g. After reading articles in this chapter, describe how national programs to reduce obesity could "uncouple healthy lifestyle behaviors from weight loss" (McAfee and Lyons) and minimize the stigma of being overweight.

Part 2: Body image, shape, projects

a. Draw a map of a woman's body. Going from head to toe, identify messages women get about "attractive" vs. "unattractive" versions of this body part, what women are encouraged to do to make that part "attractive," and what products and procedures are marketed to "improve" that part of the body.

b. "Pretty in Ink" identifies how women use tattooing "to communicate a wide range of personal and cultural messages." Based on the widest range of ways you and your friends do and do not use clothing, make-up/body art, body shaping, or body manipulation, describe your own examples of how you use your body to communicate personal and cultural messages.

The Continuum of Women and Food Relationships

Starving[16]   Large for years[15]

Anorexia[1]   Subgroup of   Weight   Up and down dieters[14]
                   weight preoccupied[2]   preoccupied[3]

Anorexia-like symptoms[4]   Compulsive eater[13]

Chronic anorexia[5]   Dieter
                                                          ex-"normal eater"[12]

Recovered anorexic[6]   Bulimorexic[8]

                                                          Thin fat people[11]

Ex-anorexic difficulties resolved[7]   Used to living on
                                                          semi-starvation diet[10]

                         Unnatural relationship
                         to food and eating[9]

1. Anorexia—Try to avoid eating as far as possible. Often have a distorted view of their bodies seeing themselves as grotesque and enormous instead of thin. Tend to be extremely close mouthed about their eating but observe others closely. (Orbach, 1984, p.30)

2. Sub-group of weight pre-occupied women. This group scored high or higher than the anorexia nervosa group on all Eating Disorder Inventory (EDI) subscales. (The EDI is designed to assess the cognitive and behavioral dimensions characteristic of anorexia and to differentiate between patients with anorexia and those without the disorder.) "It is likely that at the very least, they suffer from a subclinical variant of the disorder." (Garner, 1984, pp. 255–266.)

3. Weight preoccupied women. This group was compared to women with anorexia by the EDI (see 2). Weight preoccupied women and anorexic women were comparable on body dissatisfaction, bulimia, perfectionism, and maturity fears subscales. The EDI subscales which best differentiated weight preoccupied women from anorexics were ineffectiveness and interreceptive awareness. (Garner, 1984, pp. 255–266)

4. Women with anorexia-like symptoms. College women who scored high on Garner and Garfinkel's Eating Attitudes Test. This group was similar to the anorexia group in the proportion of subjects reporting binge eating and self-induced vomiting. This group did not show distress on a psychiatric symptom checklist. "These findings indicate that food and weight preoccupations common in anorexia nervosa do occur on a continuum, but the milder expression was not associated with psychosocial impairment." (Thompson and Schwartz, 1982, quoted in Garner, 1984)

5. Chronic anorexia—a anorexic makes a partial recovery, gains enough weight to keep her alive but maintains it at an artificially low level, sometimes for years. Her life continues to be utterly dominated by the desire to avoid food. (Lawrence, 1984, p. 108)

6. Recovered anorexic—sizeable proportion of ex-anorexics are able to live creative and independent lives but still retain some elements of their preoccupation with food and weight. (Lawrence, 1984, p. 108)

7. Ex-anorexic difficulties resolved. "The woman is no longer vulnerable to further anorexic episodes and *is no more neurotic about food than anyone else.*" (Lawrence, 1984, p. 109)

8. Bulimorexic—women often of average size, but weekly, daily, sometimes hourly, they binge on substantial amounts of food which they bring up. Very few feel comfortable talking about their way of coping. Feel purging after gorging is the only way to stay slim. (Orbach, 1984, p. 30) Estimated 15–20% of USA college women have bulimia. Only 44% sought professional help. (Potts, 1984, pp. 32–35)

9. Unnatural relationship to food and eating. For body image study, "I sought subjects with no history of psychiatric illness or eating disorder. It immediately became clear that it is a rare woman in this culture who is not eating disordered or who does not experience herself as struggling with food and weight issues. Of 114 women screened for this study 109 reported an unnatural relationship to food and eating. Of those selected as subjects—whose weights all fell within the normal range—only 1 woman was not actively waging a war against fat. This astonishing statistic suggests that weight and eating issues are inseparable from body image struggles in today's woman." "Although describing themselves as eating disordered . . . most women reported eating patterns typical of the culture as a whole, patterns that in men would never be labeled as pathological. These women are for the most part suffering not from eating disorders but from labeling disorders." (Hutchinson, 1982, p. 61)

10. Used to living on semi-starvation diet. Having grown up with the concept that thinness is identical with beauty and attractiveness . . . these women have grown used to living on a semi-starvation diet, never eating more than their bony figures show. Never having permitted themselves to eat adequately, they are unaware of how much their tension, bad disposition, irritability, even inability to pursue educational and professional goals is the direct result of chronic undernutrition. (Bruch, 1980, p. 19)

11. Thin fat people—people who stay reduced but who cannot relax. They seem as preoccupied with weight and dieting after they have become slim as before. (Bruch, 1980, p. 18)

12. "Diets turn 'normal eaters' into people who are afraid of food." (Orbach, 1984, p. 29)

13. Compulsive eating means eating without regard to physical cues signalling hunger or satisfaction. Feels out of control about what she eats. (Orbach, 1984, p. 29)

14. Women who go up and down the scale (maximum of 60 lbs), diet from time to time and binge irregularly. Open about talking about food problems. Feel that things would be better for them if they were thin. "The largest group of women." (Orbach, 1984, p. 30)

15. Women who have been large for years, who feel themselves to be fat, but are despairing about ever being able to lose weight. Experience their eating as chaotic. Discuss the topic openly. Feel things would be a lot better if they were slim. (Orbach)

16. Both starvation and dieting may produce many of the behaviors associated with anorexia. Both obese humans and starving organisms demonstrate thrifty metabolism, heightened preference for sweets and inhibition of satiety mechanisms. (Smead, 1983)

References

Bruch, H., "Thin Fat People" in Kaplan, J. R. (ed) *A Woman's Conflict: The Special Relationship Between Women and Food,* Prentice Hall, New York, 1980.

Garner, D. M., Olmstead, M. P., Polivy, J., and Garfinkel, P. E., "Comparison Between Weight-Preoccupied Women and Anorexia Nervosa", *Psychosomatic Medicine,* Vol. 46, No. 3, 1984, pp. 255–266.

Hutchinson, M. G., "Transforming Body Image: Your Body, Friend or Foe?", *Women and Therapy,* Vol. 1, No. 3, 1982, pp. 59–67.

Lawrence, M., *The Anorexic Experience,* Women's Press, London, 1984.

Orbach, S., *Fat Is a Feminist Issue 2,* Hamlyn Paperback, London, 1984.

Potts, N. L., "Eating Disorders—The Secret Pattern of Binge/ Purge", *American Journal of Nursing,* Vol. 84, No. 1, 1984, pp. 32–35.

Smead, V. S., "Anorexia Nervosa. Bulimarexia, and Bulimia: Labeled Pathology and the Western Female", *Women and Therapy,* Vol. 2, No. 1, 1983, pp. 19–35.

CHAPTER 9

Sexuality and LBT Issues

Sexuality can be a very important part of women's mental and physical health. The other way around, problems with mental or physical health often manifest themselves in a woman not being able to maximize on her sexual health and enjoyment. This chapter explores how social and cultural definitions of sexuality can be either positive or detrimental to emotional and physical health. The male emphasis on vaginal intercourse as the "real thing" limits or invalidates the experiences and preferences of many women. The question of who defines sexuality, and whether those definitions encourage or limit women's enjoyment of sexuality and maximizing on sexual health, will be central to this chapter.

"Exposed at Last: The Truth About Your Clitoris" is an appropriate way to begin this sexuality chapter. Although textbooks have often defined the clitoris as the "key" to female sexuality (the term clitoris is derived from the Greek work for key), they have also hidden it and presented it as very small, described as pea-sized. Jennifer Johnson's article notes that "the clitoris was more accurately described in some 19th century anatomy texts, but then it mysteriously shrunk into a mere speck on the anatomical map." When the clitoris is more fully and accurately described as homologous (arising from the same structure) to the penis (see Sloane's *Biology of Women* for details of the sex differentiation of the embryo), many aspects of female anatomy and sexual response make more sense. As we read this article, we should once again ask ourselves whether different things would be considered "scientifically interesting" and studied if more scientific decision-makers were women.

"How Being a Good Girl Can Be Bad for Girls," by Deborah Tolman and Tracy Higgins, gives both a societal overview and three specific adolescent girls' experiences of how "women's sexuality is frequently suspect in our culture, particularly when it is expressed outside the bounds of monogamous heterosexual marriage." In the same way that we have seen healthy women defined as passive and dependent (see "Mental Health Issues," Chapter 5), "good" women are sexually defined as "passive and threatened sexual objects" with no sexual desire. Tolman and Higgins point out that "When women act as sexual agents, expressing their own sexual desire rather than serving as objects of men's desire, they are portrayed as threatening, deviant, and bad." They look at all the no-win situations this puts girls and women in as they are held responsible for sexual gate-keeping. Within this framework, girls/women do not have permission to discover, express or enjoy their own sexual desire, but are too often held culturally or legally responsible for not stopping rape. This article starts the discussion of how such good girl/bad girl dynamics can be resisted and feminists are encouraged "to analyze the complexity of living in women's bodies within a culture that divides girls and women within themselves and against each other."

The provocative article, "The Orgasm Gap," pushes us to recognize the cultural construction of sexuality, the price women pay for this, the enormous possibilities for "making sex an act of shared, mutual pleasure" and why that must be a core component of work toward gender equality:

> Seventy-five percent of men have orgasm in partner sex on a regular basis, but only 29% of women do . . . Women are not inherently less orgasmic than men. In fact, women are physically capable of multiple orgasms, and most women who masturbate reach orgasm without fail. Women who have sex with a female partner come 83 percent of the time. Clearly, the problem lies not with women themselves, but in the way *heterosexuals* have sex.

"Women's Liberation is Coming" shows how many third-wave feminists are creating cultural changes by resisting sex-negative messages. The owner of Venus Envy Stores observes a new attitude which says, "Nobody can tell us what we can and cannot do with our bodies. Don't tell us who we should be partnered with or even that we need a partner." June Jordan's essay, "The New Politics of Sexuality," asserts the important points that freedom is indivisible, that the politics of sexuality are not the province of "special interest" groups, and that bisexuality gives an important perspective on the complexity of sexuality.

The next three articles in this chapter work together to demonstrate the urgency of both individual health practitioners and the health system as a whole learning to do better jobs of appropriately serving *all* their patients regardless of patients' sexual identity or practices. Society's homophobia is very much reflected in the medical system's homophobia, and fear and shame are recurring themes in stories of lesbian, bisexual, gay and trans people's experiences with the health system. Studies have consistently shown that a major health issue for lesbians is that they do not take care of regular routine health care, i.e., gynecological exams, because of actual or feared poor interactions with homophobic or heterosexist providers. Dr. Jennifer Potter's "Do Ask, Do Tell" relates her own story of moving from being a frightened suicidal young lesbian to being a proud, out, lesbian, physician, and educator:

> Many lesbians and gay men find it difficult to avoid internalizing some of these (society's) homophobic attitudes. As a consequence, shame and fear are common emotions, and we are more likely to be isolated; engage in risky behaviors; suffer from stress-related health conditions, substance abuse, and depression and attempt suicide.

Dr. Charles Moser's very practical, very explicit chapter, "Health Care Without Shame—Some Background for the Practitioner" comes from his book *Health Care Without Shame—A Handbook for the Sexually Diverse and Their Caregivers* (published by Greenery Press, *http://www.bigrock.com/greenery)* and is recommended as a present to every health practitioner! As you read "Trans Health Crisis: For Us It's Life or Death," think about how much more appropriate and humane Leslie Feinberg's experiences with the health system would have been if Leslie's providers, including front desk staff, had carried through the suggestions in the "Health Care Without Shame" chapter. In raising awareness about the health crisis for the trans population, Leslie's personal story demonstrates how health practitioners' ignorance and prejudice is dangerous and life-threatening for their trans patients:

> After the physician who examined me discovered I am female-bodied, he ordered me out of the emergency room despite the fact that my temperature was above 104° F. (Later hospitalized for the same undiagnosed bacterial endocarditis. . .) They place transsexual women who have completed sex-reassignment surgery in the male wards. Putting me in a female ward created a furor. I awoke in the night to find staff standing around my bed ridiculing my body and referring to me as a "Martian." The next day the staff refused to work unless "it" was removed from the floor. These and other expressions of hatred forced me to leave. Had I died from this illness, the real pathogen would have been bigotry.

The question of who defines women's sexuality is next explored in terms of issues of disability. Social attitudes about women's sexuality are also extremely problematic in their impact on women with disabilities. In "Forbidden Fruit," Anne Finger examines the strong prejudice against people with disabilities in our society—the belief that they should neither be sexual nor have children.

We close this sexuality chapter with the important classic, "The Need for Intimacy." In previous editions of this book, we placed this article in the aging chapter but we have decided that the issues raised are too important to be marginalized as an issue only for older, widowed women. Clearly, opportunities for healthy intimacy are crucial at *every* stage of people's lives: "No matter what our age, we each need intimacy in our lives—at least one other person with whom we can share both pleasure and pain." In keeping with the other questions explored in this chapter, it seems imperative to ask how the cultural definitions of sexuality limit people's opportunities for intimacy, especially for people who are not in a "socially sanctioned couple" and what can we (collectively) do to change this. The reader is asked to synthesize points made in both "The Need for Intimacy" article and Myth 4: Women Want Intimacy; Men Want Sex in "The Orgasm Gap" to come up with a comprehensive statement acknowledging the roles that both intimacy and orgasms could play in both women's and men's lives.

Exposed at Last

The Truth About Your Clitoris

by Jennifer Johnson

"At a witch trial in 1593, the investigating lawyer (a married man) apparently discovered a clitoris for the first time; he identified it as a devil's teat, sure proof of the witch's guilt. It was 'a little lump of flesh, in a manner sticking out as if it had been a teat, to the length of half an inch,' which the gaoler, 'perceiving at the first sight there of, meant not to disclose, because it was adjoining to so secret a place which was not decent to be seen. Yet in the end, not willing to conceal so strange a matter,' he showed it to various bystanders. The witch was convicted."

from *The Vagina Monologues* by Eve Ensler [Villard].

Pick up almost any medical, anatomy or biology text and you'll find something missing: the greater part of the clitoris.

The clitoris is like an iceberg; only the tip is visible on the outside, its larger mass is under the surface. The visible tip is the glans, or head of the organ. While modern medical science books stop there, the clitoris actually continues under the pelvic bone, then turns down to surround the vagina from above and on either side. The structure forms a dense pyramid of tissue, well-supplied with nerve and vascular network, and is comparable in size to the penis. Like the male organ, the clitoris is flaccid when unaroused and erect when aroused.

And yet, even in the most ponderous, detailed texts, the clitoris is described as a "vestigial organ," or "pea-sized." The diagrams typically show a diagram of a spread-legged female, with a little bulb arrowed "clitoris." The internal diagrams show her reproductive organs, but the bulk of the clitoris—the shaft (body), legs (crura), and bulbs—are missing. Next to the illustration showing the female sex organ as a bump usually appears a drawing of the male sex organ on an extremely well-hung man. Even *Gray's Anatomy*—the authoritative text of biologists—doesn't accurately depict the clitoris.

As a biologist, I first discovered this while doing an anatomical study (dissection) on a human subject. I was shocked to discover that the clitoris was far larger than I had been taught. I could not understand how such a basic—not to mention crucial—piece of biological information had been neglected. I searched textbooks, consulted doctors and professors and found all of them unaware of the actual size of the clitoris.

Of course, I was not the only student of science to discover this. When Helen O'Connell became curious about why the female sex organ was "glossed over" in the texts, she made it her business to take a closer look when she became a doctor. Now a surgeon at the Royal Melbourne Hospital in Australia, she and her colleagues

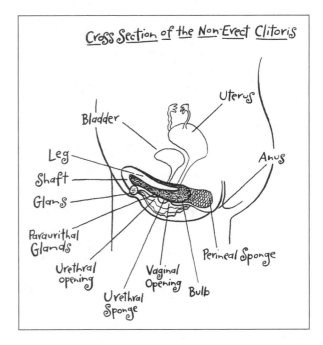

Illustration: Noreen Stevens

have been dissecting and measuring the clitoris; her findings were reported in a recent article in *New Scientist.* "Sometimes the whole structure is drawn as a dot," says Dr. O'Connell. In fact, the legs of the clitoris, called the crura, are five to nine centimeters long, extending from the body (shaft) of the clitoris and filling the space between its legs are two bulbs, one on either side of the vaginal cavity. Contrary to the belief that the urethra and clitoris are entirely separate, the clitoris actually encompasses the urethra. Dr. O'Connell believes the clitoris squeezes the urethra shut during sex, reducing the entry of bacteria.

Drawing a more accurate picture of the female sexual anatomy explains a few things. It helps explain why some women are not having orgasms, since women must first be erect before they can reach orgasm. It may also explain why Viagra appears to work for women even though it's not supposed to—suggesting that women may be impotent for the same physiological reasons as men. It also explains why women frequently report that their sex lives were damaged following some types of pelvic surgery—the nerves to the clitoris, and sometimes the organ itself, can be damaged or severed during surgery. It also sheds light on the controversy of the clitoral vs. vaginal orgasm that was debated a few years ago.

When seen as an entire complex organ, there is room for a wide range of experiences. Some women experience orgasm through stimulation of the outer glans of the clitoris; at other times they may experience a different orgasm when combined with penetration. An orgasm reached through external stimulation may feel quite different. For many women, orgasm is intense and relatively easy to reach with digital or oral contact because this is the most direct way to stimulate the large pudendal nerve which runs straight down into the tip of the clitoris (the glans). What has been referred to as "the vaginal orgasm" is a vaginal-induced orgasm, brought on by stimulating the clitoris indirectly through the vaginal walls. (Of course, it's common to add some direct pudendal stimulation on the outside.)

Then there is the G-spot. Part of the vaginal wall clinically known as the urethral sponge, the G-spot can be found by exploring the roof of the vagina. It's about a knuckle-length in—from one and a half to three inches inside. The easiest way to find it is to have your partner crook a finger or two and reach toward the belly button. The size varies from half an inch to 1.5 inches. When unaroused, it feels like the back of the roof of your mouth. If your partner presses up on this spot and you feel like you have to urinate, they've found it. When it is stroked, it will puff out and feel like a marshmallow.

While there are many differences between male and female sexual responses, there are unmistakably many

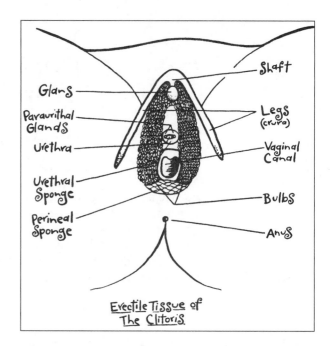

Illustration: Noreen Stevens

similarities. When the clitoris is engorged and erect, endorphins are released and induce a 'high.' The long bands of the crura become hard and flare out along the pubic bones. Vaginal blood vessels widen and fill with blood and the perineal sponge thickens. The uterus balloons forward, the tubes and ovaries swell. The broad ligament tightens, pulling up the uterus and causing the vagina to enlarge. The neck of the cervix is flexible, like an accordion, and during orgasm, the cervix moves forward and down, dipping its head in the seminal pool if a male partner has ejaculated. As well, ejaculation fluid squirts from the woman's paraurithal glands, located on either side of the urethra. This may come as news to women who haven't had a female sexual partner and therefore may not have experienced a female ejaculation first hand. The ejaculate may be a small amount and not noticeable, or it may be a copious amount that 'soaks the sheets.'

The size of the clitoris is actually not a new 'discovery' but the revealing of a secret. The clitoris was more accurately described in some 19th century anatomy texts, but then it was mysteriously shrunk into a mere speck on the anatomical map. The French, however, have been more accurately depicting the clitoris since before the turn of the century.

While doing research for this article, I contacted many sex-related organizations, including the famous Kinsey Institute, the British Association for Sexual and Marital Therapy, even the German Society for Sex Research. None had accurate information on the clitoris, and most did not believe that the clitoris is larger and more complex than medical texts indicate. In bookstores, I found current sexology books that didn't have more than a paragraph on the clitoris, some only a few lines, many did not have "clitoris" indexed at all! Even the famous British 'feminist' scientist Desmond Morris's new book, *The Human Sexes,* contains no indexed references for clitoris. Without exception, every sex book gave 'penis' all kinds of room—entire sections, chapters and references.

What does it all mean? Dr. Jennifer Berman, director of the Women's Sexual Health Clinic at Boston University, predicts that knowing the proper female anatomy will lead to research in this area of female function and dysfunction, which she says has been "grossly neglected."

In an article published with her colleagues in *The Journal of Urology* in June 1998, Dr. O'Connell and her colleagues wrote, "Since the studies of Masters and Johnson, there has been surprisingly little investigation of basic female sexual anatomy or physiology." The article describes the intricate connection between the urethra and the clitoris and says that surgeons should be made aware of the damage that can be done to the organ during urethral surgery. O'Connell says anatomy texts should be changed to accurately depict the clitoris and perineal anatomy. She is now mapping the nerves to the pelvic region innervating the female sex organ.

"They were mapped in men a decade ago," says O'Connell, "but they've never been mapped in women."

It does beg the question doesn't it? Why not? One anthropologist I spoke to explained that the size of the clitoris may have been overlooked because "the size of the male phallus" is a symbol of power; admitting women have the same size organ would be like admitting they are equally powerful. Indeed.

Sex psychologist Dr. Micheal Bailey doesn't buy into the patriarchal conspiracy theory. "There's been very little scientific interest in female sexuality," he insists. Then adds, "It's possible *we* didn't look."

How Being a Good Girl Can Be Bad for Girls

by Deborah L. Tolman and Tracy E. Higgins

Women's sexuality is frequently suspect in our culture, particularly when it is expressed outside the bounds of monogamous heterosexual marriage. This suspicion is reflected in the dominant cultural accounts of women's sexuality, which posit good, decent, and normal women as passive and threatened sexual objects. When women act as sexual agents, expressing their own sexual desire rather than serving as the objects of men's desire, they are often portrayed as threatening, deviant, and bad. Missing is any affirmative account of women's sexual desire. Yet, even while women's sexuality is denied or problematized, the culture and the law tend to assign to women the responsibility for regulating heterosexual sex by resisting male aggression. Defined as natural, urgent, and aggressive, male sexuality is bounded, both in law and in culture, by the limits of women's consent. Women who wish to avoid the consequences of being labeled "bad" are expected to define the boundaries of sexual behavior, outlined by men's desire, and to ignore or deny their own sexual desire as a guide to their choices.

The cultural anxiety precipitated by unbounded female sexuality is perhaps most apparent with regard to adolescent girls. Coming under scrutiny from across the political spectrum, girls' sexuality has been deemed threatening either to girls themselves (potentially resulting in rape, sexually transmitted diseases, unwanted pregnancy), or to society (as evidenced by the single mother, school dropout, welfare dependent). Although none of these issues is limited to teenage girls, all frequently arise in that context because of society's sense of entitlement, or, indeed, obligation, to regulate teen sexuality. Accordingly, the cultural and legal sanctions on teenage girls' sexuality convey a simple message: good girls are not sexual; girls who are sexual are either (1) bad girls, if they have been active, desiring sexual agents or (2) good girls, who have been passively victimized by boys' raging hormones. Buttressed by the real concerns that girls themselves have about pregnancy, AIDS, and parental as well as peer disapproval, the good-girl/bad-girl dichotomy organizes sexuality for young women. This cultural story may increase girls' vulnerability to sexual coercion and psychological distress and disable them from effectively seeking legal protection.

The Cultural Story of Girls' Sexuality in the Media and in Law

Sexually assertive girls are making the news. A disturbed mother of a teenage boy wrote to Ann Landers, complaining of the behavior of teenage girls who had telephoned him, leaving sexually suggestive messages. After publishing the letter, Landers received twenty thousand responses and noted, "If I'm hearing about it from so many places, then I worry about what's going on out there. . . . What this says to me is that a good many young girls really are out of control. Their hormones are raging and they have not had adequate supervision" (qtd. In Yoffe 1991). What were these girls doing? Calling boys, asking them out, threatening to buy them gifts, and to "make love to [them] all night." In the *Newsweek* story, "Girls Who Go Too Far," in which the writer described this Ann Landers column, such girls were referred to as "obsessed," "confused," "emotionally disturbed," "bizarre," "abused," "troubled." Parents described the girls' behavior as "bewilder[ing]" or even "frighten[ing]" to boys. A similar, more recent story in the *Orlando Sentinel* noted that "girls today have few qualms about asking a boy out—and they have no qualms about calling a boy on the telephone" (Shrieves 1993). Describing late-night telephone calls from girls to their teenage sons, the adults interviewed characterized the situation as "frustrating" and "shocking" and suggested that "parents should be paying more attention to what their daughters are doing." Girls' behavior, including "suggestive notes stuck to a boy's locker or even outright propositions," was deemed "obsessive."

In contrast, media accounts of boys' sexuality tend to reflect what Wendy Hollway has called the "discourse of male sexual drive," wherein male sexuality is portrayed as natural, relentless, and demanding attention, an urge that boys and men cannot help or control (Hollway 1984). Media coverage of the so-called Spur Posse in Lakewood, California, reflects this discourse. Members of the Spur Posse, a group of popular white high school boys in a middle-class California suburb, competed with one another using a point system for their sexual "conquests" (Smolowe 1993). When girls eventually complained, several boys were charged with crimes ranging

from sexual molestation to rape. Although many criticized the incident as an example of unchecked adolescent sexuality, others excused or even defended the boys' behavior. One father explained, "Nothing my boy did was anything any red-blooded American boy wouldn't do at his age." Their mother commented, "What can you do? It's a testosterone thing."

A comparison of the different boundaries of acceptable sexual behavior for girls and boys illustrates the force of the cultural assumption of female passivity and male aggression. Although the Spur Posse incident was covered as a troubling example of male sexuality out of control, the point at which adolescent sexual aggression becomes suspect is strikingly different for girls and boys. For girls, it's phone calls; for boys, it's rape. The girls' suggestive phone calling is described as shocking to the parents and even threatening to the sons, not because the desire expressed was unusual in the realm of teen sexuality, but because the agents were girls and the objects were boys. In the Spur Posse incident, the possibility of girls' sexual agency or desire shifted responsibility from the boys' aggression to the girls' failure to resist. For some observers, whether or not the boys in the Spur Posse were considered to have acted inappropriately depended upon an assessment of the sexual conduct of the girls involved. If the girls were shown to have expressed any sexual agency, their desire was treated by some as excusing and justifying the boys' treatment of them as objects or points to be collected. As one mother, invoking cultural shorthand put it, "Those girls are trash." The boys' behavior was excused as natural, "a testosterone thing," and the girls were deemed culpable for their failure to control the boys' behavior.

Through these cultural stories, girls are simultaneously taught that they are valued in terms of their sexual desirability and that their own desire makes them vulnerable. If they are economically privileged and white, they become vulnerable because desiring (read "bad") girls lose credibility and protection from male aggression. If they are poor and/or of color, or bisexual or lesbian, they are assumed to be bad, as refracted through the lenses of racism, classism, and homophobia that anchor the cultural story (Tolman forthcoming). While in some communities girls' and women's sexuality is acknowledged and more accepted (Omolade 1983), the force of cultural stories permeating the dominant cultural presses upon all girls. This constant pressure often inflames the desire of marginalized girls to be thought of as good, moral, and normal, status denied them by mainstream standards.[1] Moreover, all girls' vulnerability is compounded by the extraordinary license given to adolescent boys regarding the urgency of their sexuality. Perhaps more than any other group of men, teenage boys are assumed to be least in control of their sexuality. The responsibility for making sexual choices, therefore, falls to their partners, usually teenage girls, yet these "choices" are to be enacted through passivity rather than agency. Girls who attain good girlhood are at constant risk of becoming bad girls if they fail in their obligation to regulate their own sexual behavior and that of their partners. It is during adolescence, then, that girls are both most responsible for sexual decision making and most penalized for acting on their own sexual desires. It is also during adolescence that girls are socialized into cultural stories about being sexual and being women (Brown and Gilligan 1992; Tolman 1994a and 1994b).

The power of these cultural norms to mediate the interpretation of teen sexuality is perhaps most vividly revealed in the comments of those who would defend "aggressive" girls. Teenage girls interviewed in the *Sentinel* story explained their peers' behavior in terms of girls giving boys what the boys wanted. One suggested that "sometimes girls, in order to get certain guys, will do anything the guy wants. And that includes sex." That would include propositioning a boy "[I]f that's what she thinks *he wants*." The girl's actions are reinterpreted in terms of satisfying the boy's desire rather than her own. Explaining away the possibility of the girls' sexual desire, one counselor suggested that the girls may not really be "sex-crazed." Rather, they are probably simply "desperate for a relationship" (Shrieves 1993). Describing the girls as trading sex for relationships, the counselor reinterprets their actions in a manner that is consistent with the cultural story of male aggression and female responsibility, which is devoid of female desire. The girl gives the boy what he (inevitably or naturally) wants, negotiating her need only for a relationship by managing his drive for sexual pleasure.

The contrasting media coverage of teenage girls' and teenage boys' sexuality stands as one manifestation of a broader cultural message about gendered norms of sexual behavior. Feminists have documented and discussed this message as a theme present throughout literature, law, film, advertising, and general sources of cultural wisdom on sexuality such as self-help books, advice columns, and medical treatises. The story of male aggression and female responsibility suffuses the culture and operates to regulate human sexuality on conscious and subconscious levels in a gender-specific way. By discouraging women's sexual agency and men's sexual responsibility, these cultural norms undermine communication and encourage coercion and violence. This effect is perhaps nowhere more clear than in the legal regulation of sexuality through rape statutes and the media coverage of rape trials.

Premised on the notion of male sexual aggression and irresponsibility, the law of rape incorporates cultural norms that place upon the woman the burden of regulating sexual activity and, at the same time, penalize her for acting as a sexual subject (Henderson 1992). In so doing, the law of rape incorporates both sides of the good girl/bad girl dynamic. The good girl's attempt to exercise her responsibility to regulate male sexuality is encoded in the requirement of nonconsent to sexual intercourse. Proof of nonconsent, however, frequently depends upon establishing an absence of desire. To be a victimized good girl and therefore entitled to protection, a girl or woman must both resist *and* lack desire. A desiring bad girl, on the other hand, is often deemed deserving of the consequences of her desire.

In cases of nonstranger (acquaintance) rape, rape trials frequently hinge upon whether nonconsent is established, a standard which, as feminists have noted, takes little account of women's sexuality. As Carol Smart has argued, the consent/nonconsent dyad fails to capture the complexity of a woman's experience (Smart 1989). A woman may seek and initiate physical intimacy, which may be an expression of her own sexual desire, while not consenting to intercourse. Nevertheless, by imposing the consent/nonconsent interpretive framework, rape law renders a woman's expression of any desire immediately suspect. Expression of desire that leads to intimacy and ultimately submission to unwanted sex falls on the side of consent. As the "trashy" girls who were the victims of the Spur Posse illustrate, to want anything is to consent to everything. The woman has, in effect, sacrificed her right to refuse intercourse by the expression of her own sexual desire. Or, more precisely, the expression of her desire undermines the credibility of her refusal. Evidence that the rape victim initiated sexual interaction at any level operates to undermine her story at every stage of the process—police disbelieve her account, prosecutors refuse to press the case, and juries refuse to convict. At trial, the issue of consent may be indistinguishable from the question of whether the woman experienced pleasure. Thus, within rape law, a woman's behavior as a sexual subject shifts power to the aggressor, thereby maintaining the power hierarchy of the traditional story of male aggression and female submission. As in pulp romance, to desire is to surrender.

The centrality of the absence of female desire to the definition of rape cuts across racial lines, albeit in complicated ways. As African American feminists have pointed out, rape and race are historically interwoven in a way that divides the experiences of women of color from white women (i.e., Collins 1990 and Harris 1990; see also Caraway 1991). Nevertheless, whatever the woman's race, the absence of female desire stands as a prerequisite to the identification of a sexual act as rape.

The difference emerges as a product of the interlocking elements of the cultural story about women's sexuality which segregate white women and women of color. For example, a key element in the cultural story about women's sexuality is that African American women are sexually voracious, thereby making them unrapable—as distinguished from white women, who are asexual and thus in a constant state of rapability. The absence-of-desire standard is still applied to women of color but presumed impossible to meet. Conversely, when white women accuse African American men of raping them, the required absence of female desire is simply presumed.

If, under ordinary rape law, expression of female sexual desire takes women and girls outside the protection of the law, rendering them unrapable, statutory rape law defines female sexuality as outside the law in a different way. By criminalizing all intercourse with minors, statutory rape laws literally outlaw girls' expression of their own sexuality.[2] In terms of female sexual desire, statutory rape laws represent a complete mirroring of rape law regulating men's access to adult women—with statutory rape, absence of desire is presumed. Instead of rendering a woman unrapable or fully accessible to men, the law simply makes young women's expression of sexual desire illegal.

Both rape law and statutory rape law reinforce cultural norms of female sexuality be penalizing female sexual desire. The coverage of rape in the media, in turn, frequently heightens the focus on the sexuality of the victim, casting her as either good (innocent) or bad (desiring). For example, in the coverage of the Mike Tyson rape trial, the media referred repeatedly to the fact that Desiree Washington taught Sunday school, as though that fact were necessary to rebut the possibility that she invited the attack by acting on her own sexual desire. In an even more extreme case, the mentally disabled adolescent girl who was raped by a group of teenage boys in her Glen Ridge, New Jersey, neighborhood was portrayed both by her lawyers and by the media as largely asexual. To establish nonconsent, the prosecution argued explicitly that she was incapable of knowing or expressing her sexuality.[3] Although she was not sexually inexperienced, this strategy rendered her sexually innocent. Coverage of these two trials stands in sharp contrast to another highly publicized rape trial at the time, that of William Kennedy Smith, in which the media revealed not only the victim's name but her sexual history and her driving record. Much was made in the media of the victim's sexual history and her apparent willingness to accompany Smith home that night. Her desire to engage in flirtation and foreplay meant that her alleged refusal of intercourse could never be sufficiently credible to convict. Smith was acquitted.

As illustrated by the coverage of rape trials, the media and the law interact to reinforce the cultural story of male aggression and female passivity, reinforcing the good girl/bad girl distinction. With the suffusion of this story throughout our culture, girls and women come to understand the norms of acceptable sexual behavior—that good girls are those who are sexually innocent, meaning without sexual desire, although not necessarily without sexual experience. These girls are sexual objects, not subjects, charged with defending the boundaries of their own sexual activity by resisting male aggression. In contrast, bad girls are girls who express their desire, acting as sexual subjects on their own behalf. They are assertive girls, "girls who go too far." Vilified by the media and the culture more broadly as deviant and threatening, these girls are rendered far less likely than good girls to be able to invoke the protection of rape laws and are thus made doubly vulnerable.

Problem of Desire for Adolescent Girls

In this section, we turn to the voices of adolescent young women speaking about their experiences. We rely on a feminist method of analyzing interviews to understand how cultural stories about girls' sexuality may create vulnerability for girls rather than protect them from it.[4] This method takes women as authorities on their own experiences. We listen to what they say and how they say it so that our role as interpreters of their words is clear; that is, we do not claim the authority to say what they are saying but convey how we understand the stories they tell, given our perspective on these issues. We have drawn two case studies from a psychological study of adolescent girls' experience of desire (Tolman 1994a and 1994b),[5] and one from the legal literature. We selected the cases from the study because each of these girls chose to speak about a sexual experience with a boy who was not her boyfriend. Although each associated her experience with sexual violence, the two girls differ profoundly in their understanding of these experiences and also in their critical perspective on gender relations, the cultural story about male and female sexuality, and the good girl/bad girl dynamic. In Jenny's case, a lack of a critical perspective on these issues disables her from feeling outraged or empowered to act on her own behalf. For Pauline, such a perspective appears to enhance her sense of entitlement and ability to act. Through this contrast, we demonstrate how being a good girl can be bad for girls and, conversely, how challenging the terms of the good girl/bad girl dichotomy can be enabling. Finally, we selected the case of Sharon from the legal literature to underscore our point that denying desire in the name of good girlhood can diminish girls' ability to garner protection under the law.

Jenny: When Bad Things Happen to Good Girls

Sixteen-year-old Jenny, who lives in a suburb of a large city, looks like the quintessential good girl. She is white, has long, straight, blond hair framing a lightly freckled, fair face. She is slim, dressed fashionably yet unassumingly. She sits with her legs tensely crossed; she is polite and cooperative and smiles often. Like many girls in this study, throughout the interview Jenny describes how she lives her life by trying to stay carefully within the boundaries of good girl. She and her mother are "very close," and it is very important to her to be "nice" and a "good friend"—even if it means silencing her own displeasure or dissent in relationships.[6] Complying with conventional norms of femininity, Jenny explains that she has never experienced feelings she calls sexual desire: "I actually really don't think I've ever like, wanted anything, like sexually that bad. I mean I don't think I've ever been like sexually deprived or like saying, oh I need sex now or anything, I've never really felt that way before, so, I don't know. I don't really think that there's anything that I would, I mean want." Given Jenny's concern about and success at being a good girl in other domains of her life, it is not surprising that she does not report feeling desire. Having a "silent body" is a psychological response to the belief that good girls are not sexual (Tolman 1994a).

The vulnerability of this silence in her life is tangible in the narrative she tells about the first time she had sexual intercourse, which occurred just prior to our interview. This experience was not what she had hoped it would be:

We got alone together, and we started just basically fooling around and not doing many things. And then he asked me if I would have sex with him, and I said, well I didn't think I, I mean I said I wanted to wait, 'cause I didn't want to. I mean I like him, but I don't like him so, and I mean he sorta pushed it on me, but it wasn't like I absolutely said no, don't, I— it was sort of a weird experience. I just, I sort of let it happen to me and never like really said no, I don't want to do this. I mean I said no, but I never, I mean I never stopped him from doing anything. . . . I guess maybe I wanted to get it over with, I guess . . . I don't know. I, I just, I mean I could've said no, I guess and I could've pushed him off or whatever 'cause he, I mean, he wasn't, he's not the type of person who would like rape me or whatever, I mean, well I don't think he's that way at all. . . . I was always like, well I want to wait, and I want to be in a relationship with someone who I really like, and

I want it to be a special moment and everything, and then it just sort of like happened so quickly, and it happened with someone who I didn't like and who I didn't want a relationship with and who didn't want a relationship with me, and it was just sort of, I don't, I don't know, I regret it. . . . I wish I had just said no. I mean I could've, and I did for once but then I just let it go. And I wish that I had stood up for myself and really just like stood up and said no, I don't want to do this. I'm not ready or I want it to be a different experience. I mean I could've told him exactly how I felt. . . . I don't know why I didn't.

In this story, Jenny is unsure about how to understand her first experience with sexual intercourse. In listening to her, we, too, are unsure. When she begins this story, Jenny knows that she did not want to have sexual intercourse with this boy, although she did want to "fool around." She, in fact, said "no" when the boy asked her if she would have sex with him. There is a clarity to her no that she substantiates with a set of compelling reasons for not wanting to have sex with this boy: she "wanted to wait," she didn't "like him" or "want a relationship with him." After the fact, she is again clear that she did not want to have sex with this boy. She "regrets it." But we notice that this clarity gives way to a sense of confusion that colors Jenny's voice and gains momentum as her narrative, itself an interplay of description and assessment, unfolds. Cleaving to the convention that girls are ultimately responsible for boys' sexual behavior, she attempts to make sense of the fact that this boy behaved as though she had not said no. Assuming responsibility, Jenny suggests that she had "never stopped him from doing anything," implying, perhaps, that she had not meant the no that she had said.

Jenny's suggestion that she might have said *no* and meant *yes* raises a troubling issue for feminists who have rallied around the claim that "no means no." Although "no means no" is effective as an educational or political slogan or perhaps even as a legal norm, such norms protect girls only at the margin. Within the broader context of adolescent sexuality, girls' no must be credible both to girls and to their partners. Yet the cultural story that good girls do not have sexual desire undermines the credibility of their no, not only to others but also to themselves. When girls cannot say yes, no (or silence) is their only alternative and must express the range of their choices. Some have suggested that girls can ameliorate the problem by simply taking responsibility for communicating their desire (e.g., Roiphe 1993). This answer falls short and, in fact, leaves girls in the lurch by failing to account for the cultural sanctions on girls' expression of their sexuality. Leaving those sanctions unaddressed, so-called power feminists reinforce the assignment of responsibility to girls for sexual decision making without criticizing the constraints under which such decisions are made.

Jenny struggles within those constraints as she attempts to take seriously the possibility that she may have wanted to have sex with the boy despite having said no; the possibility that her no meant yes. Yet her reflection, "I guess maybe I wanted to get it over with, I guess" is literally buttressed by doubt. While this statement stands as a potential explanation of why she had sex even though she said no, Jenny herself does not sound convinced. The explanation sounds even less plausible when compared to the clarity of her elaborated and unambiguous statements about why she did not want to have sex. She explains, "I want to be in a relationship with someone who I really like, and I want it to be a special moment and everything."

As her story progresses, we hear Jenny's confusion about what she wanted intensify. This confusion seems to undermine Jenny's knowledge that she had actually said no to this boy. Eventually, Jenny seems to forget that she ever said no at all. Despite having just explained that she had not wanted to have sex with this boy and had told him so, Jenny starts to speak as if she had not said no. "I said no" becomes "I sort of let it happen to me and never like, really said no, I don't want to do this." She progressively undoes her knowledge that she articulated her wish not to have sex. "I mean I could've said no, I guess, and I could've pushed him off or whatever," finally becomes "I wish I had just said no." Thus, when this boy behaved as though Jenny had not said no, Jenny loses track of her knowledge and her voice, becoming confused not only about what she wanted but also about what she said.

The conditions Jenny gives for an appropriate sexual encounter—"a special relationship," someone she "really like[s]"—resonate with the cultural story that girls' sexuality is about relationships and not desire. Because the encounter she describes did not meet these conditions, she decided that she did not want to have sex and told the boy no. Yet these conditions did not supply an adequate framework for Jenny either to make a clear decision and insist that it be respected, or, if it was not respected, to identify the incident as one of violation. In this context, it is significant that Jenny makes no reference to her own sexual desire. It is only later in the interview, in response to a direct question, that Jenny reports that she "hadn't felt desire for the person I was with." She notes, however, that this absence of desire does not distinguish this encounter from any other: "I've never like had sexual feelings to want to do something or anything." We wonder whether, in the moment, Jenny was

not able to hold onto her knowledge that she did not want to have sex because her own desire has never been available as a guide to her choices. We suggest that not feeling desire is one way to cope with the good girl/bad girl dichotomy. Were Jenny not subject to the good girl standard that prevents her from attending to her own sexual feelings, perhaps she would feel desire in some situations, and her lack of sexual desire could operate as a clear signal to her, perhaps leaving her less vulnerable to such confusion.

The consequences of Jenny's confusion include physical and psychological vulnerability. Her difficulty in holding on to her no and insisting that her no be respected leaves her physically vulnerable to sexual encounters that she does not in any clear way want. Jenny's confusion makes her vulnerable psychologically as well. By discounting her own thoughts and feelings, she risks becoming dissociated from her own experience and from reality. Such dissociation makes it difficult for Jenny to be able to know and name sexual exploitation. Accustomed to being the object of someone else's sexual desire, not considering that her own sexual desire might be relevant or significant, Jenny pastes over the complexity of what did, in fact, happen with the phrase "it just sort of like happened." This "cover story" symbolizes and sustains Jenny's vulnerability in a culture that leaves out her sexual desire.

At the same time, Jenny's suggestion that "it just sort of like happened" keeps another story at bay, a story of a girl whose spoken wish was not heeded, who was coerced. Was Jenny raped? Jenny herself brings the word "rape" into her story: "I mean I could've said no, I guess and I could've pushed him off or whatever 'cause he, I mean, he wasn't, he's not the type of person who would like rape me, or whatever. I mean, well I don't think he's that way at all." She seems to wonder whether this experience might somehow be connected to rape. She may associate this experience with rape because the word signifies something about what it felt like for her, a violation. Although she stopped saying no and apparently assented nonverbally to the act, this sexual experience was not related to any feeling of yes on Jenny's part. Jenny's experience of having passively consented and of having been violated suggests the disjuncture between consent and desire in women's experience, a disjuncture that likely heightens Jenny's confusion over how to interpret what happened to her. Such confusion prevents Jenny from speaking clearly in the first instance about her desire and from later interpreting what happened in a way that acknowledges her own resistance.

Nonetheless Jenny is an astute observer of the social landscape of adolescent heterosexual relationships. She identifies some imbalances in how girls and boys behave and in how they are treated by others in response to their behavior. Later in the interview, she notes that "whenever like a girl and a guy do something and people find out, it's always the girl that messed up or, I mean, maybe the guy messed up, but the guys like get praise for it [laughing] and the girl's sort of like called, either a slut or something, or just like has a bad reputation. Which is sort of [laughing] awful." Jenny believes that "it is just as much the guy's fault as it is the girl's fault. . . . It's just like the guys and the girls make fun of the girls but no one makes fun of the guys [laughing]." What Jenny needs is an analytic framework that links the inequities she observes to cultural stories about sexuality. She suspects, but does not know, that these stories operate in a way that creates gendered power differences. Identifying the good girl/bad girl divide, Jenny tries without success to make sense of the contradiction she observes, that both girls and guys may be at "fault" in sexual situations like hers, but only girls are chastised. We notice that she does not say what she thinks about this contradiction. When she is asked directly, her constant confusion about gender relations is audible: "I really don't know."

Sharon: The Slippery Slope off Good Girlhood

The legal vulnerability created when girls become confused about their own desire is illustrated by the testimony of Sharon, the victim in the U.S. Supreme Court's statutory rape case *Michael M.* v. *Sonoma County*. In her portion of the trial transcript reproduced in the Supreme Court's opinion, Sharon, who, like Jenny, is sixteen and white, is being questioned by the defendant's lawyer about whether she wanted to have sex with the defendant, a boy who was not her boyfriend. Ordinary rape law requires that she make a clear claim that she did not want to have sex with the defendant in order to gain legal recourse. The confusion that emerges as she testifies not only renders the case problematic under ordinary rape law but also calls into question the legitimacy of the statutory rape prosecution. The lawyer's questions about Sharon's desire subtly garner the good girl/bad girl dynamic as part of a strategy to undermine the credibility of her claim that she did not want to have sexual intercourse. In the face of these questions, Sharon appears to lose her clarity about the exact parameters of her desire:

Q: Now, after you met the defendant, what happened?

A: We walked down to the railroad tracks.

Q: What happened at the railroad tracks?

A: We were drinking at the railroad tracks and we walked over to this bus and he started kissing me and stuff, and I was kissing him back, too, at first. Then I was telling him to stop—

Q: Yes.

A: —and I was telling him to slow down and stop. He said, "Ok, Ok." But then he just kept doing it. He just kept doing it and then my sister and two other guys came over to where we were and my sister told me to get up and come home. And then I didn't. . . . We were laying there and we were kissing each other, and then he asked me if I wanted to walk with him over to the park. We walked over to the park, and then we sat down on a bench, and then he started kissing me again, and we were laying on the bench. And he told me to take my pants off. I said "No," and I was trying to get up and he hit me back down on the bench, and then I just said to myself, "Forget it," and I let him do what he wanted to do and he took my pants off and he was telling me to put my legs around him and stuff.

Q: Did you have sexual intercourse with the defendant?

A: Yeah.

Q: Did you go off with [the defendant] away from the others?

A: Yeah.

Q: Why did you do that?

A: I don't know. I guess I wanted to. (Michael M. *v.* Sonoma County 450 U.S. 464 [1980]: 483–488)

Sharon begins by speaking clearly about what she did and did not want to do with the boy. She wanted to kiss him back, she wanted him to slow down and stop, and she also wanted to walk over to the park with him. However, when the sexual interaction turned from kissing or "fooling around" to "tak[ing] off [her] pants," she said "no," unequivocally and clearly and "tri[ed] to get up." We hear that her desire had specific contours: while she had wanted to "fool around," she did not want to have sexual intercourse. Nevertheless, like Jenny, she stopped saying no and "let him do what he wanted to do." In so doing, she may have given her consent legally although not emotionally or psychologically.

Initially Sharon maintains clarity about the limits of her desire. Confusion creeps into her previously straight-forward account, however, as she is asked about her motives for having gone to the park with the defendant. Implicit in the lawyer's question "[why] did you go off with [the defendant] away from the others?" is the unspoken condemnation of the actions of a bad girl, the conditional phrase *"unless you wanted to have sexual intercourse with him?"* So understood, the question is really about her desire. Having been asked to speak about her own desire, Sharon loses the clarity of her earlier explanation. She seems to suspect (along with the lawyer) that there is an inconsistency between having wanted to go to the park and having not wanted to have sex with the boy.

Confronted with the threat of bad girl status, Sharon retreats from the earlier articulation of her desire. Following on the heels of an unequivocal account that portrays the parameters of her desire, Sharon's statement of ambivalence makes her seem confused and uncertain. By responding that she does not know what she wanted, that she "guess[es]" that she "wanted to," Sharon undermines the credibility of her previous testimony. As a witness, Sharon becomes trapped within the good girl/bad girl dichotomy. Her admission of her desire to go to the park with the boy undermines the credibility of her claim that she was coerced. At this point, her reiteration of her direct statement that she wanted to go to the park coupled with her retreat from that statement render her testimony unreliable. Her mistake, as she seems to realize, was to relinquish good girl status by confessing her desire.

Paulina: Empowerment through Rejecting the Good Girl/Bad Girl Dichotomy

Paulina, a white girl who lives in an urban environment, tells stories that offer a counterpoint to Jenny's. Seventeen-year-old Paulina looks like the other adolescent girls in this study: long, dark hair frames her pretty, open face; stylish jeans and sweater clothe a slim figure. Despite her appearance, Paulina does not sound like the other girls: having immigrated from Eastern Europe several years prior to the interview, Paulina speaks with a strong accent. It is the content of her narrative, however, that distinguishes her from most other study participants. Like Jenny, Paulina is also a competent consumer of cultural stories about girls and sexuality, and can recite them without a moment's hesitation:

> They expect the woman to be pure, I mean, she has to be holy and everything, and it's okay for a guy to have any feelings or anything, and the girl has to be this little virgin who is obedient to the men. . . . usually a guy makes the first move, not the girl, or the girl's not supposed to do it, the girl's supposed to sit there going, no, no you can't. I can't do that. . . . I mean the guy expects the girl to be a sweet little virgin when he marries her, and then he can be running around with ten other women, but when he's getting married to her, she's not supposed to have any relationship with anybody else.[7]

Paulina echoes Jenny's observation about how the label "slut" is—and is not—used: "Guys, they just like to brag about girls. Oh she does this, and she's a slut because she slept with this guy, and with this guy, but they don't say that about guys. It's okay for them to do it, but when a girl sleeps with two guys it's wrong, she shouldn't do that, she automatically becomes a slut."

In contrast to Jenny's ambivalence and uncertainty, Paulina has strong opinions about the sexual double standard: "I just don't agree with it. . . . I just don't think so." A sense of entitlement, accompanied by outrage, suffuses her well-articulated view of female sexual agency: "Woman can do whatever they want to, why shouldn't they? . . . . I think that women have the same feelings as men do, I mean, I think it's okay to express them too. . . . I mean, they have the same feelings, they're human, why should they like keep away from them?" While Jenny seems unable to make sense of this inequity, Paulina grounds her dissension in an analysis linking gender and power: "I think males are kind of dominant, and they feel that they have the power to do whatever they want, that the woman should give in to them." Paulina also parts from Jenny in her detailed knowledge about her own sexual desire.

Perhaps not coincidentally, Paulina speaks of this embodied experience with an ease that reflects and underscores her belief that girls' sexual desire is normal or, in her words, "natural": "I feel really hot, like, my temperature is really hot. . . . I felt like a rush of blood like pumping to my heart, my heart would really beat fast, and it's just, everything are combined, you're extremely aware of every touch, and everything, everything together . . . you have all those feelings of want." Paulina is clear that this desire can guide her choices and that it should be respected: "To me if you have like a partner that you're close to, then it's okay. And if you feel comfortable with it, 'cause if you don't, then you shouldn't do it. You just don't want to." Thus, Paulina grounds her sexual decisions in her own feelings and beliefs—she can identify and is able to account for the presence and absence of her own desire. As a result, Paulina appears to be less vulnerable to becoming confused about what she feels and what she has said.

Like Jenny, Paulina has had a "bad" sexual experience with a boy whom she thought of as a friend. In the interview, she describes a time when this male friend tried to force her to have sex with him:

> There was one experience, the guy wanted to have sexual intercourse and I didn't. I didn't have sex with him. He, he like pulled me over to the couch, and I just kept on fighting. . . . I was just like begging him to like not to do anything, and like, I really did not have like much choice. Because I had my hands behind me. And he just like kept on touching me, and I was just like, just get off me. He goes, you know that you want to, and I said no I don't. Get off me, I hate you. . . . So he's like, well, I'll let you go if you're gonna kiss me. So I kissed him, and I'm like well I can go now. And he was like no. But um, the phone rang later on, I said I have to answer this, it's my mother. . . . So he let me answer the phone. So. And it was my friend and I just said, oh can you come over? And, since I'm Polish I spoke Polish, so I'm like oh just come over, come over as soon as you can.

Ultimately, when her friend arrived, she was able to convince the boy to leave.

Paulina's assailant attacked her both physically and psychologically, telling her, "You know that you want to." However, because Paulina had a clear understanding of her sexual feelings, she is able to speak clearly about not feeling sexual desire. In response to his coaxing, Paulina's retort is direct and unequivocal: "No, I don't. Get off me. I hate you." Unlike Jenny and Sharon, Paulina does not become confused: she has no doubt in her mind about the parameters of her own sexual feelings; she did not want any sexual interaction with this young man. Her sense of entitlement to her feelings and choices empowers her to resist the attack.

It must be emphasized that Paulina was very lucky in this situation. She was able to think clearly and take advantage of an opportunity—her friend's phone call—to protect herself from being raped. The critical point is not that she was able to avoid assault in this case, but that she was clear about the threat of violence. Had Paulina not escaped attack, it seems likely that she would have maintained her clarity about her own actions and desires, a clarity that would enable her to claim the protection the law offers.

Conclusion

In listening to three adolescent girls voice experiences with their own sexuality, we hear both how the good girl/bad girl dynamic becomes embodied and embedded in girls' psyches and relationships and how it can be resisted. We suggest that Paulina's ability to know her desire and know its absence, in contrast to Jenny's "silent body" and Sharon's confusion, is linked to her critical consciousness about how male power and dominance underpin the good girl/bad girl dichotomy. Because she rejects a cultural story about her sexuality that makes her own desire dangerous, we think she is less vulnerable to the confusion that Sharon and Jenny voice and more empowered to know and to speak with clarity about her sexual interactions and the social landscape of gendered relationships.

The voices of these three girls living (with) the good girl/bad girl dynamic suggest the necessity of what Michelle Fine terms an affirmative discourse of desire (Fine 1988) for adolescent girls. Such a discourse must recognize, reveal, and then reject the good girl/bad girl categories as patriarchal strategies that keep girls and women from the power of their own bodies and their bonds with one another. It should center on all girls' entitlement to their sexuality, rather than focus solely on the threat of lost status and respect or diminished safety. With the words and analysis to interrupt the good girl/bad girl dynamic, girls and women can identify and critique cultural stories that impair them psychologically and under the law.

The task for feminists, then, is to help adolescent girls and women to analyze the complexity of living in women's bodies within a culture that divides girls and women within themselves and against each other. It is true that the threat of sexual violence against girls and women, as well as social isolation, is real and constant, effectively keeping girls' and women's bodies and psyches filled with fear, rendering sexual desire difficult and dangerous. Yet it is also true that girls and women at this moment in history can feel profound pleasure and desire and should be entitled to rely on their own feelings as an important aspect of sexual choices. By holding the contradiction of pleasure and danger, girls and women can expose and loosen the tight weave seamlessly worked by the good girl/bad girl dynamic in society and in their individual lives.

Notes

1. Some young women are able to resist such norms by anchoring their sexual self-concept in their culture of origin (Robinson and Ward 1991).
2. Although the modern reinterpretation of the purpose of statutory rape laws is that such legislation is designed to prevent teen pregnancy, the historical justification was the protection of female virtue. For example, in 1895, the California Supreme Court explained:

    > The obvious purpose of [the statutory rape law] is the protection of society by protecting from violation the virtue of young

unsophisticated girls. . . . It is the insidious approach and vile tampering with their persons that primarily undermines the virtue of young girls, and eventually destroys it; and the prevention of this, as much as the principal act, must undoubtedly have been the intent of the legislature. (People *v.* Verdegreen, 106 Cal. 211, 214–215, 39 P. 607, 607–609 [1895]

In 1964, the same court explained that "an unwise disposition of her sexual favor is deemed to do harm both to herself and the social mores by which the community's conduct patterns are established. Hence the law of statutory rape intervenes in an effort to avoid such a disposition" (People v. Hernandez, 61 Cal. 2d 531, 393 P. 2d 674 [1964]).

As Professor Fran Olsen has argued, although the boy's conduct is punished by criminal sanction, it is the girl who is denied the capacity to consent. Under gender-specific statutory rape laws, the boy may legally have intercourse with women who are over the age of consent (Olsen, 1984).

3. The prosecution's strategy to portray the victim as asexual was controversial among advocates for people with mental disabilities. (See Houppert 1993, citing Leslie Walker-Hirsch, president of the American Association on Mental Retardation's special interest group on sexual and social concerns). Nevertheless, in this, as in many other rape trials, the surest means of establishing lack of consent was to establish the sexual innocence of the victim.

4. This method adopts the psychodynamic concept of the layered psyche in interpreting girls' and women's narratives in individual interviews conducted by women (Brown et al. 1991). Importing this clinical construct into empirical research is not by fiat a feminist act. But requiring the interpreter to focus actively on her own subjectivity and theoretical framework in the act of interpretation subverts the tendency in psychology of an authoritative, expert "voice over" of a girl or woman's words. This psychological method, called the Listening Guide, enables an exploration of ways in which internalized oppression may operate to constrain what a girl or woman says, thinks, or knows, and how she may resist such oppressions. This method asks us to consider what is not said as well as what is said and how power differences embedded in the brief research relationship may circulate through the narrative. The method obligates the interpreter to ask herself persistently how a woman's structural position in society or individual relational history may contribute to layered ways of understanding her voice—what she says, where she falters, when she is silent. The use of this method yields multiple interpretations of women's narratives by highlighting different voices or perspectives audible in a single story. Using this method means creating a dialectic between the way one girl or woman speaks and how another woman, from a distinctly feminist point of view, hears her story.

5. The study was designed to fill in a gap in the psychological literature on adolescent girls' sexuality: how girls experience their own sexual feelings, particularly their bodies. This feminist question challenged the belief that girls' sexuality is essentially a response to boys' sexual feelings and began to flesh out how sexual desire is a part of adolescent girls' lives. For her dissertation, Tolman interviewed a random sample of thirty girls from two different social contexts: they were juniors, aged fifteen to eighteen, at a suburban and an urban public high school. These girls were black, Hispanic, and white and represented a range of religious backgrounds, sexual experiences, and ethnicities. The interviews often had a conversational tone

because the feminist approach used emphasizes listening to girls, in contrast to the traditional procedure of strict adherence to a preset questionnaire. Overall these girls reported that their own desire was a dilemma for them because they were not supposed to experience sexual feelings but, in fact, did. For more on this study see Tolman 1994a, 1994b, and forthcoming. The analyses of this data have focused on class rather than race differences, due to the demographics of the sample. Both qualitative and quantitative analyses revealed similarities across class, such as in the proportion of girls who reported an absence of or confusion about desire and those who reported an awareness of their own desire, and significant class differences in the association of desire with vulnerability and pleasure. Urban girls' narratives were more likely to be about vulnerability and not about pleasure, while suburban girls' narratives were more likely to be about pleasure rather than vulnerability.

6. Brown and Gilligan 1992 and Jack 1991 describe these qualities of the "tyranny of nice and kind" and the tendency to silence or sacrifice the self's disruptive feelings as characteristic of girls' and women's descriptions of their relationships.

7. Paulina's responses have been reported previously in Tolman 1994b.

References

Brown, Lynn, and Carol Gilligan. 1992. *Meeting at the Crossroads.* Cambridge, MA: Harvard University Press.

Brown, Lynn, Elizabeth Debold, Mark Tappan, and Carol Gilligan. 1991. "Reading Narratives of Conflict for Self and Moral Voice: A Relational Method." In *Handbook of Moral Behavior and Development: Theory, Research and Application,* ed. William Kurtines and Jacob Gewirtz. Hillsdale, NJ: Lawrence Erlbaum.

Caraway, Nancie. 1991. *Segregated Sisterhood.* Knoxville: University of Tennessee Press.

Collins, Patricia Hill. 1990. *Black Feminist Thought.* New York: Routledge.

Fine, Michelle. 1988. "Sexuality, Schooling, and Adolescent Females: The Missing Discourse of Desire." *Harvard Educational Review* 58 (10: 29–53).

Harris, Angela. 1990. "Race and Essentialism in Feminist Legal Theory." *Stanford Law Review* 42: 581–592.

Henderson, Lynne. 1992. "Rape and Responsibility." *Law and Philosophy* 11 (1–2): 127–128.

Hollway, Wendy. 1984. "Women's Power in Heterosexual Sex." *Women's Studies International Forum* 7 (1): 63–68.

Houppert, Karen. 1993. "The Glen Ridge Rape Draws to a Close." *Village Voice* (March 16): 29–33.

Jack, Dana. 1991. *Silencing the Self.* Cambridge, MA: Harvard University Press.

Michael M. v. Sonoma County, 450 U.S. 464 (1980).

Olsen, Frances. 1984. "Statutory Rape: A Feminist Critique of Rights Analysis." *Texas Law Review* 63: 387.

Omadale, Barbara, 1983. "Hearts of Darkness." In *Powers of Desire: The Politics of Sexuality,* ed. Ann Snitow, Christine Stansell, and Sharon Thompson. New York: Monthly Review Press.

Robinson, Tracy and Janie Ward. 1991. "A Belief in Self Far Greater than Anyone's Disbelief: Cultivating Resistance Among African American Female Adolescents." In *Women, Girls, and Psychotherapy: Reframing Resistance,* ed. Carol Gilligan, Annie Rogers, and Deborah Tolman. New York: Haworth Press.

Roiphe, Katie: 1993. *The Morning After: Sex, Fear, and Feminism on Campus.* Boston: Little, Brown.

Shrieves, Linda. 1993. "The Bold New World of Boy Chasing." *Orlando Sentinel* (22 December): E1.

Smart, Carole. 1989. *Feminism and the Power of the Law.* New York: Routledge.

Smolowe, Jill. 1993. "Sex with a Scorecard." *Time* (5 April):41.

Tolman, Deborah. Forthcoming. "Adolescent Girls' Sexuality: Debunking the Myth of the Urban Girl." In *Urban Adolescent Girls: Resisting Stereotypes,* ed. Bonnie Leadbetter and Niobe Way. New York: New York University Press.

———. 1994a. "Daring to Desire; Culture and the Bodies of Adolescent Girls." In *Sexual Cultures: Adolescents, Communities and the Construction of Identity,* ed. Janice Irvine. Philadelphia: Temple University Press.

———.1994b. "Doing Desire: Adolescent Girls' Struggle for/with Sexuality." *Gender and Society* 8(3): 324–342.

Yoffe, Emily. 1991. "Girls Who Go Too Far." *Newsweek* (22 July): 58.

The Orgasm Gap

by Marcia Douglass and Lisa Douglass

Nikki and Joe lie naked in their bed, kissing in passionate embrace. As they caress one another, Nikki slowly glides her hand down Joe's chest and abdomen to his penis. She delights in the way it responds to her touch and savors its warm, firm feel in her hand. Joe reaches between Nikki's legs and slides his finger into her vagina. Nikki tilts her hips so that his fingertip meets her clitoris. She closes her eyes to focus on the rush of excitement his touch sends through her genitals. As Joe rubs her clitoris and kisses her neck, shoulder, and nipples, Nikki's pleasure borders on orgasm.

After a few minutes on this erotic edge, Nikki begins to worry that Joe wants to move on. She gets up, straddles him, and together they roll on a condom. Nikki massages on some lubrication then slips Joe's penis into her vagina. She caresses his penis inside her, alternately tightening and releasing her vaginal muscles. As Joe's excitement builds, Nikki senses that her own arousal is not keeping pace. The intensity of her pleasure dissipates, and she feels her orgasm slipping away. Nikki does not want to deny Joe his pleasure, so they flip over. Joe thrusts rhythmically and deeply inside her, then quickly comes. Nikki is disappointed that she has not had an orgasm, but as they rest in each other's arms, she takes pleasure in their intimacy.

For Nikki, as for most women, orgasm in sex is like a mirage: It appears on the horizon one minute, like a delicious glass of water to a thirsty traveler. But the next minute—poof!—it is gone. Sometimes, especially when she is on top during intercourse, Nikki comes, too. But at other times, she fakes orgasm. (Actually, she just lets Joe believe she has come.) Occasionally, when Joe asks, Nikki tells him, "It felt great! Really, it's OK. I love just being close to you." These are words that Joe has never uttered. He never has to: Like most men, Joe always has an orgasm when he has sex. As Joe begins to snore in satisfied slumber, Nikki lies awake trying to convince herself that it really was good for her, too.

Most men would not see the point of sex if their orgasms were so elusive. Yet Nikki and millions of other heterosexual women put up with unsatisfying sex on a regular basis, and the sexual culture—the way people in our society define sex—seems undisturbed by this fact. Both women and men expect sex to be a physically satisfying experience, but for many women it is not. Although sex virtually always includes *his* orgasm, hers is optional—nice, but not necessary.

The orgasm gap disrupts the pleasure of sex for both Nikki and Joe. When Joe comes but Nikki does not, they both feel frustrated or somehow deficient. Nikki thinks it is her mood. *I just could not let go tonight.* Sometimes she blames how she looks. *If I could just lose ten pounds.* Joe feels he has not "performed" adequately. *Maybe if I had lasted longer. Maybe if my penis were bigger.* Nikki and Joe tell themselves that orgasm is always harder for women to achieve. *Women just do not come as easily as men.*

What Nikki and Joe never blame is the *way* they have sex. For them, sex is synonymous with intercourse. They never have sex that does not include it. Intercourse gives Joe direct genital stimulation and virtually ensures his orgasm. Nikki loves the way intercourse feels, too, but most of the time it does not lead to her orgasm.

Nikki knows that she comes every time she masturbates by massaging her clitoris. But in partner sex, she never touches herself there. Joe pays her clitoris some attention during foreplay, but the stimulation he gives her usually stops short of orgasm. When they move to intercourse, the clitoris is all but forgotten. Nikki enjoys the feeling of Joe's penis inside her, but because penetration bypasses the clitoris, it does not make her come. Sometimes Nikki is tempted to ask Joe to keep his fingers on her clitoris a little longer or to give her cunnilingus. But having an orgasm from manual or oral sex is seen as inferior somehow. Both Nikki and Joe have learned that orgasm should come from intercourse. So they cut foreplay short and begin penetration, even though it is likely to mean that sex will soon culminate in his, but not her, orgasm.

The orgasm gap between women and men is not just an individual problem. Nikki's experience of hit-or-miss orgasm is typical of sex for heterosexual women in the United States today. Seventy-five percent of men have orgasm in partner sex on a regular basis, but only 29 percent of women do. Two-thirds of women have orgasms only sometimes or not at all. It is difficult to imagine men accepting sex that excluded their orgasm. Yet because women have learned to accept this double standard, the orgasm gap has hardly budged over decades of social change—the sexual revolution of the 1960s, the women's movement of the 1970s, the antisex backlash in the era of AIDS in the 1980s, and into the sexual quandary of the 1990s. The 29/75 gap continues today in a social environment that appears to be more open than ever about sex. Intimate details of sexual activity are now discussed in safer sex instruction, on television and radio talk shows, and explicit sex acts are regularly portrayed in the popular media. But the orgasm gap is rarely discussed. It is simply accepted as the way sex is.

The orgasm gap between women and men is not restricted to any particular group of people. It crosses all lines of income, race, and ethnicity. It exists not only in every region of the United States but in every society around the world. Its near universality is not, however, proof that the orgasm gap is inevitable. Women are not inherently less orgasmic than men. In fact, women are physically capable of multiple orgasms, and most women who masturbate reach orgasm without fail. Women who have sex with a female partner come 83 percent of the time. Clearly, the problem lies not with women themselves, but in the way *heterosexuals* have sex.

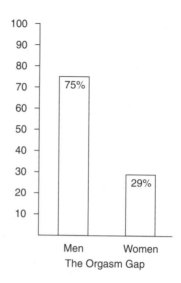

The Orgasm Gap

Most people attribute the orgasm gap to biology and ignore the fact that people learn to have sex and to have orgasms according to the beliefs of their particular culture. In the United States, people believe that there is a difference in hormones that makes men want and need sex more than women. They believe that it is natural fact that men reach their sexual peak at age eighteen, while most women's sexuality surges at thirty-five. They believe that women have a harder time having orgasms than men as a result of some evolutionary master plan of nature, when the real culprit is the way women and men are taught to have sex. It usually takes a woman decades before she figures out that the model of sex she was taught was wrong: It leaves out her orgasm.

Other people, including many sex experts, attribute the orgasm gap to women's psychology. In this view, women do not have orgasms because they have psychological hang-ups about sex. If women can just learn to relax in sex, they will have orgasms. But even the most carefree and uninhibited woman will not have an orgasm unless she gets the appropriate stimulation. Yet the sexual culture defines sex in such a way that women and men either never learn to use or are discouraged from using the kind of stimulation that works.

At the start of a new millennium, most young women face the same confusing path toward orgasm their mothers and grandmothers encountered. They must make their way through a morass of inconsistent messages about sex. The most damaging of these is that sex is essentially intercourse and every other kind of sexual activity is not the real thing, even when they are more likely to give women orgasms. The sex = intercourse message leaves a woman to flounder through a long series of unsatisfactory sexual encounters before she finally figures out that clitoral stimulation, not intercourse

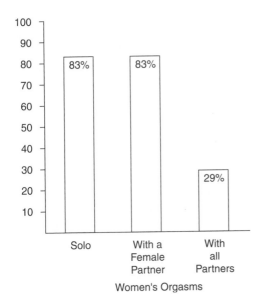

Women's Orgasms

alone, will bring her to orgasm. Although the role of the clitoris in women's orgasm is mentioned in sex manuals and sex education texts, a woman can easily miss this important fact. Most women eventually discover the clitoris-orgasm connection. But then they face the higher hurdle of making this knowledge mesh with the way their partner (and the sexual culture) expects them to have sex.

The information a woman receives about orgasm is often so garbled and contradictory that she gives up trying to have one. Orgasm should come from intercourse, she is told, yet for most women it never does. Orgasm comes from clitoral stimulation, she reads, but a woman should nevertheless try to come from intercourse. Don't worry if you have never had an orgasm or only have them sometimes, she hears. Sex is so much more than orgasm: It is romance, sensuality, emotional intimacy, and above all, an expression of love.

But love is not enough to make sex good. And bad sex can interfere with love. An intimate relationship cannot thrive and grow where the physical pleasures of sex are as unequal as they are between Nikki and Joe. Some women settle for orgasms that happen now and then, and they focus their energies on romance and intimacy. But for women who find sex more frustrating than pleasurable, more embarrassing than ecstatic, and more of a duty than an opportunity, not having orgasm takes them further away from a loved partner, not closer. When the man has an orgasm but the woman does not, sex is not only less fun, but a gap can develop between two lovers in which doubt, anger, and blame begin to fester. Some women just stop having sex. One woman told us, "I faked it for over twelve years. And then it got to a point where I felt turned off to sex altogether. I didn't even

want to deal with it because I wasn't getting anything out of it."

Men suffer from the orgasm gap, too. They have learned that it is up to them to "give" their partner an orgasm with their penis. If she does not come, they feel that it is a failure of either their own sexual prowess or a result of their partner's "frigidity." A man may tell a woman that she just needs to let go. The woman, too, believes that the problem is all in her head. They both accept the sexual culture's explanation that women's psychological hang-ups are the main cause of the orgasm gap. Yet the fault actually lies with a sexual culture that defines sex as intercourse.

Some women manage to defy the sexual culture and learn to have satisfying orgasmic sex. Some stumble upon orgasm by chance or luck. Others make a conscious effort to cultivate their sexuality. Of the women who regularly experience orgasm, some have one orgasm, some have multiple orgasms (more than one orgasm in a sexual session), and some ejaculate, a sexual pleasure most women never even learn about. Because sex is more often alluded to than honestly and openly discussed, women in our society have little chance of growing sexually unless they question the sexual culture and determine to cultivate their sexuality on their own.

There is little social support for women who challenge the sexual status quo. Even though women talk to each other about their periods, their relationships, and other intimate subjects, what they do in sex is a topic even the closest friends fear to broach. Women never take the opportunity to learn from other women about orgasm. Nor do most women talk frankly with their male partners about safer sex, much less better sex.

Nikki and Joe have never talked about what they actually do in bed. Neither of them has ever stopped to think about how they might do things differently because, in spite of their orgasm gap, they consider their sex life to be pretty good. They are equally interested in having sex, they enjoy foreplay, and when they have intercourse, it lasts longer than the national average of two and a half minutes. Yet, at some level, both of them know that sex between them could be so much better if Nikki had an orgasm, too.

Although primarily a problem for straight women, the orgasm gap also affects lesbians, bisexual women, and all men who care about gender equality and who like good sex. When the sexual culture focuses on what gives men pleasure in sex with a woman, all other sexual activities and everyone who is not a heterosexual male gets short sexual shrift. All women are pushed to the margins of sex defined as intercourse—lesbians do not have "real" sex, bisexual women "play around" with women until a man comes along, and straight women are expected to get pleasure from the same things that please men. If the sexual culture considers women's pleasure at all, it is only insofar as it fits into a model for sex designed to satisfy men.

Is Orgasm Important?

> I don't think orgasms are the be-all, end-all, but I sure as hell wouldn't want to live without them.
>
> —Betty Dodson

Most men never question the importance of orgasm—it is simply their sexual right. Many women cannot say whether or not orgasm is important, however, because they have never had one. A woman who does insist on having an orgasm may be accused of being too unromantic, too male, or too demanding. Yet no man ever has to justify his desire for orgasm. The goal of sex for women in contrast, is supposed to be intimacy, not orgasm. Yet orgasmic sex improves intimacy. When only one partner's orgasm is important, even necessary, while the other partner's is ignored or denied, true intimacy is impossible.

The Sexual Culture

The orgasm gap can be bridged only by changing the way women and men have sex. Changing the way people have sex means changing the sexual culture and confronting the assumptions upon which it is based. The first assumption is that sex is natural and that people are driven by hormones and genital urges. A person is thought to have a "sex drive" that motivates sexual behavior. Yet, as Leonore Tiefer's recent book proclaims in its title, *Sex Is Not a Natural Act.* Everyone who has ever had sex knows that it involves not only the body, but the mind and spirit. They know that it occurs in the context of complex relations with other people. Furthermore, sex is learned. And it is carried out according to the standards of a particular culture. Although sex takes place in and through the body, it is not governed by people's hormones or gonads. Sex is a social act to its very core, including in the way we define the body and sex itself.

Recognizing that sex is learned, people can act to change it. Until now, women have learned to have sex in ways that favor male pleasure, but they can unlearn those ways and invent new ones that foster more equal and satisfying sex.

To make sex as good for her as it is for him, Nikki and Joe need to examine each layer of their sexual activity to look at what they do and why. This means talking about sex. Already, sex is a popular topic of public discussion, but in the age of AIDS, the talk sometimes gets reduced to a debate about whether to "just say no" or to "do it, do it, do it," without ever asking what are we doing when we "do it"? Why are we doing it? For pleasure? Out of obligation? To demonstrate love? For all of these reasons? And why is one way of having sex considered right, and another considered wrong? The sexual culture promotes intercourse between a woman and a man as something that should "come naturally." But if intercourse "comes naturally," why is only one partner coming?

Recognizing that sex is not natural, but rather a product of culture, opens up exciting possibilities for change. Reinventing sex is a radical project that involves more than just trying new positions or buying a sex toy (although these can definitely add to the fun). Changing the way we have sex requires thinking in profoundly different ways about the body, about power relations between women and men, and about sex itself. It means developing a new language to talk about sex in more equal terms. By imagining a new sexuality, women and men will do much more than enhance their own enjoyment. Making sex an act of shared, mutual pleasure is an essential part of creating true gender equality.

Four Myths

In order to begin rethinking sex, it is useful to first consider several taken-for-granted assumptions or myths that are the foundation of the sexual culture.

Myth #1: Women = Sex

In our society, the body of a woman—a young, beautiful, revealingly dressed woman—is the symbol for sex. More precisely, certain parts of a woman's body stand for sex because they are a turn-on for heterosexual men. A woman's breast and buttocks are probably the prime icons of sex, but long legs, high heels, big hair, and a round, red mouth are also widespread cultural symbols that set up the sexual equation. The woman, like the car, the beer, or the magazine her body advertises, is an object of desire. A sexy woman is an item of consumption, and man is her consumer.

Equating sex with an idealized female image puts real women in a sexual no-person's land. The vast majority of women neither meet the criteria of what is sexy nor fit the profile of the consumer. Most women know that our sexual culture does not have them in mind when, for example, a magazine article entitled "Sex" is illustrated by a nineteen-year-old blonde in a Wonderbra, garter belt, and spike heels.

Every woman knows what it is to struggle with what one friend calls "the body thing." Women learn from the time they are young to treat their own bodies as perpetual improvement projects as they strive to emulate an externally imposed image of what is sexy. A woman's growth as a sexual person is compromised by the goal of looking sexy on the outside, and eventually a woman becomes estranged from what her body feels on the inside.

One woman told us that from the time she was a teenager, she felt she was expected to look *sexy* but never to be or feel *sexual*. She often dressed in provocative ways. "But if I went beyond a certain point," she says, "my father would call me awful names. I never had it right, and I still don't." A woman is made to feel like a performer on a tightrope who walks a fine line imposed by the demands of the audience below—an audience that eggs her on while simultaneously criticizing her as shameless for performing in the first place. Despite its perils, this performance is one that many women feel compelled to carry out.

In a sexual culture that equates sex with the female body, a woman is told that she deserves sexual pleasure only if she looks attractive. Many women get great satisfaction from dressing up, but focusing on being attractive on the outside can interfere with sexual satisfaction within. A woman may never cultivate or respond to her own feelings or desires because she develops her sexuality based on the way others see, touch, and treat her.

The sexual culture's emphasis on a woman's exterior makes it difficult for her to develop a healthy sexual self. In reinventing sex, women can turn the focus of sex to their own experience of their bodies. They can have sex on their own terms, a privilege most men take for granted. Instead of handing her sexuality over to others, a woman controls and possesses it herself. She can enjoy orgasm when and if she wants to—she is neither pressured into coming to boost her partner's ego, nor denied orgasm because of neglect. When women reinvent sex, a woman will not earn good sex because she fits a sexy physical ideal. Instead, she will deserve good sex because she is a human being.

Myth #2: Sex = Intercourse

When heterosexuals refer to "sex," they usually mean vaginal intercourse. Whether euphemism ("the sex act"), slang ("getting laid"), or profanity ("fucking"), most words for *sex* are actually words for *intercourse*. Even many women get in the habit of thinking of intercourse as the only *real* sex. A woman recently told us that she likes to use a vibrator to have an orgasm before she has "sex." Apparently, sex does not begin until a penis gets into the act.

Vaginal penetration by the penis is the defining act of sex for most heterosexuals. A recent survey found that 95 percent of heterosexuals usually or always have intercourse when they have sex. Other sexual activities, such as manual and oral sex, sometimes serve only as either a warm-up for intercourse or an imitation of it. French kissing and finger penetration are sometimes performed to mimic it more than for their own intrinsic pleasures. Even though intercourse is the way women are least likely to come, the sexual culture places the greatest value on orgasm that results from intercourse. Clitoral stimulation is overlooked in favor of penetration, and the stereotype is that women want a man who is "long, hard, and can go all night long." Even many vibrators are shaped like a penis because it is assumed that a man's source of pleasure—the penis—should also sexually satisfy a woman.

Vaginal penetration is a rite of passage in our sexual culture. It is the only sex act that can validate marriage. (Lesbians are not granted any comparable rite to validate a partnership.) It is a testament to the crucial meaning of intercourse that a woman can engage in masturbation or in manual, oral, or anal sex with a partner and have an orgasm, perhaps multiple orgasms, but she is still a "virgin" if her vagina has not been penetrated by a penis. A woman's virginity is something *only* a man's penis—and not his hands or mouth, much less the woman herself, or another woman—has the power to take away.

To "go all the way" means arriving at the ultimate destination: vaginal penetration. For most men, intercourse is the last stop on the sex train. His orgasm announces to the woman that the trip is over. Intercourse is where she should get off, too. But it leaves most women idling on the tracks, their engines still running.

It is little wonder that men come easily during vaginal penetration. Intercourse brings a man to orgasm because the male counterpart of the clitoris lies within the penis, and the penis is surrounded on all sides by massaging vaginal walls. A woman's clitoris lies mostly within her body separate from the vagina. Her clitoris is mostly untouched by intercourse. Only the exposed tip and clitoral shaft receive some stimulation from the tugs and strokes of the man's penis or from intermittent pressure from his pelvis. For some women, this is sufficient for orgasm, especially if they are "on top." Most of the time, however, expecting intercourse alone to result in a woman's orgasm is comparable to expecting Joe to be satisfied by a massage of his testicles. It feels good, but the longer Nikki does it, the more likely he is to feel annoyed than to have an orgasm.

The low rate of orgasm for women is correlated with the high rate of intercourse-oriented sex. Intercourse simply does not give enough direct stimulation to the clitoris for orgasm to occur in most women. The penis and the clitoris pass one another like ships in the night, but only the penis makes it to port. Yet amidst multiple messages that it is the high point of sex, a woman battles a lingering feeling that she *should* be able to achieve orgasm during coitus.

A woman gets caught in a catch-22. Sex consists of intercourse, which does not make her come. Oral and manual sex do make her come, but they are seen as remedial or even "deviant" forms of sex. Oral sex is only a rare offering and manual sex is confined to foreplay, if done at all.

To some, intercourse may seem an imperative of nature. The vagina and the penis appear destined for each other, or rather, the vagina is made for the penis. The penis slips so easily into the vagina, like a sword into its sheath. Indeed, vagina *means* sheath. Its very name implies that the vagina has no sexual identity of its own but only becomes a sexual organ when the penis enters it.

The act of intercourse reflects the larger cultural notion that sex is something that men do *to* women. Even women's active role in reproduction is made to seem passive. The penis in intercourse is likened to a plow that prepares the soil and presses the seed into a receptive earth. Because of its role in reproduction, intercourse is seen as the natural way to have sex. People often point to other animals: Birds "do it," bees "do it," and so do cats and dogs. Sexual intercourse is indeed the typical and optimal means for egg to meet sperm in humans. But people engage in sex for conception only a few times in their lives. Above all, they have sex for pleasure. And as anyone who masturbates knows, the most fun one can have in sex, hands down, is orgasm.

Myth #3: Women and Men Are Different and Unequal

Perhaps the most influential myth of our sexual culture is that women and men are opposite sexes. But rather than opposite and equal, men are taken as the norm, and women the deviation. Women are both men's opposites and their inferiors. The apparently greater size of men's genitals is sometimes read as evidence of their more powerful sex drive, while women's seemingly smaller genitals reflect a lesser interest in sex. Seen as inferior in so many ways, it is not surprising that women tend to come out "on the bottom" in sex.

The myth that women are sexually inferior to men is supported by three beliefs: (1) that women have a lesser sex drive than men; (2) that women do not need orgasm as men do; and (3) that women have lesser genitals than men.

Women Have a Lesser Sex Drive Than Men The sex drive is not considered the result of social conditioning or experience but as an inborn or natural gender trait. In our sexual culture, it is believed that "female hormones" (actually, the excess of female and shortage of male hormones, especially testosterone) make women less sexual. Yet hormones and other biological processes used as evidence of sex difference are always interpreted according to the terms of the culture. Women's lower levels of testosterone are said to explain why women initiate sex less often than men, but this ignores how women get decades of training to please others and are told they are "bad" if they act on their own sexual desires. Women can be so busy responding to desires of men and the sexual culture that they hardly get a chance to cultivate their own. Women's capacity for multiple orgasms, for example, rarely gets nurtured, while the qualities that contribute to men's pleasure—beauty and sexual acquiescence—are rewarded and emphasized.

The notion of a natural sex drive helps to validate men's sexual priority. It is believed that women simply never experience the same urge to have sex "right now" that men do. Indeed, some men blame their uncontrollable sex drive when they pressure women for sex ("You got me so turned on"). It explains why men visit prostitutes or cheat on their wives or girlfriends ("Men have sexual needs"). It is even used to absolve the man and blame the woman for her own rape ("He was so turned on by her, he couldn't stop"). It seems that men simply cannot help themselves when sex goes into overdrive. For a woman to express a strong sex drive, in contrast, is seen as unnatural, even immoral. A woman who expresses an urgent desire for sex risks being seen as a "slut."

That our society considers sex a "drive" at all renders it a force beyond human control. It supports the notion that there is little an individual can do to control nature's engine. But neither men's so-called sex drive nor women's apparent indifference to sex is the product of biology and hormones, for sex unfolds in a social context. In a society that organizes sex around achieving men's orgasm and that caters to men's sexual pleasure in countless other ways, it is not surprising that a woman might show less interest in sex. But it is not because they are born that way. When sex lacks the clitoral stimulation that most women enjoy to orgasm, it becomes a self-fulfilling prophecy that women are the less sexual half of the population. Yet when men have orgasms and women do not, the difference is treated as the playing out of the distinct sexual natures of females and males, rather than as the result of sex socialization by gender and the sexual culture's definition of sex as intercourse to the man's orgasm.

Women Do Not Need Orgasm as Men Do   Orgasm is practically a medical Rx for a man. If he becomes sexually aroused and does not reach orgasm and ejaculate, it is said he will suffer "blue balls." The man's visually obvious erection makes penetration (or, as many women well know, a hand job or a blow job) seem imperative. Even though a woman also experiences the equivalent of an erection, our sexual culture neither names nor recognizes this event. A woman is not described as suffering from "blue clit" if her sexual arousal does not culminate in orgasm—even though the frustration of sex that ends before orgasm is a much more common experience for women than it is for men.

To acknowledge that women need orgasms as much as men do is to suggest that women and men are much more alike sexually than different. This idea challenges the sexual culture because it implies that women are capable of and deserve pleasure no less than men.

> There are very few absolute sex differences and . . . without complete social equality we cannot know for sure what they are.
> —Anne Fausto Sterling, *Myths of Gender*

Women Have Lesser Genitals Than Men   The sexual culture focuses on the towering erection of the man's penis while it ignores the fact that the erectile tissues of a woman's clitoris and bulbs are the same size and also respond to stimulation. The organs of both sexes expand and become firm during sexual arousal, yet the event that is so significant in men, erection, is not even acknowledged in women.

The sexual culture defines erection as a purely male phenomenon and spotlights vaginal "wetness" in women. Vaginal lubrication is interpreted as a sign of female readiness for penetration (and the man's pleasure). It ignores how a woman's genitals become erect in the same process of blood engorgement and muscle tension that a man experiences.

Our sexual culture evaluates genitals based not on how people experience pleasure, but on how well they fit into a model of sex that features the penis in a starring role. When the stage is set for sex, the man's large, assertive organ appears at center stage and the vagina plays the part of its accommodating sidekick. The woman's clitoris acts only as a puny, uncredited extra who barely emerges from the wings.

Myth #4: Women Want Intimacy; Men Want Sex

An extension of the myth of gender difference is the belief that women and men want different things when they have sex: Women want decor (wine and candlelight), while men want hard core (genital sex and orgasm). Men want to penetrate and come; women want to cuddle and talk. Intimacy and genital sex are presented as opposite and irreconcilable goals. Women complain of not getting enough intimacy and attention, while men complain of not getting enough "sex." Women and men have indeed been taught to eat different halves of the sexual pie. But even after she gets her slice of closeness, and he gets his serving of orgasm, they both may be left feeling hungry. Perhaps the reason men get sex less often than they want is because women are not sexually satisfied. And women who are sexually unsatisfied turn their interests elsewhere. Susan Quilliam, who surveyed British women on sex, suggests that women may focus on intimacy to compensate for the lack of orgasms. A woman who regularly has sex without orgasms would indeed begin to think that pleasure must lie elsewhere.

With the mantra "Women want intimacy and men want sex," sexuality splits into two parts, each assigned to one gender. Author and relationship guru John Gray goes even further. He argues in his books *Men Are from Mars, Women Are from Venus* and *Mars and Venus in the Bedroom* that, when it comes to relationships and sex, women and men are from different planets. This view is popular because it reassures heterosexual couples that there is nothing wrong with them. If they feel alienated from their partner, it is because she or he truly is an alien. Gray's view encourages people to believe that the problems between women and men are a result of innate differences that cannot be changed. Gray completely ignores how the sexual culture teaches women to focus on intimacy and men to focus on sex. By characterizing women as an emotional "planet" and men as a sexual "planet," he dresses up the sexual culture's oldest stereotypes in New Age garb. In bed, the two planets remain separated by the orgasm gap.

Rather than assigning intimacy to women and sex to men, sex could be better for everyone if it included both experiences. The last time we looked, women and men both lived on Earth, a planet located midway between Venus and Mars. Here on Earth, both women and men are capable of enjoying intimacy along with orgasmic sex. In fact, instead of conflicting, the two pleasures enhance one another. Orgasmic sex and intimacy are part of a single continuum of sexual, emotional, mental, and

---

Your (Society's) Sexual IQ Test

1. What sexual activity is most likely to bring a woman to orgasm?
   a. intercourse
   (b) clitoral stimulation
   c. sex with a partner she loves
2. What shape does the female clitoris most resemble?
   (a.) a four-inch wishbone
   b. a pea
   c. a miniature penis
3. When is sex between a woman and a man usually considered over?
   a. when the woman has an orgasm
   b. when each partner is sexually satisfied
   (c.) when the man ejaculates
4. What is the most common sign that a woman is having an orgasm?
   (a.) her pelvic muscle contracts
   b. her chest flushes red
   c. she moans
5. Some women ejaculate a fluid in sex that is chemically closest to
   a. urine
   b. vaginal secretions
   (c.) prostatic fluid similar to men's

6. What is the average duration of heterosexual vaginal intercourse?
   a. one hour
   (b.) two to three minutes
   c. fifteen minutes
7. Who can masturbate to orgasm faster?
   a. men
   b. women
   (c.) women and men can be equally fast
8. Only some women have a G spot.
   T
   (F)
9. A woman's vagina always lubricates or gets "wet" when she is sexually excited.
   T
   (F)
10. When sexually excited, women experience the same engorgement and increased muscle tension that is known as "erection" in men.
    (T)
    F

ANSWERS AT THE END OF THE CHAPTER.

What Women (Do Not) Want

What do women want, Freud asked. The old fool, the charlatan. He knew what women wanted. They wanted nothing. Nothing was good enough. Everyone knew that.

—A Woman Reflecting on Sex in Carol Shields's Novel, *The Stone Diaries*

---

physical expression. When women reinvent sex, both women and men will have equal access to all the fruits in the same garden of earthly delights.

In this book, we gather together ideas and resources women can use to reinvent sex. We focus on the body and begin by rethinking women's bodies and sexuality; but a similar process for men is also needed. By considering the pleasures and desires women and men share, both can work together to debunk the myths and develop alterna-

tive, more inclusive, and more equal attitudes and activities that will make sex not just male fun, but mutual fun.

In Orgasm Denial

Reinventing sex requires that women recognize the problems of the sexual culture. Yet many women are in denial about the orgasm gap. Some ignore the problem because they have great, orgasmic sex with their partners. They say they feel no need to rethink sex, thank you very much. "Is there a problem?" asked one twenty-something college graduate who told us she has three orgasms every time she has sex. Some thirty-, forty- and fiftysomething urban professional women ask us: "Didn't we already do this in the 1970s?" And our mother tells us that she and all her World War II–generation friends figured out orgasmic sex without a hitch.

The key phrase here is "figured out." Many of these women just stumbled upon orgasm by accident or they were lucky enough to have a knowledgeable partner. Others became orgasmic in solo sex by violating the taboo against masturbation. All of them figured out how to enjoy sex not through the sexual culture, but *in spite of it*. One by one, each woman had to reinvent the sexual wheel.

There are other women, however, who are either unable or not inspired to make this effort. In a sexual culture in denial about women's orgasms, it can take a substantial effort to make partner sex satisfying. Since women's pleasure is not a topic either among women, in sex education, or even in the media, only a woman who goes out of her way to learn about sex is likely to become orgasmic. The silence surrounding female sexuality hurts even orgasmic women because it fails to acknowledge or give authority to their experiences of sex. A woman who comes with oral sex, for example, may enjoy sex less because she is wondering, "Am I coming the 'right' way?" A woman who has orgasms now and then may lack the information, opportunity, and encouragement to ask why sex is not always orgasmic. She may prefer to keep the peace rather than stir up trouble, especially when the solution challenges not only her taken-for-granted assumptions about sex, but also her relations with men.

Many women are aware of the orgasm gap but prefer not to confront it. We know women who have been married for decades, with grown children and sexually satisfied husbands, who have never had an orgasm. When they have sex they focus on the man's pleasure. Some have orgasms when they masturbate, but have not mustered the courage or developed the communication skills to talk to their partner about making orgasm a mutual part of sex together. A few have partners who refuse to change the way they have sex. For these women, orgasm looms as a rather daunting challenge rather than being something they look forward to enjoying.

Attaining orgasmic sex is sometimes so bewildering that, when a woman finally does have orgasms regularly with a partner, she may confuse what she feels with love. Or, she may stay in a relationship because she is afraid she will not find another partner who "gives" her orgasms. Good sex may enhance love, and love often enhances sex, but they are not the same thing.

Some feminists and sex therapists fear that encouraging women to strive for orgasm only adds to the women's feelings of sexual inadequacy. But in the name of protecting women's feelings, this view may inadvertently make orgasm all the more elusive for women. It implies that it is a woman's own fault that she does not have orgasms, rather than the fault of the way sex is defined. Others downplay the importance of orgasm because they believe that to celebrate orgasm is to succumb to male values. In a more female-oriented sexuality, they suggest, sensual pleasures such as caressing, kissing, and holding would supersede genital sex

and orgasm. Women can enjoy what a special 1995 issue of *Ms.* magazine referred to as "hot unscripted sex," that is, "whatever turns you on."

Widening women's options for sexual pleasure is important, but to dismiss orgasm is to throw out the baby with the bathwater. This view also falls into the gender-stereotyped orgasm-versus-intimacy trap. Leaving women's physical pleasure vaguely defined as "whatever" makes it more likely that women's natural capacity for orgasm will remain undeveloped. A woman can always choose *not* to come, but it only truly becomes a choice for her when orgasm becomes a readily available option.

Dismantling the Sex Machine

Most observers of the 1960s now agree that the sexual revolution was a boon for sex—that is, if you were a heterosexual male. Many women expected that all the commotion would revolutionize sex for them, too. Some of them believed that by simply having *more* sex, with *more* partners, in *more* intercourse positions, or *more* days of the week, sex would become as good for them as it seemed to be for men. But more sex did not necessarily mean better sex for women, because the balance of pleasure did not change. Even when oral sex came into fashion, and more men were willing to give women cunnilingus (oral sex on a woman) than ever before, rates of fellatio (oral sex on a man) rose, too, and always remained higher. The so-called sexual revolution failed women because it did not change sex in the fundamental ways necessary to make it more *equal* fun. Ultimately, the revolution only revved up the existing sex machine. It oiled the gears, when what was needed was to dismantle the engine, melt down the parts, and completely rebuild sex from the inside out of women's experience. This has not yet happened and, as a result, at the turn of a new century, many women are still stuck in the missionary position wondering, "Did the sexual revolution come yet? . . . because I haven't!"

It is now time to rethink sex in fundamental ways. Feminists and lesbian, gay, and bisexual activists of recent decades form the vanguard of a contemporary rethinking that promises a *real* revolution in sex. Like the little girl in the village crowd who announced that the emperor had no clothes, these groups are revealing the secret that women habitually keep to themselves: Sex as it is currently defined does not satisfy women.

Crucial ingredients for reinventing sex have been contributed by people such as Shere Hite, who published a study reporting what thousands of women themselves said about sex. *The Hite Report: A Nationwide Study of Female Sexuality* was a highly controversial book that revealed the discrepancy between what women were supposed to experience in sex and what they actually felt. Critics found fault with its lack of statistical method (even though the gist of Hite's findings has been borne out by other, more "scientific" studies). Some bristled at its radical views of both sex and society. But many women found that what Hite was saying rang true to their own experience. The sexual culture was not ready to hear that sex (essentially, intercourse) was not as satisfying for women as it was for men.

Out of the grass-roots women's health movement came a new view of women's bodies. Organized through community clinics and epitomized by books such as The Boston Women's Health Book Collective's *Our Bodies, Ourselves,* first published in 1969, this movement encouraged women to take charge of their own health, including their sexual health, and to resist the alienating messages of the media and the medical establishment that treated women as either objects *for* or imperfect versions *of* men. By advocating that each woman learn to examine her own cervix and breasts and to take responsibility for her own sexual pleasure, the movement helped women to gain a greater measure of control over their bodies and lives.

The rethinking of female sexual well-being continues with books such as *A New View of a Woman's Body,* by a collective known as the Federation of Feminist Women's Health Centers, which replaces the male model of sex with one based on women's own experiences, observations, and self-examinations.

Lesbians and bisexual women are among the feminists who have challenged many facets of women's role in the sexual culture. With their critique of what Adrienne Rich called compulsory heterosexuality, activists in the lesbian, gay, bisexual, and transgender movement have helped imagine a new sexual culture for both themselves and others. Their work has made it easier for young women to avoid settling into sexual roles and ways of having sex that do not have women's best interest in mind. In their assertion that "we are here," lesbians, bisexual women and men, gay men, and transgendered people have forced the whole society to question traditional assumptions about sex and sexual categories. Bisexual visibility has put flesh on sex researcher Alfred Kinsey's view of sexual orientation as a continuum by suggesting that sexuality is more fluid and open than the categories of "heterosexual" or "homosexual" allow. Mainstream popular culture now acclaims gender-bending performers, such as the androgynous k.d. lang and flamboyant drag queen Ru Paul, who undermine the sexual culture's insistence that "femininity" and "masculinity" are inherent to people who have the genitals of women and men respectively. Books such as Martine Rothblatt's *The Apartheid of Sex,* Leslie Feinberg's *Transgender Warriors,* appearances by transsexuals on

TV talk shows, and public writings by feminist scientists such as biologist Anne Fausto-Sterling (who asserts that there are five sexes at least) have created greater awareness that neither the genitals nor gender come in two neatly separated types.

The impact of these challenges on the sexual culture has been heightened by the AIDS epidemic. The need for a conscious and radical change in the way people engage in sex has rarely been more urgent than it is today when the questions are no longer simply whether to say yes or no. The questions people now face confront the very purpose and definition of sex. What is sex? Why have sex? Who is sex for? These questions force everyone to scrutinize and rethink the most taken-for-granted and fundamental aspects of sex. They unsettle sexual complacency and prepare the ground for reinventing sex for women's pleasure.

A clear alternative framework for sex has yet to be established, but it is in the process of emerging. Women are at the vanguard of this change, one that will transform not only how people have sex, but how the genitals themselves are envisioned.

It's the Clitoris, Stupid

Reinventing sex for women and men starts with outing the clitoris. The clitoris is absent from most talk about sex, especially compared to its high-profile acquaintance and alleged counterpart, the penis. References to the penis so often go without mention of its orgasm-producing counterpart in women that it sometimes seems as if the sexual culture had undergone a clitoridectomy. The vagina gets far more attention than the clitoris, and not just because it is the pathway to the uterus and conception. The vagina matters because it provides pleasure to the penis. The clitoris sometimes receives perfunctory attention as a prelude to intercourse, but that stimulation is usually neither sufficient nor appropriate for setting off a woman's orgasm.

Given its low profile, it is not surprising that the location, size, and behavior of the clitoris is a mystery for some men. One woman told us that she has considered pinning up a picture over her bed with a diagram of her genitals with arrows pointing to her clitoris and a label "Touch here."

Even men who earnestly search out the clitoris in order to pleasure their partner often have trouble finding or keeping track of it. Others have difficulty staying with it long enough to allow the woman to come, or they are not sure how to stimulate it to their partner's satisfaction. When men realize that they have a clitoris too (which, as we will show, is inside their penis), they may be better able to appreciate why it is worth finding on a woman.

Women themselves may often be unable to instruct their partner because their own familiarity with female anatomy is limited. Many women avoid touching their genitals, and few are on the same first-name basis with their own clitoris that they are with their partner's penis. Boys grow up hearing jokes and stories about the exploits of the penis, but girls hear the word clitoris so infrequently that many are not even sure where the accent falls (clí-to-ris and cli-tor'-is are both acceptable). A boy often learns from other boys what his penis can do, but a girl rarely talks about her clitoris with other girls and few get acquainted with it on their own. Indeed a woman can reach adulthood without even being aware that she has a clitoris. If a girl discovers clitoral pleasure, she often does so only by accident. The exact location of the good feeling between her legs remains a mystery to her.

Contributing to the clitoris's anonymity are sex education texts that portray it as a tiny organ that "hides" beneath its hood when erect, invoking the stereotype that women are sexually shy. Even when the sexual culture does acknowledge the clitoris, it cuts the organ down to a smaller size. Few women or men are aware that the clitoris is not a pea-sized penis, but is more than four inches long and extends inside the body.

It was decades ago that laboratory studies confirmed millions of women's own experience that the clitoris was the trigger for orgasm. Every sexologist from Hite to Masters and Johnson to Dr. Ruth has made it clear that the clitoris is the place to stimulate a woman to orgasm. Yet the sexual culture's focus on intercourse continues undeterred. Freud's contention that women who came only via clitoral stimulation suffered from a "sexual dysfunction" still infects how people talk about sex, and there is a lingering sentiment that the "vaginal orgasm" should be a mature woman's goal.

Other misconceptions haunt the clitoris as well. Updated sex manuals such as *Sex: A Man's Guide* by Stefan Bechtel, Laurence Roy Stains, and the editors of Men's Health Books and *Mind-blowing Sex in the Real World: Hot Tips for Doing It in the Age of Anxiety* by Sari Locker describe the woman's clitoris as "the only organ designed solely for pleasure." But even their inaccurate hyperbole (since men have this sensitive organ, too) does not raise the clitoris to the stature of the penis. Sex remains focused on penis-in-vagina intercourse, often to the exclusion of the kinds of sexual activity that directly stimulate the clitoris. In women's magazines, for example, articles on sex dutifully mention the importance of clitoral stimulation for women's orgasm, but rather than encouraging women to stimulate the clitoris directly, they frequently end up advising women to get on top in intercourse and hope for the best.

There are signs that the clitoris is beginning to get noticed. Many sex educators, activists, and researchers are trying to bring the clitoris out into public discussion. Humor books such as Holly Hughes's *Clit Notes* put the word on the front table of some bookstores and woman-friendly sex outlets such as Good Vibrations and Eve's Garden advertise vibrators and other sex toys in mainstream magazines. But in a sexual culture either afraid or disinclined to examine women's genitals too closely, there are still millions of women and men who remain unaware of the clitoris's orgasmic power.

It's the G Spot, Too

In 1982, a book called *The G Spot* by Alice Kahn Ladas, Beverly Whipple, and John D. Perry brought attention to another source of female sexual pleasure at a spot that can be reached through the vagina a few inches inside on the front wall. With the book, women familiar with pleasurable sensations from that area finally had their experience validated. But some feminists believed that the G spot was just a craze or a fad. Worst of all, it seemed to revive Freud's notion of the vaginal orgasm. Many women never even bothered to look for the G spot because they considered it a hoax, while others saw it as just one more sexual goal women were expected to achieve. Despite the controversy, the book helped women who were willing to explore to find their G spot. (Using the fingers works better than searching with their partner's penis.) A woman we know in her forties who never read the earlier book only found her G spot recently after reading Chapter 6 of this book. "I can't believe I've been having sex all these years and didn't know about this!" she told us.

Some researchers hypothesize that the G spot is the female prostate gland, similar to the male prostate gland. Men's prostate gland is also sexually sensitive and can be stimulated along the front anal wall, while the woman's G spot can be stimulated along the front vaginal wall. (Women can get "prostate" cancer, too, although it is less common and usually not life-threatening.) Although it is stimulated through the vagina, the G spot surrounds the urethra. Stimulating the G spot with the fingers, what we call G spotting, creates pleasurable feelings and can lead to orgasm.

G spotting also makes some women ejaculate. Like male ejaculation, female ejaculation is a pleasurable sexual experience in which fluid spurts out of the urethra. Yet women who ejaculate are often told they are "urinating." If they look female ejaculation up in books, they will find either no reference to it at all or contradictory opinions about what it is and doubts about whether it occurs. Those who have experienced or observed female ejaculation know that it occurs, and that ejaculate does not smell or look like urine. It is thought to be prostatic fluid similar to male ejaculate without the sperm. But debate persists among researchers about where it comes from and why only some women ejaculate.

The current sexual culture takes little account of either female ejaculation or the G spot because they do not fit into the existing framework for female sexuality. The current model of sex also keeps the clitoris a secret, depriving women of the information they need to enjoy orgasm. All of these secrets and misconceptions can be cleared away by reinventing sex from the inside of women's own experiences of pleasure.

Sex Transformed

Reinventing sex requires a new framework for understanding the body and sexual activity. Because the sexual culture has focused on men, and even sees women's bodies in terms of male (and, only secondarily, female) pleasure, women currently lack the concepts and words with which to talk about their sexuality. Women have neither names for genital parts nor words to describe the sexual techniques that make sex orgasmic. New words and a new language for sex will allow women to talk with and learn from one another. A new vocabulary will help women to communicate with a partner and will fundamentally change how women and men have sex.

Some new terms for *women's genitals* we develop in this book include:

- Orgasmic Crescent—This is our term for the crescent-shaped area that is women's pleasure center. The orgasmic crescent begins at the clitoris and extends back across the opening of the urethra (another sexual area) and up inside the vagina behind the pubic bone to the G spot. The labia swell when a woman is erect. Stimulating all the areas along the orgasmic crescent at the same time can give a woman a powerful orgasm. Some women also ejaculate.
- Cligeva (cli-GEE-va)—This is our name for women's genitals as a whole. No word now exists that includes all of women's sexual parts. The word combines the most important sexual parts for women's pleasure. The word combines the first syllable of each sexual part—the clitoris, the G spot, and the vagina. The final "a" also refers to the anus, an often overlooked site of pleasure. The word also has the advantage of listing the parts in the order in which many women like to be genitally stimulated.

We also use new words for *sexual techniques* that focus on women's pleasure including:

- Manual Sex—Many people use their hands in partner sex to great effect, yet they rarely use the name for it, manual sex. Manual sex is a widely practiced and highly pleasurable sexual art that has been trivialized as "foreplay" or "petting." As one of the most direct routes to orgasm for women, it deserves being promoted to a category of sex on a par with intercourse and oral sex.
- Clittage (cli-TAZH)—This is our word for the most basic kind of manual sex—manual stimulation of the clitoris. It combines clitoris and massage. Clittage or clitoral massage is the most common way women reach orgasm, yet this sexual act has no name. Fingers—one's own or a partner's—can provide orgasmic pleasure at any time, including during intercourse or in a mutually orgasmic quickie. Clittage can also be effectively performed with a vibrator.
- G spotting—Another kind of manual sex involves stroking the G spot with the fingers. G spotting can also be done with a dildo or performed by a man with his erect penis.
- Forget Foreplay—In a sexual culture that includes women's pleasure, "foreplay" will disappear. Instead of being treated as a prelude to sex, the manual and oral sex that now make up foreplay would become the central features of sex.
- Ladies First—This rule of orgasmic etiquette appears in many sex manuals but is frequently ignored in practice. Ladies first reminds a man that woman's orgasm (at least her first one) ideally comes before intercourse and always before the man ejaculates. This ensures a woman of orgasm every time she has sex with a man.
- Mutual Erection—The genitals of both women and men become erect when sexually aroused. Even though women's genitals become engorged (and therefore erect), women's erections have been ignored. Erection is as conducive to a woman's orgasm as it is to a man's. Similarly, a woman's erection is as essential for intercourse as a man's penis. Vaginal penetration is far more pleasurable for a woman when she is erect. Mutual erection makes intercourse an orgasmic experience for *both* partners.

New words and concepts for sex will enable women to bridge the orgasm gap. Sex will not longer take place solely on men's terms. Instead, it will unfold according to a new sexuality that is equally oriented toward women's pleasure.

Your (Society's) Sexual IQ Test Answers

1. b

Most women reach orgasm from direct clitoral stimulation, not from vaginal intercourse. Women who have orgasms during intercourse are probably doing so primarily because of clitoral stimulation, either from indirect pressure or from direct manual stimulation. While feelings of love certainly can enhance sexual pleasure, love does not provide the genital stimulation needed for orgasm.

2. a

The shape of the entire clitoris resembles a four-inch wishbone. It extends from the external and visible pea-sized tip, up the shaft and into the body. The legs of the clitoris inside the body split off like those of a wishbone onto either side of the vaginal walls. Men also have a clitoris inside the penis that is the same size as women's (relative to body size), but its legs are shorter. The tip of the man's clitoris cannot be touched directly because it lies underneath the head of the penis. The tip of the woman's clitoris is usually compared to the whole penis, but this is like comparing a part to a whole. The more accurate comparison is between the entire female and the entire male clitoris, from tip to legs.

3. c

Sex between a woman and a man is usually considered over when the man ejaculates (it is assumed he has had an orgasm, too). The woman's orgasm (and certainly not her ejaculation) is not a required part of sex as currently defined.

4. a

The pelvic muscle (specifically the PC or pubococcygeus muscle) usually contracts during orgasm in both women and men. Masters and Johnson observed a red flush on some women's chests during orgasm, but most women do not experience or observe this. A woman and a man can tell when a woman is having an orgasm by the buildup of her erection, her PC muscle contractions, and the subsequent release of muscle tension and blood in her genitals.

Many men expect women to make the same synthesized moans during orgasm that women perform in pornographic movies and on records. Instead, when her attention is truly riveted on the pleasure in her body, a woman may let out a scream or make no sound at all. There is no standard performance for orgasm.

5. c

It is not known what percentage of women ejaculate. It is possible that all women ejaculate but the amount of fluid is very small, so they are not aware of it. All women have a prostate gland or G spot and a urethra and therefore all are potentially capable of ejaculating. Yet because the sexual culture rarely acknowledges female ejaculation, most neither find their G spot nor learn how to ejaculate. Women who do ejaculate are sometimes told they are urinating and some women stifle their ejaculations. Others mistake the fluid as an abundance of vaginal juices. But female ejaculate comes out of the urethra, just as it does in men, and is a watery fluid chemically similar to prostatic fluid in men.

6. b

Vaginal intercourse lasts an average of two to three minutes. The average length of the whole sexual encounter is typically just fifteen minutes. Sex that begins with the man's erection and ends when he comes rarely lasts more than an hour.

7. c

It takes women and men about the same amount of time—about four to five minutes, on average—to reach orgasm. When women take longer to come than men or do not come at all, it is usually because they are not getting adequate clitoral stimulation.

8. F

Most body parts are not optional. If some women have a G spot, it is likely that all women do. Many women have never looked for their G spot because they are either unaware of it or doubt it exists. Rather than asking whether or not all women have a G spot, women should be asking why it remains a mystery instead of being treated as a pleasurable fact of a woman's sexual experience.

9. F

Some women get wet when they are sexually excited, yet all women are made to feel that vaginal lubrication is a measure of their sexual "responsiveness." Vaginal wetness is not always an accurate way to evaluate a woman's state of arousal. The more useful indicator in both women and men is the genital engorgement and muscle tension that occurs with erection.

10. T

When a woman is aroused, her genitals, including the clitoris and G spot, engorge with blood and the PC muscle becomes taut. This same process is called an *erection* in men. Women's genital erections have so far gone ignored and unnamed.

Women's Liberation Is Coming

by Jennifer O'Connor

Imagine a Tupperware party . . . or a quilting bee. Now add a harness and numerous other sex gadgets. Seven women, varying in age, size and body piercings, sit in a living room, surrounded by sex paraphernalia, safety gear and the famous 'vulva puppet'—an anatomically-correct teaching tool scaled large enough to impress any size queen. They talk about female ejaculate, why silicone lubes should not be used with silicone toys and discuss the merits of plug-in vibrators versus portable.

These women are discussing the joys of sex in the film *Please Don't Stop: Lesbian Tips for Givin' & Gettin' It,* a Sex Positive production that is the first film of its kind to be made by a cast and crew of lesbians of colour. But such adventures aren't just happening on videotape. In books, e-zines (on-line publications), performance, and activism, women are claiming their sexuality.

For Shelley Taylor, third-wave sexuality is characterized by "a much more assertive belief that we own our bodies and we can do whatever we want with them." The owner of the Halifax and Ottawa-based Venus Envy stores describes the attitude as, "Nobody can tell us what we can and cannot do with our bodies. Don't tell us who we should be partnered with or how many people we should be partnered with or even that we need a partner." The result, Taylor explains, is that it's becoming more and more acceptable and sexy to be knowledgeable and forward and assertive about sex. And if it means bending their boyfriend over, these gals know how to do it safely.

Not that it's as simple as grabbing some lube and latex. Young feminists in particular, writes Merri Lisa Johnson in *Jane Sexes It Up: True Confessions of Feminist Desire,* "feel the edges of feminist history grind against the conservative cultural contexts in which our lives unfold." They live inside the contradiction of a political movement that affirms and encourages expressions of sexuality, and the "real world of workplaces, families and communities that continue to judge women harshly for speaking of sex, much less expressing one's 'deviant' acts and complex erotic imagination."

Examples of this deviance are everywhere. Shar Rednour and Jackie Strano's S.I.R. Video Productions make films such as *Hard Love & How to Fuck in High Heels* (lesbian porn) and *Bend Over Boyfriend* (a straight couple's guide to male anal pleasure). *Bust* magazine provides readers with sex-positivity in sections such as The Sex Files, Susie Q's (an advice column By Susie Bright) and an erotica section aptly called "One-Handed Read." And women are signing up for workshops on female ejaculation and introduction to BDSM (bondage and discipline, sado-masochism) at women-focused stores, such as Good For Her in Toronto, where I've worked for the past year.

But you don't have to venture that far to find sexy-girl media. Mainstream magazines such as *Chatelaine* have a sex advice columnist and television programs such as the W Network's (formerly WTN) *Sunday Night Sex Show* are as close as your cable provider.

Of course, women didn't invent sexuality sometime around 1991. No, the stops on this tawdry tour include early feminists at the turn of the century advocating for birth control, articles about the legalization of abortion that appeared in *Chatelaine* under the editorship of Doris Anderson and, more recently, Little Sisters' battles with Canada Customs over gay porn.

However, as Lee Damsky writes in *Sex and Single Girls,* most of us don't live in this blithe bubble. As she explains, "We grew up with a mix of social-sexual contradictions: the conservative backlash and the AIDS epidemic, the queer movement and gender-fuck. We got divorced parents and 'family value,' homophobia and lesbian chic, 'Just Say No' and 'Ten Ways to Drive Him Wild.'" In short, "[W]e simply grew up surrounded by sex, where the old rules were not so much overthrown as internalized, displayed, contradicted." For all the accomplishments of feminism, women still can't be sure they'll be able to get an abortion if they choose to have one. We still see women's sexuality used to sell everything from shampoo to surfboards. And we don't talk about sensuality nearly enough, if at all.

"It is obvious that the suppression of sexual agency and exploration, from within or from without, is often used as a method of social control and domination," according to Rebecca Walker. In her essay, "Lusting for Freedom," in *Listen Up: Voices From the Next Feminist Generation,* she beckons women to reclaim their sexual power. "Witness widespread genital mutilation and the homophobia that dictatorially mandates heterosexuality; imagine the stolen power of the millions affected by just these two global murderers of self-authorization and determination."

The lesson is that the personal is still political. Continues Walker, "Without being able to respond to and honour the desires of our bodies and ourselves, we become cut off from our instincts for pleasure, dissatisfied living under rules and thoughts that are not our own. When we deny ourselves safe and shameless exploration and access to reliable information, we damage our ability to even know what sexual pleasure feels or looks like."

And there is no one description of what pleasure feels or looks like. Says Linda Capperauld, executive director of Planned Parenthood, "Heterosexual, bisexual, lesbian, two-spirited and transgendered women will define their sexuality in different ways and each individual's definition will be affected by many determinants of health."

And while there is still much work to do to promote healthy sexuality in all its forms, along with safer sex practices and reproductive choice, Capperauld says that many women are increasingly taking advantage of birth control methods. "Since women are making choices about sexually transmitted infection prevention and the postponement of pregnancy, taking charge of one's sexuality has become an integral part of many women's lives," she says.

Predictably, to provide a counterpoint to all this pro-sex revelling, we have books such as Wendy Shalit's *A Return to Modesty,* full of guard-your-hymen wisdom. "Indeed, the primary and most direct consequence of a recovery of modesty's meaning would be an end to a culture that objectifies women and inadvertently encourages the violent acting-out of any deep misogynous impulses. Yet, just as it would save many women from harm, so, too, it would confer on women a new version of an old obligation—the obligation to serve as the civilizing force in a culture that seems increasingly uncivilized."

Not everyone agrees that women should rely on Miss Modesty to protect them. No, sisters are doing it for themselves. Says Krista Jacob, editor in chief of the online journal *Sexing the Political: A Journal of Third Wave Feminists on Sexuality,* "My generation is challenging many forces that suppress our sexuality—from our puritanical culture that shames women for their sexuality, to the sexual violence of our culture that wounds our sexuality and takes our power away, to the lack of empowering sexual images within our own movement."

Sexuality is, therefore, an integral part of third-wave feminism. Jacob explains that, "Sexuality and feminism are as inextricably linked as sexuality and human nature. It's difficult to think of them as being separate in any way."

Kind of like the silver-sparkly dildo and coordinating pink vinyl harness I sold to a guy and a grrrl.

A New Politics of Sexuality

by June Jordan

As a young worried mother, I remember turning to Dr. Benjamin Spock's *Common Sense Book of Baby and Child Care* just about as often as I'd pick up the telephone. He was God. I was ignorant but striving to be good: a good Mother. And so it was there, in that bestseller pocketbook of do's and don't's, that I came upon this doozie of a guideline: Do not wear miniskirts or other provocative clothing because that will upset your child, especially if your child happens to be a boy. If you give your offspring "cause" to think of you as a sexual being, he will, at the least, become disturbed; you will derail the equilibrium of his notions about your possible identity and meaning in the world.

It had never occurred to me that anyone, especially my son, might look upon me as an asexual being. I had never supposed that "asexual" was some kind of positive designation I should, so to speak, lust after. I was pretty surprised by Dr. Spock. However, I was also, by habit, a creature of obedience. For a couple of weeks I actually experimented with lusterless colors and dowdy tops and bottoms, self-consciously hoping thereby to prove myself as a lusterless and dowdy and, therefore, excellent female parent.

Years would have to pass before I could recognize the familiar, by then, absurdity of a man setting himself up as the expert on a subject that presupposed women as the primary objects for his patriarchal discourse—on motherhood, no less! Years passed before I came to perceive the perversity of dominant power assumed by men, and the perversity of self-determining power ceded to men by women.

A lot of years went by before I understood the dynamics of what anyone could summarize as the Politics of Sexuality.

I believe the Politics of Sexuality is the most ancient and probably the most profound arena for human conflict. Increasingly, it seems clear to me that deeper and more pervasive than any other oppression, than any other bitterly contested human domain, is the oppression of sexuality, the exploitation of the human domain of sexuality for power.

When I say sexuality, I mean gender: I mean male subjugation of human beings because they are female. When I say sexuality, I mean heterosexual institutionalization of rights and privileges denied to homosexual men and women. When I say sexuality I mean gay or lesbian contempt for bisexual modes of human relationship.

The Politics of Sexuality therefore subsumes all of the different ways in which some of us seek to dictate to others of us what we should do, what we should desire, what we should dream about, and how we should behave ourselves, generally, on the planet. From China to Iran, from Nigeria to Czechoslovakia, from Chile to California, the politics of sexuality—enforced by traditions of state-sanctioned violence plus religion and the law—reduces to male domination of women, heterosexist tyranny, and, among those of us who are in any case deemed despicable or deviant by the powerful, we find intolerance for those who choose a different, a more complicated—for example, an interracial or bisexual—mode of rebellion and freedom.

We must move out from the shadows of our collective subjugation—as people of color/as women/as gay/as lesbian/as bisexual human beings.

. . .

I can voice my ideas without hesitation or fear because I am speaking, finally, about myself. I am black and I am female and I am a mother and I am bisexual and I am a nationalist and I am an anti-nationalist. And I mean to be fully and freely all that I am!

Conversely, I do not accept that any white or black or Chinese man—I do not accept that, for instance, Dr. Spock—should presume to tell me, or any other woman, how to mother a child. He has no right. He is not a mother. My child is not his child. And, likewise, I do not accept that anyone—any woman or any man who is not inextricably part of the subject he or she dares to address—should attempt to tell any of us, the objects of

This column was adapted from her keynote address to the Bisexual, Gay, and Lesbian Student Association at Stanford University on April 29, 1991.

her or his presumptuous discourse, what we should do or what we should not do.

Recently, I have come upon gratuitous and appalling pseudoliberal pronouncements on sexuality. Too often, these utterances fall out of the mouths of men and women who first disclaim any sentiment remotely related to homophobia, but who then proceed to issue outrageous opinions like the following.

That it is blasphemous to compare the oppression of gay, lesbian, or bisexual people to the oppression, say, of black people, or of the Palestinians.

That the bottom line about gay or lesbian or bisexual identity is that you can conceal it whenever necessary and, so, therefore, why don't you do just that? Why don't you keep your deviant sexuality in the closet and let the rest of us—we who suffer oppression for reasons of our ineradicable and always visible components of our personhood such as race or gender—get on with our more necessary, our more beleaguered struggle to survive?

Well, number one: I believe I have worked as hard as I could, and then harder than that, on behalf of equality and justice for African-Americans, for the Palestinian people, and for people of color everywhere.

And no, I do not believe it is blasphemous to compare oppressions of sexuality to oppressions of race and ethnicity: Freedom is indivisible or it is nothing at all besides sloganeering and temporary, short-sighted, and short-lived advancement for a few. Freedom is indivisible, and either we are working for freedom or you are working for the sake of your self-interests and I am working for mine.

If you can finally go to the bathroom, wherever you find one, if you can finally order a cup of coffee and drink it wherever coffee is available, but you cannot follow your heart—you cannot respect the response of your own honest body in the world—then how much of what kind of freedom does any one of us possess?

Or, conversely, if your heart and your honest body can be controlled by the state, or controlled by community taboo, are you not then, and in that case, no more than a slave ruled by outside force?

What tyranny could exceed a tyranny that dictates to the human heart, and that attempts to dictate the public career of an honest human body?

Freedom is indivisible; the Politics of Sexuality is not some optional "special-interest" concern for serious, progressive folk.

And, on another level, let me assure you: If every single gay or lesbian or bisexual man or woman active on the Left of American politics decided to stay home, there would be *no* Left left.

· · ·

One of the things I want to propose is that we act on that reality: that we insistently demand reciprocal respect and concern from those who cheerfully depend upon our brains and our energies for their, and our, effective impact on the political landscape.

Last spring, at Berkeley, some students asked me to speak at a rally against racism. And I did. There were 400 or 500 people massed on Sproul Plaza, standing together against that evil. And, on the next day, on that same Plaza, there was a rally for bisexual and gay and lesbian rights, and students asked me to speak at that rally. And I did. There were fewer than seventy-five people stranded, pitiful, on that public space. And I said then what I say today: That was disgraceful! There should have been just one rally. One rally: Freedom is indivisible.

As for the second, nefarious pronouncement on sexuality that now enjoys mass-media currency: the idiot notion of keeping yourself in the closet—that is very much the same thing as the suggestion that black folks and Asian-Americans and Mexican-Americans should assimilate and become as "white" as possible—in our walk/talk/music/food/values—or else. Or else? Or else we should, deservedly, perish.

Sure enough, we have plenty of exposure to white everything so why would we opt to remain our African/Asian/Mexican selves? The answer is that suicide is absolute, and if you think you will survive by hiding who you really are, you are sadly misled: There is no such thing as partial or intermittent suicide. You can only survive if you—who you really are—do survive.

Likewise, we who are not men and we who are not heterosexual—we, sure enough, have plenty of exposure to male-dominated/heterosexist this and that.

But a struggle to survive cannot lead to suicide: Suicide is the opposite of survival. And so we must not conceal/assimilate/ integrate into the would-be dominant culture and political system that despises us. Our survival requires that we alter our environment so that we can live and so that we can hold each other's hands and so that we can kiss each other on the streets, and in the daylight of our existence, without terror and without violent and sometimes fatal reactions from the busybodies of America.

Finally, I need to speak on bisexuality. I do believe that the analogy is interracial or multiracial identity. I do believe that the analogy for bisexuality is a multicultural, multi-ethnic, multiracial world view. Bisexuality follows from such a perspective and leads to it, as well.

Just as there are many men and women in the United States whose parents have given them more than one racial, more than one ethnic identity and cultural heritage to honor; and just as these men and women must deny no given part of themselves except at the risk of self-deception and the insanities that must issue from that; and just as these men and women embody the principle of equality among races and ethnic communities; and just as these men and women falter and anguish and choose and then falter again and then anguish and then choose yet again how they will honor the irreducible complexity of their God-given human being—even so, there are many men and women, especially young men and women, who seek to embrace the complexity of their total, always-changing social and political circumstance.

They seek to embrace our increasing global complexity on the basis of the heart and on the basis of an honest human body. Not according to ideology. Not according to group pressure. Not according to anybody's concept of "correct."

This is a New Politics of Sexuality. And even as I despair of identity politics—because identity is given and principles of justice/equality/freedom cut across given gender and given racial definitions of being, and because I will call you my brother, I will call you my sister, on the basis of what you *do* for justice, what you *do* for equality, what you *do* for freedom and *not* on the basis of who you are, even so I look with admiration and respect upon the new, bisexual politics of sexuality.

This emerging movement politicizes the so-called middle ground: Bisexuality invalidates either/or formulation, either/or analysis. Bisexuality means I am free and I am as likely to want and to love a woman as I am likely to want and to love a man, and what about that? Isn't that what freedom implies?

If you are free you are not predictable and you are not controllable. To my mind, that is the keenly positive, politicizing significance of bisexual affirmation:

To insist upon complexity, to insist upon the validity of all of the components of social/sexual complexity, to insist upon the equal validity of all of the components of social/sexual complexity.

This seems to me a unifying, 1990s mandate for revolutionary Americans planning to make it into the Twenty-first Century on the basis of the heart, on the basis of an honest human body, consecrated to every struggle for justice, every struggle for equality, every struggle for freedom.

Do Ask, Do Tell

by Jennifer E. Potter, MD

As a consequence of bias and ignorance within the medical profession, lesbians and gay men frequently receive suboptimal health care. Knowledge of each patient's sexual orientation and behaviors is critical for the development of a productive therapeutic relationship, accurate risk assessment, and the provision of pertinent preventive counseling. However, clinicians often forget to ask about this information, and many lesbians and gay men are reticent to reveal the truth. I present vignettes from my personal experiences as a lesbian patient and doctor to illustrate the importance of creating an environment in which such disclosure can occur and to portray the challenges and rewards of coming out as a gay physician.

I juggle many hats in my life: mother, partner, doctor, and educator. Like all my female colleagues, my experiences as a daughter, sister, patient, and student have influenced my approach to each of these roles. But I am also lesbian, and this fact has shaped my life profoundly. It underlies my decision to become a primary care doctor; select women's health as an area of clinical expertise; and commit myself especially to improving the lives of lesbians, gay men, and people from other minority groups.

It is a challenge to be lesbian in our society. People assume that a young woman is straight, will marry, can get pregnant if she is sexually active, and will have children. This progression is "normal." Anything else is different and may be perceived as abnormal, wrong, or bad. Historical and continuing records of harassment, assaults, and homicides against lesbians and gay men abound. The medical profession itself has viewed homosexuality as a disorder; aversion techniques, hormone administration, shock treatment, castration, and even lobotomy have been used as purported "treatments" (1). I feel fortunate that I have never been the target of clearly overt actions because of my sexual orientation.

Insidious effects of prejudice affect my life deeply, however. Imagine how it feels to hear yet another gay joke or to open the paper to confront yet another antigay news story. Examples include the U.S. military's "don't ask, don't tell" policy, repeated referenda that limit the civil rights of lesbians and gay men (even compared with other minority groups), and the opposition of many religious organizations. Many lesbians and gay men find it difficult to avoid internalizing some of these homophobic attitudes. As a consequence, shame and fear are common emotions, and we are more likely to be isolated; engage in risky behaviors; suffer from stress-related health conditions, substance abuse, or depression; and attempt suicide (2).

Finding help is not easy. It is hard to trust other people, even health professionals, when one anticipates disapproval. Doctors share the same biases as the rest of society and are frequently ignorant about lesbian and gay health issues. I have often been disappointed with the medical care I have received; several examples from my experience as a lesbian patient are illustrative.

As a teenager, I reacted to the emergence of attraction to other girls with a jumble of conflicting feelings: excitement, fear, fascination, and horror. When I tried to broach the topic cautiously with my family doctor, he laughed and said, "Don't worry about that; it's just a phase a lot of girls go through." He meant to reassure me, but his comment trivialized and dismissed me instead. An important opportunity was missed to explore and validate my feelings.

By age 15, I was overwhelmed and isolated and made a suicidal gesture that might have had grave consequences. The psychiatrist to whom I was referred believed that same-sex attraction was a sign of stunted psychological development. His attitude perpetuated my notion that something was wrong with me; I stifled exploration of my identity during 2 ensuing years of therapy. I eventually found the support I needed when I met a lesbian couple who listened to me, encouraged me to be myself, and demonstrated that it was possible both to be lesbian and to pursue the goals I wanted in life—a committed relationship, a family, diverse friends, and a deeply challenging and rewarding career.

In college, I consulted a physician for evaluation of vaginal symptoms. She asked if I was sexually active (yes), whether I was using contraception (no), and whether I was trying to conceive (no). Before I had a chance to explain, she began to talk about birth control options and the importance of using condoms to prevent sexually transmitted diseases. At that point, I was too embarrassed to reveal my lesbianism. I never did ask the question that was on my mind ("Could I infect my lover?") and left, uncomfortable, with an absurd prescription for the pill. Her immediate assumption that I was straight and my reticence to reveal the truth prevented the development of a productive doctor–patient relationship and resulted in inappropriate care.

Later in life, when I disclosed my lesbianism to a new internist, she told me that my risk for cervical cancer was so low that I did not need to have regular Papanicolaou smears. This advice was incorrect. She assumed that my sexual relationships were exclusively lesbian and that the chief cause of cervical cancer, human papillomavirus, cannot be transmitted by woman-to-woman sexual contact. However, sexual identity cannot be equated with sexual behavior. Some lesbians are celibate, many have male partners, and some have partners of both sexes. Moreover, emerging evidence suggests that several genital infections can be acquired during lesbian sexual activity (3). A detailed sexual history is necessary to understand the situation of each patient, ascertain risks for sexually transmitted diseases, and provide pertinent medical counseling.

As a result of my experiences with doctors who did not know how to communicate effectively, I became interested in ways to break down barriers that prevent gay and other minority patients from obtaining good care. I joined a lesbian and gay speaker's bureau and told my story to students at local high schools, colleges, and medical schools. I believe I helped to enlighten others and demolish some stereotypes. Then, after considering teaching, nursing, psychology, and medicine, I decided that my best course of action was to become a physician.

The medical establishment was an inhospitable place for gay trainees in the 1980s. As recommended by my premedical advisor, I concealed my lesbianism during the medical school application process; I question whether I would have received my "Welcome to the Harvard family" letter if I had been more forthright. Once a trainee, I faced all the challenges that every medical student and resident encounters: trying to master a huge body of knowledge, accepting the enormous responsibility of caring for people, learning to function with aplomb in emergency situations, and competing with others for advancement. In addition, I had to cope with tacit and overt advice that my lesbianism would be tolerated only as long as I kept quiet about it.

Ambivalence about being open is a problem that heterosexual persons can barely comprehend. It arises because of a continuing lack of acceptance of gays by most of the population and the fact that homosexuality is invisible, unlike the minority status of people with different skin color or language. As a consequence, disclosure is a choice left to each gay person.

On the face of it, maintaining silence makes almost everyone happy. I can interact with others without fear of prejudice, and people are spared the discomfort of responding to a sensitive proclamation. But invisibility has many downsides. Self-respect is difficult to preserve when one lies by omission. Silence implies acceptance that, as a member of a minority group, I have nothing valuable to contribute—that I am a "minus." If I selectively omit mention of involvement in activities that could identify me as gay, I cannot highlight all of my accomplishments. If I attend professional social gatherings alone, I miss the opportunity to introduce my partner of 23 years, show our example of a long-term relationship, and provide everyone with a chance to build acceptance.

Secrecy leads to isolation. Whenever I encounter new and unfamiliar situations, I am tempted to watch, wait, and figure out the lay of the land before revealing my lesbianism. Although this strategy feels safe, it produces loneliness. A subculture of lesbians and gay men exists through which clandestine identification takes place. But when secrecy is the paramount mode of operation, people are reluctant to gather together because of guilt by association. Silence limits opportunities for friendship, support, and professional collaboration not only with other lesbians and gay men but also with sympathetic people from the mainstream who share my values and goals.

Secrecy also requires an enormous expenditure of energy. Staying "in the closet" is not a passive process; constant vigilance is required to steer conversations away from personal issues. Of course, people sometimes ask directly whether I am in a relationship. If I deny that I am involved, I enter a vicious cycle of deception. If I admit to having a partner but try to conceal her sex, I have to take great care to avoid the pronouns "she" and "her" in subsequent discussion. Such behavior wastes a great deal of energy that could be channeled productively.

When I remain silent, people make assumptions about me that can be very awkward, especially if they later realize that their beliefs were wrong. When I started to practice medicine, many of my colleagues assumed that I was single because I did not talk about a boyfriend or husband or wear a wedding ring. Some concluded that I was an "old maid by choice"—a woman who had subjugated family to career. Others assumed that I was available, so I had to decline advances. When I became pregnant, nearly everyone assumed that I was married. In a particularly embarrassing moment, the chief of a major service told me in a public forum that he thought he knew my husband!

I have gradually learned that it is advantageous to be open about my sexual orientation. Disclosure is empowering: It allows me to be myself, integrate my public and private lives, voice my opinions, celebrate all of my achievements, and work passionately to increase tolerance and acceptance. I know that I deserve respect and recognize that I serve as an important role model.

Coming out is a process that never ends. Every time I meet someone new, I must decide if, how, and when I will reveal my sexual orientation. I find it simplest to be candid with colleagues from the start, but this approach can be awkward with patients, because it is considered inappropriate to mention intimate personal details in the context of a professional relationship. However, every doctor–patient interaction is built on trust, and I believe strongly that I have an obligation to be honest. Patients often ask me personal questions about my family and how I balance home life and career. Up-front disclosure of my sexual orientation avoids embarrassing people who might otherwise assume that I am straight and ask about my "marriage" or "husband" and allows patients who feel uncomfortable having a lesbian as their physician to choose a different doctor.

In general, I try to communicate who I am nonverbally, by displaying pictures of my family and having gay-friendly posters and health literature in my office. I developed and use an intake form that is inclusive of alternative lifestyles and avoids the designations "single," "married," "divorced," and "widowed." My name is listed in a lesbian and gay health guide, I give talks to lay audiences on lesbian and gay health issues, and I volunteer free health screening for lesbians and other minority groups in the community. I have also developed and teach a curriculum on lesbian and gay health to medical students and residents as well as to peers at continuing medical education conferences. When I am asked directly about my private life, I answer truthfully.

Reactions to my openness have been mixed, but my experiences coming out as a lesbian health professional have been rewarding overall. When I decided to coordinate a lesbian and gay student group in medical school, I had to identify myself to the administration in order to apply for funding and take the risk of being seen posting notices about group activities. Some flyers were defaced, presumably by other medical students, and I once saw one being removed by a dean. I tried to channel my anger into eloquence and gave a talk to my classmates. Although a few ignored me subsequently and one student began to pray for me every morning before class began, the posters were no longer disturbed and attendance at group-sponsored educational events increased.

Later, as a resident in the early AIDS era, I encountered numerous examples of homophobia in the hospital. There were many antigay jokes; some implied that gay men were getting what they deserved. Some of my peers refused to shake hands with gay patients or put on gowns and gloves before entering their rooms. My coming out stopped the jokes, at least in my presence, and seemed to result in more humane behavior toward people with AIDS-related illnesses.

Over the years, I have received a few lectures on the ills of homosexuality and even a letter stating that people like me should not be permitted to become doctors. However, several gay patients have told me that my visibility enabled them to find me and finally receive the understanding and support they craved. My openness has also allowed gay medical students and residents to identify me as a role model and mentor, and many of my straight colleagues and patients have thanked me for the opportunity to examine their assumptions and biases about gay people.

Somewhat to my surprise, my openness has not harmed my clinical practice. On the contrary, I have many referrals from medical colleagues and hospital administrators who want me to care for their wives and daughters, and I was recognized by *Boston Magazine* as a top internist for women in the February 2001 issue. Coming out has also afforded me some novel professional opportunities. I believe that my openness during an era of emphasis on cultural competence was a factor in my appointment to the Beth Israel Deaconess Hospital Board of Trustees. Likewise, my willingness to speak out has resulted in invitations to participate in a panel discussion on lesbian and gay health at the Massachusetts Department of Public Health and to serve on an advisory board to the American Cancer Society.

Despite these successes, much work still needs to be done. In recent years, Harvard Medical School has taken steps to diversify the racial and ethnic composition of its student body and to increase tolerance and acceptance of its gay community by sponsoring town meeting discussions. However, few minority faculty members have been promoted to leadership positions, and consequently, many of my values and those of minority colleagues remain poorly represented. I strive to promote further institutional change by being visible and voicing my questions and concerns.

A professor at my institution once warned that it is a mistake to "ghetto-ize" one's career in women's health. I take issue with this statement. I believe that my work is not only legitimate but of critical value. My talents include an instinctive ability to understand and empower patients from highly diverse backgrounds and a gift for changing the attitudes and behaviors of medical students and doctors. My work requires courage and resilience, and I believe that the outcomes are as important as the results of basic science research and clinical trials. Challenging clinicians' stereotypes and increasing the sensitivity with which they communicate with people from different cultures will benefit all of their present and future patients. I am proud to be a lesbian physician and educator.

Requests for Single Reprints   Jennifer E. Potter, MD, Beth Israel Deaconess Medical Center, Harvard Medical School, 330 Brookline Avenue, Boston, MA 02215; e-mail, jpotter@caregroup.harvard.edu.

References

1. Miller N. Out of the Past: Gay and Lesbian History from 1869 to the Present. New York: Vintage Books; 1995.
2. Dean L, Meyer IH, Robinson K, Sell RL, Sember R, Silenzio VMB, et al. Lesbian, gay, bisexual, and transgender health: findings and concerns. Journal of the Gay and Lesbian Medical Association. 2000;4:101–51.
3. Diamant AL, Lever J, Schuster M. Lesbians' sexual activities and efforts to reduce risks for sexually transmitted diseases. Journal of the Gay and Lesbian Medical Association. 2000;4:41–8.

Health Care without Shame

Some Background for the Practitioner

by Charles Moser, PhD, MD

(This chapter and the following chapter are adapted from two articles which first appeared in *San Francisco Medicine,* Nov./Dec. 1998, pp. 23–26.)

Physicians and other health care practitioners have just begun to address the special health and lifestyle issues of the gay, lesbian or bisexual patient. However, the medical concerns of other sexual minorities (including transgendered patients, patients with multiple sexual partners, sex workers, and patients involved in S/M and other "kinky" sexual behaviors) have received little to no attention. This chapter will, I hope, be a starting point for physicians and other health care professionals who wish to address the health concerns and needs of sexual minority patients.

The first question to answer for yourself is whether or not you really wish to treat such patients. Some physicians are unable to overcome their own issues about alternative sexual behaviors and should refer these patients. Even if you're a member of one sexual minority community, you may not be able to nonjudgmentally treat any or all sexual minority patients.

Just because you choose to refer these patients does not relieve you of the responsibility of learning at least the basics of how to care for them. I do not, and unfortunately never will, speak Japanese, so it is reasonable for me to refer new patients who only speak Japanese to a Japanese-speaking physician. Nevertheless, I have had to take care of such patients. I try to employ translators (both Japanese speakers who work in the hospital and family members). I have learned something of Japanese culture. The hospitals where I work have devised "Asian diets" (comfort food is important when you are sick) and have made other accommodations. Physicians confronted with sexual lifestyles with which they are not comfortable need to take similar actions: seek out experts and attempt to make accommodations for patient comfort.

If you decide that sexual minority patients will be a significant aspect of your practice, here are some recommendations on how to treat them effectively and respectfully.

Who They Are vs. What They Do   In treating such patients, you must distinguish between identity and behavior—a task which is not as simple as it seems. Individuals may choose to define their sexuality with a label, but their actual behavior may be very different. Medical risk is related to a patient's behavior, heredity or environment, not his or her identity. It does not matter medically whether a male patient identifies as gay, but it does matter if he has sex with men. Additionally, anal sex with a man opens him up to a different type of medical risk than anal sex with a dildo-wielding woman.

Nevertheless, identity is also an issue. A woman who self-defines as a lesbian is often subjected to a variety of stresses that a heterosexual-identified woman is not, without regard to her behavior. There are social stresses regarding partner choice ("Will my partner be allowed to visit into the MICU? What will happen when my co-workers meet my lover?"). There are also genuine physical dangers—rape, assault and even homicide—associated with being gay, lesbian, a sex worker, an S/M practitioner, or transgendered, as the crime sheet in any city can attest.

Sexual identity and behavior are both fluid. There are people who defined themselves first as gay, then straight, then bisexual. It can be hard to imagine, but there are people who are not quite sure which gender they are, people who are frustrated when no one will acknowledge their chosen gender, and people who find any gender at all intolerable. Is a woman who is happily married, but secretly desires sexual contact with other women, a lesbian or bisexual or even heterosexual? Does that orientation change if she begins an affair with another woman, if she leaves her husband, or even if she becomes celibate? There are no simple answers. Just remember that because someone identifies with one sexual orientation, it does not necessarily define their actual behavior. Acceptance of this fluidity is the first step in providing nonjudgmental health care and not alienating your patient.

Your sense of a patient's probable identity may not match up with the patient's own self-identification; you're not a mind-reader, and appearances can be deceptive. Be aware that many people, when faced with a question about someone's sexual identity, tend to categorize people into the less societally accepted roles. For example, a heterosexual man who has sex with a man is assumed to be a closeted gay, but a homosexual man who has sex with a woman is not assumed to be a closeted straight.

No Assumptions   Associating certain medical problems with specific sexual minorities acts to stigmatize that minority. We all know that unprotected anal coitus is a risk factor for HIV transmission, but it may surprise some that more heterosexuals take part in anal coitus than homosexuals. The point is: talk with *all* your patients about anal safer sex practices. The assumption that you can choose whom to advise on this issue will unfortunately be proved wrong too often.

Just as an aside, anal sexuality is an area often forgotten in our medical school education. Possibly the best piece of advice you can give to patients interested in exploring anal sex is to make sure anything inserted into the anus has a flange to prevent it from being lost in the rectum. A second safety technique, which should *also* be included, is attaching a string to the device to allow for retrieval if the flange fails to prevent the object from being lost in the rectum. Discussions of how to prevent colonic perforations (smooth soft toys, exceedingly short fingernails, quick referral for bleeding) should also be emphasized, in addition to safer sex advice. Information about sexually transmitted diseases (STDs) that can be transmitted by anal sex and oral/anal contact should also be reviewed.

How Does Your Office Appear to the Sexual Minority Patient?   Your prospective patient's first contacts with your practice are your office staff and your forms. Patient information sheets routinely ask questions that may seem simple and routine to you, but are really quite difficult. Prospective transgendered patients must choose between male and female; S/M practitioners must choose between listing their spouse or their S/M mistress as their emergency contact. How will the new doctor respond to a newly married gay couple? A new patient will judge your paperwork, before ever finding out how accepting you are.

Your office staff can also be the cause of a misunderstanding. The odd look from your receptionist . . . the nurse who does not understand the need for a male doctor to have a chaperon when examining a female-to-male transsexual . . . the medical assistant who shudders when seeing nipple rings . . . the bookkeeper who refuses to explain a charge on the bill to the patient's significant other . . . all these can represent genuine obstacles to health care for the sexual minority patient.

The somewhat unfriendly form or staff can all lead to a hostile or fearful patient. It is probably a good idea to read over your patient materials to make sure they are not inadvertently offensive. A frank discussion with your office staff, letting them know that you welcome sexual minority patients into your practice and will not tolerate any disrespect, can also be useful. Be especially aware of the staff member who is tolerant of most sexualities, but frightened or upset by a particular sexual lifestyle or behavior; perhaps some education on your part can help allay this person's qualms.

Your Own First Impression   A physician who is not knowledgeable or respectful about sexual minority practices often reveals that ignorance in the initial history and physical. To avoid a bad first impression, consider some better ways of asking questions, whether you're asking them during the initial interview or on your forms:

Rather than ask "marital status?"

Ask "Are you single, married, divorced, separated, or partnered?" The next question is "With whom do you live?"

Rather than "What form of birth control do you use?"

Ask "Do you use birth control?" If the patient says yes, ask "What methods do you use?" If the patient says no, then ask "Do you need birth control?" (If you ask the second question first, you will overlook the patient who is relying on the rhythm method.)

Rather than "Do you have any sexual problems?"

Ask, "Do you have any sexual concerns?" Then follow up with more detailed questions: there is research to indicate that the general question alone will not uncover sexual dysfunctions. You have to ask about each specific dysfunction: for example, do you have difficulty having an orgasm, getting an erection, maintaining an erection, with pain during sex, orgasm too soon, lubricate enough or long enough, do you desire sex? Also, referring to sexual "concerns" allows the patient to bring up concerns other than dysfunctions.

Rather than "With how many partners do you have sex?"

Ask, "Are you currently having sex with anyone?" If the patient says "no," you can ask "Is that a problem for you?" If the patient says "yes," you can ask "Do you have more than one partner?"

Rather than "Who beat you up?"

Ask, "How did you get those marks/bruises/welts?"

Rather than "What is your sexual orientation?"

Ask, "Do you have sex with men, women or both?"

Finish the sex-oriented part of the interview with, "Do you engage in any sexual activities about which you have health questions?"

Respecting Patients' Identity and Relationships   It seems only courteous to refer to patients as they request. Nevertheless, it can be difficult to remember to refer to your budding, but balding, male-to-female (MTF) transsexual patient as a "she"—to write "Frank" on the prescription, but refer to her as "Francesca." It can be hard to remember to do a pap smear on Dick, your female-to-male (FTM) transgendered patient.

I hope that you already include the patient's significant other in major decisions if that is the patient's desire, despite the relationship's legal status. Sometimes it is difficult to ferret out the relationships that are important to your patient. Your patient may have a wife and a master, or two significant others. It is appropriate and desirable to ask the patient who they would like present.

Dealing with the Mistrustful Patient   Many sexual minority patients mistrust traditional medicine. Some of this mistrust is understandable: many alternative sexual behaviors are also psychiatric diagnoses, and in some cases may be illegal; many patients have had less than pleasant interactions with non-accepting physicians. Reliance on alternative medicine and folk remedies, and avoidance of traditional medicine, are common. Sexual minority patients tend not to take care of health care maintenance or even simple problems. So when they finally seek medical care, there can be serious medical concerns.

For similar reasons, many sexual minority patients also mistrust mental health professionals—so a suggestion that your patient see a psychiatrist or psychotherapist may be greeted with skepticism or hostility, particularly if the patient believes that you are suggesting such therapy to "cure" the patient's sexual behavior.

I hope it goes without saying that consensual and satisfying sexual behaviors among adults that do not interfere with the patient's functioning do not need curing. Nevertheless, depression, personality disorders, stress and other psychiatric problems are at least as likely among sexual minorities as the general population. Due to the stresses of living a non-traditional lifestyle, some emotional difficulties may be more common. Illicit drug fads within (and outside) the various sexual minority communities may lead to psychiatric and medical problems. Sensitive physicians are able to assure their patients that they are recommending mental health treatment because of the psychiatric problem and not because of the sexual behavior.

Sexual minority patients are concerned, often with cause, that health care providers will pathologize them because of their sexual identity or behaviors. You will have better success with these patients if you can assure them truthfully that you do not consider their sexuality to be, in and of itself, a problem.

Trans Health Crisis

For Us It's Life or Death

by Leslie Feinberg

I'm sitting in a cardiologist's waiting room filling out my intake forms. The tip of my pen hovers above the ubiquitous binary boxes. Female or male? I was born female-bodied and I identify as female—as a lesbian butch. However, some people see me as a feminine male. And whether they guess male or female, I am always perceived as "queer" because my gender expression is very fluid and complex. I am transgender. Which box do I check to get the medical attention I need so badly right now?

I sit here recalling recent studies showing that females my age are more likely than males to die from heart attacks. The symptoms of females are not necessarily the same as those of men. Distorted through the lens of sexism, these symptoms are often not recognized or taken seriously enough. I consider all this and decide to check the "F" box, hoping the doctor will take my birth sex into account in listening to my cardiac symptoms.

One of the 2 women at the front desk takes the clipboard and flashes me a generous smile. "Have a seat, sir." Minutes later she calls out, "Miss Feinberg, do you have insurance?" I stand up; she looks bewildered. To her credit, she recovers quickly. She goes out of her way to be warm to me.

I sit back down and leaf through a magazine. The other woman at the front desk explodes in derisive laughter. She comments out loud about a patient's records: "Do you know what's on this *man's* chart? This man had a *breast* biopsy!" She snorts and snickers in a mean-spirited way. Everyone in the waiting room can hear her.

You may be appalled at that breach of patient confidentiality. But as a transgender patient, I have another take on it. I hear her backwardness about sex and gender variance, and I hear her intolerance. I feel more fearful about this appointment today. My reluctance isn't just because of how I might be treated by the front office

staff. I dread seeing a physician because of a lifetime of experiences.

Five years ago, while battling an undiagnosed case of bacterial endocarditis, I was refused care at a Jersey City emergency room. After the physician who examined me discovered that I am female-bodied, he ordered me out of the emergency room despite the fact that my temperature was above 104° F (40° C). He said I had a fever "because you are a very troubled person."

Weeks later I was hospitalized with the same illness in New York City in a Catholic hospital where management insists patients be put in wards on the basis of birth sex. They place transsexual women who have completed sex-reassignment surgery in male wards. Putting me in a female ward created a furor. I awoke in the night to find staff standing around my bed ridiculing my body and referring to me as a "Martian." The next day the staff refused to work unless "it" was removed from the floor. These and other expressions of hatred forced me to leave.

Had I died from this illness, the real pathogen would have been bigotry.

I could recount many terrible incidents that illustrate the various ways hostility to trans patients is conveyed. This is not my individual problem; it is a widespread social crisis. You may have heard of Billy Tipton, a well-known white jazz musician who died of a bleeding ulcer in 1989 rather than see a doctor. After his death, lurid headlines revealed that he had been born female-bodied.

In 1995, African American hairdresser Tyra Hunter was in a car accident in Washington, DC. Eyewitnesses reported that rescue medics suspended treatment and made ridiculing remarks after they cut open her pants to treat her and discovered she had male genitals. Onlookers shouted at the medics until they took her to the emergency room, where she died. Hunter's mother won a

---

wrongful-death lawsuit against the District, in which the jury also ruled against the emergency room physician for failing to diagnose Tyra's injuries and for not following nationally accepted standards of care.

Everyone who is living in a sex other than the one assigned to them by a stranger at birth, or who is born on the anatomical spectrum between female and male, or who cross-dresses, or who is perceived as a feminine male or masculine female, or who is gender-ambiguous or gender-contradictory, can most likely recount similar horror stories. As a result, many of us fear contact with health professionals.

Too many of us have already died unnecessarily, have been turned away from a doctor's office or a hospital, or have delayed pursuing preventive or emergency care because of previous mistreatment. And many individuals who are socially identifiable as transsexual or gender-variant are so marginalized by oppression—specifically, in the workforce—that we lack health insurance and a primary care physician. Those who do have insurance often cannot afford health care plans that allow us to choose our own doctors. Then, trans patients hesitate to go to HMOs and start over each time with a new physician who might be hostile.

There are also many people in this society who may not identify as trans but who have been humiliated because of some perceived difference in their secondary sexual characteristics or because their mode of self-expression is not considered "man" enough or "woman" enough. All of this shaming drives people underground. As a result, there is no way of knowing how large a segment of the population avoids seeking health care because they have been wounded by sex and gender oppression.

Beyond Pink or Blue

How the term "trans" is defined, and by whom, will shape the approach of public health to our population. Many communities—representing a spectrum of sexualities and a wide range of individual identities—march under the banner of trans liberation. And transsexual, transgender, and intersexual people can be found in every economic class, nationality, ethnicity, and region.

Broad generalizations about gender and sex will oversimplify this manifold segment of the population. A female who is considered feminine in her rural community may find herself harassed on urban streets for being too masculine. A Latina drag queen who has lived homeless on the streets of Manhattan since she was 10 years old does not experience the world in the same way as does a white heterosexual male who owns a corporation and cross-dresses several times a year at private parties.

I would recommend that public health professionals put aside definitions for now. They can be conceptually self-limiting.

The crisis for trans patients won't be solved by creating 2 more boxes: female-to-male and male-to-female. While that would create greater recognition of transsexual patients, it does not take into account that a diverse segment of the human population is reluctant to seek health care because of current social and medical models of what is "natural."

Sex is best viewed as a continuum. That truth is being articulated by courageous intersexual adults—those who were born on the anatomical sweep between female and male. Intersexual people have been surgically and hormonally shoehorned to fit into the either–or categories of female or male. Intersexual activists are speaking out publicly about their rights to self-determination and to make informed decisions about their own bodies. And birth biology is not the sole determinant of what it means to be a woman or a man. That is demonstrated by the bravery of transsexuals, who live in the sex that feels like home.

Gender expression is also represented most accurately by a continuum. Those pink and blue birth caps in delivery rooms are knitted with inaccurate assumptions that girls will grow up to be feminine and boys to be masculine. Trying to talk about gender articulation using only the terms widely used in English today—feminine, masculine, androgynous—is as ludicrous as trying to make yourself understood in a language composed of 3 words.

Even in this society, in which departures from the Ozzie-and-Harriet paradigms of gender are cruelly punished, I still see uniqueness and complexity, contradiction and ambiguity—what each individual has fashioned out of the social cloth they were issued. And if we are going to defend this full spectrum of self-expression, we must be prepared to defend its poles: masculinity is not rewarded in females, and femininity in a misogynist society is not a privileged gender expression in females or males.

To impose rigid social binaries on this range of human self-expression is to deny what actually exists. Evidence reveals the prevalence and acceptance of gender variance, sex reassignment, and intersexuality in societies on every continent since the earliest oral and recorded history. Historically, laws that partitioned the sexes and punished individuals who bridged or blurred the divide arose with the creation of patriarchal class divisions. The paradigm of 2 genders based on 2 biological sexes began to prevail in Western dominant culture only in the early 18th century.

This historical overview needs to be factored into any discussion about trans health care, especially because bigots use a vulgarization of the modern biological model of sex and gender to denounce any variation as "unnatural."

Experts on Our Own Oppression

For many decades, trans people have been told that the way to change the system is to talk to medical students about our bodies and identities, and even about some of the problems we've faced in accessing health care. But those individual patient narratives, introduced and framed by non-trans professionals, have not solved the problems.

The degree to which we as trans people are committed to helping change institutional patterns can be understood when I say that for us to describe to an audience what we have suffered as patients is oftentimes as painful as it is to recount a rape—a metaphor I do not use lightly. There are incidents that I have endured in health care settings that I still will not talk about.

I have spoken to classes of medical students about my overall experiences for more than 30 years. Sometimes students would later approach me on the street or in a supermarket to tell me how moved they were by my account. But in the course of those 3 decades I was not able to get a Pap test or find a primary care physician. And even the individuals who were sympathetic lacked the tools to change the systems they worked in.

Education is important. But attitudinal change is not the same as institutional change. If education is not tied to transforming systems of health care delivery, then it's as effective as putting out a forest fire with teacups full of water. Sensitivity and diversity training has to be linked to a commitment to institutional change and mechanisms for compliance.

Our standing before medical audiences to tell personal stories as patients has not been effective in ushering in change. Now we as an emerging political movement of trans communities are speaking out with a collective voice to say that we are experts on our own lives and what we need as patients.

Imagine that you discovered that male researchers and physicians—no matter how well-meaning—had written the entire body of medical literature on women's health needs, and that these articles narrowly defined "woman" and made sweeping, often erroneous, generalizations about women's psychology, experiences, and health needs. What if, as the basis for their "expertise," these men cited that they had seen some female patients and had read some books by women? Would this literature be problematic because more female patient narratives were needed? Or could this problem be solved only by the organized intervention of women?

Equal Partners in Problem Solving

Now here is a moment of truth for you. I want to talk to you as an equal partner in problem solving about how to remove institutionalized obstacles for trans people. If this is controversial, I welcome that controversy. I believe that this kind of debate will motivate the most progressive, self-confident, and compassionate members of the health care community—many of you battling your own oppression—to insist that we as trans people must be part of any dialogue or any plan about how to solve what is an urgent crisis for us.

This participation must include the most downtrodden and disenfranchised of the sex- and gender-oppressed populations, including people of color, street youths, the homeless, and prisoners. As trans grassroots organizers, we can also enlist the organizational networks established by intersexuals, cross-dressers, and trans men and women.

Will our insistence that we be included as peers create a struggle among divergent currents in the health care community? You bet! But as Frederick Douglass wisely and succinctly explained, "Power concedes nothing without a struggle."

So let me begin with a few concrete ideas that would make a big difference for us as trans people.

We need immediate changes in treatment-based situations, because those are often the most life threatening for us. We urgently need a centralized listing of trans-friendly health care providers and facilities. Those individuals and institutions need ongoing educational information and training about what constitutes sensitive care.

Some of the solutions are so easy, really. Refer to patients by their first and last names, not Mr. or Ms., sir or ma'am. Remove sex-specific signs and stick-figure symbols from single-occupancy restrooms. Provide unisex equipment, such as wide-mouth urinary devices.

We need health care providers to understand why it is so important not to ask us to remove our clothing unless it is absolutely necessary, and if it is necessary, to explain why. You may not realize how many times we have been told to strip and have suffered genital examinations and prurient questions when we were seeking treatment for strep throat or removal of a mole on the upper body.

We need written institutional standards establishing the minimum of good care for trans patients. We need health care worker competencies. We need on-site patient advocates to help us redress our grievances.

These and other actions will send up a signal flare to trans people that a transformation is taking place in health care. This signal will help us reach trans populations that are currently underground in order to do needs assessments.

Trans research should be community-based because of our specific sensitivities, understanding, experience, and consciousness. How will research be conceptualized and formulated? How will teams locate the most oppressed segments of the population? How will the results of research be interpreted? How will the findings be distributed—not only to the public health community, but also to trans communities that need that information? The quality and success of trans research will depend on how you answer these questions.

But trans needs assessment cannot be determined by community-based research alone. We also need to look at how misunderstandings or prejudices in the non-trans health care community affect needs assessment. For example, are very masculine females less likely than others to do breast self-examinations? Or are health care providers less likely to educate them about the need to do breast examinations?

We need profound changes to show the trans population that it is safe to seek care. Imagine if a prestigious group of public health educators, researchers, administrators, doctors, nurses, and health care unions issued a statement saying that sex and gender are much more complex than the currently accepted paradigm, that expressions of sex and gender are much more accurately

represented by Kinsey-type continua than by either–or boxes. Suppose these medical professionals said they were going to work with sex- and gender-variant people to create models that more accurately reflect the range of human bodies and self-expression. That would have a stunning impact on social consciousness as a whole, not just the health care community.

I believe that our trans movement will find strong allies in public health care. More than any other area of medicine, public health care has always factored in social, economic, and political impacts—specifically oppression and poverty—on community wellness.

I have brought you just a few of the ideas that I, and other trans activists, have about our health crisis. We want to hear your thoughts about how the barriers to trans health care can be removed. Now we arrive at another moment of truth: When and where will our dialogue continue?

References

List of references is available in the original source.

Forbidden Fruit

by Anne Finger

Before she became a paraplegic, Los Angeles resident DeVonna Cervantes liked to dye her pubic hair 'fun colours'—turquoise, purple, jet black. After DeVonna became disabled, a beautician friend of hers came to the rehabilitation unit and, as a Christmas present, dyed DeVonna's pubic hair a hot pink.

But there's no such thing as 'private parts' in a rehab hospital. Soon the staff, who'd seen her dye job when they were catheterizing her, sent the staff psychiatrist around to see her. Cervantes says that he told her: 'I know it is very hard to accept that you have lost your sexuality but you don't need to draw attention to it this way.' Cervantes spent the remainder of the 50-minute session arguing with him, and, in perhaps the only true medical miracle I've ever heard of, convinced him that he was wrong—that this was normal behaviour for her.

Cervantes' story not only illustrates woeful ignorance on the part of a 'medical expert'; equating genital sensation with sexuality. But it shows clearly a disabled woman's determination to define her own sexuality.

Sadly, it's not just medical experts who are guilty of ignoring the reproductive and sexual rights and needs of people with disabilities. The movements for sexual and reproductive freedom have paid little attention to disability issues. And the abortion rights movement has sometimes crudely exploited fears about 'defective fetuses' as a reason to keep abortion legal.

Because the initial focus of the women's movement was set by women who were overwhelmingly non-

From *New Internationalist,* July 1992, pp. 8–10. Copyright © 1992 by New Internationalist. Reprinted by permission.

disabled (as well as young, white, and middle-class), the agenda of reproductive rights has tended to focus on the right to abortion as the central issue. Yet for disabled women, the right to bear and rear children is more at risk. Zoe Washburn, in her poem, 'Hannah', grieves the child she wanted to have and the abortion she was coerced into: '. . . so she went to the doctor, and let him suck Hannah out with a vacuum cleaner. . . . The family stroked her hair when she cried and cried because her belly was empty and Hannah was not only dead, but never born. They looked at her strange crippled-up body and thought to themselves, thank God that's over.'

Yet the disability rights movement has certainly not put sexual rights at the forefront of its agenda. Sexuality is often the source of our deepest oppression; it is also often the source of our deepest pain. It's easier for us to talk about—and formulate strategies for changing—discrimination in employment, education, and housing than to talk about our exclusion from sexuality and reproduction. Also, although it is changing, the disability rights movement in the US has tended to focus its energies on lobbying legislators and creating an image of 'the able disabled'.

Barbara Waxman and I once published an article in *Disability Rag* about the US Supreme Court's decision that states could outlaw 'unnatural' sex acts, pointing out the effect it could have on disabled people—especially those who were unable to have 'standard' intercourse. The *Rag* then received a letter asking how 'the handicapped' could ever be expected to be accepted as 'normal' when we espoused such disgusting ideas.

Because reproduction is seen as a 'women's issue', it is often relegated to the back burner. Yet it is crucial that the disability-rights movement starts to deal with it. Perhaps the most chilling situation exists in China where a number of provinces ban marriages between people with developmental and other disabilities unless the parties have been sterilized. In Gansu Province more than 5,000 people have been sterilized since 1988. Officials in Szechuan province stated: 'Couples who have serious hereditary diseases including psychosis, mental deficiency and deformity must not be allowed to bear children'. When disabled women are found to be pregnant, they are sometimes subjected to forced abortions. But despite widespread criticism of China's population policies, there was almost no public outcry following these revelations.

Even in the absence of outright bans on reproduction, the attitude that disabled people should not have children is common. Disabled women and men are still sometimes subject to forced and coerced sterilizations— including hysterectomies performed without medical justification but to prevent the 'bother' of menstruation.

Los Angeles newscaster Bree Walker has a genetically transmitted disability, ectrodactyly, which results in fused bones in her hands and feet. Pregnant with her second child, last year, she found her pregnancy the subject of a call-in radio show. Broadcaster Jane Norris informed listeners in a shocked and mournful tone of voice that Bree's child had a 50-percent chance of being born with the same disability. 'Is it fair to bring a child into the world knowing there's two strikes against it at birth? . . . Is it socially responsible?' When a caller objected that it was no one else's business, Norris argued, 'It's everybody's business.' And many callers agreed with Norris's viewpoint. One horrified caller said, 'It's not just her hands—it's her feet, too. She has to [dramatic pause] wear orthopaedic shoes.'

The attitude that disabled people should not have children is certainly linked with the notion that we should not even be sexual. Yet, as with society's silence about the sexuality of children, this attitude exists alongside widespread sexual abuse. Some authorities estimate that people with disabilities are twice as likely to be victims of rape and other forms of sexual abuse as the general population. While the story of rape and sexual abuse of disabled people must be told and while we must find ways to end it, the current focus on sexual exploitation of disabled people can itself become oppressive.

As Barbara Faye Waxman, the former Disability Project Director for Los Angeles Planned Parenthood states, 'The message for disabled kids is that their sexuality will be realized through their sexual victimization. . . . I don't see an idea that good things can happen, like pleasure, intimacy, like a greater understanding of ourselves, a love of our bodies.' Waxman sees a 'double whammy' effect for disabled people, for whom there are few, if any, positive models of sexuality, and virtually no social expectation that they will become sexual beings.

The attitude that we are and should be asexual seems to exist across a broad range of cultures. Ralf Hotchkiss, famous for developing wheelchairs in Third World countries, has travelled widely in Latin America and Asia. He says that while attitudes vary 'from culture to culture, from subculture to subculture,' he sees nearly everywhere he travels, 'extreme irritation [on the part of disabled people] at the stereotypical assumptions that people . . . make about their sexuality, their lack of it.' He also noted: 'In Latin American countries once they hear I'm married, the next question is always, "How old are your kids?"'

Some of these prejudices are enshrined in law. In the US, 'marital disincentives' remain a significant barrier. To explain this Byzantine system briefly: benefits (including government-funded health care) are greatly reduced and sometimes even eliminated when a disabled person marries. Tom Fambro writes of his own difficulties with the system: 'I am a 46-year-old black man with cerebral palsy. A number of years ago I met a young lady who was sexually attracted to me (a real miracle).' Fambro learned, however, that he would lose his income support and, most crucially, his medical benefits, if he married. 'People told us that we should just live together . . . but because both of us were born-again Christians that was unthinkable. . . . The Social Security Administration has the idea that disabled people are not to fall in love, get married, have sex or have a life of our own. Instead, we are to be sexual eunuchs. They are full of shit.'

Institutions—whether traditional hospitals or euphemistically named 'homes', 'schools', or newer community care facilities—often out-and-out forbid sexual contact for their residents. Or they may outlaw gay and lesbian relationships, while allowing heterosexual ones. Disabled lesbians and gays may also find that their sexual orientation is presumed to occur by default. Restriction of access to sexual information occurs on both a legal and a social plane. The US Library of Congress, a primary source of material for blind and other print-handicapped people, was instructed by Congress in 1985 to no longer make *Playboy* available in braille or on tape. And relay services, which provide telecommunication between deaf and hearing people have sometimes refused to translate sexually explicit speech. In her poem, 'Seeing', blind poet Mary McGinnis writes of a woman being watched by sighted men while bathing nude:

> *. . . the guys sitting at the edge of the pond*
> *looked at her, but she couldn't see them . . .*
> *and whose skin, hair, shirts and belts*
> *would remain unknown to her*
> *because she couldn't go up to them*
> *and say, now fair is fair, let me touch the places*
> *on your bodies you try to hide,*
> *it's my turn—don't draw back or sit on*
> *your hands, let me count your rings, your scars,*
> *the hairs coming from your nose. . . .*

I have quoted poets several times in this piece; many disability-rights activists now see that while we need changes in laws and policies, the formation of culture is a key part of winning our freedom. Disabled writers and artists are shaping work that is often powerful in both its rage and its affirmation.

In Cheryl Marie Wade's 'side and belly', she writes:

> He is wilty muscle sack and sharp bones fitting my gnarlypaws. I am soft cellulite and green eyes of middle-age memory. We are side and belly trading dreams and fantasies of able-bodied former and not real selves: high-heel booted dancers making love from black rooftops and naked dim doorways. . . . Contradictions in the starry night of wars within and being not quite whole together and whole. Together in sighs we say yes broken and fire and yes singing.

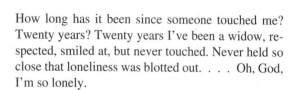

The Need for Intimacy

by Jane Porcino

How long has it been since someone touched me? Twenty years? Twenty years I've been a widow, respected, smiled at, but never touched. Never held so close that loneliness was blotted out. . . . Oh, God, I'm so lonely.

These poignant words from the poem "Minnie Remembers," by Donna Swanson, reflect one of our deepest fears about aging. No matter what our age, we each need intimacy in our lives—at least one other person with whom we can share both pleasure and pain. We hunger

for someone who will accept us as delightfully different. This other person can be female or male, young or old.

Research demonstrates that babies who never are held or touched suffer psychologically and may actually wither and die. This also is true as we grow older. And yet, an increasing number of women over 65 live alone, without partners, many of them deprived of any expression of intimacy.

One reality we will face as we grow older female is that there are more women than men; we are likely to

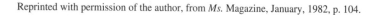

Reprinted with permission of the author, from *Ms.* Magazine, January, 1982, p. 104.

find ourselves without a male partner. In the beginning decades of this century, there were equal numbers of women and men over the age of 65. Today, there are almost 150 older women for every 100 men. Divorce after 25 to 30 years of marriage is becoming common-place, and the average age for a widow is only 56. Complicating all of this is the fact that men who are widowed or divorced in mid- or late-life quickly re-marry, most often to younger women. There are nine bridegrooms to every bride over the age 65. Not only is remarriage rare for older women, but there are few so-cial opportunities for close relationships with men. As a result, almost half of all older women live alone—many of them lonely. One woman stated the problem well when she wrote to me:

> One thing unites us all—babies, adults, and grand-mothers—our need for response from some living creature. Of course, tender loving care would be bet-ter, but we can survive without that luxury. What we cannot do without is some kind of reciprocal sharing of life experiences.

Are millions of us doomed to loneliness in old age? Not if we are willing to plan now for our later years, and not just let them happen to us. First, it is important to strengthen and nurture our friendships with women—in-deed, glory in them. Fortunately, we were encouraged to develop close female friendships, to share trust and con-fidences, and to express our feelings to one another. Many of us, even many married women whose relation-ships with their husbands lack intimacy, presently share much of our social life with women. We seek out envi-ronments in which we can express our innermost thoughts. The coffeeklatch, PTA-days have evolved to rap groups, consciousness-raising meetings, and profes-sional networking (the "old girls' club").

Collective living is one way to counter loneliness in our later years. Small groups of us can join together to share living space, incomes, companionship, thoughts, and tasks in a supportive environment. Women are successfully doing this throughout the country. There is a great deal that we can do together that we cannot do alone.

The seeking of intimacy could be encouraged even within nursing homes. My own mother lived out her last years in such a facility, where she developed a close friendship with another woman. They shared all the de-tails of their daily lives, and yet to the end, these two proper women called each other "Mrs.," and rarely touched. The friendship was so deep that when one died, the other followed in a few months.

A prevailing fear of homosexuality among many heterosexual older women may prevent them from ac-knowledging their human need for intimacy. Some women have shared sexual intimacy with other women most of their adult years. Even women who prefer het-erosexuality are moving toward intimacy with women in their later years because of the limited choices available to them. Only a few women may find sexual gratification in their female relationships. But they will find many other kinds of intimacy. Women I know say that they enjoy the companionship of other women; many say they have no desire at all to make the accommodations that would be necessary to form new heterosexual relationships. Two wrote the follow-ing to me:

> I am blessed with a few special women friendships. They are nonsexual, greatly sharing, mutually sup-portive "conversational love affairs."
>
> I've a whole circle of supportive, nutritive, loving women friends. I talk over life circumstances, prob-lems and interests with them very openly, receive a great deal of support from them, and give the same. We often have just fun together. I love them and they love me. These friendships have been the most stable thing in my life.

The upcoming generation of elderly women (those now in their late 30s and 40s—the baby-boom genera-tion) are more open to exploring different ways to be inti-mate. Those of us presently in our middle or late years can learn from them. Although we have been socialized to seek only one significant other, perhaps our search should be for a few such people in our lives—people to have fun with, to share our pleasure and pain, and to give us the physical touching we need.

Love has the potential for deepening as we age. We have years of experience behind us, and now we have the time. Sensuous grandmothers abound—women like Lena Horne, Mary Calderone, and Ingrid Bergman, whose vibrant way of being in the world draws people to them. Our only limit may be a weak imagination.

WORKSHEET—CHAPTER 9
Sexuality and LBT Issues

This worksheet needs to be optional. It asks personal questions which no one should be required to answer.

1. **Sexual preference/identity:** Society, parents, and friends give very clear messages about who one should relate to sexually, how and when! We are all aware that we are "breaking the rules" if we are sexually involved with someone of the "wrong" age, the "wrong" color, the "wrong" social status, or the "wrong" sex. Heterosexism is so prevalent that most heterosexuals never think about why they relate sexually to the opposite sex. Imagine a mother asking her 18 year old daughter to explain why she is going out with men instead of women. But most lesbians and bisexuals have had to think through, question, and explain their choices.

   Answer the following questions for yourself and a friend who would identify their sexual identity or situation as different from yours. (If you prefer not to answer these questions yourself, interview two people with different identities and compare their answers.)

   a. Briefly describe your present lifestyle and your sexual identity.

   b. Describe how you made this choice about your sexuality. Was it a gradual evolution or a sudden awareness? Has your sexuality changed or stayed the same since your first sexual identity? What factors have influenced this?

   c. Do you have a sexual partner or partners now? Would your sexual identity be the same if you did not have a partner/partners?

   d. In what specific ways do you consciously work towards a balance of power in your relationships? How equal are your relationships sexually?

   e. How does your sexual relationship(s)/identity affect your relationships with friends, both men and women, with whom you are not having a sexual relationships?

   f. How does your sexuality affect your choices regarding having children/being a parent?

g. The women's movement has emphasized that "the personal is political": the decisions we make in our personal lives and the way we live our lives are political issues. How do you see "the personal is political" relating to sexuality, sexual identity, and sexual choices?

h. Do you feel there is such a thing as "heterosexual privilege"? If so, how does this affect your life?

2. After reading "Do Ask, Do Tell," "Health Care Without Shame," and "Trans Health Crisis," think about your recent visits to health settings. Think about the illustrations on the walls and brochures, the forms you were asked to fill out, and questions you were asked in person. Was the setting and interaction designed to be equally comfortable for heterosexual, bisexual, gay, lesbian, and trans people? If yes, describe how this was accomplished. If no, give specific recommendations for how your health care setting could be made more welcoming for a diversity of patients.

3. After reading "The Need for Intimacy," give suggestions for how our society could make it easier for people of all ages to have opportunities for healthy intimacy.

4. Synthesize points made in both "The Need for Intimacy" article and "Myth 4: Women want intimacy; men want sex" in "The Orgasm Gap" to come up with a comprehensive statement acknowledging the roles that both intimacy and orgasms could play in both women's and men's lives.

KEGEL EXERCISES

The pubococcygeus (P.C.) muscles support the walls of the vagina, the urethra and rectum. Good, strong P.C. muscles can be important for childbirth, preventing stress incontinence (loss of urine when coughing or sneezing), and can enhance sexual enjoyment. Kegel exercises (developed by Dr. Arnold Kegel) are designed to strengthen the P.C. muscles. Unlike most exercises, no special clothes, gyms, etc. are required. These exercises can be done anywhere and no one else will even know you are doing them.

a. Find your P.C. muscles. When you are urinating, stop the flow of urine in midstream. The muscles you are feeling are your P.C. muscles, the muscles you want to strengthen.

b. Examples of Kegel exercises:

Flicks—Do a series of contractions as rapidly as possible. It has been suggested that one does this in time to the car's turn signals.

Squeeze and hold for as long as possible, trying to work up to holding for 8–10 seconds.

Take a slow, deep breath, squeezing the P.C. muscles as you are breathing in. Pretend you are slowly drawing something into your vagina. Imagine you are lifting weights in your vagina!

CHAPTER 10

Fertility, Infertility, and Reproductive Rights/Freedom*

Real reproductive rights would mean that a woman is able to choose when, whether, and under what conditions to have children, how many children to have, and to assume that she and her children would survive (and thrive) during pregnancy, childbirth, and the postpartum periods. What kind of health system would truly allow *all* women to have healthy babies, healthy children, and healthy families? What other societal changes need to happen for women to be able to make their own "choices" not to have children or to have the number of children they want? Too often the media, and maybe even the movements themselves, have promoted the image that the struggle for reproductive rights is about abortion and contraceptive issues. Certainly access to affordable, safe contraception, with affordable, safe abortion as a back-up, is an essential part of women being able to control their bodies and their lives, but many other issues are also part of the bigger picture of what reproductive rights and reproductive freedom* really mean.

Building on the work of the Black Women's Health Project and African-American Women for Reproductive Rights (see *The Black Women's Health Book*), other women of color groups have been actively organizing around and clearly articulating that an agenda for reproductive rights must be more broadly defined to include many issues central to their lives. The articles "For Native Women Reproductive Rights Mean" and "Latinas for Reproductive Choice" summarize more inclusive, more culturally relevant definitions of reproductive freedom and provide examples of ways Native American women and Latinas are organizing around these issues.

Connie S. Chan's "Reproductive Issues Are Essential Survival Issues for Asian-American Communities" describes how she, as a middle-class, educated, bi-lingual Asian-American, was unaware of the reproductive health issues of poor, non-English speaking immigrant women and what she learned as a translator. This article is a reminder of how easy it is not to understand what reproductive rights mean to another woman or group of women; it begs us to think through the ramifications for poor women when health care benefits are not available to them because of their immigrant status or because Medicaid benefits will not cover abortion. At its most provocative level, this article asks us to think about the many ways the health system and society have failed a woman and her children when abortion becomes the only "choice" for basic survival.

Patricia Hill Collins' "Will the 'Real' Mother Please Stand Up?" identifies how societal messages and population policies specifically give very clear messages about who is and is not considered a good mother and supported in this role:

> New reproductive technologies, dominant ideologies about motherhood promulgated in the media, and social institutions work to keep middle-class white women firmly entrenched in popular culture and scholarship as the essence of desirable motherhood that is worth protecting. Health care policies in particular reflect a fascination with increasing middle-class white women's fertility, often to the detriment of other pressing maternal and child health needs.

---

*Loretta Ross, a long-term women's health activist, uses the term reproductive rights in connection with the more white-dominated movements which have focused very much on abortion and contraceptive issues, and the term reproductive freedom for the organizations, with women of color leadership, which have worked on a much wider range of issues related to women's reproductive lives.

In contrast, she describes strong messages that working class white women are "less fit" mothers and working class African-Americans are "unfit" mothers. She then moves us to see how the present day political climate is particularly detrimental to anyone labeled a less or unfit mother:

> . . . the assault on affirmative action policies in higher education and the workplace, . . . the Personal Responsibility and Work Opportunities and Reconciliation Act, which effectively abolished AFDC . . . , the emergence of increasingly strident anti-immigration rhetoric in public discourse, and the increasing privatization of schools, health care, and selected public services can all be seen as part of an overarching framework designed to maintain differences between fit and unfit mothers.

"Contraceptive Jelly on Toast and Other Unintended Consequences of Sexuality Education" is included here to stimulate a discussion of the folklore and contemporary legends we hear about contraception (and other women's health issues) and what we can learn about people's misinformation, anxieties and fears by analyzing such stories. From my (Whatley's) perspective as a health educator and my sister's (Elissa Henken) perspective as a folklorist, "One of the clear messages sexuality educators should get from these stories is that education about contraceptives needs to be specific, concrete, and as literal as possible." The next article is a reminder of the crucial information women are not getting. The seemingly apolitical article from the *FDA Consumer,* " 'The Pill' May Not Mix Well with Other Drugs," raises very worrying questions about the politics of information when the reader realizes that very basic information with life-changing ramifications, such as "certain drugs may decrease the effectiveness of your contraceptive or your contraceptive may alter the way your body responds to other medications," is not available to many women choosing to use the contraceptive pill.

Another major political question is why are "reproductive rights" so much seen as issues for women? If we lived in a more egalitarian society or if men shared equally in the responsibility for childcare, how would that affect *all* reproductive rights and health issues? Why has almost all of reproductive research focused on finding ways to interfere with a woman's body to prevent pregnancy or understanding how a pregnant woman's environment affects fetal health? Is it fair that women have to bear the burden of nearly all the health risks associated with contraception? If safe, reliable contraceptives were available for men, how many women would trust their male partners with responsibility for contraception in their relationships? Do you think we would see more articles and research like "Eight New Nonhormonal Contraceptive Methods for Men" if more women had the power to help determine reproductive health research priorities? And very relevant to *this* book, as we now stick the "classic" symbol on to this 1992 article about so-called *new* methods for men, why have we still not heard of any of these methods over a decade later?

In an increasingly conservative climate where women's access to safe, legal abortion is constantly threatened or eroded, having accurate information on abortion issues and ramifications of restrictions is an important part of the struggle to work for what we believe is important. The three fact sheets by the Abortion Access Project summarize key information on young women and abortion, the shortage of abortion providers, and who has abortions. Working against the backlash to the reproductive rights which we have won often takes so much of our energy that we do not take time to discuss controversial and contradictory issues about abortion with other reproductive rights activists. The next article, "The Bad Baby Blues—Reproductive Technology and the Threat to Diversity," should be thought provoking enough to stimulate some healthy debates among friends or students who usually simply pride themselves on being "pro-choice." This article asks us to remember that real choice must include the choice to have a child with disabilities and to look at ways that oppressive societal attitudes about disability have an impact on pregnant women facing prenatal screening. We might ask ourselves what the role of prenatal screening would be in a society where many of the societal "handicaps" of disability had been eliminated or minimized. What would it mean if there were more social supports for people with disabilities so that individual families could "choose" to have a child with disabilities?

In working for a broader definition of reproductive rights, which includes women being able to have as many children as they choose, we need to have an analysis of how the issue of infertility has been medicalized. High tech medicine certainly promises exciting possibilities for offering some women with infertility the possibility of producing a baby. In many cities, it is already routine to offer in vitro fertilization, bypassing blocked fallopian tubes, to many heterosexual women who happen to have an extra

$5000 to try it. But, health activists have questioned who benefits, who makes money, and who is determining priorities in the rapidly growing field of infertility technology? Why is all the research emphasis on finding expensive highly technological solutions instead of looking at ways to prevent infertility (safer contraceptive methods, safer work and living environments) which could benefit far more people? Which women do and do not have access to infertility investigations and infertility treatments and should it be a goal to make these resources equally available to all women? Anne Woollett's moving personal diary (from a book by Pfeffer and Woollett) serves to remind us that there is much more to infertility than sophisticated medical technology: how does the health care system respond to many of the experiences of infertility (including the tests and treatments) that are related to self-image, sexuality, relationships, and dreams for the future? Dr. Anne Woollett and Dr. Naomi Pfeffer have written an update to their 1983 book, especially for this book. Their update answers many of the questions of students who read Anne's diary, ask how the field of infertility has changed since the early 1980's, and want to know what happened to the authors after they wrote *The Experience of Infertility*, one of the first books to explore personal feelings about infertility. Both Woollett and Pfeffer are visible, much published women's health lecturers, working in London universities. In their update, they describe how infertility technology has changed since 1983 but how many of the personal and social issues remain the same. Anne moves us to share in her thinking of herself as "childless" rather than "infertile" and trying to disentangle what it means to be a "mother" and to be a "woman."

A few more questions about who benefits from infertility technology are answered in "Grade A: The Market for a Yale Woman's Eggs." This story about a college woman *hoping* to be selected to earn $25,000 for donating eggs, is described as personally unsettling for the "candidate." We think the article may also be unsettling for readers who reflect on Patricia Hill Collins's analysis of "real" mothers:

> New reproductive technologies are emerging as central to reorganizing the experiences of all women with motherhood. Working with longstanding patterns of race and social class in the United States, these technological advances fragment the meaning of motherhood. The proliferation of reproductive technologies . . . has allowed the splitting of motherhood into three categories: genetic, gestational, and social motherhood. Genetic mothers are those who contribute the genetic material to another human being. Gestational mothers are those who carry the developing fetus in utero until birth. Social mothers care for children actually born. Traditional views of motherhood forwarded by the traditional family ideal present one middle-class white woman as fulfilling all three functions, assisted by domestic servants. But new reproductive technologies have made it possible for women to specialize in one of these mothering categories.

From the other side of the equation, choosing the sperm from a sperm bank for inseminations, "Father Knows Baste" is the story of one woman's decision to become a single mother by choice.

For Native Women Reproductive Rights Mean . . .

by Native Women for Reproductive Rights Coalition

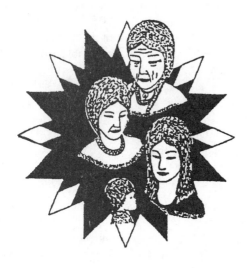

1. The right to knowledge and education for all family members concerning sexuality and reproduction that is age, culture and gender appropriate.
2. The right to all reproductive alternatives and the right to choose the size of our families.
3. The right to affordable health care, including safe deliveries within our communities.
4. The right to access safe, free, and/or affordable abortions, regardless of age, with confidentiality and free pre and post counseling.
5. The right to active involvement in the development and implementation of policies concerning reproductive issues, to include, but not limited to, pharmaceuticals and technology.

6. The right to include domestic violence, sexual assault and AIDS as reproductive rights issues.
7. The right to programs which meet the nutritional needs of women and families.
8. The right to programs to reduce the rate of infant mortality and high risk pregnancies.
9. The right to culturally specific comprehensive chemical dependency prenatal programs, including, but not limited to, prevention of Fetal Alcohol Syndrome and Effects.
10. The right to stop coerced sterilization.
11. The right to a forum for cultural/spiritual development, culturally-oriented health care, and the right to live as Native women.
12. The right to be fully informed about, and to consent to any forms of medical treatment.
13. The right to determine who are members of our Nations.
14. The right to continuous, consistent and quality health care for Native People.
15. The right to reproductive rights and support for women with disabilities.
16. The right to parent our children in a non-sexist, non-racist environment.

In order to accomplish the foregoing stated rights, the Native Women for Reproductive Rights will create coalitions and alliances to network with other groups.

Latinas for Reproductive Choice

by Latinas for Reproductive Choice

The National Latina Health Organization was co-founded by four Latinas on March 8, 1986, International Women's Day. The NLHO was formed to raise Latina consciousness about our health and health problems, so that we can begin to take control of our health and our lives. We are committed to work towards the goal of bilingual access to quality health care and the self-empowerment of Latinas through educational programs, outreach and research.

The National Latina Health Organization has been redefining reproductive issues from our very beginning. We have been actively advocating the expansion of abortion rights to include all the reproductive issues . . . family planning, prenatal care, education and information on sexuality that is culturally relevant and in our language, birth control, freedom from sterilization abuses; and above all, access to all health services. This is being done with our constituents locally and nationally.

At the beginning of 1990, the NLHO, along with other community activists, created "Latinas for Reproductive Choice", a project of the NLHO. We feel strongly that Latinas need to take a public stand on reproductive issues in the way that they affect us. We launched our project with a press conference in San Francisco on October 3, 1990, the thirteenth anniversary of the death of Rosie Jimenez. Our legislators and the general public need to become aware that we are now ready to become a very visible, public, vocal and very strong force in this historic debate that will decide the future of all women. Another very important effect of our becoming public is that other Latinas who have never openly dealt with these issues, even though they themselves may have had an abortion, will finally have the support that they need to make a personal difference. It is very historic, that Latinas are coming together in coalition to publicly take a stand on reproductive issues.

As Latinas for Reproductive Choice we propose to:

1. Break the silence on reproductive rights issues within the Latina community and provide a platform for open discussion.
2. Debunk the myths that surround Latinas through public education.
3. Include Latinas in the national reproductive rights debate by promoting Latinas on the boards of the traditional reproductive rights groups.
4. Monitor elected officials who represent Latino communities.
5. Advocate and pressure elected officials, organizations, and individuals to support reproductive choice issues for Latinas.

We are using the following letter to bring our community together on these vital issues.

. . .

Dear Amiga,

Did you know . . .

. . . Latinas make up 8.4% of women 15-44 years of age in the United States, yet 13% of all abortions are performed on Latinas in that age group?

. . . the abortion rate for Latinas is 42.6 per 1,000 compared to 26.6 per 1,000 for non-Latinas aged 15-44?

. . . it is easier today for a poor Latina to be sterilized than it is for her to receive quality family planning services and obstetrical care?

. . . In some areas of the U.S., 65% of all Latina women have been sterilized?

Do you care . . .

. . . that because Latinas have been left out of the abortion debate a myth has been promulgated by others that Latinas don't have abortions (after all, we're all Roman Catholic aren't we?)

. . . that if abortion rights are restricted, Latinas will be among the first victims of illegal abortions?

. . . that a group of Latinas has banded together to address these issues and do something about them?

We are Latinas for Reproductive Choice and we will no longer stand on the sidelines and let others decide our fate. We have come together to make sure Latina voices are part of the debate and to mobilize Latinas who are as alarmed as we are at what has been happening to our hermanas across the nation.

On October 3, 1977 a poor, young Latina died because of an illegal Texas abortion. That was the year Medicaid funding for abortions was cut. The young Latina was Rosie Jimenez, the first woman to die from such an operation following the cutoff of Medicaid funds for abortions. Lack of reproductive choice killed Rosie Jimenez. And we can't afford to lose any more Rosies to this kind of murder! Yet, there continue to be millions of young women just like Rosie Jimenez today. Right now, in 1990, most Latinas still do not have reproductive choice. If we do not fight to maintain access to safe and legal abortions thousands more young women like Rosie Jimenez will die needlessly.

Access to abortion is only half the issue for Latinas. Reproductive choice for us is much more than abortion—it is the ability to have healthy babies when, and if, we want. It means the freedom to choose to have one child or 10. Or even none. Reproductive choice means access to culturally-relevant, quality health care and information, education about sexuality and contraception for our daughters, and access to alternative forms of birth control, regardless of cost. Sterilization should not be our only choice simply because it is federally funded. Reproductive choice means the freedom to make informed choices about our bodies.

Reproductive health and abortion issues will dominate the 1990's. Candidates in the upcoming November election will be elected on the basis of their positions on reproductive issues. In recent months the United States Supreme Court has upheld more and more state restrictions on the right to an abortion and with the resignation of Justice William Brennan, the future is not encouraging. For the first time since the historic Roe v. Wade decision the Supreme Court appears willing to overturn a woman's right to a safe and legal abortion.

It is clear that if we do not speak for ourselves, no one else will. We need to ensure that Latina voices are heard in this historic debate because we have a unique perspective that has been ignored for too long.

This is why we have come together as Latinas for Reproductive Choice. Won't you join with us to make sure Rosie Jimenez did not die in vain? Help us provide a voice for all other Latinas who find themselves without choice. Help us speak out as Latinas on the most momentous issue of this decade. We can no longer afford to be silent. Add your name to the list of Latinas who are willing to take a stand.

Sinceramente,
LATINAS FOR REPRODUCTIVE CHOICE
PO BOX 7567
OAKLAND, CA 94601
(415) 534-1362

Reproductive Issues Are Essential Survival Issues for Asian-American Communities

by Connie S. Chan

When the Asian-American communities in the U.S. list their priorities for political action and organizing, several issues concerning basic survival are usually included: access to bi-lingual education, housing, health, and child care, among others. Yet the essential survival issue of access to reproductive counseling, education, and abortion is frequently missing. Why are reproductive issues perceived as unimportant to the Asian-American communities? I think there are several reasons—ignorance, classism, sexism, and language barriers. Of course, these issues are interrelated, and I'll try to make the connections between them.

First, let me state that I am not an "expert" on the topic of reproductive issues in Asian-American communities, but that I have some firsthand experiences which have given me some insight into the problems. Several years ago, I was a staff psychologist at a local community health center serving the greater Boston Asian population. Most of our patients were recent immigrants from China, Vietnam, Cambodia, Laos, and Hong Kong. Almost all of these new immigrants understood little or no English. With few resources (financial or otherwise) many newcomers struggled to make sense of life in America and to survive in whatever fashion they could.

At the health center, the staff tried to help by providing information and advocacy in getting through our confusing system. I thought we did a pretty good job until I found out that neither our health education department nor our ob/gyn department provided *any* counseling or information about birth control or abortion services. The medical department had interpreted our federal funding regulations as prohibiting not only the performance of abortions on-site, but prohibiting the dissemination of information which might lead to, or help patients to obtain an abortion.

Needless to say, as a feminist and as an activist, I was horrified. When I found out that pregnant women who inquired about abortions were given only a name of a white, English speaking ob/gyn doctor and sent out alone, this practice seemed morally and ethically neglectful. One of the nurse-midwives agreed with me and suggested that I could serve as an interpreter/advocate for pregnant women who needed to have abortions or at least wanted to discuss the option with the English-speaking ob/gyn doctor. The only catch was that I would have to do it on my own time, that I could not claim any affiliation with the health center, and that I could not suggest follow-up care at the health center.

Not fully knowing the nature of what I was volunteering for, I agreed to interpret and advocate for Cantonese-speaking pregnant women at their appointments with the obstetrician. It turned out that over the course of three years I interpreted during at least a hundred abortions for Asian immigrant women who spoke no English. After the first few abortions, the obstetrician realized how essential it was to have an interpreter present, and began to require that all non-English speaking women have an interpreter during the abortion procedure.

As a middle-class, educated, bi-lingual Asian-American woman, I was aware of the importance of having the choice to have an abortion, and the necessity to fight for the right to choose for myself, but I had been unaware of how the right to have an abortion is also a right to survival in this country if you are a poor, uneducated, non-English speaking immigrant.

The women I interpreted for were for the most part not young. Nor were they single. They ranged in age from 25–45, with a majority in their late twenties and early thirties. Almost all of the women were married and had two or more children. Some had as many as five or six children. They needed to have an abortion because they had been unlucky enough to have gotten pregnant after arriving in this country. Their families were barely surviving on the low wages that many new immigrant workers earned as restaurant workers, garment factory workers, or as domestic help.

Almost all of the women worked full-time: the ones who had young children left them with older retired family members or did piecework at home; those with older children worked in the factories or hotels. Without fail, each woman would tell me that each needed to have an abortion because her family could not afford another mouth to feed, that they could not afford to lose her salary contribution, not even for a few months, to care for an infant. In some ways, one could not even say that these women were *choosing* to have abortions. The choice had already been made for them and it was a choice of basic survival for the members of their family unit.

Kai was one of the women for whom I interpreted. A 35-year old mother of four children, ages 2 to 7, she and her husband emigrated to the U.S. from Vietnam. They had no choice in their immigration either, they were refugees whose village had been destroyed, and felt fortunate to escape with their lives and all four of their children. Life in the U.S. was difficult, but they were scraping by, living with another family in a small apartment where their entire family slept in one room. Their hope was that their children would receive an education and make it in American society: They lived with the day-to-day hope of that deferred dream for the next generation.

When Kai found out that she was pregnant she felt desperate. Because she and her husband love children and live for their children, they wanted desperately to keep the child, this one that would be born in America and be an American citizen from birth. Yet they sadly realized that they could not afford another child, they could not survive on just one salary, they could not feed another one. Their commitment was to the children they already had, and keeping their family together.

When I accompanied Kai to her abortion, she was saddened, but resigned to what she had to do. The $300 that she brought to the clinic represented almost a month of wages for her, she had borrowed the money from family and friends. She would pay it back, she said, by working weekends for the next ten weeks. Her major regret was that she would not be able to buy any new clothes for her children this year because of this unexpected expense.

Kai spoke very little English. She did not understand why she had to go to a white American doctor for her abortion, instead of receiving services from her Asian doctor at the health center. She had no understanding, really, of reproductive rights issues, of *Roe v. Wade,* or why there were demonstrators waving pictures of fetuses and yelling at her as we entered the clinic. Mercifully, she did not understand the questions they shouted at her in English, and she did not ask me what they said, remarking only that they (the protestors) seemed very angry at someone. She felt sure, I think, that they were not angry at *her.* She had done nothing to provoke anyone's anger. She was merely trying to survive in this country under this country's rules.

It is a moral crime and an injustice that Kai could not receive counseling in her language by her doctors at the Asian neighborhood health center. It is an injustice that she had to borrow $300 to pay for her own abortion, because her Medicaid benefits did not pay for it. It is a grave injustice that she had to have me, a stranger, interpreting for her during her abortion because her own doctor could not perform the procedure at her clinic. Again,

it was not a matter of choice for her to abort her pregnancy, but a matter of basic survival.

Kai will probably never attend a march or rally for choice. She will not sign any petitions. She might not even vote. But it is for her and the countless thousands of immigrant women like her that we need to continue the struggle for reproductive rights. Within the Asian American community, the immigrant women who are most affected by the lack of access to abortions have the least power. They do not speak English, they do not demand equal access to health care; their needs are easily overlooked.

Thus it is up to us who are bi-lingual, those of us who can speak English and who can speak to these issues, to do so. We need to insure that the issue of reproductive rights is an essential one in the Asian American political agenda. It is not a woman's issue; it is a community issue.

We must speak for the Kais, for their children, for their right to survive as a family. We must, as activists, make the connection between the issues of oppression based upon gender, race, national origin, sexual orientation, class or language. We can, and must lead the Asian American community to recognize the importance of the essential issue of reproductive rights for the community's survival.

Will the "Real" Mother Please Stand Up?

The Logic of Eugenics and American National Family Planning

by Patricia Hill Collins

In the United States, motherhood as a constellation of social practices, a social institution, and an American cultural icon remains central to multiple systems of oppression. Just as mothers are viewed as important to family well-being, the status of motherhood as an institution remains essential to American health and prosperity. But in a nation-state like the United States, where social class, race, ethnicity, gender, sexuality, and nationality comprise intersecting dimensions of oppression, not all mothers are created equal.

In this politicized climate, the issue of which women are "real" mothers best suited for the tasks of reproducing both the American population and seemingly American family values takes on added importance. "Real" has many meanings, such as authentic, genuine, indisputable, and true. "Real" also has physical connotations, meaning concrete, tangible, and material. Another constellation of meanings of "real" references sincerity—earnest, honest, truthful, trustworthy, and reliable. Within these intersecting meanings of "real," dichotomies emerge that construct certain groups of women of the right social class, race, and citizenship status as "real" mothers worthy and fit for the job. Affluent, white and holding American citizenship, "real" mothers are those whose authenticity lies in their biological and natural reproduction versus their social mothering; whose physicality operates via their willingness to participate in every facet of their children's lives; whose sincerity lies in beliefs about mother love; and whose surety lies in their indisputable ties to their biological offspring. Against these idealized "real" mothers, other categories of women of the wrong social class, race, and citizenship status are judged to be less fit, less worthy to be mothers. Within this intellectual framework, women deemed fit to be "real" mothers encounter population policies supporting their contributions as mothers to national well-being. In contrast, those deemed unfit to be "real" mothers experience population policies that are markedly different.

In this paper, I explore this relationship between motherhood, American national identity, and population policies. First, I examine how the traditional family ideal functions to structure notions of "real" motherhood and how this family ideal in turn frames American national identity. I suggest that not only does the metaphor of the biological, nuclear family operate to shape notions of an American nation whose health is assessed using family rhetoric, but that this American national family draws upon race for much of its meaning.

Second, I investigate how a logic of eugenics provides an intellectual context for assessing contemporary population policies by which the nation-state aims to attend to its health. Societies that embrace eugenic philosophies typically aim to transform social problems such as unemployment, increasing crime rates, childbearing by unmarried adolescents, and poverty into technical problems amenable to biological solutions. Via social engineering, societies shaped by eugenic thinking see "race and heredity—the birth rates of the fit and the unfit—as the forces that shape . . . political and social developments". Moreover, eugenics movements that seek biological solutions to what are fundamentally social problems often arise when other mechanisms of controlling subordinate populations seem no longer adequate. The United States may be experiencing such a period, and American understandings of population policies aimed at regulating the mothering experiences of women from diverse racial, social class, and citizenship groups might benefit by viewing such policies within the context of a logic of eugenics.

Finally, in order to highlight the centrality of motherhood in these relations, I survey population policies targeted toward middle-class white women, working-class white women, and working-class African-American women. These three groups of women each occupy different social locations in their ability to be "real" mothers of the nation. As a result, population policies applied to each group demonstrate how the American nation-state seeks to regulate experiences with motherhood of women from different racial, ethnic, social class, and citizenship groups in defense of nation-state interests.

"Real" Mothers in Family, Race, and Nation

As sociologist Paul Gilroy observes, "race" differences are displayed in culture that is reproduced in educational institutions and, above all, in family life. Not only are families the nation in microcosm, its key components, but they act as the means to turn social processes into natural, instinctive ones. In the United States, families constitute primary sites of belonging: the family as an assumed biological entity, the racial family or community reinforced via geographically identifiable and racially segregated neighborhoods, and the national family symbolized via images of Mom, Dad, baseball, and apple pie.

The particular model of family is germane here, for a specific family ideal frames family rhetoric in the United States. According to the American traditional family ideal, a normative and ideal family consists of a heterosexual couple that produces its own biological children. A state-sanctioned marriage confers legitimacy not only on the family structure itself but on children born in this family. This metaphor functions as a deep taproot in American social policy. Just as individuals acquire varying degrees of authority, rights, and wealth based on their mode of entry into their biological families, a nation-state's population reflects similar power relations. The nation gains meaning via family metaphors. Moreover, this family metaphor articulates both with structures of institutionalized racism and with the labor needs of capitalism, such that the American national family is defined in race- and class-specific terms in the United States.

Several features characterize the links between the biological, nuclear family and the American national family. First, presumptions of blood ties underlie both constructs. Just as women's bodies produce children that are part of a socially constructed family grounded in notions of biological kinship, women's bodies produce the population for the national family or nation-state, conceptualized as having some sort of biological oneness. In nuclear families, the legitimate sons and daughters of a heterosexual marriage, related by blood to biological parents, are contrasted to illegitimate children who, while they may also be related by blood, stand outside state-sanctioned marital relationship. In a similar fashion, those lacking the appropriate blood ties to the American nation-state are seen as outsiders, non-family-members, and are treated accordingly. "Real" mothers remain central to reproducing these genuine blood ties.

Second, family metaphors and those of nation both rely on distinctive notions of place, space, and territory. This dimension of the link can be seen through multiple meanings that people attach to the concept of home, meanings that range through levels of family household, neighborhood as family, home as the place of one's birth, and one's country as home. For example, the theme of the home as a sanctuary from outsiders and the turmoil of the public sphere creates boundaries for the biological family along lines of privacy and security. Similarly, the notion of homeland or national territory that must be defended against marauding aliens or foreigners operates in a similar fashion. Both spaces are seen as needing protection from outsiders. "Real" mothers are those who take care of the home, who provide that sanctuary that must be protected.

Third, in the same way that those born into a biologically defined family acquire certain lifelong rights and obligations to other family members, those born into the American national family as so-called natural or real citizens acquire certain rights attached to that citizenship. Citizens are also expected to fulfill certain obligations to one another. For example, people within family units routinely help members of their own families by baby-sitting, lending money, assisting relatives in locating employment and housing, or caring for economically unproductive family members such as the very young or the elderly. Family members are entitled to these benefits merely by belonging. In contrast, those who lie outside the family orbit are not entitled to such benefits—but individuals may earn them by being redefined as fictive kin or by being particularly worthy. Since citizenship is often conferred through both birth or attachment to the mother, determining the "real" mother of a child can serve as a test of citizenship and belonging.

Fourth, within biological families a pecking order or naturalized hierarchy emerges with, for example, good sons and daughters compared to their less ambitious or less fortunate siblings. This internal hierarchy parallels notions of first-class and second-class citizenship in the national family. Hierarchy may be determined by order of arrival: either birth order or immigration order. Claims that White Anglo-Saxon Protestants who migrated to the United States earlier are entitled to more benefits than more recent immigrants reflect this notion.

Or hierarchy accompanies gender. In many families, girls and boys are treated differently regarding economic autonomy and freedom to move in public space. This differential treatment serves as a foundation for sex-typing of occupations in the paid labor market and male domination of public arenas such as politics and professional sports. As is the case with all situations of hierarchy, actual or implicit use of force, sanctions, and violence may be needed to maintain unequal power relations.

Finally, families contain policies or rules regulating their own reproduction. Family planning comprises a constellation of reproductive options ranging from coercion to choice, from permanence to reversibility. Within individual families, decision-making lies with family members—technically, it is they who decide whether to have children, how many children to have, and how those children will be spaced. But can this analogy from family to nation be extended to public policies on the national level? In what ways do social policies designed to foster the health of the American nation-state, especially those concerning motherhood, follow a similar family planning logic?

Planning for the National Family: The Logic of Eugenics Thinking

Eugenics movements or movements for "racial hygiene" of the early twentieth century compellingly illustrate the thinking underlying population policies designed to control the motherhood of different groups of women for reasons of nationality and/or race. Eugenics philosophies and the population policies they support emerge within political economies with distinctive needs and within societies with particular social class relations.

Common to eugenics movements throughout the world has been the view that biology is central to solving social problems. Societies that embrace eugenic philosophies typically attempt to transform social problems into technical problems amenable to biological solutions effected via social engineering. Eugenic approaches thus combine a "philosophy of biological determinism with a belief that science might provide a technical fix for social problems" (Proctor 1988). Two sides typically exist to eugenic thinking. So-called positive eugenics consists of efforts to increase reproduction among the "aristogenic" or "fit," who allegedly carry the outstanding qualities of their group in their genes. So-called negative eugenics aims to prevent reproductions by the "cacogenic" or "unfit," those likely to have undesirable or defective offspring.

The case of population policies enforced by the Nazi nation-state offers an unsettling example of a nation-state that was able to follow the logic of eugenics thinking grounded in national family planning rhetoric to its rational conclusion. Because German scientists borrowed from eugenics philosophies developed elsewhere in Europe and in the United States, German nation-state policies during the Nazi era of 1933–1945 provide a particularly compelling case for understanding the connections among the logic of eugenics, institutionalized racism, institutionalized sexism, and social policy. The intellectual climate characterizing the Nazi German nation-state was *not* unique. Rather, it emerged from a common intellectual heritage framing Western industrialized countries, including the contemporary United States. Unlike other countries that held similar beliefs about eugenics or "racial hygiene" but were unable to implement them as fully, the Nazi German nation-state actually enforced eugenics philosophies.

Under the Nazis, eugenics thinking followed three main paths. First, the German population was racialized, with Jews and Aryans, among others, constructed as categories of immutable difference. Second, these putative racial differences were linked to issues of national identity and prosperity. Jews were blamed for failed economic and political policies and characterized as outsiders in the homeland of the German national family who hindered the nation-state's prosperity. Finally, specific population policies were designed for the worthy and unworthy segments of the general population. For example, the Jewish population encountered a continuum of policies designed to control their numbers. Stripping Jewish citizens of their property rights, legal protections, and employment opportunities; relegating the Jewish population to ghettos; deploying specific reproductive policies such as sterilization; and the so-called final solution of genocide targeted against the already born population collectively constitute eugenics as public policy.

All three elements of eugenics thinking characterize the history of American social institutions. First, because the United States has operated as a racialized state since its inception, race operates as a core concept in constructing American national identity. Despite promises of political and religious freedom for all American citizens in the Constitution, by excluding sizable segments of the population from citizenship, this same Constitution simultaneously codified race, gender, and class into the founding laws of the country. Enslaving African-Americans to exploit their labor and reproductive capacities and conducting military actions against Native Americans in order to acquire their land constituted population policies targeted explicitly for these racialized groups. Moreover, race remains important in framing the basic institutions that comprise political, economic and social institutions in the United States. While the categories of race may shift in response to changing political and economic conditions, the fundamental belief in race as a guiding principle for viewing segments of the American population remains remarkably hardy.[1]

The second element of eugenics-inspired population policies consists of associating diverse racial groups with perceived national interests. This element also has a long history in the United States. At various times, this has taken the form of restrictive immigration legislation targeted toward non-European racial and ethnic groups, a response to what was seen as the non-white threat from outside national boundaries. Slavery, de facto segregation, and other repressive policies applied to African-Americans, Latinos and other nonwhite populations within American borders also operated in response to perceived threats from nonwhite populations. While recent interconnections of racism and national policy may be more covert than in the past, operating, as sociologists Michael Omi and Howard Winant suggest, in a "hegemonic" fashion, such ties continue. Racialized discourses exist around themes that serve as proxies for race, themes such as poverty, crime, immigration, affirmative action and urban policy. While none of these terms directly refers to people of color, all have been used as codes to indicate how the presence of people of color is problematic for national unity or national aspirations.[2]

The third feature of eugenics-inspired population policies, the direct control of different segments of the population through different population control measures, also characterizes American politics.[3] Ironically, the United States pioneered the eugenics thinking actually implemented in Nazi nation-state policies. Nazi science looked to England and the United States for inspiration in crafting its eugenics policies. Francis Galton, the founder of the eugenics movement in England, claimed that "Anglo-Saxons far outranked the Negroes of Africa, who in turn outranked the Australian aborigines, who outranked nobody. Because he believed that large innate differences between races existed, Galton felt that a program to raise the inherent abilities of mankind involved the replacement of inferior races by the superior".

Galton's ideas proved popular in racially segregated United States. Preceding the sterilization laws of other countries by twenty years, American eugenics laws were seen as pioneering ventures by eugenicists of other countries. The U.S. Supreme Court's 1927 *Buck vs. Bell* decision held that sterilization fell within the police power of the state. Reflecting the majority opinion, Oliver Wendell Holmes contended,

> It would be strange if it could not call upon those
> who already sap the strength of the state for these

lesser sacrifices, often not felt to be such by those concerned, in order to prevent our being swamped by incompetence. It is better for all the world, if instead of waiting for their imbecility, society can prevent those who are manifestly unfit from continuing their kind. The principle that sustains compulsory vaccination is broad enough to cover cutting the Fallopian tubes. . . . Three generations of imbeciles is enough.

Given this intellectual context, it seems reasonable to conclude that differential population policies developed for different segments of the American population, especially those identifiable by race, citizenship status, and social class, have long existed in direct relation to any group's perceived value within the Untied States. Rather than the more familiar definition of population policies emphasizing reproductive policies, I define population policies more broadly. Population policies comprise the constellation of social policies, institutional arrangements, and ideological constructions that shape reproductive histories of different groups of women within different racial/ethnic groups, social class formations, and citizenship statuses. Examining population policies through this lens reveals the fallacy of viewing race-based policies and gender-based policies as basically regulating different forms of social relations. Current assumptions view African-Americans as having race, white women as having gender, and African-American women as experiencing both race and gender, with white men lacking both race and gender. Such assumptions dissipate when confronted with actual population policies aimed at regulating the mothering experiences of different groups of women. Since the 1970s, major changes in the American political economy, stimulated by four recessions and a declining standard of living, provided a social context fostering differential population policies for different groups of women in the United States. Given this context, how does the logic of eugenics thinking frame the population policies targeted to different groups of women?

Policies for "Fit" Mothers: Middle-Class White Women

According to the logic of eugenics, falling birth rates of the dominant group constitute "race suicide." In this situation, women of the dominant group are routinely encouraged to increase their reproductive capacities. In the United States, white women's reproduction remains central to American national aspirations. Currently, efforts to encourage white women to produce more white babies, a so-called positive eugenics goal, occur for several

reasons. First, only white women possess the genetic material necessary for creating white babies. Thus, white women hold the key to notions of racial purity central to systems of white supremacy. Second, white women remain central in socializing young white people into a system of institutionalized racism. Their activities as mothers receive praise in light of this goal. Finally, white women allegedly fulfill the symbolic function of mothers of the national family. White women have been central as symbols of the nation that must be protected and defended and as the group responsible for transmitting national culture to the young.

Overall, access to new reproductive technologies, dominant ideologies about motherhood promulgated in the media, and social institutions work to keep middle-class white women firmly entrenched in popular culture and scholarship as the essence of desirable motherhood that is worth protecting. Health care policies in particular reflect a fascination with increasing middle-class white women's fertility, often to the detriment of other pressing maternal and child health needs. Specifically, the construction of infertility as a national tragedy and the huge amounts of media attention paid to this condition reflect this preoccupation with increasing reproduction among women of the dominant group. Infertility is typically presented either as a human tragedy, the case of the unfortunate woman who cannot bear the child she so desperately wants, or, increasingly, as a personal failing—women who pursued careers, waited too long to have babies, and now find themselves childless because they turned their backs on their rightful roles as women. Middle-class women found to be infertile are assisted with a dazzling array of medical advances to cure this socially constructed tragedy. Usually insured by private insurance carriers, these women are able to defray part of the enormous costs of infertility procedures. New reproductive technologies such as in vitro fertilization, sex predetermination, and surrogate embryo transfer are routinely differentially distributed depending on the race, class and sexual orientation of women.

Popular culture and media representations play a part in both identifying middle-class white motherhood as ideal and in creating a climate where acquiring and raising a healthy white baby takes on such importance. For example, films of the 1980s and 1990s such as *The Hand That Rocks the Cradle,* whose plot centers around an affluent white woman who innocently hires a crazed nanny who tries to steal her baby, trumpet social messages that children belong at home with their "real" mothers. The mothering capacities of working mothers came under particular scrutiny. Films such as *Baby Boom,* a portrait of a successful career woman who suddenly discovers how unfulfilled her life had been when she inherits a baby, seem designed to portray the message that working mothers are acceptable just as long as motherhood comes first.

Social institutions also reflect efforts to assist middle-class white women in attaining this curiously idealized "real" mothering experience. Despite the increase in the numbers of working mothers, school day schedules that can begin as early as 7:30 A.M. and dismiss children as early as 1:30 P.M. continue to privilege stay-at-home mothers. Modest reforms designed to make the workplace accommodate the family needs of women remain more a reaction to the stated needs of middle-class white women professionals to juggle both family and career than they do any sustained national commitment to child care. While working-class mothers do benefit from corporate day care, because so many working-class women do not work for large corporations, the children of white middle-class women remain the primary beneficiaries of this upper-tier child care.

Racial segregation, and to a lesser extent social class segmentation, in American housing, education, and public services also support middle-class white mothering. The growth of gated communities and planned suburban developments designed to keep out unwelcome others speaks to the need to protect white children and their mothers. Privatizing educational and recreational experiences of white middle-class children reflects efforts to insulate this group from the perceived harm of attending school with working-class whites and working-class children of color. While the signs of racial segregation have been taken down, the results that these signs were designed to produce have not changed as rapidly. Middle-class white children still receive markedly better treatment than all other children in areas such as education, health care, housing, recreational facilities, nutrition, and public facilities such as libraries and police protection. Through public policy, ideological mechanisms, and institutional policies, their mothers receive strong messages to reproduce.

Policies for "Less Fit" Mothers: Working-Class White Women

The position of working-class white women, especially those living in poverty, differs dramatically from that of middle-class white women. On the one hand, working-class white women's ability to produce white babies renders this group "fit" to produce the biological or population base of the nation. But on the other hand, when it comes to passing on national culture, raising academically and economically productive citizens, and being symbols of the nation, working-class white women remains less "fit" for

motherhood. Public policies, popular ideology, and the structure of social institutions all work to encourage white middle-class women to fulfill their expected place as mothers of the nation by encouraging them both to have children and to raise children. In contrast, working-class white women are encouraged to have children but receive much less support for their ability to raise them.

Social policies reflect this basic contradiction. With the passage of *Roe v. Wade* in 1973, working-class and poor white women gained legal access to safe abortions. As a result, many young white women chose not to carry their babies to term. The decreasing stigma attached to single motherhood, coupled with changes in eligibility for social welfare benefits, lessened the social and economic barriers confronting single mothers of any racial background. Many white women who formerly would have given their children up for adoption chose to raise their children themselves, often alone. Together, these factors, among others, resulted in a sharp decrease in healthy white babies who formerly would have been available for adoption into white middle-class families.

Recent efforts to decrease social welfare benefits, to weaken antidiscrimination legislation against women in the workplace, and to limit access to abortion and other selected family planning services for working-class and poor women have meant that working-class white women's reproductive "choices" have changed. If working-class white women carry babies to term, the result will be an increase in the number of healthy white babies. This changing political climate suggests that young white mothers will find it more difficult to raise their children in poverty and, denied access to the choice of whether to choose to carry a child to term, will be increasingly pushed toward adoption as the best "choice."

Ideological portrayals of working-class white women as mothers must be careful to validate motherhood as a biological function yet support the notions that working-class white women do not make particularly fit mothers. In some cases, working-class white women become fit mothers by giving up their children. In her study comparing unmarried white and African-American mothers in the 1950s, Rickie Solinger reveals how working-class African-American women were actively discouraged from placing their babies up for adoption, while working-class white women encountered serious pressure to become fit mothers by releasing their children for adoption. They were told that they became good women by doing what was best for the child. Through these policies, working-class white women could gain respectability. Recent ideological representations of working-class white women must also walk this fine line between constructing them as simultaneously fit for some dimensions of motherhood, and unfit for others. Take, for example, *Roseanne* and *Grace Under Fire,* two popular American television shows of the 1990s portraying working-class white mothers. While Roseanne clearly violates many of the rules of fit motherhood, she remains married and thus gains legitimacy. In contrast, Grace, a single mother with three children, is portrayed with dignity, yet her checkered past of illicit sexuality, wife battering, and alcoholism speaks to her past transgressions. As the series continued, Grace also was revealed to have had an illegitimate child that she relinquished for adoption. Both Roseanne and Grace gain respectability within the parameters set for working-class white women.

Social institutions such as housing, schools, employment, and health care also collectively frame the mothering experiences of working-class white women. Many working-class white women are in the labor market, often in part-time work or in service jobs that offer less desirable salaries and benefits, especially health care benefits. Working-class white women thus encounter a specific constellation of population policies, ideological constructions, and social institutions. They are denied abortion services. They are denied opportunities to support their children financially. They encounter increased exposure to cultural messages that encourage them to have their biologically white babies but to give them up for adoption to "good" homes. Because they receive insufficient economic support in raising their children from the disadvantaged position of working-class white males, from their own position in the labor market, and from the insufficient government supports affecting poor people, working-class white women are increasingly encouraged to give up their babies to infertile middle-class white women.

Policies for "Unfit" Mothers: Working-Class African-American Women

Working-class African-American women, especially those who live in poverty, encounter markedly different treatment. In this section, I emphasize working-class African-American women's experiences not because I see these experiences as reflecting some sort of essential blackness, but because this group's experiences are constructed as normative for African-Americans as a collectivity by dominant groups. Whereas working-class white women's fitness for motherhood is measured against the assumed norms of middle-class white women, African-American women experience a reversal of this process. Specifically, working-class African-American women's experiences are stereotyped and labelled as deviant from

those of middle-class white women and are simultaneously considered normative for African-American women as a collectivity. In policy discussions of reproduction, middle-class African-American women are compared not to middle-class white women, but to working-class African-American women, when they are rendered visible at all.[4]

Controlling both the biological reproduction and mothering experiences of working-class African-American women has long been essential to maintaining a racialized American nationalism. In prior eras, a combination of a need for cheap, unskilled labor and the political powerlessness of black populations worked to produce population policies that encouraged African-American women to have many children. Because they did not require costly training and could be easily fired, such children cost employers little. In Southern states, for example, school years for African-American children were often shorter and adjusted to allow them to work in agriculture. Because they were denied education and social welfare benefits routinely extended to other groups, they cost the state little. Black children were viewed as expendable.

The post-World War II political economy changed all this. The mechanization of agriculture, industrial relocation out of inner-city areas, and other economic trends fostered a decreasing demand for low-skilled labor (Squires 1994). Instead, the so-called postindustrial economy required higher skilled labor requiring expensive investments in schooling and health care. During this same period, African-Americans gained political rights unavailable prior to the passage of the Civil Rights Act and Voting Rights Act in the early 1960s (see, e.g., Amott's 1990 discussion of African-American women and Aid to Families with Dependent Children) that allowed them to benefit from entitlement programs long enjoyed by whites. From the perspective of employers, a large African-American population with political rights of full citizenship became both economically unfeasible and politically dangerous. Since fewer African-Americans were needed, population policies, ideological constructions of African-American women, and the structure of social institutions combined to discourage working-class and poor African-American women from having children.

Providing lavish services to combat infertility for white middle-class women while withholding family planning services except sterilization from poor African-American women reflects contemporary population policies emerging within the logic of eugenics thinking. Currently, poor women and women of color are often *discouraged* from having children and are rewarded by government policy if they do so. In the context of lack of abortion services, government-funded permanent sterilization often becomes one of the few viable methods of birth control. The introduction of Norplant and Depo-Provera as reversible quasi-sterilization methods illustrates how population policies directed at African-American women reflect notions of their seeming unfitness to be mothers. Ideological constructions of African-American women also foster a climate in which it is claimed that they make bad mothers and thus are irresponsible if they reproduce. Long-standing images of African-American women as matriarchs or "unfit" mothers are now joined by newly emerging images that portray them as sexually irresponsible, as abusive mothers, and/or as welfare queens. Building on stereotypes of people of African descent and women as being less intellectual, more impulsive, and more emotional than whites, the image of the welfare queen in particular provides a context for quasi-coercive population policies such as Norplant and Depo-Provera. Ironically, images designed for middle-class African-American women, especially high-achieving professionals, also perpetuate views of African-American women as unfit mothers. By choosing to remain childless, such women are seen as being selfish, hoarding resources, being overly aggressive and unfeminine, and thinking only of themselves. Moreover, these new "black lady" overachievers, as Wahneema Lubiano describes them, are simultaneously constructed as affirmative-action hires, the middle-class unworthy recipients of government favors that parallel their less affluent welfare queen sisters. Within this nexus of images, while both middle-class and working-class African-American women can be constructed as the enemy within, whose reproduction or lack of it threatens American national interests, working-class and poor African-American women remain most vulnerable to attacks that result from this logic.

In this climate, where African-American women are constructed as unfit mothers, social institutions that they encounter take on a particularly punitive cast. Black working-class and poor mothers are often employed, yet are severely disadvantaged—child care remains hard to find, health benefits are limited for those in part-time or seasonal employment, and lack of job security makes it difficult to plan. A history of racial segregation mean that working-class African-American women encounter limited opportunities in their own education, housing, employment, access to health care, access to quality schools and recreational facilities for their children.

New Realities

If the nation-state is conceptualized as a national family, with the traditional family ideal structuring normative family values, then standards used to assess the contributions of family members in heterosexual, married-couple households with children become foundational for assessing group contributions to national well-being overall. The United States may be in an important historical moment where the logic of eugenics is being appropriated by interest groups who aim to reconstruct the American national family to its former glory. In understanding these new realities, several themes are of special significance.

First, the range of reproductive choices available to white women could not have occurred without the exploitation of the labor of African-American women and of other women of color. As women of the desirable group, middle-class white women have long depended on the labor of poor women and women of color in order to fulfill their responsibilities as mothers. Historically, for example, African-American women served as child care workers and performed the domestic labor that allowed middle-class white women to maintain their social positions as fit mothers. These traditional functions are more recently being taken over by new "employable mothers," namely, undocumented immigrant women of color. In her analysis of undocumented Latinas, Grace Chang notes that in the past, analyses of immigration retained a focus on male migrant laborers who allegedly stole jobs from "native" American workers. Since the mid-1980s, this concern has shifted to an emphasis on how immigrants impose a heavy welfare burden on American "natives." As Chang observes, "Men as job stealers are no longer seen as the immigrant problem. Instead, immigrant women as idle, welfare-dependent mothers and inordinate breeders of dependents are seen as the great menace". In this context, the treatment of undocumented Latina mothers and other women who lack the benefits of American citizenship closely resembles historical patterns of regulation of African-American mothers. In these cases, the notion of nonwhite mothers as employable exists alongside prevailing views that maternal employment harms children's development.

Second, the connection between welfare-state capitalism and perceived national interests remains significant, especially regarding women of varying race, social class, and citizenship groups. The welfare state mediates the conflicting demands placed on all women. On the one hand, social norms encourage women to remain in the home in order to care for their children and thus reproduce and maintain the labor force. But on the other hand, these same norms encourage women across social classes to perform traditionally female low-wage work in the paid labor force, such as teaching, secretarial work, and domestic work. By encouraging and subsidizing some women to remain at home in order to nurture the current future workforce while forcing others into low-wage work, the welfare state uses race, social class and citizenship differences among women to resolve this conflict. Working-class women of color of varying citizenship statuses bear the brunt of capitalist development. Such women are simultaneously engaged in low-wage work as paid employees doing the reproductive labor for families other than their own.

Third, new reproductive technologies are emerging as central to reorganizing the experiences of all women with motherhood. Working with longstanding patterns of race and social class in the United States, these technological advances fragment the meaning of motherhood. The proliferation of reproductive technologies in the post-World War II era has allowed the splitting of motherhood into three categories: genetic, gestational, and social motherhood. Genetic mothers are those who contribute the genetic material to another human being. Gestational mothers are those who carry the developing fetus in utero until birth. Social mothers care for children actually born. Traditional views of motherhood forwarded by the traditional family ideal present one middle-class white woman as fulfilling all three functions, assisted by domestic servants. But new reproductive technologies have made it possible for women to specialize in one of these mothering categories. With the growing technological ability to make distinctions among genetic motherhood, gestational motherhood, and social motherhood, African-Americans, Latinas and other women of color become candidates for gestational motherhood, supplementing and perhaps even supplanting white working-class women's participation as genetic and gestational mothers.

Fourth, the mother glorification targeted toward middle-class white women coexists with a heterogeneous collection of social policies designed to retain the image of motherhood as vitally important for all women while simultaneously discouraging selected groups of women from becoming mothers because they fail to attain the standards of "real" mothers. For example, mid-1990s phenomena such as the assault on affirmative action policies in higher education and the workplace, the passage of the 1996 Personal Responsibility and Work Opportunity and Reconciliation Act, which effectively abolished AFDC by placing it under the supervision of fifty individual states, the emergence of increasingly strident anti-immigration rhetoric in public discourse, and the increasing privatization of schools, health care, and selected public services can all be seen as part of an overarching framework designed to maintain differences between fit and unfit mothers. But the rhetoric of mother glorification must be tempered with a long look at how children are actually treated in the United States. Children were disproportionately hurt by social policies of the 1980s and have become the most impoverished age group in the United States. In 1974, 15 percent of American children lived below the poverty line. By 1986, 21 percent did so—a 40 percent increase in just twelve years. Approximately 40 percent of African-American and Latino children live in poverty. Yet despite these startling statistics, infertility continues to be presented as a major public health issue affecting large numbers of Americans.

Finally, the emergence of new family forms in the United States has the potential of either supporting or challenging the traditional family ideal and the entire edifice of population polices that it sanctions. For example, growing support for the categories of "biracial" and "multiracial" in the U.S. Census speaks to newly emerging family forms that defy boundaries of race. Of particular interest are the white mothers raising biracial or multiracial children, through either adoption or biological reproduction. How are we to interpret current efforts to include multiracial categories as part of government data? Are the efforts at reclassification an effort to make such children honorary whites with all the benefits that accrue to white middle-class children? Or are the efforts designed to deconstruct a system of racial classification that routinely distributes privileges based on such classification? In a similar fashion, the emergence of families organized around gay and lesbian couples with children raises similar challenges to the traditional family ideal and the complex social structures it simultaneously shapes and sanctions. The very existence of these emerging family forms and their increasing legitimacy within state agencies means that the bedrock of family as defined by the traditional family ideal can no longer serve in the same way as the glue linking systems of race, gender, class, nationality, and heterosexist oppression. What comes of these challenges remains to be seen.

Notes

1. Racial formations in the United States demonstrate a shift from theories of race based on the racist biology that characterized nineteenth-century science, and toward a cultural racism more useful in defending current racial practices. But this means neither that racism based in biology has atrophied nor that it may not take on new forms. Troy Duster (1990) offers an unsettling argument concerning the reracialization of genetic arguments in contemporary American scholarship. Duster argues that advances in genetic research show that genetic disorders are distributed differently through different racial/ethnic groups. Duster queries, "The importance of race and ethnicity in cultural history has refueled the old logic to give rise to a new question: if genetic disorders are differentially distributed by race and ethnicity, why aren't other human traits and characteristics?" (p. 3).

2. Scholarship on the welfare state reveals how state policies reflect race-, class-, and gender-specific concerns. For analyses of how social policies have had differential impact on different groups, see Mink 1990, Nelson 1990, and Gordon 1994. Gilkes 1983 and Brewer 1994 provide analyses of how race frames state policy.

3. This process is neither historical nor confined to the United States. For discussions of similar population policies, see Heng and Devan's (1992) analysis of Singapore and Kuumba's (1993) discussion of South Africa.

4. Middle-class African-American women occupy a peculiar place in the nexus of population policies targeted toward African-American women as a group. On one hand, these women clearly have the economic resources to care for their children. In this sense, African-American middle-class children will not be drains on nation-state resources. But at the same time, these children are not of the "right" genetic stock to become symbolic of the nation. They compete with the "rightful heirs" of the nation—its white children—for resources. The analogy between the king's rightful heir and the king's bastard son seems apt here—both are seen as being part of the royal family, but their status is not the same. As mothers, African-American professional women who excel in their careers and who are mothers may be cast as "bad" mothers because they do not stay at home with their children.

References

A list of references is available in original source.

Contraceptive Jelly on Toast and Other Unintended Consequences of Sexuality Education

by Mariamne H. Whatley and Elissa R. Henken

A doctor reported that he had fitted a 23-year-old woman with a diaphragm. When she returned to the doctor for a check-up, the doctor noticed a purple stain on the center of the diaphragm. When he asked the woman about it, she told him it was a stain from the jelly she used with it. He asked her what brand she was using and she answered, "Smucker's grape jelly."

A first reaction to this story is usually laughter at the punch line, followed by disbelief about this being a "true" story, and amazement that, if it is true, anyone could make such a ridiculous mistake. On one level, many of the stories in this chapter can be read as focusing on the ignorance of the client/patient, but another more useful reading is that the education/health care practitioner was at fault for presenting information in ways that facilitated misunderstandings. There are many ways, which will be explored throughout this book, in which folklore can help sexuality and health educators in their practice. This chapter focuses on one potential role of folklore—to point out the nature of errors, whether they have actually occurred or not, that can be made in educational processes. The following stories focus on attempts at contraception, so the consequences of the misunderstandings are serious—unplanned pregnancies. While the ungainly attempts are often presented humorously in the story, the results are often devastating for the woman (and man) involved. The opening story and the one following were reported by a student who heard them on her father's AutoDigest tapes of an obstetrics/gynecology conference. It is important to note that even though these stories were collected from a seemingly reliable source, they have all the earmarks of contemporary legends.

A doctor reported that another woman had been using a diaphragm, but had immediately become pregnant. When he examined the diaphragm, he found the center was cut out. Because there had been no center when she had been fitted for the diaphragm, she cut it out of hers.

A similar story was published in the journal *Hospital Pharmacy* in 1987. A student nurse reported that she had been teaching new mothers about child care and contraception:

> After giving one of the lectures on contraception, a fifteen-year-old, who had received no prenatal care, reacted in astonishment to what I said about how contraceptive jellies should be used. After explaining how the jellies needed to be applied vaginally prior to intercourse, the mother realized for the first time how she had become pregnant. She had purchased a contraceptive jelly from a retail pharmacy and routinely had been placing it on her toast at breakfast! She said that she had received no instruction on how the jelly was supposed to be used and just thought that jellies were for toast—not for intravaginal use. (Cohen, 1987, p. 956)

Although this version was reported in 1987, the story is very persistent and made a big comeback ten years later. A reader wrote to advice columnist Ann Landers (Landers, 1997):

> It seems a woman has filed suit against a small mom-and-pop pharmacy because she purchased a tube of contraceptive jelly, spread it on a piece of toast and ate it. She then had unprotected sex, believing she was "safe" and became pregnant.
>
> The contraceptive came with instructions, but the woman says the pharmacist should have put a specific warning on the box saying it wasn't effective if eaten. She is asking for a half million dollars, even though she is quoted as saying, "Who has time to sit around reading directions these days, especially when you're sexually aroused?"

One contributor to *FoafTale* News reported that this story of oral use of contraceptive jelly was circulating widely in May and June, 1997, through the media and Internet (Hiscock, 1998). The same contributor also reported an e-mail of a first-person narrative by a public health nurse that had been forwarded to him. When a pregnant woman is asked by the nurse about her contraceptive practices, the woman shows the nurse "vaginal foaming pills (about the size of a Necco wafer). She said, 'I've been taking them just like the doctor told me—every time I have sex I take one. They're hard to swallow but I manage'" (Hiscock, 1998, p. 17). Describing the pills as resembling a specific candy does help explain some of the confusion; however,

these may be more accurately described as about the size of a thumb joint and about one-half inch thick.

Another story, told as a legend or a joke, relates that a woman became pregnant after the birth control pill kept rolling out of her vagina. This is the reverse of the jelly on toast story, for in this case a woman uses vaginally what should be taken orally. Actually, hormones are well absorbed vaginally, so the vagina could work as a delivery site for birth control pills, though it would certainly not be recommended. A story reportedly told by someone working in a pharmacy also illustrates another misunderstanding of how oral contraceptives work:

> A woman kept coming in to get her birth control pills at a point where she ought to be only halfway through with them. The pharmacy workers finally got suspicious and asked her if she was taking one a day like she was supposed to and she replied, "Yes, and so is my husband."

One student reported watching a documentary on television in which young teenagers discussed sex:

> Some of the girls said they knew of other girls who would steal one birth control pill from a sister's pack. They would take the pill before having sex and think they were protected from becoming pregnant.

There are also similar condom stories. For example, one student reported that after a nurse demonstrated how to put a condom on, using her hand as a model, a couple used it by carefully covering the man's hand. This mistake was discovered after the woman became pregnant. As far as we know there have been no similar mishaps after the popular demonstrations of condom strength and elasticity that involve the educator's pulling a condom on over his or her head.

Rather than focusing on the likelihood that any of these incidents could really have happened or on the lack of understanding by the people involved of reproductive anatomy, health educators should reflect on what these examples say about contraceptive education in clinical and other settings. Many of these stories are examples of what Greenberg (1985) has named "iatrogenic health education disease," the condition in which health education has made learners less healthy. Certainly, health education that results in a woman eating contraceptive jelly and becoming pregnant would fit this definition. In the diaphragm stories, it is clear that careful and thorough explanations, with more realistic assumptions about the common understandings of terms such as jelly, could have prevented these mistakes. A description of the function of the spermicidal jelly would have made it clear both that grape jelly would be ineffective and that the jelly would need to be placed vaginally or in the diaphragm, not on toast. Even a brief explanation of the way a diaphragm works would have prevented a woman from assuming that a fitting ring was the model for an effective contraceptive. One of the clear messages sexuality educators should get from these stories is that education about contraceptives needs to be specific, concrete, and as literal as possible. If a woman were actually handed a tube of spermicide, shown how to apply it to a diaphragm (not a fitting ring), and helped to insert it vaginally (in a class, this can be done on a plastic model, though in clinical settings, the woman should get a chance to insert it in herself to gain assurance that it is in correctly), it is unlikely that any of the above errors could be made. An explanation of how to use the vaginal tablet, rather than "Use one just before sex," would be much more effective. Because these are sold over the counter, however, a purchaser would not have to see a health care practitioner, who might give some instructions and explanations. As the Ann Landers story points out, people do not always read instructions, due to low literacy, not being able to read English, too small print, assuming they know what to do, or just being in a hurry. Most people would agree that the purported lawsuit against the pharmacy is inappropriate, but it is a strong reminder to pharmacists about their potential role in health education. Explanations of how oral contraceptives work in a woman's body should certainly keep anyone from assuming that a man should take them along with his partner or that a woman should just take one before intercourse. While a model of a penis is not necessary for a condom demonstration, it is important to note that the banana, or whatever item is used, does represent a penis. Even if the previous examples are rare or even totally apocryphal, other problems could be prevented by this concrete approach. For example, a demonstration may prevent the mishap of applying so much spermicide that the compressed diaphragm flies out of the woman's fingers. In all areas of health and sexuality education, the same rules apply: be specific and concrete, with appropriate visuals and hands-on demonstrations.

Language is also very important. For example, for some people the term "contraceptive" is so closely associated with oral contraceptives (the Pill) that referring to any contraceptive may connote oral use, a meaning reinforced by such terms as jelly, cream, and tablet. Another story, recounted by a folklorist, while clearly in the joke genre, also reveals an important point about language:

> By the way, I recall from my adolescent years a story about condoms. A couple wishing to avoid pregnancy was told by their doctor to use them. A few months later they returned and told the doctor that pregnancy had occurred even though they had used condoms. When the doctor asked, "Did you follow the directions on the package?" the husband replied, "It said 'place on organ,' but we don't have an organ so we put them on the piano."

This joke/story probably served as a means for young adolescent boys to check out their own and others' knowledge about condoms and "organs," but is unlikely to have been accepted as a true story. However, it is a reminder that we can never make assumptions about the vocabulary of learners, either their knowledge of technical terms or their use of certain slang or euphemisms. It is important to make sure everyone is talking about the same thing. Often health educators will ask students to list all the words they can think of for penis or vagina or other relevant terms. Once the list is generated, they can then suggest that everyone use the same specific term (usually the correct medical or anatomical term, but in some cases it may work better to use the most common slang term). In any case, it would be clear what an individual meant when using a certain term. If an educator is unclear about what a slang word means, it is better to ask than to try to appear cool and knowledgeable, while actually being wrong. For example, in parts of the South, *cock* refers to female rather than male genitalia (Cassidy, 1985). Slang terms are very specific culturally and historically. By using the term "cool" above, we were assuming a certain common understanding of a term that, in fact, may be very out of fashion with certain age groups or meaningless for certain cultural groups. It is better to ask them to clarify a term or to say, "I think it means this but I'm not sure, so let me know if I'm wrong." They will.

Health care practitioners who complain about "noncompliance" may be neglecting their own failures to provide the kind of information that would help someone follow through on a prescription or recommendation. By collecting folklore such as these legends and using them to analyze failures of educational practice, health educators may create much more effective communication.

'The Pill' May Not Mix Well with Other Drugs

by Judith Willis

A young newlywed had been taking birth control pills several months in the early 1970s when she developed a bladder infection. She consulted her doctor, who prescribed an antibiotic. The infection cleared up quickly. But nine months later she gave birth to her first child.

Today, with proper communication between physician and patient, the inadvertent pregnancy in this mythical example would be far less likely to occur. Many interactions between oral contraceptives (OC's) containing both estrogen and progestogen and other drugs are now well-known and included in both the physician and patient labeling of the pill.

Such interactions can not only diminish the contraceptive's effectiveness, but also increase or decrease the potency of the other drug. Both those who take oral contraceptives and those who don't may find it interesting to look at what is known about the how and why of such OC-drug interactions.

Some drugs decrease contraceptive effectiveness apparently because they increase the metabolism of the contraceptives. This means that the liver breaks down the hormones in the contraceptive faster, and they are eliminated from the body more quickly. Thus, the levels of estrogen and progestogen are reduced, sometimes so much that they no longer suppress ovulation. Breakthrough bleeding is often a symptom of this reduced effectiveness. This type of interaction is of even more concern with the very-low-dose contraceptives, since the level of hormones they contain is already low.

The first drug with which that type of OC interaction was reported was rifampicin, used to treat tuberculosis. In the early 1970s, medical journals reported breakthrough bleeding and contraceptive failure in OC users taking rifampicin. Alerted to this effect with one drug, physicians over the next few years noted the possibility of this type of decreased effectiveness with many different drugs. They include:

- antibiotics such as isoniazid, ampicillin, neomycin, penicillin V, tetracycline, chloramphenicol, sulfonamides, nitrofurantoin, and griseofulvin,
- barbiturates,
- anticonvulsants such as phenytoin and primidone, and
- the anti-inflammatory phenylbutazone.

Also, some analgesics, tranquilizers and anti-migraine preparations may have this type of interaction. OC users taking such drugs are advised *to use an additional form of contraception until they discontinue therapy with the second drug.*

When it comes to the other side of the coin—OC's affecting the potency of other drugs—knowledge about such interactions is more limited. But again, the how and why seem to be tied to the way the drug is metabolized; that is, changed into a form that can be eliminated from the body.

Some drugs are metabolized in the liver primarily by oxidation, and thus are excreted through the kidneys rather than the bowels. These drugs appear to be metabolized more slowly in OC users, according to research by a group of scientists headed by Darrell Abernathy, M.D., Ph.D., and reported in the April 1, 1982, *New England Journal of Medicine.* The researchers reported that long-term use of low-dose estrogen-containing OC's may cause diazepam (Valium), a benzodiazepine anti-anxiety drug, to stay in the body longer. This means that OC users may require lower dosages of diazepam and other drugs that are metabolized in the same way. However, since not all people metabolize drugs in the same way, the patient should be monitored by her physician to see if the dose should be adjusted. Other drugs that may stay in the body longer because of OC's include: other benzodi-

From *FDA Consumer,* March 1987, Government Printing Office, by the U.S. Department of Health and Human Services.

azepines such as chlordiazepoxide (Librium); hydrocortisone; antipyrine; phenothiazines; and some tricyclic antidepressants.

In contrast, some drugs that are excreted mainly through the bowels (and at times partly through the kidneys) may be eliminated more quickly in OC users. Even though the metabolism of some benzodiazepines may be slowed by OC's, there are other benzodiazepines (such as lorazepam, oxazepam and tamazepam) whose metabolism may be enhanced, so they may be excreted more quickly in women taking birth control pills. However, information on exactly how such drugs interact with OC's is scarce. In an article in the September 1982 issue of *Obstetrics & Gynecology,* Abernathy reported that, in women using low-dose OC's containing estrogen for more than three months, acetaminophen (Tylenol) was eliminated more quickly than in non-OC users. The authors theorized that this increase in the speed at which the drug is eliminated from the body might offer some protection against liver toxicity in cases of acetaminophen overdose.

But OC users taking only the recommended dosages of acetaminophen might need a higher dosage than non-OC users. Again, because response to medication is so individual and because different combinations and dosages of estrogen and progestogen may have different effects, OC users should consult their physicians about any deviation from recommended dosages.

OC users taking other drugs may need to have the dosage monitored and possibly adjusted for a variety of reasons. Some epileptics may need a change in the dosage of an anticonvulsant drug they are taking, depending on the type of OC they're using. But other women taking the same combination may not need the dosage changed. The exact reason for this "iffiness" is not known, but it may be because OC-related changes in fluid retention could influence the frequency of seizures. Because of these difficulties, many doctors recommend that women taking anticonvulsants rely on another contraceptive than birth control pills.

A similar recommendation is often made for diabetics, because OC's may cause blood sugar levels to rise. If a diabetic does take birth control pills, she should be closely monitored to see if there needs to be a change in her diabetes medication.

Hypertension can be a problem in women on birth control pills, and elevated blood pressure has been known to occur in women not hypertensive before taking OC's. To complicate matters further, some of the medications used to control high blood pressure do not work the same way in those on The Pill as in non-OC users. In particular, the blood pressure drug guanethidine often does not adequately control hypertension in OC users. OC users taking blood pressure drugs need to be more carefully monitored.

In addition to interactions with drugs, OC's may also interact with certain vitamins. Labeling for birth control pills notes that OC users may have disturbances in the metabolism of tryptophan, an amino acid. Although such a disturbance is not considered cause for undue concern, it may result in a deficiency of pyridoxine (vitamin B6). Whether that is a cause for concern is not known. Also, in rare cases, megaloblastic anemia, a certain type of anemia due to insufficient pyridoxine, has been reported in OC users. In addition, levels of folic acid—one of the B vitamins—may be lower in women on The Pill.

Preliminary studies have shown that vitamin C may increase the bio-availability of estrogens. This means that women using birth control pills who take large doses of vitamin C may be risking increased side effects from the pill's estrogen. For this reason, some experts suggest that OC users take no more than 1,000 milligrams of vitamin C daily.

Some laboratory test results can be altered by OC use. The pathologist or other lab personnel should be informed when a woman undergoing lab tests is taking birth control pills so that this can be taken into consideration when evaluating the tests. Tests that are altered by OC use include those measuring: liver function, coagulation (clotting), thyroid function, blood triglycerides and phospholipid (fats) concentrations, serum folate, glucose tolerance, and plasma levels of some trace minerals.

In most young, healthy women, the effects of taking other drugs while using oral contraceptives are no cause for alarm and should not keep women who can benefit from the contraceptive effectiveness of OC's from taking them. The effects of OC-drug interactions may vary greatly from woman to woman. Yet women should be aware of the possibility of such interactions and tell their doctor if they are taking birth control pills so that other therapy can be properly coordinated.

Eight New Nonhormonal Contraceptive Methods for Men

by Elaine Lissner

Can you think of a male contraceptive other than the condom and vasectomy? Probably not, and for good reason: though more than eight new methods exist, some of them ready to use, none have been publicized. The methods range from simpler, safer, less surgical vasectomy to ancient "folk" methods which have performed well under scientific scrutiny. They are:

#1 No-scalpel Vasectomy According to Dr. Douglas Huber, recent medical director of the Association for Voluntary Surgical Contraception, "The no-scalpel vasectomy technique is the way all vasectomies should be done. If a vasectomy can be accomplished with this minimal surgery, then any surgeon doing more surgery should justify why more is necessary."

No-scalpel vasectomy, which has been performed for 4-8 million men in China and more than 1500 men in the rest of the world, involves gently poking and stretching a small opening in the scrotal skin rather than cutting the skin. Each vas deferens (sperm duct) is then blocked just as in a standard vasectomy. No-scalpel vasectomies bleed less and heal faster than standard vasectomies; they also eliminate the need for stitches. A list of U.S. physicians who perform no-scalpel vasectomy can be obtained from the Association for Voluntary Surgical Contraception at (212) 561-8000.

#2 Permanent Contraception by Injection In this experimental method, an injection of chemicals is used to close off the vas deferens, rather than cutting it surgically.

#3 Potentially Reversible Contraception by Injectible vas Deferens Plug Tests in China in over 512,000 men have shown a 98% effectiveness rate, and all the men who have had their plugs removed for at least a year have regained fertility. Encouraged by these results, the World Health Organization recently started tests in ten men. Continued success will reportedly lead to a trial in 3500 men around the world (and availability in some parts of the world within two years).

#4 Potentially Reversible Contraception by Surgically Implanted vas Deferens Plug Here, a soft silicone plug, or "Shug," is implanted in the vas deferens in an operation similar to vasectomy. The Shug's main advantage over injectible plugs is its two-plugs-in-one design, which gives it the potential to be more leak-free. Any sperm which leak past the first plug are likely to stay in the space between the plugs rather than continuing on their course. Currently being studied on men in the Chicago area, the Shug is proceeding slowly but steadily.

#5 Temporary Injectible Contraception The interior of the vas deferens is coated with a sperm-killing solution that keeps its effects for up to five years and can be reversed before then with a simple injection. Fertility can be restored at any time. This method has been completely safe and effective in ten years of animal trials. Human trials are beginning in India, but testing in the United States is stalled partly because the necessary polymer has not been sent to the National Institutes of Health.

#6 Wet Heat Method The deleterious effect of heat on male fertility has been known since the time of Hippocrates. Much as aspirin was "discovered" in the 1800s from a bark that Native Americans had long been accustomed to chewing to relieve pain, heat methods are now being "discovered" as a new form of male contraception. In this method, the testes are bathed in hot water every night for three weeks. Effectiveness goes up with increased temperature (hot tub temperature is not enough). At the recommended temperature, 116 degrees Fahrenheit, forty-five minutes per day provides contraceptive effect for six months. Although 116 degrees may sound very hot, one man has reported that this temperature is actually more comfortable on the testes than on any other part of the body.

Heat methods should be used in conjunction with sperm count checks (unless, for example, the heat method is just being used to enhance another method such as condoms or diaphragms). Sperm count can be checked easily at a doctor's or urologist's office.

#7 Artificial Cryptorchidism ("Jockey Method")
Special jockey shorts are worn during the day to hold the testes inside the inguinal canal (the same tube to which the testes retract naturally during cold or dangerous conditions.) This raises the testes to body temperature, thereby achieving the heat effect. Men appear to be about equally divided between those who find it a strange feeling and those who wouldn't mind it. Some men have expressed concern that this method would cause "jock itch," but this problem has not arisen for volunteers.

#8 Ultrasound Method
Ultra-short sound waves (the same type used by physical therapists to heal injuries) are applied to the testes for ten minutes once every six months, efficiently achieving the heat effect.

Ultrasound should be used only after knowing all the details, as it may also be a permanent method in much greater doses.

All of these methods are nonhormonal (and thus not as prone to complicated side effects). Two of the methods (artificial cryptorchidism and wet heat) require little or no doctor intervention and could be put to use almost immediately. In addition to providing self-determination to men, any of these methods would improve the health, economic status and survival rates of women in countries (including the United States) where inadequate medical care makes many female methods unsafe or unavailable.

Do you wonder why you've never heard of these? In addition to the hurdles which face all contraceptive development, research bias has played a large part. In the past, funding agencies have found reasons not to fund research on male contraceptives, such as claiming that men are not committed to contraception (even though vasectomy makes up 12% of the world's contraceptive use) and that new male methods shouldn't be developed because they don't prevent the spread of HIV (even though new female methods such as Norplant don't either). Simple methods with low profit-margins have re-

---

If You Want to Use These Methods

The only methods which are "ready to go" are wet heat, artificial cryptorchidism and no-scalpel vasectomy.

No-scalpel vasectomy is a small improvement on vasectomy. However, if you or someone you know is considering a vasectomy, this is the way to do it. To get a list of physicians who perform no-scalpel vasectomies, call the Association for Voluntary Surgical Contraception's general number at (212)561-8000. No-scalpel vasectomy is even safer and less invasive than the already safe vasectomy procedure.

Wet-Heat method and artificial cryptorchidism ("jockey method") are in some sense ready to use—if you are willing to be your own researcher, method user, doctor and critical thinker all rolled into one. Neither of these methods is in widespread use or well-known to doctors. Hopefully, in the near future men will be able to go to their doctors for an ultrasound treatment or for a "do's and don'ts" manual for using the other heat methods. However, until that time men and women who use these methods must take full responsibility for read-

ing up, knowing what they're doing and making a fully informed choice.

If you are interested, start by reading the original paper, **"Frontiers in Nonhormonal Male Contraceptive Research."** Then go to a medical library and photocopy all the references in that citation on heat methods in general and the specific method you're interested in. Be certain to read the Kandeel and Swerdloff paper, even though it is very technical. **Contact the Male Contraception Information Project if you need more information.**

If you decide to use the wet heat method you'll have to experiment a bit to find a way to keep the water hot. Be creative. For example, modified old-style baby bottle warmers might work. If you come up with a good idea, let us know so we can pass it on. Regarding the use of hot tubs, you should know that it would take hours of hot-tubbing every day to produce contraceptive effect. That is why the wet heat method involves testes-only bathing at higher temperatures.

—Elaine Lissner
Male Contraception Information Project

ceived even less support. With funding levels so low, even supportive researchers couldn't accomplish much.

According to a 1990 committee convened by the Institute of Medicine/National Research Council, "Unless immediate steps are taken to change public policy, the choice of contraceptives in the United States in the next century will not differ appreciably from what it is today." However, many researchers and policymakers believe men don't care about contraception.

How can this be changed? Read up on the subject and make it one of your priorities, since research will increase only when public pressure is strong enough to provide incentive. Think about these methods, talk about them, and share this article with a friend. Bias is already fading, and with eight new methods in the wings, men and women don't need to wait any longer.

Abortion Fact Sheet

Young Women and Abortion

Young women belonging to the post-*Roe v. Wade* generations have never known illegal abortion. They tend to take abortion for granted, seeing it as something they're entitled to, not something to fight for. Although 52% of all women who seek abortions are under 25,[1] young women are often unaware of the obstacles to services that are created by restrictions on abortion.

Many Young Women Face Unplanned Pregnancies, Despite Increased Contraceptive Use Nationally, 9 in 10 sexually active women and their partners use a contraceptive method, although not always consistently or correctly.[2] 76% of women used contraception at first intercourse in the 1990s, compared with 50% before 1980.[3] But contraception is not fool-proof: 6 out of 10 women who seek abortions experienced contraceptive failure.[4]

Each year, almost one million teenage women—11% of all women aged 15–19 and 20% of those who have had sexual intercourse—become pregnant.[2] 78% of teen pregnancies are unplanned, accounting for ¼ of all accidental pregnancies annually.[2] Nearly 4 in 10 teen pregnancies (excluding miscarriages) end in abortion.[2] 52% of U.S. women obtaining abortions are younger than 25: Women aged 20–24 obtain 32% of all abortions, and teenagers obtain 20%.[1]

In Massachusetts in 1996, women under 25 accounted for 44% (12,843) of all abortions. Girls 14 and under had 148 abortions; 15–19 years had 4465; 20–24 years had 8230.[5]

Restrictions on Abortion Disproportionately Affect Teenage Women 39 states, including Massachusetts, have parental involvement laws on the books for abortion. These laws are enforced in 31 states.[6] 61% of teens having abortions do so with at least one parent's knowledge.[2] Yet 27 states and the District of Columbia have laws that specifically authorize a pregnant minor to obtain prenatal care and delivery services without parental notification,[7] representing a double standard in our commitment to young women's health.

Young Women Are Unaware of Obstacles to Health Care Created by Restrictions on Abortion In 1998 the Pro-Choice Public Education Project (PEP) conducted polls with young women across the country. The PEP poll found that a majority of young women support the availability of legal abortion and consider themselves pro-choice. However, young women are often unaware of how restrictions such as parental involvement laws, a shortage of providers, a lack of funding, biased counseling requirements and mandatory waiting periods can interfere with their ability to exercise the right to choose abortion. The *Real Women, Real Choices* Campaign produced by the Abortion Access Project is one local effort to educate young women and the public about the impact of these restrictions.

Source: *Abortion Access Project*

References

1. Alan Guttmacher Institute, "Induced Abortion," 2000.
2. Alan Guttmacher Institute, "Teen Sex and Pregnancy, 1998.
3. Alan Guttmacher Institute, "Contraceptive Use," 1998.
4. Alan Guttmacher Institute, "Facts in Brief: Induced Abortion," 1996.
5. Massachusetts Department of Public Health Bureau of Health Statistics Research & Evaluation, 1997.
6. NARAL, *Who Decides: A State-by-State Review of Abortion and Reproductive Rights.* 1998.
7. Alan Guttmacher Institute, "Teenagers' Right to Consent to Reproductive Healthcare," 1997.

The Shortage of Abortion Providers

- 87% of all U.S. counties[1] and 95% of all rural U.S. counties have no abortion provider.[2]
- Half of all OB-GYN doctors who provide abortions are 50 years of age or older.[3]
- In 1983, 42% of all OB-GYN doctors offered abortion services; in 1995 only 33% did.[4]
- 2% of OB-GYNs perform the majority of abortions in the U.S.[4]
- Only 12% of OB-GYN residency programs require training in first trimester abortion.[5]
- Only 7% of OB-GYN residency programs require training in second trimester abortion.[5]
- Only 15% of chief residents in family medicine residency programs had clinical experience providing first trimester abortions.[6]
- 44 states have "physician only" provisions in their abortion laws which prevent qualified practitioners such as nurse-midwives, nurse practitioners, and physician assistants from performing abortions.[7]
- 7% of abortions are performed in hospitals, 4% are performed in private doctor's offices, 89% are performed in clinics.[1]
- Between 1992 and 1996 the number of U.S. hospitals providing abortions decreased by 18%.[1]
- There have been almost 2,400 reported instances of violence against abortion providers since 1977, including 7 murders and 16 attempted murders (actual instances are most likely higher).[8]
- Abortion is the only medical procedure with a "conscience clause" that allows medical providers to refuse to participate in the care of a patient.

References

1. S. K. Henshaw, "Abortion Incidence and Services in the United States, 2000," *Family Planning Perspectives,* 35:1. Jan/Feb 2003.
2. S. K. Henshaw, "Abortion Incidence and Services in the United States, 1995–96, *Family Planning Perspectives,* 30:6, 1998.
3. "Kaiser Family Foundation Media Briefing," 1995.
4. J. Hitt, "Who Will Do Abortions Here?" *New York Times Magazine,* January 18, 1998.

5. H. T. MacKay and A. P. MacKay, "Abortion Training in Obstetrics and Gynecology Residency Programs In the United States, 1991-1992," Family Planning Perspectives, 27: 112-115, 1995.
6. J. E. Steinauer et al., "Training Family Practice Residents in Abortion and Other Reproductive Health Care: A Nationwide Survey," *Family Planning Perspective* 29: 222–227, 1997.
7. National Abortion Federation, "The Role of Physician Assistants, Nurse Practitioners, and Nurse-Midwives in Providing Abortions," 1997.
8. National Abortion Federation, "NAF Violence & Disruption Statistics," 1999.

Who Has Abortions?

"There aren't 'women who have abortions' and 'women who have babies'. Those are the same women at different points in their lives."
Rachel Atkins, PA, MPH, Executive Director, Vermont Women's Health Center

Women of all ages, races, ethnic, economic and religious backgrounds have abortions for many different reasons every year; each reason is as compelling and legitimate as the next. Women have abortions because their contraceptive methods fail, because of their health, age, rape, because they cannot afford a child, or because they don't feel ready to become a parent at the time of the unplanned pregnancy.

- By the age of 46, 4 in 10 women in the US will have had at least one abortion.[1]
- 54% of women seeking abortions experienced contraceptive failure.[1]
- 61% of the women who have abortions have had at least one previous birth and 48% of these will have had at least one prior abortion.[1]
- 27% of women who have abortions and are open to disclosing their religion are Catholic and 43% are Protestants.[2]
- 41% of U.S. abortions are obtained by white women, 32% of all abortions are obtained by Black women, 20% by Hispanics, and 7% are obtained by other women of color.[2]
- 19% of women receiving abortions are 11–19 years old; 56% are between 20–30 years of age.[2]
- 57% of women who obtain abortions have family incomes under 200% of the poverty line. Low-income women are three times more likely to have abortions than those who are financially better off.[2]
- About 13,000 women have abortions each year following rape or incest.[1]
- 61% of minors who have abortions do so with at least one parent's knowledge; 45% of parents are told by their daughter. The great majority of parents support their daughter's decision to have an abortion.[3]

References

1. Facts in Brief. Induced Abortion," Alan Guttmacher Institute, 2001.
2. "Patterns in the Socioeconomic Characteristics of Women Obtaining Abortions in 2000–2001," Rachel K. Jones, Jacqueline E. Darroch and Stanley K. Henshaw, *Perspectives on Sexual and Reproductive Health* 34 (5) 2002.
3. Henshaw S. K. and Kost K., "Parental involvement in minors' abortion decisions," *Family Planning Perspectives,* 1992, 24 (5); 196–297 & 213.

The Bad Baby Blues

Reproductive Technology and the Threat to Diversity

by Lisa Blumberg

The public discourse we need has been stalled—even in the disability community—because when people discuss the implication of the new reproductive technology at all, they tend to do so within the framework of their views on abortion. Yet these issues transcend the abortion controversy.

It was my feminist leanings superimposed on my disability orientation that fueled my interest in the implications of reproductive technology. In 1980, a woman I worked with who was pregnant told me she was having amniocentesis. "I really don't want the test," she said. "I don't know what I'm supposed to do if there is a problem. I don't want to make a decision about having the child." When I asked why she was having it, she said, "I'm 37, and my doctor told me every expectant mother over 35 needs to have it. He wouldn't feel comfortable if I refused."

I just said "good luck" (as is usually the case, the test revealed nothing) without telling her that her doctor's stance made me uncomfortable. Until then, I thought that whether to have prenatal tests was a decision that prospective parents made for themselves, based on their own attitudes on pregnancy, disability, family life and a host of other things. Without being able to articulate why, I thought it was dangerous for a doctor to impose an obligation on a woman to learn beforehand whether her child might be disabled.

A few years later, I was a watching a news story on the merits of a predictive test for spina bifida. A woman explaining why she had gotten an abortion after test results had been positive said, "I defy any woman, no matter how much she wants a child, to continue a pregnancy after they show her a picture of a deformed baby and tell her that 'this is going to be yours.'"

I thought about that woman a lot. What concerned me was not so much the choice she made as the approach of her medical advisors. What a baby with an untreated medical problem looks like does not indicate what a person with a disability can become. Was it fair to urge people to make such a profound decision as to whether to bring a particular type of child into world on the basis of such a firsthand visceral response?

I started seeing articles in news magazines suggesting that if prenatal testing were used widely and women were then "willing" to abort fetuses found to be "defective," the incidence of children with certain types of disabilities could be significantly reduced.

The word "willing" always jumped out at me. Amniocentesis had originally been touted as a way to expand pregnant women's options, but now it seemed that women were expected to use the knowledge that could be gained by prenatal testing in a way that satisfied others.

In the past decade, prenatal testing has become a multi-billion dollar industry, with hundred of conditions now capable of pre-birth detection. Screening methods, some invasive and some not, are constantly evolving. Ultrasound, which used to just measure fetal growth and position, is giving way to targeted ultrasound which can zero in on a specific body part of the fetus such as the face. In most cases (but by no means in all) when a fetus is diagnosed as having a permanent disability, the pregnancy is terminated.

It is amazing that there has been scant public debate about this revolutionary new technology that allows us for the first time in all of human history to ascertain certain medical facts before one is even a person. Nothing that earlier generations dealt with during pregnancy was in any way comparable. In what varying ways can we react as individuals? How should we react as a society? What are legitimate public health goals? Can we view all people as equals and still feel that it is important to identify some traits prenatally? These are some of the questions that we must start addressing or else we could find ourselves drifting toward a society where there is little tolerance for either physical diversity or diversity in decision-making.

Disability activists need to be aggressive in initiating and framing the debate because our interests, along with those of women, are the most directly involved.

There are differences between ordinary abortion and selective abortion. Most abortion occurs because the pregnancy is unexpected and the prospect of parenthood itself is creating a crisis for the woman. Selective abortion, which constitutes a tiny fraction of all abortions, occurs when the pregnancy is planned but the fetus is perceived as having undesirable characteristics. In other words, selective abortion involves judgments about people. Indeed, women who abort due to fetal "defect" are often urged to get pregnant again quickly.

Almost everyone, regardless of how pro-choice they are, has views on where a moral line should be drawn in selective abortion. Where the difference in opinion arises is the positioning of that line. Many feminists express misgivings over abortion based on sex. Most medical ethnicists would oppose abortion based on eye color. The idea that a couple who share an inherited trait such as some types of deafness might want to end a pregnancy involving a fetus that did not have the same gene and "try again" out of the belief that their family will work better if all members have the same characteristics is controversial even in the disability community.

Without suggesting there should be restrictions on abortion, it is legitimate for disability activists to question the general public consensus that fetal disability is one of the "best" reasons for abortion—right up there with rape or incest and what right-to-lifers call "hard cases." It is not inevitable that prenatal diagnosis must change a wanted future baby into a "defective" fetus about which a decision must be made. As Adrienne Asch, a professor at Wellesley College has written,

"suppose Down syndrome, cystic fibrosis or spina bifida were depicted not as an incalculable, irreparable tragedy but as a fact of being human? Would we abort because of those conditions or seek to limit their adverse impact on life?"

The disability rights movement in the quarter century it has been in existence has been successful on some nuts-and-bolts access issues. Important civil rights laws have been passed. However, basic attitudes towards disability really have not changed. It is a premise of the movement that a person with a disability is limited more by society's prejudices than by the practical difficulties that may be created by the disability. Unfortunately, by and large, nondisabled people don't believe it. Most people, to the extent they must think about disability at all adhere to the medical model of disability. Under the medical model, a person's disability is seen to be the cause and sum of that person's problems, with the paramount question therefore being whether the impairment can be alleviated.

Nowhere is the medical model more entrenched than with medical professionals. And it is medical professionals, and in particular genetic counselors, who help prospective parents evaluate their options after prenatal diagnosis.

The role of genetic counselors is to give prospective parents advice about how their child's expected condition can affect people—so the parents can make an informed decision regarding whether to continue the pregnancy. Genetic counseling is intended to be "nondirective," and most counselors do refrain from telling their clients what their decision should actually be. However, when counselors provide prospective parents with merely a list of deficits their future child may have (or may not have, since the same diagnostic label can reflect itself in different individuals in widely disparate ways), they are only telling half of the story. The other half is how people cope with these limitations and what other factors may influence their lives.

Perhaps the most serious limitation of genetic counseling is that counselors rarely offer clients the opportunity to meet persons with disabilities similar to those their child might have or to talk with parents of disabled children. Indeed, some genetic counselors resist the idea out of the belief that this would increase the discomfort of their clients. Yet clients who did not want to accept the offer could just say so. We can and must urge that the sources of information people have access to within the genetic counseling process be broadened.

Persons affected by disability are the most qualified to provide insight on the lifestyle concerns that prospective parents will have after prenatal diagnosis. We cannot tell others what they can personally cope with, but we can tell them how it is for us—and we can share with them our individuality and the range of our views. We can suggest that it is alright to embark on an endeavor which sometimes may be hard, which may make one an outsider and where there are few signposts. We can point out that it is OK to do the unusual thing.

On a more general social level, consideration also needs to be given to how the emphasis on prenatal testing and the perceived need to make decisions after diagnosis affect people's relations with one another. A prominent newspaper columnist once described the reactions she got to her veto of her doctor's age-based recommendation that she have amniocentesis. She chose to forego the option of termination in the unlikely event the fetus was disabled, she said, because of the children she already had. She did not know how she could find the words to explain to them a decision not to have a child who might use a wheelchair or always need special guidance, she said, and still affirm for them her view that differences in people should be accepted.

She pointed out that this was not a snap judgment but something she had reflected upon at length. However, she said, people she thought knew her well dismissed her desire to contemplate older motherhood without prenatal tests with an "Oh, it must be because you're Catholic." She is, in fact, pro-choice.

The woman had hit upon something important. In an open letter to genetic counselors published in a professional journal, one woman described the aftermath for her family of a decision to end a pregnancy involving a fetus with Down syndrome. Her school-aged children disturbed by their parents' grief, asked what was so bad about this type of disability.

Their father, said the letter writer, then had to instruct the children on the realities of life with a "handicapped child"—or at least what he thought the realities were. He asked them to imagine what it would be like to be trying to cross a street and always get confused about whether red meant "go" or green meant "go."

Later, when the children were asked to write down their feelings about what had happened, the older one told how sad it had been, and said "the only good thing is not having a child like that in our family." One wonders how children specifically encouraged to see disability as an all-encompassing burden both for the person who has it and for others will interact with the people with noticeable disabilities that they will most certainly meet in life.

Genetic counselors should be urged to help parents who do decide to abort after prenatal diagnosis to find "disability neutral" ways to talk about their decision with children—discussions which focus on the limitations or competing priorities of the family, rather than on assumptions about the potential of people with disabilities.

Reproductive technology can be divisive. It can reinforce prejudices.

There is another side of prenatal testing though. At a conference designed to start a dialogue between disability rights activists and the medical community, I listened as a parent recounted how, after her first child died from Tay-Sachs, she chose to have Tay-Sachs screening in her subsequent pregnancies. All she wanted was children who would live, she said; and eventually she had them. She told us, "I was given an option which I would not otherwise have had—the option to have a family." Another woman with a family history of cystic fibrosis had a predictive test when she was pregnant because, if her child were affected, she wanted to get on a particular doctor's roster right away. There are people who do want the tests, and people who have benefitted from them.

However, it is one thing to acknowledge a couple's right to make a personal and private decision to use prenatal testing based on their own unique circumstances, it is quite another thing for there to be a general expectation that every pregnant woman over 35 will go on defect alert.

What scares me is not the individual decisions people make—although I may disagree with some of these decisions—but the fact that society has latched onto the new reproductive technology as a lead weapon in a simplistic war against "birth defects." It is chilling to read decisions in wrongful birth and wrongful life suits where judges opine that avoiding the births of disabled children is a social good. It is equally chilling to hear public health analysts debate whether the abortion rate of "defective fetuses" will be high enough to make state-sponsored prenatal programs cost effective and efficacious. The legislature of at least one state (Alabama, in a law first passed in the late 1970s) has declared it to be state policy "to encourage the prevention of birth defects and mental retardation through education, genetic counseling and amniocentesis . . ."(Section 22-lOA-l of the Alabama statutes).

How easily ignored is the ethical imperative placed on genetic counselors to be nondirective! And how easily blurred is the critical distinction between preventing persons from *having* disabilities and preventing persons *with* disabilities! Most frightening in my view, though, are the articles in legal and medical journals suggesting that carrying a disabled fetus to term constitutes "fetal abuse" on the part of the woman.

Ruth Hubbard, professor emeritus of Biology at Harvard, has written, "my problems with amniocentesis stem mostly from my concern about how it creates eugenic thinking. We act as if we can look at a gene and say 'Ah-ha, this gene causes this . . . disability' when in fact the interactions between the gene and environment are enormously complex. It moves our focus from the environmental causes of disabilities—which are terrifying and increasing daily—to individual genetic ones." This misplaced focus will not only result in individuals acquiring disabilities unnecessarily: it will undermine the status of people with disabilities, regardless of the origins of their disabilities, and of women.

The new reproductive technology represents a boon for some and terror for others.

It is startlingly new but it invokes feelings that are age-old. I believe that the public discourse that we need has been stalled—even in the disability community—because when people discuss the implication of the new reproductive technology at all, they tend to do so within the framework of their views on abortion. Yet these issues transcend the abortion controversy, even as they cut across both sides of that debate. Somehow, we must begin to think more creatively and learn to meld together different world views. It is only then that we will have the hope of solving the conundrums created by the new reproductive technology in ways that will respect the individuality of us all.

Discovering That You Are Infertile
One Woman's Experience
by Naomi Pfeffer and Anne Woollett

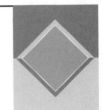

'Well,' they said, 'If you're going to have a baby you should start soon. You're not getting any younger you know.'

It took me a long time to decide that I wanted a child. I started thinking about it perhaps four years ago. I thought about it. I talked to other women. I listened to other women, to mothers and women without children. I found out about childcare arrangements. I thought about my job and how having a child would influence my work. I talked to the man I live with about a child and the effects one might have on our lives and on our relationship. We thought about when would be a good time to have a child. A baby born in the spring or summer would fit in well with my work.

April 1978   I put my cap away.

August 1978   We go away on holiday.

September 1978   Period two days late and breasts feel very tender. Are they normally tender just before my period? I become much more sensitive to my body. I live inside myself, my centre of gravity seems to be somewhere inside my uterus. I feel full, preoccupied, pleased that I might be pregnant. Then blood. No pregnancy. No baby. Perhaps next month.

1 October 1978   Perhaps next month.

30 October 1978   Blood, period, perhaps next month.

Why am I not getting pregnant? I begin to ask questions about my body. I've been taking my temperature for several months and I know that I am ovulating. How long does it normally take to get pregnant? I had assumed it could take up to six months and we have been trying for that time.

People reassure me. Sometimes it takes a long time. I'm given advice, information, details about how other people did it. I'm consoled, never mind, you'll make it. I'm trying to grapple with the idea that perhaps I won't make it. That idea creeps into my mind and I want to discuss it. But it's not something people are willing to discuss. A friend gets pregnant. It didn't take her long. She gets bigger. We discuss home confinements, epidurals, baby clothes, names. The world seems to be full of pregnant women, in the streets, holding babies, pushing prams. I'm surrounded by pregnant women. I read up on conception and find that infertility tests begin with an examination of the man's sperm.

4 December 1978 A friend, a nurse, arranges for us to have a sperm test. She provides us with the plastic container in its brown box, complete with instructions. 'The sperm must be produced by masturbation and reach the laboratory within four hours.' So today, the alarm goes off, I get up and make a cup of tea while Paul produces the specimen (how quickly we get into the jargon) and we rush it up the road to my friend who takes it to the lab at work.

The same friend arranges for us to attend the fertility clinic attached to the birth control clinic where she works. This is the same clinic I have been attending for years. The appointment is for after Christmas. We hope that I get pregnant over Christmas so that we won't need to keep the appointment. In the meantime I read up on infertility investigations.

5 January 1979 Our first appointment. Our medical histories are taken and we are both examined physically. We are seen by the consultant separately and then he talks to us together. 'Yes, everything seems quite normal.' But we are told that the sperm count is not terribly high, about thirty million, but high enough. Conception is possible with lowish sperm counts. Paul is told to give up his Y-fronts and to wear boxer shorts. This may increase the sperm count. I'm told that from my charts it looks as though I'm ovulating. I'm to continue taking my temperature but I must use the official forms rather than bits of graph paper. We are told that the next step is the post-coital test for which I am to make an appointment after my next period has started.

In some ways I feel quite elated after this first appointment. Our problem has been recognized and something is being done for us. We go straight to Marks and Spencers to buy the shorts, feeling that things had started, that we had acquired some kind of control.

7 January 1979 Period begins. I start my new temperature chart on the official form and ring the hospital to make an appointment for a post-coital test. At this particular clinic post-coital tests are done only on Tuesday mornings.

16 January 1979 First post-coital test. Attending the clinic is a depressing experience. A feeling of heaviness comes over me as I get closer to the clinic. I walk past the Family Planning clinic which I've attended for many years, down the corridor, past the row of women waiting their turn, to the door marked 'Subfertility Clinic'. I am redefined. I am now infertile, a woman with a problem. I announce my arrival, show my card with my new num-

ber on it. When I was fertile I was E34976. Now that I'm infertile, I'm 4032.

I wait my turn, sitting by myself, getting lower and lower, trying to fight the tears, and the feelings of self-pity. It is my turn. I go in and undress, and lie on the couch as instructed. A doctor, a woman, not the one we'd seen previously, inserts a speculum and then using a long rubber tube takes a sample of my cervical mucus. While I get dressed, she goes over to the other side of the room to examine my mucus under a microscope. 'I don't like this at all,' she says. I panic. What have I done? Hadn't we followed the instructions? I feel like a naughty child and I start to cry. The tears stream down my face and they continue unabated for the rest of my appointment. It transpires that what she doesn't like is the way the sperm and the mucus are getting along. There aren't enough sperm and they don't seem to be surviving well in my mucus. The doctor suggests that Paul sprays his testicles twice a day with cold water using one of those small indoor plant sprays. I don't know how he will take to that. If this spraying is such a good idea, then why hadn't the doctor suggested it on our first visit when Paul was there. That way at least he'd have been told directly. Now it was up to me to tell him. I'd brought his sperm to them and now I was taking bad news back home. My mucus didn't meet with her approval either. It was described on my form as 'tacky.' I am given a prescription for some oestrogen tablets and told to come back next month for another post-coital test.

There are lots of questions I want to ask. But the tears are still streaming down my face and I feel far too distraught to ask them. So I fumble around for my coat and bag and leave, while the doctor talks into her tape recorder about my case.

The force of my feelings and my inability to cope with them surprises me. During the next month I think a great deal about what happened and how I might cope in the future.

8 February 1979 Period starts. I feel depressed. I've got to go back to the clinic again. I ring up to make an appointment. Tuesdays arrive this cycle either on day eight or day fifteen of my cycle. The nurse thinks that I should go for the earlier date. I take the oestrogen tablets in preparation for the appointment.

16 February 1979 Second post-coital test. This time I feel much stronger. When the doctor appears and calls my name my stomach turns over. I force it back into place and I follow her into the room. I try to attend very carefully to what she does. Both the procedure and the doctor are the same as before. 'Well, the mucus is better, but the sperm are much the same as before.' She writes this down. I confess that Paul has refused to spray his testicles. The doctor points out that this is quite important as the present emphasis is to get the balance right between my mucus and his sperm. She suggests that I douche myself with a solution of bicarbonate of soda just before intercourse during the fertile days. This may make my vagina more conducive to the survival of Paul's sperm. I tell her that I am puzzled. Should I take the oestrogen tablets for my mucus to coincide with my clinic appointments or around ovulation as the two days are a week apart? Am I undergoing tests or treatment? The doctor says that, as she has an empty slot the following Tuesday, I can return for another post-coital so she can check the sperm and the mucus nearer to ovulation and after I have been using the douche. When she'd got the mucus right, she'd move on to other things, in particular, on to checking whether my tubes were unblocked. I'm even more puzzled. Why bother spending months checking my mucus if we then discover that my tubes are blocked? Why is only one test done at a time? I suppose I'd expected the investigation to be more like an MOT, where your car is given a whole range of tests at one go, and so you know what's wrong fairly rapidly. I tell the doctor how depressed I feel and that I'm worried that the investigations might destroy the relationship into which the child would be born. But any talk of emotions is brushed aside with the comment that some people feel quite heartened to think that treatment is being offered and that some couples are willing to go to the most elaborate extremes to have a child. I take the hint and shut up.

The clinic nurse shows me how to use the douche. She is much more cheery and tries to boost me by telling me how successful the doctor is at getting women pregnant.

The visit is over. The tension gradually subsides. At least this time I didn't collapse and I did manage to ask most of my questions. Now I have to go home with my collection of bits and pieces, instructions and information and prepare us for the next appointment.

I tell Paul what the doctor said about spraying his testicles, that he must do it to improve motility. He refuses. She made it clear that this is the next step in the proceedings. If he's not prepared to do it then we've reached a stalemate. Will they be prepared to continue the investigations if he's uncooperative? I feel cross with him. I've had to go to the clinic, go through the humiliating examinations and face the doctor and now he won't do his share. Later he agrees to try. Our sex life has taken on new elements: Paul sprays his balls twice a day; just before intercourse I pop into the bathroom and spend five minutes with the douche.

20 February 1979 Third post-coital test. My mucus has remained good and the number of sperm has im-

proved but their motility is still low. The doctor suggests I continue with the current regime of tablets, douche and spray. We now move on to other things: an X-ray of my Fallopian tubes. A form is filled in and I am told to ring the hospital's X-ray department when my next period arrives to make an appointment for day ten of my cycle. Via me, Paul is advised to see the semenologist, in six weeks' time.

26 February 1979 My fertile period is over and so the rites can cease for a while till next month. I can stop gently bullying Paul for a while, and relax. My friend has had her baby and I go to see it. I feel very thrilled for her. But after the excitement wears off I feel very sad. If I'd got pregnant quickly my baby would be almost due. I realize how much I'd stopped thinking about children and babies. My goal now is conception.

13 March 1979 Period starts. It is about three days late and I'd just begun to feel really hopeful. Yesterday I'd had moments of discomfort; and stomach ache but I'd ignored them till I saw the blood today. I feel weak and tearful. All the strength I thought I'd acquired just seems to have drained away. The discomfort serves as a reminder of my failure. So much for menstruation as a sign of femininity and the potential for motherhood. All it signifies to me is my failure.

21 March 1979 To the hospital for an HSG (X-ray of my Fallopian tubes). I had rung them beforehand to find out how long it would take and whether I would feel well enough to go back to work afterwards. I'm nervous so I've asked my friend to come with me. In the X-ray department, I undress completely and put all my clothes into a brown paper bag and cover myself with one of the hospital's green overalls. I'm shown into the X-ray room and told to sit on a long table with the equipment all around and above it. The doctor and radiographer, both men, arrive. My friend who is a nurse and works at the hospital is allowed to stay. The doctor tells me what will happen. I can watch the proceedings on a TV screen. The insertion of the dye may feel like a period pain. He inserts the dye. It is very painful and the pain gets worse. I pass out. When I come round the doctor shows me the X-ray. I try to concentrate but I can't take in what he's saying. The left tube appears to be clear but my right tube has gone into spasm. I fear there may never be a baby. I am put on to a trolley and wheeled into the corridor where I lie in pain for some time. Gradually the pain begins to ease and I am able to get dressed. My friend finds a taxi, takes me home and puts me to bed with a hot water bottle. By the evening I feel better.

The investigations seem to be taking so long. A day does not pass by without my thinking about them and my infertility. I feel I must go on with the tests, and all the pain they cause, because I need to know if I will ever be able to have a child, and because there is no other source of help for my infertility to which I can turn.

19 April 1979   Appointment with the semenologist. The appointment is at 3:40 and so at 2:30 Paul produced his sperm sample into the little plastic container provided by the hospital. We then rush to the hospital, clutching the sample. The doctor looks at some of the sperm under the microscope and sends the rest to the lab for a sperm count. He thinks that the count and motility are increased, but this will be confirmed by the laboratory test. That's it basically. It's heartening to think there's an improvement. The spraying must be working so Paul will continue with that. We fix another appointment with the semenologist to see whether the improvement has continued.

26 April 1979   I'm in contact with children who have German measles so I have a blood test to see whether I am immune to German measles.

1 May 1979   Appointment at the Infertility Clinic to hear the results of the HSG. The doctor tells me the same tale as I was told in the X-ray room. One tube is definitely clear but the result is uncertain for the other. This tube may be blocked or it might be a technical problem which made it difficult for the dye to get through. My agony is reduced to a technical hitch. If I have not conceived in three months time, I am to have a laparoscopy. This will involve a short stay in hospital. The waiting list is long so she will put my name down on it the next time I see her, in three months' time. Why do I have to wait till then? Why can't my name be put on the list now? Meanwhile, the doctor suggests I try an insemination cap. I am to return to the clinic in two days to be shown how to use it. I am to use it in the middle of the cycle and then come back to her with it in place to see if I am using it properly and to check whether it's improving the sperms' chances of survival. This calls for another new element in our sex life: I take the oestrogen tablets around the time of ovulation; then before 'intercourse' I am to spend five minutes in the bathroom with the douche after which I am to insert the insemination cap. Meanwhile Paul is masturbating into the hospital's plastic pot, with his balls nicely chilled twice daily. I am then to syringe his sperm into the tube which dangles from the insemination cap. What erotic excitement!

3 May 1979   To the hospital to learn how to use the insemination cap. It's a bit fiddly and difficult to get into place.

19 May 1979   Fourth post-coital but with insemination cap in place. The results seem exactly the same as for the test we had in February. Mucus is okay, sperm count is fine, but the motility is low. The insemination cap has not made any difference so the doctor doesn't think it's worth continuing with it. I indicate my relief at that news. We are sent back to the semenologist for a sperm-mucus compatibility test to see if my mucus is killing off Paul's sperm.

12 June 1979   Second appointment with semenologist. We go together with a sperm sample in a little container. The semenologist examines it and pronounces his approval of both the count and motility. We then persuade him to do the sperm-mucus compatibility test which is the reason we came to see him. He seems happy with the result. I feel totally confused. One doctor says the motility is low. Another says it's fine. One tells me to douche. The other says that it's unnecessary. How am I to deal with this lack of consensus? The only response seems to be to feel cheerful. At least someone has said we're okay. I may not be pregnant but any ray of hope is to be appreciated.

1 August 1979   Appointment to see the consultant. He puts me on the list for a laparoscopy. I should have an appointment within six months. It's just a question of waiting. And because my cycle is somewhat irregular, he decides to put me on an ovulation-inducing drug. I am given one month's supply. Am I to go back each month for another prescription?

10 August 1979   We go on holiday. It is the second holiday we've taken since trying to get pregnant. Events like this remind me of time passing.

On our return from holiday, we decide to buy a house. We had been thinking for some time about where we were going to live. The flat was a bit small for a child. We had no garden and getting up and down the stairs would not have been easy with a small baby. When we first started trying to conceive, our plan had been to move out soon after the baby's birth. But as the months passed with no signs of a baby, we put this plan to one side. It just did not seem possible to make any decisions about where we were to live until we knew more about whether we were likely to have a baby. How much longer could we go on delaying plans and decisions because one day there might be a baby? So many aspects of our lives were becoming controlled by our frustrated attempts to become parents. We went ahead and bought a house. It is a large house—one that gives us plenty of space for us and for children.

15 October 1979   Receive a card from the hospital telling me to fix the date for a laparoscopy in the second half of my next cycle.

7 November 1979   I enter hospital for a laparoscopy the next afternoon. I have never been in hospital before and I am nervous. It is much jollier than I expected. There are thirteen women in the ward and we quickly discover who we all are. Six of us are to be operated on tomorrow. As we have all come in for different operations, we each have different anxieties, but we are great company for one another, laughing and joking together. I realize how much more pleasant it is to have other women around you while going through tests, someone to share the worries and the news. There are two other women on the ward who are having problems in conceiving. It is good to talk to them, to compare notes about the tests and their reactions to infertility. I realize that I did not know anyone who had been through the investigations or who is infertile. While a lot of women have been very kind and listened to my tales of tests and anguish, none of them have been through similar experiences or had similar feelings. This is the first time I've spoken to women who've said, 'Yes, they did that to me,' or 'Yes, I felt like that too'. I see that I've become very careful about the people I get close to. I am only relating to close friends and relatives who know about my problem. I feel very vulnerable about stepping outside of that group into the great beyond of those who don't know.

9 November 1979   The doctor comes round to tell us all about the results of our operations. He confirms that I am ovulating and that my tubes, ovaries and uterus are okay. So I am proclaimed fit and told to report back to the consultant in six weeks' time.

I feel now as though I have done the rounds. A series of tests have revealed little that was seriously wrong with either Paul or myself. I imagined that at the next appointment I would be told that medical science had its way with us and that now it was up to us to go away, to forget the hassles we had been through, to relax and conceive.

24 November 1979   Period starts.

22 December 1979   It comes again. Another Christmas passes and I'm not pregnant.

4 January 1980   Appointment to see the consultant. This is the anniversary of my first appointment at the Infertility Clinic. The consultant looks at the report of my laparoscopy, reads all the notes and thinks. He suggests a blood test to check my progesterone level.

This is fixed for 13 January as it has to be done late in my cycle. I'm also told to make an appointment for a fifth post-coital test to check that everything is still all right there.

13 January 1980   I have a blood sample taken for the progesterone test. I delay making the appointment for a fifth post-coital.

2 February 1980   We move into our new house. It requires a lot of work which the builders have started. At first I organize the rooms around a child. One room is to be a nursery. Later that same room becomes my study.

8 May 1980   I make an appointment for a post-coital test.

20 May 1980   Fifth post-coital test. I have taken the oestrogen tablets for the first time in months. I had a hard job finding them. When I arrive at the clinic, I feel that I need to explain to the nurse why I hadn't come sooner. The doctor, however, either doesn't notice or doesn't ask about the long delay. So I say nothing. I take off my knickers. I get on the couch. It's all so familiar, I feel positively light-headed. A seasoned traveller. The result seems the same as ever. The sperm are there but not very motile. So one year and a half later, we are back where we started. The results of the progesterone test are not too encouraging. I am ovulating, but not very well. To improve my ovulation, I am given Clomid as well as oestrogen tablets. I am also sent off to have a blood test to see if I have antibodies to sperm.

I go away feeling fed-up. It seems as if a whole lot of new problems are coming up—low progesterone, sperm antibodies. If they are significant factors, why were they not looked for months ago. I've had a number of blood tests. Why hadn't these been included then? And I don't understand why the motility of Paul's sperm is a matter of differing opinions. If it is a significant factor in our infertility then why put me on Clomid? We seem to be going round in circles, backtracking over ground that I thought we'd explored. I feel like a detective story, with the doctors sniffing round for clues, going over old suspects as well as checking on esoteric possibilities. Nevertheless, I take the Clomid in my next cycle as well as the oestrogen tablets.

20 June 1980   I feel very ill.

4 July 1980   Period starts. It's fourteen days since I felt so ill so I feel sure that it was due to the Clomid. Why hadn't I been warned of the side-effects? Also, how am I to know if the Clomid is working? No tests are being done to check on my defective progesterone levels. I am depressed.

31 July 1980 Period starts. I've run out of oestrogen tablets. The hospital no longer dispenses them so I have to go to my GP. Since I moved, I haven't found a new GP. By the time I work all this out, it's too late to take Clomid this cycle.

This summer is the third since we tried to conceive. We work on the house. I find out through my friend at the hospital that the test showed that I do not have antibodies to Paul's sperm. It dawns on me that I have decided by default not to continue with the Clomid or with the tests. I feel uneasy about giving up the investigations. Having gone so far it seems silly not to continue. The next test might be the one which gives me the answer. They might just find something that works for me. But then I remember what the tests were like and I feel loathe to go back to the hospital and try again.

I feel the key question is changing slowly. I am asking less why am I infertile. Instead, I am thinking about how to reconcile myself with my infertility, and how I can move forward into a life in which children may not have a central role. I feel that this is where I prefer to put my energies, and that continuing with the tests will interfere with this. So I do not go back to the clinic.

Update to "Discovering That You Are Infertile:

One Woman's Experience"

by Anne Woollett and Naomi Pfeffer

"Discovering that You Are Infertile" was written some years ago. In a number of respects infertility, its impact for women and their reproductive decisions have changed considerably. Treatment options have increased, so that while many of the investigations mentioned in the diary continue to be part of their experiences, the decisions infertile men and women now commonly make include those which relate to the new techniques of assisted conception, such as IVF and surrogacy (Franklin, 1997).

These techniques are complex and expensive and so are available only to those who can afford the costs of treatment and associated drugs, travel and accommodation. In the US, they are rarely covered by health insurance (King and Meyer, 1997). These techniques of assisted conception are seen as producing new treatment opportunities (and career and financial opportunities for medical and scientific staff). The first child conceived by IVF was born in 1978 and we have, as yet, little evidence about the effects and long term psychological development of children conceived in these ways (McMahon and Ungerer, 1998). There is now more recognition of the emotional and psychological costs of treatment for women and partners (Sandelowski, 1993), but there is still little discussion about and research into the effects on the long term health of women of IVF and especially drugs employed to stimulate ovulation (Klein and Rowland, 1989).

The techniques of assisted conception have opened up treatment options and fertility choices for some women and their partners. However, these treatments still have a low success rate, and hence result in the birth of a live baby for only a minority of infertile couples (Pfeffer, 1993). For many women, therefore, coming to terms with infertility and finding ways of relating to others as infertile/ childless women remains as much of an issue as when this diary was written (Franklin, 1997).

The new techniques of assisted conception have changed considerably the ways in which infertility is represented and written about. There is now more discussion of infertility in professional accounts (medical, bioethical, psychological, sociological) and in popular culture. These suggest that while women may find it easier to recognize infertility as a 'problem', many

This update was written specifically for *Women's Health: Readings on Social, Economic and Political Issues.*

women still experience a strong desire to become mothers and motherhood is viewed as a central, 'normal', and expected role for women (Phoenix, Woollett and Lloyd, 1991; Morrell, 1994). As Mardy Ireland (1993) argues, within this framework infertility continues to be construed as a shock, a loss, and as a lack of reproductive choice. A different representation of infertile women (but not infertile men) has emerged in the debates about the ethics of the new techniques. Women prepared to become mothers by means of these unconventional routes are said to threaten the stability of the nuclear family. Yet, ironically, it is the nuclear family which many of these women are seeking to create.

However, in spite of greater public recognition, there are still many unasked and unanswered questions about infertility. One concerns the diversity of women's lives, their social and economic situations, and ideas about motherhood and mothering (Collins, 1994) hence how they view infertility and being childless (Woollett, 1996). Another concerns the ways in which women's ideas about infertility change over time. The diary points to some ways in which one woman's thinking about infertility changed over time: from concerns about being a mother and how motherhood would fit into her life and relationships, to concerns about her body, why she was not getting pregnant, what 'the problem' was, and about the swings in her mood during her menstrual cycle. Since writing that diary, Anne's thinking about infertility has changed considerably. She decided to step off what felt like an emotionally draining and isolating roundabout of infertility investigations. This meant thinking of herself not so much as 'infertile' as 'childless' (Woollett, 1996).

Professionally she became more interested in how women resist representations of themselves as 'mad', 'sad' or 'desperate'. Drawing on research such as that of Morell (1994) and Ireland (1993) she began to think about the identities, activities and ways in which childless women relate to others, and to disentangle what it means to be a 'mother' and to be a 'woman'.

References

Collins, P. H. (1994) Shifting The Centre: Race, Class and Feminist Theorizing about Motherhood. In E. N. Glenn, G. Chang, and L. R. Forcey (eds) Mothering: Ideology, Experience and Agency. New York. Routledge.

Franklin, S. (1997) Embodied Progress: A Cultural Account of Assisted Conception. London. Routledge.

Ireland, M. S. (1993) Reconceiving Women: Separating Motherhood from Female Identity. New York. The Guilford Press.

King, L. and Meyer, M. M. (1997) The politics of reproductive benefits: US insurance cover of contraceptive and infertility treatments. Gender and Society, 11, 3–30.

McMahon, C. A. and Ungerer, J. A. (1998) Parenting and infant development following conception by reproductive technology. In C. A. Niven and A. Walker (eds) Current Issues in Infancy and Parenthood. Oxford. Butterworth Heinemann.

Morell, C. (1994) Unwomanly Conduct: The Challenge of Intentional Childlessness. London. Routledge.

Pfeffer, N. (1993) The Stork and The Syringe: A Political History of Reproductive Medicine. Cambridge. Polity.

Phoenix, A., Woollett, A. and Lloyd, E. (eds) (1991) Motherhood: Meanings, Practices and Ideologies. London. Sage.

Sandelowski, M. (1993). With Child In Mind: Studies of the Personal Encounter with Infertility. Philadelphia. University of Pennsylvania Press.

Woollett, A. (1996) Infertility: From 'Inside/Out' to 'Outside/In'. Feminism Psychology, 6, 74–78.

Grade A

The Market for a Yale Woman's Eggs

by Jessica Cohen

When a Yale undergraduate explored becoming an egg donor for a wealthy couple willing to pay top dollar to the right candidate, she didn't realize how unsettling the process of candidacy would prove to be

Early in the spring of last year a classified ad ran for two weeks in the *Yale Daily News:* "EGG DONOR NEEDED." The couple that placed the ad was picky, and for that reason was offering $25,000 for an egg from the right donor.

As a child I had a book called *"Where Did I Come From?"* It offered a full biological explanation, in cartoons, to answer those awkward questions that curious tots ask. But the book is now out of date. Replacing it is, for example, *Mommy, Did I Grow in Your Tummy?: Where Some Babies Come From,* which explains the myriad ways that children of the twenty-first century may have entered their families, including egg donation, surrogacy, in vitro fertilization, and adoption. When conception doesn't occur in the natural way, it becomes very complicated. Once all possible parties have been accounted for—egg donor, sperm donor, surrogate mother, paying couple—as many as five people can be involved in conceiving and carrying a child. No wonder a new book is necessary.

The would-be parents' decision to advertise in the *News*—and to offer a five-figure compensation—immediately suggested that they were in the market for an egg of a certain rarefied type. Beyond their desire for an Ivy League donor, they wanted a young woman over five feet five, of Jewish heritage, athletic, with minimum combined SAT score of 1500, and attractive. I was curious—and I fit all the criteria except the SAT score. So I e-mailed Michelle and David (not their real names) and asked for more information about the process and how much the SAT minimum really meant to them. Then I waited for a reply.

Donating an egg is neither simple nor painless. Following an intensive screening and selection process the donor endures a few weeks of invasive medical procedures. First the donor and the woman who will carry the child must coordinate their menstrual cycles. Typically the donor and the recipient take birth-control pills, followed by shots of a synthetic hormone such as Lupron; the combination suppresses ovulation and puts their cycles in sync. After altering her cycle the donor must enhance her egg supply with fertility drugs in the same way an infertile woman does when trying to conceive. Shots of a fertility hormone are administered for seven to eleven days, to stimulate the production of an abnormally large number of egg-containing follicles. During this time the donor must have her blood tested every other day so that doctors can monitor her hormone levels, and she must come in for periodic ultrasounds. Thirty-six hours before retrieval day a shot of hCG, human chorionic gonadotropin, is administered to prepare the eggs for release, so that they will be ready for harvest.

The actual retrieval is done while the donor is under anesthesia. The tool is a needle, and the product, on average, is ten to twenty eggs. Doctors take that many because "not all eggs will be good," according to Surrogate Mothers Online, an informational Web site designed and maintained by experienced egg donors and surrogate mothers, "Some will be immature and some overripe."

Lisa, one of the hosts on Surrogate Mothers Online and an experienced egg donor, described the process as a "rewarding" experience. When she explained that once in a while something can go wrong, I braced myself for the fine print. On very rare occasions, she wrote, hyperstimulation of the ovaries can occur, and the donor must be hospitalized until the ovaries return to normal. In even rarer cases the ovaries rupture, resulting in permanent infertility or possibly even death. "I must stress that this is very rare," Lisa assured prospective donors. "I had two very wonderful experiences . . . The second [time] I stayed awake to help the doctor count how many eggs he retrieved."

David responded to my e-mail a few hours after I'd sent it. He told me nothing about himself, and only

---

briefly alluded to the many questions I had asked about the egg-donation process. He spent the bulk of the e-mail describing a cartoon, and then requested photos of me. The cartoon was a scene with a "couple that is just getting married, he a nerd and she a beauty," he wrote. "They are kvelling about how wonderful their offspring will be with his brains and her looks." He went on to describe the punch line: the next panel showed a nerdy-looking baby thinking empty thoughts. The following paragraph was more direct. David let me know that he and his wife were flexible on most criteria but that Michelle was "a real Nazi" about "donor looks and donor health history."

This seemed to be a commentary of some sort on the couple's situation and how plans might go awry, but the message was impossible to pin down. I thanked him for the e-mail, asked where to send my pictures, and repeated by original questions about egg donation and their criteria.

In a subsequent e-mail David promised to return my photos, so I sent him dorm-room pictures, the kind that every college student has lying around. Now they assumed a new level of importance. I would soon learn what this anonymous couple, somewhere in the United States, thought about my genetic material as displayed in these photographs.

Infertility is not a modern problem, but has created a modern industry. Ten percent of American couples are infertile, and many seek treatment from the $2-billion-a-year infertility industry. The approximately 370 fertility clinics across the United States help prospective parents to sift through their options. I sympathize with women who cannot use their own eggs to have children. The discovery must be a sober awakening for those who have always dreamed of raising a family. When would-be parents face this problem, however, their options depend greatly on their income. All over the world most women who can't have children must simply accept the fact and adopt, or find other roles in society. But especially here in the United States wealth can enable such couples to have a child of their own and to determine how closely that child will resemble the one they might have had—or the one they dream of having.

The Web site of Egg Donation, Inc., a program based in California, contains a database listing approximately 300 potential donors. In order to access the list interested parties must call the company and request the user ID and the password for the month. Once I'd given the receptionist my name and address, she told me the password: "colorful." I hung up and entered the database. Potential parents can search for a variety of features, narrowing the pool as much as they like according to ethnic origin, religion of birth, state of residence, hair color, eye color, height, and weight. I typed in the physical and religious characteristics that Michelle and David were looking for and found four potential donors. None of them had a college degree.

The standard compensation for donating an egg to Egg Donation is $3,500 to $5,000, and additional funds are offered to donors who have advanced degrees or are of Asian, African-American, or Jewish descent. Couples searching for an egg at Egg Donation can be picky, but not as picky as couples advertising in the *Yale Daily News*. Should couples be able to pay a premium on an open market for their idea of the perfect egg? Maybe a modern-day Social Darwinist would say yes. Modern success is measured largely in financial terms, so why shouldn't the most successful couples, eager to pay more, have access to the most expensive eggs? Of course, as David illustrated in his first e-mail, input does not always translate perfectly into output—the donor's desirable characteristics may never actually be manifested in the child.

If couples choose not to find their eggs through an agency, they must do so independently. An Internet search turned up a few sites like Surrogate Mothers Online, where would-be donors and parents can post classified ads. More than 500 classifieds were posted on the site: a whole marketplace, an eBay for genetic material.

"Hi! My name is Kimberly," one of the ads read. "I am 24 years old, 5'11" with blonde hair and green eyes. I previously donated eggs and the couple was blessed with BIG twin boys! The doctor told me I have perky ovaries! . . . The doctor told me I had the most perfect eggs he had ever seen." The Web site provided links to photographs of Kimberly and an e-mail address. Would-be parents on the site offered "competitive" rates, generally from $5,000 to $10,000 for donors who fit their specifications.

About a week after I sent my pictures to David and Michelle, I received a third e-mail: "Got the pictures. You look perfect. I can't say this with any authority. That is my wife's department." I thought back to the first e-mail, where he'd written, "She's been known to disregard a young woman based on cheekbones, hair, nose, you name it." He then shifted the focus. "My department is the SAT scores. Can you tell me more about your academic performance? What are you taking at Yale? What high school did you attend?"

The whole thing seemed like a joke. I dutifully answered his questions, explaining that I was from a no-name high school in the Midwest, I couldn't do math or science, and my academic performance was, well, average; I couldn't help feeling a bit disconcerted by his particular interest in my SAT score.

Michelle and David now had my educational data as well as my photos. They were examining my credentials and trying to imagine their child. If I was accepted, a harvest of my eggs would be fertilized by the semen of the author of the disturbing e-mails I had received. A few embryos would be implanted; the remaining, if there were any, would be frozen; and then I would be out of the picture forever.

The modern embryo has been frozen, stolen, aborted, researched, and delivered weeks early, along with five or six instant siblings. The summer of 2001 was full of embryo news, and the first big story was President Bush's deliberation on stem-cell research. The embryos available for genetic research include those frozen by fertility clinics for later use by couples attempting in vitro fertilization.

Embryos took the spotlight again when Helen Beasley, a surrogate mother from Shrewsbury, England, decided to sue a San Francisco couple for parental rights to the twin fetuses she was carrying. The couple and Beasley had agreed that they would pay her $20,000 to carry one child created from a donated egg and the father's sperm. The agreement also called for selective reduction—the abortion of any additional embryos. Beasley claimed that there had been a verbal agreement that such reduction would occur by the twelfth week. The problem arose when Beasley, who had discovered she was carrying twins, was told to abort one, but the arrangements for the reduction weren't made until the thirteenth week. Fearing for her own health and objecting to the abortion of such a highly developed fetus, she refused. At that time she was suing for the right to put the babies up for adoption. She was also seeking the remainder of the financial compensation specified in the contract. The couple did not want the children, and yet had the rights to the genetic material; Beasley was simply a vessel. The case is only one of a multitude invited by modern fertility processes. On August 15, 2001, *The New York Times* reported that the New Jersey Supreme Court had upheld a woman's rights to the embryos that she and her ex-husband had created and frozen six years before. A strange case for child-custody lawyers.

Nearly ten years ago, at the University of California at Irvine's Center for Reproductive Health, doctors took the leftover frozen embryos from previous clients and gave them without consent to other couples and to research centers. Discovery of the scam resulted in more than thirty prosecutions: a group of children had biological parents who hadn't consented to their existence and active parents who had been given stolen goods. Who can say whether throwing the embryos away would have been any better?

Even if Michelle and David liked my data, I knew I'd have a long way to go before becoming an actual donor. The application on Egg Donation's Web site is twelve pages long—longer than Yale's entrance application. The

first two pages cover the basics: appearance, name, address, age, and other mundane details. After that I was asked if I'd ever filed for bankruptcy or ever had counseling, if I drank, what my goals in life were, what two of my favorite books were, what my paternal grandfather's height and weight were, what hobbies I had, what kind of relationship I would want to have with the parents and child, and so forth. A few fill-in-the-blanks were thrown in at the end: "I feel strongly about__. I am sorry I did not__. In ten years I want to be __." Not even my closest friends knew all these things about me. If Egg Donation, offering about a fifth what Michelle and David were offering, wanted all this information, what might Michelle and David want?

Michelle and David were certainly trying hard. On one classified-ad site I came across a request that was strangely familiar: "Loving family seeks exceptional egg donor with 1500 SAT, great looks, good family health history, Jewish heritage and athletic. Height 5'4"–5'9", Age 18–29. We will pay EXTREMELY well and will take care of all expenses. Hope to hear from you." The e-mail address was David and Michelle's familiar AOL account. Theirs was the most demanding classified on the site, but also the only one that offered to pay "EXTREMELY well."

I kept dreaming about all the things I could do with $25,000. I had gone into the correspondence on a whim. But soon, despite David's casual tone and the optimistic attitude of all the classifieds and information I read, I realized that this process was something I didn't want to be a part of. I understand the desire for a child who will resemble and fit in with the family. But once a couple starts choosing a few characteristics, shooting for perfection is too easy—especially if they can afford it. The money might have changed my life for a while, but it would have led to the creation of a child encumbered with too many expectations.

After I'd brooded about these matters, I received the shortest e-mail of the correspondence. The verdict on my pictures was in: "I showed the pictures to [my wife] this AM. Personally, I think you look great. She said ho-hum."

David said he might reconsider, and that he was going to keep one of my pictures. That was it. No good-bye, no thanks for my willingness to be, in effect, the biological mother of their child. I guess I didn't fit their design; my genes weren't the right material for their *chef d'oeuvre*. So I was rejected as a donor. I keep imagining the day when David and Michelle's child asks where he or she came from. David will describe how hard they both worked on the whole thing, how many pictures they looked at, and how much money they spent. The child will turn to them and say, "Ho-hum."

Father Knows Baste

by Tamar Abrams

"**D**A" was Hannah's first and favorite sound. When she said it, at nine months old in the pediatrician's waiting room, another mother told me she must be thinking of her daddy. Frankly, I doubt it. Hannah's daddy has a number, not a name. He is 741, an anonymous Los Angeles law student who, in 1992, was paid about $50 to produce the sperm that helped create my beautiful daughter.

I arrived at the decision to become a single mother by choice fairly quickly and without a great deal of angst. My twenties and early thirties were spent focusing on my career, and I prided myself on my independence. A series of boyfriends came and went, leading my father to declare, when I was only 28, that I was too picky with men and would likely never find one I could settle down with.

He was smarter than I thought. One day I woke up and realized that I was 34 and alone. I lived in a condo that I owned in Washington, D.C. I had no houseplants, no pets, nothing that required constant care and nurturing. My job for Planned Parenthood entailed nonstop travel. It was exciting and exhilarating, but I was painfully aware of my abandoned childhood plan to marry and have at least four children.

Weeks of soul-searching led me to the conclusion that I could live without regret if I never was a wife, but I couldn't be happy if I were never a mother. And that's how, in August of 1991, I ended up in the offices of Dr. Belinda Marascalco, then with Columbia Hospital for women in Washington, D.C. She offered no lectures on the inadequacies of single motherhood, no judgments. I realized as she spoke how little I knew of the reproductive process and how much I would have to learn. I also realized how committed I was to bearing and mothering a child.

I left the clinic with a list of donors from California Cryobank—a Los Angeles-based sperm bank—and a sense of tremendous anticipation. California Cryobank was one of two choices available to me; the other sperm bank was in Louisiana. I stuck with the California Cryobank because it has an excellent reputation for screening donors, and because I liked the idea of my East Coast baby-to-be having some California blood in her or him.

In those days, you would begin by looking through a donor book of more than 100 listings. Each listing gave the basics—blood type, ethnic origin, hair color and texture, height and weight, educational background, general medical history, family history, and some essay questions. Once you found a few you were interested in, you could request a more comprehensive 20-page listing that included medical histories going back several generations. Today the process has been brought into the 21st century: you can peruse the lists online, listen to an audio tape of the donor, ask Cryobank staff to find a donor who looks like a family member and even ask a panel to rank the attractiveness of your chosen donor.

But back then, it was just me and a few pieces of paper. I combed the listings, not sure what I was looking for. Finally, I decided that I wanted a donor who could give the child all the physical characteristics I could not—long legs, a tall, slender body, and good eyesight. I screened out anyone with a relative who had died of cancer or other possibly genetic diseases. I didn't care about religion or hair color, although I admit that SAT scores were marginally significant. One donor was eliminated because he listed tuna casserole as his favorite food.

Over the course of the next six months, I attempted to conceive twice a month with four different donors. I did this with the help of Dr. Marascalco, a basal body thermometer and monthly parties. The parties involved my girlfriends—and the occasional red-faced male—who would listen as I read donor information sheets, and vote on their choice for Donor of the Month. Fueled by wine and the upbeat mood of the parties, we had a blast and I always ended up with a donor.

Once I had determined that ovulation had just occurred, I would race over to the clinic for my insemination. The room was clinical, the procedure involved a syringe and about ten seconds of the doctor's time—but it was a magical time for me. I would lie in the room for half an hour afterwards, visualizing conception. It was peaceful and invariably hopeful.

In December, however, my most fertile day happened to fall on the day of Columbia Hospital's holiday party. As a result, the doctor wasn't going to be available to do the insemination. Instead, arrangements were made for me to visit the clinic between 8:30 and 9 that morning to pick up a vial of my donor's sperm to take home. The woman working in the andrology lab showed me where the specimens were stored and even put a tiny bit of the sperm under a microscope so I could see all the activity. She seemed happy to have the company and cheerfully explained the do-it-yourself insemination. I should have paid more attention.

Placing the vial in my bra to keep it warm, I pushed the D.C. speed limit and reached my Capitol Hill home in record time. In the kitchen, I successfully emptied the vial into the syringe I was given—but I lost most of the sperm down the sink while trying to tap out any air bubbles. Literally, $150 and a lot of hope went down the drain.

Like failing to become pregnant in more conventional ways, failing with donor insemination is accompanied by disappointment and fear that infertility is one's lot in life. At the time, one of my friends commented that the process of trying to conceive was no fun my way. I disputed that. While it wasn't soft lights and Luther Vandross ballads, there was an element of fun and anticipation. Several times during the six months it took me to conceive, I would spend an hour or more in the fertility center's conference room poring over lists of donors. Sometimes nurses on their lunch breaks would help me. It was a bit like shopping—starting out with a good idea of what you want, but finding yourself distracted by the unexpected.

The search ended and the journey began on March 8, 1992—my father's birthday—when my darling daughter was conceived. By this time I had begun to lose patience with the process. To speed things along, I had been taking Clomid, a fertility drug. And in the end, the donor wasn't even chosen by my friends or by me—he was selected by a nurse at the fertility center who said he was a "sure thing." And so I was matched with 741. The Prince of Fertility. Mr. Super Sperm Count. He was no slouch in other departments, either: green eyes, curly red hair, a law student who scored 1400 on his SATs.

His essay-question responses looked like he was in a hurry to complete the form, but he did manage to write about himself: "fun-loving, active, patient, athletic, enjoy life, hard-working, driven, intellectually stimulated." He's someone I think I would have liked knowing.

On March 8, 741's defrosted sperm registered a 4-plus on the fertility scale—the highest possible rating. Those little guys were ready to party. Thanks to Clomid, I had produced five eggs just waiting for the music to begin.

By this time, I had spent about $2,000 of my own money, six months of my life and a great deal of time praying. But in the end, it was worth every penny and every second. On December 1, 1992 at 3:38 a.m., the lovely Hannah Lily Abrams was born into the world by emergency C-section. Through the haze of drugs and fatigue, I looked at this tiny, puffy child and knew with certainty that this was the greatest accomplishment of my life. The lack of a husband in no way diminished the pride and joy of that moment. We were now a family.

More than nine years later, I can still recall the moment of my daughter's birth. Sometimes she's even willing to cuddle in my arms while I tell her the story of her conception and birth, though more often she rolls her eyes and runs off to ride her bike. This story is hers now, not mine. But I protect it and cherish it until she's ready to take it from me.

Hannah's life is indistinguishable from that of her friends. She's a Brownie knocking on doors to sell Girl Scout cookies. She's a child who has had the same best friend since they met in Montessori school seven years ago. Our house is filled with light and toys and books and videos and, increasingly, CDs of Britney, the Backstreet Boys, and a few Broadway musicals. For the Brownies' Father/Daughter Snowflake Ball in February, Hannah donned a burgundy velvet-and-taffeta gown, and beamed as her beloved grandpa slid a corsage onto her wrist.

My child has grown up knowing the story of how she came to be. I began telling her about it while she was still too young to understand, because I wanted the words to be familiar to her. We never talked about "father" or "daddy," but about "donor" instead. This led to the time, when she was two, that she told her friends that her father was a "doughnut." But familiarity doesn't ease the way entirely.

When Hannah was three and we were driving somewhere in the dark, she suddenly announced that she knew who her father really was. Despite the frequency with which she stated eternal truths while riding in the back seat of the car, I was shocked. As calmly as I could, I asked who her father really was and she replied, "Peter Pan." It made sense to me—eternally youthful, wearing green tights, able to fly, and of course living somewhere far away in Never Neverland. She stuck with that story for several months.

At four, she began crying in the tub and exclaimed fiercely, "But I want a daddy! All my friends have one!" It was a moment I had anticipated and dreaded in equal measure. I said the first thing that came to mind, "I'm so sorry you don't have a daddy. I know you want one." Later, following the advice of a much wiser single mom, I asked Hannah what she would do if she had a

Daddy. She thought long and hard and said, "I don't know. Just stuff."

That conversation has evolved over the years. It was punctuated by her request at the age of six to know more about the donor. In a nod toward full disclosure, I sat beside her on the couch and handed her the long form donor profile. She was excited to read it and full of self-discovery. "He likes math like I do!" she yelled. "He likes music too." She read each page carefully and then announced she wanted to call him . . . immediately.

We both wept as I explained that we couldn't call him, that he was deliberately anonymous to us. But she could write him a letter that would be delivered to him when she turned 18. That was perhaps the hardest day of this journey for me. She was so bitterly disappointed and all the positive reasons that I chose to have her on my own could not, in that moment, compensate for the obvious negatives. I cried long after she stopped.

To Hannah's credit, though, she has handled her difference with grace and dignity. When her preschool friends would ask why there was no daddy in her home, she would state in a matter-of-fact-tone, "I don't have one. I have a mommy and a grandma and a grandpa and an aunt and a cat." To those who challenged her by pointing out that everyone has a father, she would reply, "I don't."

As she gets older, Hannah seems almost bored by the fact that she is the child of a single mother. Perhaps it's because she's puzzling through larger issues—why she has to practice the violin so often, why boys can excite and repel her at the same moment, why she can't be a famous actress right now. I am relieved that embarrassment and shame are not the legacies of her unusual beginning.

Hannah tells her story to friends patiently and slowly. She starts by saying, "My mom really wanted to have a baby but didn't have a husband. So she found a nice doctor who got her some seeds . . ." I've received a few calls from parents who were not happy that their children were getting this explanation, but it seems reasonable to me.

More unexpected have been the reactions of men to my method of having a child. I didn't begin dating again until about a year ago. It wasn't from lack of interest, but more a lack of time and energy. As Hannah gets older, she needs my time a little less. And I've found myself missing the intimacy and love of a mature relationship. Most of the men I've gone out with have been divorced fathers. So their assumption is universally that Hannah's dad is lurking somewhere in the background.

I never introduce the topic of donor insemination, but am always ready to discuss it if a man asks where Hannah's father is or when I got my divorce. I assumed initially that men would be disgusted by the idea of donor insemination or threatened by my assertiveness in having a child on my own. I was wrong. They have all been fascinated and even delighted. It means that there is no bitter divorce in my past, no shared custody, no complications. And they seem to admire my courage in doing it my way. One man said he was attracted to me because I never chose the conventional path to getting what I wanted in life. Who knew?

But there are complications with having a child through donor insemination that are unique to the process. For example, during the time that Hannah's donor was actively "giving," he may have fathered several dozen children. We have met and formed a relationship with one of them. Sam is three years younger than Hannah and lives in New York. I told her about him when she was five and she has since claimed him as a "half-brother." They exchange letters and photos that show some remarkable physical similarities. Last summer we spent the day together in Manhattan. The two children walked down Ninth Avenue, huddled together under an umbrella and talking in conspiratorial terms. We have claimed Sam and his mom as family.

So many of Hannah's friends are adopted or the children of divorced parents or even the children of single mothers by choice that it barely registers anymore that she has only one parent. I'm not naïve enough to expect that it won't become a much bigger issue for Hannah as she cruises into adolescence. I'm as prepared as I can be. And I'm entirely comfortable with the choices I made that led to her birth. No regrets.

I'm also very careful to speak respectfully of marriage when Hannah is around. I have never wanted her to infer that I became a single mom because of some deep-seated animosity toward men or marriage. She announced when she was four or five, "Mom, I hope you don't mind, but I think I'd like to be married before I have children." I was thrilled!

I still hold out hope that one day I may marry. But I'm not desperate for it. I've discovered that my journey is a circuitous one, filled with happiness and drama. When I first came to the conclusion that being a mother was important, I was realistic enough to know that there would be moments of great loneliness and loss and rigorous hurdles. I know now that I had no idea of the depth and breadth of the joy I would experience with my child, or the sometimes haunting loneliness. I had only the slightest inkling of the patience, fortitude, and humor that parenting requires—even when one is part of a couple. The requirements are doubled when you're doing it on your own.

Sometimes I meet women who are considering becoming single mothers by choice. I tell them there are no bad motivations for making that choice. Reproduction is inherently a selfish act, no matter how many people are involved. But those single mothers who seem to be the happiest have thought through the ramifications of their decision. They look beyond the sweet-smelling infant to the cranky toddler and the demanding fifth grader and the impossible adolescent. They understand that dating will be difficult and saving money is a pipe dream. They know that in achieving one dream, they are also letting go of another.

It has been ten years since I made one of the most important decisions of my life. The theme of these years has been gratitude. Every night since my lovely daughter was born, I wash up and get ready for bed. Just before I turn out the light, I quietly sneak into Hannah's room. Standing by her bed, I rearrange any covers she's kicked off. I check that the room temperature is appropriate. I bend low over her sleeping body and ensure that I see her chest rising and falling. I kiss my fingertip and lay it on her cheek. And then I thank God, Columbia Hospital for Women, the donor, my parents, and the universe for giving to me the child I once dreamed of. Only then can I sleep.

WORKSHEET — CHAPTER 10
Fertility, Infertility, and Reproductive Rights/Freedom

1. Three situations are described below. Make a list of all possible contraceptives which are options in the situations and briefly comment on the pros and cons for each contraceptive option. Be sure to include the widest range of contraceptives and specifically comment on how the choice of contraception will be affected by or impact on protection against sexually transmitted infections.

Linda and Larry

Linda and Larry are 22. They have been married for one year and want a family someday. Linda feels it is very important that she does not get pregnant while she is supporting both of them because Larry (a scientist) is unemployed. Because of their shared religious beliefs, Larry is not happy about Linda using birth control and both feel very strongly against abortion. Linda does not feel comfortable about her own body and does not have much understanding of the menstrual cycle or the process of fertilization.

Betsy and Bob

Betsy and Bob are 22. They have been married for one year and want a family someday, but want to wait until they are older. Betsy and Bob are working towards equality in their relationship so both are working half time and going to school half time. Although Betsy and Bob hope to prevent an unplanned pregnancy, they have the money and views which would permit abortion as a back-up to failed contraception. Both Betsy and Bob feel comfortable with their bodies and both recently got A's in a women's health course.

Susie and Sam

Susie and Sam are 22. Susie identifies as bisexual. She is mostly sexually active with women, but once in awhile she is still sexually active with her old boyfriend, Sam. Both Susie and Sam are responsible and well informed about sexual relationships. Both Susie and Sam feel strongly that their infrequent sexual encounters should not result in a pregnancy.

2. We get used to thinking about ways a woman can control her fertility to limit the number of children she has. As reflected in the articles in this chapter, true reproductive freedom means being able to have as many or few children as desired. List a wide range of factors which would enable women to have as *many* children as they wish. (What would be the factors to enable men to have as many children as they wish?)

3. After reading "The Bad Baby Blues," identify some of the ramifications of routine prenatal genetic testing.

   a. Give a reason why a woman might choose to have prenatal genetic testing even if she knew she would not choose to have an abortion.

   b. What could our society do to make it easier for women, couples, and families to choose to have a child with a disability?

4. Identify ways in which reproductive freedom and being valued by society are closely related issues. List specific examples of how a lack of reproductive freedom is related to racism, homophobia, ageism, poverty, and other issues.

5. After reading "Contraceptive Jelly on Toast and Other Unintended Consequences of Sexuality Education," identify an example of folklore—a joke, belief, or urban legend—you have heard about sexuality, contraception, or pregnancy. What is the point of the story and how does it reflect social values, misinformation, or people's anxieties?

CHAPTER 11

Childbirth and Lactation

Many of the problems in the relationship between women and the health care system are clearly visible in the area of childbearing. The paternalism, the reliance on technology, and the performance of unnecessary surgery characterizing certain aspects of the medical profession in the U.S. are all evident. On a positive note, this is also an area in which organized movements by women have had a major impact in improving care for women and their babies, and increasing their options. It is an area of continuing struggle, in which apparent victories may actually weaken the movement for more fundamental changes. For example, in some cases, "birthing centers" are merely hospital rooms decorated to look like home, with families allowed to be present for the birth, sometimes with a nurse midwife attending, but with the same medical interventions and little change in who makes the decisions. Such birthing centers may "pacify" some women who would otherwise work for major changes.

As with organizing around any women's health issue, activists for increasing choices for women during pregnancy and childbirth have had to take into account the ways different women benefit from different choices. For example, many women have worked to increase the availability of home births, but this is certainly not an option for homeless women or women in other living situations. Similarly, many women have worked to have husbands, boyfriends, and female partners present during childbirth but this now routine practice may not be appropriate for a battered woman because battering often begins or escalates during pregnancy. A theme of this book is the importance of activism to make information and choices available so women can empower themselves and have more control over the decisions affecting their health. However, as we read critiques of the medicalization of childbirth, me must remember that at a time when childbirth killed many women, women wanted more, not less, intervention, and medicalization along with improved hygiene and a better understanding of disease processes played an important role in making childbirth safer for women and their babies. Also, it is important to remember that consumer lawsuits are a driving force in pushing health care providers to "over" medicalize childbirth and that not all women are equally enthusiastic about being involved in medical decision-making.

Doris Haire's classic paper, "The Cultural Warping of Childbirth," was first published in the *International Childbirth Education Association News* in 1972. It was a very influential article, comparing the experience and outcomes of childbirth in the US with that of other countries. It identified common pathologically oriented practices throughout the entire pregnancy and postpartum period that "served to warp and distort the childbearing experience in the United States." The specific issues defined in this paper became many of the key issues around which childbirth activists organized for the next thirty years.

Although childbirth remains one of the most medicalized areas of women's lives, midwives offer an alternative, though not as accessible in the US as supporters would like. The question raised in the title of the article "Routine Midwifery Care: Why Not Here?" is an important one. Leah Hyder points out that "the majority of healthy women in Europe use professionally trained midwives," and compares that to the barriers midwifery encounters in the US. The two fact sheets, "Midwifery Facts" and "Caesarean Section in the United States" provide information that demonstrates the benefits of midwifery.

Infant mortality rates (IMR) provide one good way to evaluate the health of a nation, while maternal mortality (MM) provides another measure. As Deborah Maine points out in "How Do Socioeconomic Factors Affect Disparities in Maternal Mortality?" these two measures may be affected by socioeconomic factors in different ways, with the US relatively better off than other countries in the latter (MM) than in the former (IMR). While there have been major decreases in maternal mortality in the US, there are still major disparities, as, for example, African American women have much higher MM than white women. Understanding the factors affecting MM can help reduce the gaps among groups.

One of the issues related to pregnancy that is often overlooked is that of miscarriage, and those who experience this loss often do not receive the support they need. "Understanding Distress in the Aftermath of Miscarriage" provides useful information about reactions by the woman, her partner, and society to miscarriage, and how these relate to support and treatment. Another psychological dimension related to childbirth that remains insufficiently studied is postpartum depression. Leslie Tam presents a summary of the risk factors and possible interventions.

The remaining articles in this chapter focus on issues related to breastfeeding, which is an important factor in infant health and also reduces risk of breast cancer in the mother. The first two, "Formula for Profit" and "From TV to Real Life," explore the marketing of infant formula and how that reduces breastfeeding and directly affects the health of infants. The next article explores the practice of breastfeeding among new immigrants in the US, showing the interaction among many factors, including the marketing discussed in the previous article, traditional beliefs, religious beliefs, and education to promote breastfeeding. The final article gives a more theoretical presentation of how certain "female" body fluids are constructed in this culture (this could also have been included in the chapter on menstruation) and ties back into the theme of marketing that undermines breastfeeding.

The Cultural Warping of Childbirth

by Doris Haire

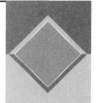

While Sweden and the Netherlands compete for the honor of having the lowest incidence of infant deaths per one thousand live births, the United States continues to find itself outranked by fourteen other developed countries.[1] A spokesman for the National Foundation March of Dimes recently stated that according to the most recent data, the United States leads all developed countries in the rate of infant deaths due to birth injury and respiratory distress such as postnatal asphyxia and atelectasis. According to the National Association for Retarded Children there are now six million retarded children and adults in the United States with a predicted annual increase of over 100,000 a year. The number of children and adults with behavioral difficulties or perceptual dysfunction resulting from minimal brain damage is an ever growing challenge to society and to the economy.

While it may be easier on the conscience to blame such numbing facts solely on socioeconomic factors and birth defects, recent research makes it evident that obstetrical medication can play a role in our staggering incidence of neurological impairment. It may be convenient to blame our relatively poor infant outcome on a lack of facilities or inadequate government funding, but it is obvious from the research being carried out that we could effect an immediate improvement in infant outcome by changing the pattern of obstetrical care in the United States. It is time that we take a good look at the overall experience of childbirth in this country and begin to recognize how our culture has warped this experience for the majority of American mothers and their newborn infants.

As an officer of the International Childbirth Education Association, I have visited hundreds of maternity hospitals throughout the world—in Great Britain, Western Europe, Russia, Asia, Australia, New Zealand, the South Pacific, the Americas, and Africa. During my visits I was privileged to observe obstetric techniques and procedures and to interview physicians, professional midwives, and parents in the various countries. My com-

panion on many of my visits was Dorothea Lang, C.N.M. (Certified Nurse-Midwife), Director of Nurse-Midwifery for New York City. Miss Lang's experience as both a nurse-midwife and a former head nurse of the labor and delivery unit of the New York–Cornell Medical Center made her a particularly well-qualified observer and companion. As we traveled from country to country certain patterns of care soon became evident. For one, in those countries that enjoy an incidence of infant mortality and birth trauma significantly lower than that of the United States, highly trained professional midwives are an important source of obstetrical care and family planning services for normal women, whether the births take place in the hospital or in the home. In these countries the expertise of the physician is called upon only when the expectant mother is ill during pregnancy, or when labor or birth is anticipated to be, or is found to be, abnormal. Under this system, the high-risk mother—the one who is most likely to bear an impaired or stillborn child—has a better opportunity to obtain in-depth medical attention than is possible under our existing American system of obstetrical care where the obstetrician is also called upon to play the role of midwife.

Deprivation, birth defects, prematurity, and low birth weight are not unique to the United States. While it is tempting to blame our comparatively high incidence of infant mortality solely on a lack of available prenatal care and on socioeconomic factors, our observations indicate that, comparatively, the prenatal care we offer most clinic patients in the United States is not grossly inferior to that available in other developed countries. Furthermore, the diet and standard of living in many countries which have a lower incidence of infant mortality than ours would be considered inadequate by American standards.

As an example, when one compares the availability of prenatal care, the incidence of premature births, the average diet of various economic groups, and the equipment available to aid in newborn-infant survival in two such diverse countries as the United States and Japan, there are no major differences between the two countries. The differences lie in (a) our frequent use of prenatal and obstetrical medication, (b) our pathologically oriented management of pregnancy, labor, birth, and postpartum, and (c) the predominance of artificial feeding in the United States, in contrast to Japan.

If present statistics follow the trend of recent years, an infant born in the United States is more than four times more likely to die in the first day of life than an infant born in Japan. But a survival of the birth process should not be our singular goal. For every American newborn infant who dies there are likely to be several who are neurologically damaged.

Unfortunately, the American tendency to warp the birth experience, distorting it into a pathological event rather than a physiological one for the normal childbearing woman, is no longer peculiar to just the United States. In my visits to hospitals in various countries I was distressed to find that some physicians, anxious to impress their colleagues with their "Americanized" techniques, have unfortunately adopted many of our obstetrical practices without stopping to question their scientific or social merit.

Few American babies are born today as nature intended them to be.

It is not unlikely that unnecessary alterations in the normal fetal environment may play a role in the incidence of neurological impairment and infant mortality in the United States. Infant resuscitation, other than routine suctioning, is rarely needed in countries such as Sweden, the Netherlands, and Japan, where the skillful psychological management of labor usually precludes the need for obstetrical medication. In contrast, in those European countries, such as Belgium, where the overall pattern of obstetrical care is similar to our own, the incidence of infant mortality also approaches our own.

Obviously there will always be medical indications which dictate the use of various obstetrical procedures, but to apply the following American practices and procedures routinely to the vast majority of mothers who are capable of giving birth without complication is to create added stress which is not in the best interests of either the mother or her newborn infant.

Let us take a close look at some of our common obstetrical practices from early pregnancy to postpartum which have served to warp and distort the childbearing experience in the United States. While not all of the practices below affect infant mortality, it is equally apparent that they do not contribute to the reduction of infant morbidity or mortality and therefore should be reevaluated.

Withholding Information on the Disadvantages of Obstetrical Medication   Ignorance of the possible hazards of obstetrical medication appears to encourage

the misuse and abuse of obstetrical medication, for in those countries where mothers are not told routinely of the possible disadvantages of obstetrical medication to themselves or to their babies the use of such medication is on the increase.

There is no research or evidence which indicates that mothers will be emotionally damaged if they are advised, prior to birth, that obstetrical medication may be to the disadvantage of their newborn infants.

Requiring All Normal Women to Give Birth in the Hospital   While ICEA does not encourage home births, there is ample evidence in the Netherlands and in Chicago (Chicago Maternity Center) to demonstrate that normal women who have received adequate prenatal care can safely give birth at home if a proper system is developed for home deliveries. Over half of the mothers in the Netherlands give birth at home with the assistance of a professional midwife and a maternity aide. The comparatively low incidence of infant deaths and birth trauma in the Netherlands, a country of diverse ethnic composition and intermarriage, is evidence of the comparative safety of a properly developed home delivery service.

Dutch obstetricians point out that when the labor of a normal woman is unhurried and allowed to progress normally, unexpected emergencies rarely occur. They also point out that the small risk involved in a Dutch home delivery is more than offset by the increased hazards resulting from the use of obstetrical medication and obstetrical tampering which are more likely to occur in a hospital environment, especially in countries where professionals have had little or no exposure to normal labor and birth in a home environment during their training.

Elective Induction of Labor   The elective induction of labor (where there is no clear medical indication) appears to be an American idiosyncrasy which is frowned upon in other developed countries.

The elective induction of labor has been found almost to double the incidence of fetomaternal transfusion and its attendant hazards.[2] But perhaps the least appreciated problem of elective induction is the fact that the abrupt onset of artificially induced labor tends to make it extremely difficult for even the well-prepared mother to tolerate the discomfort of the intensified contractions without the aid of obstetrical medication. When the onset of labor occurs spontaneously, the normal, gradual increase in contraction length and intensity appears to provoke in the mother an accompanying tolerance for discomfort or pain.

Since the British Perinatal Hazards Study found no increase in perinatal mortality or impairment of learning ability at age seven among full-term infants unless gestation had extended beyond forty-one weeks,[3] there would appear to be no medical justification for subjecting a mother or her baby to the possible hazards of elective induction in order to terminate the pregnancy prior to forty-one weeks' gestation.

Separating the Mother from Familial Support During Labor and Birth   Research indicates that fear adversely affects uterine motility and blood flow,[4] and yet many American mothers are routinely separated from a family member or close friend at this time of emotional crisis.

In most developed countries, other than the United States and the Eastern European countries, mothers are encouraged to walk about or to sit and chat with a family member or supportive person in what is called an "early labor lounge." This lounge is usually located near but outside the labor-delivery area in order to provide a more relaxed atmosphere during much of labor. The mother is taken to the labor-delivery area to be checked periodically, then allowed to return to the labor lounge for as long as she likes or until her membranes have ruptured.

Confining the Normal Laboring Woman to Bed   In virtually all countries except the United States, a woman in labor is routinely encouraged to walk about during labor for as long as she wishes or until her membranes have ruptured. Such activity is considered to facilitate labor by distracting the mother's attention from the discomfort or pain of her contractions and to encourage a more rapid engagement of the fetal head. In America, where drugs are frequently administered either orally or parenterally to laboring mothers, such ambulation is discouraged—not only for the patient's safety but also to avoid possible legal complications in the event of an accident.

Shaving the Birth Area   Research involving 7,600 mothers has demonstrated that the practice of shaving the perineum and pubis does not reduce the incidence of infection. In fact, the incidence of infection was slightly higher among those mothers who were shaved.[5] Yet this procedure, which tends to create apprehension in laboring women, is still carried out routinely in most American hospitals. Clipping the perineal or pudendal hair closely with surgical scissors is far less disturbing to the mother and is less likely to result in infection caused by razor abrasions.

Professional Dependence on Technology and Pharmacological Methods of Pain Relief   Most of the world's mothers receive little or no drugs during pregnancy, labor, or birth. The constant emotional support provided the laboring woman in other countries by the nurse-midwife, and often by her husband, appears greatly to improve the mother's tolerance for discomfort. In contrast, the American labor room nurse is frequently assigned to look after several women in labor, all or most of whom have had no preparation to cope with the discomfort or pain of childbearing. Under the circumstances, drugs, rather than skillful emotional support, are employed to relieve the mother's apprehension and discomfort (and perhaps to assuage the harried labor attendant's feeling of inadequacy).

Routine Electronic Fetal Monitoring   The wisdom of depending on an experienced nurse using a stethoscope to monitor accurately the effects of obstetrical medication on the well-being of the fetus has been demonstrated by Haverkamp.[6] No one knows the long-term or delayed consequences of ultrasonic fetal monitoring on subsequent human development. The fact that some electronic fetal monitoring devices require that a mother's membranes be ruptured and the electrode be screwed into the skin of the fetal scalp creates hazards of its own. Current research indicates that obstetrical management which reduces the need for such monitoring is advisable.

Chemical Stimulation of Labor   Oxytocic agents are frequently administered to American mothers in order to intensify artificially the frequency or the strength of the mother's contractions, as a means of shortening the mother's labor. While chemical stimulation is sometimes medically indicated, often it is undertaken to satisfy the American propensity for efficiency and speed. Hon suggests that the overenthusiastic use of oxytocic stimulants sometimes results in alterations in the normal fetal heart rate.[7] Fields points out that the possible hazards inherent in elective induction are also possible in artificially stimulated labor unless the mother and fetus are carefully monitored.[8]

Shortening the phases of normal labor when there is no sign of fetal distress has not been shown to improve infant outcome. Little is known of the long-term effects of artificially stimulating labor contractions. During a contraction the unborn child normally receives less oxygen. The gradual buildup of intensity, which occurs when the onset of labor is allowed to occur spontaneously and to proceed without chemical stimulation, appears likely to be a protective mechanism that is best left unaltered unless there is a clear medical indication for the artificial stimulation of labor.

Delaying Birth until the Physician Arrives   Because of the increased likelihood of resultant brain damage to the infant the practice of delaying birth by anesthesia or physical restraint until the physician arrives to deliver the infant is frowned upon in most countries. Yet the practice still occurs occasionally in the United States and in countries where hospital-assigned midwives do not routinely manage the labor and delivery of normal mothers.

Requiring the Mother to Assume the Lithotomy Position for Birth   There is gathering scientific evidence that the unphysiological lithotomy position (back flat, with knees drawn up and spread wide apart by "stirrups"), which is preferred by most American physicians because it is more convenient for the *accoucheur,* tends to alter the normal fetal environment and obstruct the normal process of childbearing, making spontaneous birth more difficult or impossible.

The lithotomy and dorsal positions tend to:

1. Adversely affect the mother's blood pressure, cardiac return, and pulmonary ventilation.[9]
2. Decrease the normal intensity of the contractions.[10]
3. Inhibit the mother's voluntary efforts to push her baby out spontaneously[11] which, in turn, increases the need for fundal pressure or forceps and increases the traction necessary for a forceps extraction.
4. Inhibit the spontaneous expulsion of the placenta[12] which, in turn, increases the need for cord traction, forced expression, or manual removal of the placenta[13]—procedures which significantly increase the incidence of fetomaternal hemorrhage.[14]
5. Increase the need for episiotomy because of the increased tension on the pelvic floor and the stretching of the perineal tissue.[15]

Australian, Russian, and American research bears out the clinical experience of European physicians and midwives—that when mothers are supported to a semi-sitting position for birth, with their feet supported by the lower section of the labor-delivery bed, mothers tend to push more effectively, appear to need less pain relief, are more likely to want to be conscious for birth, and are less likely to need an episiotomy.[16]

The increased efficiency of the semisitting position, combined with a minimum use of medication for birth, is evidenced by the fact that the combined use of both forceps and the vacuum extractor rarely exceeds 4 percent to 5 percent of all births in the Netherlands, as compared to an incidence of 65 percent in many American hospitals. (Cesarean section occurs in approximately 1.5 percent of all Dutch births.)

The Routine Use of Regional or General Anesthesia for Delivery   In light of the current shortage of qualified anesthetists and anesthesiologists and the frequent scientific papers now being published on the possible hazards resulting from the use of regional and general anesthesia, it would seem prudent to make every effort to prepare the mother physically and mentally to cope with the sensations and discomfort of birth in order to avoid the use of such medicaments. Regional and general anesthesia not only tend adversely to affect fetal environment pharmacologically, which has been discussed previously herein, but their use also increases the need for obstetrical intervention in the normal process of birth, since both types of anesthesia tend to prolong labor.[17] Johnson points out that epidural and spinal anesthesia significantly increase the incidence of midforceps delivery and its attendant hazards.[18] Pudendal block anesthesia not only tends to interfere with the mother's ability effectively to push her baby down the birth canal due to the blocking of the afferent path of the pushing reflex, but also appears to interfere with the mother's normal protective reflexes, thus making "an explosive" birth and perineal damage more likely to occur.

The Routine Use of Forceps for Delivery   There is no scientific justification for the routine application of forceps for delivery.[19] The incidence of delivery by forceps and vacuum extractor, combined, rarely rises above 5 percent in countries where mothers actively participate in the births of their babies. In contrast, as mentioned previously, the incidence of forceps extraction frequently rises to as high as 65 percent in some American hospitals.

Routine Episiotomy   There is no research or evidence to indicate that routine episiotomy (a surgical incision to enlarge the vaginal orifice) reduces the incidence of pelvic relaxation (structural damage to the pelvic floor musculature) in the mother. Nor is there any research or evidence that routine episiotomy reduces neurological impairment in the child who has shown no signs of fetal distress or that the procedure helps to maintain subsequent male or female sexual response.

The incidence of pelvic floor relaxation appears to be on the decline throughout the world, even in those countries where episiotomy is still comparatively rare. The contention that the modern washing machine has been more effective in reducing pelvic relaxation among American mothers than has routine episiotomy is given some credence by the fact that in areas of the United States where life is still hard for the woman pelvic relaxation appears in white women who have never borne children.

In developed countries where episiotomy is comparatively rare the physiotherapist is considered an important member of the obstetrical team—before as well as after birth. The physiotherapist is responsible for seeing that each mother begins exercises the day following birth which will help to restore the normal elasticity and tone of the mother's perineal and abdominal muscles. In countries where every effort is made to avoid the need for an episiotomy, interviews with both parents and professionals indicate that an intact perineum which is strengthened by postpartum exercises is more apt to result in both male and female sexual satisfaction than is a perineum that has been incised and reconstructed.

Why then, is there such an emotional attachment among professionals to routine episiotomy? A prominent European professor of obstetrics and gynecology recently made the following comment on the American penchant for routine episiotomy, "Since all the physician can really do to affect the course of childbirth for the 95 percent of mothers who are capable of giving birth without complication is to offer the mother pharmacological relief from discomfort or pain and to perform an episiotomy, there is probably an unconscious tendency for many professionals to see these practices as indispensable."

Interviews with obstetrician-gynecologists in many countries indicate that they tend to agree that a superficial, first degree tear is less traumatic to the perineal tissue than an incision which requires several sutures for reconstruction. There is no research which would indicate otherwise.

Early Clamping or "Milking" of the Umbilical Cord
Several years ago De Marsh stated that the placental blood normally belongs to the infant and his or her failure to get this blood is equivalent to submitting him or her to a rather severe hemorrhage. Despite the fact that placental transfusion normally occurs in every corner of the world without adverse consequences, there is still a great effort in the United States and Canada to deprecate the practice. One must read the literature carefully to find that placental transfusion has not been demonstrated to increase the incidence of morbidity or mortality in the placentally transfused infant.[20]

Delaying the First Breast-feeding
The common American practice of routinely delaying the time of the first breast-feeding has not been shown to be in the best interest of either the conscious mother or her newborn infant. Clinical experience with the early feeding of newborn infants has shown this practice to be safe.[21] If the mother feels well enough and the infant is capable of suckling while they are still in the delivery room then it would seem more cautious, in the event of tracheoesophageal abnormality, to permit the infant to suckle for the first time under the watchful eye of the physician or nurse-midwife rather than delay the feeding for several hours when the expertise of the professional may not be immediately available.

In light of the many protective antibodies contained in colostrum it would seem likely that the earlier the infant's intake of species specific colostrum, the sooner the antibodies can be accrued by the infant.

Offering Water and Formula to the Breast-fed Newborn Infant
The common American practice of giving water or formula to a newborn infant prior to the first breast-feeding or as a supplement during the first days of life has not been shown to be in the best interests of the infant. There are now indications that these practices may, in fact, be harmful. Glucose water, once the standby in every American hospital, has now been designated a potential hazard if aspirated by the newborn infant, yet it is still used in many American hospitals.

Restricting Newborn Infants to a Four-hour Feeding Schedule and Withholding Nightime Feedings
Although widely spaced infant feedings may be more convenient for hospital personnel, the practice of feeding a newborn infant only every four hours and not permitting the infant to breast-feed at all during the night cannot be justified on any scientific grounds. Such a regimen restricts the suckling stimulation necessary to bring about the normally rapid onset and adequate production of the mother's milk. In countries where custom permits the infant to suckle immediately after birth and on demand from that time, first-time mothers frequently begin to produce breast milk for their babies within twenty-four hours after birth. In contrast, in countries where hospital routines prevent normal demand feeding from birth, mothers frequently do not produce breast milk for their babies until the third day following birth.

Overdistention of the breast or engorgement is a hospital acquired condition which does not occur to any comparable degree in cultures where mothers are permitted to breast-feed their babies on demand from birth.[22]

Preventing Early Father-child Contact
Permitting fathers to hold their newborn infants immediately following birth and during the postpartum hospital stay has not been shown by research or clinical experience to increase the incidence of infection among newborns, even when those infants are returned to a regular or central nursery. Yet only in the Eastern European countries is the father permitted less involvement in the immediate postpartum period than in the United States.

Research has consistently confirmed the fact that the greatest sources of infection to the newborn infant are the nursery and nursery personnel.[23] One has only to observe a mother holding her newborn infant against her bathrobe, which has probably been exposed to abundant hospital-borne bacteria, to realize the fallacy of preventing a father from holding his baby during the hospital stay.

Restricting Intermittent Rooming-in to Specific Room Requirements Throughout the world great effort is made to keep mothers and babies together in the hospital, no matter how inconvenient the accommodations. There is no research or evidence which indicates that intermittent rooming-in should be restricted to private rooms or to rooms which have a sink, or which provide at least eighty square feet for mother and baby. Such requirements are based on conjecture and not on controlled evaluation.

Restricting Sibling Visitation The common American practice of prohibiting toddlers and children from visiting their mothers during the hospital stay is an emotional hardship on both the mothers and their children and is unsupported by scientific research or evidence. Experience in other countries and in several hospitals here in the United States suggests that where sibling visitation is permitted, a short explanation as to the importance of not bringing suspect illnesses into the hospital seems to be effective in controlling infection.

Summary

As mentioned previously, most of the practices discussed above have developed not from a lack of concern for the well-being of the mother and baby but from a lack of awareness as to the problems which can arise from each progressive digression from the normal childbearing experience. Like a snowball rolling down hill, as one unphysiological practice is employed, for one reason or another, another frequently becomes necessary to counteract some of the disadvantages, large or small, inherent in the previous procedure.

The higher incidence of fetal, neonatal, and maternal deaths occurring in our large urban hospitals, as opposed to our smaller community hospitals,[24] is undoubtedly due, in part, to the greater proportion of high-risk mothers in the urban areas. But we in the United States must stop looking for scapegoats and face up to the fact that by individualizing the care offered to maternity patients, much can be done immediately to improve infant outcome without the slightest outlay of capital.

There is currently an increasing emphasis on consolidating maternity facilities. However, we in ICEA do not see the consolidation of community obstetrical facilities as being always in the best interest of the vast majority of mothers who are capable of giving birth without

complications. There should, of course, be centers where those mothers who have had no prenatal care or who are anticipated to be obstetrical risks can be properly cared for. But to insist that every healthy mother must go to a major maternity facility which is unnecessary for her needs and inconvenient for her family, and where she is very apt to be "lost in the crowd," will only spur the growing trend in the United States toward professionally unattended home births.

Throughout the United States the current inclination of many expectant parents is to seek out, to "shop around" for the type of physician and hospital they feel they need in order to have the type of childbearing experience they want. They not only want a doctor who will support them in their efforts to have a prepared, natural birth, with a minimum of or no medication; they also want a hospital which offers education for childbearing and a supportive family-centered atmosphere. These expectant mothers appreciate the availability of such facilities as an early labor lounge, a dual purpose labor-delivery room, a mother-baby recovery room, and a children's visiting room if they have older children. But most of all they want a supportive atmosphere in which they can share the childbearing experience to the extent that they desire, and one which makes an effort to meet the individual needs of the mother, the father, and their newborn baby as they form their family bonds during the hospital stay.

Notes

1. H. Chase, "Ranking Countries by Infant Mortality Rates," Public Health Reports 84 (1969): 19–27; M. Wegman, "Annual Summary of Vital Statistics—1969," *Pediatrics* 47 (1971): 461–64.
2. A. Beer, "Fetal Erythrocytes in Maternal Circulation of 155 Rh-Negative Women," *Obstet. & Gynec.* 34 (1969): 143–50.
3. N. Butler, "A National Long-Term Study of Perinatal Hazards," Sixth World Congress of the Federation of International Gynecology & Obstetrics, 1970.
4. J. Kelly, "Effect of Fear Upon Uterine Motility," *Am. J. Obstet. & Gynec.* 83 (1962): 576–81.
5. R. Burchell, "Predelivery Removal of Pubic Hair," *Obstet. & Gynec.* 24 (1964): 272–73; H. Kantor et al., "Value of Shaving the Pudendal-Perineal Area in Delivery Preparation," *Obstet. & Gynec.*[25] (1965) 509–12.
6. Haverkamp, A. D., Thompson, H. E., McFee, J. G. et al., "The Evaluation of Continuous Fetal-Heart Monitoring for High Risk Pregnancies." *Am. J. Obstet. & Gynec.* 125, no. 3 (June 1, 1926): 310–20.
7. E. Hon, "Direct Monitoring of the Fetal Heart," *Hospital Practice* (September 1970): 91–97.
8. H. Fields, "Complications of Elective Induction" *Obstet. & Gynec.* 15 (1960): 476–80; H. Fields, "Induction of Labor: Methods, Hazards, Complications, and Contraindications," *Hospital Topics* (December 1968): 63–68.
9. C. Flowers, *Obstetric Analgesia and Anesthesia* (New York: Hoeber, Harper & Row, 1967); L. S. James, "The Effects of Pain

Relief for Labor and Delivery on the Fetus and Newborn," *Anesthesiology* 21 (1960): 405–30; A. Blankfield, "The Optimum Position for Childbirth," *Med. J. Australia 2* (1965): 666–68.

10. Blankfield, "The Optimum Position for Childbirth"; F. H. Howard, "Delivery in the Physiologic Position," *Obstet. & Gynec.* 11 (1958): 318–22; I. Gritsiuk, "Position in Labor," *Ob-Gyn Observer* (September 1968).

11. Blankfield, "The Optimum Position for Childbirth"; Howard, "Delivery in the Physiologic Position"; N. Newton and M. Newton "The Propped Position for the Second Stage of Labor," *Obstet. & Gynec.* 15 (1960): 28–34.

12. Newton and Newton, "The Propped Position for the Second Stage of Labor."

13. M. Botha, "The Management of the Umbilical Cord in Labour," *S. Afr. J. Obstet.* 6, no. 2 (1968): 30–33.

14. Beer, "Fetal Erythrocytes in Maternal Circulation of 155 Rh-Negative Women."

15. Blankfield, "The Optimum Position for Childbirth."

16. Ibid.; Newton and Newton, "The Propped Position for the Second Stage of Labor."

17. L. Hellman and J. Pritchard, *Williams Obstetrics,* 14th ed. (New York: Appleton-Century-Crofts, 1971).

18. W. Johnson, "Regionals Can Prolong Labor," *Medical World News,* October 15, 1971.

19. Butler, "A National Long-Term Study of Perinatal Hazards."

20. S. Saigal et al., "Placental Transfusion and Hyperbilirubinemia in the Premature," *Pediatrics* 49 (1972): 406–19.

21. H. Eppink, "Time of Initial Breast Feeding Surveyed in Michigan Hospitals," *Hospital Topics* (June 1968): 116–17.

22. M. Newton and N. Newton, "Postpartum Engorgement of the Breast," *Am. J. Obstet. & Gynec.* 61 (1951): 664–67.

23. H. Gezon et al., "Some Controversial Aspects in the Epidemiology of Hospital Nursery Staphylococcal Infections," *Amer. J. of Public Health* 50 (1960): 473–84; R. Ravenholt and G. LaVeck, "Staphylococcal Disease—An Obstetric, Pediatric & Community Problem," *Amer. J. of Public Health* 46 (1956): 1287–96.

24. E. Bishop, "The National Study of Maternity Care." *Obstet. & Gynec.* (1971): 745–50.

Routine Midwifery Care
Why Not Here?
by Leah Hyder

In our ever-changing fast paced system of health care delivery, many women feel that they receive little personal attention, especially during pregnancy and childbirth. Into this breach step midwives, who have a long history of providing women with holistic care during pregnancy and childbirth. Despite the high quality of care that midwives provide to expectant mothers, American women have few opportunities to use the services of midwives and to have those services covered by their health insurance plans. Clearly, midwifery in the Untied States faces more barriers than most other countries.

Midwifery Is Welcomed in Europe

The United States is lagging behind other nations of the world in fully integrating midwifery into its health care system. While midwives deliver only 6% of the approximately 220,000 babies in the United States each year, midwives in other countries attend up to 80% of their countries' births. Barriers against and support for midwifery vary from country to country.

The majority of healthy women in Europe use professionally-trained midwives. Most European countries have passed laws regulating midwives and publicly support midwifery schools and professional organizations. Most midwives in Europe work for governmental health services.

Austria, Sweden, the United Kingdom (UK), and particularly the Netherlands possess sound systems of midwifery. In Austria, the law requires that a midwife be present at every birth. In Sweden, midwives provide more than 80% of prenatal care and family planning services. Midwives in the UK attend 70% of all births and also provide the vast majority of care to women who want home births. They also provide a high proportion of care between pregnancies. The midwives in England are independent practitioners, responsible for the full

Certified Nurse-Midwives (CNMs)—CNMS are Registered Nurses (RNs) who complete training to become certified in nurse-midwifery by the American College of Nurse-Midwives (ACNM). In the US, CNMs care for 5% of all births and 95% of all births delivered by midwives.

Certified Midwives (CMs)—CMs are not registered nurses, but are accredited by the ACNM and have graduated from an ACNM accredited midwifery school.

Certified Professional Midwives (CPMs)—Midwives who are certified by the North American Registry of Midwives (NARM).

Licensed Midwife—A legal term denoting state-licensed direct-entry midwives.

Direct-Entry Midwives—Direct-entry midwives have completed a formal midwifery education program or are licensed to practice in their state or local jurisdiction or are certified by a local or state organization.

Birth Attendants—Birth attendants assist the primary birth attendant, usually a CNM or physician. This term is also used by some non-CNM midwives who practice in states where midwifery is illegal unless practiced by a CNM or a physician.

Granny and Lay Midwives—Granny and lay midwives are other types of midwives which have existed in the U.S. but that are virtually nonexistent today. Midwives historically called lay or professional midwives often call themselves traditional or independent midwives today.

spectrum of care for healthy women. The Netherlands is the only industrialized country where the majority of women have home births.

Midwifery in the Developing World

Midwifery is also prevalent in developing countries, though standards of practice are not at the same level as European nations. Developing countries often use lay midwives to complement the sparse distribution of physicians. Often, the only training midwives have is observation of relatives and physicians. In most third-world countries, the care midwives provide includes treatments which reflect cultural practices such as fasting, prayers, herbal medicines, and sacrifices to appease gods.

Further, midwives in developing countries face unique challenges, such as lack of information about and access to proper sanitation measures, illiteracy, scarcity of training programs and the means to attend them, and the lack of financial resources to sustain their own practice. Often, even where physicians are available, women prefer midwives because of economic and sociocultural reasons.

Midwifery in the United States

Barriers to midwifery care in the United States are numerous and imposing. They include physician opposition, public perception of midwives as substandard, state and federal regulations, the current economic and political environment, lack of training programs, strife between midwifery groups, lack of access to malpractice insurance, and lack of acceptance among third-party payers, including Medicaid.

Physician Opposition

Although some physicians encourage midwifery, others adamantly oppose it. While Ob-Gyns are specialists trained in interventions which are sometimes necessary in complicated or high-risk pregnancies, midwives' training emphasizes skills which help women have healthy outcomes with as little intervention as possible. A common perception is that women are safer in a hospital, with a doctor. In fact, studies show that both mothers and babies are safer with midwives. Births attended by certified Nurse-Midwives (CNMs) produce fewer cesarean sections, infant abrasions, complications, perineal lacerations, postpartum hemorrhage, and vacuum- or forceps-assisted deliveries than physicians. CNMs also cost approximately $1000 less than physicians per birth and most develop a strong relationship with the mother. Is it any wonder that many physicians oppose midwives? Midwives treat normal pregnancies as the natural processes that they are. Midwives need to fight this physician opposition and medicalization, as well as the accompanying public perceptions.

Regulatory Barriers

Often regulations pose another barrier to midwifery care. Laws governing midwifery care vary from state to state and often do not comply to the national standards of practice set by the American College of Nurse-

Midwives (ACNM). Laws that require midwives to practice in hospitals or be supervised by a physician limit the midwives' scope of practice. This often means that women in rural areas who, without such restricting laws, would have convenient access to local midwives must instead travel for miles to reach a hospital or physician. In addition, the Joint Commission on Accreditation of Health Care Organizations (JCAHCO), a regulatory organization overseeing activities of most healthcare organizations in the United States, requires that physical examinations of women be done only by physicians. Because eligibility requirements for health care providers to have hospital privileges often include completing physical examinations, which non-physicians cannot do per JCAHCO standards, midwives would not be allowed to practice in a hospital.

Economic Woes

Midwives face economic barriers as well. Although they do similar work, midwives are paid thousands of dollars less per year than physicians. Medicare reimburses CNMs up to 65% of the physician fee schedule which means that physicians earn over 1/3 more than nurse-midwives for the same services. Many third-party payers adopted this payment policy, making the injustice more widespread. In this session of Congress, U.S. Rep. Edolphus Towns (D-NY) is proposing "The Certified Nurse-Midwives Medicare Services Act" to increase this reimbursement to 95%, which although progressive, fails to address the similar needs of midwives who are not CNMs. Additionally, many free-standing birth centers receive no coverage in numerous state and federal Medicaid programs at all. Midwives also disproportionately render care to underserved populations who often do not have insurance and can not pay out of pocket for services.

Access to Liability Insurance

Midwives often lack available and affordable malpractice insurance. This is a primary impediment to maternity care by midwives. As a result of the liability insurance crisis of the 1980s, many Ob-Gyns and midwives left practice because they could not find adequate malpractice insurance. Most CNMs now obtain insurance from their employers, the ACNM, or from local insurance companies. Some problems with obtaining malpractice insurance include its increasing cost, restrictions related to the place of birth, and medical management of pregnancy and childbirth as the accepted standard.

Dearth of Education Programs

Access to midwife education and training is challenging. Midwifery programs across the U.S. are filled to capacity due to the demand for midwives, which is greater than the supply. One reason so few schools educate midwives is lack of funding. Additionally, the U.S. is still very physician-oriented. But because the public demand for physicians is higher than it is for midwives, funding for the training of physicians receives more attention than that for midwives. As women increasingly use midwifery services, leverage may be created for funding of midwifery programs.

Barriers to U.S. Subpopulations

Barriers to midwifery care exist for subpopulations of the general public in the U.S. as well. Historically, poor, rural, Hispanic, African-American, and Native-American women have used midwives the most frequently. This prevalence was often due to the cost of care, exclusion by white hospitals, and transportation problems. Because of these factors of inequality, these women often felt that they were given inferior care when treated by a midwife. Midwives have fought this perception of the quality of their care.

Building Bridges in U.S. Midwifery

Although midwives currently face these political barriers, various groups are working for change. The American College of Nurse-Midwives (ACNM) is a professional organization for CNMs. It speaks for its membership on issues affecting education, practice, recognition, and reimbursement. A second professional group, MANA (the Midwives Alliance of North America), welcomes and hopes to unite all midwives, including both lay and certified midwives. While MANA focuses on direct-entry midwives, their agenda includes all midwives.

Although some tension among the groups exists, different groups have taken measures to unify all midwives. The Bridge Club is an organization of the nurse-midwives who want to unify the ACNM and MANA, which sometimes have conflicting views. The Midwifery Communication and Accountability Project (MCAP) of Boston, Massachusetts, has midwives work together on the community level to raise money for policy issues, hoping that working together towards a common goal would help unify the midwives. MANA welcomes all midwives and encourages dialogue among the groups.

Despite their varying educational backgrounds, all midwives have much in common and many realize that working together to promote the causes of midwifery will help them all as well as the women they serve.

Future Prospects of Midwifery in the United States

While some third-party payers are apprehensive about using midwives because of liability issues, other third-party payers utilize midwives because of their cost-effectiveness. It remains to be seen whether the trend in third-party payers will be to utilize midwives in the name of cost efficiency or not to utilize them because of their liability. As more women demand midwifery services and the professional reputation of midwives grows, more third party payers may utilize midwives.

The barriers to midwifery in the U.S. are substantial, but midwives constantly work to lessen them. Yet we can look to European countries for a good model and to show us areas in which we could improve to make midwifery affordable, accessible, and acceptable in the U.S.

To learn more about midwifery or its advocacy, contact the ACNM at (202) 728-9860, the Massachusetts Friends of Midwives at (508) 369-1468, or MANA at (931) 964-2589.

I would like to thank Doris Haire, Linda Holmes, and Carol Sakala for their input into this article.

Leah Hyder was a summer Network intern.

References

A list of references is available in the original source.

Cesarean Section in the United States

by Midwifery Task Force

- The most common major operation performed in the United States is a cesarean section. (1)
- Sixteen U.S. hospitals had cesarean section rates of 45% or higher in 1994. (1)
- 106 U.S. hospitals had cesarean section rates of 37% or higher in 1994. (1)
- About half of the cesareans done in the U.S. in 1991 were unnecessary. This cost Americans more than $1.3 billion. (1)
- The World Health Organization states there is no justification for having a cesarean section rate higher than 10–15%. (2)
- The risk of maternal death associated with cesarean section is 2 to 9 times that associated with vaginal births. (3,4)
- Midwife-attended birth is associated with low rates of cesarean section. (5,6)
- Obstetricians who work with midwives have low rates of cesarean section. (7)

- The World Health Organization states that the countries with some of the lowest perinatal mortality rates in the world have cesarean rates under 10%. (2)
- Evidence and peer education do not change standards of practice. (8,9–11)
- Between 2 to 6% of babies delivered by cesarean operation suffer accidental lacerations during the surgery. (12)
- Twenty percent of women having cesarean section suffer fever after the surgery, primarily because of iatrogenic infections. (13)

References

1. Gabay M, Wolfe S. *Unnecessary Cesarean Sections: Curing a National Epidemic.* Public Citizen's Health Research Group, May 1994.
2. WHO Consensus Conference on Appropriate Technology for Birth, Fortaleza, Brazil, 22–26 April 1985.

3. Petitti DB et al. In-hospital mortality in the United States: time trends and relation to method of delivery. *Obstetrics & Gynecology* 1982;59:6–11.

4. Hall M, Bewley S. Maternal mortality and mode of delivery, *The Lancet* 1999;354:776.

5. Durand AM. The safety of home birth: the Farm study. *American Journal of Public Health* 1990;82(3):450–453.

6. Rooks J et al. Outcomes of care in birth centers: the national birth center study. *New England Journal of Medicine* 1990;321(26):1804–1811.

7. Pel M and Heres MHB. OBINT: a study of obstetric intervention. The Hague: CIP-Koninklinike Bibliotheek.

8. Goer H. *Obstetrical Myths Versus Research Realities* 1995, Bergin & Garvey.

9. Porreco RP. Meeting the challenge of the rising cesarean birth rate. *Obstetrics & Gynecology* 1990:75(1):133–136.

10. Lomas J et al. Do practice guidelines guide practice? The effect of a consensus statement on the practice of physicians. *New England Journal of Medicine* 1989;321(19):1306–1311.

11. Dillon WP et al. Obstetric care and cesarean birth rates: a program to monitor quality of care. *Obstetrics & Gynecology* 1992;80(5):731–737.

12. Smith J et al. Fetal laceration injury at cesarean delivery. *Obstetrics & Gynecology* 1997;90:344–346.

13. Enkin M, Enkin E, Chalmers I, Hemminki E. Prophylactic antibiotics in association with caesarean section, in *Effective Care in Pregnancy and Childbirth,* eds: I Chalmers, M Enkin, M Keirse, 1989, Oxford University Press.

Midwifery Facts

by Midwifery Task Force

- The percentage of countries providing universal prenatal care that have lower infant mortality rates than the United States: 100%
- The percentage of U.S. births attended principally by midwives: 5% The percentage of European births attended principally by midwives: 75%
- Number of midwives practicing in the U.S.: 3,000–4,000 direct entry midwives; 3,500 certified nurse-midwives
- Number of midwives needed in the U.S. to meet European levels: 120,000
- The World Health Organization (WHO) states that the preferred location for most births is outside the hospital, either at home or in a birthing center, and that out-of-hospital birth should be implemented and maintained as the basic standard for all midwifery education and training programs.
- According to two recently published studies, direct entry midwife-attended home births were accomplished with safety comparable to that of conventional births. In fact, physician-attended hospital birth has never been shown to be safer than midwife-attended home birth for women with normal pregnancies. (American Journal of Public Health 1992;82:450-453; Birth, 1994;1:141–148)
- Most home births in the United States are attended by direct entry midwives.
- Americans could save $13 billion to $20 billion annually in health care costs by developing a network of midwifery care providers, demedicalizing childbirth, and encouraging breastfeeding. (Frank A. Oski, M.D., professor and director, Department of Pediatrics, John Hopkins University School of Medicine, Baltimore)

How Do Socioeconomic Factors Affect Disparities in Maternal Mortality?

by Deborah Maine, DRPH

Socioeconomic factors affect nearly every cause of death, but not always in the same ways. Understanding which components of socioeconomic development were responsible for the great declines in maternal mortality in the United States and Britain can help us design effective programs in developing countries. The literature shows that maternal mortality is most strongly influenced by women's access to medical care for complications of pregnancy. In addition to international disparities in maternal mortality, there are still great disparities among racial groups in the United States. Here, too, analysis of the factors at work may be helpful in tailoring interventions. (*JAMWA*. 2001;56:189–190)

Nearly every disease varies with socioeconomic status—among countries and among social groups within countries. But that does not mean that all causes of death are affected by the same factors. After all, socioeconomic status is composed of a variety of elements, including education, nutrition, income, social status, and access to medical care, that influence health and disease in different ways. Therefore, although infant and maternal mortality (MM) may both vary with socioeconomic status or stage of development, they may actually be affected by quite different forces. Examining historical patterns of mortality can help us identify which elements of socioeconomic status have the greatest influence on particular causes of death. This can, in turn, assist us in designing more effective programs to improve health.

Although maternal deaths are now very rare in developed countries, they are still everyday events in the developing world. More than half a million women die each year of complications of pregnancy and childbirth, 99% of them in developing countries. As Table 1 shows, MM ratios are estimated to be nearly 100 times higher in Africa than in North America. This is the greatest disparity between developed and developing countries of any commonly used public health indicator.

Clearly, MM shines a spotlight on the vast disparities in health between people in developing and developed countries. It also highlights some disparities in developed countries. For example, black women in the United States have had higher levels of MM than white women for as long as data have been available, and the gap widened during the 20th century.

One of the great truths of public health is that medical care is not the most important influence on the health status of populations. It was not an important factor in the steep decline in mortality in the 19th and early 20th centuries. Instead, improved living conditions in Europe and North America resulted in sustained and impressive declines in infant mortality long before medical technology to prevent or treat the major causes of death was developed. For example, there were more than 1200 deaths from measles among children in the United Kingdom in 1860. By 1940, the number of deaths had dropped to about 100, even though immunization was

TABLE 1 Estimated Maternal Deaths and Maternal Mortality Ratios, Selected Regions and World, 1995*

Area	Maternal Deaths, n	MM Ratios[†]
Africa	272 500	1006
Asia	217 000	276
Europe	2 200	28
North America	500	11
World	514 500	397

*Data from Hill et al.
[†]Maternal deaths per 100 000 live births.

From *Journal of the American Medical Women's Association*, Fall 2001, Vol. 56, No. 4. Copyright © 2000 by the American Medical Women's Association. Reprinted by permission.

not introduced until decades later. Better food and living conditions are presumed to have improved the ability of infants to survive infection.

In contrast, MM did not decline during this period. From 1840 (when the first MM statistics were available) to the mid-1930s, MM remained as high in Britain as it is today in many developing countries. This shows that nutrition, education, and general standard of living are not the major factors in MM. These factors had improved and are credited with causing the drastic declines in infectious diseases.

Then, after nearly a century of stagnation, MM declined so sharply that within 15 years it was no longer a major public health problem. This was largely because the technology to treat obstetric complications—including antibiotics (first sulfa drugs and then penicillin), banked blood, and safer surgical techniques—became available. In 1934, there were 441 maternal deaths per 100,000 births in England and Wales. By 1950, there were 87, and in 1960 there were only 39. Similar patterns are found in other European countries and in the United States, despite the great variety in patterns of care. For instance, in the United Kingdom, general practice physicians managed most deliveries, whereas in the Netherlands midwives played an important role, and the United States increasingly relied on obstetricians.

Not only was the decline in MM *not* the result of improvements in the general standard of living, but the usual relationship of mortality to social class was also reversed. For most causes, death is higher in disadvantaged groups. As Table 2 shows, in the early 1930s, the usual social class gradient was reversed in England and Wales, with the highest classes having the highest MM. In fact, this pattern persisted from at least the end of the 18th century through the early 20th century, although each time such statistics were published the reaction was usually "surprise bordering on disbelief."

The main explanation for this rare pattern is the practice of interventionist obstetrics among the physicians who delivered upper-class women. During the late 19th and early 20th centuries, for example, "the use of chloroform and forceps in ordinary domiciliary deliveries was often as high as 50% or even 70%." Consequently, at that time the death rate was higher among women delivered by physicians than among those delivered by midwives. As Table 2 shows, not only did the level of MM decline dramatically by the latter half of the 20th century, but the usual social class gradient was also restored.

Why spend so much time on the history of MM? Because much of it is relevant to present-day developing countries. Maternal deaths in developing countries are not caused by exotic conditions. They are caused by the same complications that were responsible for high levels of MM in now-developed countries. In fact, many women in industrialized countries still develop these complications, but very few die of them because they receive prompt, adequate treatment.

As Table 3 shows, hemorrhage, sepsis, and hypertensive disorders are still leading causes of MM in the United States. The major differences in causes between developed countries (represented here by the United States) and the world (composed mostly of developing countries) are in deaths from abortion, obstructed labor, and embolism. The availability of safe, legal abortion has virtually eliminated mortality from abortion complications. Unfortunately, in most developing countries abortion is either legally restricted or unavailable. There are almost no deaths from obstructed labor in the United States because almost all women deliver in medical facilities, where cesarean sections are readily available.

Thus, the literature strongly demonstrates that medical care—specifically, treatment of life-threatening

TABLE 2 Maternal Mortality by Social Class in England and Wales, 1930–1932 and 1979–1981*

Social Class	MMR, 1930–1932[†]	MMR, 1979–1981[‡]
1 & 2 (highest)	444	12
3	411	15
4 (or 4 & 5)	416	17
5	389	. . .
Worst/best ratio	1.14	1.42

*Data from Loudon and Turnbull et al.
[†]Maternal deaths per 100 000 births.
[‡]Maternal deaths per 100 000 legitimate, live births.

TABLE 3 Direct and Indirect Obstetric Deaths, by Cause: Global Estimates, 1993 and United States, 1987–1990*

Cause of Death	World 1993, %	United States 1987–1990, %
Hemorrhage	25	29
Embolism	[†]	20
Sepsis	15	13
Hypertensive disorders of pregnancy	12	18
Obstructed Labor	8	[†]
Unsafe abortion	13	[†]

*Data from WHO and Berg et al.
[†]Negligible.

complications—is the key to reducing MM in developing countries. Application of this knowledge varies, however. In many parts of the world, the first step is to make sure that care is available and accessible. Consider the example of cesarean section. Although this procedure is overused in some countries, it is necessary to save the lives not only of women with obstructed labor, but also of women with eclampsia and other complications. The World Health Organization and other agencies have estimated that 5% to 15% of deliveries should be done by cesarean section in order to preserve maternal and infant health.

In many countries in African and Asia, however, a sizeable proportion of government hospitals do not provide the full range of obstetric services. A study of 20 district hospitals in Bangladesh, for example, found that 6 of these hospitals had performed no cesarean sections at all during the previous year, even though each district had more than a million residents. Surveys have shown that the proportion of deliveries by cesarean section is well below the minimum in India (2.5%), Indonesia (4.3%), Morocco (2.0%), Nigeria (2.5%), and Pakistan (2.7%). The problem is especially serious in rural areas. For example, 5.7% of births among urban women in India in 1992-1993 were by cesarean section, compared to only 1.6% among women in rural areas, and MM ratios are much higher in rural areas.

In most countries, improving the availability of emergency obstetric care does not require building new hospitals or even increasing the ranks of health personnel. A substantial proportion of the need for emergency obstetric care could be met if existing facilities (such as district hospitals) functioned as they were meant to and if existing personnel were deployed more equitably. Furthermore, in some countries laws and regulations designed to "protect" women's health actually serve as barriers to health care. For example, in Morocco, general physicians are not permitted to perform surgery, even though many provincial hospitals do not have obstetricians. Similarly, in many countries midwives are not permitted to perform such critical functions as manual removal of retained placenta. For women who live far from functioning hospitals and experience postpartum hemorrhage, this can make the difference between life and death.

As noted earlier, racial disparities in MM are still a problem in the United States. As Table 4 shows, MM has been higher among nonwhite than white women in the United States since 1915 (the first year for which records exist), when the nonwhite/white MM ratio was 1.76. (This is higher than the gap between the lowest and highest classes in the United Kingdom, shown in Table 2.) Moreover, as the 20th century progressed, the

TABLE 4   Maternal Mortality Ratios in the United States, by Race, 1915–1990*

Year	Nonwhites[†]	Whites[†]	Nonwhite/White Ratio
1915	1056.0	601.0	1.76
1930	1174.0	609.0	1.93
1945	455.0	172.0	2.65
1950	222.0	61.0	3.64
1990	26.7[‡]	6.5	4.11

*Data from USDHEW and Berg et al.
[†]Maternal deaths per 100 000 live births.
[‡]Data are for "black," not "nonwhite."

gap between races in the United States grew ever larger, until by 1990 the MM ratio was more than 4 times higher among black women than among white women.

The meaning of these data is not immediately clear. It might be that factors other than medical care are responsible for the racial disparity. For example, it might be due to a higher prevalence of risk factors (such as greater age or parity) among black women. However, a recent study found that these factors did not explain the racial difference. In fact, among women classified as high risk, black and white women had similar rates of death; it was among the low-risk women that the racial disparity was found. Furthermore, there was no major difference in leading causes of MM. Thus, health problems known to be more common in black women, such as heart disease, did not explain the difference. One can speculate that part of the racial disparity in the United States may be due to poorer quality of care for minorities, which has already been demonstrated for such conditions as congestive heart failure, pneumonia, and colorectal cancer.

Although MM generally reflects disparities in socioeconomic level, it does not automatically reflect women's status in the society, as the historical data from Britain (and the current low level of MM in Saudi Arabia) show. However, it does reflect women's access to treatment of obstetric complications. This, in turn, may provide us with insights into the values and priorities of a society. India, for example, has a vast medical system and a wealth of physicians, but large proportions of the population lack access to life-saving care for obstetric emergencies. And the fact that the racial disparity in MM in the United States not only persists, but has increased, is a national shame.

References

A list of references is available in original source.

Understanding Distress in the Aftermath of Miscarriage

by Pamela A. Geller, PhD

Our culture typically associates pregnancy and child-birth with positive emotions and with motherhood, but this is not the case for all pregnancies or for all women. When a reproductive loss occurs, our society does not encourage women and their partners to discuss their experience, and in many cases even tends to minimize the loss.

Rates and Risk Factors

Miscarriage involves the spontaneous termination of an intrauterine pregnancy that results in fetal death. Although studies have varied widely in how they distinguish miscarriage from later reproductive loss, most studies define miscarriage as the unintended termination of pregnancy before 27 completed weeks of gestation.

Because many pregnancies end in miscarriage before the mother even knows she is pregnant, some estimates suggest that as many as 45 to 50 percent of all pregnancies end in miscarriage. Of clinically recognized pregnancies, however, 10 to 20 percent end in miscarriage. Risk appears to vary substantially by age; for example, rates are 9 percent for women age 20 to 24 years, but 75 percent for women older than 45. Stillbirth, defined as late fetal death with a fetus weighing more than 500 grams, has about a 1/1000 risk in singleton pregnancies and higher risk in multiple pregnancies.

Risk factors can be broadly classified as environmental (e.g., caffeine, nicotine and other drug use; toxins; electro-magnetic fields; stressful life events) or biological (e.g., genetic, including chromosomal abnormalities; endocrinologic; anatomic; immunologic; microbiologic).

Common Psychological Reactions

For many women, miscarriage constitutes an unanticipated, traumatic experience that can bring considerable physical pain and discomfort, and may even pose a serious threat to the life of the woman. Physiologically, miscarriage marks the end of a pregnancy, and psychologically, a myriad of reactions are possible, including sadness, distress, guilt, self-reproach, fear and even relief. Other typical responses can include loneliness; anger at oneself, family members, insensitive friends and often God; jealousy towards pregnant women or others with children; and physical sensations like tightness in the chest or hollowness in the stomach. When continued, these reactions can impact long-term adjustment and functioning. These include an intense "yearning" for the lost pregnancy and lost baby, and preoccupation with the loss.

Women who have miscarried may also be anxious about a number of issues, such as continued bleeding or discharge, possible underlying medical illness or genetic factors that may have contributed to the loss, and fears about their ability to carry a subsequent pregnancy to term. Anxiety symptoms may be even greater than depressive symptoms immediately post-miscarriage, and there may be an increased risk for posttraumatic stress disorder or a recurrent episode of obsessive-compulsive disorder.

Several issues make miscarriage a unique loss. First, it is usually untimely and unexpected; children are not expected to die before their parents. Miscarriage also is an "ambiguous loss" since it involves mourning what *would* have or *could* have been. Because the loss is early and the embryo has not fully developed, miscarriage is even less defined as a loss than is a stillbirth, neonatal or sudden infant death. Moreover, many social and legal definitions suggest that the fetus was never an actual human being. Regardless, it is still a baby in the mind of the parents.

Partner's Reaction

A severely neglected area of miscarriage research is that of the partner's reaction to the loss. To date, there had been little rigorous research addressing the impact on male partners, and no published research regarding the female partner's response in the case of lesbian couples. Initial uncontrolled studies suggest that although males may be affected by miscarriage, their depression and anxiety may be shorter-lasting than women's. In addition, they may have difficulty relating to their partner's intense emotional grief, their coping strategies may differ from those of women, and they may express their grief and distress somewhat differently. For example, men appear to cry less, want to talk less about the loss, express more anger, and attempt to cope by returning to work as soon as possible and using such maladaptive behaviors as substance use. Men who have seen an ultrasound scan of the living fetus may have greater difficulty coping and demonstrate greater despair compared to men who have not seen an ultrasound. Researchers hypothesize that men's coping difficulties are related to the demands of being the "comforter," compounded by feelings of inadequacy aroused by their inability to influence events while insufficiently attending to their own emotional response.

This emerging area of interest sorely needs systematic work that employs appropriate comparison groups and male as well as female partners of women who have miscarried, with greater numbers of lesbian couples making the decision to have children. In addition to addressing the female partner's responses to the loss itself (and how these responses may differ from those of male partners), researchers should also address other issues unique to lesbian couples (e.g., if the choice for one partner to conceive was made only after the other partner miscarried).

Societal Reactions

Society still sees miscarriage as an "unfortunate event," but one that is less tragic than the loss of a child. Women who have miscarried are often told that they can "try again," which suggests that the lost baby is interchangeable with another, something rarely expressed when an older child dies. Parents whose first child has died before birth are often not considered to be parents, making it more difficult to feel their grief is justified. In addition, this type of loss tends not to be socially legitimized or supported, as many people expect the grief to be mild and transient and do not understand that parents can grieve as intensely for a reproductive loss as for any other loss. For most parents, the relationship to the child begins long before birth, creating a host of expectations, hopes and feelings to grieve.

Since miscarriage involves a loss that often remains unknown to all but a woman's most intimate confidants and her health care providers, the grieving process may be compounded by limited social support and the challenge of managing feelings associated with the loss of a *potential* child. There are few memories and stories to share with others, so the parents are often isolated and may avoid social contact out of shame and others' discomfort. In addition, the mother may feel she has failed. Unlike other experiences that get easier to handle with repetition, multiple miscarriages challenge coping resources to an even further degree.

Societal reactions may also differ by gender, with women's sense of self-identity more deeply affected than men's. Society pressures women, regardless of socioeconomic status, ethnic-racial status and religion, to view motherhood as our primary adult role. Violating these societal norms and expectations has both social and personal consequences. The stigma associated with childlessness involves social definitions of women as selfish, unfeminine, unnatural and inadequate— ideas that many women incorporate into their own self-concept.

Treatment Issues

Although supporters often struggle to find the "right thing to say," practically every empirical study has emphasized the *ability to listen over the ability to say something*. Speaking about loss aids in healing. To counteract the social negation of miscarriage, supporters should allow the parents to express their grief for what they lost individually, as a couple and as a family, regardless of the gestational age at loss. Because women may cope by socially isolating themselves, they need frequent reminders that someone is ready to listen and cares how they are feeling. Parents often require some validation and confirmation of the child's existence. They may need to remember and review their thoughts and feelings about the child from the very beginning of the pregnancy to make it seem real, and save mementoes or plan a farewell ritual to begin to feel some resolution. Additionally, since couples often attribute the miscarriage to something they have done, factual information about the probable cause of the miscarriage should be provided when possible.

Debate continues as to whether clinicians should advise women who have miscarried to try to conceive right away or to wait until their grief and depressive symptoms have resolved. Recent studies conclude that while women may be justifiably distressed or anxious during a subsequent pregnancy about the prospect of yet another loss, a subsequent pregnancy is in fact healing for many parents. Parents are encouraged to discuss their individual situation with their clinician and reach their own decision, particularly since a sense of choice and control is often a welcome relief in itself.

As a whole, little clinical attention has been paid to treating the grief and psychological distress associated with miscarriage, despite the fact that treatment in the early weeks after loss may help offset more serious psychological and psychiatric consequences. Since there is no systematic treatment protocol in place for women who have miscarried and their families, mental health referrals are varied and depend on the particular treating physician or hospital. This may be because health care providers generally have little understanding of the needs of these women and have limited training in grief counseling, along with time constraints and general discomfort with psychological issues. Compounding these issues is the reality that women who have miscarried often adopt a coping strategy of avoidance, further preventing them from receiving treatment.

Our national resource for information and support is SHARE: Pregnancy & Infant Loss Support Inc. (800-821-6819; *www.nationalshareoffice.com*).

References

A list of references is available in the original source.

What Is Postpartum Depression?

by Leslie W. Tam

It's not what Andrea Yates, the Texas woman who drowned her five children, had. It appears that she was afflicted with postpartum psychosis, a much more severe postpartum illness. However, with the sensationalistic and often inaccurate media coverage that followed, it seems more important than ever to clarify what is meant by these often misunderstood disorders. The umbrella term "postpartum distress" or "PPD" actually refers to a range of postpartum mental disorders. These include the "baby blues," depression, anxiety and, in the worst cases, psychosis. Every woman who contemplates a pregnancy should be educated about the risks of these psychiatric complications and empowered to manage her particular situation with appropriate interventions.

Definitions

Most new mothers will experience the **"baby blues."** On the third or fourth day postpartum, 80 percent of women notice a brief period of mild weepiness, irritability and depressed mood. With the abrupt change in hormone levels once the baby and placenta are delivered, the baby blues are thought to be related to the biological changes taking place. Especially since they are so ubiquitous, the baby blues are considered a normal and self-limiting postpartum symptom, and their symptoms usually resolve within a week or two.

When the blues persist beyond two weeks or generalize to encompass sleep and appetite changes, frequent crying, disinterest in the infant or feelings of being overwhelmed, then the diagnosis is more likely to be major depression with postpartum onset. **Postpartum depression** occurs in 10 to 15 percent of new mothers and can actually have its onset at any time in the first postpartum year. Like the blues, postpartum depression is thought to be related to hormonal changes brought on by sleep deprivation, weaning and the resumption of the menstrual cycle. Prior or family history of depression also increases a woman's risk.

It is also common for **anxiety disorders,** such as panic disorder, generalized anxiety disorder or even obsessive-compulsive disorder (OCD), to present or recur in the postpartum period. Postpartum OCD is typically characterized by a mother's hypervigilance about possible harm to her baby, which then becomes a recurrent, unwanted thought or obsession. The mother may become compulsively protective of her infant to the extent that her functioning is impaired, or she may wish to avoid her baby or situations in which she fears she might do it harm.

The most serious and fortunately the most rare postpartum mental illness is **postpartum psychosis.** Unlike the other disorders, postpartum psychosis is thought to be primarily biologically based and related to hormonal changes in the immediate postpartum period.

Psychosis usually presents within a few day of giving birth, though there have been reports of later onsets. Women with underlying psychotic disorders are at heightened risk, but postpartum psychosis also can occur in women who seem to have no risk factors. The psychosis is most often an affective psychosis resembling acute mania. Affected women tend to have difficulty sleeping, are prone to agitation or hyperactivity, and intermittently experience delusions, hallucinations and paranoia.

Most concerning are psychotic thoughts that may include the wish to harm themselves or their infant. These symptoms wax and wane, making this disorder particularly difficult to diagnose. However, postpartum psychosis represents a medical emergency and usually requires hospitalization.

Risk Factors

Other factors that may play a role in the development of postpartum depressive or anxiety symptoms include an unexpected birth outcome, marital stress, lack of support and a troubled relationship between the new mother and her own mother. Mothers who have a traumatic or unsatisfying birthing experience also may blame themselves or feel that they have failed. Also, mothers who find themselves unable to breastfeed, for whatever reason, may experience disappointment or a sense of inadequacy.

The birth of a premature or severely compromised infant also can trigger symptoms; interestingly, however, the onset is usually after the baby's situation has been stabilized. It is as if the mother puts herself on hold to deal with the crisis of her severely ill newborn, and only when the crisis is over does she react to the psychological as well as biological stressors.

Marital or relationship stress can have a major role in the onset of postpartum symptoms in vulnerable women. The arrival of an infant tests a relationship in many ways. Fathers or partners can feel left out when an infant seems to monopolize the new mother's time and affections. Also, fathers or partners may have to take on more household responsibilities that the new mother

may be unable to perform. Even in gay, lesbian or adoptive couples, this shift of responsibilities can breed resentment and foster discord.

By whatever means a woman becomes a parent, she will experience sleep deprivation, ambivalence and several other stressors that are part of the adjustment. New mothers require added support to meet the physical and emotional demands of parenthood; those who do not receive adequate support may be at risk for symptom development.

In my practice of reproductive psychiatry, I meet with couples before the baby arrives and help them consider the many types of assistance that may be needed: care for other children, house-cleaning, meal preparation, laundry, etc. In other cultures it is common for other women from the family, neighborhood or tribe to take over the new mother's responsibilities for the first 40 days or so after childbirth, freeing her to rest, recover and bond with her infant. Most western societies offer new mothers nothing of the sort!

What Postpartum Depression Isn't

In our society we operate under the assumption that new mothers can take care of their infants, continue to function in their previous roles and adjust in stride to all the changes that new motherhood brings. Many women I have treated sought help from their health care providers for what turned out to be postpartum depression but were told that their symptoms were a normal part of new motherhood, or that they would pass. Neither is true. Many women feel they are unable to live up to society's, their family's or their own expectations and so view themselves as having a character flaw or as just not trying hard enough. In reality, they are suffering from a postpartum illness that, when treated, resolves and allows them to return to their previous level of functioning. Attitudes and perceptions are extremely important in dealing with this population.

What Can Be Done?

In working with women with postpartum disorders, it has become clear to me that health care providers and others who advocate for greater awareness of postpartum mental health issues have a long way to go. The level of ignorance among providers about these disorders is astonishing. Several organizations work to educate the public and providers about these illnesses (see addenda). Education should also be a part of prenatal education. So many patients have told me they wish they had known that such illnesses were even a possibility.

We also need to empower women to make good decisions regarding their own health as well as that of their children. There are times, for instance, when it probably isn't advisable for a new mother to breastfeed. Even though advocates remind us that "breast is best," some women are too depressed, psychotic, fatigued or uncomfortable with their own bodies to breastfeed. Sometimes it is appropriate to treat pregnant or nursing mothers with medications, and yet many women are led to believe that no medications are safe. Yes, medication use can be risky for this group of women. However, it's best to weigh the risks and benefits to mother and baby of both the medication and the illness.

Despite the prevalence of postpartum disorders, there is no formal screening mechanism in the present standard of U.S. health care. Very adequate screening questionnaires could be administered to new mothers at follow-up visits with obstetricians, at the pediatrician's office or in other systems that interface with them. It is encouraging to note that the U.S. House of Representatives passed a resolution (HR-163) to mandate screening for postpartum mental illness. However, it remains to be seen just how and when the screening will be implemented.

Recently, Rep. Bobby Rush (D-Illinois) introduced further legislation with the Melanie Stokes Postpartum Research and Care Act (HR-2380), which would appropriate more funding for postpartum research and treatment. The addendum lists a few organizations that provide further information about these disorders and that advocate for education and awareness.

As stated above, it is likely that Andrea Yates had a severe case of postpartum psychosis. In her confession, she stated that for weeks prior to the incident she believed that she was a terrible mother, that she had done irreparable harm to her children and that she should kill them to spare them further pain. These were clearly delusional thoughts. Fortunately, some of the media (see *Newsweek,* July 2, 2001) took the time to clarify the difference between depression and psychosis. Even so, I received several calls from depressed patients wondering if something like that might happen to them. All the more reason for the public and professionals to become informed about these serious and potentially dangerous disorders.

Selected References

Cox JL, Holden JM, Sagovsky R. "Detection of Postnatal Depression: Development of the 10 Item Edinburgh Postnatal Depression Scale." *British Journal of Psychiatry* 1987; 150: 782–86.

O'Hara M, Zekoski E. "Postpartum Depression: a Comprehensive Review." In R. Kumar and I. F. Brockington, Ed. *Motherhood and Mental Illness.* Wright, 1988; 17–63.

Miller LJ, ed., *Postpartum Mood Disorders,* American Psychiatric Press, 1999.

Sichel D and Driscoll JW, *Women's Moods: What Every Woman Must Know about Hormones, the Brain, and Emotional Health,* William Morrow & Co., 1999.

Further Reading

This Isn't What I Expected, by Karen R. Kleiman, MSW and Valerie D. Raskin, MD, Bantam Books, 1994.

Mothering the New Mother, by Sally Placksin, Newmarket Press, 1994.

Postpartum Survival Guide, By Ann Dunneworld, PhD and Dian G. Sanford, PhD, New Harbinger Publications, 1994.

The Postpartum Husband, by Karen R. Kleiman, MSW, Xlibris Corporation, 2001.

Advocate Organizations

Postpartum Support International, 927 N. Kellogg Avenue, Santa Barbara, CA 93111. Phone: 805-967-7636, fax: 805-967-0608, email: *jhonikman@ earthlink.net, web: www.postpartum.net.*

Depression After Delivery, PO Box 1282, Morrisville, PA 19067. Phone: 215-295-3994 or 800-944-4PPD, web: *www.behavenet.com.*

Formula for Profit
How Marketing Breastmilk Substitutes Undermines the Health of Babies

by Jennifer Coburn

Because of the strident societal and economic impact wielded by the formula industry, bottle-feeding has today become the social norm in the US. Fewer than half of all US babies are exclusively breastfed during their first day or two in the hospital. By the time they are six months old, only 19 percent of US babies receive any breastmilk, and only 2 percent of one year olds. Contrast this with the average age of weaning worldwide, which is 4.2 years. This country's societal hostility towards breastfeeding is such that many states have had to pass laws protecting a mother's right to breastfeed her child anywhere that she is otherwise permitted to be.

The very need for such legislation is a sad commentary on the lack of appreciation for the broad range of health, social, and environmental benefits of breastfeeding. Nevertheless, the slogan "breast is best" is no exaggeration. Breastmilk contains 400 nutrients that cannot be recreated in a laboratory, and several studies suggest that breastfeeding reduces the risk of sudden infant death syndrome. An absence of breastfeeding has been linked to an increased risk of hospitalization, childhood cancer, diarrheal diseases, lower respiratory illness, ear infections, bacterial infections, diabetes, infant botulism, Crohn's disease, ulcerative colitis, and even cavities. In *Milk, Money and Madness: The Culture and Politics of Breastfeeding,* Naomi Baumslag, MD, MPH, asserts that breastfed babies also have lower incidence of allergies, urinary tract infections, obesity, learning, behavioral and psychological problems, later-life heart disease, pneumonia, neonatal sepsis, and giardia infection.

Children are not the only ones who benefit from breastfeeding. Nursing mothers enjoy a reduced risk of premenopausal breast cancer, ovarian cancer, and osteoporosis. Breastfeeding is advantageous for people who are outside the mother-baby unit, when you consider healthier babies mean lower health insurance premiums for everyone, and lower absenteeism among working parents. The production of formula, bottles, plastic nipples, and formula cans, not to mention cleaning artificial feeding supplies—all create pollution and in some cases hazardous waste. Finally, breastmilk is also free and convenient, considerations that should give pause to families faced with an average yearly cost of $800 per baby if they choose to formula feed.

The economic implications of formula are certainly significant. The industry generates $5 to $6 billion in sales each year, and its executives reap huge profits—the CEO of Abbott Labs earns more than $4 million per year; his counterpart at Bristol-Myers Squibb (makers of Enfamil), nearly $13 million. Part of the reason the industry is so profitable is the fact that every dollar formula makers charge their retail distributions outlets costs them a mere 16 cents on production and delivery. Formula is, in short, big business—the result of a complex social marketing campaign that began half a century ago, one that has speciously managed to define artificial feeding as a convenient, liberating, and "modern" way of feeding one's infant.

Science Crushes Nature

"At the beginning of the 20th century, basically women breastfed, had a wet nurse or their babies died," says Mary Lofton, spokesperson for La Leche League International (LLLI). Insofar as artificial baby milk became available as a life-saving alternative to breastmilk, it was deemed a blessing. "The crucial social phenomenon," Lofton adds, "was the shift from home to hospital in childbirth. . . . Women were given anesthesia, babies were taken away, schedules were rigid, and all those interferences led to problems with breastfeeding."

Considering formula to be nutritionally equal to breastfeeding, doctors began recommending it to patients. Tangentially our society experienced a burgeoning captivation with science and technology, and became increasingly enamored with an efficiency-model of infant feeding and care. The advent of World War II encouraged women to work outside the home, which only furthered the reliance on artificial feeding. By the 1950s, infant formula gained the widespread endorsement of the pediatric community, and artificial feeding increasingly became seen as equal—if not superior—to nursing.

Marian Tompson, one of the founding mothers of LLLI, thinks the 1950s doctor acted out of ignorance. "I think anyone with half a brain would realize that human milk is species-specific," she says. "No one ever suggests that I feed my kittens with milk from the cocker spaniel next door." Nevertheless, with its decidedly scientific-sounding name, formula fit right into the landscape of an America mesmerized by the march of modernity, leisure, and ease. Measuring formula, sterilizing bottles, the modern mom became a domestic chemist. Bottle-feeding became a symbol of modern living, prosperity, and progress—indeed, healthful living! In contrast, breastfeeding took on the aspect of a primitive, retrograde thing to do.

The Role of the Medical Establishment

The campaign to normalize artificial feeding gains a great deal of its effectiveness from an unholy alliance between the pharmaceutical industry and the medical establishment. To promote artificial feeding, formula manufacturers spend millions of dollars securing exclusive distribution deals for formula samples, at a yearly average of $6,000 to $8,000 per doctor. They donate $1 million annually to the American Academy of Pediatrics in the form of a renewable grant that has already netted the AAP $8 million. The formula industry also contributed at least $3 million toward the building costs of the AAP headquarters.

The American College of Obstetrics and Gynecology received $548,000 from two of the four major formula makers in 1993. The American Medical Association television program is sponsored by the makers of Similac. Moreover, the American Dietetic Association, the National Association of Neonatal Nurses, and the Association of Women's Health, Obstetric and Neonatal Nurses all receive generous funding from the formula industry. A 1994 study that was published in the *Journal of the American Medical Association* exposes the influence the formula industry wields over the medical estab-

lishment. "By giving physicians money," the authors found, "the [formula] companies are successful in influencing doctors to recommend their product."

Formula manufacturers play hardball to get hospital business. Take the example of Canada, where Mead Johnson secured an exclusive contract with Toronto's Women's College Hospital that pays the hospital $1 million the first year and $350,000 per subsequent year for a decade. Abbott Labs and Bristol-Myers Squibb got into a bidding war over the right to promote formula through Grace Hospital in Vancouver, Canada's largest birthing facility. Ross Labs offered to pay the Doctor's Hospital in Canada $1 million for a contract which would require that the hospital would give their product to all mothers in take home packages, supply breastfeeding mothers with Ross's instructions on nursing, and make sure mothers had "access" to Ross architectural services for nurseries.

Jack Newman, MD, author of *Dr. Jack Newman's Guide to Breastfeeding,* a book on the politics of formula use, characterizes the relationship between the pharmaceutical industry and medical establishment as bribery. From large donations to the "myriad of other little 'useful' items" such as pens, paper pads, measuring tape, growth charts, and coffee cups (all of which feature formula advertising), Newman considers these contributions wholly unethical.

Physical separation of hospital nurseries and maternity wards begin to erode the breastfeeding relationship right from the start. James McKenna, PhD, director of University of Notre Dame Mother-Infant Behavioral Sleep Laboratory, told me "Our studies of breastfeeding mother-baby pairs, where infants were about four months, reveal that proximity to mother, particularly the types of intimate contact that occur during bed-sharing that permit the infant to smell its mother's milk, doubles the amount of breastfeeding episodes, and triples the amount of nightly breastfeeding time."

Perhaps the most coveted payoff for formula makers, however, is the opportunity to exclusively distribute their products through hospital maternity wards. When a mother is released from a hospital or birthing center, she is often given a discharge gift basket that includes free formula. Research shows this tacit endorsement on the hospital's part is so effective in establishing brand loyalty that 93 percent of mothers who artificially feed continue using the brand of formula given to them by the hospital. Research suggest that exposure to formula advertising during pregnancy seriously undermines a future breastfeeding relationship.

Even more egregious than subjecting a mother to a barrage of formula advertising is veiling formula marketing as a form of health service, as the Nestle corporation has done. In past decades the company deployed sales staff, posing as "milk nurses," to promote artificial feeding to mothers in developing nations, compensating the sellers commensurate with the amount of artificial baby milk sold. To save money on the costly formula, mothers often diluted the mix. This on its own would have a deleterious, nutrition-depleting effect on the babies, but compounded with the lack of access to sterilized water, the use of formula in these countries led to many infant deaths. Formula use is still associated with the deaths of one and a half million children each year—both overseas and in the US.

Ross Laboratories' Mother's Survey

The formula industry's insistence on framing the debate on infant feeding even extends to their endeavor to collect and publish "national breastfeeding statistics." Barbara Heiser, executive director of the National Alliance for Breastfeeding Advocacy (NABA) says Ross Laboratories' role in tracking breastfeeding rates creates a conflict of interest. "We wouldn't ask the tobacco industry for statistics on lung cancer," she says. Daven Lee, a breastfeeding advocate and writer, says Ross is the only group that tracks national breastfeeding statistics—via a survey generated by their Marketing Department, and subsequently presented as unbiased research. "This way," Lee states, "Ross wins credibility and is cited as a resource in the media."

Clearly, Ross and other formula makers are competing not with each other, but with breastfeeding itself. In that light, breastfeeding mothers are caught in the crossfire. Heiser points out that mothers who purchase nursing pads often receive coupons for free formula. "Just recently a man was in renting a breast pump for his wife and he asked for two receipts because he could get a $10.00 coupon for formula with every breast pump rental receipt he sent in" to the formula makers, she remarks, an irony that lactation consultant and childbirth educator Linda Smith has also witnessed. "The breastfeeding mother gift packs companies give mothers," Smith says, "often contain breast pumps that are "uncomfortable and usually ineffective—along with bra pads and formula samples. These are very popular with mothers and nurses." And, for a new mom, sleep-deprived, and struggling to meet her baby's needs, tempting.

Indeed, an interesting inverted rationale exists whereby formula feeding is considered by some to be a pro-woman, even feminist practice. By aligning themselves with the feminist ideal of flexibility—including the freedom to return to work or to pursue personal interests—the formula was originally embraced by the feminist movement. Marion Tompson says since then,

however, "We've seen a total turnaround." In fact, she says, as far back as 1975 attorneys for the National Organization for Women (NOW) successfully fought to eliminate inquiries about a mother's breastfeeding status from the unemployment eligibility questionnaire. Prior to this, a nursing mother's commitment to finding employment was questioned and benefits could be denied.

More recently, women's groups have fought for public breastfeeding laws, unpaid time off to pump breastmilk, insurance coverage for lactation specialists, and the Family and Medical Leave Act, which allows a new mother to take a 12-week maternity leave without threat of losing her job. Not all of these measures were approved, but feminists signed on to every effort. So although formula makers are trying to link arms with the feminist movement, the courtship is arguably one-sided. In reality, it is extraordinarily paternalistic to withhold information from mothers about the profound inferiority of artificial feeding. Feminist ideals demand informed choice.

The WHO Code

The aggressive marketing of infant formula stands in direct conflict with the directives of the World Health Organization (WHO) and United Nations International Children's Education Fund (UNICEF), which jointly adopted an International Code of Marketing of Breastmilk Substitutes in 1981. The objective of the WHO Code is "to contribute to the provision of safe and adequate nutrition for infants, by the protection and promotion of breastfeeding and by the proper use of breastmilk substitutes, when these are necessary, on the basis of adequate information and through appropriate marketing and distribution." The code carries ten main provisions:

- No advertising of breastmilk substitutes
- No free samples of breastmilk substitutes to mothers
- No promotion of products through healthcare facilities
- No company-appointed "nurses" to "advise" mothers
- No gifts or personal samples to health workers
- No words or pictures idealizing artificial feeding, including pictures of infants, on the labels of the products
- Information to health workers should be scientific and factual
- All information on artificial feeding, including the labels, should explain the benefits of breastfeeding and the costs and hazards associated with artificial feeding
- Unsuitable products, such as sweetened condensed milk, should not be promoted for babies
- All products should be of high quality and take into account the climatic and storage conditions of the country where they are used

Tompson, part of the group that drew up the guide-lines in Switzerland, proposed that formula labels include health hazards of artificial feeding like the surgeon general's warning on cigarettes—a suggestion that the group, comprised of about 50 representatives of nongovernmental organizations (NGOs), as well as executives from the formula industry, rejected. Yet Tompson still thinks warning labels are a good idea. "Today when you see an ad on television for a drug, a soft voice lists all of the contraindications. . . . You don't hear that soft voice telling you all that can go wrong with formula," she adds. Nevertheless, the US' reluctance to sign onto the voluntary code—ten years after most other nations did—under-scores the fact that, however well intended, the WHO Code is as toothless as the infants it aims to benefit.

The Baby-Friendly Hospital Initiative

WHO and UNICEF have experienced greater breast-feeding promotion success with the Baby-Friendly Hospital Initiative (BFHI), established in 1991 to help hospitals and birthing centers create an environment that is conducive to breastfeeding. Resting on the foundation of the WHO Code and the Innocenti Declaration (a resolution prepared at an international breastfeeding conference for international policy makers in Innocenti, Italy, in 1990), the BFHI was drafted to encourage hospitals to educate mothers about the benefits of breastfeeding.

Although the ten criteria for baby-friendly status are easily attainable, the US lags behind: of 14,000 baby-friendly hospitals worldwide, only 23 are in the US, says Judy Lannon, project manager for the Baby-Friendly Hospital Initiative (BFHI). To earn this standing, a hospital "may not distribute gift packages to new mothers that contain formula" adds Lannon. The other requirements are that hospitals do the following:

- Have a written breastfeeding policy that is routinely communicated to all healthcare staff
- Train all healthcare staff in skills necessary to implement this policy
- Help mothers initiate breastfeeding within an hour of birth
- Show mothers how to breastfeed and how to maintain lactation, even if they should be separated from their infants
- Give newborn infants no food or drink other than breastmilk, unless medically indicated
- Practice "rooming in" by allowing mothers and infants to remain together 24 hours a day
- Encourage breastfeeding on demand
- Give no artificial teats, pacifiers, dummies, or soothers to breastfeeding infants

- Foster the establishment of breastfeeding support groups and refer mothers to them on discharge from the hospital or birthing center

Seventy-five US hospitals are currently holding "certificates of intent," meaning they are preparing to be reviewed for BFHI status in the near future. Lannon says that if a hospital fails to meet the criteria the first time, they are given recommendations and urged to reapply. There is no limit on how many times a hospital may apply, she adds.

In other nations, the BFHI has led to tremendous breastfeeding successes. In Chile, only 4 percent of infants were exclusively breastfed in 1985. By 1991, less than one year after the BFHI was launched, the rate had risen to 25 percent. Six years after Cuba adopted the BFHI, the rate of mothers who were breastfeeding at the time of hospital discharge jumped from 63 percent to 98 percent. In Iran, it took only five years for the rate of exclusively breastfeed infants to rise from 10 to 53 percent. China experienced comparable success: 6,300 hospitals reached baby-friendly status by 1996, along with regulations on the marketing of formula. A 1994 survey found that in just two years, breastfeeding rates increased from 10 percent to 48 percent for infants in urban areas; it rose from 29 percent to 68 percent in rural areas.

The Tobacco Connection

The formula industry's marketing tactics have been likened to big tobacco companies that give away free samples, and place their products in popular movies and television shows, while denying that their products are addictive. Likening formula marketing to tobacco marketing is an argument that gains credibility when one considers that 4,000 babies worldwide die every day because they are not breastfed. (According to the American Lung Association, 1,180 people die from smoking-related illnesses every day in the US.) Many Americans falsely believe that the alarming number of formula-related infant deaths is solely due to unsanitary water and overdilution in developing nations. But formula feeding increases babies' health risks everywhere. In the US, four of every 1,000 infants born die because they are not breastfed. Healthcare savings would reach an estimated $2 to $4 billion annually if every child in the US were breastfed for as little as three months.

Smith says that there are some similarities in marketing formula and tobacco, but she's not sure the two are parallel. A significant difference, she believes, is that "there is a limited need for formula for some babies and mothers." In her work as a lactation consultant, Smith says she sees one case about every few years where "a loving and wonderful mother tries absolutely everything and she simply isn't able to breastfeed." Although formula does serve an important function for a small minority of children, it is clear that formula makers have every baby in their sights as they wage their aggressive marketing efforts. And the vast majority of mothers who experience insurmountable obstacles to breastfeeding have simply been failed by the medical establishment. Like prescription drugs, formula should be administered judiciously.

Formula Recalls

Artificial milk's health risks to young children are only compounded by the frequent occurrence of product recalls, of which there were 22 "significant" ones between 1982 and 1994. Seven of these were classified as Class I, potentially life threatening. Salmonella contamination, vitamin deficiencies, and bacterial contamination were among the most serious health risks, with the presence of glass particles from bottle chipping among the less serious, but not negligible, offenses.

In 1999, 120,000 cans of Mead Johnson's ProSobee formula were recalled for labeling errors after a parent called the company to inquire why the product smelled strange. It was discovered that cans labeled as infant formula contained, in fact, Vanilla Sustacal—an adult nutritional supplement that, if consumed by infants, could lead to what the Mead Johnson Corporation itself calls "severe medical problems." The formula in question was shipped to stores at least six months prior to the recall.

Nevertheless, Mead Johnson termed the recall an "extra precautionary" measure. Wouldn't extra precaution be to have caught the labeling error before the formula left the factory and spent half a year on supermarket shelves? We will never know how many mothers fed their babies the defective product, threw away the can, and later had no idea why their infants became ill.

Dr. Derrick Jelliffe, in a 1980 interview with the *Wall Street Journal,* characterizes the history of formula production as "a succession of errors." He adds, "Each stumble is dealt with and heralded as yet another breakthrough, leading to further imbalances and then more modifications."

The Food and Drug Administration (FDA) fact sheet on formula, titled the "Overview of Infant Formulas," maintains that "the composition of commercial formula is carefully controlled and the FDA requires that these products meet very strict standards." Further, the document boasts that the quality of formula is "ensured" by the Infant Formula Act, a law which gives the FDA authority to create and enforce formula production standards. This is a bold—and grossly inaccurate—

statement about a product that has a track record of health-threatening production errors.

The Infant Formula Act was signed into federal law in 1980 after deficient formula hit the market and caused infant deaths, says Baumslag. Realizing that there were no guidelines to oversee formula production, Congress introduced this law and gave the FDA authority to set the standard for—and monitor—formula production.

But however well intended the Infant Formula Act may have been when introduced, it has not prevented significant health risks in formula production. In fact, in standardizing production methods, the IFA did not account for which ingredients were healthiest for infants. It simply considered which were most commonly used. This forced several smaller companies with alternative, perhaps healthier, ingredients out of the market. The legislation created an opportunity for major pharmaceutical companies to dominate formula sales.

How to Reverse the Trend

If doctors or parents ever had any questions about the cause and effect relationship between formula marketing and declining breastfeeding rates, they now can reference the first randomized, controlled study investigating the issue. Recently published by the *Journal of Obstetrics and Gynecology,* the "Office Prenatal Formula Advertising and Its Effects on Breastfeeding Patterns" concludes that prenatal exposure to formula advertising "significantly increased early termination of breastfeeding." Women who did not receive direct marketing materials from formula makers were more successful at maintaining the breastfeeding relationship.

The American Academy of Pediatrics policy on breastfeeding, which was revised in 1997, is "a huge step in the right direction," adds Smith. She says, "It shows that the AAP is now solidly on board with breastfeeding." The statement encourages doctors to learn more about human lactation and promote breastfeeding as the optimal source of nutrition for babies. It also made headlines by encouraging women to breastfeed for a minimum of one year. Smith adds that over the last five years she's also seen an emergence of lactation consultants in pediatric offices, another indication that the medical community is moving in the right direction. Still, this leaves the question of the economic ties between the medical establishment and formula makers.

The social marketing campaign launched by the formula industry has been a successful one, but this doesn't mean the trend is irreversible. The US can return to being a breastfeeding culture if healthcare providers, policy makers, and families make it a national priority.

First, the medical establishment must financially disentangle itself from formula makers. The WHO Code must be enforced, and artificial baby milk must not be marketed through medical facilities. Second, birthing centers and hospitals should strive to meet the criteria of the BFHI and create a setting that is conducive to breastfeeding. Distribution deals and formula promotion in medical settings must cease because when mothers receive formula samples from trusted health providers, they assume artificial feeding offers health benefits, instead of considering the risks associated with infant formulas. The medical community has an ethical obligation not to violate their patients' trust or compromise their health for economic gain.

Finally, our entire culture must support breastfeeding. All workplaces should be equipped with lactation stations. Health insurance ought to provide coverage for lactation consulting. And no woman should ever be chided for breastfeeding in public or "too long." Then our culture will not just say breast is best. We'll act like it.

References

A list of references is available in the original source.

From TV to Real Life
Lack of Education Causes Tragic Results
by Jennifer Coburn

Part of the resistance to breastfeeding in the US stems from the popular culture's portrayal of nursing and bottle-feeding. A fall 1998 episode of the TV show *Chicago Hope* featured a couple whose baby died of dehydration and malnutrition because his breastfeeding mother, who suffered from insufficient milk syndrome, refused to supplement with formula. One hospital staff member finger-wagged at the irresponsible parents. The baby-friendly hospital was chided for pressuring the mother to nurse.

Pharmaceutical Research and Manufacturers of America (PhRMA), whose members include major formula-makers like Abbott Labs, American Home Products, Bristol-Myers Squibb Company, Johnson & Johnson, and Wyeth-Ayerst International, were quite open about financially backing several episodes of the hospital drama, through what was called the Living with Hope project. This project, a collaborative effort between John Hopkins Medicine, PhRMA, CBS Television, and Twentieth Century Fox, was to sponsor a season of episodes, although PhRMA chose to fund only "three or four," according to their spokespeople.

PhRMA vice president of public affairs, Alixe Glen, said in a written statement that the partnership "allows our message to be associated with high-quality programming that deals with information on medical conditions in a responsible way." The press statement also says that this project is "part of a broader campaign strategy for the pharmaceutical association, aimed at placing PhRMA's message in positive and trusted 'health settings.'"

Although PhRMA spokespersons Alexandra Bickel and Meredith Hart say the press statement was not issued by their organization, neither deny its content. Bickel says, though, that the organization's involvement in the show "should not be taken out of context," and says PhRMA had "no idea" what the subject matter of the show was before it aired. "We were just aligning ourselves with the program, we do not have any control over its content." she asserts. Neither could affirm whether PhRMA would have withdrawn its support if it had had prior knowledge of the antibreastfeeding theme of the episode. Hart cannot recall the amount her organization paid to support their portion of the Living with Hope project, but stated that PhRMA has a "large budget for image advertising." The Living with Hope project was, she says, PhRMA's sole endeavor in the world of pure entertainment.

A CBS spokeswoman, who asked that she not be named, says *Chicago Hope* did not formally notify

PhMRA about the topic of the shows beforehand. However, the network website lists story lines, and breastfeeding advocates around the country were well aware of the show's content before it aired. "La Leche League was up in arms and issued a press release days before the episode aired because they were very concerned about the content," she says. Baumslag recalls seeing press releases about the episode before it aired. She, along with other breastfeeding advocates who distrust PhRMA's feigned innocence, questions why the major sponsors of the show would have no prior knowledge of the content when plenty of outsiders had the information.

The media onslaught against breastfeeding continues. In February 2000, NBC's legal drama *Law & Order* aired an episode that also featured insufficient milk syndrome and a baby's death. In a move that was, perhaps, even more irksome to breastfeeding advocates than the CBS drama, this show featured a lactation consultant who was portrayed as a heavy-handed drill sergeant devoid of practical advice for her client. The episode frustrated Kim Cavaliero, public relations director at LLLI. "We are here to support and educate, but we certainly don't intimidate people into breastfeeding." she says. "It seemed they pulled out every possible negative stereotype about lactation consultants and exaggerated them just for the fun of it."

Representatives at the *Law & Order* Advertising and Promotions Department, Publicity Office, production team, and Network Office all say they don't know who funded the episode, but some breastfeeding activists (aka "lactivists") say the antibreastfeeding message was too well crafted to have been uninfluenced by formula makers. Dia L. Michels, co-author of *Milk, Money and Madness,* says whether formula makers had

a hand in the show is irrelevant. "There doesn't need to be a finger pointing at formula makers every time because their influence is everywhere," she says.

Given the fact that breastmilk production typically follows Mother Nature's law of supply and demand, the more a child nurses, the more milk the mother will produce. Conversely, if a mother is feeding her baby formula, she will produce less breastmilk. In frustration, she may rely even more on artificial baby milk, starting a process that often culminates in insufficient milk syndrome, a condition whose real life consequences are extremely serious.

Tabitha Walrond, a young Bronx, New York, mother, was tried for manslaughter when her seven-week old, exclusively breastfed son died of malnutrition. In September 1999, Walrond was convicted of criminally negligent homicide and was given five years probation. Walrond's milk supply may have been diminished by prior breast reduction surgery. Or, because she was taking medication for several days, she may have nursed less frequently and decreased her milk supply. Her case is a clear example of why pediatricians and ob/gyns need adequate training in human lactation, so that they may better advise mothers to breastfeed more frequently and pump milk to increase their supply.

Highly publicized cases like Walrond's, coupled with hysterical antibreastfeeding television entertainment, go a long way in scaring new and expectant mothers. Glaringly absent from these messages is the fact that infants are far more likely to suffer health problems—and die—if they are artificially fed.

References

A list of references is available in the original source.

Nutrition, Breastfeeding, and Ethnicity
Understanding Maternal and Child Health
Beliefs among New-Wave Immigrants
by Caroline Westbrook Arnold

Introduction

While African Americans remain the largest of the "old" minority groups in the United States, in recent years there has been a marked increase in the growth of Hispanic and Asian populations, largely because of immigration. Given the declining birth rate of the native-born American population, immigrants now comprise a greater percentage of the nation's total population growth than they have since the first two decades of the twentieth century: approximately 25 percent of the population increase. Even conservative estimates indicate that Hispanic and Asian populations are likely to double, to thirty and ten million, respectively, by the end of this century. Unlike the older immigration from Canada and Europe, new-wave immigrants come increasingly from the Third World. Of all immigrants who have entered this country after 1970, for example, 78 percent came from Latin America and Asia. At present, the predominant sources of immigration to the United States are Asia, the Caribbean, and Central and South America. A decade ago, the leading countries of origin for immigrants were Mexico, the West Indies, Vietnam, the Philippines, Cuba, Korea, the Dominican Republic, China, and India, in that order.

Historically, immigrant populations have been highly susceptible to adverse health and social consequences and attendant problems of displacement. Yet despite inordinate need, these highly vulnerable groups receive less efficacious health care than native-born majority groups. Although considerable progress has been made in recent years to lessen disparities, children who are born to mothers who are poor, non-English-speaking, minority immigrants or refugees are at the greatest risk for health deficits. Immigrant minority mothers are more likely than non-immigrants to suffer from poor nutritional status; greater maternal morbidity, infection, and mortality; a lack of prenatal and over-all medical care; and greater exposure to occupational diseases and health hazards due to lack of protection in employment, poor environmental and living conditions, and substandard housing. They are also more likely to experience the adverse social consequences of low educational attainment, low income, and underemployment. Children born to immigrant minority mothers are more likely to be underweight, premature, or suffer from birth abnormalities than children in the population at large.

Because maternal and infant risk factors are sensitive indicators of individual, family, and community health status, the imperative to respond to these issues among immigrant populations is clear. Moreover, the health care system and other institutions of society must be called upon to reflect the pluralism and diversity of the nation and move to elevate the health status and well-being of all its peoples.

The Significance of Nutrition and Breastfeeding in Elevating the Health Status of New-Wave Immigrant Groups

Nutrition is one important way to address concerns about maternal and infant health deficits among immigrant groups, specifically the problems of high infant mortality rates and low birth weights. Improving nutritional status before, during, and after pregnancy greatly improves the viability of the fetus during gestation, the health of the newborn during the critical first year of life, and the well-being of the child during its formative

Reprinted from *Wings of Gauze: Women of Color and the Experience of Health and Illness*, eds. Barbara Bair and Susan E. Cayleff, Wayne State University Press, 1993 with permission of Wayne State University Press.

years. Another key way of promoting greater health and survival rates is to encourage the practice of breastfeeding among immigrant mothers.

There is much evidence that the fetus is sensitive to the pre-pregnancy and gestational nutrition of the mother. There is also considerable proof that maternal under-nutrition and malnutrition in pre-pregnancy and during pregnancy significantly affect the birth weight of the new-born and the health of the infant up to six to nine months of age, as well as the nutritional health of the child during the critical transition to preschool, up to three years of age. A nutritional diet in pregnancy is beneficial to both mother and fetus. It lowers the risk of small-size infants resulting from fetal malnutrition by increasing the levels of fetal stores of nutrients such as vitamin A, ensuring optimal nutrient stores in both the fetus and the mother, and laying down adequate lactation reserves during pregnancy in the form of fat needed as a major source of calories, fatty acids, and subsequent breast milk production.

Breastfeeding can best be understood as nutritional, psychological, biological interaction and communication between mother and offspring, with each affecting the other. While the dyadic link, both transplacentally and in breast milk, between mother and fetus would appear to be biologically obvious, much of the practical significance and mutually beneficial nature of the breastfeeding process is still under-appreciated. The newborn can be thought of as an external fetus, with the breast taking the place of the placenta as the primary source for meeting nutrition needs. Indeed, the complex, species-specific nature of the nutritional and immunological components of breast milk are uniquely suited to meet the changing needs of the infant and are impossible to duplicate.

There is no way to replicate the ever-changing physiological, psychological, and developmental interaction which occurs between the nursing mother and her offspring. The superiority of human milk and breast-feeding over formula and bottle-feeding applies to rich and poor families alike and persists whether the family lives in a wealthy community or a poor inner-city neighborhood. Until recently the relative consequences of the two methods of feeding were considered to be of no real importance in urban societies. We now know, however, that recognition of the public health significance of breastfeeding and of human milk can make a particularly positive difference in poor urban communities. In 1981, 57.6 percent of American newborns were reported to be breastfed when discharged from the nursery. More mothers are continuing to breastfeed for as long as six months. However, this increase is not particularly evident in lower socioeconomic groups and among women of color. One study shows wide differentials in breastfeeding practices between ethnic groups—43.5 percent

for whites; 9.2 percent for blacks; 22.6 percent for Hispanics; and 42.1 percent for others. Another study shows a smaller variance, concluding that "blacks were less likely to breastfeed than whites by 21 percent and 26.8 percent respectively."

Research on patterns of breastfeeding among immigrant women indicates striking urban-rural differences in the number of women who breastfeed, the duration of breastfeeding, and the child's age at weaning. It appears that the abandonment of breastfeeding is principally an urban phenomenon, often not so much because urban mothers work as because bottle-feeding is one of the sophistications of city life adopted by immigrants. This phenomenon is evident both within the United States and in areas where large numbers of immigrants to the United States originate. The case of Haitian migrants is illustrative of this point. In rural areas of Haiti almost all mothers breastfeed their children up to twelve months, but in Port-au-Prince, nearly 23 percent have stopped breastfeeding before the child is a year old. In both urban and rural areas younger women wean their children earlier than do older women. Women in urban areas are more likely to wean children before one year, or to never begin breastfeeding at all, in comparison with rural women. Likewise, data on Southeast-Asian women show that their infants tend to be weaned early from breast to formula. This practice is partly related to the mother's need to work outside the home and partly because of the perceived association of higher status and formula.

This trend is especially disturbing given the decided benefits of breastfeeding for both mother and infant. For example, there is convincing evidence that in contrast to formula, breastfeeding establishes a bond between mother and child, helps ward off or minimize postpartum depression, helps the uterus resume normal size, and delays ovulation, thus contributing to the spacing of children and aiding in the restoration of the physique. Breast milk provides antibodies and friendly bacteria that help babies resist infection and fortifies the immune system through the transfer of antibodies, hormones, enzymes, and other biologic substances, a process crucial to early physical and mental development. Breastfed babies have fewer illnesses and are particularly less likely to have allergies and diarrhea, the leading cause of hospitalization of infants. They are also less likely to be overweight in infancy and later as well. Breast milk is easily digested and contains the nutrients that babies need in the correct proportions. Importantly, it is a steady and ready supply of sterile fluid of exactly the right composition and ideal temperature. Thus it helps mothers avoid having their infants contract diseases associated with non-sterilized bottles or watered down formula tainted by unsafe or contaminated water supplies.

In communities where food supplies are inadequate, or where there is little money for the purchase of food, breastfeeding costs nothing and aids in the mobility of mothers and infants. While breastfeeding has these positive consequences, the use of powdered milk and formula in bottles can have disastrous results for infant health, including problems associated with nursing-bottle syndrome—severe dental caries, oral malocclusions, and nutrient deficiencies.

Health Education, Outreach, and Cultural Awareness Regarding Breastfeeding and New-Wave Immigrant Patients

The promotion of breastfeeding is, of course, a multifaceted process. It includes the need for programmatic services and activities designed to inform, educate, and advocate breastfeeding among health workers, health care institutions, and public policy makers. Providers and facilities must modify their attitudes, approaches, and policies to recognize and respond to the high-risk need of immigrant populations. They must make the promotion of breastfeeding an integral component of their maternal and infant health ideology.

Results of current surveys demonstrate that this is not presently the case. For example, a 1986 survey conducted in Boston-area hospitals showed that " . . 15 of 28 area hospitals routinely distribute formula milk gift packets to all new mothers, including those mothers who intend to breastfeed." The results of another study conducted at Boston City Hospital and reported in the April 1986 edition of the *American Journal of Disease of Children* were equally disturbing. This study showed that women who were given commercial packets of formula were less likely to breastfeed, regardless of their intent when they first entered the hospital, than women who were given non-commercial packets containing breast pads and health education pamphlets which advocated breastfeeding. The study also found that when bedside lactation counseling supplemented the non-commercial packets and there was follow-up telephone counseling after discharge—accompanied by encouragement and support of the decision to breastfeed—the likelihood that mothers would begin and continue to breastfeed is even greater.

According to A. Naylor, the promotion of breastfeeding is a multifaceted process; health care providers who understand the complexities of lactation and suckling, are trained to convey this understanding to women, possess supportive attitudes, and are staunch proponents of the practice are essential to the socialization of mothers. Unfortunately, such training is uncommon, and any clinical exposure to the subject is coincidental. While other areas of medical or nursing education have undergone numerous revisions in response to the many advances made during the past three decades, attention to lactation and breastfeeding declined to near-extinction. Obstetrics instruction taught students how to inhibit lactation and speed the postpartum involution of the breast, while pediatrics training concentrated on the fine points of providing infants with artificial formula. The breast became a topic discussed primarily in pathology classes and surgical clerkships, where the details of how to temporarily or permanently eliminate its basic function were the focus. Nothing was taught about how to encourage and enhance its normal processes, nor how to prevent, diagnose, or treat deviations from normal functions. As a result, most physicians remain uneducated, untrained, indifferent, or ambivalent about breastfeeding. They embark upon their practice unprepared to assist the nursing mother, and they often give advice and carry out procedures that lead directly to breastfeeding problems and failures.

Social support from key influential people, family members, and friends can be important in a woman's decision to begin and continue breastfeeding, and this has implications for outreach programs and policies. A study which examined the influence of social support systems and the decision to breastfeed found that among Anglo-American mothers, the male partner is clearly the single most important source of support in promoting breastfeeding. In this group, support from a best friend was influential, but not as great as from the male partner. In contrast, among African Americans the most influential person was the best friend. The male partner had little influence among Mexican-American families, where the mother of the birthing mother was the primary source of social support for breastfeeding. Reaching the people who are most influential in the birth mother's support system can have implications for the ways in which programs and services to promote and encourage breastfeeding are devised among various ethnic groups. For example, programs targeted to Anglo-American families should include male partners, whereas educational programs targeted to blacks should involve female peers, including school, social, or church groups. Among Mexican Americans groups which involve prospective grandmothers are good places to promote breastfeeding.

Many myths, misconceptions, and superstitions have been perpetuated about breastfeeding, both within and without the medical establishment. Understanding the cultural implications of illness and health care is crucial when dealing with new minority groups coming from cultures alien to traditional American health ideology. Health care providers need to know about the health problems of immigrants that might differ from those they ordinarily encounter. They also need to be aware of the traditional health practices and cultural and religious beliefs of the immigrants, and how these might affect their ability to receive and maintain care.

It is well, for example, to consider the cultural mystique surrounding breastfeeding and breasts within American culture among American women. Despite the fact that a growing number of American women breastfeed, breasts are still more closely associated with eroticism than with reproduction and infant feeding. A widely held belief is that large breasts are a measure of sexuality and denote greater sexual responsiveness. For many women, the size and shape of the breasts are a defining component of their self-concept, self-image, and self-worth as sexual beings. Because of such cultural interpretations, many women have feelings of inadequacy and self-consciousness about their bodies, even if nursing, and experience discomfort and shame if their breasts are exposed in public to nurse their children.

When patients come from a different country, culture, or social milieu, health workers must know something about how they conceive and conceptualize their condition in order to communicate with them effectively about a treatment regime. Practitioners must familiarize themselves with patients' views of etiology and therapeutics and develop a special understanding of the cultural constructs and context of traditional and folk beliefs and practices.

Traditional Health Belief Systems and Ideas of Well Being and Illness

For many newcomers traditional and folk health belief systems and Western medicine are not mutually exclusive. For example, central to the folk systems of Latin America, Haiti, and Southeast Asia is the concept of humoral medicine, which has its roots in Hippocratic, Western medicine. In this belief system, illnesses are classified as either hot or cold. Food and medicine, also classified this way, are used to restore the body's natural balance. Embodied in the concept of humoral medicine is the notion of health as a state of opposing forces: balance/imbalance, positive/negative, male/female, hot/cold, Yin/Yang. For example, H. G. C. Wiese describes traditional Chinese beliefs about humoral medicine as follows:

> Although the particulars of humoral theory vary widely among various cultural groups, the underlying premise remains the same. The concept rests on the assumption that the elements exist naturally in a state of binary opposition and the effects of one element upon the other equalizes the balance of each. One common manifestation of humoral medicine is

a hot/cold classification of foods. This classification does not depend on any physical property of heat or cold, but rather on an innate quality of that food to generate heat or cold on or within the body. The classification of foods is just one aspect of humoral medicine; the classification of body states and illnesses is another. Like that of foods, this system varies considerably among cultures. The premise upon which it is based, however, is the same: the equilibrium between hot and cold. Maintenance of health in such cultures is believed to depend upon meticulous care of this balance in everyday activities. Where these humoral classification systems intersect, they greatly affect behavior.

In many Latin-American cultures, the hot/cold (*caliente/frio*) dimension of the humoral concept dominates traditional medicine. Diseases are grouped into hot/cold classes, while medications and foods are trichotomized as hot, cold, or an intermediate category, "cool" (*fresco*). Cold-classified illnesses are treated with hot medicines and foods, while hot illnesses are treated with cold or cool substances thought to neutralize them. Although the terminology of the hot/cold system suggests that it is based on temperature, the thermal state in which food or herbal medicines are taken is not relevant to the classification scheme. When new foods are introduced into the diet or medications are prescribed, they are incorporated into the hot/cold system according to the effect they have on the body.

The hot/cold classification has implications for maternal and infant health care. For example, during pregnancy a Latin-American woman is careful to avoid hot foods or medications to prevent her baby from being born with an "irritation" (a rash or red skin). An important consequence of the avoidance of hot substances during pregnancy is that many women will not take "hot" iron supplements or vitamins. However, to "cool" or neutralize these "hot" medicines women can be encouraged to take them with fruit juices or herbal teas. Another example of food avoidance concerns post-partum practices. A. Harwood reports that, "Many women avoid eating cool foods after delivery on the grounds that they impede the flow of blood and therefore prevent complete emptying of the uterus and birth canal." As discussed previously, like most other minority mothers, Hispanic mothers tend not to breastfeed. Therefore, perhaps the most important implication of the hot/cold system concerns the feeding of infants and the use of commercial formula. Evaporated milk, the formula base usually recommended to mothers upon leaving the hospital, is considered a hot food, whereas whole milk is considered cool. Because "hot" evaporated milk is thought to cause rashes in the infant, mothers prefer to feed their infants "cool" whole milk and almost immediately begin the transition from evaporated milk to whole milk. This transition can be abrupt or gradual, using cool substances such as barley water, magnesium carbonate, and mannitol to supplement the formula and neutralize the effects of evaporated milk. Health workers should be alert to this practice, because these neutralizing foods have a cathartic and diuretic effect when taken in sufficient quantity and may cause dehydration, diarrhea, and other side effects in infants.

Similarly, the hot (cho)/ cold (fret) system is a salient feature of traditional medicine in Haitian culture. In addition to being a classification system for illness, medications, and cures, the system ascribes qualities of "light" and "heavy" to foods, and the method of preparation affects food groupings. According to Haitian tradition, there is a belief that not all foods are good at all times for the human body; the use of food must be in harmony with the individual life cycle. There are foods for babies, foods for adults, foods for menstruating women, foods for the sick, and foods for the elderly. Some foods are forbidden to people at different stages of the life cycle. Pregnant women are particularly subject to food taboos or special food practices. They are permitted to "eat for two" (*manger pour deux*) and therefore gain considerable weight during pregnancy. They are also cautioned to avoid spices, but red fruits and vegetables (for example, beets or pomegranates) are thought to build up the baby's blood. Another example of Haitian food taboos relative to maternal and infant nutrition is eating "cool" tomatoes or white beans after childbirth, because they are believed to induce hemorrhage. The body of a woman is believed to be "hot" during the weeks after childbirth. Lactating women are thought to be particularly susceptible to illness, and any illness, it is believed, affects their milk in various ways. The milk of a lactating mother is believed to be stored in her breast, and the mother must eat very well to be able to produce healthy milk for her child. Although breast milk is believed to be a nutrient for both mother and baby, it can also be detrimental to the health of both if it is too "thin" or too "thick." If milk is too thick, it is said to cause impetigo (*bouton*) in the child. It is believed that breast milk can become thick when a mother is frightened, which causes the milk to move to her head, inducing acute headaches or postpartum depression in the mother and imparting diarrhea to the baby. Breast milk itself is classified as neutral, neither hot nor cold, and is thought to have a balanced effect on infants. If, however, an infant develops a condition—such as a rash—which is considered hot, mothers supplement breastfeeding with "cool" liquids—such as herbal teas or fruit juices—to restore humoral balance.

Among Southeast-Asian cultures the humoral notion is evidenced in the concept of Yin-Yang, which postulates that the universe, and consequently each human being, is composed of two opposing forces: male, positive energy, or Yang, that produces light, warmth, dryness, and fullness; and Yin, or female, negative energy that produces darkness, cold, wetness, and emptiness (Manderson and Matthews 1981). An illness or imbalance is attributed to metaphysical forces. Therapeutic adjustment of the diet requires consideration of the hot/cold qualities of food, cooking methods, and the nature of the illness. Although among Oriental cultures notions of hot-cold are similar to those in the Hispanic and Haitian cultures discussed above, Asian systems are more difficult to decipher and translate with precision. However, in general, most fruits and vegetables, along with fish, duck, and other things that grow in water, are considered "cold'; most meats, sweets, coffee, and spicy condiments, such as garlic, ginger, and onion, are "hot." "Hot" foods and beverages are believed to replace and strengthen one's blood; therefore, after surgery or childbirth, "hot" drinks are preferred and cold drinks, jello, and juices are avoided (Muecke 1983). Pregnant women are encouraged to eat special herbs and food to insure the babies' health as well as their own. Various "health" foods are carefully prepared and provided for the mother. One such health food is ginseng herb, which is believed to be a general-strength tonic for both the expectant mother and the postpartum mother.

Religious Belief and Health Practices

Traditional and religious beliefs and practices are intertwined with health belief systems. Often there is not a clear distinction between orthodox religion, folk religion, folk healing, and Western medicine. For example, although Catholicism is the predominant, official religion of Haiti, many Catholic Haitians strongly hold and combine the beliefs and practices of Vodum (voodoo)—a complex system of beliefs and rituals derived from African traditions—with Catholicism. They experience no contradiction in the simultaneous practice of both systems. Moreover, the distinction between physical and spiritual healing is not fully drawn. Disease and illness are frequently attributed to supernatural causes and possession by spirits (*mystere*). Therapeutics and cures may be sought singularly or in combination from parish priests, vodum priests (*Houngon*) and priestesses (*Mambo*), spiritual doctors, healers, readers, or diviners, as well as Western medical doctors.

Catholicism in Latin American cultures combines with traditional healing systems. Depending upon the nationality and ethnic group, the folk-healing system includes the practice of *Espiritismo* (a religious cult of

European origin based on an ethical code which is concerned with communication with spirits and the purification of the soul through moral behavior) or *Santeria* (a blend of African beliefs and Catholic practices which, unlike Espiritismo, takes no moral position). The leader, or *santero,* works solely on behalf of the practitioner of the faith, and his activity can be beneficial, of no import, or harmful to others.

Less familiar to Anglo-Americans are the non-Christian, non-Western religions prevalent in Asian cultures where conversion to Christianity has been minimal. The majority of Southeast Asians identify with the orthodox religions indigenous to Oriental cultures. According to Hoang, *Buddhism,* the main religion of Southeast Asia, is much less a matter of organized and institutional orthodoxy than a state of mind. Buddhism teaches that suffering is a reality of life and can be seen as a divine punishment for wrongdoing, and therefore it is not universally accepted as a symptom of disease. Adherence to this belief system can lead to undue delay in seeking medical care. Further, *Confucianism* is described as a code of ethics emphasizing hierarchy in society and stressing the worship of ancestors. The opinion of the elders of the family is sought in making decisions about medical care. Taoism or *Naturalism* advocates taking no unnatural action to achieve conformity with the "Tao," or creative principle, that orders the physical universe. When things are allowed to take their natural course, they move toward perfection and harmony. This belief reinforces passivity and procrastination in seeking medical care. And finally, Hoang describes *Animism* or Animistic belief as the philosophical system most commonly practiced by the hill tribes of Laos. The Laotians believe in gods, demons, and evil spirits as a way of life, and they feel they must communicate with the spirits of deceased ancestors to obtain their beneficial protection. When illness occurs, cures are sought through the rituals of shaman or by wearing symbolic objects on the body to ward off harmful spirits.

It should be noted that within each of these major religions, there is much variation and diversity. Additionally, variations occur in different forms among various nationalities and ethnic groups, as well as within each ethnic group of Southeast Asia.

Religious, dietary and health beliefs are inextricably related, and the food habits of any group of people must be seen systematically as an integral part of their social matrix. It is important to recognize that in almost every society there are close associations between food and religious symbolism, food and the body as it relates to states of health, and food as it is interpreted through the disciplines of medicine and nutrition. And while people bring their food habits with them when they move from one country to another, their eating patterns are inevitably disturbed. This is especially true when the countries are as different as the United States and the countries of Southeast Asia, the Caribbean, and South and Central America in terms of culture, climate, and the availability of foodstuffs, in ways of preparing, purchasing, and storing food, and so forth. In addition, factors such as taste, smell, and appearance strongly influence the acceptability of new foods. These elements must be taken into account by health care practitioners who hope to encourage the introduction of new foods among people with traditional eating habits.

There is substantial evidence that immigrants and refugees are in general more likely to suffer from deficits in nutrition status and that the adverse effects of inadequate nutrition are intergenerational. Similarly, since food preferences—and, often, the poverty that limits food choices and availability—are continued through generations, nutrition status becomes a part of family history. In the same way, social class, and the economic and political factors that condition it, are also integral to family history. Inadequate diet is not only a question of personal volition, but, rather more likely, a factor of social status. Because food, diet, and eating habits are a learned way of life and are passed on from generation to generation, conditions fostered by six or eight generations of inadequate diet cannot be completely remedied by the current generation of mothers breastfeeding their infants and revising their own and their families' diets. Nutrition status can be improved, however, and good nutrition does make a difference in overall health and well-being.

At the same time, there is substantial support and precedence for the view that American health care workers should be obligated to become aware and knowledgeable about, but not necessarily to alter, the food ideologies of other cultures. To do otherwise, either by design or default, severely compromises the ultimate effectiveness and diminishes the quality of the health enterprise. Moreover, it is imperative that the American health care system take culture and ethnicity (including the social and economic character of newly-arrived consumers' lives and the environmental conditions that influence them) into account and make an effort to translate cultural considerations into clinical practices, treatment protocols, and institutional policies. Indeed, to encourage heightened cultural literacy in the health care system poses no contradiction. It is both desirable and appropriate that the system reflect the diversity and differences of all the people whom it serves.

References

A list of reference is available in the original source.

Blood and Milk

Constructions of Female Bodily Fluids in Western Society

by Ros Bramwell, PhD

Abstract. This paper explores ways in which these essentially 'female' bodily fluids are constructed in Western societies. It first reviews the context of menstruation and lactation in modern Western societies. It next considers menstruation and breastfeeding as affirmations of womanhood, and then the extent to which breast milk and menstrual blood are considered 'good,' 'different' to other milk and blood, sexual and disgusting. Finally, it discusses pressures which arise from the marketing of related products. The paper suggests that women's belief in their ability to nourish their infant from their own body may be undermined by negative constructions of women's bodily fluids which 'product'-based promotion of breast milk may fail to address. *[Article copies available for a fee from The Haworth Document Delivery Service: 1-800-342-9678. E-mail address: <getinfo@haworthpressinc.com> Website: <http://www.HarworthPress.com> © 2001 by The Haworth Press, Inc. All rights reserved.]*

This paper presents an exploration of the ways in which two essentially 'female' body fluids—milk and menstrual blood—are constructed in our society. It draws on a variety of different disciplines and types of material to explore similarities and contrasts in the ways in which menstrual blood and breast milk—and the processes of menstruation and lactation—are represented and experienced. It is part of the nature of this material, and of the different representations of menstruation and lactation within Western culture, that the representations and experience of lactation and menstruation are analysed in different sources targeted at different readerships. Much of the available published literature on breast feeding recognises the health benefits of breast feeding and discusses ways in which breast feeding rates might be improved. In both drawing on this literature and discussing negative constructions of breast milk and the impact these may have on breast feeding behaviour, this paper may seem to seek to criticise women who use formula milks. This is not, however, the intention. Rather, by examining the complex constructions of breast milk, this paper places infant feeding behaviour in an explicitly public rather than private context, and demonstrates ways in which bottle feeding may be a more appropriate behaviour within this culture.

It is a truism that the representations of and our feelings towards our bodies are multi-faceted and diverse. A review such as this necessarily over-simplifies the issues, and suggests of homogeneity of attitude which is obviously far from the reality.

The health benefits of breast feeding for both mother and baby are continually re-affirmed in the literature, as is survey data demonstrating that health promotion initiatives have failed to reverse a social trend towards bottle feeding. Analyses such as that presented here may be of real practical importance in the promotion of breastfeeding. Whilst Henderson, Kitzinger and Green affirm that sociocultural factors are believed to play a part in women's decisions about breastfeeding, Hoddinott and Pill have pointed to the limitations of the health promotion model and the need for more sociocultural models for understanding how women make decisions about infant feeding.

Such sociocultural models might build on existing analyses of women's understanding and feelings towards their bodies and bodily processes. Negative representations of menstrual blood may arguably undermine attempts to promote breast milk and breastfeeding. For instance, it may affect women's confidence, and lower confidence in ability to breastfeed has been shown to predict failure to meet one's own goals for breastfeeding. Moreover, such negative constructions of female bodily fluids may produce negative attitudes which are little changed by positive information about the benefits of breast milk which de-contextualise the milk from the female body, and fail to address the underlying negative constructions of female body fluids.

Previous Work

Menstrual blood and breast milk may initially be seen as antithetic markers of women's reproductive capacity: Martin discusses the ways in which menstruation is described as 'failed' pregnancy by medical texts, whereas lactation (usually) follows the birth of a child. Following birth, however, women do both lactate and discharge the blood-coloured lochia from their vagina, and Laws found that at least some British men would identify menstrual blood with discharges following childbirth.

Potential connections between menstrual blood and breast milk have a long history. Walker describes how Aristotle, in the 4th century BC, argued that lactating women converted menstrual blood into breast milk. More recently other authors writing about breast feeding, such as Palmer have recognised potential parallels between menstrual blood and breast milk, but the topic remains relatively under-researched. The only empirical work which has touched directly on the relationships between women's perceptions of their menstrual flow and breastfeeding behaviour was a study sponsored by Farleys. Unfortunately, this seems to have only ever been published as an in-house publication, of which new copies are no longer available, which lacked proper explanation of methodology. This, combined with the unacceptability of research sponsored by companies producing formulas to many researchers and practitioners in the breastfeeding field, means the research has received little attention.

Context

Western women living in the late 20th century have an experience of both breastfeeding and menstruation which is unique in time and place, largely because contraception and a social norm of small families means that the average number of pregnancies and children is lower than for most of the recorded history of the Western world, and than that experienced in most other countries of the world today. Of course, there have always been celibate women, and some Western women today still have many children, but combined with an earlier experience of menarche, and a generally high calorie intake, the low incidence of pregnancy and birth means that a majority of modern Western women can expect to experience menstrual bleeds literally tens or hundreds of times more often than a majority of women in other times and other places. This does not, however, mean that menstruation is very visible in our society, indeed a number of authors have argued that menstrual bleeding is an event women are encouraged to conceal.

These same changes in patterns of reproductive behaviour which have increased the number of menstrual bleeds have dramatically decreased our exposure to breastfeeding. The large families and extended family life characteristic of some current non-Western cultures, and of Western cultures in the past, would have meant that most women could have grown up familiar with the sight of female relatives (or those they employed as wet nurses) breastfeeding infants. In the West today small, nuclear families and the popularity of bottle feeding mean that many young women will not have any comparable experience. Coupled with the low tolerance for breastfeeding in public spaces, and the few representations of breastfeeding in the media, many young Western women today will only ever have caught fleeting glances of breastfeeding mothers. (The potential impact of this lack of experience is shown in Hoddinott and Pill's finding that positive experiences of having seen a close friend or relative breast feed were associated with first time mothers' commitment and confidence in their own ability to breastfeed.) Of course, birth rates are low or falling in many non-Western societies, and bottle feeding is gaining ground internationally. Nevertheless, as a generalisation, the uniqueness of modern Western women's experience in time and place is that most will have far more experience of menstrual bleeding and far less experience of breastfeeding than would be the norm across time and around the world.

Affirmation of Womanhood

Both breastfeeding and menstruating are exclusively female activities. In a culture which sees menstruation almost entirely negatively, one of the positive aspects is its affirmation of womanhood. For instance, one of the few truly positive items in the Menstrual Attitudes Questionnaire is 'Menstruation is a reoccurring affirmation of womanhood.' Similarly, the image of the mother holding a child to her breast is a defining icon of idealised motherhood in Western culture. This is seen, for instance, in the many Christian paintings of the Madonna and Christ. This image is repeated through centuries of religious art from the elite to the vernacular right up to present-day Christmas cards (although it is noticeable that although the mother holds the child to her breast, an actual naked breast is not usually visible). The dissociation of this ideal from what is acceptable behaviour in actual women is wittily satirised in a Posy Simmonds cartoon reproduced in Palmer, which shows the same individuals both admiring the idealised image of madonna and child and turning away in embarrassment and disgust from an actual breastfeeding woman.

'Goodness'

Blood and milk produce strong cultural resonances in Western society. Blood can be seen as representing kinship and relatedness (as in 'blood ties,' 'blood brothers'), but is also a symbol of violence, war and conflict. Christianity, as a dominant cultural force, has at the heart of its mystery and ritual a paradoxical representation of cleansing blood, as the human sin is described as being washed away by the precious blood of the crucified Son of God. The blood of a murdered victim, often seeing as leaving an indelible stain, is here the agent which removes the indelible stain, a miraculous paradox. Menstrual blood, on the other hand, is almost universally presented as bad. Advertising stresses the potential for staining clothes, and particularly the potential embarrassment caused by any leaking and staining (see section on 'difference' below). Blood can be a symbol of power and strength (as in a 'red-blooded male' indicating a strongly passionate man, or 'my blood was up' indicating anger), and its loss in menstruation is represented as draining and robbing the body, and the menstruating woman as drained and weak.

In contrast, milk is seen as symbolic of purity and of motherhood, symbolism which includes an ideal of milk as 'white,' a colour which our society also associates with goodness and purity. The essential 'goodness' of milk is evident in phrases like 'the milk of human kindness' (see, for instance, Shakespeare's play 'Macbeth,' Act I Scene V), and its richness and wholesomeness in the Biblical description of the 'Promised Land' as 'flowing with milk and honey' (Exodus iii 8). The promotion of breast milk in current health promotion campaigns also heavily emphasises its natural goodness, and its nutritional and protective qualities. However, women may lack confidence in the ability of their own bodies to produce this 'ideal' milk, and there is evidence that they do compare the appearance of their own breast milk to formula milk (which in turn is probably carefully formulated to correspond as far as possible to mothers' expectations). However, the primacy of a woman nursing her baby as a defining symbol in our culture may already be eroded: Henderson et al. argue, on the basis of a study of media portrayals of infant feeding, that bottle feeding has become a symbol for babyhood in British society.

'Difference'

Against the background of the general perception of milk and blood within out culture, the 'specialness' and 'difference' of menstrual blood and human breast milk is often emphasised. For instance, Martin has documented the ways in which descriptions of menstruation in physiology and medical texts emphasise the idea of menstrual blood as 'waste,' and the presence of other 'dead' tissue in the menstrual flow. Laws found that many of the men she interviewed saw menstrual blood as unlike other blood, as containing 'impurities' or 'discharges.'

Promotion of human breast milk has emphasised its 'humanness' to distinguish it from formula milk, emphasising the ways in which it meets the specific needs of human infants in both its nutritional content and in terms of the protective antibodies it contains. However, the current promotion of formula milk de-emphasises its 'animal' origins in favour of its 'scientific' formulation (at a recent conference on infant feeding, a delegate reported that she had encountered clients who were unaware that formulas were based on cows' milk).

Sexual

Both breast milk and menstrual blood are uniquely female bodily fluids, and both leave the body by parts which our society identifies as 'sexual.' The vagina, through which menstrual blood is lost, is very much seen as a sexual part of the body, and it is likely that this is an important element in the embarrassment which surrounds menstruation. However, breasts also are seen largely as for the purposes of sexual allure and pleasure. Van Esterik proposes that "Breastfeeding challenges views of the breast as primarily a sex object." That this produces immediate practical problems for breastfeeding women is well-documented, because the taboos in our society against breasts being seen in public produces restrictions on where women can breastfeed, and Henderson et al. found that a key theme emerging from an analysis of media representations of breast feeding was the sexuality of breasts.

More subtly, however, it has the potential to produce deep-seated conflicts in women as to who and what her breasts are for—are they for her own and (even more important in our society?) her partner's sexual pleasure? Can she 'share' her breasts between her baby and her partner, or is this an inappropriate mingling of role and function, or a potential source of jealousy? Some women express concerns that lactation has made their breast ugly. Suckling a baby may produce feelings of pleasure in the mother which are similar to those experienced in sexual pleasure and orgasm. Whilst such feelings may be expected to encourage breastfeeding, they may in fact be a source of great confusion and distress to the mother because such feelings seem so inappropriate to her relationship with her infant in a society which sees 'mother love' as entirely distinct from sexual passion.

Western writers have long identified 'taboos' against sexual intercourse during both lactation and menstruation in 'other' cultures, but some commentators have critiqued tendencies to make generalisations about the attitudes and actions of individuals in 'other' cultures, and to make simplistic assumptions about the meaning and function of 'taboo.' Laws explored the taboos surrounding menstruation in our British culture, and found some apparent fundamental contradictions. Whilst much of men's talk about menstruation seemed to emphasise menstruation as an interruption to sexual activity, many of the men she interviewed had and did engage in penetrative sex with their female partners during menses. Whilst this could be seen as a more 'liberated' attitude to menstruation, and was experienced as such by many of her respondents, Laws argued that whilst a new ideology of sexuality and menstruation is, indeed, emerging in British culture, it expresses equally oppressive ideas about women. She argues that women's bodies have, in fact, been further 'sexualised,' and that women's control over their own bodies has not been increased by the breaking of a taboo which men saw as limiting their sexual access to women's bodies.

There is no comparably detailed study of the taboos surrounding sexual intercourse and breastfeeding in a Western society, but the potential tensions are recognised by many commentators, and it is suggested that this may be an important reason why many women choose, or soon switch to, formula feeding.

Disgusting?

As a society, we tend to view all bodily secretions as more or less disgusting and embarrassing, although there are degrees of disgust. Some bodily secretions and excretions are more disgusting than others, and the secretions of those we love or are close to are less disgusting than those of strangers (e.g., we might share a toothbrush with a lover or close friend, but not with someone we don't know or like). It may be argued that menstrual blood is especially so. It tends to be positioned alongside faeces and urine as a waste product, rather than with secretions such as saliva and mucus. It is also likely that the 'sexual' nature of menstrual blood contributes to this disgust, given that Western society, which has such deeply ambiguous views on sex, often views sex as 'dirty.' It is also a symptom of the way in which menstrual blood is viewed as very different to other blood. Almost all of us would suck our own finger if we cut it and, excepting possible fears about infections such as HIV, would probably suck, lick or kiss a wound on someone else close to us if necessity required or out of affection (like 'kissing better' a grazed knee for a child). Some of us eat animal blood, within the meat itself (visibly so, in the case of a rare steak), or in products such as black pudding or boudins, although some religions have strong taboos against this. The idea

of tasting menstrual blood, even our own, would, however, probably arouse disgust. Greer wrote 'If you think you are emancipated, you might consider the idea of tasting your menstrual blood—if it makes you sick, you've a long way to go.' In Jong's feminist novel 'Fear of Flying,' the female protagonist describes cunnilingus during menstruation as a 'Hells' Angels' initiation ritual, and suggests that an ideal partner would be one who was prepared to engage in oral sex with her while she was menstruating. Here again, our society shows some deep ambiguities.

Animal milks, especially cows' milk, and their products are widely consumed in modern Western societies. Again, our view of human breast milk is highly ambiguous, despite the promotion of its benefits to the infant. In the concluding scene of Steinbeck's classic novel 'The Grapes of Wrath,' written in the 1930s, Rose-of-Sharon, whose baby has died, encouraged by her mother, suckles a chance-met starving stranger in order to save his life. The scene may be seen as depicting the triumph of human love in the face of dispossession and inhuman industrialisation, and certainly the book celebrates the centrality of women and motherhood in maintaining family life and a caring society. It may be that our attitudes to breastfeeding have changed since this scene was written over half a century ago. The scene may also have undertones of sexual fantasy, as the recipient of this charity is a man, and Rose-of-Sharon insists that they must withdraw into the privacy of a barn.

Nevertheless, Steinbeck's scene contrasts strongly with anecdotes of the revulsion which the idea of an adult ingesting human breast milk evokes. For instance, a colleague recounted to me her disgust when, as a midwife making a post-natal home visit, she was given a cup of tea containing human breast milk. Palmer describes how telling junior doctors that the tea they had just drunk contained expressed breast milk was a popular 'joke.' Why should we, as human adults, feel that milk from cows, sheep and goats is acceptable to drink, and yet the milk of our fellow-humans is not?

The Pressure for Profit

Our course, modern Western women experience both menstrual bleeding and breastfeeding in the context of a capitalist culture. There are clearly substantial profits to be made from the so-called 'sanitary' products which women use to soak up their menstrual flow, but these can be increased by producing products with ever more 'value added' features. These include the ability to increase the invisibility of periods by using internal 'protection,' products which are specially wrapped for discretion, etc. Further threats to discretion are identified in the form of possible odours which can be counteracted or neutralised by particular products, and panty-liners and disposable pants are marketed as further safeguards against staining of clothes. Treneman presents an analysis of the ways in which advertising of 'sanitary' products both make use of and reinforce negative messages about menstruation. Berg and Block Coutts conclude that panty liner advertisements imply that women are always in a state of uncleanness and need to protect against their normal bodily discharges every day. Furthermore, generic items like clothes-washing agents can include in their marketing the product's ability to remove blood stains, although the possible source of such stains in menstrual flow is not made overt. Further marketing opportunities exist in products such as dietary supplements, herbal remedies and painkillers to alleviate symptoms associated with the pre-menstrual and menstrual phases of the cycle, and Eagan presents an analysis of 'who profits from marketing PMS.'

There is obviously money to be made from selling marketing formula milk, and the economic forces which underpin the promotion of formula and the undermining of breastfeeding have been well identified. What is perhaps less well documented are the ways in which 'aids' to breastfeeding are also being marketed. Some are to 'treat' problems: Nipple shields and creams for sore nipples, and devices to draw out inverted nipples. Research evidence for the efficacy of these products is often weak or lacking, and many breastfeeding experts would argue that problems like sore nipples would be best addressed by good advice and support to achieve proper attachment of the baby to the breast. Breast pumps are presented as 'liberating' women from the need to be with their baby so much, allowing them to pursue a more culturally normal lifestyle, although again it can be argued that women can learn hand expression techniques instead of using electric pumps. Breast pads 'protect' women against the fear of embarrassing staining of their clothes by 'leaking' breast milk. Key messages in marketing of both formula milks and many of these 'aids' is that the woman's body is inadequate to the task of feeding the infant, or that devices are needed to allow women to integrate breastfeeding into modern life without embarrassment or inconvenience. There are therefore clear parallels with the marketing of menstruation-related products—women's bodies need help to function, and women need help to liberate them from their enslavement to their bodily processes.

Against this, many health services and health professionals are now promoting breastfeeding. Part at least of the motivation to do this is the research evidence for improved health outcomes, in the short and long term, in breastfed babies—which for health services represents an economic saving in future health care service use.

Conclusion

Clearly, only tentative conclusions can be drawn from such a preliminary exploration of some very diverse sources. Furthermore, any conclusions must be hedged by a recognition of the diversity and ambiguity of the ways in which menstrual blood and breast milk are described and understood. If, however, any generalities can be drawn, it would seem that menstrual blood is seen largely negatively. Views of breast milk, however, are more ambiguous. Alongside traditional, highly positive images of the nursing mother may be placed the difficult contradictions created by a highly sexualised view of female breasts, and the negative connotations of leaking breasts staining clothes. It may be that there has been, and perhaps still is, an ongoing shift towards more negative constructions of breast milk. The decline in breastfeeding is clearly documented, but causal links with negative constructions of human breast milk are much less clear.

In comparing attitudes to menstrual blood and breast milk, this paper has made an explicit exploration of the possibility that the two may be linked. That discourses which position female bodily processes as problematic, and uniquely female bodily fluids as disgusting, have implicit messages for breast milk as well as for menstrual blood. If women internalise views that their bodies are disgusting, that they need to buy products to be 'liberated' from the constraints of their biology, that their bodies can be defined in terms of their capacity to provide male sexual pleasure, such views will form an important component of their attitude to breast feeding. Perhaps even more importantly, they inform the attitudes of the society within which women seek to make and act upon decisions about how to feed their infants. Such a society may both stigmatise individual mothers for not giving their infants the superior product of breast milk, whilst simultaneously stigmatising other women for exposing their breasts in public.

So far, health promotion campaigns to increase breast feeding rates have largely focused on emphasising the health benefits of breast feeding and teaching about appropriate management (such as timing of feeds) and skills (such as how to position the baby at the breast). Such initiatives may do little to counter subtle, long-standing attitudes towards women's bodies which are constantly reinforced through a multitude of discourses. The results of this preliminary analysis would suggest that some of the theoretical frameworks and methodologies which have been applied to furthering our understanding of the construction of menstrual blood might usefully be applied to breast milk. Further, that breastfeeding might become a topic for wider research, analysis and debate within the social and behavioural sciences, rather than being seen as a largely applied issue.

References

A list of references is available in the original source.

WORKSHEET—CHAPTER 11
Childbirth and Lactation

1. Doris Haire's "The Cultural Warping of Childbirth" identified many common obstetrical practices from early pregnancy to postpartum that "served to warp and distort the childbearing experience in the U.S."

   a. List ten (10) of the practices Haire identified.

   b. Choose two (2) of these practices. For these two, discuss the known health benefits/risks of each; describe how this practice has changed or not since Haire wrote this article in 1972.

   In thinking about this question, it might be helpful to ask the woman or women you interview for question #2 about her/their experiences with these specific practices.

2. Interview two women who have given birth or one woman who has given birth at least twice. (If you have given birth, you are encouraged to answer these questions.) Ask the following questions about each pregnancy and birth.

   a. How was she treated in pregnancy by health providers and others? Was she healthy during the pregnancy? Did she have access to regular pre-natal care? During her pregnancy, did she have strong ideas about what she wanted her childbirth experience to be?

Birth 1	Birth 2

   b. For the birth event: Where was the birth? Who assisted in the delivery? What kind of birth was it (natural childbirth, some intervention, Ceasarean section)? Try to be specific about the interventions if there were any.

Birth 1	Birth 2

   c. Did the woman feel she had control in the process and did she have the childbirth experience she has hoped for?

Birth 1	Birth 2

3. For the two pregnancy and birth experiences described above, identify social and economic factors that you think influenced similarities and differences in the two experiences.

4. Many people think of childbirth experiences as one extreme (doctor assisted, with a great deal of medical intervention, birth in a hospital) or the other (non-doctor woman assisted, with no medical intervention, birth at home). However, it should be possible to negotiate all three factors: who assists; type of delivery, including interventions; location of the birth.

   Make up your own scenario of a birth plan, including the three factors above for a woman who does not want to have either of the extremes. Describe the advantages and disadvantages of each aspect of this plan as compared to the "extremes."

5. The introduction to this chapter emphasizes that increasing choices for women during childbirth must take into account that different women will benefit from different choices. Identify two examples of a "choice" in childbirth that some women might want, but that might not be desirable or appropriate for other women. Give a brief explanation if the explanation is not obvious.

CHAPTER 12

Aging, Ageism, Mid-life and Older Women's Health Issues

A core theme of this book is to remember that different women have different chances of being healthy and/or having access to health services appropriate to their needs. This chapter looks specifically at a few issues for mid-life and older women. Aging is certainly a woman's issue because almost all people have more health concerns and call upon the health system more as they grow older. As women outnumber men in a ratio of 2:1 in the over 75 age group, health issues of aging are disproportionately women's health issues. Both because of women's roles and status in society and because of their longer life expectancy, women have very different experiences of aging and being old than men. Older women's incomes are on average 58% of the income of older men; women over 65 are almost twice as likely to have incomes below the poverty line as men over 65 (Ruth Sidel, "The Special Plight of Older Women" in *Women and Children Last.*) Men are much more likely to be cared for by a loved one in their dying days; women are much more likely than men to spend their last days or years in nursing homes.

When young people suggest that the issues of aging are not relevant to their lives, it is very appropriate to point out that we are all, constantly, in the process of aging! Patsy Murphy's article "Ageing" brings this point home by looking at the issues of aging from the vantage point of a 43-year old. Questions on the worksheet try to guide students of all ages to an awareness that aging is a lifelong process and that taking care of our bodies in our younger years may be the best investment we can make to maximize on our old age. In the case of osteoporosis, young people who do weight-bearing exercise and eat a diet that promotes healthy bones literally build for their future; reaching age 35 with the strongest bones possible does more to prevent osteoporosis than most decisions made after 35. There is increasing evidence that the time between a woman's first period and her first pregnancy is the time when her body is most vulnerable to carcinogens. The decisions a woman makes in her teens and early twenties about exercise, fat consumption, alcohol use, and exposure to radiation, pesticides or other environmental hazards (often not a choice at all) influence her chances of developing breast cancer later in life more than decisions she makes later. There is evidence that girls involved in athletics in high school and college have a decreased risk of breast cancer. Susan Love, breast cancer specialist, concludes, "A theory has been very seriously put forth that I find delightful: put public health funding into high school athletics for girls - not a bad use of our resources. This would likely decrease breast cancer; also it strengthens bones and helps prevent heart disease" (*Dr. Susan Love's Breast Book,* 1995, p. 239). Rose Frisch's work has shown that women involved in college athletics not only have a significantly lower lifetime prevalence of breast cancer but also have a lower rate of uterine, ovarian, cervical and vaginal cancers, and benign tumors of the breast and reproductive system than non-athletic peers. Very relevant to this chapter on aging, Frisch emphasizes, "It's not too late to start exercising . . . Regular exercise has so many advantages that it is a lifestyle to adopt at any age." (Rose E. Frisch, *Female Fertility and the Body Fat Connection,* 2002, p. 120.) The importance of *starting* health promotion at any age is most inspiringly described by Natalie Angier in *Women: An Intimate Geography:*

> Muscle is gracious. It does not hold grudges. Even an elderly woman who never learned to do cartwheels or bothered to join a fitness club in early adulthood can, in her oxidized age, become a mighty virago. Her muscles will be there for her. Miriam Nelson, a physiologist at Tufts University, has taken women in their seventies, eighties, and nineties, women who couldn't leave their apartments or rise from their chairs, women in nursing homes, and she trained them twice a week with weights the way weightlifters in gyms train with weights - not timidly, not holding back for fear of their frailty or fear that they might, heavens, "bulk up," but with intensity, using as high a weight as the woman can manage. After only four months in the program, these women, these sedentary, often arthritic women with dowager's humps and hummingbird bones, grew astonishingly strong, were as though healed by a carnival preacher, tossing aside canes and walkers, getting down on their hands and knees to garden, canoe(ing), shovel(ing) snow . . . they doubled or trebled their strength. They became stronger than they had been in middle age. (pp. 319–320.)

In addition to the physical health issues related to the aging process and being older, ageism is, of course, a mental health issue for older women. In "Women and Ageing: The Dreaded Old Woman Fights Back," Madge Sceriha identifies how sexism and society's lack of respect for older people come together in anophobia, the fear of old women. Although she describes this powerful social, economic, and political issue, as the title of her article suggests, she also emphasizes how older women are actively organizing and fighting against this oppression. Similarly, building on the theme that even women's movements have too often ignored the issues of older women, in "An Open Letter to the Women's Movement," Barbara Macdonald identifies ways we can all work against our own ageism.

Readers are requested to read the next four articles ("More Selling of HRT," "Now the Truth Is Known," "HRT: An Overview," and "Hormone Therapy: Six Steps Toward a Better Future") together and note that "More Selling of HRT" was updated in late 1999 before the important "news" (July, 2002) that hormone replacement therapy increased breast cancer, heart attack, stroke, and blood clots. The other three articles are written in response to that 2002 announcement.

"More Selling of HRT" can be viewed as an introduction to the basic issues of menopause and the medicalization of menopause and an introduction to an analysis of how the HRT story represents wider recurring themes about women's health and the marketing of products. In the words of the National Women's Health Network, HRT is symbolic of "the triumph of marketing over science." Instead of letting the "dangers of HRT" news get framed as being about one particular product at one particular moment in time, it is important that women's health students identify the many ways that the HRT story is not unique. HRT is symbolic of a recurring pattern of untested, unneeded products being marketed to healthy women for pharmaceutical company inspired "medical conditions." Both the media and the medical profession have managed to present the dangers of HRT as shocking, totally unpredictable news, but, in fact, no one should have been surprised to learn that HRT did not prevent heart disease and that its long term safety was questioned. Many researchers and activists had been saying this for over a decade. Since 1989, the National Women's Health Network (NWHN) has been publishing *Taking Hormones and Women's Health,* an accessible summary and critique of all the (midlife) hormone studies. (This book started being published and distributed by Prima Publishers, as *The Truth About Hormone Replacement Therapy: How to Break Free from the Medical Myths of Menopause* in 2002.) This regularly updated publication continually warned that the benefits of hormones had not been proven and that the long term risks were not fully understood. The NWHN played a key role in the early 1990s in advocating and lobbying for a large randomized trial (which eventually became the Women's Health Initiative [WHI]) to study the risks and benefits of estrogen and HRT. As we now recognize the importance of this study, it is crucial to remember that the study almost didn't happen: "At various times, the trial is opposed by members of Congress who think it is too expensive, by epidemiologists who think the design is too complicated, and by leading gynecologists who think the heart disease benefit is so well proven that it is unethical to ask women to accept the possibility that they might get randomized to a placebo!" (*The Truth About HRT,* p. 180). The WHI's findings on the dangers of HRT need to be a reminder of the importance of having large randomized trials for *all* products, especially for products which are marketed to healthy people.

The "HRT: Overview" fact sheet summarizes information for personal decision-making in light of the 2002 WHI findings and recommends books and websites for keeping up to date with the scientific studies on this topic. "Hormone Therapy: Six Steps Towards a Better Future" offers important policy recommendations to increase the role of science over marketing in ensuring that women's health products are safe. "Now That the Truth is Known," a NWHN response to the 2002 WHI finding, ends with the important question, "Who knows what is coming next? It is not hard to imagine that one of the new drugs people are taking today, believing that it makes them healthier, will be the HRT bombshell of tomorrow." (These words ring particularly true as this book goes to press in March, 2004, and the WHI has today announced that estrogen alone does not prevent heart disease but "the increased risk of stroke with estrogen alone outweighs any benefits found in the study.") In the months following the 2002 announcement about the risks of HRT, the media has been full of stories focusing on a number of new products women could try to "replace" their "replacement hormones." The obvious irony is that HRT has been widely used since the early 1980's but the crucial questions about its safety were only recently answered. The important thing to remember about new products is that they are *new*. (Recent changes in federal laws now require the Food and Drug Administration and pharmaceutical companies to work together to get new products to the market sooner, so long term safety studies have not been done on most new products when they reach the market.)

In light of worries about HRT and other pharmaceutical products, many women are turning to "alternative medicine" and nutritional supplements. Because there is considerably less regulation of "alternative medicine" and nutritional supplements than of pharmaceutical drugs, it is just as important that consumers make informed decisions about these products. Dr. Adriane Fugh-Berman's excellent *Alternative Medicine: What Works* (Odonian Press, 1996) and her chapter on alternatives to HRT in *The Truth About HRT* are recommended. We include her "Phytoestrogens: A New Alternative for Women?" as an example of the kinds of information women need to know in making decisions about whether to use plant products with estrogenic effects for menopausal concerns and disease prevention.

In the same way that many women's health issues have been medicalized, there is a new trend to medicalize older men's issues. In an era where we are no longer surprised to find erectile dysfunction ads on our prime time tv or in our Sunday newspaper magazines, should we be surprised that older men are being encouraged to worry about their decreasing testosterone levels? "Hormones for Men" demonstrates the parallels between marketing HRT to women and a new trend to market testosterone "replacement" to men and concludes, "It would be a shame to make the same mistake again." Maybe it is time for a men's health movement!

Ageing

by Patsy J. Murphy

I cried bitterly when I reached my twenty-third birthday because everyone else in my year in college was nineteen or thereabouts and I felt life passing me by. I dreaded thirty with a passion which in retrospect was idiotic—I had the happiest time of my life between thirty and thirty-five. I walked the beach at Dunquin on my fortieth birthday on a lovely June day and felt terrific, and when asked at forty-three to write on ageing I felt resentful—it's hip to be over forty in New York and ageing is something I wasn't thinking about anyway. Now I've been thinking about it for the last month and what I feel about ageing is GUILT. Lots of Guilt and mostly about the things that I haven't done that I thought I would have—I haven't written a book, made a movie, seen Vienna—I haven't, in short sorted out my life and it's time I did. . . . On the other hand, I've enjoyed myself, reared a daughter (almost), supported us both and today I am starting to sort out my life.

I believe that most of the time ageing isn't so dreadful. A friend of mine told me crisply that ageing is what other people notice about you—you don't monitor its progress. My daughter used to carefully count the lines on my forehead when I was thirty-three and I know they've increased and multiplied, but I remain unaware of it until I pass a shop window and see this Winnie-the-Pooh-shaped middle-aged woman and then I reel in horror at the vision that is me.

But the vision isn't as dreadful as the guilt, which has to do with things I've left undone. At my back I always hear time's winged chariot. I've run a questionnaire amongst some of my contemporaries, who are, as a French woman I know puts it, 'happy in their skin'—that is doing what they want to do and liking themselves. They don't mind ageing. I asked the cleverest woman I know how she felt about it and she said that 99 percent of the time she was totally unconscious of ageing—ageing was no bother But the one percent was the awful, awful nostalgia about the past. I'll come back to the past later, but 99 percent is OK. The message for me is to do things that make me like myself and avoid the many, many things that make me hate myself—drinking too much, not making dental appointments. The message is the same for us all, sisters.

I asked a psychologist about guilt—it's normal he says, but it's useless: 'Take it out into the back garden and get rid of it,' he says. So, guilt apart, what does ageing mean? It means the body ain't what it used to be, but what the hell—the mind has more information and the body more experience. Ageing means that situations don't scare you as much as they did when you were young. I no longer feel terror when I walk into a room full of people. I no longer dread having to speak in public. I no longer think that someone else is going to sort out my life for me though I often wish that someone would.

For many women ageing brings freedom—a time to do things for themselves, by themselves, things that family responsibilities excluded for years. You don't have to be twenty to be knocked out by Venice, and the southern sun beams as benignly on your back at forty as at eighteen. A good book is still a good book. A glass of wine is still a glass of wine.

I've convinced myself that ageing has its compensations, but I'm still frightened of old age. I'm frightened of all the things that I presume everyone fears, being on my own, having no one to love, no one loving me, not being able to manage, the fear that the whole structure that one calls one's life, which I often feel I have small control over, will collapse around me and that I won't have the health or the energy to put it together again. Old age is not a subject one hears discussed. People on the radio and in books talk to the old, not about being old, but about their past, their part in the revolution, their girlhood, their village long ago. My fear of old age is the fear of death, which I have only experienced as the loss of other people, particularly the dreadful loss of my father. I couldn't bear his death—I hated to think of him in the cold ground. I still cannot face the idea of my own death.

I can face the more immediate horrors, though. I don't believe that the menopause is such a big deal or that it's going to make me feel useless. I imagine it must be quite a relief—no more periods—and it can hardly make me more evil-tempered than I can be now. So what is it that worries me? I'm back where I started. I'm

Reprinted with permission from *Personally Speaking*, ed. Liz Steiner-Scott, Attic Press, Dublin, Ireland 1985.

back with my friend talking about the awful nostalgia. I'm there in my past looking at a photograph of us all sitting on a wall in Paris in 1958, skinny, happy, hopeful. . . . Or I'm back in a place of which I can say, like Edna O'Brien's green-eyed girl, 'I was happy here' and I feel my ghost, I see my former self, before motherhood, before mortgages, before security mattered. This is agony, the skewer in the heart and it has to be borne. Yeats felt it, Dylan Thomas, Simone de Beauvoir . . . we all feel it, bear it, hate it. Sometimes I want it back, my lovely lost past. Well, it's gone.

When I was young, I read a lot. I've continued to do so, and I will always do so, and if I'm blind I'll ask someone to read to me because books at any age are a passport to freedom. Once, in a very gloomy period of my existence, I kept sane by reading Simone de Beauvoir's series of autobiographies. I would mechanically get through my horrid day and then, clutching twenty cigarettes, get under the blanket and live a different life, a life that became more real than my own. Unhealthy, you may say, but it got me through a bad time in my life and I imagine that books will have to and will get me through more bad times. I don't have enough life left to read all that remains to be read. Apart from such old pleasures I've found new ones in middle age—gardening, listening to opera. The pleasures of the flesh? To be candid I haven't experienced them for some time but I don't think they have disimproved and I suppose everyone's life has lulls in sensuality.

Last week I saw David Shaw Smith's TV film on the life of Pauline Bewick, an artist whose work is a total celebration of womankind. In a very beautiful film, the thing that touched me most was her triumphant feeling about her future and her work now she's fifty. She looked to her future with such a shout of confidence. I would like to be like that, although I'm not.

Our friends are the most important source of pleasure. I still have the same friends that I had in my twenties, and the friendship of women is something that improves with time, because women share their sorrows, drink over them, laugh over them, grow close over them. I hope when we're old we'll be laughing more than crying.

My friends and I laughed a lot in our twenties, we got up late, looked out the window with a cup of coffee and a fag in hand and surveyed the long carefree day ahead. Then, as it was the sixties, we all got jobs we loved, and had love-lives and money and lots of crack. Then we got pregnant, and the hassles and stratagem and patchwork that are the lot of women who bring up children—especially on their own—followed. But we survived and we still enjoyed ourselves, frazzled, broke and unperceptibly ageing. We survived. What we lost with youth was freedom, the freedom, as one friend says wistfully, just to fling stuff into a rucksack and go. I was never one for rucksacks, but I know how she feels.

So I sit here at the typewriter aged forty-three and how I do feel? I think that I have not done all that I should with my life. There are moments when I feel panic-stricken and desolate: 'What if this or that happens?' 'What if it doesn't?' There are times when I trail home from work clutching the shopping and sink in front of the telly, immersed in *Hill Street Blues,* and scream silently to myself 'Is there a life out there in the world?' And yes, I know there is and I'm going out to tackle it one of these days. Perhaps I'll tackle it today. I'll put the photograph of our hopeful selves sitting on a wall in Paris in 1958 back in the album and I'll go out and confront this grey city and my life ahead.

Questions for Discussion

1. How do you feel about getting old?
2. What are the things that bother you the most about getting old? What are the things that make you feel good about ageing?
3. How does society treat older women? With respect? With indifference? With contempt? Why?
4. What relationship, if any, do younger women have with older women outside their families? Do you think that this is a source of worry for young and old?
5. Imagine yourself when you are old. What will you look like? What will you be doing? Where will you be living? With whom? How do you think you will feel?
6. Why do we try to stay 'looking young' for as long as possible? Why are we so concerned with the signs of ageing: getting grey hair, wrinkles, loose skin, etc.?
7. What effect does the menopause have on women? Do you think it is a cause of depression in women?
8. Do you think that your attitude towards sexuality will change when you're old? How?
9. What place do older women have in the women's movement? What role should they have?
10. If you are taking care of an elderly woman, how do you feel about her? How does she feel about you? Why is there so much guilt and resentment built into these relationships? What can be done about it?

Suggested Reading

Jane Barker and Rosie Graham, 'Change of Life?' *Spare Rib,* No. 51 (London: October 1976) pp. 41–3.

Colette, *Earthly Paradise: An Autobiography drawn from her lifetime writings,* Edited by Robert Phelps, (Harmondsworth: Penguin 1974).

Simone de Beauvoir, *All Said and Done* (Harmondsworth: Penguin 1977). *Old Age* (Harmondsworth: Penguin).

Barbara Macdonald with Cynthia Rich, *Look Me in the Eye: Old Women, Aging and Ageism* (London: The Women's Press 1984).

Adrienne Rich, *Of Woman Born. Motherhood as Experience and Institution* (London: Virago 1977).

Virginia Woolf, *A Room of One's Own* (Harmondsworth: Penguin 1963).

Women and Ageing

The Dreaded Old Woman Fights Back

by Madge Sceriha

Introduction

Ageism is one sociopolitical issue which has been conspicuously absent from the agenda of mainstream feminism over the years since its second wave surged some thirty years ago. For those feminists like myself who are presently facing the challenge of growing old, there is an immediacy to our concern that this omission be addressed. One compelling reason is that, while older women are increasingly evident in demographic data describing our ageing population, they are virtually *invisible* elsewhere in literature about women except as depressed, despairing, demented burdens.

Over the last decade, however, there has been a vocal and determined resistance movement gathering momentum among older women. To a large extent this represents a grassroots rebellion against the socially invalidating experience of older women's virtual invisibility within white, male-dominated western societies. Many within this movement have brought a feminist consciousness to the analysis of their experience and this has contributed to a more encompassing awareness of the effects of all forms of oppression on women throughout their lives. (Anike & Ariel 1987; Ford & Sinclair 1987; Job 1984; Rosenthal 1990; Scutt 1993; Walker 1985). Pioneers of second-wave feminism and public figures such as Germaine Greer (1991), Betty Friedan (1993) and Robin Morgan, the woman who coined the slogan 'the personal is political' and who is now editor-in-chief of *Ms Magazine,* have joined the ranks too and added strength to the movement.

It is still early days though, and inspiring women who are ageing to challenge the stereotype of the 'old woman' is no easy task. This chapter will highlight the insidiousness of ageism as it affects women: the 'links between the social devaluation of women and their own self deprecating beliefs' (Fook 1993, 15).

Anophobia

When I am an old woman I shall wear purple . . .'
(Jenny Joseph, cited in Martz 1991, 1)

These opening words from Jenny Joseph, in the now familiar poem 'Warning', sound as if they were written especially for feminists growing old. It certainly is a poem of protest against conventional role expectations for women and paints a picture of the old woman as defiant and outrageous. Yet such is the power of ageism that it is more than likely that the woman who emulates this poem's urgings would be ridiculed and her purpose in rebelling ignored or trivialised.

Most older women are not overtly rebellious. Instead they have learned to step out carefully amid the minefields of patriarchal capitalism and ever more so as they negotiate the added dangers of ageism. Were they to look more closely at ageism though, they would see that their experience of it is neither gender neutral nor new. In a different form, which Germaine Greer (1991, 2) has called 'anophobia', it has stalked them throughout their lives as women.

'Anophobia' means 'the irrational fear of old women'. This is the fear that has made being called an 'old woman' one of the most insulting things that can be said by one man about another man. This is the fear which, because it is internalized by women from an early age, complicates their own inevitable ageing experience. This is the fear that is in effect yet another way in which women are systematically oppressed in our white, male supremacist society. Anophobia is the fuel which feeds sexist ageism.

Anophobia is a most effective social control mechanism every time it silences the rage and pain of old women's existence as they struggle to survive against the constraints of economic, social and political marginalisation. It is effective too when it perpetuates divisiveness among women of different ages. Perhaps the worst outcome of all is its effectiveness in reinforcing fear and a sense of helplessness in women as ageing progresses and their capacity to serve others diminishes. For many, all that seems to be left for them is to passively serve out their time till death comes as a welcome release.

Serving and servicing others still characterises the work women do in the home and in the paid workforce and, although this 'women's work' has traditionally been devalued as low status in a male-defined model of work, it has provided many older women with a role identity over their lifetime. Where there is unquestioned commitment to this role, it can drain women physically and emotionally. An example of this is the work older women do in caring for a partner who is dying or who has some lingering illness requiring constant care. This work is all too easily taken for granted because most women in traditional marriages:

> . . . honour their commitment to selfless caregiving in line with religious beliefs as well as sex role expectations . . . [at the cost of] social isolation and problematic return to life outside family relations [when the caring role ends]. (Rosenthal 1990, 4)

The exploitation of women this represents is seldom if ever recognised on a societal basis nor is the work costed and thereby included as contributing to the economy. To have the courage to reject the caring role is not without its costs either, for the woman who fails to fulfil her role in selfless serving is all too often labelled selfish. This negative label is particularly effective as a means of social control when applied to women, especially those who are conditioned to put others' needs before their own.

The women's movement certainly has challenged structural inequalities with respect to work because such inequalities discount the value of what women do and consequently deny women as a social group access to economic power and independence. These structural inequalities have, however, not yet yielded to change fast enough or far enough for this to be reflected in major changes to women's identification with traditional roles. Ageing women therefore face an identity crisis when they contemplate a future in which they are increasingly likely to need the services of others rather than being the ones providing the services.

This identity crisis is exacerbated by the stereotypes which have been perpetuated under anophobic influence; stereotypes which infiltrate our awareness from an early age in fairy tales, legends, books, movies and television. Think about these all too familiar examples:

- the wicked witch with superhuman powers, sharp featured, hunched over her evil brew, cackling to herself or shrieking curses;
- this is not far removed from the feared and reviled matriarch who, with her razor-sharp tongue and control of the purse strings emasculates the males of the household and enslaves the females;
- in contrast there's the pathetic, useless, dried up, shabby shadow of a woman who is the ultimate form of female passivity and powerlessness, huddled in a lonely room waiting to die;
- then there's the old maid who, unfulfilled without a man and children in her life, is portrayed as an object of scorn or pity;
- for a good opportunity to ridicule think of Dame Edna Everage, an image created and exploited by a man which gives it just that extra impact;
- and of course there's Maggie in 'Mother and Son' whose image reminds us of our fears of becoming a burden, of losing our memories and doing outrageous things which shame our families and we're meant to laugh *at* her not *with* her;
- the best that is offered is the idealised grandmother image, but it is an image of a paragon of smiling, ever-available sacrifice whose own needs are always secondary to those of family and community.

Words too which are typically associated with old women are loaded with derision: 'dithering', 'dotty', 'doddering', 'little old lady', 'shrivelled shrew' and 'old bag' are telling examples. Woe betide her too if she's sexual because then she's grotesque or disgusting, especially if her partner is a younger man or, even more unspeakable, a woman.

Then there are the doom and gloom projections about the future sensationalised by the media which tell us that 'by the year 2021, 17% of our population will be over the age of 65' (Cross 1992, 13). We are warned that this will burden the young and strain the health services to say nothing of all the other services which will be clogged with these dependent, decrepit drains on the public purse. Let's face it though, the bulk of the older persons likely to be affected by such messages are women. It is women who are likely to spend most of our years supposedly 'past our prime' for it is suggested that 'women get pushed into the category of non-persons our society calls older people twenty years or so before men do.' (Cross 1992, 14). Because women also live longer on average than men, we are likely to experience the loss of status associated with ageing as a double burden—it starts earlier and lasts longer. Anophobia ensures also that we are likely to experience it more intensely.

This gender dimension has until recently been largely ignored in the literature on ageing as indeed has race and ethnicity. 'Very few Aboriginal people or Torres Strait Islanders survive to old age' we are reminded in a recent report. This report reminds us also of the 'growing numbers of migrants in the older population who are increasingly . . . from non-English speaking backgrounds,' (Davison, Kendig, Stephens & Merrill 1993, 16-17). These two facts can very easily be ignored when neither of the groups concerned has yet a voice (least of all a female voice) that commands attention in male-dominated, white, English-speaking Australian society.

The dominant societal voice is rather one that sounds out loudly and clearly that to be an old woman is the pits in the destiny stakes. Searching for an identity as an old woman is therefore fraught with anxiety when selfless sacrifice appears to be the only alternative to her more blatantly negative stereotypes. All too often we defend ourselves against this anxiety with denial, and fall back on the belief that age is a state of mind not a matter of chronological years. This belief is reflected in the observation that 'most people perceive themselves as essentially younger than they are' (Greer 1991, 272) and is exploited by advertisers every time they target older people and promote their products with images that evoke fantasies of passing for or emulating youth.

Every time we succumb to such propaganda we reinforce our own internalised anophobia. This is evident with regard to health and self-care products and procedures which are promoted through association with youthful attractiveness and youthful desirability. The success of sales of pills and potions from the health food stores, pins and tucks from cosmetic surgeons, the creams and dyes from the cosmetic houses, to say nothing of weight control regimes, is founded on unrealistic expectations for miracles of repair, restoration, reconstruction and, in terms of weight, reduction. What publicity there has been about the costs in economic terms, emotional anguish and often enough, the traumatising physical consequences of these examples of the pursuit of beauty has not had a marked impact on the thriving beauty industries which benefit from women's fear of growing old.

The Beginning of the End or the End of the Beginning

It hasn't been so easy though to deny the menopause which marks the end of women's reproductive years and, it is suggested, the end of her 'prime time' as well (Cross 1992, 14). Not so easy that is until the advent of the menopause industry. Working on the premise that menopause is an endocrine deficiency disease, the medical profession with quite a little help from the media has effectively promoted the idea that what women need to carry them through the 'dreaded change of life' is a steady dose of medicalisation in the form of hormone replacement therapy (HRT). It'll calm them down, keep them cool, and even allow them to have a bleed once a month if they want.

It's certainly a lot easier for the medical profession to prescribe pills than it is for them to deal with the social reality that this is likely to be a particularly stressful time in many women's lives. One such stressful social reality is the powerful influence of anophobia. Small wonder then that the 'quick fix' promise of HRT is so widely taken up when it is presented as providing the possibility 'of eliminating menopause and keeping all women both appetising and responsive to male demand from puberty to the grave [thereby] driving the dreaded old woman off the face of the earth forever' (Greer 1992, 2).

Women are certainly not expected to think about the fact that HRT is a very lucrative product for the drug companies if they can be assured of a population of consumers with some thirty years of consuming to do from menopause to death. We're not expected to think either about the costs to women (economic, emotional and physical) of a regime of HRT. Nor perhaps are we expected to remember that, before HRT, a woman at menopause who experienced symptoms which led her to seek out help was likely to be dismissed or trivialised, whereas now, as a potential consumer of HRT, the midlife woman is much sought after.

Nowhere is this more obvious than in the marketing of osteoporosis. In *The Menopause Industry* Sandra Coney cautions us to question the motives of that industry, in particular the pharmaceutical companies, that would have us believe that osteoporosis is a 'silent epidemic' with the potential to leave us all deformed past midlife. 'Osteoporosis sells things' she reminds us, like calcium supplements and HRT and its sales success is based on our fear of the little old lady who may turn out to be even 'littler' than our worst fears could imagine (Coney 1991, 105ff). Fear is the enemy as much as any potentially debilitating condition though, especially if we allow ourselves to be 'persuaded to feel anxious, fragile and prey to a host of unpleasant diseases [thereby] . . . worrying ourselves half to death,' (Coney 1991, 277).

We might otherwise recognise that osteoporosis could have as much to do with chronic dieting and overexercising and the tendency some women have to wear themselves out or starve themselves half to death because of an obsession with slenderness. It appears that there is advantage in the presence of a little padding as we grow older provided we also keep fit. Not only does carrying this weight benefit bone structure, it cushions any falls that could lead to fractures as well. It appears also that this padding is involved in the process of oestrogen production in our bodies after menopause. This process involves the conversion of androgens, which are produced by the ovaries and the adrenal glands, into a form of oestrogen called oestrone and this process takes place primarily in the fat of women's breasts and stomach (Coney 1991, 85, 149).

It is significant too that anophobic obsession with the idea that the young female is the yardstick of what is worthwhile and desirable in a woman is divisive and keeps women in competition with each other between and within age groupings. We must remember though that it is a particular image of the young female which is idealized. An image which, furthermore, is elusive because it is created by the media in collusion with advertisers who have no scruples about using the airbrush and computer technology to shape their models to their whim. Magazines, we are told,

> ignore older women or pretend they don't exist . . . [and] consciously or half consciously, must project the attitude that looking one's age is bad because $650 million of their ad revenue comes from people who would go out of business if visible age looked good. (Wolf 1990, 82–4)

That age is airbrushed off the faces of any older women who do happen to be featured 'has the same political echo that would resound if all positive images of blacks were routinely lightened, . . . that less is more' (Wolf 1990, 82–4).

Even within the covers of those magazines which target an older female population, the emphasis is on the message that 'it's all right to get older as long as you look as young as possible' (Gerike 1990, 42). Thus, although there are many articles featured in these magazines which take up social issues of concern to older women, they appear alongside a proliferation of advertisements in which the models are young, trim and trendy. For good measure there are the occasional accounts of celebrities like Elizabeth Taylor who at sixty still appear ever young and ravishing. It isn't surprising therefore that so many women find comfort and reassurance from being told that they've 'worn well' or they 'don't look their age' and who dread being judged as having 'let themselves go.'

There are limits to what is tolerated in the effort to pass as or emulate the young though, and this has been very clearly demonstrated in the widespread controversy attendant on the news that two post-menopausal women have given birth after undergoing fertility treatment in an Italian clinic. Reports about the international uproar these events have caused focus on concerns for the future welfare of children of an elderly mother who might die or, for some other reason, not be able to care for her children (*Townsville Bulletin,* 31 December 1993). The double standard this represents is ignored, for males past 'their prime' who father a child are more than likely to get a pat on the back because what they've done shows that there's 'life in the old dog yet'.

Within the politics of reproduction, reproductive technology has emerged as a new frontier for the women's movement in its protracted struggle against patriarchal-capitalist power and control. 'Science and commercial enterprises (forms of institutional power) join forces with ideological forms of power (the control myth of woman as mother) in their attempt to control woman's procreative power' (Rowland 1988, 163–64). Reproductive technology stands alongside the medicalisation of childbirth and menopause, the radical invasive surgery of hysterectomy and the castration of women through oophorectomy as sociopolitical issues about which we need to develop a rigorous woman-honouring 'reproductive consciousness' (Rowland 1988, 165).

We certainly need such a consciousness to counteract complacency about the effects of the removal of a woman's uterus, cervix and ovaries when she is close to menopause. The removal of these organs is often justified on the basis of the argument that they are 'useless organs, sources of potential disease and decay' (Schumacher 1990, 58). Yet evidence is accumulating that, far from being useless, these organs have lifelong structural and functional significance for women's health and well-being other than that associated with reproduction. Not least of the functional aspects is the part these organs play in woman's sexual pleasure from arousal to orgasm. Women have been too easily persuaded to accept the 'take it all out' technique and then later, when they experience the very real sexual losses this entails, to accept that '[s]ex is all psychological' anyway (Schumacher 1990, 55).

Seldom though have we heard it suggested that we name the indiscriminate use of medical practices and procedures that experiment on, invade, mutilate and manipulate women's bodies for what they are—another form of sexual abuse (Schumacher 1990, 64). Seldom too do we reflect on the marked contrast there is in our attitudes to the prospect of hysterectomy as opposed to mastectomy. "Hysterectomy is trivialised where mastectomy is dramatised; the visible mutilation . . . is dreaded in the same irrational proportion as the internal mutilation is courted' (Greer 1992, 52). Prescriptive body image beliefs and the sexual objectification of women once again triumph when we fail to make such connections.

Women still trust the male-dominated medical profession to give them authoritative advice. Perhaps though we should remind ourselves of the absurdity of such authority about women's reproductive processes as it fuelled nineteenth-century arguments that women should not be admitted to universities. Then it was said that women's monthly bleeding would rob their brains 'of the constant and substantial flow of blood . . . required for intellectual activity' (Scutt 1993, 3). Keeping them out once menopause removed this impediment to participation was then left to other mechanisms of social control, not least of which was anophobic-driven sexist-ageism. Even today when menopause could be perceived as the beginning of another developmental stage in women's lives, prevailing medical authority favours a deficiency-disease diagnosis.

Medical authority is a form of institutionalised power which can influence our beliefs about ourselves. Where that authority influences us to believe the ageing woman's body is deficient and her once valued organs of reproduction are useless, it becomes another source of tacit legitimation for the continued medicalisation of women's lives and the social practices which devalue older women on the basis of their perceived biological inferiority. It is as if '[o]ur society has the idea that the value of women over 40 starts dropping rapidly and makes it a reality by turning the assumptions into facts' (Anike 1987, 26).

The Dreaded Old Women Unmasked

Devaluing is a form of social abuse which is 'so systematic that it . . . is considered normal by the society at large' (Dworkin 1988, 133). Its purpose is to marginalise and disempower and it is most successful when it generates feelings of revulsion and fear of the devalued group. Anophobia is such an abuse. Its obvious expression is in the pathological representation and negative stereotyping of women's ageing. It is much less obvious and therefore more difficult to confront when it takes the form of patronising tolerance. Worst of all though is when women start to feel that they are invisible, as this tends to silence them as well. It is not uncommon for women to remark that they really became aware of feeling old when they were ignored in shops and bumped into in the street as if they weren't there. Experiences of that sort soon erode self-esteem and self-confidence, especially if there were little of either at the outset.

The life expectancy of women in white Australian society has increased by some thirty years over this century and women outnumber men in all age groups after the age of 65 (Parliamentary Report 1992, 18–19). Women are the majority of the aged population and will be into the future and that population is projected to increase dramatically.

Alarmist reports in the media about the consequences of this demographic phenomenon refer to a '. . . "time-bomb" that threatens to blow the economy to pieces' (Parliamentary Report 1992, 52). It isn't difficult to see how the fear this has generated already in our society will attach to women in particular because they live longer. The double standard which persists in granting males as they age greater status and privilege than women accentuates this possibility. It is not that males are immune to ageist oppression but there is no male equivalent of anophobia nor is the image of unattractiveness, asexuality, passivity, dependency and incompetence associated with being old thrust upon them so early nor so destructively.

A 1992 Parliamentary Report observes,

> Demographic change may expose inadequacies in economic and social institutions and practices, but the former is not in itself the problem . . . The debate over how best to run an economic system is not primarily an ageing discussion . . . the ageing of populations may have little to do with the outcome. (Parliamentary Report 1992, 68, 70)

We must therefore maintain a critical consciousness of how easily the aged (and most particularly women) could be scapegoated when politicians blame welfare spending for the country's economic crises. Our society would have more to fear if older women were to withdraw the unpaid caring work they do within family networks and as volunteers in the community which is a contribution they are likely to make as long as they are able. Research indicates that

> older people are more likely to be providers than recipients of any kinds of support . . . [In addition it seems that more than 60% of the over 65 population have no limit on their functional ability and about 30% report only some minor restrictions to their activity. (Edgar 1991, 17)

There is a danger in focusing on 'use value' as a justification for older women's right to more visibility and respect though, especially where it is so closely linked to privatisation of service provision within the family structure. Such a view constrains women who want to 'retire' from such role expectations and venture into other pursuits which interest them and negates those women who are frail or disabled. These issues are among the many which increasing numbers of older women are coming together to confront as part of an older women's movement which has the potential to become as politically significant as any of the radical movements which developed in the 1960s.

Accounts of this movement worldwide are proliferating. The Older Women's League (OWL) in America, The Older Feminist's Network and the Growing Older Disgracefully Collective in the United Kingdom, the Older Women's Network (OWN) in Australia and the Raging Grannies in Canada are examples of action groups that are inspiring older women to be who they are with courage, openness and a commitment to living more fully than they have ever before been allowed to think possible. These groups offer support and encouragement for women to explore their potential without imposing expectations for dramatic change. In such an environment it is more possible to become aware of internalised anophobia and all other forms of oppression which ageist prejudice exacerbates. They are not about establishing new stereotypes for old women for not all women have secret burning desires to abseil or bungee jump or even to join in direct social action. Not all women could, even if they wanted to, because of frailty, disability and/or economic constraints.

Many of these groups are encouraging women to write their own stories, to join in theatre workshops, to learn public speaking, to lead discussions, to learn self-defence, to be involved in environmental and peace is-

sues and to link in with younger women's groups for events like International Women's Day and Reclaim the Night marches and rallies. Through involvement in such activities and action women can break down the barriers isolating them from each other within and between age groups, break the silence about their concerns and discover that the world of the young woman is no utopia nor is the world of the old woman necessarily a hell on earth.

That it is a hell on earth for too many is a fact that all women, both young and old, have a stake in addressing. We know that old women are likely to be victims of socio-economic violence (or what has been more euphemistically labelled the 'feminisation of poverty') because structural inequalities in our society continue to disproportionately disadvantage women throughout their lives. We know from the burgeoning literature on elder abuse that old women are often victims of emotional, physical and sexual violence just as their younger sisters are. We know that many feel isolated, lonely, hopeless and helpless because poverty, prejudice and powerlessness confine them to the margins of societal concerns. There is good reason, therefore, for all women to be actively anti-ageist and, in particular, anti-anophobic for it is an investment in their own future.

For references, see the original.

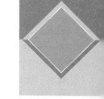

An Open Letter to the Women's Movement

by Barbara Macdonald

The following suggestions conclude a longer article entitled "An Open Letter to the Women's Movement" which deals with the widespread ageism in the women's community. The book from which this article is taken, *Look Me in the Eye,* is about women and ageing.

The following are a few suggestions to all of us for working on our ageism:

1. Don't expect that older women are there to serve you because you are younger—and *don't think the only alternative is for you to serve us.*

2. Don't continue to say "the women's movement," . . . until all the invisible women are present—all races and cultures, and *all ages* of all races and cultures.

3. Don't believe you are complimenting an old woman by letting her know that you think she is "different from" (more fun, more gutsy, more interesting than) other older women. To accept the compliment, she has to join in your rejection of old women.

4. Don't point out to an old woman how strong she is, how she is more capable in certain situations than

you are. Not only is this patronizing, but the implication is that you admire the way she does not show her age, and it follows that you do not admire the ways in which she does, or soon will, show her age.

5. If an old woman talks about arthritis or cataracts, don't think old women are constantly complaining. We are just trying to get a word in edgewise while you talk and write about abortions, contraception, premenstrual syndromes, toxic shock, or turkey basters.

6. Don't feel guilty. You will then avoid us because you are afraid we might become dependent and you know you can't meet our needs. Don't burden us with *your* idea of dependency and *your* idea of obligation.

7. By the year 2000, approximately one out of every four adults will be over 50. The marketplace is ready now to present a new public image of the aging American, just as it developed an image of American youth and the "youth movement" at a time when a larger section of the population was young. Don't trust the glossy images that are about to bombard you in the media. In order to sell products to a burgeoning population of older women, they will tell you that we are all white, comfortably middle class, and able to "pass" if we just use enough creams and hair dyes. Old women are the single poorest minority group in this country. Only ageism makes us feel a need to pass.

8. Don't think that an old woman has always been old. She is in the process of discovering what 70, 80, and 90 mean. As more and more old women talk and write about the reality of this process, in a world that negates us, we will all discover how revolutionary that is.

9. Don't assume that every old woman is not ageist. Don't assume that I'm not.

10. If you have insights you can bring to bear from your racial background or ethnic culture—bring them. We need to pool all of our resources to deal with this issue. But don't talk about your grandmother as the bearer of your culture—don't objectify her. Don't make her a museum piece or a woman whose value is that she has sacrificed and continues to sacrifice on your behalf. Tell us who she is now, a woman in process. Better yet, encourage *her* to tell us. I wish you luck in your beginning. We are all beginning.

More Selling of HRT

Still Playing on the Fear Factor

by Nancy Worcester and Mariamne H. Whatley

Introduction

For decades, women's health activists were critical of the medical system's lack of interest in older women's issues. Osteoporosis and heart disease were excellent examples of the problematic relationship between the medical system and women who use it. These prevalent, serious, life threatening conditions were characterized by an almost total lack of information and research. Until the early 1980s, most women had never heard of osteoporosis, and cardiovascular disease was so consistently labelled as a 'men's' disease that the major studies included tens of thousands of men and *no* women.

The situation has changed dramatically in the last decade. Osteoporosis and heart disease can no longer serve as examples of neglect of older women's issues. Osteoporosis has become a household word (clearly indicated by the fact that we no longer have to teach our students how to spell it), there must not be a woman in the industrialized world who has not seen a headline announcing 'heart disease is the number one killer of women', and the prevention of

---

This is an updated version (1999) of "The Selling of HRT: Playing on the Fear Factor" by Nancy Worcester and Mariamne H. Whatley which was published in *Feminist Review* (London, England) no. 41, summer, 1992, pp. 1–26.

both osteoporosis and heart disease in women has become 'hot' research.

It might seem that feminist activists should be applauding this response of the medical establishment. Any woman approaching menopause is likely to receive information from her health care practitioners on the dangers of osteoporosis and heart disease. So why are we complaining? Aren't feminists ever satisfied?

Prevention Consciousness

The interest in older women's issues is directly related to the fact that the medical establishment and the drug industry have 'discovered' that healthy menopausal and post-menopausal women represent a huge market. The selling of hormones and services which promote or follow up on them fits neatly into the needs of the drug industry, as well as health service providers and consumers. Restrictions by the government and insurance companies in the US have meant the health system cannot make enough money on sick people and women are not having 'enough' babies; the health system has had to search for previously untapped markets of healthy people. Consumers may feel the health system is finally responding to their needs if services and products are marketed to play on their new found prevention consciousness.

Contemporary US and British societies, especially the middle classes, have become highly health conscious. Advertisements in which bran cereals are pushed to prevent cancer, low cholesterol foods to reduce heart attack risk, and exercise machines to promote 'wellness' reveal the dominance of the prevention ideology in health awareness. Sometimes the meaning is sufficiently clouded that it seems that the appearance of health may be an end in itself rather than a means towards a higher quality life.

The focus on prevention and self-help is a part of an overall trend among consumers away from the sick-care model of the medical industry which devotes few resources to environmental and occupational issues, disease detection and control, or medical education, and instead prioritizes drugs, surgery, hospitals and high-technology equipment. This sick-care model may do an impressive job of patching up accident victims or putting a new heart into someone who has eaten the typical high fat, low fiber, western diet, but it does practically nothing to keep us well. The initial resistance to the medical model was often political, based, for example, on the analysis generated by the women's health movement; prevention was a way of wrestling control away from doctors and returning it to consumer.

However, it took the medical establishment and others little time to coopt the emphasis on prevention. This

consciousness has been intentionally constructed to be very individualistic—'take care of *yourself*' (i.e. don't expect society, the government or the health system to take care of you)—and victim-blaming—'it's their fault if they choose to live unhealthy lifestyles'. As major consumers in the health care system, responsible for their own health and that of other family members, women quickly were targeted as the major customers of prevention services. In her seminars on how to market women's health, Sally Rynne, consultant to for-profit women's health centers throughout the USA, noted that 18 percent of women's medical visits are preventative, that women are the major subscribers to the prevention/wellness type magazines and that the audiences at health promotion programs are predominantly women (Whatley and Worcester, 1988). Ironically, though the emphasis on prevention originated as a way to become less dependent on the medical establishment, it is now being used as a marketing technique to attract people back into the system: you cannot prevent osteoporosis or heart disease with HRT without having a doctor's prescription and surrounding services to monitor your 'progress' toward prevention!

Selling the Fear Factor

In order to maximize the market value of 'prevention', the condition to be avoided must be sufficiently serious or highly undesirable. Individuals must view the condition in question as highly prevalent or believe themselves to have a high level of personal susceptibility. Fear can become an important selling point for either true prevention or early detection tests.

As diseases become 'popular', there is a time of intense interest, during which we are inundated with media coverage of the newest plague, whether it is genital herpes, toxic shock syndrome, premenstrual tension, or chlamydia. Accurate and complete information is needed about these issues; increased awareness is essential for all individuals who want to have some control over their health. However, sensational media coverage often does little besides create fear, as the early media coverage of AIDS clearly demonstrated. Those who benefit from this fear-based media coverage are those who offer prevention, tests for diagnosis, or treatment, whether they are effective or not.

The marketing of hormone products to menopausal and postmenopausal women is particularly sadistic in the way that it plays not only on the fears of specific disabling or life-threatening conditions but also on women's fear of ageing. Disabling or life-threatening conditions are frightening enough in themselves, but ones totally associated with the ageing process, growing older or *being old,* take on an increased meaning for women in an ageist society which particularly devalues older women. It is no coincidence that *Feminine Forever* was the name of the 1966 book which first popularized the notion that a wonder drug (estrogen) could prevent the ageing process in women.

Swallowing HRT and Forgetting Its History

Feminine Forever, whose author was funded by Wyeth-Ayerst, the manufacturer of the menopausal estrogen product Premarin, promised that estrogen could keep women young forever and prevent the natural 'decaying' process of ageing. It is not surprising that by 1970 Premarin had become one of the top four prescription drugs in the USA (Eagan, 1989). By the mid-1970s, there were cities in the US where more than half of the menopausal women were taking estrogen (Sloane,1985). But, by the mid-1970s, studies were starting to show a marked increase in endometrial (lining of the uterus) cancer in women who had taken menopausal estrogens. While Wyeth-Ayerst denied the estrogen-endometrial cancer link and even resorted to sending 'Dear Doctor' letters to all gynecologists in the US (Waterhouse, 1990), women became afraid of menopausal estrogen, doctors feared lawsuits if they prescribed it, and at least another fifteen studies proved that estrogen use was associated with a marked increase in endometrial cancer (Sloane, 1985). By 1979, a consensus conference of the National Institutes of Health had rejected almost all claims which had been made for the physical or psychological benefits of estrogen replacement therapy. The conference committee concluded that of all the presumed symptoms of menopause, there were only two which could be established as uniquely characteristic of menopause and that are uniformly relieved by estrogen therapy. Estrogen is only effective for controlling hot flashes (vasomotor instability) and changes in the genitals (which text books refer to as genital atrophy—no wonder women will resort to anything to avoid this condition!)

One might think that would be the end of a product which lived up to few of its claims, in which consumers and physicians had lost confidence and which was known as a cancer-causing agent. But, drug companies had tasted the potential of marketing products to menopausal women: in the US more than 28 million prescriptions for estrogen had been filled in 1975. (National Prescriptions Audit).

The 1980s saw two changes in the marketing of estrogens: 1) Public relations firms were hired to promote estrogen products in the same way that candy, breakfast cereals or soaps are advertised, and 2) estrogens were reintroduced onto the market in combination with progestins.

Feminist health activists have found the mass marketing of estrogen products to be irresponsible. Starting in 1985, Premarin's manufacturer, Wyeth-Ayerst, hired a public relations firm to conduct a public education campaign aimed at encouraging *all* women over thirty-five years to consider estrogens to prevent osteoporosis instead of targeting the twenty-five percent of women at high risk of suffering consequence of osteoporosis. Later, Ciba Geigy, manufacturer of an estrogen patch, began mass direct mail solicitations promoting their patch to women throughout the US. Testifying before the Food and Drug Administration against the mass promotion of estrogens, Cindy Pearson stated, 'The National Women's Health Network is outraged that a potentially risky drug is being promoted with the same techniques used by Publishers Clearinghouse Sweepstakes' (Pearson, 1991).

By the drug companies' criteria, such promotion of estrogen products must seem phenomenally successful. In 1985, when Wyeth-Ayerst first started its 'education' campaign on osteoporosis, a survey found that 77 percent of women had not heard of this condition (Dejanikus, 1985). Now, women have not only heard of osteoporosis, they are also frightened by the seeming inevitability of postmenopausal hip fractures or of becoming like the elderly woman with the severely bent spine they have seen in advertisements. Having dropped to approximately 15 million prescriptions per year in the US in 1979/80, estrogen prescriptions were back up to nearly 32 million by 1989 (National Prescription Audit). According to federal health statistics, as many as half of all postmenopausal American women take some form of hormone 'replacement' at some time and at least 15 percent are taking the drugs at any one time (Michael Specter, 1989). A recent telephone survey of 500 women ages 50–74 in the US found that 38% currently used estrogen (Keating et al, 1999).

Packaging as HRT or ERT

Consumers are now faced with a 'choice' of hormonal products. By the early 1980s estrogen was often prescribed in combination with a progestin. It was believed that the progestin component would protect against the risk of endometrial cancer which was associated with estrogen on its own.

For the rest of this paper two different terms will be used to identify the two different forms in which estrogen is most commonly prescribed. **HRT (hormone replacement therapy)** will be used in reference to products or regimes where a woman is given *both* an estrogen and a progestin hormone. **ERT (estrogen replacement therapy)** will be used when a woman is given estrogen on its own. At this stage of the debate about postmenopausal hormones, it is absolutely essential that we keep track of whether we are talking about HRT or ERT.

It is accepted that ERT is related to an increase in endometrial cancer, whereas HRT is not associated with that cancer and may even have a protective effect against endometrial cancer. Any woman with a uterus (i.e. women who have not had a hysterectomy) should be informed of this and offered HRT instead of ERT if HRT is believed to fulfill the purpose for which she is considering hormones. If a woman with a uterus chooses to take ERT instead of HRT (for example, some women find they feel depressed and/or less sexually responsive on progestins), it will be essential that she have regular endometrial biopsies to check for endometrial cancer. As this paper will discuss, it is a confusing moment in history for women to be making choices about postmenopausal hormones. Many of the studies have been done with ERT, but not on HRT. As the studies have not been done, it is simply too early to know whether the progestin component of HRT diminishes or reverses effects expected of estrogen. The Women's Health Initiative, the largest randomized, controlled study ever done on women, is monitoring many thousands of women from diverse populations for the effect of ERT, HRT, or placebo (no hormone) on heart disease, cancers, osteoporosis and cognitive function (including dementia.) But, the results from this important study will not be available until 2007. As Kathleen MacPherson (1987) points out in her important article "Osteoporosis: The New Flaw in Women or Science?", some physicians will not prescribe the HRT combination because: 1) research on its long term effects is scant, 2) progestins in the contraceptive pills increased the risk of hypertension and strokes, and 3) postmenopausal women may not want to have break through bleeding which occurs monthly if they take the estrogen-progestin combination.

Women who are considering taking ERT, estrogen on its own, should be informed that in addition to the approximately five to fourteen fold increase in endometrial cancer (National Women's Health Network, 1989), women on this regimen also increase the risk of abnormal bleeding 7.8 times, need dilation and curettage 4.9 times as often, and have hysterectomy rates 6.6 times higher, than non-users (Ettinger, 1987). Women who take estrogens after menopause also have a two to three fold increase in their risk of gallbladder disease (National Women's Health Network, 1989).

Clearly the goal of estrogen manufacturers is to find a way to package estrogens so that women are willing to stay on them for their *entire postmenopausal life:*

> We are still learning ways to administer estrogen and progestogen to obtain maximum effectiveness with minimum side effects. New formulations of estrogens and progestogens, new routes of administration, and improved dosage schedules should provide more convenient and acceptable long term hormone replacement, one that women can use for their entire postmenopausal life time without the inconvenience of menstrual bleeding and concern about possible side effects. (Ettinger, 1987: 36)

In contrast to the drug manufacturers' goal to have women stay on hormones from perimenopause until end of life, there is much evidence that many menopausal women who "try" hormones do not stay on them long term. Short term use of low dose hormones are safer than long term use of higher doses of hormones, so it will often be appropriate for women to use hormones to ease the transition through menopause. However, women using hormones to reduce osteoporosis or heart disease will lose any protective effect soon after they stop taking hormones. The "yo-yo" effect of going on and off hormones can *cause* hot flashes and other menopausal symptoms by artificially creating the hormone fluctuations which cause these symptoms. Additionally, there is some question whether "on and off" use of hormones might actually increase bone loss. This paper will emphasize the importance of deciding *when* to take hormones as well as deciding *whether* to take them.

Hormones Dominate the System Both Physiologically and Politically

Hormones hold potential for improving quality and quantity of life for some menopausal and postmenopausal women. It will be important to come back to this point and question how feminists can better look at the potential for these hormones. Unfortunately, we seldom have the luxury of being able to do this because major forces are so persistently pushing hormones and because most information is so pro-hormones. In an effort to "balance" the discussion, feminist health activists have often ended up as lone voices critiquing the premature, routine prescribing of these drugs of unknown safety. It is interesting to note that anyone asking for this more "balanced" view of hormones (trying to shift the emphasis to asking which particular women will most benefit from which hormones and when) gets labelled as being "anti-hormones." Ironically, although postmenopausal hormones are increasingly pushed as something *all* women need, in reality, it is predominately white middle and upper class women who even get to make choices about hormones. Few low or no income women have access to hormones and with the important exception of the new Women's Health Initiative, women of color have been noticeably missing from other hormonal studies.

Even if women have *all* the available information on postmenopausal hormones, with the present state of knowledge it is extremely difficult to weigh the potential benefits and the unknown risks. But, in fact, very few women 'choosing' to embark upon hormone treatment even know that the drugs they are taking are controversial and possibly hazardous. The information women get in the lay press is very much biased towards the use of hormones. A survey of thirty-six menopause articles in the most popular women's magazine found that three-quarters of the articles were clearly pro-hormone and half the articles did not even mention any risks of hormone use (Pearson, 1991). The information women get from their doctors may be nearly as biased: over 75 percent of US gynecologists routinely prescribe hormones to all menopausal women.

Even the smallest doses of ERT or HRT have very powerful effects on a woman's body and totally dominate her body's own regulation and production of hormones. How desirable or safe this is physiologically is a question which remains to be answered. What is known at this time is that the way hormones are being promoted is very dangerous for women politically and must be seen as the part of the purposeful medicalization of women's lives.

Feminists have long been critical of the ways in which normal, healthy processes such as contraception, pregnancy and childbirth have been medicalized. We used to criticize the fact that real health issues such as premenstrual tension, infertility, and osteoporosis were ignored by the health system. Now that women's health issues have been 'discovered' and there are money-making drugs or technologies to offer, we see an expansion into medicalizing whole new areas of women's lives. We are already witnessing what this means. The medical profession is taking control over more aspects of women's lives, more conditions are being labelled as illness and used against the equality of women, drugs or high technology procedures have been identified as the solution to newly targeted 'problems' and, in the name of prevention, more women are being hooked into a medical system which does not meet their needs.

The medicalization of menopause means that menopause and postmenopause are defined as 'deficiency illnesses'. Even the terms 'hormone replacement therapy' and 'estrogen replacement therapy' wrongly imply that something is missing which must be replaced. The fact that this misinformation can so easily be used as a selling point for products is a sad reflection on how little information most women have about their own bodies. As the National Women's Health Network's position paper on hormone therapy puts it, **'We object to the view of normal menopause as a deficiency disease. Menopause does not automatically require "treatment".'** (National Women's Health Network, 1999)

Menopause is a normal, healthy transition phase of a woman's life when her body has within it all the mechanisms necessary to gradually change from dealing with demanding reproductive cycles to meeting the different, post-reproduction, physiological needs of post-menopause. The postmenopausal woman is still capable of making the estrogens she needs: the older woman's body needs less estrogen and makes it in a different way. During the reproductive years, a woman's ovaries will be the main producers of estrogens and relatively high quantities of estrogens will be produced. Menopause is the time when the ovaries gradually decrease their production of estrogens, with the dominant form of estrogen changing from estradiol to estrone, and the estrogens produced by the adrenal glands and converted from androgens by fat and muscle tissue become the major estrogens in a woman's body. Menopause should be viewed as the healthy transition from premenopause to postmenopause in the same way that puberty is recognized as the time when young women make the transition from pre-reproduction to being capable of reproduction.

Viewing menopause as a normal, healthy transition does not imply that transition is easy for all women. Although many of the problems faced by menopausal women are social rather than physiological, woman may experience symptoms such as hot flashes when or if their estrogen levels drop rapidly (which is what happens if a woman's ovaries are surgically removed). Taking ERT or HRT works to *delay* the transition by keeping hormone levels artificially high. If a woman suddenly stops taking hormones she can experience the same or worse symptoms than the ones for which she was taking hormones. If a woman chooses to take ERT or HRT to relieve hot flashes or genital changes, to *ease* the transition she would want to take gradually reduced amounts of hormones for as short a period of time as possible for specific complaints (National Women's Health Network, 1999).

The medicalization of menopause is particularly dangerous in that *all* attention has become focused on hormones as the 'answer' to whatever is identified as the menopausal/postmenopausal 'problem'. While some women may benefit from hormones, many or most women will be able to go through the transition phase and minimize osteoporosis and heart disease risks with less hazardous measures such as a healthy diet, appropriate physical exercise, and using alternatives to hormones. Whether in determining research priorities or influencing the information the mass media should give to empower women through informed decision making, much more attention needs to be focused on healthy alternatives to hormones. As Kathleen MacPherson (1987: 60) puts it,

> To recommend widespread use of HRT as a public health measure to prevent osteoporosis without assessing the needs of individual women would be the same as recommending that everyone take antihypertensive drugs because so many people have high blood pressure. For no other condition is anything as potentially dangerous as hormones being recommended as a preventative measure.

Osteoporosis

Creating the Fear of Osteoporosis

In order to create markets for their products, both drug companies and calcium manufacturers effectively used the media to introduce people to osteoporosis, a previously ignored condition, and to scare them into buying products which promised to prevent this. Both prevention consciousness and fear of aging contributed to the success of osteoporosis-related advertising. Many advertisements played on both of these, such as the spot for a calcium supplement which showed a healthy thirty year old transformed to a stooped sixty-five year old within thirty seconds (Giges, 1986). Such an image not only capitalizes on the fear of losing youthful beauty, it also draws on even deeper fears of disability leading to loss of independence. In another very recent advertisement, Merck used a similar scare tactic before their drug (Fosamax) to treat osteoporosis was even available. The advertisement did not name a specific product but helped build on women's fears of disability and aging; the image was of a young woman riding a bicycle and the large shadow cast—that of a wheelchair. The information on hip fractures has been presented in an even more frightening way. For example, a popular guide to preventing osteoporosis states: 'The consequences of hip fractures can be devastating. Fewer than one-half of all women who suffer a hip fracture regain normal function. Fifteen percent die shortly after their injury, and nearly 30 percent die within a year' (Notelovitz and Ware 1982: 37). The deaths are not inevitable and are related to complications such as pneumonia but they certainly serve as a useful scare tactic.

Because the lethality of hip fractures has been used so effectively as a scare tactic in the marketing of a whole new range of products to prevent, treat, or identify osteoporosis, it may be useful to know a little more about hip fractures. What happens to a healthy vigorous 80 year old who breaks her hip and what happens to a frail, unhealthy 80 year old who breaks her hip are as different as the women's health conditions were before the hip fractures. In her *Dr. Susan Love's Hormone Book,* Susan Love contrasts ramifications of hip fracture on her step mother and mother-in-law. The healthy woman broke her hip while traveling in Cambodia, flew home to have the hip fracture nailed, recovered promptly, and a year later returned to Cambodia to "finish" her trip. In contrast, the frail woman became less and less independent after a broken hip and a year later broke her other hip; as she was becoming less and less healthy her hip fracture(s) were the last straw (Love, 1997). Instead of simply seeing that adults often have major life threatening problems after suffering a hip fracture, it is important to question whether hip fractures initiate or reflect the process of health deterioration (Wolinsky, 1997). Osteoporosis researcher Steven R. Cummings, University of California Medical Center, San Francisco, has summarized the situation as, 'Hip fractures may often be a marker and not the cause of declining health and impending death. Most patients who suffer a hip fracture have severe concomitant illness that accounts for much of the increased mortality after hip fractures' (Cummings, 1990: 4). Ironically, even though the fear of hip fractures has been used primarily to market products to white women, this population is the least likely to die after hip fracture. In a study of 712,027 persons covered by Medicare, white women experienced the lowest mortality rate following a fracture of the hip, 17.2 per 1000 person months, in contrast to 22.9 for Black women, 33.5 for Black men, and 33.7 for white men (Jacobsen, 1992).

The information about complications of osteoporosis as a major 'killer' of women in their 80s and the linking of osteoporosis with menopause in such a way that osteoporosis practically becomes identified as a symptom of menopause, can be further connected to imply that menopause itself is a killer unless hormones are taken to stop this process.

In fact, osteoporosis and how it affects people are much more complicated and unpredictable than the hormone and calcium promoting information suggest. Osteoporosis is not an 'all or nothing' condition, it is 'not a disease like tuberculosis that a person either has or does not have' (Parfitt, 1988). Indeed, there is much controversy over how osteoporosis should even be defined. The World Health Organization (WHO) defines osteoporosis as a value for bone mineral density (BMD) which is 2.5 standard deviations or more below the mean peak bone density in young adults (aged 25–40.) A definition this broad means that a very high proportion of older women eventually get defined as having a disease. The National Women's Health Network says, "This is a case where a definition has created a disease!" (NWHN, 1999). The National Women's Health Network believes that "low" bone density levels should be determined for older women by comparing older women to healthy older women rather than to the standard of a 25–40 year old reaching their optimum lifetime bone mass.

A statement like, 'It would appear inevitable that if a person lives long enough, he or she will suffer from osteoporosis' (Kirkpatrick, 1987) may help British or American women put their newly created fear of osteoporosis into perspective. However, taking a more cross-cultural approach such as, 'osteoporosis is not a natural part of aging and does not occur all over the world, even among the elderly'(Brown, 1988) will be more useful for understanding that osteoporosis is not inevitable, is very much related to industrialized/western diets and lifestyles, and that *real* prevention has nothing to do with hormones.

> Looking at cross-cultural data, we see that blaming osteoporosis on an estrogen deficiency is just a little less absurd than blaming heart attacks on a deficiency of by-pass surgery. Surgery might solve the problem for a while, but it is not a deficiency of the operation that caused the problem. (Brown, 1988:6)

Osteoporosis often is billed as a major health issue for all older women, when, in fact, some women are much more at risk than others. The fact that lighter complexioned women with ancestors from northern Europe or Asia are much more likely to develop osteoporosis than darker complexioned women with African, Hispanic, Mediterranean or Native American ancestry probably accounts for this condition finally receiving the attention it has. Real pressing health needs of 'minority' older women as defined by the women themselves still tend to get ignored.

However, while critiquing the misinformation that osteoporosis is equally an issue for all older women, it is also important to emphasize that just because certain groups have lower rates of osteoporosis that does not mean that no one in those groups is at risk. Osteoporosis may have different impacts on white women and women of color, as is the case with other diseases. For example, it has long been noted that Black women have a lower incidence of breast cancer than white women but a disproportionately high percentage of Black women compared to white women die of breast cancer and five year

breast cancer survival rates are considerably lower in Black women than white women. An unpublished study by Lian Partlow (1991) traces how Black women gradually got left out from the osteoporosis literature. She cites earlier studies which concluded that 'hip fractures are three times greater in white women than Negro women' or 'Black women in the US have age-specific incidence rates for hip fractures of about half of those of white women.' However, by the 1980s and 90s when osteoporosis became a major research topic, those important though not equal rates of osteoporosis in Black women disappeared and almost all scientific articles included a statement such as, 'Black women were excluded from this study because of their low risk for hip fracture' (Cauley, 1995). Osteoporosis, like breast cancer, seems to be less common in Black women than white women, but potentially more lethal for Black women than white women. (See hip fracture mortality rates above.)

Fractures Are Not Synonymous with Osteoporosis

Disabling or life-threatening fractures must not be seen as synonymous with osteoporosis. Not all women with osteoporosis have fractures, not all women with fractures have osteoporosis, studies have shown that women with and without hip fractures had similar bone densities, and women in other cultures have low rates of bone fractures even with low bone density (National Women's Health Network, 1999).

The *real* health issue for women is the prevention of fracture and the best way to prevent fractures is to prevent falls. Falls are the immediate precipitating factor for approximately 90% of hip fractures and 80% of other fractures in women (Cummings, 1993). Factors such as impaired vision (including poor depth perception), muscle strength, balance, flexibility, obstacles in the home, having to walk on icy sidewalks, and advancing age have been demonstrated to influence the chance of fracture more than the density of bone mass (Whatley, 1988a, Atkins, 1996). Dr. Carol Frey (1998), Director of the Foot and Ankle Center at the Los Angeles Orthopedic Hospital, says that avoiding falls can often be as simple as choosing appropriate shoes for different situations. Her research has found that 28% of falls in older people were blamed on the "wrong" shoes: 60% wearing sneakers fell because their shoes caught or dragged on the floor and 40% had fallen in situations where their athletic shoes became too slippery. Falls among elderly people are known to be significantly greater for those using antidepressants, sedative/hypnotics and vasodilators (drugs that dilate blood vessels) (Myers, 1991;

Tromp, 1998) and modification of medications has been shown to be an effective method of reducing falls and fractures in both community and nursing home settings (Wolfe, 1991a; Close, 1999). Even a simple home-based exercise program for elderly women also significantly reduced the risk for falls and resulting fractures (Campbell et al, 1997). So, in many cases reducing, rather than increasing, drugs, and taking fairly simple measures will be the key preventative issues for minimizing complications of osteoporosis in elderly women.

A more creative and caring, less profit-motivated approach might come up with some very interesting ideas about what to do about osteoporosis (Whatley, 1988). For example, Kathleen MacPherson emphasizes that health policies must reflect the need for bold structural changes in our society instead of the usual incremental or "bandaid" policies suggested as osteoporosis prevention (MacPherson, 1987: 61). Her recommendations are for policies to "alleviate the feminization of poverty, a living wage, pension plans, social security, benefits for homemakers, and a national health care plan to provide ongoing health promotion and maintenance for all citizens." Ending violence against women so that more women felt safe walking and running and getting a wide range of exercise in various settings would certainly improve more than just bone mass!

It is now accepted that standard doses of ERT and HRT slow loss of bone mass in most women and can reduce the risk of hip fractures while it is taken (Writing Group for PEPI, 1996; Cauley, 1995; Assessment of Fracture Risk, WHO, 1994). Articles also refer to estrogen increasing bone density up to 5% (Genant, 1997, Libanati, 1999) but *Dr. Susan Love's Hormone Book* (1997, p. 94) emphasizes that, 'estrogen appears to halt or slow bone resorption rather than actually building bones: thus the 5% represents a filling in of resorption pits rather than the development of new bones.'

Now that osteoporosis is a 'hot' topic, the market is being flooded with a range of new products promising to be miracle drugs for preventing or treating osteoporosis. Because of recent changes in Food and Drug Administration (FDA) regulations, it is easier to get new products onto the market than it used to be and drug companies are allowed to advertise their products directly to consumers rather than just to physicians and other health practitioners with prescribing privileges. Consumers need to be aware that most new products have been tested for only short term effects and safety.

Two osteoporosis treatment products deserve mention because of the aggressive marketing and attention they are getting. Calcitonin, a version of the hormone produced by the parathyroid gland, is now available as the nasal spray, Miacalcin. Fosamax (alendronate) is a

bisphosphonate that works to inhibit resorption and increase bone density. Comparing the two products, *The Medical Letter* (January 5, 1996) concluded, 'Miacalcin offers the least concern about safety, but its effectiveness is limited. Fosamax is probably more effective, but its long term safety remains to be established.'

Fosamax is being marketed very aggressively by its manufacturer, Merck, but in its first years on the market there have been a very high number of adverse drug reactions reported against it (Annual Adverse Drug Experience Report, 1996) and the FDA Regulatory Review Office had to contact Merck more than once about misleading claims in violation of the Federal Food, Drug and Cosmetic Act (Reb, 1997). It should be emphasized that Fosamax is for *treating* not preventing osteoporosis and anyone taking Fosamax has to follow a very strict regimen (i.e. take the drug with sufficient water but absolutely no other food or drugs and do not lie down for at least one half hour) (Cummings, 1998b).

Women wanting to make decisions about osteoporosis prevention and treatment will want to keep in mind a number of issues. Some methods (Miacalcin and Fosamax) work only on the bone and do not provide other health benefits. ERT and HRT work to reduce bone loss and may have additional benefits but benefits need to be weighed against risks, particularly breast cancer. In contrast, appropriate dietary and physical activity changes may reduce osteoporosis and provide other health promotion benefits (particularly in relation to heart disease and fracture reduction) without risks. For many women, a major issue will be whether they can afford the method(s) they would like to use. The following information is given as the name of the drug or product, the suggested dose per day, and the average wholesale cost per month (Freeman, 1998):

1. Vitamin D = 400 units = $0.30–0.75
2. Calcium Carbonate = 1000mg = $2.25
3. Estrogen pills = 1.0mg - 0.625mg = $10.00
4. Estrogen patches = 0.05mg/week = $20.00
5. Estrogen/progestin combined = 0.625/2.5 = $17.60–19.20
6. Alendronate (Fosamax) = 10mg = $52.00
7. Calcitonin injection = 100 units = $96.00
8. Calcitonin spray (Miacalcin) = 100 units = $100.00

Osteoporosis Screening

Detecting osteoporosis also gets deliberately confused with preventing the condition. In the US and Canada, osteoporosis screening has been widely promoted. Finding a noninvasive way to predict a woman's risk for fractures may seem a benefit of medical science with which few could find fault. Certainly the prevalence and potential consequences of osteoporosis are serious enough to justify screening.

An editorial in the *Journal of the American Medical Association* observed, 'The field of osteoporosis has been overwhelmingly focused on bone mass, both because imagers can measure it and because clinicians can affect it' (Heaney, 1998: 2119). However, just because you can measure and change something doesn't mean that that's the most important or even appropriate procedure to follow! It is not a coincidence that much of the information on the dangers of osteoporosis and the value of bone screening and much bone screening equipment are paid for by pharmaceutical companies with osteoporosis products. How many people know that the work of the National Osteoporosis Foundation (including their toll free hotline and research) is largely funded by Merck? An evaluation of bone mass measurements as a screening procedure reveals serious limitations in what can be learned from bone density readings (Napoli, 1988; Whatley and Worcester, 1989). In the most comprehensive review and evaluation of the literature on bone density issues, the British Columbia Office of Health and Technology (1997) concluded, "Research evidence does not support whole populations or selective bone mineral density (BMD) testing of well women at or near menopause as a means to predict future fractures. On some issues, evidence is insufficient because the research has not been done. Existing research evidence, though imperfect, indicates substantial limitations of BMD testing."

Several techniques are currently being used to detect osteoporosis and these techniques vary in availability, cost, accuracy, reproducibility, and what they actually measure. But, there are certain problems with all of them and the most available techniques are the least reliable. Speakers at a recent osteoporosis conference noted that the pace of technological change in the bone density field is such that women are being screened today with technology which will be out of date by the time she has a second screening. ("Emerging Approach" 1997)

While screening can show that bone mass has been lost, screening cannot predict how rapidly someone will be losing bone and cannot predict whether or not someone is at risk for osteoporosis. Bone loss is neither constant nor predictable. Knowing someone's bone mass at one age does not help predict how fast that women will lose bone mass; a woman with a low bone mass may end up losing at a very slow rate and a woman with a much higher bone mass might end up losing rapidly (Whatley, 1988). Screening is even limited in its ability to identify full-blown cases of the disease. While bone density screening would be expected to differentiate between those who do and do not have osteoporosis related hip fractures, these measurements are of little use in the most at-risk elderly population because, 'if the highest bone mass seen in patients with fractures is designated as the "fracture threshold", then nearly all women over 70 will by definition have osteoporosis' (Ott, 1986, p. 875). Bone density of one bone does not necessarily predict bone density elsewhere. For example, many right handed women have higher bone mass in their right wrist than their left wrist. Measurements of the wrist do not necessarily reflect bone density at the hip (Ott, 1986; Riggs and Melton, 1986). One study found a 150% increase in the number of women who would be defined as having osteoporosis if they took BMD measurements at two sites per woman rather than just one site because bone densities are so different from one part of the body to another (Abrahamson, 1997).

It must be emphasized that techniques for measuring bone mass are extremely useful for research purposes. However, at this stage, unreliable but sophisticated, expensive screening has little to offer the consumer. Requiring regular monitoring of bone mass, osteoporosis screening offers enormous potential for clinics as a profitable procedure and enormous risk to women that it will hook them into a system which has little to offer them except hormone prescriptions (Worcester and Whatley, 1988). There is now considerable evidence that BMD measurement is useful, and used, to convince women to use hormones. Because women do not necessarily have the information they need to make informed decisions about what BMD results mean, studies show 'screening for low bone density significantly increases the use of HRT . . . but without any immediate adverse or positive effects on the quality of life' (Torgerson, 1997: 2121–2125; Silverman, 1997). The sentiment, 'Women who refuse HRT for osteoporosis prevention should be offered a BMD measurement' ("Emerging Approach, 1998, p. 590), which shows up in the medical literature, may be common in clinical practice. Another study which demonstrated that bone density screening can be influential in pushing women to use hormones also showed that women who were told they had low BMD became fearful of falling and began to limit their activities to avoid falling (Rubin, 1992). Bone screening could be counterproductive if it results in less physical activity by exactly the women who might most benefit from physical activity to strengthen bone mass!

Role of Diet

There is plenty of evidence that western/industrialized lifestyles and diets are responsible for the prevalence of osteoporosis and the fact that it affects women much more than men. Britain and the US report much higher rates of osteoporosis than less industrialized/ western-ized countries. For example, the US rate is 24 times higher than that of some other countries. People in Singapore, Hong Kong, certain parts of Yugoslavia and the Maori of New Zealand have very low rates of osteoporosis caused fractures and Africans and people living traditional indigenous lifestyles have been described as 'almost immune' to osteoporosis (Brown, 1988).

Osteoporosis as a male disease in Britain and the US gets very little attention (because no one has figured out how to convince men that their problems are all due to 'estrogen deficiency'?) despite the fact that (US) men suffer one-sixth the spinal fractures and approximately one-half the hip fractures as women. In other parts of the world, i.e. Hong Kong, some parts of Yugoslavia, and in the South African Bantu, it has been documented that men experience osteoporosis and fractures at the same or higher rates than women. Medical anthropologist Susan Brown (1988) gives the following explanations for the excessive development of osteoporosis in western women: 1) as a group, women have less exposure to sunlight which helps the body make vitamin D which is essential for calcium absorption, 2) women are not encouraged to be as physically active, 3) women use more prescription drugs, 4) women are more subject to removal of the sex hormone producing gonads, the ovaries (i.e. if the testes are removed, men also develop osteoporosis), and 5) men generally consume a higher quality/ more nutritional diet than women.

Western diets contribute to the development of osteoporosis both by not providing enough calcium in the first place, and more importantly, by "wasting" the calcium which is ingested. The typical western diet encourages a heavy imbalance in the ratio of phosphorus (high levels in carbonated beverages and high protein foods, including meats) to calcium which can cause a loss of bone calcium, low levels of vitamin D and high levels of fiber, oxalates, and phytates interfere with calcium absorption and high intakes of caffeine and alcohol also significantly contribute to excessive bone loss (Abelow, 1992, Campbell, 1997, Finn, 1987 and Brown, 1988, and Hu, 1993). Instead of dealing with anything as complex as the calcium-wasting effects of our diet, or questioning high consumption of foods like meat which are central to our diet and economy, calcium has been promoted as something one can simply add to what one already consumes. Retail sales of calcium supplements grew from $18 million in 1980 to $166 million in 1986, a calcium-fortified sugar-free drink mix was marketed, and the sales of the diet cola, Tab, tripled when calcium was added. Jumping on the calcium bandwagon and hoping it would make people forget their cholesterol concern, the dairy industry launched a campaign with the theme 'dairy foods: calcium the way nature

intended' (Giges, 1986). In the 1990s, calcium-fortified orange juice has become readily available.

It is well established that because bone mass peaks at age 35 years, the greatest benefit from calcium occurs in the years from birth to age 35 (Finn, 1987). However, it is discouraging to see how, in the push towards hormones, the role of calcium for menopausal and post-menopausal women has been ignored or discounted. In explaining why recommended intakes of calcium for older women had not been increased in the Food and Nutrition Board's latest (10th edition) *Recommendation for Daily Nutrient Allowances,* the director stated, 'because estrogen is more effective in preventing osteoporosis than calcium.'

That answer is much too simplistic and totally ignores the risks of estrogens and the fact that many women cannot or will not take hormones. Most importantly, such attitudes influence research and policy agendas so that the potential of calcium alone or in sufficient quantities to reduce the amount of estrogens needed, are not being explored despite work showing the merit of this approach. In a study believed to be the first one looking at both lifelong and current calcium intake in normal postmenopausal women not taking estrogens, researchers found a protective effect of calcium on bone density in women who reported high calcium intakes *both* throughout their lifetime and presently (Cauley, 1988). The excellent review article, 'Calcium for Prevention of Osteoporotic Fractures in Postmenopausal Women' by Robert G. Cumming and Michael C. Nevitt (1997) summarizes results from 37 calcium studies published between 1966 and early 1997. Using meta-analysis techniques (combining information from many studies) these authors found that 1000 mg/day of dietary calcium was associated with a 24% reduction in hip fracture risk, and stated, 'Our conclusion is that calcium supplements and dietary calcium probably reduce the risk of osteoporotic fractures in older women. The consistency in effect size between small randomized trials and pooled observational studies (after adjustments for measurement error) is particularly impressive. Our systematic review of the evidence supports the current clinical and public health policy of advising older women to increase their calcium intake' (Cumming and Nevitt, 1997, p. 1329).

Even Bruce Ettinger (1987: 33–34), previously quoted as supporting the goal of keeping women on estrogens for their entire postmenopausal lives, gives us reason to remind pro-hormone scientists that calcium deserves more attention. He states, 'Although calcium given alone is incapable of maintaining skeletal mass, high intakes of calcium allow estrogen to be more effective; by simply augmenting calcium intake to 1,500 mg. per day, women may be adequately protected while taking half the usual dosage of estrogen . . . It has also been suggested but not proven that very low intake of calcium—perhaps less than 300 mg. per day—can also diminish or abolish estrogen's protection.'

Thinking of *real* osteoporosis prevention is a useful case study of how life long interactions of social, economic, and political issues affect women's health and how factors in a young woman's life affect her chances of being able to maximize on her full potential. With 'femininity' so closely associated with an obsession with thinness and the conflicting, never appropriate messages given to young women about physical activity, sex role socialization and gender identity have to be seen as causal agents of osteoporosis. The obsession with thinness and fear of fat promote osteoporosis in several different ways. First, avoiding high calcium foods because of caloric content, dieting that results in nutritional deficiencies or nutritional imbalances, fasting, and purging can be identified as behaviors which interfere with calcium absorption and contribute to low peak bone mass (Kirkpatrick, 1987). The benefits of increased calcium intake for young women was demonstrated in a study on the effect of increased milk intake in adolescent girls (median age 12.2), which found that, compared to the control, the increased milk group gained a significant amount of bone mineral with no other significant changes, such as in weight or fat mass (Cadogan et al, 1997). Secondly, low body weight reduces the mechanical forces applied to the skeleton by gravity and muscle contraction so there is less 'built-in' stimulation for bone formation. As a generalization, heavier people tend towards more bone mass (Goodman, 1987). Additionally, it is well established that fat tissue in a woman's body produces estrogen and the more fat a woman has, the more estrogen she will produce. But how many women know this or can listen to the message if they hear it? Society so consistently pushes thinness and hormones, that contradictory healthy advice such as that in Mary Kirkpatrick's 'A Self Care Model for Osteoporosis' is seldom mentioned:

> Ironically, midlife may be a good time to have a little extra weight to act as a protective mechanism against osteoporosis. If fat tissue provides more estrogen, the bone loss at menopause may be slowed. Also, body weight can act as a loading factor and can produce necessary stress on the bony structure to form bone mass. (Kirkpatrick, 1987, pp.48–49)

Physical Activity

Numerous studies have shown that exercise, particularly of the weight-bearing type, can promote bone strength in women under 35 and help maintain bone mass in women over 35. But, how often do women, particularly young women, get useful, sensible advice about the health benefits of moderate exercise? Too often women get only one of two equally inappropriate messages: don't exercise or do too much of it!

When tested for physical performance, girls and boys are matched up to ages 10 to 12. Thereafter, they receive very different messages about what is 'lady like' or 'masculine' and after age 12, boys tend to increase in strength and cardiovascular fitness more than girls who are discouraged from being physically active (Whatley, 1988b). The young women who resist the pressure to be sedentary, are often encouraged to go to the other extreme. Both the 'cosmetic athletes' who obsessively exercise to achieve 'beauty' and the serious athletes who exercise too strenuously, can delay menarche or cause amenorrhea which can be detrimental to building bone density (Goodman, 1987).

Interestingly, the relationship of 'athletic amenorrhea' to osteoporosis started attracting quite a bit of media attention as more young women have begun to explore their athletic capabilities. Physiologically, the explanation and consequences of amenorrhea may be the same whether caused by athletic training, ballet dancing or extreme dieting. However, as western cultures find ballet and dieting to be ideal 'feminine' activities, the media attention has focused almost exclusively on the potential osteoporotic risks of athletic amenorrhea. Regular, moderate, weight-bearing exercise is undoubtedly a healthier approach to osteoporosis prevention. Further research is needed to determine the type, intensity, duration, and frequency of physical activity which best builds and maintains bone mass (Goodman, 1987).

When to Start Hormones?

The emphasis on taking hormones at perimenopause or menopause to prevent bone loss has been based on the thinking that the most rapid bone loss takes place during the first six years after menstruation ceases so that hormonal 'treatment' would have the greatest impact on reducing bone loss if begun within three years after natural menopause. However, recent studies show that when and how women lose bone mass is far less predictable. The importance of preventing bone loss at menopause seems to have been overemphasized. One longitudinal study of bone loss in postmenopausal women described two quite distinct groups: although one third of women lose significant bone mineral (the 'fast losers'), two-thirds lose only a minor amount of bone mineral (Riis, 1995). Other longitudinal studies have shown that bone loss continues or even accelerates with increasing age

(Ensrud, 1994). 'It is becoming clear that, at least at sites other than the spine, bone loss continues unabated into the oldest age ranges and probably accelerates at the hip, the most important region for predicting hip fractures' (Black, 1995: 2A–69S).

Even people who promote hormones for osteoporosis prevention debate whether hormones should be started before or after menopause. Since bone loss similar to normal loss during menopause years sets in as soon as the hormones are stopped, estrogen started at menopause, even if taken for as long as ten years, does not protect women into their late seventies. Serious fractures are most common in the elderly: the average age of hip fracture is 80 (Cauley, 1995). As a result, treatment started at menopause would need to continue lifelong, possibly for 30 or more years with all the associated risks.

Starting estrogen before menopause may increase breast cancer risks without increasing osteoporosis benefits. A meta-analysis of studies on ERT found that studies in which estrogen therapy was started before menopause showed a much greater increase in breast cancer than studies of women who started estrogen after menopause (Steinberg, 1991).

A woman's decisions regarding hormones for osteoporosis prevention can be made many years after menopause. The emphasis on menopause as a time for intervention has more to do with it being an easily identifiable marker in a woman's life than that it is the optimal time for intervention. It may also have to do with the fact that women at the age of menopause are more likely to be covered by health insurance that covers prescription drugs than are elderly women. The Rancho Bernardo Study of 740 women over 60 found that there was no significant difference in bone mineral density between women who started estrogen at menopause and those who started after 60 (Schneider, 1997).

Although the Osteoporotic Fractures Research Study (a study of 9704 women) emphasized that estrogen is most effective if initiated soon after menopause and continued indefinitely, the conclusion of the study was that current use of estrogen in women 65 years of age and older, whether started 'early' (up to 5 years after menopause) or 'late' (more than 5 years after menopause) reduces the risk for fractures (Cauley, 1995). Dr. Dennis Black, UC-San Francisco, has argued that 'stopping bone loss at age 65–70 can still prevent most instances of very low bone mass in women over 80, that screening at age 65 can more precisely identify risk of hip fracture at age 80, and that treatment beginning at age 65 may be more cost-effective than earlier screening and treatment' (Black, 1995).

In terms of osteoporosis prevention, it is more effective for a woman to delay her decision about starting hormones rather than going on and off hormones. Theoretically, going on and off hormones post-menopausally could mean the body goes through accelerated 'transitional bone loss' more than once.

Heart Disease

Women may have become saturated with information about ERT and osteoporosis; a new angle has been necessary to raise anxiety to the point at which a new group of women will actively seek ERT prescriptions. The long overdue attention to *prevention* of heart disease in women has provided exactly the right focus for an expanded ERT market, giving physicians an additional rationale to prescribe it. The new media coverage of women and heart disease has helped generate fears and then ERT has been offered as the solution.

This contrasts with approaches in the past when very little attention had been paid to either prevention or treatment of heart disease in women, for it has traditionally been viewed as a man's disease. While men experience heart disease at younger ages and have more heart attacks than women, women account for 47 percent of the heart attack deaths in the United States, making it the leading cause of death for women (Winslow, 1991). In addition, women who suffer a heart attack are more likely to die than men (39 percent vs. 31 percent) and more likely to suffer a second heart attack within four years (20 percent vs. 15 percent) (Winslow, 1991). However, these high risks for women have not been reflected in treatment. For example, in one study of patients hospitalized for coronary heart disease, men were 28 percent more likely to have angiography, a procedure to determine the extent of arterial blockage, and 48 percent more likely to have bypass surgery or balloon angioplasty. In another study of men and women hospitalized for major heart attacks, men were nearly twice as likely to have angiography and bypass surgery (Winslow, 1991). This study also found that, before the heart attack, chest pains and other symptoms were more disabling for women than men. One of the authors of the latter report emphasized her concern that women who continued to have chest pains after their heart attacks still do not receive angiography (Kolata, 1991a).

These studies and others document the lack of attention by the medical profession to heart disease as a major women's health issue, but the fact that these studies exist at all is a sign that there is finally some concern. If heart disease is the leading killer of women in the United States, why has there been so little emphasis on it before? Why do so many women fear breast cancer but are apparently unaware of their risks of heart disease? Without going into reasons for past neglect, it is possible to offer some explanations for the new-found hype of heart disease as '#1 killer of women.' One view is that the market is fickle and there needs to be a 'disease of the month' to capture the interest of the media, consumers, practitioners, and the people (politicians included) who control research funding. However, with an old disease, only a new angle, preferably with something to sell, will generate the necessary interest. For example, there was considerable media attention when a study suggested that aspirin reduced the risk of heart attacks in men (Steering Committee of the Physician's Health Study Group, 1989). Aspirin manufacturers must have been delighted by the press aspirin received, especially after the earlier negative publicity about Reye syndrome, a potentially fatal condition in children caused by aspirin being given during a viral infection such as flu or chickenpox. However, the media reports rarely mentioned that the study was done on men only and could not be extrapolated to women. In response to the gap in the research, a study reported that women who took one to six aspirin a week experienced a 25 percent reduction in risk of heart attack compared to women who took no aspirin (Manson, Stampfer, and Colditz, 1991). The results are hardly conclusive, however. The study, which included only nurses, was an observational study (the women made their own choices about aspirin and reported it, while the researchers just looked for the effects), not an experimental one. This leads to the strong possibility of confounding variables, for the groups may vary in much more than the factor of aspirin use (Appel and Bush, 1991).

In spite of the flaws, this study received a lot of publicity and generated more interest in women and heart disease, providing a good opening for calling attention to the role of ERT in preventing heart disease. In an apparent attempt to expand their market, Wyeth-Ayerst, the manufacturers of Premarin, the most commonly prescribed oral estrogen, requested that the U.S. Food and Drug Administration (FDA) allow promotion of Premarin for the prevention of heart disease, at least for women who have had hysterectomies (Rovner, 1990). The FDA Advisory Committee concluded, after listening to much conflicting testimony, that 'the cardiovascular benefits of estrogen replacement therapy with Premarin in women without a uterus may outweigh the risks, considering the individual patient's risk for various estrogen-related diseases and conditions' (Rovner, 1990: 9). Dangerously, this statement, as it has been reported and repeated has been reduced to a simple 'benefits outweigh the risks;' in addition, the distinctions between ERT and HRT are rarely clarified.

In terms of the research itself, the results are not clear-cut. Generalizability is limited because almost all

the subjects have been white and middle-class. As with the aspirin study, these studies have been observational; the researchers did not control the choice of treatments but merely observed the results based on the women's choices. A major confounding factor is that the women who *choose* Premarin may be at reduced risk for heart attack anyway. For example, a co-author of the major lipid study cited in the FDA hearings, Elizabeth Barrett-Connor said that women who used Premarin were also less likely to smoke, were thinner, and were better educated than non-users, all of which might have been factors in reducing risk (Rovner, 1990). One of the clearest ways to emphasize that users and non-users may represent different populations is the result of one study which found users of estrogen had lower mortality rates, not only from heart disease, but also from accidents, suicide, and homicide. As Cindy Pearson, of the National Women's Health Network, asked, when she was testifying *against* FDA approval for Premarin being promoted for the prevention of heart disease, 'Does this mean we can conclude that estrogen use protects one from being murdered?' (Rovner, 1990, p. 9).

Until recently, no study has been without the major flaw of lack of comparability between users and non-users of ERT. This is well illustrated in a study published after the FDA hearings, which was heralded as more good news about ERT. The study of 49,000 post-menopausal women showed 44 percent fewer heart attacks and 39 percent reduced risk of heart attack death in those who took ERT (Kolata, 1991b). However, the study was on nurses, 98 percent of whom were white, who had made their own choices about use of ERT. As an example of this problem, a very heavy woman, who might be more at risk for heart attack, might also be less likely to select ERT because she would also be *less* likely to experience menopausal changes for which ERT is recommended. A nurse who considered herself at risk for heart disease might not have taken ERT because physicians in the 1970s were discouraging women at risk of heart disease from taking estrogen at all (Sojourner, 1991). Up until recently, all the evidence for the role of estrogen in preventing heart disease was based on non-randomized observational studies. In 1998, an important randomized study on HRT compared to placebo in postmenopausal women with preexisting coronary disease was published (Hulley et al, 1998). While the lipid profile was better in the HRT group, there was no difference in cardiovascular outcomes at the end of the study and, in the first year, there were more heart attacks and deaths from heart disease in the HRT group. The results do not preclude possible benefits to women with no known coronary disease, but they do raise questions about the benefits of estrogen, which it was assumed would be especially beneficial to the group of women in the study.

Besides the studies directed at heart attack risks, much of the support for the role of ERT in preventing heart disease comes from data on HDL (high density lipoprotein) and LDL (low density lipoprotein). *Higher* HDL and *lower* LDL are favorable to reduced risk of heart disease. A review article by Bush and colleagues (Bush et al, 1988) provides a good summary of the factors affecting these lipoproteins in women. These include genetics, diet, obesity, exercise, alcohol, cigarette smoking, oral contraceptives.

The data on oral contraceptives is particularly interesting. All formulations increase LDL, the 'bad lipoprotein.' The largest increases in LDL occur with the lowest estrogen dose and the strongest anti-estrogenic progestin. As the potency of progestin increases, HDL, the 'good' lipoprotein decreases. The implications from the oral contraceptive data for the use of ERT as compared to HRT are borne out by the studies on estrogens as menopausal therapy. According to Bush and colleagues (Bush et al, 1988), use of unopposed and synthetic estrogens leads to the more favorable HDL/LDL profile. However, cyclic estrogen-progestin therapy (HRT) has either a minimal or adverse effect on lipoproteins, depending on the progestin used. In other words, while estrogen therapy by itself may have very positive effects, the addition of progestins at least partially negates those effects. HRT, therefore, in the best case, provides little benefit in terms of HDL/LDL profile, the main route by which ERT is believed to have a protective effect against heart disease. However, many women take HRT to avoid the increased risks from ERT in terms of endometrial cancer. If the progestin component protects against endometrial cancer but at least partially undoes the protective effects against heart disease, women may have to make difficult decisions about which disease they fear most.

The lipoprotein data also provides some interesting results about alcohol. Bush et al., (1988) state that moderate alcohol consumption is strongly related to increased HDL levels in men and women. A recent report suggested that moderate alcohol consumption has a protective effect against heart disease in men, which supports previous work finding benefits for men and women. If estrogen manufacturers are allowed to say their products reduce heart disease, why shouldn't beer and wine companies request that the FDA allow them to promote their products as reducing risk of heart disease? Such a claim would surely be countered with the argument that the risks of alcohol consumption outweigh the benefits. But do we really know that benefits of ERT outweigh the risks?

While much of the discussion has focused on the effects of HDL and LDL, recently more attention is being paid to high levels of triglycerides as a possible risk factor for heart disease. It is now theorized that in women high triglycerides are more predictive of risk than high total cholesterol and that high HDL cannot counter the negative effects of high triglycerides. In discussions of the effects of estrogen on the lipid profile, it is often not emphasized that ERT *increases* triglycerides, thereby potentially *increasing* risk of heart disease.

Some of the answers about ERT and HRT should come from the Women's Health Initiative, mentioned previously. When the data from this study is analyzed completely, it may be appropriate to make some recommendations about HRT and ERT. In the meantime, while we wait for the data to come in, perhaps it would be more appropriate to focus on what we do know about preventing heart disease in women and provide education about diet, exercise, smoking, and treating high blood pressure (Wolfe, 1991b).

Breast Cancer

In the attempt to reduce the risk of heart disease or osteoporosis by taking ERT or HRT, women may be replacing one disease with another. There is strong evidence that estrogens increase the risk of breast cancer, but the issue seems to be how big a risk that really is. A Swedish study, published in 1989, showed a 10 percent increased relative risk of breast cancer in women on estrogens, with the risk increasing with length of treatment. After nine years of use, there was an excess risk of 70 percent. The addition of progestins did not reduce the risk and may even have increased it slightly (Bergkvist et al, 1989). The differences in the estrogen of choice in the US and Sweden was apparently one reason why this study did not receive more press, as well as the fact that the risk was seen as only slightly increased.

A later study from the United States received more attention but also was presented as showing a slight risk. In a study that followed over 12,000 nurses for 10 years, Colditz and colleagues found that women taking estrogen were 30 to 40 percent more likely to develop breast cancer than those who did not (Colditz et al, 1990). This might be seen by many as a serious risk in a disease that is said to strike one out of eight women in the United States. However, the media coverage played down the effects as slight. For example, referring to the increased risk of 30 to 40 percent, one article claimed, 'But this risk is considered small; it is only about half the risk a woman faces if her mother had breast cancer' (Kolata, 1990: A11). This is hardly reassuring for women considering ERT who have other risk factors, particularly the woman whose mother had breast cancer. The one note that women may actually find reassuring is that the additional risk seems to disappear a year after stopping estrogens. However, that does not help much for women who are on the long-term plan for estrogen to maintain the reduced risk of osteoporosis and heart disease until death.

A large number of studies on ERT and breast cancer were evaluated using meta-analysis, a statistical method to evaluate data from a number of studies, which can give a more accurate picture than a single study (Steinberg et al, 1991). The data suggest an increased risk of breast cancer for women who used estrogen for more than five years. Women with a family history of breast cancer had a markedly increased risk. A particularly interesting finding was that the studies in which estrogen therapy was started before menopause showed a much greater increase in risk than those which included only women who started estrogen after menopause. The duration of estrogen therapy is clearly related to risk and going off it seems the only way to reduce the risk. While progestins may protect these women against endometrial cancer, it will apparently do nothing to reduce breast cancer risks. The most recent studies conclude that there is an increased risk of breast cancer with ERT/HRT. In 1997 a detailed analysis of data from 51 studies involving large numbers of postmenopausal women concluded that breast cancer risks were increased a small but significant amount, with increased duration of use increasing risk (Collaborative Group, 1997). It is important to note that with one out of eight women in the US developing breast cancer, even a small percentage increased risk leads to many more women with cancer.

In weighing up the risks of breast cancer versus the possibility that ERT or HRT can prevent osteoporosis or heart disease, women essentially need to decide which disease they fear the most. Dr. Lynn Rosenberg, a Boston epidemiologist, says that most women decide whether to take estrogen by a sort of fear meter, asking themselves which diseases or discomforts they most dread (Kolata, 1991c). Even more to the point, Dr. Adriane Fugh-Berman (1991, p. 3), speaking on behalf of the National Women's Health Network puts it,

> We are concerned that the concept of disease prevention may be expanded to include the concept of disease substitution.

Dr. Fugh-Berman's statement was made in reference to tamoxifen, a totally different topic, but one which we mention here for the purpose of emphasizing the complications and unknowns of menopausal/postmenopausal hormones. Tamoxifen is a drug which has been recognized for its effectiveness in prolonging the disease-free interval in postmenopausal women with estrogen receptor-positive breast cancer. However, now, tamoxifen is being experimented with in both England and the US as a way to *prevent* breast cancer in normal healthy women. In the US, the National Women's Health Network was the only organization to present testimony to the Food and Drug Administration Committee on Oncology Drugs opposing the trial. This is not the place to detail why the trial was 'premature in its assumptions, weak in its hypotheses, questionable in its ethics, and misguided in its public health ramifications' (Fugh-Berman, 1991:3). Relevant to this paper is the fact that tamoxifen is known to be effective as breast cancer treatment because it works as an *anti*-estrogen: it blocks the effect of estrogen on the breast. Researchers justified studying the effects of tamoxifen on healthy women because they felt there was sufficient evidence to suggest that blocking the effects of estrogen on the breasts may be a way of preventing (delaying?) breast cancer.

The irony of the situation must be obvious to anyone reading this paper. How can it be that at this particular moment in history, in the name of 'prevention', huge numbers of women are being given estrogen products and another group is being studied with anti-estrogens? *All* the women taking either estrogens or anti-estrogens are part of massive experiments which should help us learn more about hormones but do *nothing* to support health-promoting methods of disease prevention.

The tamoxifen as 'prevention' trial received a great deal of attention recently because of the apparent success in reducing the risk of breast cancer. However, in the flurry of announcements about tamoxifen as preventing breast cancer, it was not well-publicized that there was an increase in endometrial cancer, pulmonary embolism, and stroke in the tamoxifen group (Fisher et al, 1998). In fact, Fugh-Berman's prediction of 'disease substitution' was correct.

'Designer Estrogens'

Tamoxifen is now being marketed by its manufacturer, Zeneca, in a direct to consumer advertising campaign that implies that it can be taken by healthy women to prevent cancer (*Network News*, 1999a), but tamoxifen is only the beginning of a new approach to estrogens. It is one of a group of drugs called selective estrogen receptor modulators or SERMs, also known as 'designer estrogens.' These are being developed with the goal of having all the beneficial (proven or alleged) effects of estrogens, with none of the negative effects, that is, having both estrogenic and anti-estrogenic effects. Tamoxifen, for example, may reduce the risk of breast cancer but it still has the estrogenic effect of increasing the risk of endometrial cancer. Another SERM, raloxifene, manufactured by Eli Lilly under the name Evista, has been widely promoted in direct to consumer advertising, in magazines such as *Parade*. Raloxifene has been approved by the FDA for prevention of osteoporosis in postmenopausal women. Though the research is still in a relatively early stage, the popular media coverage of this drug suggests that it has the estrogenic effects of reducing osteoporosis and promoting a good lipid profile, while having anti-estrogenic effects of reducing risk of breast cancer and not stimulating the endometrium. At this point there is simply insufficient data and the studies have not been conducted for a long enough period to draw conclusions about the benefits, risks, or safety of raloxifene. As of 1999, there are plans for a large study comparing tamoxifen and raloxifene in reducing risk of breast cancer. In the mean time, both Lilly and Zeneca have direct to consumer campaigns, some of which have been identified as misleading. In fact, in response to complaints by the National Women's Health Network to the FDA, both companies have had to pull some of their ads (*Network News,* 1999b). As more of these drugs are developed and tested, consumers will be bombarded with advertising that tries to convince them that one form or another of estrogen or 'designer estrogens' is the real 'answer' to their fears about osteoporosis, bone density, heart disease, etc.

Conclusion

HRT raises large questions for individual women trying to decide whether to take it and for women's health movements which must analyze why it is that once again huge numbers of women are swallowing a product of unknown safety. There are no simple answers for either individual women or for feminist health activists.

The marketing of ERT/HRT has escalated in the 1990s as new research suggests—but has not proven—new benefits from these hormones. For example, women are now being told that ERT will prevent memory loss and dementia, including Alzheimer's disease. Certainly, the threat of losing our mental capabilities and memory is a powerful scare tactic. The fear of Alzheimer's disease may easily outweigh fear of other risks, since there are no other 'answers' for preventing this serious condition. The media has hyped the benefits of estrogen in this area and the manufacturers of Premarin have, without going beyond what they legally can, suggested in advertisements that estrogen may help. However, even though the media may accept estrogen as a proven prevention or treatment for loss of cognitive function, especially Alzheimer's disease, right now there is no proof for these benefits.

Two detailed thorough reviews of the literature conclude that the evidence does *not* support recommending estrogen for prevention or treatment of dementia or loss of cognitive function (Haskell et al, 1997; Yaffe et al, 1998).

This paper has covered many of the issues which individual women will want to weigh as they make their own decisions. At some level, it is a very personal decision to balance known and unknown risks with the narrow range of choices available. Each woman will want to make today's and tomorrow's decisions based on her own personal hormone history. Most of the studies which have been done have been on women for whom oral contraceptives were not available. It remains to be seen how much different formulations of oral contraceptives taken for different lengths of time influence issues related to ERT or HRT. Much research will be done on many aspects of hormone use in the next few years. Any woman taking, or considering, hormones should find a source of information which she trusts such as the National Women's Health Network. Excellent health check ups, including pelvic exams, mammography and physical breast exams, pap smears, monitoring of blood lipids and blood pressure, and endometrial biopsies, must be available to all women who are or have been on hormones for any length of time.

HRT raises enormous challenges for women's health movements. Many of us have lived through the tragedies of DES, the Dalkon Shield, thalidomide, and toxic shock syndrome. One of the biggest questions must be, why aren't the lessons from the immediate past more central to our present debates? Why do large numbers of women not know about, or choose to ignore, the tremendous risks involved in taking drugs whose long term safety is not known? An even trickier question is why are so few people questioning the long term safety of hormonal products for menopausal and postmenopausal women? A number of people who have been allies in the struggle for safer contraceptives are not involved in evaluating and critiquing the mass marketing of ERT and HRT. Is ageism a factor? Are we willing to accept a few more side effects in a product designed specifically for older women? Are we willing to lower our standards just a little bit for products which promise to interfere with the ageing process?

The HRT debate—or more accurately, the *lack* of debate—serves as a reminder of the urgency of empowering *all* women to understand their own bodies and having access to appropriate (language, reading level, relevant to own issues) information for the 'choices' they face. One of the biggest lessons in the marketing of HRT has been that many women still do not know enough about the normal healthy workings of their bodies to resist a mass manipulation of the fear factor.

ERT and HRT are very valuable products to have available. They will definitely make a difference in the quality and length of life for *some* women. However, they will probably never be products which should be given to *most* women for a long length of time. If these products are as valuable as the manufacturers say, these products should be available to the women who would most benefit from them rather than the present situation where it tends to be the healthiest groups of women with easy access to the medical system which are given hormones.

To answer any of the questions raised in this paper, long term, controlled studies which look at multiple parameters and the interactions of many factors must be done with diverse groups of women. Without a clearer understanding of the actual value and risks of ERT and HRT, the mass marketing of these products is certainly premature. A renewed focus on *real* prevention and self help as a way of wrestling control *for* the consumer, *away* from the medical system and makers of highly profitable products, continues to be a most urgent priority for women's health movements.

References

Abelow, B. J., et al., study reported in *Calcified Tissue International,* January, 1992, referred to in Health Facts (Center for Medical Consumers) vol. 22, no. 10, October, 1997, pp. 4–5.

Abrahamsen, B, T.B. Hansen, L. Bjorn Jensen, A.P. Hermann, and P. Eiken (1997) "Site of Osteodensitometry in Perimenopausal Women: Correlation and Limits of Agreement Between Anatomic Regions," *Journal of Bone and Mineral Research,* vol. 12, no. 9, pp. 1471–1479.

Appel, Lawrence J. and Bush, Trudy (1991) 'Preventing Heart Disease in Women. Another Role for Aspirin' *Journal of the American Medical Association,* vol. 266, (pp. 565–566).

Annual Adverse Drug Experience Report, 1996, http://www.fda.gov/cder/dpe/annrep96/index.htm

Assessment of fracture risk and its application to screening for postmenopausal osteoporosis, WHO Technical Report Series 843. Geneva: WHO, 1994 cited by John A. Kanis, "Treatment of Osteoporosis in Elderly Women" in *The American Journal of Medicine,* vol. 98 (supple 2A), February 27, 1995a, p. 2A–60S.

Atkins, D., telephone interview with Atkins, reported in *HealthFacts* [Center for Medical Consumers] July 1996, vol. XXI, no. 206, pp. 1 & 4)

Bergvist, L. et al (1989) 'The Risk of Breast Cancer after Estrogen and Estrogen-progestin Replacement' *The New England Journal of Medicine,* vol. 321. no. 5, (pp. 293–297).

Black, Dennis M., "Why Elderly Women Should be Screened and Treated to Prevent Osteoporosis" in *The American Journal of Medicine,* vol. 98, suppl 2A, February 27, 1995, pp. 2A–67S–2A–75S.

Brown, Susan (1988) 'Osteoporosis: An Anthropologist Sorts Fact from Fallacy', unpublished longer version of article which was edited and appeared as 'Osteoporosis: Sorting Fact from Fallacy' in (National Women's Health Network) *Network News,* July/August, (pp. 1, 5–6).

Bush, Trudy, Fried, Linda P., and Barrett-Connor, Elizabeth (1988) 'Cholesterol Lipoproteins and Coronary Heart Disease in Women' Clinical Chemistry, vol. 34. no. 8(B), (pp. B60–B70).

Cadogan, J. et al (1997) 'Milk intake and bone mineral acquisition in adolescent girls: Randomised, controlled intervention trial' *British Medical Journal,* vol. 315 (Nov 15) (pp. 1255–1260).

Campbell, J. et al (1997) 'Randomised controlled trial of a general practice programme of home based exercise to prevent falls in elderly women' *British Medical Journal,* vol. 315 (Oct 25) (pp. 1065–1069).

Campbell, T. Colin, interview in *Health Facts* (Center for Medical Consumers) vol 22, no. 10, October, 1997, pp 4–5.

Cauley, Jane A. (1988) and Gutai, James P., Kuller, Lewis H., Ledonna Dorothea, Sandler, Rivka B., Sashin, Donald, and Powell, John G. (1988) 'Endogenous Estrogen Levels and Calcium Intakes in Postmenopausal Women' *Journal of the American Medical Association,* vol. 260, no. 21, (pp. 3150-3155).

Cauley, Jane A., Dana G. Seeley, Kristine Ensrud, Bruce Ettinger, Dennis Black, and Steven Cummings, for the Study of Osteoporotic Fractures Research Group, "Estrogen Replacement Therapy and Fractures in Older Women" *Annals of Internal Medicine,* vol. 122, no. 1, January 1, 1995, pp. 9-16

Cedar Rapids Gazette (1991) 'Estrogen Cuts Heart Disease Risk: Study' *Cedar Rapids (Iowa) Gazette,* September 12.

Close, Jacqueline, Margaret Ellis, Richard Hooper, Edward Glucksman, Stephan Jackson, and Cameron Swift, "Prevention of Falls in the Elderly Trial (PROFET); A Randomised Controlled Trial, *Lancet,* vol. 353, January 9, 1999, pp. 93-97.

Colditz, G. A. Stampfer, M. J., Willett, W. C. *et al* (1990) 'Prospective Study of Estrogen Replacement Therapy and Risk of Breast Cancer in Postmenopausal Women' *Journal of the American Medical Association,* vol. 264, (pp. 2648–2653).

Collaborative Group on Hormonal Factors in Breast Cancer (1997) 'Breast cancer and hormone replacement therapy: Collaborative reanalysis of data from 51 epidemiologic studies of 52,705 women with breast cancer and 108,411 women without breast cancer' *Lancet,* vol. 350 (Oct 11) (pp. 1047–1059).

Cumming, Robert G. and Michael C. Nevitt (1997) "Calcium for the Prevention of Osteoporotic Fractures in Postmenopausal Women," *Journal of Bone and Mineral Research,* vol. 12, no. 9, pp. 1321–1329.

Cummings, S. R., "Bone Mass and Bone Loss in the Elderly: A Special Case?" *Int. J. Fertil Menopausal Stud,* 38 Supple 2, 1993, pp. 92–97.

Cummings, Steven R., in *Annals of Internal Medicine,* 15 October, 1990 article, quoted in *HealthFacts,* vol. XXI, no. 206, July 1996, p. 4.

Cummings, Steven R., Dennis M. Black, Desmond E. Thompson, William B. Applegate, Elizabeth Barrett-Connor, Thomas A. Musliner, Lisa Palermo, Ronald Prineas, Susan M. Rubin, Jean C. Scott, Thomas Vogt, Robert Wallace, A. John Yates, Andrea Z. Lacroix, for the Fracture Intervention Trial Research Group, "Effect of Alendronate on Risk of Fracture in Women with Low Bone Density but Without Vertebral Fractures," *Journal of the American Medical Association,* vol. 280, no. 24, December 23/30, 1998, pp. 2077–2082.

Dejanikus, Tacie (1985) 'Major Drug Manufacturer Funds Osteoporosis Education Campaign' (National Women's Health Network) *Network News,* May/June, (pp. 1, 3).

Eagan, Andrea Boroff (1989) 'Hormone Replacement Therapy Overview' (National Women's Health Network) *Network News,* May/June, (pp. 1, 3)

"An Emerging Approach to Osteoporosis Prevention" discussion at Clinical and Economic Considerations in the Prevention of Osteoporosis Among Postmenopausal Women Conference, September 19, 1997, reported in *The American Journal of Managed Care,* February, 1998, vol. 4, No. 2, Sup., pp. S85–S93.

Ensrud KE, Palermo L, Black DM, et al. Hip bone loss increases with advancing age: longitudinal results from the study of osteoporotic fractures. In: LG Raisz, ed. *Sixteenth Annual Meeting of the American Society for Bone and Mineral Research.* Kansas City, Missouri: Mary Ann Liebert, 1994; S153, cited in Dennis M. Black, "Why Elderly Women Should be Screened and Treated to Prevent Osteoporosis" in *The American Journal of Medicine,* vol. 98, suppl 2A, February 27, 1995, pp. 2A–67S–2A–75S.

Ettinger, Bruce (1987) 'Update: Estrogen and Postmenopausal Osteoporosis 1976–1986' Health Values, Vol. 11, no. 4, (pp. 31–36).

Finn, Susan (1987) 'Osteoporosis: A Nutritionist's Approach' *Health Values,* vol. 11, no. 4, (pp. 20–23).

Fisher, B. et al (1998) 'Tamoxifen for prevention of breast cancer: Report of the National Surgical Adjuvant Breast and Bowel Project P-1 Study,' *Journal of the National Cancer Institute,* Vol. 90, no. 18, (pp. 1371–1389).

Freeman, Ruth, "The Management of the Patient with Osteoporosis— A Modern Epidemic," *American Journal of Managed Care,* February 1998, vol. 4, no. 2, sup, pp S94–S107.

Frey, Carol—article to be published in *Biomechanics* in 1998, cited in Jane E. Brody's "When the Elderly Fall, Shoes May Be to Blame," *New York Times,* February 24, 1998, p. C7.

Fugh-Berman, Adriane (1991) 'Tamoxifen in Healthy Women: Preventative Health or Preventing Health?' (National Women's Health Network) *Network News,* September/October (pp. 3–4).

Genant, Harry K., Johna Lucas, Stuart Weiss, Mark Akin, Ronald Emkey, Heidi McNaney-Flint, Robert Downs, Joseph Mortola, Nelson Watts, Hwa Ming Yang, Niranyan Banav, John J. Brennan, and Joseph C. Nolan, for the Estratab/Osteoposis Study Group, "Low Dose Estrified Estrogen Therapy," *Archives of Internal Medicine,* vol. 157, December 8/22, 1997, pp. 2609–2615.

Giges, Nancy (1986) 'Calcium Market Shrugs Off Study' *Advertising Age,* vol. 59, (pp. 49, 56).

Goodman, Carol E. (1987) 'Osteoporosis and Physical Activity' *Health Values,* vol. 11. no. 4 (pp. 24–30).

Haskell, S.G., Richardson, E.D., and Horvitz, R.I. (1997) 'The effect of estrogen replacement therapy on cognitive function in women: A critical review of the literature' *Journal of Clinical Epidemiology,* vol. 50, no. 11, (pp. 1249–1264).

Heaney, Robert D., 'Bone Mass, Bone Fragility, and the Decision to Treat,' *Journal of the American Medical Association,* vol. 28, no. 24, December 23/30, 1998, pp. 2119–2120.

Hu, J-F., Zhao, X-H., Jia, J-B., Parpia, B., Campbell, T.C. 'Dietary Calcium and Bone Density Among Middle-aged and Elderly Women in China,' *Am. J. Clin. Nutr.* 58: 219–227, 1993.

Hulley, S. et al (1998) 'Randomised trial of estrogen plus progestin for secondary prevention of coronary heart disease in postmenopausal women' *Journal of the American Medical Association,* vol. 280 (Aug 19) (pp. 605–613).

Jacobsen, Steven J., Jack Goldberg, Toni P. Miles, Jacob A. Brody, William Stiers, and Alfred A. Rimm, "Race and Sex Differences in Mortality following Fracture of the Hip," *American Journal of Public Health,* August 1992, vol. 82, no. 8, pp. 1147–1150.

Keating, N.L. et al (1999) 'Use of hormone replacement therapy by postmenopausal women in the United States' *Annals of Internal Medicine,* vol. 130, (pp. 545–553).

Kirkpatrick, Mary (1987) 'A Self Care Model for Osteoporosis' *Health Values,* vol. 11, no. 4, (pp. 44-50).

Kolata, Gina (1990) 'Cancer Risk in Estrogen is Slight, Study Asserts' *New York Times,* 28 November, (p. A11).

———(1991a) 'Women Don't Get Equal Heart Care' *New York Times,* 25 July, (pp. A1, A9).

———(1991b) 'Estrogen After Menopause Cuts Heart Attack Risk, Study Finds' *New York Times,* 12 September, (pp. A1, A13).

———(1991c) 'Women Face Dilemma Over Estrogen Therapy' *New York Times,* 17 September.

Libanati, Cesar, "Prevention and Treatment of Osteoporosis," *Primary Care Reports,* vol. 5, no. 5, February 22, 1999, pp. 27-4.

Love, Susan, with Karen Lindsey, *Dr. Susan Love's Hormone Book,* Random House, New York, 1997.

Macpherson, Kathleen I. (1987) 'Osteoporosis: The New Flaw in Woman or in Science?' *Health Values,* vol. 11, no. 4, (pp. 57–61).

Manson, J.E., Stampfer, M.J., Colditz, G.A. *et al* (1991) 'A Prospective Study of Aspirin Use and Primary Prevention of Cardiovascular Disease in Women' *Journal of the American Medical Association,* vol. 266, (pp. 521–527).

The Medical Letter, January 5, 1996 report on osteoporosis products, reported in *HealthFacts,* Center for Medical Consumers, February 1996, vol. XXI, no. 201, pp. 3–4.

Myers, Ann H., Baker, Susan P., Vannatta, Mark L., Abbey, Helen, and Robinson, Elizabeth G. (1991) 'Risk Factors Associated with Falls and Injuries among Elderly Institutionalized Persons' *American Journal of Epidemiology,* vol. 133, no. 11, (pp. 1179–1190).

Napoli, Maryann (1988) 'Screening for Osteoporosis: An Idea Whose Time Has Not Yet Come' (pp. 115–119) in Worcester, Nancy and Whatley, Mariamne H. (1988) *Women's Health: Readings on Social, Economic, and Political Issues,* Dubuque, Iowa: Kendall/Hunt Publishing Company.

National Prescriptions Audit, IMS America Ltd., prepared for the National Women's Health Network (hormones and breast cancer files) by the USA Food and Drug Administration Staff, February, 1990.

National Women's Health Network (1999) *Taking Hormones and Women's Health* (available from the NWHN, 514 10th St., N.W., Suite 400, Washington D.C. 20004)

Network News (National Women's Health Network) (1999a) 'Tamoxifen approved for risk reduction: Network criticizes first ad' January/February (p. 4).

Network News (National Women's Health Network)(1999b) 'Zeneca vs. Lilly vs. Zeneca: Will lawsuits lead to better information?' March/April (p. 6).

Ott, Susan (1986) 'Should Women Get Screening Bone Mass Measurements?' *Annals of Internal Medicine,* vol. 104, no. 6 (pp. 874–876).

Parfitt, M. (1984) 'Definition of Osteoporosis: Age-related Loss of Bone and its Relationship to Increased Fracture Risk', presented at the National Institutes of Health Consensus Development Conference on Osteoporosis, Bethesda, Maryland, April 1-2, quoted in MacPherson (1987).

Partlow, Lian (1991) Personal communication.

Pearson, Cindy (1991) Testimony before the USA Food and Drug Administration Select Committee on Aging, Subcommittee on Housing and Consumer Interests, 30 May.

Reb, Anne M., (Regulatory Review Officer, Division of Drug Marketing, Advertising, and Communications, Food and Drug Administration) letters dated (approximately) April 14, 1997 and

July 2, 1997, to Ellen R. Westrick, Senior Director, Office of Medical/Legal Issues, Merck.

Riis, Bente Juel, 'The Role of Bone Loss' in *The American Journal of Medicine,* vol. 98, suppl 2A, February 27, 1995, pp. 2A–29S–2A–32S.

Riggs, B. Lawrence and L. Joseph Melton (1986) 'Involutional osteoporosis,' *New England Journal of Medicine* 314, no. 26: 1, 676–684.

Rovner, Sandy (1990) 'Estrogen Therapy: More Data, Less Certainty' *Washington Post Health,* 4 September, (p. 9).

Rubin, S.M. and S.R. Cummings, 'Results of Bone Densitometry Affect Women's Decisions About Taking Measures to Prevent Fractures,' *Annals of Internal Medicine,* vol. 116, no. 12 pt 1, June 15, 1992, pp. 990–995.

Schneider, Diane L., Elizabeth L. Barrett-Connor, Deborah J. Morton, 'Timing of Postmenopausal Estrogen for Optimal Bone Mineral Density' *JAMA,* February 19, 1997, pp. 543–547.

Silverman SL, Greenwald M, Klein R, Drinkwater BL. 'Effect of Bone Density Information on Decisions about Hormone Replacement Therapy: A Randomized Trial,' *Obstet Gynecol* 1997; 89: 321–325., referred to in Robert Lindsay, Nelson B. Watts, and Donna Shoupe, symposium presentation "Current Approaches to Osteoporosis Prevention" in *The American Journal of Managed Care,* vol. 4, no. 2, sup, pp. S64–S69.

Sloane, Ethel (1985) *Biology of Women,* New York: John Wiley.

Sojourner (1991) 'Debating Estrogen Replacement Therapy' *Sojourner—The Women's Forum,* November, (pp. 13–14).

Specter, Michael (1989) 'Hormone Use in Menopause Tied to Cancer' *Washington Post,* 3 August, (p. 1).

Steering Committee of the Physician's Health Study Group (1989) 'Final Report on the Aspirin Component of the Ongoing Physician's Health Study' *New England Journal of Medicine,* vol. 321, (pp. 129–135).

Steinberg, Karen, Thacker, Stephen, Smith, Jay *et al* (1991) 'A Meta-analysis of the Effect of Estrogen Replacement Therapy on the Risk of Breast Cancer' *Journal of the American Medical Association,* vol. 265, (pp. 1985–1990).

Torgerson, David J., Ruth E. Thomas, Marion K. Campbell, David M. Reid, 'Randomized Trial of Osteoporosis Screening: Use of Hormone Replacement Therapy and Quality of Life Results,' *Arch Intern Med,* vol. 157, Oct. 13, 1997, pp. 2121–2125.

Tromp, A.M., J.H. Smit, D.J.H. Deeg, L.M. Bouter, and P. Lips, 'Predictors for Falls and Fractures in Longitudinal Aging Study Amsterdam,' *Journal of Bone and Mineral Research,* vol. 13, no. 12, 1998, pp. 1932–1939.

Whatley, Mariamne H. (1988a) 'Screening is Calculated Exploitation', (National Women's Health Network) *Network News,* January/February, (pp. 1, 3).

——(1988b) 'Women, Exercise and Physical Potential' in Worcester, Nancy and Whatley, Mariamne H. editors, *Women's Health:*

Readings on Social, Economic, and Political Issues, Dubuque, Iowa: Kendall/Hunt.

Whatley, Mariamne H. and Worcester, Nancy (1989) 'The Role of Technology in the Co-optation of the Women's Health Movement: The Case Study of Osteoporosis and Breast Cancer Screening' (pp. 199-220) in Ratcliff, Kathryn Strother, et. al., *Healing Technology—Feminist Perspectives,* Ann Arbor, Michigan: University of Michigan Press.

Winslow, Ron (1991) 'Women Face Treatment Gap in Heart Disease' *Wall Street Journal,* July 25, (pp. B1, B4).

Writing Group for the PEPI Trial, 'Effects of Hormone Therapy on Bone Mineral Density—Results from the Postmenopausal Estrogen/Progestin Interventions (PEPI) Trial', *JAMA,* November 6, 1996, vol. 276, no. 17, pp. 1389–1396.

Wolfe, Sidney M., editor, (1991a) 'Risk Factors for Falls in the Elderly' (Public Citizens Health Research Group) *Health Letter,* nol. 7, no. 8, (p. 10).

——(1991b) 'New Evidence that Menopausal Estrogens Cause Breast Cancer; Further Doubts About Prevention of Heart Disease' (Public Citizens Health Research Group) *Health Letter,* June (pp. 4–6).

Wolinsky, Fredric D., John F. Fitzgerald, & Timothy E. Stump, 'The Effect of Hip Fracture on Mortality, Hospitalization, and Functional Status: A Prospective Study,' *American Journal of Public Health,* March 1997, vol. 87, no. 3, pp. 398–403.

Worcester, Nancy and Whatley, Mariamne H. (1988) 'The Response of the Health Care System to the Women's Health Movement: The Selling of Women's Health Centers' (pp. 117–130) in Rosser, Sue V. (1988) *Feminism Within the Science and Health Care Professions: Overcoming Resistance,* Oxford: Pergamon Press.

Yaffe, K. et al (1998) 'Estrogen therapy in postmenopausal women—Effects on cognitive function and dementia' *Journal of the American Medical Association,* vol. 279, no. 9 (pp. 688–695).

Acknowledgement

The authors want to acknowledge the work of the National Women's Health Network's Hormone Education Campaign in providing the key leadership for US women in the evaluation and critique of menopausal hormones. The excellent publications and testimonies before Food and Drug Administration Committees have been extremely valuable in preparing this paper. *Taking Hormones and Women's Health* is available from The National Women's Health Network, 514 10th Street, N.W., Suite 400, Washington D.C., 20004 (USA).

Now the Truth Is Known

by Amy Allina and Cindy Pearson

Editor's note: On July 9, 2002, 16,000 participants in the Women's Health Initiative (WHI) were told to stop taking hormone replacement therapy. The bombshell announcement, made because women had elevated chances of breast cancer, heart attack, stroke and blood clots after five years of using HRT, vindicated the Network's long effort to draw attention to the dangers of HRT and of aggressive pharmaceutical marketing. The following is excerpted from an article that appeared in the San Jose Mercury News within days of the WHI announcement.

In 1966, *Feminine Forever* was published and quickly became a bestseller. The book, by Dr. Robert Wilson, promoted estrogen as a wonder drug that could counter the changes of menopause and keep women young, attractive, sexually vital and happy.

Wilson set up a foundation and traveled around the country, preaching the gospel of estrogen and describing the experience of menopause in frightening, Gothic terms: warning that "no woman can be sure of escaping the horror of this living decay." Menopausal women, whom Wilson called an "inter-sex" because they supposedly are no longer truly female, could, however, save themselves by taking estrogen. It would make them "more pleasant to live with" and prevent them from becoming "dull and unattractive."

Estrogen had been in use since the 1930s to treat hot flashes and other menopause symptoms. But Wilson's claims were grander, playing on aging women's desire for longevity and on their fear of losing beauty and health. By 1975, Ayerst-manufactured Premarin, the leading estrogen pill, was one of the top five most-prescribed drugs in the United States.

It was only years later that the public became aware that Wilson's book and his foundation were financed secretly by Ayerst, which merged with, and is now known as, Wyeth.

Now, more than 35 years later, drug companies are still selling hormones to menopausal and postmenopausal women who fear loss of their youth and the onset of age-related illnesses. The marketing is more sophisticated today, but the underlying message is the same: There's a pill that will make you healthy, happy and beautiful—never mind whether it has been scientifically proved.

A Larger Problem

The WHI news highlights a story that affects us all. It is a cautionary tale about our desire to believe that pills can keep us healthy and youthful, and the lengths to which drug companies exploit our desire for that silver bullet.

The first big scare about taking estrogen came in December 1975, when two studies linked estrogen to endometrial cancer, in the lining of the uterus. Estrogen prescriptions dropped off until the 1980s, when research showed that risk of uterine cancer was reduced when estrogen was combined with a second hormone, progestin.

The popularity of hormone therapy exploded as doctors and many women embraced it enthusiastically. Although the drugs are now available together in one pill, many women still take estrogen and progestin in separate dosages. Estrogen pill sales rose from 13.6 million prescriptions in 1982 to 31.7 million in 1992. In 1995, Premarin estrogen pills were the top-selling brand-name pharmaceutical in America. Sales of progestin pills rose fivefold in the same period, to 11.3 million.

But there were some women who remained skeptical and, in 1990, they found justification in the results of a new study. The Nurses Health Study, then the largest U.S. women's health study, found that women with breast cancer had a moderately greater chance of having used estrogen than women without breast cancer. It didn't prove that estrogen caused breast cancer, but it was a strong association.

Hormone proponents responded by assuring women the combination HRT drug was not associated with increased risk of breast cancer, and by asserting that hormones offered benefits that far offset the small increased risk of breast cancer. Both of these arguments have now been proved false.

Drug-company ad campaigns have played paradoxically to feminist sensibilities even as they promoted the idea that it's important for aging women to look young. Well-meaning doctors also were misled by sales pitches crafted to look like scientific information. It was, effectively, the marketing of theory as fact. Manufacturers of HRT drugs also paid for favorable research about the drug and to disseminate the results to doctors. They footed the bill for medical-journal supplements that resembled peer-reviewed studies.

The drug makers and their defenders were taking legitimate scientific hypotheses and presenting them as proven conclusions—without doing the time-consuming work of clinical trials. In day-to-day life, it is normal to take leaps of faith to act on a hypothesis without proof. But in health care, the stakes are higher. Drugs are powerful and carry the possibility of harm. To prescribe them based on faith instead of science is a big risk. In this case, the leap of faith has exposed millions of women to increased risk of breast cancer, heart attack and stroke—all of which can kill.

Alternatives Available

There are alternatives to HRT that have been found by the Food and Drug Administration to safely prevent bone loss and fractures. Bisphosphonate drugs and raloxifene prevent fractures, although they are new and no long-term safety data is yet possible. Moreover, the National Institutes of Health has found strong evidence that calcium and vitamin D help preserve strong bones and that regular exercise contributes to developing bone mass and reducing the risk of falls in the elderly.

The mere fact that the government was willing to pay for an expensive medical study of HRT should have been enough to let everyone know that HRT was unproven for long-term use and disease prevention.

But women's hopes for a bulwark against aging, combined with decades of drug-company marketing, had done their work. Most women and most doctors prescribing hormones to their patients believed they were safe and prevented everything from heart disease to wrinkles. Now the truth is known.

But the ways Americans view medicine, and the marketing methods of the drug industry, have not changed. Who knows what is coming next? It is not hard to imagine that one of the new drugs people are taking today, believing that it makes them healthier, will be the HRT bombshell of tomorrow.

HRT

Overview

by National Women's Health Network

The widespread popularity of hormone replacement therapy (HRT) in the United States is a triumph of marketing over science and advertising over common sense. Drug companies and many health care providers present menopause as a disease. In fact, it is a normal transition that occurs in all women.

For decades, we've been told that the use of estrogen alone or the use of estrogen/progestin together will protect women from age-related disorders and help women look and feel younger. Despite these claims, there is no valid scientific evidence that estrogen prevents Alzheimer's disease, incontinence or wrinkles, or improves memory, mood and energy. And recent large randomized trials have proven that an estrogen/progestin combination taken every day causes heart attack, blood clots, stroke, breast cancer and makes women feel worse.[1, 2] A similar study of estrogen taken alone is continuing, as there is not yet clear evidence of strong benefit or risk.[1]

There is evidence that taking hormones at menopause reduces the symptoms of the menopausal transition and delays bone loss. Estrogen and progestin in a combination reduces the risk of fractures and colon cancer. But in the largest and most rigorous study, the risks of the combined hormones outweighed the benefits for healthy women.

Hormones Have Not Been Shown To

1. prevent wrinkles or other natural signs of aging
2. cure urinary incontinence
3. help moodiness or depression
4. improve sexual desire or responsiveness
5. improve memory
6. prevent Alzheimer's disease

Should I or Shouldn't I?

There is really no single answer to the conundrum should I or shouldn't I take hormones. Alleviating hot flashes or vaginal dryness and preventing fractures are all proven benefits of HRT. However, the decision must be individualized for each woman, taking into account her medical history, preferences and concerns. There are no scientific studies that support the routine use of hormones in healthy menopausal and perimenopausal women.

Currently, scientific evidence supports the use of HRT only in the following cases:

- for women who have had both ovaries surgically removed at an early age
- for short-term use by women with severe hot flashes, night sweats, or vaginal dryness
- as one option for maintaining bone density and reducing the risk of fractures in women at high risk for osteoporosis

We recommend that women who experience troublesome hot flashes or vaginal dryness try non-hormonal therapies as the first line of treatment. If a woman chooses hormones, we suggest she take the lowest dose that alleviates her symptoms for as short a time as possible.

The Bottom Line

To us the bottom line is clear. Some health care providers, influenced by drug company promotions, are pressuring women to take hormones as soon as their regular menstrual cycles start to change. Much information in the popular media also echoes the interests of drug companies and encourages women to think of menopause as a disease—an estrogen deficiency state—and to begin taking hormones as soon as possible.

Both groups make it sound as though the cessation of normal menstrual cycles does lasting harm to the body within days or weeks of its onset. The truth is that it doesn't. Most women have months or years to make decisions about whether or not hormones make sense for them and to reevaluate their decisions as their situations change or as new scientific information becomes available. We urge you to take all the time you need to make an informed decision about starting or continuing hormones.

Resources

For a good overview of women's health at midlife that disentangles menopause and other conditions associated with aging, we recommend *Ourselves, Growing Older*, Simon & Schuster, 1994, $20.

For more information about menopause, HRT and alternatives, try the Network's recent book *The Truth About Hormone Replacement Therapy* Prima, 2002, $15.95 and *Dr. Susan Love's Hormone Book*, Three Rivers Press, 1998, $15.

Websites sponsored by groups that have no financial ties to drug companies include

http://www.womenshealthnetwork.org;

http://www.susanlovemd.com;

http://www.ourbodiesourselves.org; and

http://www.4woman.gov.

References

1. Writing group for the Women's Health Initiative investigators. Risks and benefits of estrogen plus progestin in healthy postmenopausal women. Principal results from the Women's Health Initiative randomized controlled trial. *JAMA*, July 17, 2002; 288: 321-333.
2. Hlatky, MA, Boothroyd, D, Vittinghoff, E, et al. Quality-of-life and depressive symptoms in postmenopausal women after receiving hormone therapy. Results from the Heart and Estrogen/Progestin Replacement Study (HERS) trial. *JAMA*, February 6, 2002; 287: 591–597.

Hormone Therapy

Six Steps Toward a Better Future

by Cindy Pearson

On October 24, 2002, Network Executive Director Cindy Pearson discussed the implications of the Women's Health Initiative at a Scientific Workshop on Menopausal Hormone Therapy at the National Institutes of Health. More than 500 physicians, researchers and activists were in the audience. Before concluding with the recommendations excerpted below, Pearson warned that drug companies, professional societies, women's groups, policy makers and government agencies had all been complicit in creating a "climate of enthusiasm for hormone therapy" and allowing the needless suffering of tens of thousands of women.

To consider the implications for future research, we need to consider current research. The Women's Health Initiative's controlled trials of hormone therapy took place in the context of massive off-label use of hormone therapy. Millions of healthy women were taking long-term hormone therapy for a preventive benefit not yet proven because medical practice was determined under the influence of industry rather than the influence of evidence. . . .

To prevent more tragedies like this, and to make sure that future research is able to make as big an impact as possible, significant changes are needed in policy and practice within the regulatory agencies, media, professional societies, consumer groups with financial ties to industry, and the behavior of industry itself.

Future research will be undercut before it is underway unless we as a society muster the necessary will to take the following steps:

- Get drug company money out of medical education.

- Give the FDA the authority to pre-approve direct-to-consumer advertisements for prescription medications.
- End industry payments to physicians for writing papers that appear in medical journals.
- Stop quoting medical experts in media reports on health without reporting on their financial relationship with industry.
- Clean up consumer groups' health education efforts so that the all-too-common and dangerous influence of drug company money is replaced with a healthy skepticism.
- Bar anyone with significant financial ties to industry from involvement in the development of professional guidelines.

The National Women's Health Network calls on the policy makers, researchers, clinicians and leaders assembled here to take steps to make these changes a reality.

Phytoestrogens

A New Alternative for Women?

by Adriane Fugh-Berman, MD

Phytoestrogens, or plant estrogens, are much weaker estrogens than our own bodies make. Phytoestrogens are only about 1/200th the strength of endogenous estrogens. There are two main kinds of phytoestrogens: lignans and isoflavones. Foods that contain lignans include oily seeds, especially flaxseed (also called linseed) and also cereal grains, beans, vegetables and fruits. Premenopausal women fed 10 grams a day of flaxseed powder multiplied their lignan excretion 3 to 285 fold. Isoflavones are less common, occurring mainly in soybeans, chickpeas, and other legumes (Knight). Some phytoestrogens are also found in black cohosh, clover and other medicinal herbs, but these are different than phytoestrogens found in food plants and should not be treated the same in terms of safety.

Hot Flashes and Vaginal Dryness

Whole grains and beans (especially soybeans) are the most commonly eaten source of phytoestrogens. Asian women complain less of hot flashes than Western women do, and it may be that eating soy products serves as a type of hormone replacement therapy (Adlercreutz). There is evidence that supplementing with phytoestrogens can help hot flashes and vaginal dryness. A study of 145 Israeli women with menopausal symptoms found that the 78 women assigned to a phytoestrogen-rich diet had fewer hot flashes and less vaginal dryness than the 36 women in the control group who did not change their diet (Adlercreutz 1997). The study lasted twelve weeks and women in the treatment group substituted phytoestrogen-rich foods (including tofu, soy drink, miso, and flax seed) for approximately one fourth of their daily caloric intake (Brzezinski).

Two studies have looked at whether supplementing the diet with phytoestrogens resulted in estrogenic changes in vaginal cells. One study found a positive result (Wilcox) and the other a negative result (Baird), but the study that did not find an effect used an unusual method of collecting vaginal cells that may have underestimated estrogenized cells (Knight).

Breast Cancer Prevention

What is the effect of phytoestrogens on breast cancer risk? Although there has not been a prospective study on this, studies of different populations show that groups that consume a lot of phytoestrogens have a lower rate of breast cancer. A recent case control study found that women with breast cancer excreted much lower amounts of phytoestrogens in their urine than women without breast cancer (Ingram).

However, this protective effect may be strongest in premenopausal women. Soybeans are quite high in phytoestrogens, and there is a high intake of soy products in some Asian countries, especially China, Japan, and Korea. A study of Chinese women in Singapore found that soy product intake seemed to protect premenopausal women, but not postmenopausal women, from breast cancer (Lee).

Different Effects in Premenopausal and Postmenopausal Women

The above result is not all that surprising because phytoestrogens may have opposite effects in premenopausal and postmenopausal women. Premenopausal women have nominally higher estrogen levels than postmenopausal women. In premenopausal women who eat a lot of plant estrogens, the weak plant estrogens perform some of the same functions as our own, stronger estrogens. Chemical messengers regulate estrogen in our bodies by determining when more or less estrogen is needed; when weak plant estrogens are meeting our estrogen needs, our own hormone factories take a break. So premenopausal women with normally high estrogen levels who eat plant estrogens everyday have a constantly lower rate of production of homegrown estrogens, and the total estrogen effect on their bodies (lower internal estrogen production plus weak plant estrogens) is lower. So in premenopausal women, the effect of a diet high in phytoestrogens is actually anti-estrogenic.

"Background" estrogen levels are already low in postmenopausal women, so eating phytoestrogens boosts the estrogen levels. So for postmenopausal women, phytoestrogens may have an estrogenic effect. This estrogenic effect may affect different organs differently. A high soy intake appears to protect against endometrial cancer in both premenopausal and postmenopausal women (Goodman).

Different Menopausal Experiences in Asian and Western Women

Some people theorize that hot flashes and other menopausal symptoms may be due less to low estrogen levels than to a sudden drop in estrogen levels. According to this theory, Asian women complain less of hot flashes and other menopause-related complaints because decades of eating soy products may have lowered estrogen levels sufficiently that the menopausal drop, especially cushioned by continued high intake of phytoestrogens, may be an easy hormonal descent. Westerners start at a higher estrogen level and fall to a lower level; we plummet over a hormonal cliff.

Other factors may be equally important, of course; it is difficult to determine the importance of the fact that Asians respect age while Westerners worship youth. The transition to menopause in the West might be very different if we looked forward to an honored place in society rather than discrimination and poverty.

If You Have Breast Cancer

Phytoestrogens in food have been consumed for thousands of years by Asian women, who have a lower risk of breast cancer than Western women at all ages, and the idea that these foods are dangerous is clearly absurd. For premenopausal women with breast cancer, phytoestrogen would be expected to lower circulating estrogen levels and thus be beneficial.

For postmenopausal women with breast cancer the situation is more complicated. Soybeans contain substances that are estrogenic and substances that are anticancer. It is not clear whether the estrogenic properties of soybeans could cause breast cancer to grow. In cultured breast cancer cells, both estradiol and a phytoestrogen stimulated cell growth, but when added together, little to no growth stimulation occurred. But in an immunocompromised mouse model, phytoestrogen implants caused estrogen receptor positive (but not estrogen receptor negative) breast cancer implants to grow (Helferich).

On the other hand, phytoestrogen supplementation in postmenopausal women markedly increased sex hormone binding globulin (SHBG) (Brzezinski). High levels of SHBG are associated with lower breast cancer risk.

The Network believes that supplementing one's diet with phytoestrogens makes sense for premenopausal women. Whether postmenopausal women with breast cancer should avoid supplementing with phytoestrogens is an open question. The Network believes that there is no need for postmenopausal women with breast cancer to actively avoid phytoestrogens, which are consumed in quantity in many countries with low breast cancer rates, and are found in many foods with high nutritive value. Whether or not to actively supplement a diet with phytoestrogens is a different story.

Some people argue that Asian women have lower breast cancer rates at all ages than Westerners, so phytoestrogen intake can't be harmful. But Asians consume high levels of phytoestrogens throughout their lifetime, and this may create a very different hormonal situation than a Western woman who has a low phytoestrogen intake premenopausally and then suddenly increases her phytoestrogen intake postmenopausally. It is theoretically possible that that scenario increases her lifetime exposure to estrogens. Also, other factors may contribute to a lower rate of breast cancer in Asian women, who generally consume a low-fat, high-fiber diet, and have different exposures to environmental factors. A case can be made for postmenopausal women with breast cancer to maximize or minimize phytoestrogen intake, but there is not adequate evidence to justify a strong recommendation either for supplementing or avoiding phytoestrogens.

Should breast cancer patients who are being treated with the hormonal drug tamoxifen supplement with phytoestrogens? These two substances have similar effects in terms of having some estrogenic and some antiestrogenic properties. There are no studies on what the effects are of combining the use of phytoestrogens and tamoxifen. The Network believes that once again, a case can be made either for supplementing or avoiding phytoestrogens, and that the most prudent decision may be to do neither.

Cardiovascular Disease

Soybeans also may have a beneficial effect on cardiovascular disease. A meta-analysis of 38 controlled clinical trials found that eating a lot of soy protein was associated with reduced cholesterol (9.3% less than controls), reduced LDL cholesterol (12.9%), reduced triglycerides (10.5%). HDL cholesterol was unaffected (Anderson).

Osteoporosis

The effect of phytoestrogens on bone has not been well studied, but there is reason to believe that there may be some effect on bone. Asians have a lower rate of osteoporotic bone fracture than Western women do, despite the fact that the bones of Asian women are thinner and their calcium intake is far lower than Western women. And genistein, the predominant isoflavone in soybeans, helps to maintain bone in rats that have had their ovaries removed (Knight).

If You Want to Supplement with Phytoestrogens

Soybean products are the most widely consumed source of isoflavones and also contain some lignan precursors. Chick peas (garbanzo beans), lima beans, other beans, and peas are also good sources of isoflavones.

In Asia, consumption of legumes (soybeans, lentils, other beans, and peas) provides 25–45 mg of total isoflavones a day, compared with Western countries, where less than 5 mg/day is eaten. In Japan, where soy consumption is very high, up to 200 mg/day of isoflavones are consumed (Knight).

Not all soy products are equal in terms of phytoestrogen content. Soy oil and soy sauce don't have measurable amounts of phytoestrogens in them.

Tofu (soy bean curd) comes in many different textures and is almost tasteless on its own; it easily takes on other flavors. "Silken" tofu is the softest and is best for blending; try making shakes with fruit juice or substituting it for oil in your favorite salad dressing recipe. Very firm tofu can be cut up and put into soups and curries or marinated and stir-fried with vegetables.

An added bonus for eating tofu is that many brands are made with calcium sulfate and can supply a significant amount of this important nutrient. According to the USDA, ¼ block (116 mg) of tofu made with calcium supplies 406 mg. of calcium, and ¼ block of firm tofu (81 gm) supplies 553 mg of calcium. Read the label to see if your brand of tofu is made with calcium.

You can increase your intake of lignans by eating more whole grains (especially rye) and eating flaxseed. Several breakfast cereals are made with flaxseed. It tastes nutty when toasted and can be sprinkled on hot or cold cereal, yogurt, etc.

Summary

The Network believes that phytoestrogens are safe and beneficial to the health of premenopausal women, and may alleviate menopausal symptoms in postmenopausal women, but that the safety of supplemental phytoestrogens in postmenopausal women with breast cancer has not been clearly established.

References are available from the office of the National Women's Health Network.

Hormones for Men

Is Male Menopause a Question of Medicine or of Marketing?

by Jerome Groopman

It goes by many names. "Male menopause" is perhaps the most popular, but "andropause" is the term that many doctors favor, and PADAM ("partial androgen deficiency in aging men") has its partisans, too. The condition may afflict millions of Americans, and, if they do not yet recognize the symptoms, a public-awareness campaign has been launched to help them. A two-page ad that ran in *Time* not long ago showed a car's gas gauge pointing to Empty and beside it the words "Fatigued? Depressed mood? Low sex drive? Could be your testosterone is running on empty." The ad explains that "as some men grow older, their testosterone levels decline," and that such men should consult their doctors about testosterone therapy. At the bottom of the page, the gas gauge points to Full.

Physicians have been targeted with similar ads. One that appeared in a recent issue of a primary-care journal calls on them to "identify the men in your practice with low testosterone who may benefit from clinical performance in a packet." The photographs are eye-catching: there's a well-built fellow in his middle years beside the words "improved sexual function"; a smiling man in shorts and a T-shirt who is standing next to a mountain bike ("improved mood"); a policeman directing traffic ("increased bone mineral density"). Doctors are told to "screen for symptoms of low testosterone" and "restore normal testosterone levels."

These ads were paid for by Unimed, a division of the Belgian conglomerate Solvay. Unimed makes AndroGel, a drug that was approved by the F.D.A. two years ago, and is the fastest-growing form of testosterone-replacement therapy for men. Pills, introduced in the sixties, often caused liver damage. Intramuscular injections, particularly favored by bodybuilders and competitive athletes, produce a sharp spike of the hormone, and then a fall, and these fluctuations are often accompanied by swings in mood, libido, and energy. In the late eighties, a transdermal patch was developed, and its use is still widespread. The patch provides safer and steadier

dosing, but often causes skin irritation, and sometimes falls off during exercise. AndroGel, by contrast, delivers testosterone in a colorless, drying gel that is simply rubbed on an area of the body—usually the shoulders—once a day. It has thus made testosterone available in a form that almost any man can use conveniently.

If hormone-replacement therapy for andropause becomes as common as such therapies have been for menopause—and this seems to be the ambition of some drug companies—the consequences, both medical and financial, could be dramatic. Given the popular desire to reverse human aging with a simple nostrum and the growing intimacy between commercial and clinical concerns, the trend may prove to be irresistible. The pharmaceutical industry is, of course, in the business of inventing treatments. Some people wonder whether it may help invent diseases, too.

To be treated for andropause, you first need physicians who can confidently make the diagnosis. One of them is Dr. Abraham Morgentaler, the director of Men's Health Boston. He is forty-six years old, with thick black hair and deep-set eyes. Trained as a urologist, he specializes in male sexual dysfunction and infertility. He views testosterone deficiency in older men as a silent epidemic, and worries that, of the perhaps five million American men who suffer from it, ninety-five percent go undiagnosed. Replacing missing testosterone, he believes, will help restore youthful muscle tone, bone strength, potency, and general vigor. He recently put an ad in the Boston Globe urging men who were experiencing "low sex drive" or "low energy" to have their testosterone level tested at his clinic. The costs of both the ad and the tests were underwritten by a Unimed educational grant.

Men's Health Boston is in a modern brick-and-glass office building at a busy intersection in Brookline. It has a well-appointed waiting room with soft lighting and upholstered chairs; photographs of famous local athletes adorn the walls. The men who came to see Morgentaler on a recent afternoon had all been given a questionnaire provided by Unimed:

1. Do you have a decrease in libido (sex drive)?
2. Do you have a lack of energy?
3. Do you have a decrease in strength and/or endurance?
4. Have you lost height?
5. Have you noticed a decreased "enjoyment of life"?
6. Are you sad and/or grumpy?
7. Are your erections less strong?
8. Have you noticed a recent deterioration in your ability to play sports?
9. Are you falling asleep after dinner?
10. Has there been a recent deterioration in your work performance?

Among the patients was a real-estate broker in his late fifties. He had answered "Yes" to questions 1, 2, 3, 5, 7, and 10. "I'm just exhausted by the end of the afternoon," he said, after Morgentaler gave him a physical. "And my brain often feels foggy." He likes to shoot pool, and he remarked that his game wasn't what it used to be.

"Have you noticed any change in sexual performance?" Dr. Morgentaler asked.

"Well, I'm not a kid anymore," the patient said, but he had no real complaints.

Morgentaler then showed the man the results from his blood assay. His testosterone levels were "somewhat low," Morgentaler said, "Now, if I had a magic wand and I could do anything for you, what would it be?"

"Fix the energy thing."

"I have good news for you," Dr. Morgentaler said, "There is an excellent chance that giving you testosterone will help to restore your energy. And, in terms of being foggy, I can't promise, but I have several men in my practice who are professors. They take testosterone, and they say it makes their brains much sharper."

Dr. Morgentaler explained that, while testosterone would not cause prostate cancer, if the patient had a hidden tumor the hormone would "act like food, nourishing the cancer." For that reason, his P.S.A. (prostate-specific antigen) level would be checked, and Morgentaler would take six biopsy samples of the prostate gland to make sure that there was no malignancy.

"I'll give you a prescription now, and you can get started once we complete these tests," Dr. Morgentaler said. "When I give men back testosterone, some say 'Whoa!'"

The patient liked the sound of that. "Maybe I'll be a stallion again," he said.

Testosterone, an androgen, is a steroid hormone derived from cholesterol. It is produced primarily by the testes, but the signal to produce it comes from the pituitary gland, in the form of two other hormones, which ar-

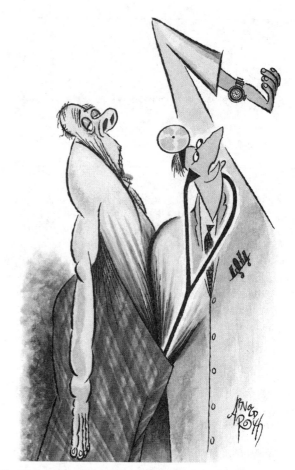

Should a seventy-year-old have the testosterone levels he had at twenty?
Arnold Roth: The New Yorker.

rive in pulses at certain times of the day. As men age, the response of testes becomes more muted; for men over the age of forty, the levels of testosterone in the bloodstream decline, on average, by about 1.2 percent each year.

Morgentaler's next patient was a construction worker in his forties. The man was on cardiac medication and had an implanted defibrillator, because he was prone to life-threatening arrhythmias, and occasionally he received electric jolts from the device. His wife had died some three years before, but in the previous six months he had been in a stable relationship. He had come to the clinic because he had difficulty reaching orgasm.

Morgentaler asked about other symptoms.

"I used to be able to play racquetball non-stop, but I'm tired now after four games."

Morgentaler nodded. "We caught it just at the right time."

"But my primary-care doctor checked my testosterone and said it was 800, which is normal. He told me he couldn't do anything about my problem."

Morgentaler looked at the results of the man's blood assay. Total testosterone was in the normal range, at 509 nanograms per decilitre. But his free testosterone, Morgentaler told him, was another matter. At any moment, about two percent of circulating testosterone is "free"—unbound to any protein—and thus biologically active. The patient's free testosterone was a little under the lower limit of normal. ("Normal" testosterone levels refer to what's normal for men in their twenties.)

"If I had a magic wand and I could do anything for you, what would it be?" Morgentaler asked.

"Get rid of the problem with orgasm."

"Well, I believe we have a very good chance of helping you." Morgentaler wrote out a prescription for AndroGel. "We'll check your P.S.A. today, but we don't need to do biopsies of your prostate gland until after the age of fifty. So you can get started right away."

"I can't thank you enough," the patient said.

When the F.D.A. decides to permit the sale of a new drug, it specifies a list of "indications"—particular medical conditions for which the drug has been approved. "The F.D.A. never approved AndroGel for andropause," says Dr. Dan Shames, the director of the Division of Reproductive and Urological Drug Products at the F.D.A. "We're not sure what 'andropause' is. The intention was that AndroGel would be for people with conditions like Klinefelter's and pituitary dysfunction." Klinefelter's syndrome is a congenital disorder in which men have an extra X chromosome and underdeveloped testes. Other suitable candidates for therapy are men whose testes have been scarred by viral inflammation. Still others have had a tumor that damaged the hypothalamus or the pituitary gland, so the brain no longer sends activating signals to the testes. In such men, muscle strength, libido, and bone density are diminished, and testosterone replacement is an effective treatment.

The trouble is that there aren't very many of these people—they number only in the tens of thousands. But there are some thirty-five million men in the United States over the age of fifty, and, if the andropause movement takes off, annual revenues for the producers of testosterone-replacement drugs could reach billions of dollars. Estrogen-replacement therapy in menopausal women—a comparable market—had generated more than two billion dollars a year in revenue, largely for Wyeth, the maker of Premarin, the most popular estrogen-replacement drug.

This is where marketing and medical science may part ways. Pharmaceutical companies often obtain F.D.A. approval of a new product for a niche population with a relatively rare disease, hoping to expand later to a larger and more profitable market. Once a drug is approved for sale, a physician can legally prescribe it for any clinical condition

he thinks would benefit from it. The F.D.A. prohibits drug companies from advertising "off label" uses—those other than the approved indications—but they can pursue alternative strategies. They can run ads that "raise awareness" of a condition without mentioning the proprietary therapy by name. And they can align themselves with so-called "opinion leaders," well-known physicians whose views are thought to have influence among their peers, by financing their research, say, or offering them consulting agreements.

If you're hoping to expand the medical "indications" for a drug regimen, there are few greater boons than the endorsement of a major medical society. Unimed's andropause campaign won a considerable victory when the Endocrine Society—a prestigious organization of hormone specialists—convened its First Annual Andropause Consensus Conference, in April of 2000, just six weeks before AndroGel came on the market. The conference, which was held in Beverly Hills, set out to define andropause and decide how it should be treated. The chair was Dr. Ronald Swerdloff, an endocrinologist at Harbor-U.C.L.A. Medical Center, and he assembled a panel whose task was to come up with recommendations for clinical practice. These recommendations were distributed at this year's annual meeting of the Endocrine Society, in June, and undoubtedly they will have considerable influence in the medical community.

The panel acknowledged that the benefits of testosterone replacement in aging men hadn't been established, but it nonetheless recommended that all men over the age of fifty be screened for testosterone deficiency. Screening should start with a questionnaire, like the one that Unimed had provided for Morgentaler. Patients who had symptoms, whose morning testosterone levels were under the lower limit of normal, specified as 300, and who had no conditions that would rule out testosterone replacement, like prostate cancer, "would likely benefit from treatment," the panel stated. A table accompanying the recommendations suggested that low testosterone levels would be found in more than ten percent of men over fifty, and nearly thirty percent of men over seventy—in perhaps as many as seven million Americans.

There's no doubt that the panel reached its conclusions in good faith; the androgen enthusiasts are nothing if not sincere. But it's also the case that a Unimed/Solvay educational grant was the sole source of funding for the Beverly Hills conference. According to Scott Hunt, the Endocrine Society's executive director, Unimed even suggested some of the panel's members. And, of the thirteen panelists in the final group, at least nine, including Swerdloff and his co-chair, had significant financial ties to the drug company, in the form of research grants, consulting arrangements, or speaking fees. The recommendations made reference to the educational grant but not to the panelists' ties to Unimed.

The bid to medicalize middle age may be well supported by the pharmaceutical industry, but it remains poorly supported by scientific research. Is the decline in testosterone levels really responsible for most of the symptoms of aging in men? What levels of testosterone are, in fact, "normal"? Does andropause even exists? The limits of medical knowledge are starkly evident when you visit a research center like the one run by Dr. William Crowley, the chief of the Reproductive Endocrine Unit at Massachusetts General Hospital, and his associate Dr. Frances Hayes. In a laboratory crowded with centrifuges, chemical hoods, and spectrophotometers, they and their team spend hours double-checking sensitive chemical assays for hormones produced by the hypothalamus and the testes, as well as the pituitary and adrenal glands. In an adjoining clinical-research center, volunteer human subjects are hooked up to I.V.s and insulin clamps.

Several years ago, Dr. Crowley realized that, in order to study hypogonadal men, he needed a clear definition of normal testosterone levels. So he inserted catheters into the veins of healthy young subjects in their twenties and drew blood samples every ten minutes in the course of twenty-four hours. He still sounds amazed by what he found.

"We measured the size of their testes, evaluated body hair, erectile function, sperm count, muscle mass, bone density, pituitary function," Crowley recalls. "These men were completely normal from every parameter. And it was incredible: fifteen percent had testosterone levels during the day that were well below what is set as the lower limit of normal—more than fifty percent below the cutoff."

Why do testosterone levels among healthy men vary so much? Hayes speculates that some men may have highly efficient testosterone receptors—cellular traps that grab the free hormone in the blood—so that what appears to be an abnormally low testosterone level is all the hormone they need. But even an individual's testosterone levels can be markedly different at different times. One factor may be stress, which seems to reduce levels of sex steroids. Drug interactions, too, might alter testosterone levels in unpredictable ways. And much of the variation simply eludes explanation. Crowley studied several young men whose initial test results showed testosterone levels ranging from 150 to 200—well below the 300 cutoff—over twenty-four hours. "They had a perfectly normal testosterone profile," Crowley says. "There can be a funny disconnect between one measurement and a later one"—which means that testosterone deficiency may be easily overdiagnosed.

"This variability in testosterone levels was really a physiological curiosity until AndroGel was approved," Crowley continues. "Now every time the testosterone level is below 300 the question of prescription is raised." As for the often quoted figure of four or five million "andropausal" men—the figure touted in the Unimed ads—Hayes says, "Frankly, I don't know where that number comes from or how real it is."

What makes things more confusing is that the usual commercial tests that physicians use to measure testosterone levels are notoriously unreliable. The andropause movement has made laboratory assays a lucrative business, and all kinds of patented kits have come on the market. But, as Swerdloff's panel discovered, the results tend to be inconsistent. "It's really a big problem," Swerdloff says. "Practicing doctors have a great belief in the numbers, but in the past few years the assays have deteriorated." If you assayed blood samples from normal men with one proprietary test, you might find values between 300 and 900, while another test would give values between 160 and 700. So men whose tests report low total testosterone levels—like the real-estate broker Morgentaler saw—might actually have normal levels. The tests for free testosterone seem to be even less accurate.

Not every practitioner finds reason for concern. "The tests aren't as reliable as we want them to be, but it doesn't matter," says Morgentaler, who sometimes even prescribes AndroGel "preventatively" for middle-aged men whose testosterone levels are in the lower quarter of the normal range. "It's not credible that we aren't helping these men by giving them testosterone. The truth is, there's a deep emotional issue in some people who oppose hormone-replacement therapy, because it asks the question 'Is there hope of achieving eternal youth?' There are those who don't want to oppose Mother Nature."

And there are those who don't want to wait for scientific validation. Last year, a panel organized by the National Institutes of Health—maybe the closest thing we have to a voice of independent scientific consensus—released a paper concluding that the andropause hypothesis is unproved. The report that Swerdloff's group released at the Endocrine Society meeting in June contains references to sixty-two relevant publications, but omits any reference to the N.I.H. report.

Swerdloff and his colleagues reviewed the half-dozen controlled studies available on giving testosterone to healthy aging men, and were evidently impressed by those which found that it increased lean muscle mass, strength, and bone-mineral density in the spine. Unfortunately, most of these studies were small, involving forty or fifty men. The reported improvements were far from dramatic, and different studies have had contradictory findings. In fact, the largest and longest-term study, of a hundred and eight men over three years, showed no improvements in energy level, sexual performance, or strength.

So there's a lot of uncertainty about the effects of the age-related lowering of testosterone. "There appears to be a threshold level of testosterone below which libido and sexual function are impaired," Hayes says. "Boosting above this threshold doesn't seem to enhance sexual performance." The role that testosterone plays in maintaining strong bones in healthy elderly men is highly controversial, too. Dan Shames, of the F.D.A., says, "Just because you are increasing bone density doesn't mean you prevent fractures." Even in studies that found a positive correlation between testosterone levels and bone strength, the hormone accounted for only about five percent of age- and weight-adjusted differences. Men with severely low testosterone levels showed improvement in the spine, but no change was observed in the hips—and it is mainly hip fractures that debilitate the elderly.

"Each pharmaceutical company wants to get up and say, 'This is the magic bullet for aging,'" Crowley says. "But it's overly simplistic to attribute such a complex process as aging to the change in the level of a single hormone like estrogen or testosterone."

If the benefits of treating "andropause" are in doubt, so, more worrisomely, is the safety. The known side effects of testosterone therapy include gynecomastia (abnormal enlargement of the breasts) and testicular shrinkage (as gonads compensate by making less of the hormone). Testosterone also raises the level of circulating red blood cells; if this level is excessive, the blood becomes viscous, which can lead to congestive heart failure or stroke. And among men who received a 100-milligram daily dose of AndroGel over a year, nearly twenty percent developed some sort of prostate disorder, such as prostatic hyperplasia.

More troubling is how testosterone accelerates the growth of prostate cancer. The majority of men over the age of sixty-five have clusters of cancer cells in their prostate glands which are both "occult" and "indolent": they're hard to find, and they grow so slowly that they're unlikely to create any trouble by themselves. Here the perils are twofold. On the one hand, unnecessary biopsies can lead to unnecessary surgery, aimed at eradicating cancers that might have remained inactive. On the other hand, biopsies can easily miss cancers that, under a regimen of testosterone replacement, become more aggressive than they otherwise would be. Not surprisingly, Dr. Shames says that the F.D.A. has "issues of concern over the safety" of prescribing testosterone-replacement therapy for men whose hormone levels fall as part of normal aging.

Even Dr. Swerdloff acknowledges these uncertainties. "I agree that currently there are insufficient data on the long-term effects of testosterone-replacement therapy on the heart or on the development of prostate cancer, but the benefits seem considerable," he says. The andropause panel he chaired was aware that the N.I.H. is thinking of doing rigorous, placebo-controlled clinical studies that would span six or more years. "If the answer is yes, that replacement therapy causes heart damage or sparks emergency of prostate cancer, then you will know in six years or so," he says. "But older people in this age group won't wait six to ten years to have solid answers. Clinical practice will move at one rate, and the data will trail."

This is precisely what concerns many scientists. "Pharmaceutical marketing is the drive, not physiology," Crowley complains of the andropause movement. "Maybe we're *meant* to lower our testosterone levels—maybe it's healthy and protects us from developing prostate cancer. Of course, that's pure conjecture, but it's something that needs to be carefully addressed." When you elevate the testosterone levels in a seventy-year-old man to those he had at twenty, are you really returning him to "normal"? Crowley says, "I worry that this widespread prescription of testosterone for aging men is going to precipitate an epidemic of prostate cancer."

Of course, it will not be the first time that hormones have been heavily marketed—in advance of the scientific evidence—as a way to recapture youth. In the late sixties, estrogens were touted to women as their chance to be "feminine forever." And initial data from small or uncontrolled studies were encouraging. Estrogen therapy was believed to help sustain sexual health, and mood, while protecting bones form osteoporosis and the heart from arteriosclerosis. The media were flooded with ads for estrogen therapy, and publishers churned out books celebrating its benefits. Nearly forty percent of postmenopausal women have been prescribed hormone-replacement therapy.

As we now know, conventional H.R.T. not only increases the risk of breast cancer but can lead to heart attacks, strokes, and blood clots. A nationwide trial of sixteen thousand women—part of the Women's Health Initiative—was recently terminated when the therapy was linked to a twenty-six percent increase in invasive breast cancer and a significant increase in cardiovascular disease as well. A hormone regimen meant to reverse the effects of aging has proved to accelerate serious disease. As Dr. Swerdloff put it, the data trailed clinical practice.

Meanwhile, testosterone-replacement therapy is becoming increasingly popular. Last year alone, sales of transdermal testosterone doubled. An estimated quarter of a million American men are now taking the hormone. If the current rates continue, that number will rise to nearly a million within two years—and, with the newly conferred imprimatur of the Endocrine Society, the rates could surge.

To date, the best published safety data we have on AndroGel as a treatment for andropause comes from a study of sixty-seven men who took the drug for an average of twenty-nine months. An accurate assessment of its effects on the heart, blood vessels, and prostate would require many years of observing many thousands of men—a male counterpart to the Women's Health Initiative. Until then, the attempt to reverse the gradual decline in testosterone levels in aging men can't be considered the treatment of a disorder: it amounts to a vast, uncontrolled experiment, whose consequences remain uncertain. As Hayes says, "It would be a shame to make the same mistakes again."

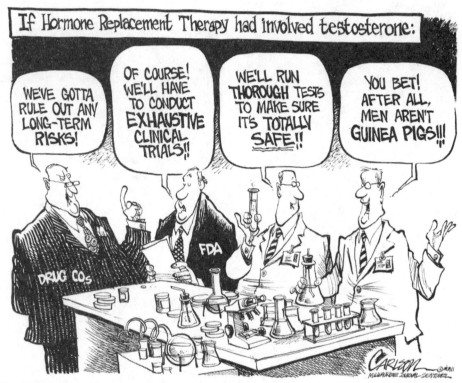

Copyright © Journal Sentinel. Reprinted by permission.

WORKSHEET—CHAPTER 12
Aging, Ageism, Mid-life and Older Women's Health Issues

1. Compare who you are physically, emotionally, and intellectually today to the person you were 5 years ago. Which of the changes are positive? Which changes are negative? How do you think the changes of the last 5 years are similar and different than the changes you will go through in the next 5 years? How do the issues you have identified compare with those Pasty J. Murphy identifies in "Ageing?"

2. It is often hard to think about aging when we are young. However, there are many lifestyle factors throughout our lives that can have an impact on the health we experience when we get older. (Be sure to read the introduction to this chapter and the articles before completing these questions.)

    a. Examine your own health-related behaviors (nutrition, exercise, use of drugs, etc.) to see how these might affect risks for both osteoporosis and heart disease.

    b. What changes could you make now to decrease these risks? Be specific!

    c. Do you think the answers for question B will be different for a 20 year old, a 40 year old, and a 60 year old?

    d. How could health policies and health education for young people be most appropriate for maximizing the possibility for a healthy old age?

3. Pretend you are a health educator designing a poster for mid-life (35–65 year old) women to encourage positive images and health promotion. Describe what your poster could look like.

4. Healthy mid-life women are a huge market. Observe how products and lifestyle issues are marketed to this group in magazines, in tv ads, and talk shows. What messages do women get about aging? What information is given about specific products? Do you think woman have the information they need to evaluate whether they "need" a product and whether it is safe?

5. Read the information on HRT in this chapter. (Better yet, read the scientific report from the Writing Group for the Women's Health Initiative in *JAMA*, 2002, 288(3), 321–333, and scientific articles on the March, 2004 reports.) Compare the scientific information on findings about HRT with how that information got covered in the popular press at that time.

6. Interview two older women about the following issues and summarize their answers.

    a. Ask them their age and ask them to think about how one or two women's health issues have changed in their lifetimes. How do they think women's health issues are different for today's 20–30 year old women than they were when they were that age?

Woman 1	Woman 2

    b. Ask them to describe their attitudes and experiences of menopause and what they think influenced their attitudes and experiences? Were they surprised by the "news" that estrogen and HRT have serious health risks? How has that "news" and other information influenced their decisions about medication for menopause symptoms and for osteoporosis and heart disease prevention?

Woman 1	Woman 2

    c. Ask them to identify key health issues in their lives today. How secure do they feel about being able to meet their health needs in the next five years and for the rest of their lives?

Woman 1	Woman 2

    d. Compare the answers you heard from these two women. In comparing their answers, think about how differences or similarities in age, race, class, sexual identity, education, religion, or other issues may have impacted on the differences or similarities in their answers.

CHAPTER 13

The Politics of Disease

The politics of disease can be seen in the decisions made by government agencies, pharmaceutical companies, and the health care industry regarding priorities in funding, research, services, and education. Another aspect of the politics of disease is how women interact as both consumers and practitioners with these systems to fight for the priorities we identify. The first section of this chapter focuses on breast cancer, which it is estimated that one out of eight women in the United States will develop. The excerpt, "Breast Cancer: Power vs. Prosthesis," from *The Cancer Journals* by Audre Lorde, an extraordinary writer who died of breast cancer, examines the complexities around Lorde's decision not to use a prosthesis after mastectomy. The reader is encouraged to think about ways this article illustrates a number of themes in this book. While some women feel the use of a breast prosthesis or implants will be an important part of their coping with or healing from breast cancer, other women will identify with Lorde in not wanting to hide the battle they are fighting or have won. Thus Lorde's "Power vs. Prosthesis" can be considered a critique of a medical system which too often assumes "one size fits all." Similarly, this important classic symbolizes body image issues where there is too narrow a definition of what women should look like and there is enormous pressure for women to "fit" this image no matter how inappropriate it is for their health and well-being. (Also see Lorde's essays in Chapter 6, pp. 74–84: "Age, Race, and Sex: Women Redefining Difference" and "There Is No Hierarchy of Oppression.")

We draw your attention to Rita Arditti and Tatiana Schreiber's "Breast Cancer: The Environmental Connection" because it so eloquently asks us to think about what it would mean to *prevent* breast cancer rather than merely detect it or treat it. The worksheet encourages students to compare what is known about the prevention, diagnosis, and treatment of cancers. Students are always surprised and disappointed with how little they can find about the prevention of cancers compared to what is known about detection and treatment. This certainly demonstrates the priorities and funding for cancer research and this reflects the pressure for researchers to be able to design quick fix studies, which will get measurable, statistically significant findings in the short time frame of most funding cycles. Contrast that to the reality of how cancer works. In the excellent *Dr. Susan Love's Breast Book,* Dr. Love suggests that breast cancer rates could be reduced by 25% by reducing the amount of fat in the diet and decreasing obesity in a population but she quotes a researcher who has acknowledged "that the changes in the diet would probably have to start at age five, and would have a 20 year lag until an effect would even be seen, and (it would be) 80 years until the maximum effect would be realized" (Love, 1995, p. 235).

A crucial question about breast cancer, and all other diseases, is how can we shift the medical interest and funding from detection and treatment to primary prevention? The importance of this question and *not* confusing prevention, detection, and treatment are demonstrated in other articles. The frightening articles on mammograms argue that instead of looking at the complexities of breast cancer, the public has been duped into simplistically accepting that mammography is always good and that early detection will save lives. These articles, addressing the possible dangers of mammography for premenopausal women, are not intended to scare women. We hope they increase awareness of the limitations of mammography, the dangers that when people "strongly believe in something, (they) don't waste time looking at evidence that challenges their beliefs," and the urgent need to shift action and research to breast cancer prevention. There is now a whole pink-ribbon, mammography-promoting culture which has grown up around the inaccurate slogan, "early detection is your best prevention." Few know that this slogan and National Breast Cancer Awareness Month were conceived of and promoted by Imperial Chemical Corporation, now Zeneca, the manufacturer of tamoxifen and one of the world's largest producers and users of chlorinated products which are believed to increase breast cancer. The medicalization of prevention is examined in Rita Arditti's article on tamoxifen. She critiques that this drug, with powerful side effects (including endometrial cancer), previously successfully used for breast cancer *treatment,* is now being marketed to healthy women to supposedly prevent breast cancer: "It is frightening to think that our most influential scientists and physicians doing cancer research have bought into the cancer industry's definition of breast cancer prevention. The whole concept of prevention has been distorted to fit the needs of greedy companies . . . exchanging breast cancer for other life threatening problems will be considered a success." While breast cancer affects all groups of women, incidence, mortality rates, and survival rates vary considerably. Some of these differences may reflect access to and appropriateness of health care, though there certainly are other factors such as diet and exposure to environmental carcinogens which impact differently on different groups of women. The four fact sheets produced by the National Women's Health Network on breast cancer issues for Asian American, Native American, Latina, and African American women highlight these differences and remind us that, in analyzing any health issue, we need to keep in mind the different issues for different groups of women.

Heart disease in women has become a "hot" topic for media coverage, but "A Survey of Attitudes and Experiences of Women with Heart Disease" demonstrates that the "Wear Red Day" (first Friday in February) for women's heart disease awareness is as much about image rather than substance as those pink ribbons encouraging mammograms for breast cancer *prevention*. Despite the media attention on heart disease as the leading cause of both disability and death in women, it turns out that health care practitioners are not good at recognizing the seriousness of heart disease in women and identifying it or treating it appropriately. Heart disease deserves attention for symbolizing that despite decades of women's health research and activism, the medical system still fails to meet the needs of women: "heart disease tends to be delayed or missed more often in women than in men and women are less likely than men to receive proven therapies or to be treated according to established clinical guidelines." In this survey of women with heart disease, "more than half expressed dissatisfaction with their health care, most often because of physician-related knowledge and communication."

Donna Kiefer's article on chronic fatigue syndrome examines a health issue which disproportionately affects women and is often trivialized or assumed to be "all in her head." As a former high powered attorney, she describes learning to live with her disability, "struggling just to make breakfast or take a shower" and the importance of both a support group for women with CFIDS and finding her inner strengths. Similarly, "Vagina Dialogue" describes what it is like to go from being a radio host to someone living on disability benefits because chronic vulvar pain controls so much of Caroline Moore's life, including whether she can even sit down. Both articles emphasize the isolation and frustration of having a disease which is not taken seriously or is not talked about.

Endometriosis used to be one of the conditions which was not understood or talked about, but the Endometriosis Association (1-800-992-3636) certainly changed that. The Endometriosis Association has long been one of the best examples of consumer activism and an organization built around giving voice to women with the issue. This group has been able to influence the health system by providing information about endometriosis, as learned from women who experience this disease, as well as providing support and information for women with endometriosis. "Endometriosis: New Developments" highlights the Association's increasingly visible role in drawing attention to the connections between environmental issues and endometriosis and supporting research on increased risks associated with endometriosis.

Silence about diseases takes on additional meanings when we are talking about diseases which can be spread from one person to another. The last four articles in this chapter address different aspects of the politics of sexually transmitted infections (STIs.) "What to Ask Your Gynecologist" resembles an STI-specific, updated version of the classic, "How to Tell Your Doctor a Thing or Two" in Chapter 1, p. 24. "What to Ask" looks at the hit and miss, mostly totally inadequate, way U.S. health practitioners address STIs despite the fact that "the U.S. has the highest infection rate of any industrialized nation: one out of 4–5 people will have an STI in their lifetime, and STIs are a major cause of cervical cancer, pelvic inflammatory disease, ectopic pregnancy, and infertility for women." While the answer of providing routine effective screening and treatment seems obvious, Molly M. Ginty identifies barriers (people not having insurance, insurance not covering screening, lack of consistent protocols, physicians' attitudes) which too often prevent this, so she gives women a list of ways to be more active patients around their sexual health. Both "What to Ask" and "Waging War on STDs" look at the good news that important new STI prevention and detection products are being developed. However, the misguided priorities around disease economics is most apparent when we read that more than 21 million American women (and billions around the world) say they are eager to use microbicides to prevent STIs, but "the major obstacle to microbicide development is a lack of funding and support from large pharmaceutical companies" who have decided microbicides won't make enough money.

"With or Without the Dam Thing: The Lesbian Safer Sex Debates" is an all-too-rare article both because it specifically addresses lesbian sexual health and because it addresses (HIV) disease prevention in a sex-positive, explicit manner, which looks at risks associated with specific activities. The material in this article will be useful or at least thought-provoking for anyone who is sexually active with a partner or partners.

"The Gendered Epidemic: Women and the Risks and Burdens of HIV" presents a global, gendered analysis demonstrating why "a gender dimension needs to be a central part of all AIDS strategies . . . (and) that AIDS needs to be a part of all gender strategies." Whether we're looking at why women contract HIV more easily than men, how their expected caretaking roles mean AIDS epidemics fall disproportionally as an extra burden for women, or how violence against women relates to HIV, Peter Plot reminds us that:

> The impact of AIDS is gendered in its every aspect. Women's HIV vulnerability derives particularly from contexts in which they have little control over sex, whether as a consequence of the predominating power relations between men and women or as a function of the economic and life choices available to them.

Breast Cancer

Power vs. Prosthesis

by Audre Lorde

On Labor Day, 1978, during my regular monthly self-examination, I discovered a lump in my right breast which later proved to be malignant. During my following hospitalization, my mastectomy and its aftermath, I passed through many stages of pain, despair, fury, sadness and growth. I moved through these stages, sometimes feeling as if I had no choice, other times recognizing that I could choose oblivion—or a passivity that is very close to oblivion—but did not want to. As I slowly began to feel more equal to processing and examining the different parts of this experience, I also began to feel that in the process of losing a breast I had become a more whole person.

After a mastectomy, for many women including myself, there is a feeling of wanting to go back, of not wanting to persevere through this experience to whatever enlightenment might be at the core of it. And it is this feeling, this nostalgia, which is encouraged by most of the post-surgical counselling for women with breast cancer. This regressive tie to the past is emphasized by the concentration upon breast cancer as a cosmetic problem, one which can be solved by a prosthetic pretence. The American Cancer Society's Reach for Recovery Program, while doing a valuable service in contacting women immediately after surgery and letting them know they are not alone, nonetheless encourages this false and dangerous nostalgia in the mistaken belief that women are too weak to deal directly and courageously with the realities of our lives.

The woman from Reach for Recovery who came to see me in the hospital, while quite admirable and even impressive in her own right, certainly did not speak to my experience nor my concerns. As a 44-year-old Black lesbian feminist, I knew there were very few role models around for me in this situation, but my primary concerns two days after mastectomy were hardly about what man I could capture in the future, whether or not my old boyfriend would still find me attractive enough, and even less about whether my two children would be embarrassed by me around their friends

My concerns were about my chances for survival, the effects of a possibly shortened life upon my work and my priorities. Could this cancer have been prevented, and what could I do in the future to prevent its recurrence? Would I be able to maintain the control over my life that I had always taken for granted? A lifetime of loving women had taught me that when women love each other, physical change does not alter that love. It did not occur to me that anyone who really loved me would love me any less because I had one breast instead of two, although it did occur to me to wonder if they would be able to love and deal with the new me.

In the critical and vulnerable period following surgery, self-examination and self-evaluation are positive steps. To imply to a woman that yes, she can be the 'same' as before surgery, with the skillful application of a little puff of lambswool, and/or silicone gel, is to place an emphasis upon prosthesis which encourages her not to deal with herself as physically and emotionally real, even though altered and traumatized. This emphasis upon the cosmetic after surgery reinforces this society's stereotype of women, that we are only what we look or appear, so this is the only aspect of our existence we need to address. Any woman who has had a breast removed because of cancer knows she does not feel the same. But we are allowed no psychic time or space to examine what our true feelings are, to make them our own.

Ten days after having my breast removed, I went to my doctor's office to have the stitches taken out. This was my first journey out since coming home from the hospital, and I was truly looking forward to it. A friend had washed my hair for me and it was black and shining, with my new grey hairs glistening in the sun. Colour was starting to come back into my face and around my eyes, I wore the most opalescent of my moonstones, and a single floating bird dangling from my right ear in the name of grand asymmetry. With an African kentecloth tunic and new leather boots, I knew I looked fine, with that brave new-born security of a beautiful woman having come through a very hard time and being very glad to be alive.

The doctor's nurse, a charmingly bright and steady woman of about my own age who had always given me a feeling of quiet no-nonsense support on my other visits, called me into the examining room. On the way, she asked me how I was feeling.

'Pretty good,' I said, half-expecting her to make some comment about how good I looked.

'You're not wearing a prosthesis,' she said, a little anxiously, and not at all like a question.

'No,' I said, thrown off my guard for a minute. 'It really doesn't feel right,' referring to the lambswool puff given to me by the Reach For Recovery volunteer in the hospital.

Usually supportive and understanding, the nurse now looked at me urgently and disapprovingly as she told me that even if it didn't look exactly right, it was 'better than nothing,' and that as soon as my stitches were out I could be fitted for a 'real form'.

'You will feel so much better with it on,' she said. 'And besides, we really like you to wear something, at least when you come in. Otherwise it's bad for the morale of the office.'

I could hardly believe my ears! I was too outraged to speak then, but this was to be only the first such assault on my right to define and to claim my own body.

A woman who is attempting to come to terms with her changed landscape and changed timetable of life and with her own body and pain and beauty and strength, that woman is seen as a threat to the 'morale' of a breast surgeon's office!

Yet when Moishe Dayan, the Prime Minister of Israel, stands up in front of parliament or on TV with an eye patch over his empty eye socket, nobody tells him to go get a glass eye, or that he is bad for the morale of the office. The world sees him as a warrior with an honourable wound, and a loss of a piece of himself which he has marked, and mourned, and moved beyond. And if you have trouble dealing with Moishe Dayan's empty eye-socket, everyone recognises that it is your problem to solve, not his.

Well, women with breast cancer are warriors, also. I have been to war, and still am. So has every women who had had one or both breasts amputated because of the cancer that is becoming the primary physical scourge of our time. For me, my scars are an honorable reminder that I may be a casualty in the cosmic war against radiation, animal fat, air pollution, McDonald's hamburgers and Red Dye no. 2, but the fight is still going on, and I am still a part of it. I refuse to have my scars hidden or trivialised behind lambswool or silicone gel. I refuse to

be reduced in my own eyes or in the eyes of others from warrior to mere victim, simply because it might render me a fraction more acceptable or less dangerous to the still complacent, those who believe if you cover up a problem it ceases to exist. I refuse to hide my body simply because it might make a woman-phobic world more comfortable.

Prosthesis offers the empty comfort of 'nobody will know the difference'. But it is that very difference which I wish to affirm, because I had lived it, and survived it, and wish to share that strength with other women. If we are to translate the silence surrounding breast cancer into language and action against this scourge, then the first step is that women with mastectomies must become visible to each other. For silence and invisibility go hand in hand with powerlessness. By accepting the mask or prosthesis, one-breasted women proclaim ourselves as insufficients dependent upon pretence.

In addition, we withhold that visibility and support from one another which is such an aid to perspective and self-acceptance.

As women, we cannot afford to look the other way, nor to consider the incidence of breast cancer as a private or secret personal problem. It is no secret that breast cancer is on the increase among women in America. According to the American Cancer Society's own statistics on breast cancer survival, of women stricken, only 50% are still alive after three years. This figure drops to 30% if you are poor, or Black, or in any other way part of the underside of this society. We cannot ignore these facts, nor their implications, nor their effect upon our lives, individually and collectively. Early detection and early treatment is crucial in the management of breast cancer if those sorry statistics of survival are to improve. But for the incidence of early detection and early treatment to increase, American women must become free enough from social stereotypes concerning their appearance to realize that losing a breast is infinitely preferable to losing one's life (or one's eyes, or one's hands . . .).

Although breast self-examination does not reduce the incidence of breast cancer, it does markedly reduce the rate of mortality, since most early tumours are found by women themselves. I discovered my own tumour upon a monthly breast exam, and so report most of the other women I know with a good prognosis for survival. With our alert awareness making such a difference in the survival rate for breast cancer, women need to face the possibility and the actuality of breast cancer as a reality rather than a myth, or retribution, or terror in the night, or a bad dream that will disappear if ignored. After surgery, there is a need for women to be aware of the possibility of bilateral recurrence, with vigilance rather than terror. This is not a spread of cancer, but a new occurrence in the other breast. Each woman must be aware that an honest acquaintanceship with and evaluation of her own body is the best tool of detection.

The greatest incidence of breast cancer in American women appears between the ages of 40 to 55. These are the very years when women are portrayed in the popular media as fading and desexualised figures. Contrary to the media picture, I find myself as a woman of insight ascending into my highest powers, my greatest psychic strengths, and my fullest satisfactions. I am freer of the constraints and fears and indecisions of my younger years, and survival throughout these years has taught me how to value my own beauty, and how to look closely into the beauty of others.

There is nothing wrong, *per se,* with the use of prostheses, if they can be chosen freely, for whatever reason, after a woman has had a chance to accept her new body. But usually prostheses serve a real function, to approximate the performance of a missing physical part. In other amputations and with other prosthetic devices, function is the main point of their existence. Artificial limbs perform specific tasks, allowing us to manipulate or to walk. Dentures allow us to chew our food. Only false breasts are designed for appearance only, as if the only real function of women's breasts were to appear in a certain shape and size and symmetry to onlookers, or to yield to external pressure. For no woman wearing a prosthesis can even for one moment believe it is her own breast, any more than a woman wearing falsies can.

Attitudes towards the necessity for prostheses after breast surgery are merely a reflection of those attitudes within our society towards women in general as objectified and depersonalised sexual conveniences. Women have been programmed to view our bodies only in terms of how they look and feel to others, rather than how they feel to ourselves, and how we wish to use them. As women, we fight this depersonalisation every day, this pressure towards the conversion of one's own self-image into a media expectation of what might satisfy male demand. The insistence upon breast prosthesis as 'decent' rather than functional is an additional example of that wipe-out of self in which women are constantly encouraged to take part. I am personally affronted by the message that I am only acceptable if I look 'right' or 'normal', where those norms have nothing to do with my own perceptions of who I am. Where 'normal' means the 'right' colour, shape, size, or number of breasts, a woman's perception of her own body and the strengths that come from that perception are discouraged, trivialised, and ignored.

Every woman has a right to define her own desires, make her own choices. But prostheses are often chosen, not from desire, but in default. Some women complain it is too much effort to fight the concerted pressure exerted by the fashion industry. Being one-breasted does not mean being unfashionable; it means giving some time and energy to choosing or constructing the proper clothes. In some cases, it means making or remaking clothing or jewelry. The fact that the fashion needs of one-breasted women are not currently being met doesn't mean that the concerted pressure of our demands cannot change that.

Some women believe that a breast prosthesis is necessary to preserve correct posture and physical balance. But the weight of each breast is never the same to begin with, nor is the human body ever exactly the same on both sides. With a minimum of exercises to develop the habit of straight posture, the body can accommodate to one-breastedness quite easily, even when the breasts were quite heavy.

Women in public and private employment have reported the loss of jobs and promotions upon their return to work after a mastectomy, without regard to whether or not they wore prostheses. The social and economic discrimination practised against women who have breast cancer is not diminished by pretending that mastectomies do not exist. Where a woman's job is at risk because of her health history, employment discrimination cannot be fought with a sack of silicone gel, nor with the constant fear and anxiety to which such subterfuge gives rise. Suggesting prosthesis as a solution to employment discrimination is like saying that the way to fight prejudice is for Black people to pretend to be white. Employment discrimination against post-mastectomy women can only be fought in the open, with head-on attacks by strong and self-accepting women who refuse to be relegated to an inferior position, or to cower in a corner because they have one breast.

Within the framework of superficiality and pretence, the next logical step of a depersonalising and woman-devaluating culture is the advent of the atrocity euphemistically called 'breast reconstruction'. It should be noted that research being done on this potentially life-threatening practice represents time and research money spent—not on how to prevent the cancers that cost us our breasts and our lives—but rather upon how to pretend that our breasts are not gone, nor we as women at risk with our lives.

Any information about the prevention or treatment of breast cancer which might possibly threaten the vested interests of the American medical establishment is difficult to acquire in the country. Only through continuing scrutiny of various non-mainstream sources of information, such as alternative and women's presses, can a picture of new possibilities for prevention and treatment of breast cancer emerge.

The mortality for breast cancer treated by conventional therapies has not decreased in over 40 years (Rose Kushner, *Breast Cancer,* Harcourt, Brace & Jovanovitch, 1975, p. 161). Since the American medical establishment and the ACS are determined to suppress any cancer information not dependent upon western medical bias, whether this information is ultimately useful or not, we must pierce this silence ourselves and aggressively seek answers to these questions about new therapies. We must also heed the unavoidable evidence pointing towards the nutritional and environmental aspects of cancer prevention.

Cancer is not just another degenerative and unavoidable disease of the ageing process. It has distinct and identifiable causes, and these are mainly exposures to chemical or physical agents in the environment. In the medical literature, there is mounting evidence that breast cancer is a chronic systemic disease. Post-mastectomy women must be vigilantly aware that, contrary to the 'lightning strikes' theory, we are the most likely of all women to develop cancer somewhere else in the body.

Every woman has a militant responsibility to involve herself actively with her own health. We owe ourselves the protection of all the information we can acquire about the treatment of cancer and its causes, as well as about the recent findings concerning immunology, nutrition, environment and stress. And we owe ourselves this information *before* we may have a reason to use it.

It was very important for me, after my mastectomy, to develop and encourage my own internal sense of power. At all times, it felt crucial to me that I make a conscious commitment to survival. It is physically important for me to be loving my life rather than to be mourning my breast. I believe it is this love of my life and myself, and the careful tending of that love which was done by women who love and support me, which has been largely responsible for my strong and healthy recovery from the effects of my mastectomy. But a clear distinction must be made between this affirmation of self and the superficial farce of 'looking on the bright side of things'.

Last week I read a letter from a doctor in a medical magazine which said that no truly happy person ever gets cancer. Despite my knowing better, and despite my having dealt with this blame-the-victim thinking for years, for a moment this letter hit my guilt button. Had I really been guilty of the crime of not being happy in this best of all possible infernos?

The idea that the cancer patient should be made to feel guilty about having had cancer, as if in some way it were all her fault for not having been in the right psychological frame of mind at all times to prevent cancer, is a monstrous distortion of the idea that we can use our psychic strengths to help heal ourselves. This guilt trip which many cancer patients have been led into (you see, it is a shameful thing because you could have prevented it if only you had been more . . .) is an extension of the blame-the-victim syndrome. It does nothing to encourage the mobilisation of our psychic defenses against the very real forms of death which surround us. It is easier to demand happiness than to clean up the environment. The acceptance of illusion and appearance as reality is another symptom of this same refusal to examine the realities of our lives. Let us seek 'joy' rather than real food and clean air and a saner future on a liveable earth! As if happiness alone can protect us from the results of profit-madness.

Was I wrong to be working so hard against the oppressions afflicting women and Black people? Was I in error to be speaking out against our silent passivity and the cynicism of a mechanized and inhuman civilisation that is destroying our earth and those who live upon it? Was I really fighting the spread of radiation, racism, woman-slaughter, chemical invasion of our food, pollution of our environment, the abuse and psychic destruction of our young, merely to avoid dealing with my first and greatest responsibility—to be happy?

The only really happy people I have ever met are those of us who work against these deaths with all the energy of our living, recognising the deep and fundamental unhappiness with which we are surrounded, at the same time as we fight to keep from being submerged by it. The idea that happiness can insulate us against the results of our environmental madness is a rumour circulated by our enemies to destroy us. And what Woman of Colour in America over the age of 15 does not live with the knowledge that our daily lives are stitched with violence and with hatred, and to naively ignore that reality can mean destruction? We are equally destroyed by false happiness and false breasts, and the passive acceptance of false values which corrupt our lives and distort our experience.

The idea of having a breast removed was much more traumatic for me before my mastectomy than after the fact, but it certainly took time and the loving support of other women before I could once again look at and love my altered body with the warmth I had done before. But I did.

Right after surgery I had a sense that I would never be able to bear missing that great well of sexual pleasure that I connected with my right breast. That sense has completely passed away, as I have come to realise that that well of feeling was within me. I alone own my feelings. I can never lose that feeling because I own it, because it comes out of myself. I can attach it anywhere I want to, because my feelings are a part of me, my sorrow and my joy.

I would never have chosen this path, but I am very glad to be who I am, here.

30 March 1979

Breast Cancer

The Environmental Connection

by Rita Arditti and Tatiana Schreiber

Today in the United States, we live in the midst of a cancer epidemic. One out of every three people will get some form of cancer and one out of four will die from it. Cancer is currently the second leading cause of death; by the year 2000, it will likely have become the primary cause of death. It is now more than two decades since the National Cancer Act was signed, yet the treatments offered to cancer patients are the same as those offered 50 years ago: surgery, radiation, and chemotherapy (or slash, burn, and poison, as they are called bitterly by both patients and increasingly disappointed professionals). And in spite of sporadic optimistic pronouncements from the cancer establishment, survival rates for the three main cancer killers—lung, breast, and colo-rectal cancer—have remained virtually unchanged.

In the '60s and '70s, environmental activists and a few scientists emphasized that cancer was linked to environmental contamination, and their concerns began to have an impact on public understanding of the disease. In the '80s and '90s, however, with an increasingly conservative political climate and concerted efforts on the part of industry to play down the importance of chemicals as a cause of cancer, we are presented with a new image of cancer. Now it is portrayed as an individual problem that can only be overcome with the help of experts and, then, only if one has the money and know-how to recruit them for one's personal survival efforts. This emphasis on personal responsibility and lifestyle factors has reached absurd proportions. People with cancer are asked why they "brought this disease on themselves" and why they don't work harder at "getting well."

While people with cancer should be encouraged not to fall into victim roles and to do everything possible to strengthen their immune systems (our primary line of defense against cancer), it seems that the sociopolitical and economic dimensions of cancer have been pushed completely out of the picture. "Blaming the victim" is a convenient way to avoid looking at the larger environmental and social issues that form individual experiences. Here we want to talk about environmental links to cancer in general and to breast cancer in particular, the kinds of research that should be going on, why they're not happening, and the political strategies needed to turn things around.

Extensive evidence exists to indicate that cancer is an environmental disease. Even the most conservative scientists agree that approximately 80 percent of all cancers are in some way related to environmental factors. Support for this view relies on four lines of evidence: (1) dramatic differences in the incidences of cancer between communities—incidences of cancer among people of a given age in different parts of the world can vary by a factor of ten to a hundred; (2) changes in the incidence of cancer (either lower or higher rates) in groups that migrate to a new country; (3) changes in the incidence of particular types of cancer with the passage of time; and (4) the actual identification of the specific causes of certain cancers (such as the case of beta-naphthylamine, responsible for an epidemic of bladder cancer among dye workers employed at du Pont factories). Other well-known environmentally linked cancers are lung cancer, linked to asbestos, arsenic, chromium, bischloromethyl ether, mustard gas, ionizing radiation, nickel, polycyclic hydrocarbons in soot, tar, oil, and of course, smoking; endometrial cancer, linked to estrogen use; thyroid cancer, often the result of childhood irradiation; and liver cancer, linked to exposure to vinyl chloride.

The inescapable conclusion is that if cancer is largely environmental in origin, it is largely preventable.

Our Environment Is a Health Hazard

"Environment" as we use it here includes not only air, water, and soil, but also our diets, medical procedures, and living and working conditions. That means that

From *Sojourner: The Women's Forum,* (December, 1992). Copyright © 1992 by Sojourner, Inc. Reprinted by permission.

the food we eat, the water we drink, the air we breathe, the radiation to which we are exposed, where we live, what kind of work we do, and the stress that we suffer—these are responsible for at least 80 percent of all cancers. For instance, under current EPA regulations as many as 60 cancer-causing pesticides can legally be used to grow the most commonly eaten foods. Some of these foods are allowed to contain 20 or more carcinogens, making it impossible to measure how much of each substance a person actually consumes. As Rachel Carson wrote in *Silent Spring* in 1962, "This piling up of chemicals from many different sources creates a total exposure that cannot be measured. It is meaningless, therefore, to talk about the 'safety' of any specific amount of residues." In other words, our everyday food is an environmental hazard to our health.

Recently, a study on the trends in cancer mortality in industrialized countries has revealed that while stomach cancer has been steadily declining, brain and other central-nervous-system cancers, breast cancer, multiple myeloma, kidney cancer, non-Hodgkin's lymphoma, and melanoma have increased in persons aged 55 and older. Given this context, it is not extreme to suspect that breast cancer, which has reached epidemic proportions in the United States, may be linked to environmental ills. This year, estimates are that 180,000 women will develop breast cancer and 46,000 will die from it. In other words, in the coming year, nearly as many women will die from breast cancer as there were American lives lost in the entire Vietnam War. Cancer is the leading cause of death among women aged 35 to 54, with about a third of these deaths due to breast cancer. Breast cancer incidence data meet three of the four lines of reasoning linking it to the environment: (1) the incidence of breast cancer between communities can vary by a factor of seven; (2) the risk for breast cancer among populations that have migrated becomes that of their new residence within a generation, as is the case for Japanese women who have migrated to the United States; and (3) the incidence of breast cancer in the United States has swelled from one in twenty in 1940 to one in eight in the '90s.

A number of factors have been linked to breast cancer; a first blood relative with the disease, early onset of menstruation, late age at first full-term pregnancy, higher socioeconomic status, late menopause, being Jewish, etc. However, for the overwhelming majority (70 to 80 percent) of breast cancer patients, their illness is not clearly linked to any of these factors. Research suggests that the development of breast cancer probably depends on a complex interplay among environmental exposures, genetic predisposition to the disease, and hormonal activity.

Research on the actual identification of causal factors, however, is given low priority and proceeds at a snail's pace. We still don't know, for example, the effects of birth control pills and the hormone replacement therapy routinely offered to menopausal women. Hormonal treatments are fast becoming the method of choice for the treatment of infertility, while we know nothing about their long-range effects. And the standard addition of hormones in animal feed means that all women (and men) are exposed to hormone residues in meat. Since there is general consensus that estrogen somehow plays a role in the development of breast cancer, hormonal interventions (through food or drugs) are particularly worrisome.

A startling example of the lack of interest in the prevention of breast cancer is the saga of the proposed study on the supposed link between high-fat diets and breast cancer. The "Women's Health Trial," a fifteen-year study designed to provide conclusive data about the high fat-cancer link, was denied funding by the National Cancer Advisory Board despite having been revised to answer previous criticisms and despite feasibility studies indicating that a full-scale trial was worth launching. Fortunately, it now appears that the study will be part of the Women's Health Initiative, a $500-million effort that will look at women's health issues. This success story is a direct result of women's activism and pressures from women's health groups across the country.

But even if the high fat-breast cancer correlation is established, it is unlikely to fully explain how breast cancer develops. The breast is rich in adipose cells, and carcinogens that accumulate in these fat tissues may be responsible for inducing cancer rather than the fat itself or the fat alone. Environmental contamination of human breast milk with PCBs, PBBs and DDE (a metabolite of the pesticide DDT) is a widely acknowledged phenomenon. These fat-soluble substances are poorly metabolized and have a long half-life in human tissue. They may also interact with one another, creating an additive toxic effect, and they may carry what are called "incidental contaminants": compounds like dibenzofurans, dioxins, etc., each with its own toxic properties.

Among the established effects of these substances are: liver dysfunction, skin abnormalities, neurological and behavioral abnormalities, immunological aberrations, thyroid dysfunction, gastrointestinal disturbances, reproductive dysfunction, tumor growth, and enzyme induction. Serious concerns have been raised about the risks that this contamination entails for infants who are breast-fed. But what is outrageous in the discussion about human breast-milk poisoning is that little or no mention is made of the possible effects on the women themselves, particularly since it is known that most of these substances have *estrogenic* properties (that is, they behave like estrogen in the body). It is as if the women, whose breasts contain these carcinogens, do not exist. We witness the paradox of women being made invisible, even while their toxic breasts are put under the microscope.

The Pesticide Studies

Very recently, some scientists have at last begun to look at the chemical-breast cancer connection. In 1990, two Israeli scientists from Hebrew University's Hadassah School of Medicine, Elihu Richter and Jerry Westin, reported a surprising statistic. They found that Israel was the only country among 28 countries surveyed that registered a real drop in breast cancer mortality in the decade 1976 to 1986. This happened in the face of a worsening of all known risk factors, such as fat intake and age at first pregnancy. As Westin noted, "All and all, we expected a rise in breast cancer mortality of approximately 20 percent overall, and what we found was that there was an 8 percent drop, and in the youngest age group, the drop was 34 percent, as opposed to an expected 20 percent rise, so, if we put those two together, we are talking about a difference of about 50 percent, which is enormous."

Westin and Richter could not account for the drop solely in terms of demographic changes or improved medical intervention. Instead, they suspected it might have been related to a 1978 ban on three carcinogenic pesticides (benzene hexachloride, lindane, and DDT) that heavily contaminated milk and milk products in Israel. Prior to 1978, Westin said, "at least one of them [the three pesticides] was found in the milk here at a rate 100 times greater than it was in the U.S. in the same period, and in the worst case, nearly a thousand times greater." This observation led Westin and Richter to hypothesize that there might be a connection between the decrease in exposure following the ban and the decrease in breast cancer mortality. They believed the pesticides could have promoted enzymes that in turn increased the virulence of breast cancer in women. When the pesticides were removed from the diet, Westin and Richter speculated, there was a situation of much less virulent cancer and the mortality from breast cancer fell.

Westin and Richter are convinced that there is a critical need to increase awareness about environmental conditions and cancer. Health care clinicians, for example, could play an important role in the detection of potential exposures to toxic chemicals that might be missed in large studies. This is a refreshing view since it encourages individual physicians to ask questions about work environments, living quarters, and diet, the answers to which could provide important clues about the cancer-environment connection.

In the United States, only one study we know of has directly measured chemical residues in women who have breast cancer compared to those who do not. Dr. Mary Wolff, a chemist at New York's Mount Sinai School of Medicine, recently conducted a pilot study with Dr. Frank Falck (then at Hartford Hospital in Hartford, Connecticut) that was published in *The Archives of Environmental Health.* In this case-controlled study, Falck and Wolff found that several chemical residues from pesticides and PCBs were elevated in cases of malignant disease as compared to nonmalignant cases.

The study involved 25 women with breast cancer and the same number of women who had biopsies but did not have breast cancer. The results showed differences significant enough to interest the National Institute for Environmental Health Sciences, which will fund a larger study to look at the level of DDT and its metabolites in the blood samples of 15,000 women attending a breast cancer screening clinic in New York. A recent report just released by Greenpeace, entitled "Breast Cancer and the Environment: The Chlorine Connection," provides further evidence linking industrial chemicals to breast cancer.

In the United States, levels of pesticide residues in adipose tissue have been decreasing since the 1970s (following the banning of DDT and decreased use of other carcinogenic pesticides) while the breast cancer rate continues to rise. This observation would seem to contradict the pesticide hypothesis. However, it is important to remember that the chemicals could act differently at different exposure levels, they are unlikely to act alone, and the time of exposure may be important. For example, if a child is exposed during early adolescence, when breast tissue is growing rapidly, the result may be different than exposure later in life.

Radiation and Mammography

Another area that demands urgent investigation is the role of radiation in the development of breast cancer. It is widely accepted that ionizing radiation at high doses causes breast cancer, but low doses are generally regarded as safe. Questions remain, however, regarding the shape of the dose-response curve, the length of the latency period, and the importance of age at time of exposure. These questions are of great importance to women because of the emphasis on mammography for early detection. There is evidence that mammography screening reduces death from breast cancer in women aged 50 or older. However, Dr. Rosalie Bertell (director of the International Institute of Concern for Public Health, author of *No Immediate Danger: Prognosis for a*

Radioactive World [1985] and well-known critic of the nuclear establishment) raises serious questions about mammography screening. In a paper entitled "Comments on Ontario Mammography Program," Bertell criticized a breast cancer screening program planned by the Ontario Health Minister in 1989. Bertell argued that the program, which would potentially screen 300,000 women, was a plan to "reduce breast cancer death by increasing breast cancer incidence."

Bertell's critique of mammography suggests that the majority of cancers that would have occurred in the group could have been detected by other means. A recent Canadian mammography study on 90,000 women looked at cancer rates between 1980 and 1988. Preliminary results show that for women aged 40 to 49, mammograms have no benefits and may indeed harm them: 44 deaths were found in the group that received mammograms and 29 in the control group. The study also suggests that for women aged 50 to 69, many of the benefits attributed to mammography in earlier studies "may have been provided by the manual breast exams that accompanied the procedure and not by the mammography," as Bertell noted in her paper. Not surprisingly, the study has been mired in controversy. As study director Dr. Anthony Miller remarked, "I've come up with an answer that people are not prepared to accept."

According to Bertell, the present breast cancer epidemic is a direct result of "above ground weapons testing" done in Nevada between 1951 and 1963, when 200 nuclear bombs were set off and the fallout dispersed across the country. Because the latency period for breast cancer peaks at about 40 years, this is an entirely reasonable hypothesis.

Other studies have looked at the effect of "low-level" radiation on cancer development. A study investigating the incidence of leukemia in southeastern Massachusetts found a positive association with radiation released from the Pilgrim nuclear power plant. (The study was limited to cases first diagnosed between 1978 and 1986.) In adult cases diagnosed before 1984, the risk of leukemia was almost four times higher for individuals with the greatest potential for exposure to the emissions of the plant. Other types of cancer take a greater number of years to develop, and there is no reason to assume that excessive radiation emission was limited to the 1978-to-1986 time frame. In other words, as follow-up studies continue, other cancers (including breast cancer) may also show higher rates.

The Surveillance Theory

Current theory supports the concept that cancerous mutations are a common phenomenon in the body of normal individuals and that the immune system intervenes before mutated cells can multiply. Known as the "surveillance" theory of cancer, the basic premise is that cancer can develop when the immune system fails to eliminate mutant cells. Carcinogenic mutations can be induced by radiation or chemicals, for instance, and if immunological competence is reduced at a critical time, the mutated cells can thrive and grow.

Given the apparent importance of the immune system in protecting us from cancer, we ought to be concerned not only with eliminating carcinogens in our environment but also with making certain that our immune systems are not under attack. Recent evidence that ultraviolet radiation depresses the immune system is therefore particularly ominous. At a hearing on "Global Change Research: Ozone Depletion and Its Impacts," held in November 1991 by the Senate Committee on Commerce, Science, and Transportation, a panel of scientists reported that ozone depletion is even more serious than previously thought. According to the data, the ozone layer over the United States is thinning at a rate of 3 to 5 percent per decade, resulting in increased ultraviolet radiation that "will reduce the quantity and quality of crops, increase skin cancer, *suppress the immune system,* and disrupt marine ecosystems" [our emphasis]. (The report also states that a 10 percent decrease in ozone will lead to approximately 1.7 million additional cases of cataracts world-wide per year and at least 250,000 additional cases of skin cancer.) As the writers make chillingly clear, since this is happening literally over our heads, there is no place for us to run.

In addition, dioxin (an extremely toxic substance that has been building up steadily in the environment since the growth of the chlorinated-chemical industry following World War II) can produce alterations that disrupt the immune system. "Free radicals" created by exposure to low-level radiation can cause immune system abnormalities. In other words, our basic mechanisms of defense against cancer are being weakened by the chemical soup in which we are immersed.

It follows that an intelligent and long-range cancer-prevention strategy would make a clean environment its number one priority. Prevention, however, is given low priority in our national cancer agenda. In 1992, out of an almost $2 billion National Cancer Institute (NCI) budget, $132.7 million was spent on breast cancer research but only about 15 percent of that was for preventive research. Moreover, research on the cellular mechanism of cancer development, toward which much of the "prevention" effort goes, does not easily get translated into actual prevention strategies.

In his 1989 exposé of the cancer establishment, *The Cancer Industry,* Ralph Moss writes that until the late '60s, the cancer establishment presented the view that "cancer is . . . widely believed to consist of a hereditable, and therefore genetic," problem. That line of thinking is still with us but with added emphasis on the personal responsibility we each have for our cancers (smoking and diet) and little or no acknowledgement of the larger environmental context. In a chapter appropriately titled "Preventing Prevention," Moss provides an inkling of why this is so.

The close ties between industry and two of the most influential groups determining our national cancer agenda—the National Cancer Advisory Board and the President's Cancer Panel—are revealing. The chair of the President's Cancer Panel throughout most of the '80s, for example, was Armand Hammer, head of Occidental International Corporation. Among its subsidiaries is Hooker Chemical Company, implicated in the environmental disaster in Love Canal. In addition, Moss, formerly assistant director of public affairs at Memorial Sloan-Kettering Cancer Center (MSKCC), outlines the structure and affiliations of that institution's leadership. MSKCC is the world's largest private cancer center, and the picture that emerges borders on the surreal: in 1988, 32.7 percent of its board of overseers were tied to the oil, chemical and automobile industries; 34.6 percent were professional investors (bankers, stockbrokers, venture capitalists). Board members included top officials of drug companies—Squibb, Bristol-Myers, Merck—and influential members of the media—CBS, the *New York Times,* Warner's Communications, and *Reader's Digest*—as well as leaders of the $55-billion cigarette industry.

Moss's research leaves little doubt about the allegiances of the cancer establishment. Actual cancer prevention would require a massive reorganization of industry, hardly in the interest of the industrial and financial elites. Instead of preventing the generation of chemical and toxic waste, the strategy adopted by industry and government has been one of "management." But as Barry Commoner, director of the Center for the Biology of Natural Systems at Queens College in Brooklyn, New York, put it rather succinctly, "The best way to stop toxic chemicals from entering the environment is to not produce them."

Instead, the latest "prevention" strategy for breast cancer moves in a completely different direction. A trial has been approved that will test the effect of a breast cancer drug (an antiestrogen, tamoxifen) in a healthy population, with the hope that it will have a preventive effect. The trial will involve 16,000 women considered at high risk for breast cancer and will be divided into a control group and a tamoxifen group. The National Women's Health Network (a national public-interest organization dedicated solely to women and health) is un-

equivocal in its criticism of the trial. Adriane Fugh-Berman, a member of the Network board, wrote in its September/October 1991 newsletter, "In our view the trial is premature in its assumptions, weak in its hypothesis, questionable in its ethics and misguided in its public health ramifications." The criticisms center on the fact that tamoxifen causes liver cancer in rats and liver changes in all species tested and that a number of endometrial cancers have been reported among tamoxifen users. Fugh-Berman points out that approving the testing of a potent, hormonal drug in healthy women and calling that "prevention" sets a dangerous precedent. This drug-oriented trial symbolizes, in a nutshell, the paradoxes of short-sighted cancer-prevention strategies: more drugs are used to counteract the effect of previous exposures to drugs, chemicals or other carcinogenic agents. It is a vicious circle and one that will not be easily broken.

Cancer, Poverty, Politics

Though it is often said that affluent women are at higher risk for breast cancer, this disease is actually on the rise (both incidence and mortality) among African-American women, hardly an "affluent" population overall. The African-American Breast Cancer Alliance of Minnesota, organized in October 1990, has noted this steady increase and the limited efforts that have been made to reach African Americans with information and prevention strategies. People of color often live in the most polluted areas of this country, where factories, incinerators, garbage, and toxic waste are part of the landscape. Native American nations are particularly targeted by waste-management companies that try to take advantage of the fact that "because of the sovereign relationship many reservations have with the federal government, they are not bound by the same environmental laws as the states around them."

Poverty and pollution go hand in hand. The 1988 Greenpeace report *Mortality and Toxics Along the Mississippi River* showed that the "total mortality rates and cancer mortality rates in the counties along the Mississippi River were significantly higher than in the rest of the nation's counties" and that "the areas of the river in which public health statistics are most troubling have populations which are disproportionately poor and black." These are also the areas that have the greatest number of toxic discharges. Louisiana has the dubious distinction of being the state with the most reported toxic releases—741.2 million pounds a year. Cancer rates in the Louisiana section of the "Chemical Corridor" (the highly industrialized stretch of river between Baton Rouge and New Orleans) are among the highest in the nation. Use of the Mississippi River as a drinking-water source has been linked to higher than average rates of cancer in Louisiana. The rates of cancer of the colon, bladder, kidney, rectum, and lung all exceed national averages. Louisiana Attorney General William J. Guste, Jr., has criticized state officials who claimed that people of color and the poor *naturally* have higher cancer rates. You can't "point out race and poverty as cancer factors," said Guste, "without asking if poor people or blacks . . . reside in less desirable areas more heavily impacted by industrial emissions."

It follows that African-American women, living in the most contaminated areas of this country, would indeed be showing a disproportionate increase in breast cancer incidence. However, widespread epidemiological studies to chart such a correlation have not been undertaken. For instance, given the evidence implicating pesticides in the development of breast cancer, studies of migrant (and other) farm workers who have been exposed to such chemicals would seem imperative.

Women's groups around the country have started organizing to fight the breast cancer epidemic. A National Breast Cancer Coalition was founded in 1991. Its agenda is threefold: to increase the funding for research, to organize, and to educate. All of the recently organized groups consider prevention a priority, and one of their tasks will undoubtedly entail defining what effective prevention really means. In Massachusetts, the Women's Community Cancer Project, which defines itself as a "grassroots organization created to facilitate changes in the current medical, social, and political approaches to cancer, particularly as they affect women," has developed a Women's Cancer Agenda to be presented to the federal government and the NCI. Several demands of the agenda address prevention and identification of the causes of cancer. The group has received endorsements of its agenda from over 50 organizations and individuals working in the areas of environmental health, women's rights, and health care reform and is continuing to gather support. This effort will provide a networking and organizing tool, bringing together different constituencies in an all-out effort to stop the cancer epidemic.

Cancer *is* and needs to be seen as a political issue. The women's health movement of the '70s made that strikingly clear and gave us a road map to the politics of women's health. In the '80s, AIDS activists have shown the power of direct action to influence research priorities and treatment deliveries. In the '90s, an effective cancer-prevention strategy demands that we challenge the present industrial practices of the corporate world, based solely on economic gains for the already powerful, and that we insist on an end to the toxic discharges that the government sanctions under the guise of "protecting our security." According to Lenny Siegel, research director of the Military Toxic Network, the Pentagon has produced more toxic waste in recent years—between 400,000 tons and 500,000 tons annually—than the five largest multinational chemical companies combined.

Indeed, if we want to stop not only breast cancer but all cancers, we need to think in global terms and to build a movement that will link together groups that previously worked at a respectful distance. At a worldwide level, the Women's World Congress for a Healthy Planet (attended by over 1500 women from 92 countries from many different backgrounds and perspectives) presented a position paper, Agenda 21, at the 1992 United Nations Earth Summit conference in Brazil. The paper articulates a women's position on the environment and sustainable development that stresses pollution prevention, economic justice, and an end to conflict resolution through war and weapons production, probably the greatest force in destroying the environment.

On February 4, 1992, a group of 65 scientists released a statement at a press conference in Washington, D.C., entitled "Losing the 'War against Cancer'—Need for Public Policy Reforms," which calls for an amendment to the National Cancer Act that would "re-orient the mission and priorities of the NCI to cancer causes and prevention." The seeds of this movement have been sown. It is now our challenge to nourish this movement with grassroots research, with demonstrations, and with demands that our society as a whole take responsibility for the environmental contamination that is killing us.

Author's note: Many thanks to the women of the Women's Community Cancer Project in Cambridge, Massachusetts, for their help and support. A longer version of this article with complete footnotes and references appeared in the Resist *newsletter (May/June 1992).*

National Women's Health Network Fact Sheet

Breast Cancer and Women of Color

Breast Cancer and Latina Women

Incidence

The breast cancer incidence for Latinas is lower than for White or African American women. In any one year, 70 out of every 100,000 Latinas are diagnosed with breast cancer. In comparison, 112 out of every 100,000 White women, and 95 out of every 100,000 African American women are diagnosed with breast cancer. However, the incidence is increasing faster for Latinas than for other women. (1)

Mortality

The breast cancer mortality rate for Latinas is lower than for White or African American women. In any one year, 15 out of every 100,000 Latinas die of breast cancer. In comparison, 27 out of every 100,000 White women, and 31 out of every 100,000 African American women die of breast cancer. The lower number of Latinas who die of breast cancer reflects the lower number of Latinas who get it. (1)

Survival

However, those Latinas who do get breast cancer are less likely to survive for five years after diagnosis than are White women. The five-year survival is 70% for Latinas, 84% for White women, and 69% for African American women. (1) Little research has been done on the poor survival of Latinas diagnosed with breast cancer, but it may be because Latinas are more likely to be diagnosed after the disease has spread.

Mammography Screening

Latinas are as likely as White women to have had at least one mammogram. According to a National Health Interview Survey in 1992, the percentage of Latinas who had ever been screened was 70%, for White women 69%, and for African American women 64%. (1) Being screened just once does not reduce the likelihood of dying from breast cancer, though, and research has not been done to identify how many Latinas are getting regular screening.

Further Considerations

The Latino population represents a diverse community including Cuban, Puerto Rican, Mexican, and other Central and Latin Americans. Cancer statistics are almost always reported for Latinos as a whole. Therefore, the overall rate of breast cancer in Latinas may mask higher or lower rates in certain sub-populations. The length of time in the United States may also influence the likelihood of developing breast cancer so, although the numbers look lower overall, sub-groups of Latinas may have risks similar to White women.

More needs to be done to ensure that Latinas participate in regular mammography screening and receive the appropriate treatment for breast cancer in a timely fashion. Currently, barriers exist that keep Latinas from achieving survival rates on a par with White women. Although most Latinas get at least one mammogram, lack of knowledge that regular screening is necessary, absence of encouragement by physicians, and limited access to mammography screening services are problems faced by many Latinas. (1)

In order to continue to increase the rates of mammography screening and thus reduce the number of cancer deaths in Latinas, there must be outreach education efforts and culturally appropriate cancer control interventions delivered in Spanish. (2) In addition, as the Latino population is too often understudied and underserved, continued research in this population is critical. (3)

Breast Cancer and Native American Women

Incidence

The breast cancer incidence for Native American women varies depending on region. Incidence rates are lower among American Indian women living in Arizona and New Mexico, as well as Alaska Native women, than among White and African American women. In any one year, 32 out of every 100,000 American Indian women, and 79 out of every 100,000 Alaska Native women are diagnosed with breast cancer. In comparison, 112 out of every 100,000 White women, 95 out of every 100,000 African American women, and 70 out of every 100,000 Latina women are diagnosed with breast cancer. Native Hawaiian women have a breast cancer incidence comparable to White women at 106 per 100,000 women, and higher than other Native American women, African American women and Latinas." (1) American Indian women living in the northern states have higher rates in comparison to other Native American women. (2)

Mortality

The breast cancer mortality rate for most Native American women is lower than for White and African American women, and Latinas. In any one year, 9 out of every 100,000 American Indian women, and 13 out of every 100,000 Alaska Native women die of breast cancer. In comparison, 27 out of every 100,000 White women, 31 out of every 100,000 African American women, and 15 out of every 100,000 Latinas die of breast cancer. Similar to incidence rates, regional variability exists in mortality rates for Native American women. The mortality rate for Native Hawaiian women, at 38 per 100,000 women, is higher than for other Native American women, White and African American women, and Latinas. (3) The Billings IHS Area mortality rate is comparable to White women at 25 per 100,000 women. Many Native Americans believe the incidence and deaths caused by certain diseases are underestimated due to the misclassification of ethnicity in health statistics. (4)

In a study of Native Americans in selected states, the breast cancer mortality rates for most of the areas showed a clear increase in the late 70s and after. The overall U.S. rate during this time was comparatively unchanged.

Survival

The five-year breast cancer survival rate for American Indian women is lower than all other ethnic and racial groups living in the United States. For Native Hawaiian women the survival rate is higher than for American Indian and African American women, but lower than for White women. The five-year survival is 49% for American Indians, 69% for Native Hawaiian women, 84% for White women, 69% for African American women, and 70% for Latinas. (1,3)

Insurance and Access to Services

Although Native Americans are eligible for free comprehensive health care through the Indian Health Service (IHS), only half choose or are able to use it. Some Native Americans do not use the IHS because they have other medical insurance. However, many Native Americans find that no IHS facility is accessible to them. For example, no IHS facilities exist in California which is the state with the second largest population of Native Americans and IHS usually does not cover the cost of care provided outside its system. The establishment and maintenance of breast cancer/mammography outreach efforts and clinical services for Native American women is important.

Further Considerations

In 1989, 30.9% of American Indians and Alaska Natives lived at or below the poverty level. In the same year only 9.8% of whites and 13.1% of the total U.S. population were living in poverty. Racial information is no longer standard on many forms used in hospitals. When it is requested, the health care provider often assumes and records race by visual observation. This can result in a misclassification of Native Americans as white or Hispanic. The extent of this varies from state to state and from area to area. (2)

Breast Cancer and Asian American Women

Incidence

Statistics documenting the breast cancer incidence in Asian American women living in the United States have only recently been published. For Chinese women the reported incidence is 55 per 100,000 women, for Japanese women 82 per 100,000 women, for Filipino women 73 per 100,000 women, Korean women 29 per 100,000, Vietnamese women 38 per 100,000, and Native Hawaiian women 106 per 100,000. In comparison, White women had a reported incidence of 112 per 100,000 women. (1)

Mortality

The mortality rate in Asian-American women is the lowest of the main ethnic population in the United States. Asian-American women have a combined mortality rate of 13 deaths for every 100,000 women. (2) This compares to a rate of 27 out of every 100,000 White women, 15 out of 100,000 Latina women who die from the disease. Among Asian-Americans, the mortality ranged from 7 per 100,000 for Korean and Southeast Asian women, to 12 for Filipino and 13 for Japanese women. For Chinese women the deaths were 11 per 100,000. (1) The lower number of Asian-American women who die of breast cancer reflects the lower incidence of the disease cited above.

Survival

The population of Hawaii is comprised of five major ethnic groups: Japanese, White, ethnic Hawaiians, Filipinos, and Chinese. According to a study of breast cancer in Hawaii the Japanese and Chinese women in this population were more likely to have their breast cancers diagnosed an earlier stage, therefore resulting in a better survival rate for these women. In contrast, a later stage of breast cancer at the time of diagnosis was more common for Filipino and Hawaiian women. (3)

Further Considerations

According to a national study on reproductive health, Asian women are the least likely to have an annual gynecological exam, or to ever have had a mammogram. (4) Numerous barriers affect access to medical screening and treatment for Asian women, including cultural beliefs and practices, mistrust of Western medicine, and socioeconomic factors. (5)

It is important to note that when Asian women migrate to the United States their risk of breast cancer rises considerably, a six fold increase compared to the women in their native countries and the rates approach those of White women. (6) Exposure to Western lifestyles, particular diet and nutrition, has most frequently been cited as an explanation for the dramatic differences in incidence rates for Asian women living in the United States and in Asia. (7) A recent study found that changes in reproductive patterns do not explain the increased risk of Asian-American women compared to Asian women. Thus, the overall lower incidence of breast cancer among this population can mask the sub-groups who may have risks similar to White American women.

For more recent immigrants, a further problem of language barriers and residency status influences the willingness to seek care, which may lead to late diagnosis. Continued outreach education and intervention efforts are needed that are culturally sensitive to the special considerations of Asian-American women.

Breast Cancer and African American Women

Incidence

The breast cancer incidence for African American women is lower than White women, and higher than Latinas. In any one year, 95 out of every 100,000 African American women are diagnosed with breast cancer. In comparison, 112 out of every 100,000 White women, and 70 out of every 100,000 Latinas are diagnosed with breast cancer. (1) However, up to age 40 African Americans have a higher incidence than Whites. (2)

Mortality

Like the overall U.S. population, the site with the second highest cancer mortality rate for African American women is the breast. The leading cancer killer among women is lung cancer. (3)

The breast cancer mortality rate for African American women is higher than for White women and Latinas. In any one year, 31 out of every 100,000 African American women die of breast cancer. In comparison, 27 out of every 100,000 White women, and 15 out of every 100,000 Latinas die of breast cancer. (1)

Between 1989 and 1992 there was approximately a 5% decrease in mortality rates for White women with breast cancer, but approximately a 2% increase for African American women. (4)

Survival

The five-year breast cancer survival rate for African American women is lower than for White women and Latinas. The five-year survival is 69% for African Americans, 84% for White women, and 70% for Latinas. (1)

There are several reasons for the lower survival rate in African American women:

1. Late diagnosis; i.e. African American women are more likely to be diagnosed after the cancer has spread. (5)
2. Poverty; i.e. low income cancer patients are less likely to survive, even when diagnosed early. (5,6,7)
3. Under-treatment; African American women are less likely than White women to receive appropriate treatment. According to a study in the American Journal of Public Health, in younger as well as older patients, and in earlier as well as later stages, African American patients were more likely than White patients to be untreated and to be treated by non-surgical methods. (7)
4. Cancer nature; A recent study found that the actual tumor cells in African American women grow more

rapidly, leading to more aggressive cancers at an earlier age. The differences seen in this study also led to breast cancer that was less responsive to hormone treatment. (8)

Further Considerations

Mammography rates for African American women are lower than White women and Latinas, but are increasing steadily. (1) Several barriers to getting mammograms exist for African Americans such as office visit and screening procedure costs, physicians' failure to discuss mammography with women, misconceptions that screening is unnecessary, and/or lack of health insurance. (5) The biggest unmet need for African American women is early recognition of the disease.

There are many unanswered questions concerning African American women and breast cancer. Why is it more common in younger women? Do the reasons above fully explain the worse survival rate? Further research in this population is necessary to answer these questions. In addition, there must be increased access to appropriate prevention, detection, and treatments for African American women.

It's Breast Cancer Awareness Month
Read This Before You Have a Mammogram

Last month, the Canadian National Breast Screening Study published follow-up results showing, once again, that mammography screening did not reduce the breast cancer death rate for women in their 40s (*Annals of Internal Medicine,* 9/3/02). Mammography proponents have criticized the Canadian Study ever since it first published the same unpopular finding more than a decade ago. The Study now has 11 to 16 years worth of follow-up. *HealthFacts* interviewed its deputy director, Cornelia J. Baines, MD, about the fact that—in the early years of this trial—there were more breast cancer deaths among women given mammograms. This was initially thought to be a statistical fluke when it first showed up. Now some researchers are having second thoughts.

HF: When you published your seven-year results, there were more breast cancer deaths (38) in the mammography-screened women, compared with those in the control group who had no mammograms (28). Were there any surprises now that you have 11–16 year results?

CB: No, I knew by 1983 that more breast cancer deaths were occurring in the mammography-screened group rather than the control group. Of course, that's not what we expected. When we started out, we were sure that we were going to show a major benefit. After all, the HIP Study [the first mammography trial conducted in the 1960s] had shown a benefit to women ages 50–59, and we assumed that the only reason a benefit wasn't shown for younger women was that the mammography was archaic by today's standards.

HF: When I interviewed you at the time you published the seven-year results, you said that the difference in breast cancer deaths was not statistically significant.

CB: You are quite right it's not statistically significant, but what is disturbing is that it has happened in three different countries in three other trials. 1985 was a landmark year for mammography screening trials. A Swedish study headed by Lazlo Tabar was published in *The Lancet* (4/13/85). When you read the abstract [summary] of that study, it says that women ages 40–74 showed a 31% reduction in breast cancer deaths. But if you look in the text of the article, you see that the number of deaths in the [small subset of] women in their 40s given mammograms was higher than in the control group. Similar results were observed in the Stockholm and HIP trials. The consistency of this trend demands further evaluation.

HF: Is anyone looking into it?

CB: When we published our first results in 1992, it never entered my head that the people who have been promoting mammography would try to completely destroy the credibility of our study and ignore this phenomenon which had been clearly shown in Tabar's study and which had also been shown in the HIP study. I started out saying that this needs investigating at the basic science level and believing that screening researchers would pay attention to these trends. Well, was I ever out to lunch. People, when they strongly believe in something, don't waste time looking at evidence that challenges their beliefs. That's just not human nature.

HF: But some researchers are investigating the biological mechanism underlying this mortality paradox.

CB: Yes, a meta-analysis [of all trials] shows a peak in excess deaths occurs at three years after screening, and this rise in deaths corresponds to the time when breast cancer tends to kill women. Breast cancer mortality rates show two peaks: one occurs three years after diagnosis, the other at nine years. After that, they seem to survive quite well. Increasingly, some researchers speculate that something associated with biopsy or surgery in some women stimulates growth factors, which for women with micrometastases [undetectable spread of cancer outside the breast] ends up stimulating them and then they die. This seems to support the presumption made by Bernard Fisher [America's leading breast cancer researcher] a long time ago—that micrometastases has already occurred in 90% of all breast cancers before clinical or radiological detection.

HF: Are you talking only about women in their 40s?

CB: The increase was also seen in older women in Tabar's study.

Surgeon Who Headed a U.K. Mammography Program Becomes One of Its Strongest Critics

Michael Baum, MD, emeritus professor of surgery at University College in London, U.K., has been a breast cancer surgeon for 30 years. After leaving the Breast Screening Programme for the National Health Service in the southeast of England, Dr. Baum became an outspoken critic of mammography screening, particularly for women in their 40s.

In this interview with HealthFacts, Dr. Baum is asked to comment on the new Canadian Study results. In doing so, he argues for a new paradigm for how and why breast cancer spreads. Dr. Baum champions the ideas of the famed Boston-based researcher, Judah Folkman, whose work is associated with angiogenesis. This natural process, which is controlled by certain chemicals produced in the body, leads to the formation of new blood vessels. In adults, angiogenesis is involved in wound healing and menstruation. Angiogenesis can also have negative effects. Tumor growth is dependent on blood and oxygen supplied by these newly formed blood vessels, which also provide a means by which cancer cells can travel to distant organs and form new tumors.

HF: What do you make of the increase in breast cancer deaths shown in the women given mammograms in the Canadian Study?

MB: I believe that it is a real phenomenon and not simply an artifact of this study. It appears in all the studies

HF: In all the studies, not just four?

MB: Yes, to a lesser extent in all the other trials.

HF: There were more than twice as many cases of *ductal carcinoma in situ* [Latin for cancer in place] in the mammogram group. What do you make of that?

MB: I'm very influenced by Judah Folkman's work. He believes that *in situ* is probably not a good word, and we should call it latent cancer. These latent cancers, particularly in premenopausal women, are grossly overrepresented [in those given mammograms]—something like five times more, compared to what you would expect. This suggests that if left to their own devices, these latent cancers might never trouble a woman. But if you identify these latent cancers and biopsy them, you have traumatized the area. You immediately trigger the natural healing mechanisms, and natural healing mechanisms involve angiogenesis. So, effectively, the biopsy could be considered an angiogenic switch. You take a latent cancer that would never hurt a woman, biopsy it, turn on the angiogenic switch, and it ceases to be latent. A latent disease becomes an aggressive disease.

HF: Is this true only for breast cancer?

MB: You see this in other cancers. The most notorious is renal cell cancer. If you find a symptomless renal tumor by chance, and operate, [then] in no time the patient is riddled with metastasis. This happened to a dear friend of mine. I think that an angiogenic switch might be an explanation. It's really scary.

HF: And this is that what you suspect happened to some women in the mammography trials.

MB: My explanation sounds a bit farfetched, but it is strongly supported by basic science that is coming out of the work on angiogenesis. There are profound cyclical changes going on in the premenopausal breast, and these changes can also be seen in premenopausal breast cancer. So just by happenstance, you might get a surgical insult at a time in the menstrual cycle that favors the cancer cells. It's all quite alarming.

HF: In the Canadian Study, 71 cases of *ductal carcinoma in situ* (DCIS) were diagnosed in the mammogram group, compared to 29 in the no-mammogram group.

MB: That tells you two things: (1) It emphasizes the quality of the study. If they had not detected so many cases of DCIS, then the screening zealots would say that the screening techniques in the Canadian Study were bad; (2) It demonstrates, yet again, that all screening programs will show an excess of cancers. And the excess is mostly DCIS. In women given a manual breast exam, only about 3% of cancers detected are DCIS; whereas in mammography-screened women, 20% of the cancers are DCIS.

HF: The breast cancer death rate was the same for both groups in the Canadian Study. Doesn't that indicate that early detection is of no benefit to any women with DCIS?

MB: Yes, I think so. I don't know if any lives are saved by screening, frankly. But the one argument about which I cannot be shaken is that women invited to screening should know these things. I was one of the people given the job of setting up a screening program in 1987–88 in the U. K. Then it gradually dawned on me that this was state interference with public health, and it was coercion.

I resigned in disgust from the National Screening Committee because they were intentionally deceiving women [about the harms]. They went on record saying, "We mustn't let women know this because it might deter them from coming to screen." So I decided to work outside the system to inform women about the truth of screening. I can see how some women, fully informed, would accept screening over the age of 50, but to promote mammography to women under the age of 50 is absolutely unethical.

HF: The American Cancer Society has been promoting mammography starting at age 40 for many years now.

MB: Either the ACS is funded by the screening industry, or they've backed themselves into a corner and can't admit they've been wrong all this time. The message is so seductive: "The secret to cancer is catching it early." That's rubbish. It's so naïve. The only thing that influences cancer mortality is better treatment, as far as I'm concerned. The word "early" has no meaning to a scientist.

HF: Do you have an equivalent to the ACS in your country overselling the early detection message?

MB: No, but we have "Black October," which is what I call Breast Cancer Awareness Month, when lots of fine young women have these campaigns with runway models advising breast self-examination every month. And that gets across two false messages: (1) that self-examination is of any value; and (2) that the role model for breast cancer patients is skinny girl of 23.

HF: Any parting thoughts about mammography research?

MB: It ceases to be medical science now—it's egos. A proper scientist should learn that you go through life being humiliated again and again. You have prepared yourself to admit you were wrong. That's the very mech-anism of science. Scientific truths are only temporary expressions of reality that serve us for the time being. There's no such thing as scientific truth. It's all an approximation to reality. A true scientist has to accept that his version of reality will be overturned in the fullness of time. If you can't accept that, you're not a scientist.

Tamoxifen

Breast Cancer Prevention That's Hard to Swallow

by Rita Arditti

The recent announcement from the National Cancer Institute that tamoxifen prevents breast cancer in women at high risk has resulted in a veritable media frenzy. "Researchers Find the First Drug Known to Prevent Breast Cancer," (*The New York Times,* April 7); "Breast Cancer Breakthrough," (*New York Times* editorial, April 8); "Study Finds Breast Cancer Treatment Also Prevents It," (*Boston Globe,* April 6). Dr. Harold Varmus, director of the National Institute of Health, calls the study "a big deal." To this, we must ask: "A big deal for whom?"

Tamoxifen, an antiestrogen synthetic hormone, is one of the most widely prescribed drugs for prevention of breast cancer recurrence, and is used in treating post-menopausal women at practically all stages of breast cancer. The Breast Cancer Prevention Trial involved 13,388 women considered at high risk for breast cancer—based on personal history, family history or age. Half took tamoxifen while the other half were given a placebo. Tamoxifen cut the rate of breast cancer almost in half, according to the National Cancer Institute Press Office. The trial was stopped fourteen months short to allow the untreated women the "benefits" of tamoxifen. British scientists criticized the decision to stop the trial because it will now be harder to establish the long-range effects of the treatment. Their skepticism is quite reasonable since there are already a number of serious problems emerging from this study.

Maryann Napoli, Associate Director of the Center for Medical Consumers in New York, has pointed out that a closer look at the data reveals that there were five deaths in the group taking the drug—three from breast cancer, two from pulmonary embolism—and five in the group taking the placebo—all from breast cancer. (See Napoli's letter to the editor, *New York Times,* April 13, 1998). *In other words, both groups had the same number of deaths.* The two women who died from pulmonary embolism did not develop breast cancer; they died from "side effects" of the drug. The study showed seventeen cases of blood clots in the lung for the treated group and six for the control, and thirty cases of blood clots in major veins for the treated versus nineteen in the control. Total: 47 blood clots versus 25, almost twice as many for those taking tamoxifen.

Uterine cancer is another main "side effect" of tamoxifen: 33 cases in the treated group versus 14 in the control. Apparently, these cases were treated successfully through hysterectomy, though there is evidence that the type of tumors that develop while a woman is taking tamoxifen are very aggressive. In light of this it is hard to swallow comments like the one by Dr. Judy Garber at Dana Farber Cancer Institute. She says, "The drug is proven to prevent breast cancer, and the endometrial cancer risk is manageable. It's the blood clot risk you're left with, and this may seem like the [least] of several evils for many women." (*Boston Globe,* April 13, 1998).

But blood clots and uterine cancer are only the most visible of the "side effects" of tamoxifen. In their book *Tamoxifen and Breast Cancer,* Michael W. DeGregorio, professor of medicine, and Valerie J. Wiebe, assistant

From *Sojourner: The Women's Forum,* July 1998, Vol. 23, No. 11, p. 32. Copyright © 1998 by Sojourner. Reprinted by permission.

professor of medicine and pharmacy at the University of Texas Health Science Center, San Antonio, devote a chapter to the side effects of tamoxifen. The most common side effect of tamoxifen is hot flashes. Other effects reported are menstrual irregularities, vaginal bleeding and vaginal dryness or itching; mild nausea with or without vomiting, loss of appetite, constipation, diarrhea, edema and weight gain. Tamoxifen has also been associated with depression or irritability and other psychological symptoms associated with menopause. For a small percentage of women, it has a suppressive effect on the bone marrow, leading to a decrease in the number of platelet and red and white blood cells.

Two more areas of concern are liver cancer and eye problems. In animal studies, rats fed low doses of tamoxifen developed liver tumors in approximately 11.5 percent of the cases, and at higher doses, 71.2 percent developed liver cancer. As DeGregorio and Wiebe point out, "although no direct link to liver cancer has been made, accounts of liver complications from tamoxifen are on the rise." As for eye problems, 6.3 percent of patients reported both corneal and retinal changes, which did not disappear when tamoxifen was discontinued.

In spite of these problems, it is estimated that 2.9 million healthy women would be "potentially eligible" for preventive treatment of tamoxifen. This includes all women over 60, and many younger women whose personal or family history suggests a high risk (even though no one knows how long the treatments should be continued or its effect on women of color who comprised only 3 percent of the women in the study.) At a cost of $80 to $100 for a monthly supply, this is unquestionably "a big deal" for Zeneca, the company based in Wilmington, Delaware who manufactures the drug under the brand name of Nolvadex. On the first day of the announcement

of the trial results, the shares of Zeneca closed at $147 on the New York Stock Exchange, a gain of $9.75. Zeneca will now apply to the FDA to have the drug approved as preventive therapy for breast cancer. Zeneca also makes money owning and managing eleven cancer-treatment centers in the U.S., where they prescribe the drugs they make. On top of this, Zeneca is the primary sponsor of October as Breast Cancer Awareness Month, and has veto power on the materials produced. Not surprisingly, the literature of Breast Cancer Awareness Month never mentions the word "carcinogen" and it relentlessly emphasizes mammography as the "best protection" for women. Next October, we can expect tamoxifen to be included in the list of recommendations. Zeneca is also the producer of a carcinogenic herbicide, acetochlor, and has been involved in litigation stemming from environmental damage in California harbors.

The other corporation that stands to profit is Myriad Genetics, Inc., of Salt Lake City, Utah, which does the genetic tests for the mutated genes BRCA1 or BRCA2, which increase breast cancer risk. Blood samples from women in the study will now be tested for these genes. If it is found that tamoxifen lowers the risk, the demand for gene tests will increase. Unquestionably, another "big deal."

It is frightening to think that our most influential scientists and physicians doing cancer research have bought into the cancer industry's definition of breast cancer prevention. The whole concept of prevention has been distorted to fit the needs of greedy companies. We need to open up a national debate about what prevention really means. Otherwise, God help us all, this "big deal" will encourage the development of other "prevention" strategies in which, as in this case, exchanging breast cancer for other life-threatening problems will be considered a success.

Pinstripes to Pullovers

Learning to Live with Chronic Fatigue Syndrome

by Donna Kiefer

I sat at the wide conference table on the tenth floor of an office building in downtown Boston. Half a dozen other attorneys ringed the table. We were there on a bitter January day to settle the U.S. Environmental Protection Agency's multimillion-dollar lawsuit against one of New England's most flagrant polluters.

As the lead attorney, I had spent most of my first two years at the EPA, including many evenings and weekends, researching and preparing to file this suit. Now, a year and a half later, we were finally negotiating a settlement. I wore what I considered my most imposing suit, a charcoal pin-striped blend of wool and silk.

My life was at a high point. I had finally found my niche in the legal world. Part of a solid circle of friends, I was also close to my two brothers and sister, often babysitting my nieces. I had just come out as a lesbian, and my family and closest friends were generally accepting.

But amidst my pride, I was also aware of a deep exhaustion that, along with headaches, sore throats, and low-grade fevers, had beset me for two months. It seemed to be a persistent flu. Weeks later, when the symptoms showed no sign of abating, I consulted a specialist. She diagnosed me with a common virus and could not predict how long I would be sick, saying there was no treatment except rest. I took a two-month leave to recover, but the exhaustion, sore throats, and headaches persisted. Desperate for answers, I returned to the specialist. After performing an array of blood tests, she diagnosed me with Chronic Fatigue Immune Dysfunction Syndrome (CFIDS).

This left me feeling even more lost than before. Very little is known about CFIDS. I was told again: rest, rest, rest. Other than that, there were treatments intended to relieve symptoms. The only way to determine if a certain treatment might be helpful was to try it.

One of the first treatments I tried was acupuncture. A year after falling ill, I still had hopes of being cured—hopes fed by my acupuncturist, who assured me I would burst with energy within months. Three times a week, I drove 30 minutes each way in rush-hour traffic to lie on a gurney and let my body be punctured by very thin needles. As I lay there gazing up at the skylight, gentle flute music drifting over me, I did feel a bit more vital and clear-headed. But that vitality vanished within an hour of leaving my doctor's office. Four months and more than a thousand dollars later, I was not any healthier

At least acupuncture did not make me sicker, which is more that I can say for blue-green algae. After hearing stories of people recovering from CFIDS with the help of algae, I plunked down hundreds of dollars, this time for an entire algae nutritional regimen. After a week, my fatigue and mental fog were worse than ever. The distributor assured me that this was a normal reaction, and would soon subside. Exhausted and skeptical though I was, I hung on. But after another three weeks, even the distributor had to acknowledge that the algae was not helping me.

Even more pressing than my frustration over treatment options were my fears about how the illness would affect my future. My main worry was whether I could continue working, but I also wondered whether I would ever be able to travel or swim again. I remember the look in my first doctor's eyes when I told her I was planning a trip to Peru. So sad, so remote. She shook her head and said I could not take such a trip. In her eyes, I saw a diminishment of my life beyond what I could imagine.

The course of CFIDS varies greatly. Some people recover, some cycle between periods of relatively good health and illness, and some gradually worsen over time. Others remain the same, while some improve gradually but never fully recover. There was no way of knowing which of these categories I would fall into.

The not knowing made so much of life a challenge. For instance, I had to decide what sort of accommodations to request from the EPA. First, I took the two-month break. Then, feeling better, I began working out of my home; I transferred my big case, taking work that was less time sensitive and required fewer meetings. But even with this new setup, my headaches, sore throats, and exhaustion worsened. Over the next ten months, to cope with these worsening symptoms, I was gradually forced to weaken my connection to the EPA, first cutting back on work, then taking extended leave. Finally, a year and a half after first falling ill, I had to admit that I would not be able to return to work as a lawyer. Not in the near future; perhaps never.

In a way, my resignation from the EPA came as a relief. I could stop fighting to keep my job and focus on guarding my health. But a whole new set of worries appeared. How would I support myself? Was I eligible for disability benefits?

When everything is in question, waking up in the morning feels like disappearing into a black hole. The healthy, athletic body I had once known, along with my job, my future as a lawyer, my ability to spend time with friends and family, and my very identity had all vanished. I started wondering what my purpose was. I could no longer contribute by suing polluters or by babysitting my nieces and giving support to friends and family.

Indeed, on many days I remained in sweat pants and a beat-up pullover sweater all day, struggling just to make breakfast or take a shower. After sleeping ten restless hours, I awoke feeling as though 50-pound weights were attached to my limbs. Just as disturbing to me as the utter exhaustion was the mental fog that enveloped me. I began to have trouble balancing my checkbook or remembering how to get to places that I had been to many times before. I would walk into the kitchen and discover the I had left the refrigerator door open. Many days I could not read even one newspaper article. I began to bounce checks, forgetting to deposit money into my account—something that had never happened to me before.

One day when this fog was particularly dense, I sank into the plush green armchair where I spent much of my time and picked up a paper clip. I held it between my thumb and forefinger, staring. I absolutely could not remember the name of this object. After a minute, the word "clip" came to me, but that only led to "clipper," and, finally, "nail clipper." I gave up. Only later that afternoon was I able to retrieve from my brain the words "paper clip."

While many of these concerns—loss of identity, uncertainty about the future, fear of financial ruin—are common to anyone with a disabling illness, ignorance about CFIDS made my situation especially difficult. Medical experts debated how serious an illness this was, and whether its origins were physiological or psychological. People often simplified these issues, saying those with CFIDS "are just depressed." The press further stigmatized the illness by christening it the "yuppie flu." That people with CFIDS often do not "look" sick and may have symptoms that wax and wane for no apparent reason makes it harder for others to take seriously.

The impact that this stigma had on me was powerful. I had internalized so much of the social doubt that if I were having a relatively "good" day—one in which I could cook a full meal for myself and read for more than two minutes—I would start to question whether I was indeed sick. Could I be imagining the severity of my symptoms?

Unfortunately, my self doubt was mirrored in those around me. When I met with my supervisor upon returning from my first leave he smiled from behind his desk, asking, "So, did you use this break to write the Great American Novel?" I was shocked at his misunderstanding of my condition. Yet, I also struggled with the question—could I have written that novel if I had really tried? At that moment, feeling relatively good, I forgot the days when I could not finish an article or recall the name of ordinary objects. My specialist also minimized the severity of my illness. One day after I had sat for more than an hour in her waiting room she confided that she was running late because a person with AIDS had died that day. "Now *that's* an illness you don't want to get," she said.

Since those first days of fear and uncertainty, my life has improved. I was granted disability benefits and began two treatments that have improved my energy level. One is a medication that helps me to get refreshing sleep. The other is mega-doses of vitamin B-12 that I inject to increase my stamina.

Just as important, I found greater means of coping with the illness. Much of that came through joining a support group for women with CFIDS. I immediately saw that these women were quite sick, although they too struggled with denial. Gradually I was able to build my belief in the severity of their conditions into the conviction that I also must be seriously ill. Eventually I learned to hold onto this conviction even when I was having a "good" day. I grew to like and respect all of these women. I saw that although their daily activities were limited by chronic illness, the meaning and value of their lives was not. This helped me to value my own life as it is, rather than measure it against the standard of what it had once been. I was even eventually able to let go of the need to know what my life would be like in the future. I began to see that no one—whether chronically ill or in robust health—can know what life holds in store.

Now, six years after falling ill, I volunteer with several activist groups, pulling together meetings and organizing files. While it is a far cry from negotiating multimillion-dollar lawsuits, it gives me the sense that I am making a contribution. I have also begun exploring creative writing. As I sit in jeans and pullover sweatshirt typing these words into my home computer, just a few feet away hangs the pinstriped suit that was once a symbol of my status in the world. I don't know if I'll ever wear it again, but I have learned that status, like good health, is ephemeral. I was born with one and attained the other, only to see them both stripped away.

I first reacted to my losses with sadness and anger, further fueled by the ignorance and insensitivity that I encountered. Yet, although I never would have chosen it, I have mostly made peace with my disability. It is a part of who I am, and I have accepted it in order to value my life and move forward. I have established new priorities; status is not among them. Instead I strive for honesty, compassion, and openness to each moment—qualities that come from the inside and cannot be taken from me.

A Survey of Attitudes and Experiences of Women with Heart Disease

*by Elsa Marcuccio, BA, Nancy Loving,
Susan K. Bennett, MD, and Sharonne N. Hayes, MD*

Objective. Cardiovascular disease is the leading cause of death in women, but little is known about the attitudes and experiences of the 6.4 million American women who have a diagnosis of heart disease. We assessed the knowledge, attitudes, and experiences of women with heart disease and the effect of the disease on their lives.

Subjects. A total of 204 women with a self-reported diagnosis of heart disease were the subjects.

Methods. A telephone survey with open-ended questions was used to ask women about their diagnoses, symptoms, interactions with the health care system, knowledge of risks and symptoms, satisfaction with care, and the effect of the disease on their lifestyle, psychosocial well-being, finances, interpersonal relationships, and spirituality.

Results. Most of the women (73%) had a diagnosis of coronary artery disease (CAD), with the remainder having diagnoses of other cardiac diseases. Most women took multiple medications and had undergone several diagnostic and therapeutic interventions. Almost half the women had been unaware that they were at risk of CAD and, after the condition was diagnosed, almost one-fourth of the respondents did not seek additional information about their diagnosis or treatment options from their physicians. More than half expressed dissatisfaction with their health care, most often because of physician-related knowledge and communication problems. Many women reported that they were unable or unwilling to make appropriate lifestyle changes after the diagnosis was made because of insufficient social, medical, or educational support. Educational opportunities may have been limited because less than 60% of women with CAD received cardiac rehabilitation services. Respondents reported significant changes in their interpersonal relationships, mental health, and financial and spiritual well-being as a result of having heart disease.

Conclusion. Heart disease affects many aspects of women's lives. A significant percentage of surveyed women continue to have adverse consequences long after the diagnosis is made. Furthermore, proven beneficial lifestyle changes may not be implemented, most likely because of dissatisfaction with care, lack of educational and rehabilitative resources, symptoms of depression and anxiety, and suboptimal social support. This study identifies several problems that may help explain why women with heart disease have poorer medical outcomes than men with heart disease. Further investigation and better definition of these problems may help improve outcomes among women.

Keywords: Cardiovascular diseases, Coronary disease, Health care surveys, Heart disease, Myocardial infarction, Women's health, Risk factors, Patient satisfaction

Introduction

Cardiovascular disease is the leading cause of death and disability in women, causing more than 500,000 deaths and approximately 450,000 myocardial infarctions each year. In the United States, 6.4 million women have a history of myocardial infarction or angina, or both. However, most women do not perceive heart disease as a major personal health threat, and in a 1999 Gallup poll only 55% of primary care physicians correctly identified coronary heart disease as the greatest health risk of women older than 50 years. Other surveys have found that many women are unaware that they have risk factors for cardiovascular disease or that they have symptoms consistent with heart disease.

As a result of these misconceptions among women and their physicians, the diagnosis of coronary heart disease tends to be delayed or missed more often in women than in men, and women are less likely than men to receive proven therapies or to be treated according to established clinical practice guidelines. Compared with men, women undergo fewer coronary revascularization procedures and, despite having a higher prevalence of risk factors, receive less preventive counseling and pharmacologic therapy to reduce their risks. After a myocardial infarction or coronary artery bypass grafting, women experience more depression, anxiety, and disability than men but often are not referred to cardiac rehabilitation services or psychological counseling. These disparities exist despite evidence that women receive at least as much benefit from these therapies and services as men receive.

Our report is based on the findings of a Women-Heart telephone survey of American women who have heart disease. The object of the study was to comprehensively assess women with heart disease, including their views of their diagnosis and treatment, the effect of heart disease on their lives, and their strategies to help other women. A qualitative approach was necessitated by the magnitude of the problem, the lack of prior relevant research, and the value of understanding subtle differences among the views of the participants.

WomenHeart: The National Coalition of Women with Heart Disease was founded in 1997 by female patients to provide education, support, and advocacy for women with heart disease. WomenHeart comprises a large coalition of patients, national and local nonprofit organizations, and health care providers. To assess baseline characteristics and needs of its members and of women living with heart disease, a telephone survey was devised and implemented. The survey asked American women with heart disease about their diagnosis, treatment, and risk awareness, and the effect of heart disease on their lives.

Subjects and Methods

The Survey

The questionnaire had 22 items. The topics of the questions included the type of heart disease and specific treatments that respondents had received, components of the patient-physician interaction, the level of satisfaction with care, and how the diagnosis of heart disease had affected the women's lifestyles and relationships. The questionnaire was structured to elicit initially the respondents' perspectives without bias by avoiding references to gender. Accordingly, initial questions were phrased broadly, asking respondents to report their own views. Later questions were structured but allowed open-ended responses on more specific issues. The questionnaire was formatted to elicit insights that were not foreseen by the researchers. The responses were evaluated to identify recurrent themes, and relevant passages were collated verbatim. Limited demographic data were obtained (age and state of residence).

Analysis

Individual responses were tabulated and grouped according to specific answers and general themes. Respondents could give more than one response to a question, so that absolute numbers and percentages are reported rather than frequencies.

Subjects

Survey participants were selected randomly from a list compiled by WomenHeart. These women either had joined WomenHeart or had previously requested information from WomenHeart. Interviews were performed by one author (E.M.). During July and August 2001, 311 phone numbers were dialed. Of those numbers, 107 were excluded: 8 women reported that they did not have heart disease, 38 phone numbers were invalid (such as disconnected lines and fax machine numbers), 47 women were not available when called, and 14 women declined to be interviewed. A total of 204 women completed the survey.

Results

Participant Characteristics

The interviewees lived in 41 states, with the majority of the women living in the Northeast (32%) and Southeast (25%). Except for one woman who lived in Canada, the other women lived throughout the United States: North Central (17%), Southwest (10%), Northwest (8%), and South Central (7%). The ages of the participants ranged from the 20s to the 80s; 52% were between 40 and 59 years, and 32% were between 60 and 79 years (Table 1). When asked about their cardiac diagnosis, 136 women reported ischemic heart disease, including "coronary artery disease" (CAD), "blockages," and "heart attack." An additional 12 women who did not identify CAD as their diagnosis were included in this category because they had undergone a revascularization procedure, for a total of 148 women (73%) with CAD. Some women with CAD reported additional diagnoses, including congestive heart failure (5%), high levels of cholesterol (12%), hypertension (12%), arrhythmias or valvular heart disease (7%), and "other" (32%). These diagnoses were also cited as the primary or sole diagnosis by 56 women. The 22 women who responded with a sole diagnosis of "other" indicated that they had an uncommon condition, had not been told their diagnosis, or did not remember the diagnosis.

Because so many women had CAD and because therapy for CAD was most likely different from therapy for other reported conditions, data were analyzed separately for the groups of women with and without CAD and for the entire group. Nearly all respondents (93%) were treated with prescription medication or aspirin or both. Almost two-thirds of all women and 71% of women with CAD took 2 to 5 medications per day, and 14% of all women and 14% of women with CAD took 6 or more. Only two women with CAD were taking no medication.

TABLE 1	Ages of Survey Participants	
	Participants*	
Age, y	No.	%
20–29	2	1
30–39	8	4
40–49	55	27
50–59	51	25
60–69	39	19
70–70	26	13
80–89	7	3

*$N = 204$; data were unavailable for 16 patients (8%).

Eighty-six women reported that they had experienced a heart attack, defined as either a symptomatic or silent myocardial infarction. Seventy percent of respondents had undergone coronary angiography. More than half the women had undergone one or more revascularization procedures (39% percutaneous intervention; 26% coronary artery bypass surgery). An additional 30 women had undergone angiography without a revascularization procedure. One patient had had cardiac transplantation.

Risk Awareness

Of the 204 women, 113 knew that they were at risk of heart disease before their diagnosis: 62% of these women reported that a family history of cardiac disease put them at risk; 19% identified personal cardiac risk factors such as diabetes or unhealthy lifestyle choices such as obesity, smoking, lack of exercise, and poor nutrition; and 20% identified both inherited and lifestyle factors. For the remaining 91 women, the diagnosis "came as a complete surprise." Many indicated that heart disease occurred among men in their families, but the women did not realize that they could inherit that risk. Many women said that heart disease was "a man's disease" rather than one that women should worry about. No differences in perceived risks were observed between women with and without CAD.

Virtually all survey respondents (92%) reported experiencing one or more symptoms related to heart disease. Although most women reported typical symptoms of ischemic heart disease, such as chest and arm pain, a squeezing sensation in the chest, and shortness of breath, atypical symptoms, including dizziness, nausea, fatigue, and pain or pressure between the shoulder blades, were reported as additional or sole symptoms almost as frequently. The remaining women (28%)

reported "other" symptoms, such as headaches, numbness, and motor skill and cognitive impairment. Women with CAD were significantly ($p < 0.05$) more likely than women without CAD to have experienced chest pain (35% vs. 20%), chest squeezing (25% vs. 11%), and pain between the shoulder blades (14% vs. 2%) and less likely to have reported "other" symptoms (45% vs. 61%)

Diagnosis

Only 66 women (35%) who reported symptoms and 68% of their physicians correctly recognized their symptoms as potentially related to the heart. Many women cited frustration, anger, and resentment because their physicians did not consider a cardiac diagnosis.

When participants were asked whether they had asked their physicians any questions about heart disease at the time of initial diagnosis, 23% reported that they did not ask any questions, usually because they were satisfied with the information from the physician, they were intimidated by the physician, or they had insufficient knowledge to ask appropriate questions. In contrast, 76% of the participants reported asking one or more questions, usually about the cause of their symptoms or disease (23%), secondary prevention (19%), prognosis and expected effects and limitations on their physical and emotional states (27%), general information about their disease and how it might differ from the disease in men (18%), and treatment options (11%). Nineteen percent asked "other" questions, including specific questions about their medical conditions. Similarly, 72% of the women had asked their physicians questions about recommended therapy or interventions, such as a detailed explanation of the treatment, its side effects and risks, and alternative treatment options (Table 2). However, 37% did not ask any questions about the recommended treatment.

Satisfaction with Treatment

When the women were asked whether they were satisfied with their overall medical experience, including services provided by health care professionals and hospital staff, treatment options, and any rehabilitation or social support offered, 52% expressed dissatisfaction. Slightly more women with CAD than without CAD reported dissatisfaction (56% vs. 42%; $p = 0.08$). When respondents were asked the source of their dissatisfaction, 58% cited physician-related problems: insensitivity, poor communication skills (described as rudeness, condescension, abruptness, and inattentiveness), and ignorance about

TABLE 2   Responses to "What questions did you ask your physician about treatment you received?"

Question	Participants (N = 204)	
	No.	%
Will it work? Is it working?	20	10
What are the side effects and risks?	29	14
Will I ever stop taking medication? Is the therapy permanent?	27	13
Could you explain the treatment more thoroughly?	37	18
What will my prognosis and life be like after treatment?	18	9
Are there other treatment options?	20	10
Other questions	37	18
None	76	37

recognizing heart disease in women. Eleven percent expressed dissatisfaction related to delayed and missed diagnoses, often stating that neither they nor their physicians had recognized their symptoms, and, as a result, their conditions were diagnosed as panic disorder, stress- or menopause-related conditions, or hypochondria. Other participants were unhappy about the lack of information or the poor quality of information given to them on their disease or its treatment (18%), the lack of available support systems (13%), and other concerns (17%). Women with CAD and women without CAD reported similar sources of dissatisfaction except that women with CAD were more likely to have "other" concerns (21% vs. 4%; p < 0.03).

Satisfaction with Physicians

Most women (91%) were cared for by both a cardiologist and a primary care physician, and all but three women had a primary care provider. Two women reported that they were not cared for by a physician. More than one-fourth of the women were dissatisfied with their interactions with their physicians. However, when asked whether their physician listened attentively and responded to their concerns appropriately, 72% of the women reported that their primary care physician did and 73% felt that their cardiologist did. There was no difference in satisfaction levels on the basis of physician gender.

Cardiac Rehabilitation

A total of 113 participants (69% of those with CAD and 22% of those without CAD) indicated that they had been referred to a cardiac rehabilitation program; of those referred, 84% from both groups attended. Of the women who received a referral but did not attend, most indicated a desire to enroll but cited several barriers to participation, including lack of insurance coverage, inconvenient location, and lack of transportation. When asked to describe their cardiac rehabilitation experience, 50% rated it "very positive," with several participants indicating that they "loved it" and would highly recommend it; 34% rated it "satisfactory," describing their experience as "helpful, but lacking in selected areas," such as exercise education and a suitable support system; 10% rated it "negative" and said that it was "insufficient and inadequate," lacking in several fundamental areas, or a "waste of time"; 7% had no opinion about their rehabilitation experience.

Lifestyle Changes

When asked questions about the effects of heart disease on their lifestyle, 27% of the women with CAD and 11% of the women without CAD reported that they had not changed their eating habits, either because no changes were recommended or because they were unable or unwilling to adapt a heart-healthy diet to their lifestyle. Only a few of these women felt that they had sufficiently healthy diets before their diagnoses were made. Sixty-four percent of respondents (59% with CAD; 78% without CAD) reported making minor changes in their eating habits, and 13% indicated that they had made major changes. In response to questions about physical activity, 22% of the women said that they had decreased or ceased all physical activity because of their heart disease, 31% said that they had not changed their level of physical activity, and 37% indicated that they had increased their activity by only minor amounts (this group mainly consisted of women who could increase their activities to only a limited extent because of a handicap or other comorbidity). A few women felt they were sufficiently active before their diagnosis. There were no significant differences in reported changes in physical activity between women with CAD and women without CAD.

Employment and Financial Changes

A significant number of women (42%) who were in the workforce before their diagnosis indicated that they had changed their work schedules as a result of their cardiac event or diagnosis. Of these, 58% said that they stopped working completely, either temporarily or permanently, 38% said that they had reduced the number of hours they worked, and 5% reported altering their work schedule in other ways, such as working from home or finding a less stressful job. The presence or absence of CAD did not affect changes in work schedules. Many women who reported no changes in work status indicated that they did not work outside the home or were retired. Thirty-six percent reported experiencing financial strains as a result of their heart disease. Of these, 43% had general financial difficulties, 35% cited health insurance coverage problems, and 20% experienced both problems or other types of problems. Women with CAD reported slightly more financial concerns than did women without CAD, but this difference was not statistically significant.

Interpersonal Relationship Changes

When asked how their heart disease had affected their interpersonal relationships with family and friends, 42% of the women indicated that their relationships had changed, with half saying they had improved. Some of these women commented that many people had been supportive and that although the patients were often distraught at the idea of no longer being able to be the primary caretaker at home, most family members accepted the change. Some of the 27% who indicated that their relationships worsened could no longer fulfill the family caretaker role and their families became resentful or unsupportive, or they had accused the patient of exaggerating her illness.

More women reported deterioration in their relationships with friends than with family. In particular, they said that physical limitations or decreased energy levels prevented them from spending as much time with their friends or doing some of the activities they used to do together. Some felt they had less in common with their friends who could not understand the serious nature of heart disease or who did not sympathize with what the patient was experiencing. Among the women who said their relationships had changed, 22% could not specifically describe the change and instead characterized their new relationships as "different." For example, some said that during their illnesses they had made new friends who had become more valued than their long-standing friends. Others found that their friends' increased concern for their well-being was overly confining or controlling.

Mental Health Changes

Mental illness, such as anxiety or clinical depression, associated with their heart disease was reported by 57% of the women. The presence or absence of CAD did not affect the frequency of positive responses. Many women said they felt socially isolated or without social support systems and that no one understood what they were experiencing. Although 24% did not disclose the nature of their mental illness, 38% reported clinical depression, 17% reported increased anxiety, and 21% said they experienced both.

After receiving a diagnosis of heart disease, 40% of the survey participants indicated that their spiritual life had changed. Of these, 84% said that their spiritual life had improved and that their illness had made them more reflective and thankful, 6% reported losing faith, and 10% were unable to describe how their spiritual life had changed.

Life Changes

When women were asked whether heart disease had changed their lives, only 21 reported no life changes related to their heart disease diagnosis; there were no differences in the frequency of responses on the basis of the presence or absence of CAD. The remaining 183 women gave 263 responses (Table 3). The change cited most frequently was in the women's outlook on life. These women said that they learned to "put things in perspective" and "no longer dwell on the trivial things." Also, some women said that their illness had made them "more aware of their bodies" and "increased their sense of vulnerability." Only 14% of the changes that women reported were related to diet and exercise. Eleven women responded that "everything" had changed.

TABLE 3 Responses to "Has heart disease changed your life in any way?"

Response	No. of Women
No	21
Yes	
Life perspective or outlook	64
More aware of health	57
Physical limitations	35
Diet or physical activity	29
Personality changes	27
More frightened	18
"Everything" has changed	11
Lowered my stress level	9
Other	13
Total "yes" responses	263*

*Some of the 204 women gave more than 1 response.

Advice for Others

When the women were asked what advice they had for other women who have heart disease, 199 women gave 363 suggestions. The most common advice was "Educate yourself and ask questions." These women felt that they had not been well informed about their disease, yet they felt uncomfortable asking "stupid" questions until they better understood their condition and its treatment. A second suggestion was "Find doctors who are attentive, understanding, and knowledgeable about heart disease in women—and listen to their advice." These women often felt that, had their physicians been more attentive, responsive, and knowledgeable, their experiences would have been more positive, their recovery hastened, and some of their psychological trauma avoided. A third suggestion was "Listen to your body and don't ignore your symptoms." Many of these women said they had experienced symptoms that were vague or atypical for heart disease. They felt they were too easily misled by primary care physicians who misdiagnosed the condition.

Discussion

Previous surveys have assessed attitudes, knowledge, and behaviors of the general female population toward heart disease. The purpose of the current study was to better understand the highest risk group, the 6.4 million women who have heart disease. On the basis of the results of this survey, heart disease has a significant and unique effect on the physical, mental, financial, interpersonal, and spiritual lives of women.

Attitudes and Awareness of Heart Disease Risk and Symptoms

Unlike women in the other surveys about heart disease, the women in the current study identified themselves as having a diagnosis of heart disease. Several previous surveys reported that relatively few women perceived heart disease as a significant personal health threat; most women felt that cancer, and breast cancer in particular, was more frightening. In a 1995 study of Stanford University graduates aged 48 to 52 years, most women grossly underestimated their lifetime risk of having heart disease; twice as many women reported worrying about breast cancer than heart disease (59% vs. 29%). In a survey of more than 1,000 women reported by Legato et al. in 1997, women were most interested in improving their health and fitness; their interest in health increased with age. However, although 74% of these women perceived themselves as being fairly or very knowledgeable about heart disease, almost half felt that it was somewhat or very unlikely that they were at risk of a heart attack.

Similarly, in a recent study of more than 1,000 women by the American Heart Association, only 8% of the surveyed women identified heart disease and stroke as their greatest health concerns and less than 33% identified heart disease as the leading cause of death in women. Women in this study also reported worrying less about heart disease or heart attack than about cancer or breast cancer. Despite reporting that they were "knowledgeable" about heart disease, the participants had a low level of awareness of the warning signs of a heart attack and of risk factors for heart disease. Similarly, almost half of our participants were unaware that they were at risk of heart disease before their diagnosis.

Although 55% of our respondents had a relatively high level of awareness of their personal cardiac risks, only 36% of the women recognized that their initial symptoms were cardiac. Correspondingly, one-third of the women felt that their physicians missed the diagnosis of heart disease. Other studies have shown that even when risk factors are present and self-reported, the patients do not necessarily have better knowledge of cardiac disease symptoms or earlier presentation for treatment. Lower socioeconomic status and lower educational status have also been identified as risk factors for poor knowledge of heart disease risks and symptoms, leading to the conclusion that there are opportunities to educate patients who have these risk factors.

Lifestyle and Behavior Changes after Diagnosis

The current survey found that more than 85% of women with heart disease have not made significant lifestyle changes or healthy adaptations to their diet or activity program in response to their diagnosis. The beneficial cardiovascular effects of lifestyle changes in high-risk patients should not be underestimated. Data show that a structured exercise program and a Mediterranean-style diet reduce the risks of a second ischemic event. Many women in the current survey reported that they did not receive adequate counseling to make these changes. Other studies confirm that women frequently report that they have not been counseled or informed about heart disease by their health care providers. In the American Heart Association study, less than 30% of the women reported that their physicians discussed heart disease with them. In the survey reported by Legato et al., although 86% of the women reported seeing a physician regularly and, of those, 84% indicated that they were comfortable discussing heart disease with their physician, almost

60% reported that they had never received counseling about risk factors.

Little is known about why women in particular find it difficult to make lifestyle changes. Surveys in which patients self-report recollections of discussions with providers are often criticized because of concerns about recall bias. One survey of risk factor and health behavior counseling by providers (National Ambulatory Medical Care Survey by the Centers for Disease Control and Prevention) avoided this limitation by analyzing thousands of primary care visits. This study found that there were low overall levels of counseling for physical activity, diet, and weight reduction for all patients and that a smaller percentage of women than men received this type of counseling.

Furthermore, women who receive counseling about their risks and about the benefits of lifestyle changes do not necessarily implement new behaviors. Other factors, including social and medical support systems, health literacy, motivation, socioeconomic status, race and ethnicity, psychological health, and other barriers, may contribute to suboptimal adherence to recommendations. Women, in particular, may be excessively burdened by problems with depression and a negative change in personal relationships after a diagnosis of heart disease, making lifestyle changes extremely difficult. In our survey, 57% of patients reported mental illness such as anxiety or depression, and 27% said their interpersonal relationships had changed for the worse since their heart disease was diagnosed. The inability of women to feel positive about themselves and their ability to change behaviors likely play a key role in keeping them at high risk for declining cardiovascular health.

There are few data about effective programs that have helped women at risk achieve success in making and maintaining healthy behavior changes. In a recent review of health interventions, most studies included both men and women and did not tailor the program to the needs of a population with a high prevalence of anxiety and depression as seen in women with a diagnosis of heart disease.

Only 10% of our respondents felt they had maintained a substantial increase in physical activity after their diagnosis of heart disease even though most participated in the initial positive behavior of attending a cardiac rehabilitation program with a structured exercise program. Again, susceptibility to depression and deteriorating personal relationships may be important factors in creating additional barriers for high-risk women.

Strategies and interventions to increase long-term physical activity may include efforts in worksite and community settings, although few programs have specifically assessed the unique problems of women, especially those with cardiovascular disease. Programs based in worksites have proven beneficial. One program involved frequent and structured prompting, as well as home exercise, and resulted in increased functional capacity, as assessed by maximum oxygen consumption (Vo_2max) after 6 months. Although some women with heart disease no longer work, 57% of the women in our study were of typical working age (younger than 60 years). In our survey, 38% of the respondents reduced the number of hours they worked and 24% quit work entirely, thus lessening the potential influence of worksite programs.

With so few studies addressing the population of women at risk, clearly more research needs to be done to treat women more effectively. Further assessment of the barriers and motivators to achieving healthy and lifesaving behaviors in women with heart disease is indicated to provide more effective interventions.

Interaction with the Health Care System

Although overall satisfaction with their own physicians was high, the surveyed women were frequently dissatisfied with another aspect of their health care experience. Physician attitudes and interactions were the sources of most of the disappointments. Women frequently felt that they were not taken seriously enough, which resulted in delayed or missed diagnoses. They also perceived that in the health care system they were unable to receive the type of information that they needed. Previous reports have indicated relatively higher levels of dissatisfaction with health care among women than men. In the 1993 Commonwealth National Survey of Women's Health, 41% of women and 27% of men had changed physicians because of dissatisfaction. The most commonly cited cause of dissatisfaction was communication (32%), with women more frequently than men reporting paternalistic or dismissive attitudes of their physicians (25% vs. 12%) or being told that the conditions was "all in your head" (17% vs. 7%). With the emphasis on women's health during the past decade, this situation may be improving. In the follow-up 1998 Commonwealth Survey, women were more likely to give their physicians excellent ratings and to feel that their physicians "really cared about them and their health" than in 1993. However, in that survey only 7% of all women and 21% of women older than 65 years had heart disease.

Female patients, perhaps more than male patients, are affected by patient-provider communication. In a study of physician assessment of chest pain symptoms in women, the patient's presentation style significantly affected physicians' diagnostic impressions. In this study, a scripted history was presented by a woman with chest pain symptoms and was related in three ways to general internists. An actress presented her symptoms both in a "histrionic" and in a "business-like" manner to two groups of physicians. A third group of physicians read a verbatim transcript of the history. Physicians viewing the business-like portrayal were almost four times more likely to feel that a cardiac diagnosis was possible than those who viewed the histrionic portrayal. Even after reviewing identical laboratory data, physicians were almost twice as likely to recommend further cardiac evaluation for the woman with a business-like demeanor than the same actress with the more flamboyant presentation style, despite similar estimates for the likelihood of CAD. These marked differences in diagnostic approaches, solely on the basis of communication style, should be sobering to both physicians and the women they care for. In addition, physician attitudes perceived by patients influence women's willingness or reluctance to ask questions and to participate in making medical decisions. Lack of participation by patients in making medical decisions is associated with lower levels of satisfaction with care.

Although many women prefer female providers rather than male providers for their medical care, our survey did not find a higher level of satisfaction among women cared for by female physicians. This finding may be due, in part, to patients' expectations that same-gender interactions will be better, as well as to the relatively few patients cared for by female providers. It has also been suggested that bias of physicians may be responsible for some of the observed differences in the use of cardiac procedures between male and female patients. In a recent study, however, older women were less likely than men to undergo cardiac catheterization after a myocardial infarction regardless of whether they were cared for by female or male physicians. The authors concluded that if, in fact, the observed disparities between sexes are due to physician attitudes and beliefs, these attitudes are present in both male and female physicians. In the current study, satisfaction was much more closely linked to positive patient-provider interaction than to the sex of the physician.

Cardiac Rehabilitation

In our survey, 16% of women who were referred to a cardiac rehabilitation program did not attend, most frequently because of logistical barriers. Similar barriers have been identified in other studies, and they are more often a factor for women than men. One of the most powerful predictors of participation is the patient's perception of the strength of the treating physician's recommendation. Among patients with heart disease, older women are less likely than older men to participate but are also less likely to be given a strong recommendation by their physicians than men. Consequently, older women may be doubly disadvantaged: they have the lowest baseline functional status for fitness and psychosocial states, and thus would benefit the most from rehabilitation programs, but they are less likely to be strongly urged to participate.

In the current study, 31% of women with CAD were not referred for rehabilitation services. Although data are not available to show whether this group had contraindications to, or lack of indication for, participation in a rehabilitation program, women who have strong indications for cardiac rehabilitation have consistently been shown to be underreferred. Cardiac rehabilitation programs reduce morbidity and mortality and improve symptoms, exercise tolerance, lipid levels, and overall psychosocial health. Women who are eligible for rehabilitation services, however, are fundamentally different from their male counterparts because the women are older and more likely to be depressed, and they have more comorbid conditions, lower baseline functional status, and fewer psychosocial supports. Therefore, it is not surprising that programs primarily designed for middle-aged men do not always meet the needs of women. Moore surveyed female cardiac patients' preferences about their rehabilitation experiences. Women most valued peer group support, close monitoring during exercise, and variety in their exercise choices; they were bored with treadmills and cycling. They were fearful of exercise sessions causing pain and disliked frequent weight checks. They expected program staff to be interested not only in their physical well-being but also in their emotional health. Because nearly half the current survey participants experienced modest or significant deficiencies during their cardiac rehabilitation experience, and because the benefits of participation are great, further efforts should be made to meet the unique needs of women to enhance their outcomes.

Limitations

The current study has several limitations that should be considered. First, the survey population was drawn from women who had previously contacted WomenHeart. Therefore, a measure of selection bias is most likely present. This bias and the limited demographic information collected limit the generalizability of our findings.

A follow-up study incorporating more sophisticated sampling methods and more complete demographic information is planned.

One strength of the study is that its design with open-ended questions revealed a true "voice" of the women. However, this same design, by its dependence on self-reported diagnoses, medical data, and treatment, limits comparisons among subjects and quantification of the severity of illness. Both severity and the duration of time from event or diagnosis are variables known to affect answers to several survey questions. The results of the current survey should be confirmed and expanded upon in future assessments of women with heart disease.

Conclusion

This survey reports the experiences and perceptions of women with heart disease. It raises several important issues and concerns that will be critical to address if efforts to reduce death and disability and improve the outcomes of women diagnosed with heart disease are to be successful. Women with heart disease were often unaware of their risk and frequently did not recognize their symptoms as being cardiac related. Women cited frustration in their interactions with the health care system, largely from physician-related communication problems. Their experiences with cardiac rehabilitation, including frequency of referral and satisfaction with their program, bear further study, especially in light of the low levels of appropriate lifestyle changes made after receiving the diagnosis of heart disease. The diagnosis of heart disease has wide-ranging effects on virtually all aspects of women's lives. Improved understanding of these issues will help focus efforts to enhance earlier diagnosis, improve communication with providers, and ultimately lead to better health outcomes and quality of life.

Acknowledgments

This survey was funded by WomenHeart: The National Coalition for Women with Heart Disease. Dr. Bennett is a member of the speaker's bureau for AstraZeneca, Sankyo Pharmaceuticals, and Bristol Meyers Squibb Medical Imaging. The other authors have no financial affiliations to disclose.

References

A list of references is available in the original source.

Endometriosis
New Developments

by Andrea DuBrow

Endometriosis is a puzzling, painful disease that may be linked to environmental toxins. As with any complicated disease, there are numerous aspects that deserve attention: hormonal, surgical, and alternative treatments; (in)fertility issues; pain control; coping strategies; and research directions are among a few. Long-time readers of *The Network News* may remember that we raved about *The Endometriosis Sourcebook* in 1996, a comprehensive reference that finally addressed background and emerging issues for women with endometriosis. We still recommend this book for practitioners and women's health advocates, and particularly for anyone experiencing endometriosis. The purpose of this article is to highlight some of the potential connections between endometriosis and environmental causes, and to draw attention to new research showing a heightened risk of some cancers for women with endometriosis and their families.

What Is Endometriosis?

Endometriosis occurs when some of the tissue that usually lines the uterus also grows in other parts of the body. This extra endometrial tissue is most frequently found in the pelvic area: on the ovaries, external surface of the uterus, ligaments, or fallopian tubes. These growths may build up and bleed during menstrual periods. They respond to the hormonal influences of the menstrual cycle, and because the tissue has no way to leave the body, it may cause internal bleeding and scarring, inflammation, and/or the formation of cysts and scar tissue. Typical symptoms of endometriosis include chronic pain (particularly in the pelvic region), pain when menstruating, pain with sex, infertility, and painful bowel movements or urination. Interesting new findings reported by the Endometriosis Association also link endometriosis to chronic fatigue and chemical sensitivities and/or allergies.

What Causes Endometriosis?

Originally thought of as a disease of the endocrine system, new theories are emerging that may link endometriosis to immune dysfunction. In 1992, the Endometriosis Association published an article reporting on research that showed a very high rate of endometriosis in rhesus monkeys exposed to dioxin. The study sparked additional interest in the possible link between dioxins, PCBs (polychlorinated biphenyls) and endometriosis. Dioxins and PCBs are organochlorines, made from combining chlorine with organic substances, such as petrochemicals. Organochlorines can take hundreds of years to break down completely and are stored in fatty tissues of animals and humans. Banned in the U.S. in 1979, PCBs were used widely as electrical insulators, and in the manufacture of paint and inks. Discharged by industrial plants as wastewater, PCBs now contaminate water and soil. Dioxin, another environmental pollutant, is created from the incineration of toxic waste and municipal garbage, and the manufacturing and use of certain herbicides, pesticides, and solvents. In animals, dioxin is known to cause immune suppression, cancer, and birth defects. Over the past several years, increasing attention has been paid by the scientific community to the possibility that dioxin exposure may be linked to endometriosis. Articles have appeared in *Science* magazine, *Scientific American,* and other scientific publications on the dioxin-endometriosis connection, and studies are being conducted to explore this further.

Immunological Findings

Recent studies suggest another link among endometriosis, environmental pollutants, and changes in the immune system. The Endometriosis Association's research registry tracks health problems that are reported by women with endometriosis and their families. This tracking shows higher rates of immune-related problems and diseases than are found in the general population, ranging from allergies and chemical sensitivities to severe autoimmune disorders such as lupus. Some studies suggest that endometriosis is associated with changes in systemic immunity and, that cytokines (substances produced by cells in the immune system) may influence the ability of endometrial growths to spread and flourish where they don't belong. A fairly recent realization is that environmental pollutants like dioxin also have profound immunological impacts. While the precise impact of environmental pollutants on humans is unknown, endometriosis may be the first human disease definitely linked to hormonal and immunological disruption due to pollutants. The Endometriosis Association asserts that if dioxins, which are known carcinogens, are capable of causing endometriosis, perhaps women with endometriosis (and their families who shared their environmental exposures) might be at risk for cancer, too.

Higher Risks of Cancer and Autoimmune Diseases

The Endometriosis Association registry has collected reports which show that women with endometriosis, and their families, are more likely to be diagnosed with a number of cancers and other health problems, including breast cancer, melanoma, ovarian cancer, non-Hodgkin's lymphoma, and diabetes than would be expected in the general population. For example, 26% of the women with endometriosis in the registry have a family member with breast cancer. Even though endometriosis is very common, there are relatively few published studies that look at its possible link with other diseases. A Swedish study of 20,686 women with endometriosis found an increased risk of breast and ovarian cancer and non-Hodgkins lymphoma. A study conducted at Harvard Medical School found an increased risk of melanoma. Other conditions which were reported statistically significantly more often by women with endometriosis and their families in the registry included thyroid disorders, and autoimmune diseases such as rheumatoid arthritis, lupus, multiple sclerosis and Meniere's disease. According to the Endometriosis Association, many of the women in these studies may face even higher risks for cancer. This is because the study participants with endometriosis tend to be younger women (in their teens, 20s and 30s), and most cancers occur more frequently in older age groups. Therefore, they may become even more common as the study population ages.

In an effort to advance research on endometriosis and related health problems, the Endometriosis Association is entering a partnership with Vanderbilt University School of Medicine to conduct additional research on endometriosis, including the immunological aspects of the disease. This is the first time that a major medical institution has committed $2 million in funding, along with institutional support and laboratory facilities dedicated to studying the endocrine, immune, and environmental elements that may contribute to endometriosis.

For more information, readers may contact the Endometriosis Association at 8585 N. 76th Place, Milwaukee, WI, 53223, or call toll-free 1-800-992-3636.

References

Endometriosis Association newsletter, Volume 13, No. 2, 1992.
Ballweg, M. (1996). *The Endometriosis Sourcebook*. Contemporary Books: Chicago, IL.

Vagina Dialogue

One Woman's Battle with a Mysterious Illness

by Tenaya Darlington

Caroline More strolls in wearing cowboy boots. She has an all-American, Marcia Brady smile, an infectious laugh and a fast-talking style that can make your head spin, until you notice the way she anxiously wrings her hands and wrinkles up her nose to giggle, which is maybe also her way of wincing. This is the vagina monologue you never heard. This is the story of a woman who cannot sit down.

More's condition, known as vulvodynia—chronic vulvar pain—is a little-known phenomenon that reportedly affects 15% of women, many of whom are too private to divulge the fact that their privates are killing them. More, a former Chicago radio host who now lives in Monticello, in Green County, is more than willing to come forth as a spokeswoman, if only because media attention may eventually mean a cure for a condition that has plagued her for more than 10 years.

We're talking about a woman who cannot wear pants, a woman who has to apply an anesthetic cream in order to walk her dogs. Sex? Ha! More hasn't had intercourse in more than a decade. It's the sort of story that's so horrific it almost sounds made up, which is exactly the perception More and others are fighting against. Until vulvodynia was given a name in the '80s, many women who complained of chronic vaginal pain were dismissed as crazy.

More, who is on disability due to the condition, takes comfort in knowing that she is not alone. In October 2001, *Self* ran an article entitled "The Gyno Nightmare No One Talks About," in which author Susanna Kaysen (*Girl, Interrupted*) came out with her story on vulvodynia. The next month, a similar article ran in *Redbook*.

Dr. Sheldon Wasserman, an OB-GYN at St. Mary's Hospital in Milwaukee (and also a state representative) calls vulvodynia "a very serious disease." On March 15, he'll be the keynote speaker at a vulvodynia education forum at Meriter Hospital from 10:30 a.m. to 2 p.m., which More has been instrumental in organizing.

Wasserman, who first heard about vulvodynia as a medical intern in the late '80s, says, "It's such a horrible condition, and what's sad is that it's something people often can't discuss—it becomes a joke."

So what causes vulvodynia? There's the problem—the cause is still unknown, though suspected triggers include environmental allergens or irritants, repeated infections (such as yeast) and gynecological surgery. In November 2000, the National Institutes of Health announced provisions for funding the first vulvodynia research.

More believes her condition stems from a gynecological procedure she had in 1990, when she was 28. After a slightly abnormal Pap smear, her Chicago gynecologist treated her with cryosurgery, followed by 18 rounds of Efudex, a topical salve designed for solar keratoses (skin lesions), as a form of chemotherapy.

The package insert suggested that there could be an inflammatory reaction if the salve was used with an occlusive ("airtight") dressing. More says her gynecologist ignored the warning and inserted a tampon after each application of the salve. Eventually, she says, "My vagina closed up. I couldn't walk, I couldn't drive. I couldn't stand anything touching me there without thinking it was cutting me."

More has since discovered 92 registered complaints against Efudex, including severe cervical burns and spontaneous abortion. She is currently a plaintiff in a lawsuit against her former gynecologist and Efudex manufacturer Hoffman-La Roche.

Still, none of this solves More's biggest problem, which is that that she cannot lead a normal life. "I had a great job and a beautiful condo in Winnetka, Illinois, and I had to pack my things and walk away," More says, shaking her head. "I've literally had to do a chin-up for my life."

Today, More has relocated to a rural setting, where a quiet apartment gives her the peace she needs. She spends most of her time trying to cope with her pain, which she describes as "short, jagged and moving all the time." She juggles three hot baths a day with doctors' appointments and meetings with the local vulvodynia support group.

From *Isthmus*, Feb. 21, 2003, Vol. 28, No. 8, by Tenaya Darlington. Copyright © Isthmus Publishing Co. Inc. 2003. Reprinted by permission.

She begins her day with four doses of Neurontin, a drug that replaces the morphine she used to take, and continues to try alternative therapies, from Reiki to physical therapy to hypnosis. "I've tried everything," she says, and, in a moment of pure candor at the end of our interview: "I'm honestly not sure how much longer I can go on like this."

Two seconds later, though, she's laughing in that wincing way of hers. "Sometimes I just have to turn off the phone and put on some Chopin and climb in the bath!" She shifts her stance: "It's a psychological form of terror to have vulvar pain. I was never a feminist before this. Now I'm a screaming feminist. I want my life back."

What to Ask Your Gynecologist

by Molly M. Ginty

Eileen Duffy* was baffled by the bumps. Suddenly appearing around her vagina, they looked innocent and harmless enough: small, round, white, and soft to the touch. But they tingled and itched, so shortly after finding them, she shut the bedroom door of her off-campus apartment and called home hoping for help. When her mother couldn't peg the cause of the problem, Duffy dashed to the health clinic at her East Coast college.

"After the doctor examined me, she said, 'My God! You have genital warts!' in the most offended voice possible," Duffy remembers. "She didn't offer any advice. She didn't offer any information. She responded with complete disgust. I was shocked as I sat in her office, and I cried when I went home. Being told you have an STD is bad enough. But my doctor offered me no compassion or help whatsoever."

At the time, Duffy was 20 years old and had had less than a handful of sexual partners. Now 31 and a graduate student at the University of California, Berkeley, she has learned to live with the threat of recurring genital warts and with the incurable but treatable human papillomavirus (HPV) that causes them. But, like the millions of women in this country who have sexually transmitted infections—and the millions more who are at risk for them—she's still waiting for adequate and comprehensive care when it comes to her sexual health.

According to the Kaiser Family foundation (KFF), a nonprofit organization that tracks health care policy, 15.3 million STDs are contracted annually in this coun-

try. The U.S. has the highest infection rates of any industrialized nation. Every year, STDs cost more than $8.4 billion in treatment. Experts say we could slash this expense (and eliminate untold pain and suffering) if we pledged to take one simple step: provide effective screening and treatment during medical exams.

"Many women don't know what they're getting when they go in for a gynecological exam," says Dr. Lisa Gilbert, director of the women's health program for the American Social Health Association (ASHA), a nonprofit organization devoted to STD education. "They don't realize that a Pap smear detects changes in cervical cells without testing for any specific diseases. They don't realize that practically every STD requires a separate diagnostic. Because they don't understand the difference between a Pap smear, a pelvic check, and an STD test, they walk away thinking they've had all their STD tests when, in reality, they've had none."

Tests for common STDs include cervical swabs for chlamydia and trichomoniasis, follow-up testing of abnormal Paps for HPV, and blood tests for herpes, HIV, and hepatitis B. Patients don't realize they're not getting these tests, and doctors aren't coming out and telling them. Recent surveys show that this silence is widespread. KFF found that 40 percent of women aren't asked about their sexual histories on pre-exam questionnaires. And according to the Commonwealth Fund, 84 percent of women and 72 percent of teenage girls hadn't discussed STDs with their doctors in the year preceding the survey.

Why do so many patients fall through the cracks? Experts point to a lack of public awareness. People fail

*Her name has been changed

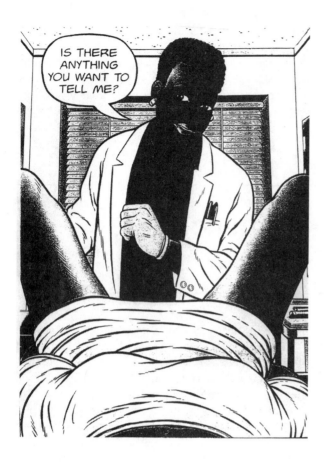

to grasp the fact that STDs are a real threat: transmitted through oral sex as well as intercourse, lurking in the systems of the mutually monogamous, and often asymptomatic or unnoticeable (which is the case with chlamydia, herpes, and HIV). People don't learn how to best protect themselves: condoms and dental dams are the most effective methods, followed by diaphragms, cervical caps, or spermicides. According to a KFF study, 74 percent of men and 69 percent of women who are of reproductive age seriously underestimate the prevalence of STDs, guessing that one in ten Americans will become infected during his or her life. Although one in ten seems scary, the truth is even more alarming: the real number is one in four. Says Tina Hoff, director of public health information for KFF, "People seem to believe that it just can't happen to them. There is such denial that it's really astounding."

Patients fail to do their part in prevention for a number of reasons. Some get tested only for HIV because it has the biggest public profile. Some discover they have rashes or discharges but then just shrug them off. Still others make the mistake of assuming they can't be at risk. "I had never been sexually active before my ex-husband, so STDs were the furthest thing from my mind," says Elaine Sweet, a 37-year-old policy analyst from Phoenix who has a strain of HPV that causes cervical cancer. "It never occurred to me that his past would come back to haunt me."

And then there's the stigma and shame of STDs. "We don't have famous people coming forward and saying, 'Can I be the poster child for herpes?'" says Gilbert. "STDs are very hidden, secret, and mysterious; and that's helping these germs replicate like crazy." Afraid of discovering that they are infected—or of being pegged as promiscuous—patients may be too timid to broach the subject with their doctors. Doctors, in turn, may be reluctant to step forward and make the first move. One KFF survey found that they were even less likely to broach the topic than their patients. "Some patients get insulted if you ask about STDs," says Dr. Robert Hagler, chair of the gynecological practice committee for the American College of Obstetricians and Gynecologists. "You run the risk of offending them, and this can make discussing STDs difficult."

Your Money or Your Life

As always, money complicates the issue. Many insurance companies refuse to cover testing that they don't deem "medically necessary." But if an STD is asymptomatic, "necessary" becomes a slippery slope. As Hagler points out, most HMOs set a ceiling fee for routine gynecological exams. If the cost of STD screening exceeds that limit, patients have to reach into their own pockets to pay for each $20 to $60 test. Add to that the fact that there are 44 million people in the U.S. that have no health insurance at all.

According to a survey by the Commonwealth Fund, women with no insurance and those who rely on Medicaid are more likely to discuss STDs with their doctors than women who see private physicians. But patients who rely on neighborhood clinics aren't necessarily getting better care. "At some public clinics in some states, the government won't pay for adequate screening," says Dr. Michael Burnhill, vice president for medical affairs at Planned Parenthood Federation of America. "These clinics use tests that have been around 20 years and aren't the most accurate or sensitive ones on the market." According to the Alan Guttmacher Institute, a reproductive rights advocacy group, the public sector spends $1 to prevent STDs for every $43 spent on treatment.

Yet another hurdle is the lack of set protocols. Each HMO has its own guidelines for STD screening. And that's just one set of marching orders. The American College of Obstetricians and Gynecologists, American Medical Association, Centers for Disease Control and

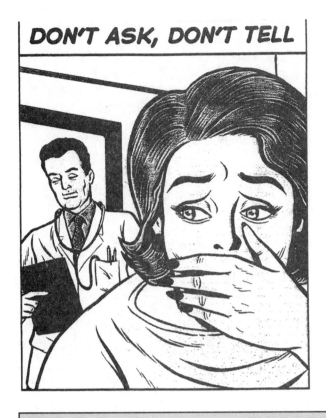

DON'T ASK, DON'T TELL

Prevention, National Committee for Quality Assurance, and ASHA all have separate recommendations. None of these wield the force of law and no two are exactly alike.

Without set protocols, doctors are left to their own devices to assess which patients are at risk. If they're in the Southeast, they might test for syphilis, which is more prevalent in that part of the country. If they're examining a patient who's under 25, they may test her for chlamydia and gonorrhea, which are more common in younger women. Beyond that, it's a matter of guesswork. "Often doctors have little more than appearance to base their screening decisions on," says Gilbert. "But it's impossible to look at someone and know if they're really at risk. STDs don't discriminate. You can't tell someone's STD status based on age, race, or socioeconomic factors."

Until modern medicine makes sense of the muddle, women must take charge of their own STD screening. Our very lives depend on it. We're more likely than men to suffer long-term health consequences: HPV can lead to cervical cancer; chlamydia can cause infertility and ectopic pregnancy; and, left untreated, HIV can be fatal.

STDS: The Good News

Recent Breakthroughs

- The addition of annual chlamydia screening for all sexually active women in the Health Plan Employer Data and Information Set (HEDIS) protocols for HMOs. These protocols, established by the National Committee for Quality Assurance, are almost always followed by HMOs. This is the first time STD screening has been included in HEDIS.
- New urine tests for chlamydia and gonorrhea that are simpler, quicker, and just as accurate as their predecessors. They test DNA and use the tiniest amount of bacteria to get an accurate diagnosis.
- New HPV tests that also use DNA, screening vaginal secretions for strains of the virus that leads to cervical cancer. They are approved as follow-ups for abnormal Paps.
- Three new herpes tests that are faster than their predecessors and are type-specific: the POCkit HSV-2 Rapid Test, the Premier Type-Specific HSV-11gG ELISA Test, and the Premier Type-Specific HSV-2 IgG ELISA Test. The POCkit test results are available immediately, sparing patients the wait of lab tests.

In the Works:

- Colorless, odorless, tasteless microbicides in the form of gels, creams, or foams that a woman can insert in her vagina before intercourse. In addition to STD protection, some prevent pregnancy as well.
- A tampon that would allow women to test themselves for several STDs.
- The first effective herpes vaccine, which could be available within two years.
- Topical antiviral therapies for herpes and HPV that work by activating the body's immune system and are now in clinical trials.
- HPV vaccines that are now in phase two clinical trials.
- HPV tests that allow a woman to swab cells from her vagina and bring them to the doctor for DNA analysis. Tested in South Africa, these are nearly as accurate as traditional Pap smears. In the future, swabs could also be used to detect chlamydia and gonorrhea.
- Rapid HIV blood tests that patients can take at home.

Women also face the added threat of transmitting infections to their unborn children. The tragic consequences can include premature birth, low birth weight, conjunctivitis, blindness, pneumonia, neurological problems, and congenital abnormalities.

To avoid these disasters, women need to step forward and get routine annual STD screening. Health advocates urge every woman to do the following:

- Get tested if you've had multiple partners, sex without a condom, or a partner who may have put you at risk.
- Get tested before having sex with someone new instead of checking for infection after the fact.
- Find out whether your health plan covers STD screening and head to a public clinic if it doesn't.
- Jot down questions before your appointment and review them with your doctor when you're most comfortable (sitting in an office chair instead of strapped in metal stirrups). *Which STDs will you be screened for?* (The answer should be the eight most common ones, which are, in order of incidence, HPV, trichomoniasis, chlamydia, herpes, gonorrhea, hepatitis B, syphilis, and HIV.) *How up-to-date are your doctor's tests?* (The answer should be no more than five years old.) *Is your doctor aware of new advances in screening?* (See sidebar.) *Will any of these be available to you?*
- Discuss your frequency of condom or dental dam use, number of past and present partners, and whether you engage in risky practices like anal sex. 'Fess up to all the nitty-gritty, and never succumb to embarrassment.
- Head back for annual testing as long as you remain sexually active. Take charge of scheduling your appointments: if you don't, your doctor may not.

Find that your doctor isn't cooperative? Find that she or he shrugs off STDs? Then, like Eileen Duffy, you may want to consider switching health care providers. "We live in an age where a woman can't assume she's not at risk," says Amy Allina, program director for the National Women's Health Network. "There are life-threatening STDs out there, and protecting your life should be something that your health care provider is concerned about."

Waging War on STDs—and Drugmaker Apathy—with Microbicides

by Elizabeth Suiter

On March 13, a coalition of scientists and advocates for women's health and HIV prevention from around the world gathered in Washington, D.C., to deliver a message to Congress: It's time to increase federal support for research into microbicides. The following day kicked off Microbicides 2000, the first international scientific conference on microbicides. Both events coincided with our production schedule, preventing us from reporting on their outcome, but here's a glimpse behind the scenes of this critical women's issue.

Inadequate means of protecting against sexually transmitted diseases (STDs) risk the lives and health of women around the world every day. For that reason, research is underway now to develop products known as microbicides, which enable women to protect themselves from HIV and other STDs but don't necessarily block conception.

Although not yet commercially available, microbicides will be similar to spermicides. They will be applied in the vagina as a foam, film, cream, suppository or gel, and will work in one of three ways: killing the organisms (or microbes) that cause HIV and other STDs, creating a barrier to block infection, or preventing the organisms from replicating after infection has occurred.

The Ideal Microbicide

What do women want in a microbicide? In acceptability research, prospective users have identified several characteristics as important for an "ideal" microbicide, including the following:

- It will be scentless and tasteless.
- It will not be messy.
- It will be long acting, making it unnecessary to apply immediately before sex.
- It will not be irritating. (This is particularly important, as vaginal irritation may both reduce microbicides' appeal and increase vulnerability to infection.)

Additionally, women's health advocates argue that microbicides should be available either with or without spermicidal capability. After all, in communities where HIV/STD prevalence is high, women cannot have children without putting themselves at risk for infection. In theory, non-spermicidal alternatives will give women the option of becoming pregnant while still protecting themselves against HIV or other STDs.

The Power of Control

STDs are one of the most important health concerns for women—and one of the least discussed. An estimated one in five people in the United States has an STD, with more than 15 million new infections occurring each year.[1] In addition to physical discomfort and social stigma, STDs are also a leading cause of infertility, cervical cancer, pelvic inflammatory disease, ectopic pregnancy and even death.

Sadly, many women cannot protect themselves from STD infection, as male condoms are the only protection proven to be effective. Heterosexual women depend on their partners to agree to use condoms, but if the partner is unwilling and the woman lacks power in her relationship, she may be unable to avoid unprotected sex. Even the female condom, another means of protecting against STDs, usually cannot be used with an unwilling partner.

Men and women alike might find microbicides more acceptable than condoms. If necessary, women could even use microbicides without their partners' knowledge.

What's more, studies show that when women control the contraception, they're much more likely to use it consistently and effectively than when they depend on their partners. Researchers expect that this pattern could hold true for STD prevention as well.

Finally, women want an option they can control. A recent survey by the Alan Guttmacher Institute (AGI) estimated that 21.3 million U.S. women ages 18 to 44 would be interested in using microbicides.[2]

Not Just for Women

Microbicides will benefit men as well as women, researchers say. A bi-directional protective effect means that women using them are less likely to infect their male partners.

Microbicides that can be used in the rectum will help to protect both men and women who have anal sex. HIV/AIDS researchers have emphasized the importance of this area of microbicide research, noting that any product approved to prevent HIV transmission in vaginal sex almost certainly will also be used for anal sex. Furthermore, anal sex is much more common among heterosexuals than is realized, particularly among adolescents who see it as a way to avoid unintended pregnancy.

Barriers to Market Availability

The major obstacle to microbicide development is a lack of funding and support from large pharmaceutical companies. Based on comparisons to spermicides, which do not make a lot of money for their manufacturers, the major drugmakers have decided not to invest a great deal of time or research in microbicide development.

Advocates argue that the spermicide comparison underestimates potential demand for microbicides. Given the demonstrated need worldwide for improved STD/HIV prevention tools, advocates say, the microbicide market could include every sexually active woman. And the AGI study showed that even women who are not worried about STDs express some interest in using microbicides.

Another concern for potential manufacturers is liability, since microbicides probably will not be 100% effective in protecting against potentially fatal diseases. However, this concern is not unique to microbicides. Moreover, some pharmaceutical representatives acknowledge that this concern will fade if the products become sufficiently profitable.

Other skeptics worry about safety. Microbicides are not, and will likely never be, as effective as condoms in preventing STDs. For instance, most of the products currently in development do not offer universal protection; instead, each is specific to one or a few types of STDs.

Researchers expect to deal with this obstacle by developing combination products that bring together components that work collectively against a broad spectrum of infections. For example, since physical barriers like diaphragms and cervical caps seem to offer some protection simply by covering the cervix, it may be possible to infuse physical barriers with microbicidal substances that also provide protection in the rest of the vagina.

What You Can Do to Bring Microbicides to the Market

Funding for research is the major obstacle to microbicide development, so the best step you can take is to help elicit support from both the public and private sectors.

- Ask your members of Congress to support expanded federal microbicide research.
- Contact pharmaceutical companies and tell them there is a market for microbicides.

- Help us gather signatures on a petition calling for greater international investment in STD prevention options for women.

To request copies of the petition or additional educational materials about microbicides, please contact our Women's Health Information Clearinghouse at 202/628-7814.

For their part, some public health advocates fear that use of microbicides could lead to lower condom use. However, preliminary studies in Thailand and surveys in the United States and Europe have shown that this is not likely to be the case, as women who are interested in microbicides often use no protection. For these women, microbicides will be a definite improvement.

Another issue is whether cost will be a barrier. Again, while microbicides may be more expensive than condoms, surveys in the United States, Europe and a number of developing countries have shown that most women are willing to pay more than twice the cost of condoms for protection they can control.

From Concept to Product

Despite low interest from large pharmaceutical companies, a number of small companies as well as governmental and nonprofit research entities are conducting research into microbicides. More than 60 different microbicide products are at various stages of testing. Approximately two-thirds are contraceptive as well as antimicrobial; the remainder act only against infection.

Products in development include:

- A buffer gel that works by maintaining the natural pH of the vagina, an environment too acidic for HIV to survive, thus countering the alkaline environment created by semen.
- A gel derived from seaweed that coats the vagina, preventing HIV transmission. (The same substance is also used as a thickening agent in ice cream.)
- A suppository that re-colonizes the vagina with normal lactobacilli bacteria that produce lactic acid and, in some species, hydrogen peroxide. Lactobacilli help keep the vaginal environment healthy and acidic.
- Genetically engineered plants that produce human antibodies against STDs, including HIV.

Some optimists estimate that a microbicide could be available to the public within three to four years. However, given the lack of funding and need for long-term research, a longer time frame is more realistic.

References

1. American Social Health Association, *Sexually Transmitted Diseases in America: How Many Cases, and at What Cost?* Research Triangle Park, NC: ASHA, 1998, Table 2, p. 17.
2. Darroch, Jacqueline and Jennifer Frost. "Women's Interest in Vaginal Microbicides." *Family Planning Perspectives.* v 31, n 1, January/February 1999, p 16.

With or without the Dam Thing
The Lesbian Safer Sex Debate

by Carol Camlin

I have a rare lesbian safer sex poster on my office wall that shows two young white women embracing, naked and wet, in a steamy public bath. One woman sits on a tiled ledge with her legs spread, hair tossed in her face, smiling blissfully. The other is on her knees, leaning into her lover's open thighs, her head arched back. The text, in lavender, reads: "Wet your appetite for safer sex."

As a lesbian HIV/AIDS educator at the AIDS Action Committee of Massachusetts, I pay keen attention to the few safer sex messages and images produced for lesbians by national and international HIV/AIDS service organizations. For one thing, this environment brimming with gay male erotic safer sex posters would make any healthy lesbian long for a few pictures of nude women. I also pay attention to keep abreast of the raging debate about lesbian sexual transmission of HIV—the so-called dam debate—among those who advocate either for or against the use of dental dams for oral sex (dental dams are small latex squares available at your local dental supply store: just masquerade as a dentist and ask for the 100-pak).

The lesbian safer-sex poster on my wall is different from gay male posters in one significant way. The scene evokes the eroticism of wetness, and seems to encourage comfort with bodily fluids. Wetness is sexy but, in the context of HIV, has come to seem dangerous. Although the poster would probably be a turn-on for most lesbians, I would imagine that The Terrence Higgins Trust (THT), the British AIDS service organization that produced the poster, has taken some flak for this one. The poster introduces the idea that there is such a thing as lesbian safer sex, without directly advocating the use of dental dams.

Carrying this message one step further, at the VIII International Conference on AIDS in July, THT unveiled a poster that directly advocates that lesbians *not* use dental dams. "Very low risk in oral sex," it advised, "so ditch those dental dams. Don't bother with gloves unless it turns you on." The poster immediately unleashed a storm of protest. Dozens of ACT UP members (most of them men) zapped the THT display booth, chanting "Shame!," spray painting it and modifying the poster with messages like "This poster is killing lesbians."

The intense controversy surrounding woman to woman sexual transmission of HIV is largely due to the fact that a very little HIV-prevention education information is geared to lesbians, despite our involvement in all aspects of the epidemic.

How many lesbians either harbor exaggerated fears of HIV or assume they're at no risk of HIV infection (or any other sexually transmitted disease)? How many lesbians are tacitly restricting their sexual practices, and so their sexual pleasure, out of fear of the unknown? How many HIV-positive lesbians know what they can safely do with their HIV-negative girlfriends? How many HIV-negative lesbians worry about how to have sex with their HIV-positive girlfriends without putting them at risk of an immune-threatening infection? Why this dearth of information?

In her July 1992 *Herizons* article, "Damned If You Do, Damned If You Don't," Lesli Gaynor of the AIDS Committee of Toronto argues: "The exclusion of lesbians and lesbian sexuality from AIDS education is not only a reflection of homophobia within mainstream education, but also a sign of the systematic sexism that exists within the gay community."

Lesbians need and deserve to get the facts abut AIDS, but the rare attempts to define safer sex for lesbians have focused almost exclusively on the use of dental dams. As a result, many lesbians have a vague idea that they should be using these devices, yet as Nancy Solomon notes in her Spring 1992 *Out/Look* article, "Risky business", very few women do—including lesbian safe sex educators who issue public pronouncements about dental dams.

Given the lack of availability of dental dams and their sexual unattractiveness, is it any surprise that we're not using them? I've heard the "damn dams" described as "about as sexy as a pair of rubber pants for the diaper wearing set" in Jenifer Firestone's "Memoirs of a Safe

Sex Slut" (in *Bad Attitude*) and cunnilingus with a dam described as "chewing on a rubber tire."

Most lesbian health educators acknowledge that the three-inch-by-three-inch dental dams are small and difficult to use. How do you know when your spit ends and her fluids begin, unless you're really alert? Some educators advocate plastic wrap as an option for oral sex, because it's convenient, and it's larger. "Also," as one plastic-wrap aficionado puts it, "you can see through it, and that's nice."

Still others question barrier use in the first place. Louise Rice, a lesbian health educator and nurse at the AIDS Action Committee observes in her August 1992 *Sojourner* article, "Rethinking Dental Dams": "Barrier protection against HIV in vaginal fluids has no proven efficacy. Dental dams provide false security for an activity (going down) that already carries a relatively low risk."

Instead of broadening the topic of lesbian safer sex, the dam debate has sometimes obscured a deeper and more detailed discussion about the range of behaviors and activities which put lesbians at highest risk for infection with HIV and other STDs. After all, cunnilingus is not *all* we do. Do we focus on the use of dental dams because that's all we know how to talk about? Do we avoid discussion about the behaviors which put us at highest risk because of deep-seated taboos within the lesbian community?

Most HIV-positive lesbians became infected by sharing injection drug needles, or having sex with men without a condom. Several studies have shown that at least one-third of lesbians in the 20 to 35 year-old age group have slept with men, even after coming out. Simply having a lesbian identity does not make you "immune" to HIV: Our community must come to terms with the facts that lesbians sometimes use IV drugs and sometimes have sex with men.

Although these two risk factors are primarily responsible for the incidence of HIV among lesbians, it is possible for HIV to be transmitted sexually from woman to woman. Even those who aren't lesbian latex zealots agree that we are not "God's Chosen People." Lesbian sexual transmission of HIV is very rare—but just how rare, exactly how it happens, and how to prevent it are all points of debate. The information available to lesbians about what constitutes safer sex for lesbians is ambiguous and diverse in opinion.

AIDS service organizations offer advice to lesbians ranging from "stock up on latex condoms or dams" to AIDS Committee of Toronto's provocative suggestion "a little more sex, a little more leather, a little more lace, a little LESS LATEX." Somewhere in the middle of this, a growing number of lesbian health educators argue that, well into the second decade of this epidemic, enough is known about HIV transmission to suggest that HIV prevention education for lesbians need not include the "dental dams at all times under all circumstances" message. What exactly are the HIV transmission risks with woman to woman sex?

Let's review the facts. For someone to get infected, HIV not only has to get OUT of one person, via an infected body fluid, it also has to get INTO another person's bloodstream, via the mucous membranes or a break in the skin.

How the Virus Leaves the Body   The highest concentration of HIV can be found in blood, and the next highest in semen. In vaginal fluid and pre-seminal fluid (or pre-cum, the fluid that men emit before ejaculation), the concentration is much lower. In some fluids such as tears or saliva, the concentration of HIV is so low or non-existent that there's no risk of infection.

The Chance of Infection via Oral Contact with Vaginal Fluid Is Very Low, and It Depends on the Presence of Blood Products   However, several factors can increase the likelihood of the presence of HIV: menstrual blood, vaginal infections (such as yeast) and sexually transmitted diseases (such as herpes and chlamydia) can elevate levels of HIV in vaginal fluid, because all would contain white blood cells which harbor HIV. In later stages of HIV disease all bodily fluids contain higher concentrations of HIV. Also, the pH, or level of acidity, of the vaginal fluid can influence whether HIV is present. The pH of vaginal fluid is normally low, or acidic, and "inhospitable" to HIV (the pH of semen, on the other hand, is higher, or alkaline—and therefore more "hospitable" to HIV). Vaginal fluid is more alkaline during menstruation and ovulation.

How the Virus Enters the Body   You can become infected with HIV if someone else's infected body fluid enters your bloodstream via breaks in the skin or via mucous membranes. Mucous membranes line the rectum, vagina and mouth (and in men also the urethra and glans—the tip of the penis); they're also found in the inside of your nose and eyelids. Some mucous membranes are thick and strong, and others are thin, and easier for the virus to pass through. The rectum is the most vulnerable because the walls of the rectum are very thin and there are tiny blood vessels at its surface which are easily ruptured during anal intercourse. The walls of the vagina are tougher and thicker, therefore less vulnerable to fissures and tears (with well-lubricated penetration and trimmed fingernails). The mucous membranes in the mouth are thicker than either the rectum or the vagina. It's therefore difficult for HIV to enter the bloodstream through your mouth. Moreover, saliva has a neutralizing effect on HIV, making it harmless when present in a low concentration, such as in vaginal fluid.

Reducing Your Risks   "Lesbians do everything from nibbling on each other's ears to fisting—and in between there are a lot of things that are safe and some things that aren't," notes Amelie Zurn, Director of Lesbian Services at the Whitman-Walker Clinic in D.C. "The point is, risk is relative . . . for some people, any risk at all is unacceptable. For other people, more risk is okay."

The key to safer sex is communication: defining your limits and talking to your partner about what you want. To assess your risks and decide what to do, communicate with your partner.

Get to Know Your Vagina   "Vaginal fluids have not been studied enough," Louise Rice acknowledges, "but women are capable of doing the studying. Getting to know your vagina, your discharges and smells, and those of a partner, can alert you to changes and potential infections. Unrecognized and untreated infections are a concern for all women, not just those with HIV. When HIV is present, an infection can quickly become disabling."

Get to Know Your Mouth   Remember, even if you go down on a woman and she is menstruating or has a vaginal infection, the virus still has to find its way into your bloodstream. You may want to use a barrier under those circumstances—but if you don't there are ways to make oral sex even safer than it is, without having to use a barrier.

If you have a cold sore, or bleeding gums, or a cut on your tongue, "wait until you've healed so that you don't have to waste time and needless worry," Lesli Gaynor of Toronto advises. "If you have a contagious mouth condition like herpes, it's only courteous to consider the other person's health."

Gaynor offers an additional tip for safe licking: "Don't brush [or floss] your teeth before oral sex—use mouthwash to get that just-brushed fresh feeling." If your partner is HIV-positive, you may want to use mouthwash as a matter of course, to protect her from germs in your mouth.

You also may want to go down on your partner BEFORE you penetrate her with your hand or a sex toy. This will reduce the chance of there being blood present in the vaginal fluid.

Gaynor also suggests, "Take a closer look at what you're about to eat. If there are sores or areas of concern, don't panic but avoid contact. Kiss the surrounding areas lovingly."

Rimming   Oral contact with the anus isn't a risk for HIV transmission unless the rectum contains blood (such as following "rough" anal penetration, and even then bleeding may not necessarily occur). But, you could contract another kind of infection via rimming, such as hepatitis A or amoebas. It's a good idea to use a barrier for rimming.

Fingerfucking or Using a Dildo   HIV can be transmitted if menstrual or other blood of an HIV-positive woman gets into the vagina or anus of her partner. The safest option is to use your own toy. Wash thoroughly after each use with soap and water. If you share toys, use a condom and put on a new condom (with plenty of water-based lubricant) before you share. Or, wash thoroughly before sharing.

Remember, **intact skin is a good barrier against HIV infection.** If you have open cuts on your fingers and she's menstruating or has a vaginal infection, use latex or vinyl gloves or finger cots when penetrating her. A message to all you "Lee-Press On" femmes: trim those finger nails if you're planning to fuck her! The lesbian fashion of trimmed, smooth fingernails is in place for good reason: you don't want to cut or tear the lining of the vagina.

If you or your partner is HIV-positive, latex or vinyl gloves serve the function of not exposing an HIV-positive woman to bacteria and other germs under the fingernails, and reducing the risk of a cut in your or her vagina which could allow the germs to pass through to the bloodstream.

Fisting   This can result in fissures or tears in the vaginal (or rectal) lining, which can result in both the presence of blood and access to the bloodstream. Fisting is an activity which can place both partners at risk, since tears may occur on the skin of the person doing the fisting. Use latex or vinyl gloves with plenty of water-based lubricant when fisting, and if you plan to go down on her, either do so before you penetrate her or use a barrier.

Piercing, Cutting and Other S/M Activities   Let the above principles of HIV transmission, and common sense be your guide in assessing risks and taking precautions with S/M activities. Invest in your own favorite equipment: latex or rubber toys, leather goods or metal equipment. The surest and safest guide is to not share equipment at all. If, however, it's not possible for you to supply your own, every precaution should be taken by you and your partner to make sure that equipment is properly cleaned prior to any sexual scene: 1) wash your equipment thoroughly, 2) soak it for several hours in a solution of one-part bleach to ten-parts water, and 3) rinse it thoroughly several times to be sure that all the bleach has been removed. These guidelines are adapted from the brochure "AIDS-Safe S/M," distributed by the

AIDS Action Committee of Mass. For further information about S/M safety, see Pat Califia's *The Lesbian S/M Safety Manual: Basic Health and Safety for Woman-to-Woman S/M* Denver: Lace Publications, 1988.

Do I think cunnilingus is an effective way of spreading HIV? No . . . and the reason is that cunnilingus is not an effective way of spreading things which are much more infectious, like hepatitis B, which has 100,000 times more viral particles per cubic milliliter of blood than HIV. There has never been a single reported case of woman-to-woman transmission of hepatitis B via oral sex. In addition, given the number of lesbians infected with HIV, we would be seeing many, many cases of women getting infected via oral sex with other women—and we aren't

When HIV/AIDS educators talk to gay men about oral sex, most say, "Oral sex is very low risk. You can make it safer by not taking his come into your mouth. To be absolutely safe, you can use a condom." Very few gay men use condoms for oral sex, yet studies have shown that only about two dozen gay men worldwide, of the millions infected with HIV, have become infected via oral sex—and in those cases, almost all the men had taken ejaculate in the mouth, there were usually severe dental or gum problems, and often a high number of sexual partners (in the hundreds).

Dental dam advocates argue that data on lesbian transmission is fragmentary, since the Centers for Disease Control (CDC) doesn't include woman-to-woman transmission among the risk factors they normally track. Any well-informed AIDS activist knows that the CDC AIDS surveillance system is faulty, because it is based on the identity rather than the behavior of the person with AIDS. The sexual orientation of a person with AIDS does not explain how they became infected. The category "male homosexual/bisexual" doesn't tell us, for example, whether a man had insertive or receptive anal sex. The "heterosexual" category doesn't differentiate between those who became infected via anal or vaginal intercourse.

Although the right questions are not asked, the surveillance data is based on a hierarchy of transmission grounded in medical research and the real experience of people who've become infected with HIV. Sharing injection drug needles will put you in the "IV Drug User" category whether you are a gay or straight woman. Having unprotected intercourse with a man will put you in the "Heterosexual" category even though you identify as a lesbian. Both of those behaviors are much more likely to have caused your infection with HIV than going down on your girlfriend, because HIV is transmitted very efficiently and easily via blood to blood or semen to blood contact. To know the scope of the epidemic in the lesbian

community at large, we need among other things a national seroprevalence survey of self-identified lesbians.

Most lesbian health educators acknowledge that although lesbians with HIV haven't been studied well, several lesbian health studies do exist. In studies of hundreds of lesbians with AIDS, only four cases of woman-to-woman transmission of HIV via sex have been reported in the medical literature. In the first case, both partners reported oral, anal and a vaginal contact with blood during sex (*Annals of Internal Medicine,* vol. 105, no. 6). The second case involved a woman whose female partner, an injection drug user, was in the late stages of HIV disease (*Annals of Internal Medicine,* vol. 111, no. 11). In the final two cases the HIV-positive lesbians' sexual partners were HIV-negative, and they reported no IV drug use or sex with men (*The Lancet,* 7/87 and *AIDS Research,* vol. 1, 84). The problem with these last three cases is that it is not reported exactly how the women became infected. There are several other anecdotal, word-of-mouth reports of sexual transmission of HIV between women. We may never know the full story with those cases, but we need only return to what we know about HIV transmission to be able to assess risks and make decisions about what we want to do sexually.

HIV prevention education for gay men is usually very sex-positive. Why do we reserve all of our sexual conservatism for lesbians, by passing out dams and gloves and issuing blanket statements to lesbians such as "oral sex on a woman is risky" and "putting your fingers inside her can be risky"? Most HIV/AIDS educators wouldn't dream of telling a heterosexual man to wear a glove when putting his fingers in his girlfriend's vagina.

Many lesbian educators and activists are feeling that lesbians already have so much stacked against our sexual pleasure and freedom: internalized homophobia, racism and sexual abuse drain our self-esteem and sexual power; sexism and the puritan tradition subtly pervade how we think about sexuality and our bodies; our parents inculcated sexual shame in most of us, and that shame and guilt is only multiplied when we realize that we are queer.

Coming out can be an explosion of that shame into delight and power—and yet well-publicized phenomena such as "Lesbian Bed Death" and the general perception hat lesbians do it less than everybody else ("Bullshit!" some of us say; "Well quantity and quality are two separate things," other of us say) are signs that these various forms of oppression have taken their toll on our community.

The implicit question asked by many lesbian educators is: Do we want to be a part of what's keeping lesbians from getting it on and enjoying themselves, by exacerbating fears and encouraging lesbians to restrict themselves sexually? Absolutely not. We do need to continue to get the information out about what's risky and what's not.

"Every day, women make decisions about the risk of different activities," Louise Rice noted, "Most of these activities (smoking or driving a car, for example) carry a far greater risk than cunnilingus. Thousands of lesbians' lives could be saved if we were to devote half the attention to mammograms and breast self-awareness that has been focused on dental dams."

Having put out all of this provocative information, I'd like to suggest that we turn our political focus outward and turn our activism towards improving the lives of ALL women with AIDS—not just lesbians with AIDS. In the United States, women with AIDS make up only 4 percent of all clinical trials, although women make up 13 percent of all people with AIDS (and that's an underestimate of about 28 percent). Fourteen million women still don't have access to health insurance. The CDC case definition of AIDS still doesn't include life-threatening gynecological manifestations of AIDS. The number-one HIV transmission risk for women is IV-drug use: We need to make clean needles available and drug treatment accessible. All of these issues are lesbian health issues. And we can achieve victories on many of these fronts if we ACT UP louder and in greater numbers. Meantime, let's talk about sex—and have as much as we want.

A Gendered Epidemic
Women and the Risks and Burdens of HIV
by Peter Piot, MD, PhD

The world has known about acquired immune deficiency syndrome (AIDS) for 20 years, and during that time, the severity of the epidemic has continued to surpass even the most pessimistic predictions. Despite the devastation that human immunodeficiency virus (HIV) has already caused, it is now clear that we are still in the early stages of the epidemic. As the epidemic has progressed, it has also become clear that it is fueled by the forces of inequality, social exclusion, and economic vulnerability.

This progression is most evident in the increasing impact of HIV on women. Where the HIV epidemic has been established longest and spread furthest, women represent an increasing proportion of those infected. Today, women make up just less than half the global total of nearly 34 million adults living with HIV, 55% of the 24 million adults living with HIV in sub-Saharan Africa, and 30% of total adult infections in the rest of the world.[1]

The largest gender difference is at younger ages: Average infection rates among teenage girls in sub-Saharan Africa are more than 5 times higher than those among teenage boys and in some countries of the region as much as 16 times higher. Women in their early 20s in sub-Saharan Africa are infected on average at 3 times the rate of men their age.[1]

The disproportionately high rates of infection among girls and young women is accounted for in large part by age mixing: younger women with older male sex partners. Not only are older male partners more likely to be infected than age-equivalent partners would be, but the relative immature genital tracts in younger women make them more susceptible to infection.

Women have come to comprise the majority of the HIV-infected population in sub-Saharan Africa because the rate of women's infection peaks at a younger age than men's, younger age groups are a large proportion of the population, and those infected at younger ages tend to survive longer. Elsewhere in the world, rates of HIV infection among women are continuing to rise. Parts of the Caribbean are characterized by longstanding epidemics and similar age mixing to that found in sub-Saharan Africa, with similar consequences. In parts of Central America, where heterosexual transmission of

From *Journal of the American Medical Women's Association,* Summer 2001, Vol. 56, No. 3 by Peter Piot. Copyright © 2001 by the American Medical Women's Association. Reprinted by permission.

HIV predominates and is exacerbated by economic and race-based disparities, the epidemic is becoming generalized across populations, and women are increasingly affected. Antenatal testing has found HIV prevalence of 3% to 7% in several of Caribbean littoral countries.[1]

Women are an increasing proportion of the epidemic in many high-income countries. Over time, the epidemic follows patterns of social disadvantage, so that in many cases, the women who have been most affected are those from disadvantaged or minority ethnic populations.

The rapidly growing epidemic in Eastern Europe, where transmission through injection drug use predominates, is also rapidly spreading to the sex partners of injection drug users. The epidemic in Asia is affecting women who are particularly vulnerable, such as sex workers, and those whose lives do not fit conventional notions of "risk." For example, 93% of 400 female attendees at a sexually transmitted diseases clinic in Pune, India, were married, and 91% had never had sex with anyone but their husbands, yet 14% were infected with HIV.[2]

The burden of HIV/AIDS on women continues to increase. Women bear a disproportionate burden of HIV-related care. The growing number of AIDS orphans—at least 13 million worldwide, mainly in Africa—have, in many communities, already exceeded the capacity of extended families to cope. Women in some African villages are helping child-headed households to cope, by ensuring that the house door is locked at the end of the day, for example.[1]

The HIV/Aids epidemic is driven by the interlocking dynamics of risk, vulnerability, and impact. The immediate risks of HIV exposure through sex or injection drug use are structured by underlying forces of HIV-related vulnerability—the extent to which individuals have the capacity to control their risks. Women's HIV vulnerability derives in particular from contexts in which they have little control over sex, whether as a consequence of the predominating power relations between men and women or as a function of the economic and life choices available to them.

In turn, the impact of the epidemic itself creates additional HIV-related vulnerabilities. Populations suffering the stresses of a substantial AIDS toll have weakened resources to resist further spread of the epidemic. Women and girls from families whose productive capacities have been weakened by AIDS may have to resort to risky sex for their livelihoods. And planning for the future becomes a more distant goal in the face of current devastation.

Breaking the vicious cycle of HIV risk, vulnerability, and impact requires a systematic, sustained, and multisectoral AIDS response. Addressing the social and economic circumstances of women and girls is key to the effectiveness of a sustained AIDS response, as are strategies that address relations between men and women.

For some time, UNAIDS, together with many other governmental and non-governmental agencies, has argued that a gender dimension needs to be a central part of all AIDS strategies. It is now time to add that AIDS needs to be a part of all gender strategies.

AIDS constitutes a global development crisis. In the worst-affected countries, AIDS is turning life expectancy back by decades, cutting economic production by 1% to 2% a year, and putting development goals out of reach. Elsewhere, it has the potential to cause similar damage, unless sustained intervention holds the epidemic in check.

The precise form of effective, society-wide AIDS responses will differ in different settings, but there are a number of conditions of success that are both universally applicable and that will bring rapid results.

Women's organizations and women-led civil society responses are vital building blocks of the AIDS response, demonstrated repeatedly in contexts as diverse as the care, support, and prevention services of The AIDS Support Organization in Uganda and the empowerment of female sex workers in Sonagachi in Calcutta. Increasingly important are organizations that provide a direct voice for HIV-positive women.

Voluntary counseling and testing is the entry point for HIV care. Its effectiveness in preventing the spread of HIV is greatly enhanced where it addresses both men and women, and, especially, couples.

Preventing HIV transmission from mother to infant has become technically feasible and relatively inexpensive, yet more than 1 million infants are born with HIV annually, because their mothers do not have access to antenatal or postnatal care, HIV testing, antiretroviral therapy, or safe alternatives to breastfeeding. Extending the reach of care to prevent transmission from mother to child should also be the platform for extending HIV care to women as the necessary infrastructure for HIV testing and care is made more widely accessible.

Keeping girls in school addresses HIV risk, vulnerability, and impact. As epidemics mature, HIV prevalence has been found to be associated with lower levels of education. The most effective school-based interventions simultaneously address both the skills children need and their social context. Tanzania, for example, is extending successful approaches that combine life-skills education, peer involvement, school-based AIDS committees (including parents), and guardian schemes to protect girls from sexual harassment.

Micro-finance initiatives, mainly involving women, are increasingly addressing AIDS by countering the social exclusion that makes some women particularly vulnerable. Micro-finance institutions have community education infrastructures that provide a venue for HIV-related community education. Micro-finance can be integrated into community coping mechanisms, as for example in the Uganda Women's Effort to Save Orphans, where micro-finance assists the caretakers of AIDS orphans.

The impact of AIDS is gendered in its every aspect: in conflict and emergency situations where rape is used as a weapon and in situations of extreme privation where sex is one of the only commodities; in the application of inheritance law where AIDS widows can lose their capacity to maintain family livelihood; in prevention commodities where female condoms, having proven acceptable, now need to become accessible; and in research where public subsidy is needed to accelerate the development of an effective microbicide, which would place a major HIV-prevention tool under women's control.

The recent UN General Assembly Special Session on AIDS saw nations sign on to a comprehensive set of AIDS targets, including a commitment to the participation of women in national AIDS strategies, reducing HIV prevalence in young people by 25%, a 20% reduction in transmission to infants by 2005 and a 50% reduction by 2010, as well as commitments to strengthened responses in relation to care, vulnerability, and conflict.

These commitments set a new benchmark of accountability for national and global AIDS responses. They will remain unachievable until and unless responding to AIDS becomes a central plank in worldwide efforts to empower women and, correspondingly, that gender becomes a central consideration across the totality of AIDS responses.

References

1. *Report on the Global HIV/AIDS Epidemic*. Geneva: UNAIDS;2000. UNAIDS/00.13EO
2. Gangakhedkar RR, Bentley ME, Divekar AD, et al. Spread of HIV infection in married monogamous women in India. *JAMA*. 1997; 278:2090-2092.

W O R K S H E E T — C H A P T E R 1 3

Politics of Disease

1. Fill in the chart below, showing what is available in terms of prevention, detection, and treatment for each of the three cancers listed.

Cancer	Prevention	Detection	Treatment
Breast			
Cervical			
Endometrial			

2. Think about what you learned from doing question # 1. Was it easier to find some information than other information? What do you think this represents in terms of the priority given to prevention, detection, and treatment of cancers?

3. Why do you think it is dangerous for there to be confusion about prevention vs. detection for cancers? How could health education and health policies emphasize prevention?

4. Several articles identify the silence around certain diseases as being a problem. The author of the chronic fatigue article identifies how important her support group was for her and the Endometriosis Association is an example of an organization which has brought women together throughout the world to talk about their condition and support each other. Identify the roles that self-help support groups could have for women. Pick a specific disease or condition around which you might organize a support group. Describe how you might find other people to join the group and imagine the topics the group might discuss. Identify advantages and disadvantages of doing this in person or through the internet.

5. Combine ideas from this chapter's "What to Ask Your Gynecologist" and Chapter 1's "How To Tell Your Doctor a Thing or Two" (p. 24) to design a poster or leaflet for college women on "Be an Active Patient to Prevent, Detect, and Treat STIs."

6. One of the most rapidly growing groups of people infected with HIV is that of adolescents, many of whom become infected through heterosexual intercourse.

   a. If you were to design an educational program for high school students to help prevent transmision of HIV, what specific information would you want to include?

   b. What obstacles might there be to presenting this information in the public schools? Discuss how you might present an argument for inclusion of the prevention program.

   c. Discuss any ideas you might have for overcoming adolescents' belief in their own invulnerability ("It can't happen to me") when teaching about HIV/AIDS.

   d. "With or Without the Dam Thing" addresses HIV-prevention in a sex-positive, explicit manner, addressing risks associated with specific sexual activities. Can you imagine using ideas from this article to design information for heterosexual, gay or lesbian teens?

7. "Women's HIV vulnerability derives particularly from contexts in which they have little control over sex, whether as a consequence of the predominating power relations between men and women or as a function of the economic and life choices available to them." Discuss how this statement specifically about HIV in "The Gendered Epidemic" could be expanded to talk about women's vulnerability to other sexually transmitted infections and unwanted pregnancies.

Resource Information

The following resources have been used in drawing together this collection of readings and are examples of the wide range of publications which now cover women's health issues from a diversity of perspectives.

(**NOTE:** The following publications which produced articles reprinted here are no longer regularly published:

Bread and Roses

Changing Men

The Coalition for the Medical Rights of Women

Sojourner: The Women's Forum.

We will particularly miss *Sojourner* which stopped publication as we were preparing this fourth edition of the book. *Sojourner* was a long-term activist paper committed to, and successful at, publishing women's health articles from a diversity of women, always looking at how women's health and health care delivery are influenced by interlocking systems of oppression.)

Abortion Access Project
552 Massachusetts Avenue, Suite 215
Cambridge, MA 02139
(617) 661-1161
Fax: (617) 492-1915
Website: www.abortionaccess.org
Website: info@abortionaccess.org

American Public Journal of Public Health
American Public Health Association
800 I Street, N.W.
Washington, D.C. 20001-3710
(202) 777-2742
Website: www.ajph.org

American Medical Student Association
(800) 767-2266
Website: amsa@www.amsa.org

Annals of Internal Medicine
American College of Physicians
American Society of Internal Medicine
Website: www.annals.org

Atlantic Monthly
77 North Washington Street
Boston, MA -2114
(617) 854-7700

Boston Women's Health Book Collective
c/o Boston University School of Public Health
715 Albany Street, W-1, Room 120
Boston, MA 02118
(617) 414-1230
Fax: (617) 414-1233
Website: www.ourbodiesourselves.org

Bust
Bust, Inc.
78 5th Avenue
New York, NY 10011

The Capital Times
1901 Fish Hatchery Road
Madison, WI 53713
(608) 252-6480

Common Ground—Different Planes (The Women of Color Partnership Program Newsletter)
100 Maryland Avenue, NE
Washington, D.C. 20002

Council on Interracial Books for Children
1841 Broadway, Room 500
New York, NY 10023

Domestic Abuse Intervention Project
202 East Superior Street
Duluth, MN 55802
(218) 722-2781
Fax: (218) 722-0779

Essence Magazine
1500 Broadway
New York, NY 10036
(212) 642-0600
Fax: (212) 921-5173
e-mail: info@essence.com

FDA *Consumer*
Department HHS, FDA
5600 Fishers Lane, Room 15A19
Rockville, MD 20857
(310) 827-7130
Fax: (301) 827-5308
Website: www.fda.gov

Feminist Review
Palgrave Macmillan Journals
Houndmills
Basingstoke
Hampshire RG21 6XS
UK
Phone: +44 (0) 1256 329242
Fax: +44 (0) 1256 320109
e-mail: feminist-review@unl.ac.uk
Website: www.feminist-review.com

Frontiers: A Journal of Women's Studies
c/o Sue Armitage-Editor
Washington State University
Pullman, WA 99164-4032
(509) 335-7268
Fax: (509) 335-4377
Website: www.wsu.edu

Gender and Society
Sociologists for Women in Society
c/o Sage Publications
2455 Teller Road
Thousand Oaks, CA 91320
e-mail: order@sagepub.com

Health Facts
Center for Medical Consumers
130 Macdougal Street
New York, NY 10012-5230
Website: www.medicalconsumers.org

Health Values
PNG Publications
Box 4593
Star City, WV 26504-4593

Herizons
Herizons, Inc.
PO Box 128
Winnipeg, MB, B3G 2G1, Canada
(204) 774-6225
Fax: (204) 786-8039

Indigenours Woman
Publication of the Indigenous Women's Network
PO Box 174
Lake Elmo, MN 55042-0174

*International Journal of Childbirth Education
(Quarterly)*
International Childbirth Education Association
Box 20048
Minneapolis, MN 55420-0048
(952) 854-8660
Fax: (952) 854-8772
Website: www.icea.org

Isthmus
101 King Street
Madison, WI 53703-3313
(608) 251-5627
Fax: (608) 251-2165
Website: www.thedailypage.com

Journal of American College Health
Heldref Publications
1319 Eighteenth Street NW
Washington, D.C. 20036-1802
(202) 296-6267
Fax: (202) 296-5149

Journal of American Medical Women's Association
801 North Fairfax Street, Suite 400
Alexandria, VA 22314
(703) 838-0500
Fax: (703) 549-3864
Website: www.jamwa-doc.org

Journal of Gay and Lesbian Social Services
Harrington Park Press
Haworth Press, Inc.
10 Alice Street
Binghamton, NY 13904
(800) 429-6784
Fax: (800) 895-0582
Website: www.haworthpress.com

Journal of Health Care for the Poor and Underserved
Sage Publications
2455 Teller Road
Thousand Oaks, CA 91320
e-mail: order@sagepub.com

Journal of Women's Health
1651 Third Avenue
New York, NY 10128

Lilith Magazine
250 West 57th Street, Suite 2432
New York, NY 10107
(212) 757-0818 or (888) 254-5484
Fax: (212) 757-5705
Website: www.lilithmag.com

MS Magazine
Liberty Media for Women
1600 Wilson Blvd, Suite 801
Arlington, VA 22209
Website: www.msmagazine.com

Midwives Alliance of North America
(888) 923-6262

The Nation
33 Irving Place
New York, NY 10003
(212) 209-5400
Fax: (212) 982-9000
Website: www.thenation.com

National Academy Press
(800) 624-6242
Website: www.nap.edu

National Latina Health Organization Newsletter
c/o National Latina Health Organization
PO Box 7567
Oakland, CA 94601-7567
(510) 534-1362
Fax: (510) 534-1364
Website: www.latinahealth.org

Network News
National Women's Health Network
514 10th Street, NW, Suite 400
Washington, D.C. 20004
(202) 347-1140
(202) 628-7814 (Information Clearinghouse)
Fax: (202) 347-1168
Website: www.womenhealthnetwork.org

New Internationalist
PO Box 1143
Lewiston, NY 14092

New Yorker
4 Times Square
New York, NY 10036-6592
Website: www.newyorker.com

New York Times
(888) NYT-NEWS
Website: www.nytimes.com

Office on Women's Health
Department of Health and Human Services
200 Independence Avenue, SW Room 730B
Washington, DC 20201
(202) 690-7650
Fax: (202) 205-2631
Website: http://www.4woman.gov/owh

The Progressive Magazine
409 East Main Street
Madison, WI 53703
(608) 257-4626

Ragged Edge (The Disability Experience in America)
c/o Advocado Press
PO Box 145
Louisville, KY 40201-0145
e-mail: editor@raggededgemagazine.com
Website: www.raggededgemagazine.com

Sex Roles: A Journal of Research
Kluwer Academic Publishers
PO Box 322
3300 A H Dordrecht
The Netherlands
Website: www.kluweronline.com/issn/0360-0025

Social Policy
Union Institute
25 West 43rd Street
New York, NY 10036

Society for Menstrual Cycle Research Newsletter
c/o Society for Menstrual Cycle Research
Website: www.pop.psu.edu/smcr

The Survivor Project
PO Box 40664
Portland, OR 97240
(503) 288-3191
Website: www.survivorproject.org

Teen Voices
Women Express, Inc.
PO Box 120-027
Boston, MA 02112-0027
(888) 882-TEEN
Fax: (617) 426-5577
Website: www.womenexp@teenvoices.com

Violence Against Women
Sage Publications
2455 Teller Road
Thousand Oaks, CA 91320
(805) 499-0721
Fax: (805) 499-0871
Website: www.order@sagepub.com

Wisconsin Medical Journal
State Medical Society of Wisconsin
330 Lakeside Street
Madison, WI 53715
(800) 362-9080
Website: www.wismed.org

Women and Children Horizon/Pathways of Courage
1511 56th Street
Kenosha, WI 53140
(262) 656-3500
Fax: (262) 656-3402
Website: poc@pathwaysofcourage.org

Women and Health
Haworth Medical Press
10 Alice Street
Binghamton, NY 13904-1580

Women's Health Issues
Publication of the Jacobs Institute of Women's Health
Elsevier Science
PO Box 945
New York, NY 10010
(212) 633-3730
Fax: (212) 633-3680
e-mail: usinfo-f@elsevier.com

Women's Studies International Forum
c/o Elsevier Health Sciences
Journals Division
625 Walnut Street, Suite 300
Philadelphia, PA 19106
(215) 238-7800
Website: www.elsevier.com

Index